EMERGENCY NURSING
Principles and Practice

EMERGENCY NURSING
Principles and Practice

SUSAN BUDASSI SHEEHY, RN, MSN, CEN

Trauma Clinical Nurse Specialist
Dartmouth-Hitchcock Medical Center
Lebanon, New Hampshire
Instructor in Clinical Surgery
Dartmouth Medical School
Hanover, New Hampshire

THIRD EDITION

with 452 illustrations

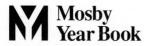
Mosby
Year Book

St. Louis Baltimore Boston Chicago London Philadelphia Sydney Toronto

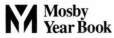
Mosby
Year Book
Dedicated to Publishing Excellence

Executive Editor: Don Ladig
Developmental Editor: Robin Carter
Project Manager: Patricia Tannian
Production Editor: Mary McAuley
Book and Cover Design: Gail Morey Hudson

Mosby–Year Book, Inc.
11830 Westline Industrial Drive, St. Louis, MO 63146

Library of Congress Cataloging in Publication Data

Emergency nursing : principles and practice / [edited by] Susan
    Budassi Sheehy.—3rd ed.
       p.   cm.
    Includes bibliographical references and index.
    ISBN 0-8016-6248-6
    1. Emergency nursing. I. Sheehy, Susan Budassi
    [DNLM: 1. Emergencies—nursing. WY 154 E5235]
  RT120.E4E48 1992
  610.73′61—dc20
  DNLM/DLC
  for Library of Congress   91-34895
                                               CIP

92 93 94 95 96 GW/VH 9 8 7 6 5 4 3 2 1

Contributors

CYNTHIA ABEL, MSN, RN, CEN

Instructor
University of Texas Health Sciences Center
School of Nursing
Houston, Texas

DEBORAH M. AMOS, MSN, RN, CCRN

Clinical Nurse Specialist, Intensive Care
Eastern Maine Medical Center
Bangor, Maine

LISA MARIE BERNARDO, MSN, RN

Clinical Nurse Specialist, Emergency Department
Children's Hospital of Pittsburgh
Pittsburgh, Pennsylvania

MARTHA M. BOHNER, MSN, RN, CEN

Head Nurse, Emergency Department
Harbor General Hospital
Torrance, California

VICKY BRADLEY, MS, RN, CEN

Divisional Director of Emergency Services
Albert B. Chandler Medical Center
University of Kentucky
Lexington, Kentucky

JEAN R. CALLUM, MHSA

Administrator, Ambulatory Services and Oncology
Eastern Maine Medical Center
Bangor, Maine

LINDA C. CARL, RN, FNC

Linda C. Carl, RN, Inc.
Washington, D.C.

DANIEL J. COBAUGH, PharmD

Coordinator, Toxicology Treatment Program
University of Pittsburgh Medical Center
Assistant Professor
Department of Pharmacy and Therapeutics
University of Pittsburgh School of Pharmacy
Pittsburgh, Pennsylvania

SUSAN R. CULLEN, RNC

Intensive Care Unit Staff Nurse, Resource Nurse
Eastern Maine Medical Center
Bangor, Maine

DIANNE DANIS, MS, RN, CEN

Clinical Nurse Specialist
Emergency Nursing Service
Massachusetts General Hospital
Boston, Massachusetts

NORMAN M. DINERMAN, MD, FACEP

Chief of Emergency Services
Eastern Maine Medical Center
Bangor, Maine

LYNNE GAGNON, BS, RN, CEN

Head Nurse, Emergency Department
Eastern Maine Medical Center
Bangor, Maine

NANCY HOGAN GROVER, MSN, RN

Associate Professor of Psychiatric Nursing
Husson College School of Nursing
Bangor, Maine

DEBORAH P. HENDERSON, MSN, RN, CEN

California EMS for Children Project Director
Harbor General Hospital
Torrance, California

BARBARA BENNETT JACOBS, RN, MPH

EMS Educator, Researcher
Hartford Hospital
Hartford, Connecticut

CINDY LeDUC JIMMERSON, RN

Trauma Coordinator
St. John's Hospital
Longview, Washington

MARILYN JOHNSON, RN, CEN

Child Protection Team
Primary Children's Hospital
Salt Lake City, Utah

SUSAN ENGMAN LAZEAR, MSN, RN

Nurse Consultant, Educator
Honolulu, Hawaii
Former Chief Flight Nurse
Airlift Northwest
Seattle, Washington

PATRICIA LENAGHAN, MS, RN, CEN

Clinical Nurse Specialist
Emergency Department
Nebraska Methodist Hospital
Omaha, Nebraska

ESTELLE R. MacPHAIL, MS, RN, CEN, CNA

Director, Emergency Services
Nashua Memorial Hospital
Nashua, New Hampshire

ANNE MANTON, PhD, MS, RN, CEN

Assistant Professor, Graduate Programs in Nursing
Massachusetts General Hospital
Institute of Health Professions
Boston, Massachusetts

JANET A. MARVIN, MN, RN

Director of Nursing
Shriner Burn Institute
Galveston, Texas

PEGGY McCALL, MSN, RN, CEN

Former Director of Emergency Services
Ben Taub Memorial Hospital
Houston, Texas

MARGARET M. MILLER, RN, MEd

Nurse Consultant
Indianapolis, Indiana

PAUL PARIS, MD, FACEP

Director, Emergency Department
University of Pittsburgh Hospital
Medical Director, Pittsburgh EMS
Associate Professor of Emergency Medicine
University of Pittsburgh
Pittsburgh, Pennsylvania

MARY ELLEN McNALLY PEDERSON, BS, RN, CPTC

Donation Coordinator, New England Organ Bank
Northern Maine Office
Bangor, Maine

JAY RANKIN, MSN, MT (ASCP)

Project Manager, Patient Information Systems
Eastern Maine Medical Center
Bangor, Maine

MARILYN RICE, BSN, RN, CEN, CNNA, MPA

Assistant Director, Inpatient Services
Freeport Memorial Hospital
Freeport, Illinois

KATHLEEN SCIABICA ROBINSON, RN, CEN

Trauma Program Coordinator
Geisinger Medical Center
Danville, Pennsylvania

SIDNEY SALVATORE, BS, RN, CEN

Nurse Manager, Emergency Department
Mount Desert Island Hospital
Bar Harbor, Maine

SUSAN BUDASSI SHEEHY, MSN, RN, CEN

Trauma Clinical Nurse Specialist
Instructor in Surgery
Dartmouth-Hitchcock Medical Center
Hanover, New Hampshire

JOAN KELLEY SIMONEAU, RN, CEN

Consultant in Emergency Nursing
San Pedro, California

PATRICIA SOUTHARD, MN, RN, CEN, JD

Attorney-at-Law
Program Coordinator, Trauma
Oregon Health Sciences University
Portland, Oregon

TERESA WILLETT STEELE, MS, RN

Associate Professor of Psychiatric Nursing
Husson College School of Nursing
Bangor, Maine

CYNTHIA L. STEMPER, MSN, RN, CEN

Director, Emergency Department
Oregon Health Sciences University
Portland, Oregon

MOLLY STROUT, BSN, RN, CIC

Nurse Manager, Infection Control
Eastern Maine Medical Center
Bangor, Maine

JANET TAYLOR, DSN, RN, OCN

Interim Director, School of Nursing
William Carey College
Hattiesburg, Mississippi

JOE E. TAYLOR, PhD, RN, CEN, CNNA, NREMT-P

Vice President, Clinical Support Services
South Central Regional Medical Center
Laurel, Mississippi

DONNA OJANEN THOMAS, MSN, RN, CEN

Nursing Director, Emergency Department
Primary Children's Hospital
Salt Lake City, Utah

BARBARA WELDON TONE, RN

Management Consultant
Simi Valley, California

DEBORAH TRAUTMAN, MSN, RN, CEN

Nurse Manager, Emergency Department
University of Pittsburgh Hospital
Pittsburgh, Pennsylvania

PATRICIA VARVEL, MSN, RN

Nursing Supervisor, Obstetrics and Gynecology
St. Luke's Episcopal Hospital and Texas Children's Hospital
Houston, Texas

THERESA WAGGONER, RN, CEN

Trauma Program Coordinator
Benedum Pediatric Trauma Program
Children's Hospital of Pittsburgh
Pittsburgh, Pennsylvania

To
JOHN

Preface

Emergency nursing's knowledge base has grown exponentially over the past two decades. Each edition of this book brings a bigger and more comprehensive collection of printed information. As you can tell from the trim size of this book, this third edition brings much new material. When planning for this edition, it became clear that several chapters had to be expanded and that several new ones had to be added. Many of you were asking for more physiology, more nursing process, and more chapter topics.

As I began to make notes and lists in preparation for this edition, it became increasingly clear that I was becoming less of an expert in *all* of emergency nursing because the core information was becoming voluminous. It was time to call in the experts. The people who have contributed chapters to this edition of *Emergency Nursing* are truly experts. I am so very pleased and excited about what they have written.

When I began the process of editing the first drafts of the chapter manuscripts, I faced the difficulty of trying to edit each manuscript so that all chapters would be in the same writing style, as is customary with most books: the idea is that, even though there are multiple authors, it looks as though one person wrote the book. That idea did not appeal to me. I intentionally did not provide a structured outline to the authors because I felt that each author was an expert in her or his topic and she or he would write it as she or he thought best to convey the information. So you will find that each chapter is unique in both content and style, written by an expert.

Many chapters have been added to the third edition: Quality Assurance and Risk Management, Interfacility Transport, Aeromedical Transport, Certification, Pain Management, Tissue and Organ Donation, Child Abuse and Neglect, Pediatric Trauma, and Pediatric Medical Emergencies. Most of the other chapters have been significantly revised, expanded, or rewritten.

I have been told that *Emergency Nursing* has become a standard on your bookshelf. I hope that the information contained within has added a new dimension to your practice of emergency nursing and that the patients you care for have benefited as well.

Susan Budassi Sheehy

Acknowledgments

As this third edition of *Emergency Nursing* goes to press, I would like to take this opportunity to acknowledge the many people who have made the completion of the manuscript possible.

A great deal of thanks goes to all the chapter authors for their expertise and for taking the time to put it in writing. Their chapter contributions have added a level of sophistication to this text that I alone would not have been able to accomplish.

Cathy Bernier was invaluable with her manuscript preparation skills. She always met my "impossible" deadlines with work that was beautifully done.

A very special thank-you to the staff at Mosby–Year Book, most especially to Don Ladig, my longtime editor who has seen me through so many projects, and to Robin Carter, my developmental editor, who has the patience of Job. She has always managed to get me back on the manuscript preparation track when my schedule became extremely hectic. She was most supportive and always there for me. Thanks, too, to Mary McAuley, Gail Hudson, and the production and design staff for a great job.

My professional colleagues at Dartmouth-Hitchcock Medical Center are a constant inspiration to me. Special thanks to a great group of clinical nurse specialists (there are 12) and unit teachers: their high energy level and clinical excellence are contagious. I have received unfailing support from the medical center's administration, most particularly from Melissa Miccolo and Kay Clark. Any voice of thanks to my colleagues would not be complete without mention of the staff nurses of the emergency department, postanesthesia recovery unit, intensive care unit, and pediatric intensive care unit. They give excellent care to our patients, are active participants in the formation, governance, and direction of nursing practice, and are a source of energy and pride for me on a daily basis.

There are many people who have given me special friendship, collegiality, and support. I would like to publicly thank them: Barbara Stettin, Judy Sawatzky, Jim and Ane Fulcher, Dave Schatz, Al Downing, Jean Callum, Mary Day, Rick Carlin, Deborah Dorley, Lisa McCabe, and most especially, Gail Lenehan.

Thank you to my Mom, Dad, and brother Steve for their encouragement and love. Most important of all, a very big warm hug for my son, John Patrick, who has had to put up with breakfasts-on-the-run, late-night peanut butter and jelly sandwich dinners, and the "mechanical babysitter" (the VCR) while Mom wrote "one last sentence" so many times.

Contents

Detailed Contents

50 Child Abuse and Neglect, 691

Marilyn Johnson

PRINCIPLES

Overview of Emergency Nursing and Emergency Care

Estelle R. MacPhail

Historically the specialty of emergency nursing may have begun in the Florence Nightingale era, but the specialty practice of emergency nursing as a discipline has occurred during the last 20 years.

Emergency nursing by definition is the care of individuals of all ages with perceived or actual physical or emotional alterations of health that are undiagnosed or require further interventions. The care is episodic, primary, and usually acute. This definition has undergone a remarkable evolution in the last decade.

The core of emergency nursing addresses the essence of emergency practice, the environment in which it occurs, and the consumers of emergency nursing. The dimensions of emergency nursing specify those roles, behaviors, and processes inherent in emergency nursing practice and delineate those characteristics unique to emergency nursing. Just as the profession of nursing is diverse, so too is the specialty of emergency nursing. Most specialty nursing groups are identified by one of the following:

Specific body system

Specific disease process or problem

Specific care setting

Specific age group

Specific population, such as women's health care

Emergency nursing crosses all these specifications and includes the provision of care that ranges from disease and injury prevention to lifesaving and limb-saving measures. Unique to emergency nursing practice are the nursing assessment, intervention, and management of cases in which patients require resuscitation and stabilization for a variety of illnesses and injuries.

The scope of emergency nursing practice involves assessment, diagnosis, treatment, and evaluation of perceived, actual or potential, sudden or urgent, and physical or psychosocial problems that are primarily episodic or acute and occur in a variety of settings.[7] These problems may require minimal care or life support measures, patient (and significant other) education, appropriate referral, and knowledge of legal implications.

Emergency patients are people of all ages with diagnosed,

undiagnosed, or misdiagnosed problems of varying complexity. Emergency nurses also interact with and care for families, communities, and preconsumers.

Emergency nursing occurs in various health care settings (primary, secondary, and tertiary) and exists whenever and wherever an emergency patient and an emergency nurse interact. The practice of emergency nursing also includes the delivery of care to consumers through education, research, and consultation. Emergency nursing practice can occur in hospital emergency departments; prehospital and military settings; clinics, health maintenance organizations, and ambulatory services; business, educational, industrial, and correctional institutions; and other health care environments. Emergency care is delivered where the consumer lives, works, plays, and goes to school.[6]

Emergency nursing is multidimensional. The dimensions include the responsibilities, functions, roles, and skills that involve a specific body of knowledge. These dimensions are manifested through emergency nursing characteristics, roles, processes, and behaviors (see box below).

Characteristics unique to emergency nursing environments include unplanned situations requiring intervention, allocation of limited resources, need for immediate care as perceived by the patient or others, and contextual factors. Contextual factors are the variety of geographic settings, unpredictable numbers of patients, and unknown patient variables that include severity, urgency, and diagnosis.[6]

Nursing roles include those of patient care, research, administration and management, education, consultation, and

---

CHARACTERISTICS UNIQUE TO EMERGENCY NURSING PRACTICE

Assessment, diagnosis, and treatment of urgent, and
  nonurgent situations involving individuals of all ages,
  often with a limited patient data base
Triage and prioritization
Disaster preparedness

advocacy. The specialty practice of emergency nursing is defined through the implementation of specific role functions, which are delineated in documents such as the Emergency Nursing Association's (ENA's) *Core Curriculum,*[3] *Scope of Practice Statement,*[6] *Standards of Emergency Nursing Practice,*[7] *Trauma Nursing Core Course,*[8] and *Prehospital Core Curriculum.*[5]

STANDARDS

A standard is an acknowledged measure of quantitative or qualitative value. It is the minimally acceptable practice that is reflected in a competency level outcome. Excellence is practice that surpasses the competency level and ultimately is that which contributes to the growth of the specialty and to the advancement of emergency nursing care.

In 1983 the *Standards of Emergency Nursing Practice* was published and provided a springboard for growth within a dynamic emergency nursing environment. The *Standards* continues to be used for such varied purposes as criteria-based job descriptions and performance evaluations, policies and procedures, standardized care plans, development of orientation and education programs, quality assurance activities, and research projects. It is also used as a resource document for a variety of other professional disciplines. The *Standards* represents a philosophy and, as such, is a compilation of recommendations and general guidelines that contain outcome criteria against which to measure and evaluate performance. Standards reflect the ongoing changes in practice and clarify the distinction between competence and excellence. Standards of practice are a measure by which the consumer of emergency health care views emergency nursing performance and to which nurses are held accountable.

Emergency nursing practice is systematic and includes nursing process, decision making, analytic and scientific thinking and inquiry, and triage. Professional behaviors inherent in emergency nursing practice are the acquisition and application of a specialized body of knowledge and skills, accountability and responsibility, communication, autonomy, and collaborative relationships with others.

Nursing diagnosis has become a component in the nursing process. In concert with a national direction for professional nursing growth, the taxonomic listing of nursing diagnoses developed by the fifth conference of the North America Nursing Diagnosis Association (NANDA) was incorporated in the ENA's *Core Curriculum* revision in 1987.[3] However, to reflect current emergency nursing practice, the use of nursing diagnosis in the *Core Curriculum* is modified to reflect identification of problems that can be influenced by both independent and interdependent nursing actions. The purpose of modification has been to integrate nursing diagnosis into the traditional phases of emergency nursing care: assessment, planning, intervention, and evaluation. Certification in emergency nursing validates this defined body of knowledge of emergency nursing practice.

RESEARCH IN EMERGENCY NURSING

The purpose of promoting research in our practice is to add to the knowledge base of emergency nursing. Emergency nurses must be committed to the generation of new knowledge, which contributes to the soundness of clinical nursing decisions. By supporting research activities, nurses expand and validate knowledge related to emergency nursing. Nurses need to value research as a methodology that furthers emergency nursing practice and join in collaborative research endeavors within the broad scope of emergency nursing care. The ENA *Code of Ethics* for emergency nurses, published in 1989, provides a distinctive set of ideals and standards of conduct regarding research activities.[2] Ethical principles serve as the moral bond linking the professions, the patient they serve, and the public.

SPECIALTY PRACTICE
Emergency Nurse Practitioner

Federal and private foundation grants supporting nurse practitioner training have created and sustained nearly 150 expanded-role programs for nurses that offer certificates or advanced degrees. Certification programs last from 16 to 68 weeks. These programs are designed to prepare the advanced nurse practitioner. Approximately 10 programs are designated "emergency nurse practitioner." Master's degree programs last from 44 to 72 weeks.[1] These curricula provide content dealing with acute and nonacute emergency situations.

Clinical Nurse Specialist

By definition the emergency clinical nurse specialist (CNS) is a registered nurse who, through advanced study of scientific knowledge, and supervised advanced clinical practice at the master's or doctoral level, has become an expert in emergency nursing. The emergency CNS demonstrates this acquired expertise through innovative, comprehensive, and high-quality performance in emergency nursing.[4] The emergency CNS is responsible and accountable for the development and application of standards and research to enhance the quality of care to the patients, their significant others, communities, and potential consumers in need of emergency care. The ultimate goal of the emergency CNS is the improvement of patient care and treatment outcomes.

The emergency CNS exemplifies professional nursing practice through the role functions of both direct and indirect patient care. These role functions include those of expert clinical practitioner, educator, consultant, researcher, and administrator or leader. Within each of these role functions, the emergency CNS is a role model, patient advocate, change agent, and cost-effective practitioner.

Because emergency health care systems are being adversely affected by the national health care problems of limited human and financial resources, a need exists for a multidimensional nursing approach within the diversity of the emergency care systems. The emergency CNS is uniquely prepared to make a significant contribution to this complex situation.

Subspecialties Within a Specialty

Another sign of the times is specialization. With the explosion of information and technology, more specialization becomes necessary and natural. "A nurse is a nurse is a nurse" has never been less true. As health care becomes more complex, so does nursing and the emergence of subspecialties within emergency nursing. In the 1980s many subspecialty groups evolved, such as flight nurses, pediatric emergency nurses, trauma nurses, prehospital nurses, and mobile intensive care nurses.

Subspecialty groups are areas within emergency nursing that have unique needs related to education, practice issues, and networking. A subspecialty group by definition is a group of nurses who work in special environments, work with specialized patient groups, perform special functions, or have special interests related to the specialty of emergency nursing. Recognition of the unique and diverse contribution of the various subspecialties to the practice of emergency nursing strengthens the practice of all emergency nurses.

EMERGENCY CARE

A characteristic inherent in emergency care is the integrated nature of the emergency health care team. The quality of care depends on the team concept. Emergency personnel include physicians, nurses, physician's assistants, paramedics, and emergency medical technicians, as well as first responders and base hospitals. In no other place in the health care system are teamwork and mutual respect more important. All members of the emergency team must function as colleagues so that optimal patient care is delivered to the injured or ill patients to decrease morbidity and mortality.

Specialty of Emergency Medicine

The first postgraduate program in emergency medicine began in July 1970 at the University of Cincinnati Medical Center. Since that time many residency programs have been developed. In late 1979, emergency medicine was formally recognized as a specialty by the American Board of Medical Specialists through the efforts of the American College of Emergency Physicians. Having emergency medicine recognized as a specialty was a positive step toward providing consumers with optimal care delivered by specialists in the field of emergency medicine. Many physicians are now board certified in emergency medicine and deliver care in various health care settings.

Certified Emergency Nurse

In September 1979 the Emergency Nurses Association (ENA) established a certified emergency nurse (CEN) certification program that is now administered by the Board of Certification for Emergency Nursing (BCEN). The first ex-

amination was given in July 1980. Since January 1986 the BCEN has been separately incorporated and is now solely responsible for this certification examination.

A certification examination for emergency nurses is a mechanism by which knowledge and skills for safe and competent practice can be measured. The purpose of the BCEN is to promote the health and welfare of those who have episodic illness that is emergent, urgent, or nonurgent by advancing the science and art of emergency nursing through the certification process. This statement is consistent with current definitions of certifications that emphasize the importance of consumer protection. The purpose of these programs is to ensure that certified individuals offer a particular level of experience and expertise that provides protection for the consumer. The CEN certification has become a coveted credential because of the level of expertise it represents. A nurse with this credential has demonstrated knowledge in the specialty of emergency nursing. Certification in emergency nursing is available through the BCEN. Certification is valid for 4 years, at which time the nurse must retake and pass the examination to retain certification for another 4-year period and be recognized as a CEN.

Prehospital Care

As emergency medicine and emergency nursing have come into their own in the last two decades, so has prehospital care. In the 1950s and 1960s it was common practice for funeral homes to provide ambulance service for transport to emergency rooms at the local hospital. These ambulances were more often than not poorly equipped and staffed.

Police officers, fire fighters, and practitioners of first aid provided prehospital care at the first-aid level. Emergency care needs became more and more apparent. Agencies and organizations began to engineer a plan to prevent prehospital deaths caused by illness and injury by bringing medical care to the streets. First, mobile coronary care units were established to bring coronary care to the streets in the hopes of preventing deaths outside the hospital caused by myocardial infarction and cardiac arrest. It soon became apparent that care should be delivered to victims who were ill or injured from various causes. This realization formed the basis for the currently popular paramedic ambulances, which are equipped for the management of trauma and obstetric, pediatric, psychiatric, and medical emergencies. In 1966 the National Highway Safety Act authorized the Department of Transportation to establish emergency medical service (EMS) guidelines. By this law, funds were allocated by statewide plans for the purchase of ambulances, the installation of communication networks, and the development of emergency medical technician (EMT) and paramedic training programs. The 81-hour EMT training program soon became the minimum standard for prehospital care providers. Other training programs were designed, and the sophistication of prehospital care began to grow.

**ELEMENTS OF AN EMS PROGRAM
RECOMMENDED BY THE EMERGENCY
MEDICAL SERVICES SYSTEMS
ACT OF 1973**

1. Personnel
2. Training
3. Communications
4. Transportation
5. Facility categorization
6. Critical care units
7. Public safety agencies
8. Consumer participation
9. Accessibility to care
10. Transfer of patients
11. Standardized patient record keeping
12. Public education and information
13. Independent review and evaluation
14. Disaster linkages
15. Mutual aid agreements

In June 1970 the National Registry of Emergency Medical Technicians was organized to unify requirements, examinations, and certification requirements for EMTs on the national level. Both EMTs and paramedics must meet specific requirements for continuing education in most states to ensure competency for recertification. The National Association of Emergency Medical Technicians was organized to meet the special needs of the EMT.

The Emergency Medical Services Systems Act of 1973 was designed to encourage regional EMS programs in the integration of 15 elements into a standard system (see box above).

The EMS division of the Department of Health and Human Services divided the country into approximately 300 EMS regions. States have been rapidly demonstrating their own interest in maintaining and improving their systems through funding, personnel licensing and certification, and facilities planning.

The national emergency telephone number (911), available in many communities, is the result of a concerted effort to improve the consumer's access to EMS. Concurrent with the growth of EMS has been a steady increase in the number of physicians, nurses, and other specialists whose primary concern is the delivery of emergency care.

EMS PERSONNEL

Personnel needs in the EMS system must include a cadre of first responders who can establish basic life support procedures. Police officers and fire fighters and other citizens may fall within this group. A call for help must be relayed by a trained EMS dispatcher, who triages the call, dispatches personnel and equipment, and provides instruction for first responders about what they should do until advanced help arrives. Advanced responders may be EMTs, paramedics, nurses, respiratory therapists, or physicians, depending on the type of call and the community-accepted protocol. For example, aboard specialized units such as helicopters or neonatal mobile intensive care units it is typical to find that respiratory therapists, transport nurses, and physicians accompany the victim, especially if the distance from the receiving facility to the transport facility is great. In many rural areas of the United States, terrain and weather conditions may present unusual problems, so other rescue workers may join the medical team to ensure safety and efficiency in the rescue effort and transport. The Military Assistance to Safety and Traffic program links the Department of Defense and other federal departments (Human Services and Transportation) and provides helicopters, fixed-wing aircraft, and military paramedic personnel to aid civilians with on-site transport efforts.

The quality of prehospital care depends on a team effort. The outcome of care in the hospital is greatly influenced by the field team's effort during initial stabilization and transfer and by ongoing communications.

HOSPITAL EMERGENCY DEPARTMENT

There have been dramatic changes in emergency department settings in the past two decades. Emergency rooms have become emergency departments, which in turn have incorporated prehospital care and flight programs, ambulatory care, occupational health programs, overnight or holding units, "fast track" care areas, satellite units, and more. Times have changed radically: since World War II, hospitals have become acceptable places in which to receive care. With the knowledge and technology gained during World War II, physicians realized the value of centralized treatment facilities. These wartime experiences changed the delivery of emergency care in the United States. Two other major events changed forever the delivery of emergency care: the 1965 Medicare Act and the 1966 Medicaid Act enabled millions of people to have access to health care, and trauma was recognized in 1966 as a major cause of morbidity and mortality, which led to the development of trauma systems. Federal grants led to the development of emergency medical systems and were a source of financial support for advancing the management and delivery of emergency care. Special units such as the pediatric emergency department emerged, as did the role of supervisory nurses, who now have become sophisticated managers with broad responsibilities. Hospital emergency departments are now reviewed regularly by the Joint Commission on Accreditation of Healthcare Organizations. Standards of care are evaluated and measured according to the level of care provided. Emergency medical evaluation or initial treatment is properly assessed by qualified individuals, and appropriate services are provided through a well-defined plan based on community need and the defined capabilities of the hospital.

Emergency departments provide care to millions of people each year. The emergency department has the only private physician many people ever know. Emergency departments serve not only as receiving centers for critically and seriously ill people but also as 24-hour clinics and as shelters for people who are frightened and have nowhere else to go. The number of individuals who receive medical care at emergency departments has grown during the last decade. Perhaps this census increase is caused by the lack of accessibility to private physicians. Persons with low income probably use the emergency department as a primary resource because it is convenient and because they are assured of receiving care if it is needed regardless of their inability to pay. Also, few primary care physicians have office hours in the evenings, on weekends, or on holidays, and many health insurance plans favor paying for emergency department visits over regular office visits to a physician. The emergency department is also convenient for individuals who prefer an unscheduled approach to health care delivery: an appointment is never necessary in the emergency department. Because emergency departments are available at all times to the public, an expectation has been created of an open system and treatment for all conditions.

Today's emergency departments are considerably more sophisticated in their management of medical and trauma cases than were the "emergency rooms" of two or three decades ago. Statewide programs for facility categorization have ensured that the services available in any emergency department are, for the intentions of the unit, of the highest quality and that the health care industry is making good use of the various types of unique capabilities (for example, a burn unit, a trauma center, or transplant facilities). Criteria for categorization concern physical facilities, specialized equipment, medical subspecialties, types of services available, numbers and types of personnel, and amount of training required to maintain currency in a specialized area. The number of available key personnel must also be documented according to their full-time, part-time, and on-call statuses.

The results of the categorization provide a clear indication of the capabilities of a facility so that all involved in EMS are more effectively able to use the services for limited emergencies, major emergencies, trauma cases, and the like. Many states have adopted unique schemes for grouping hospital emergency facilities. For example, facilities may be grouped by size, geographic location, number of medical and surgical residents, and specialty availabilities.

Disaster Preparedness

Emergency departments must have a well-defined disaster plan in which resources can be mobilized in the event of a natural or human-made disaster. Planned procedures for the management of victims of a disaster provide better preparedness for these emergencies. The plan should be comprehensive and should include the basic principles of medical and nursing care in the emergency department. Representatives from state and local prehospital provider agencies

and federal, state, and local agencies should collaborate in the development of response plans, and the contributions of these agencies should be incorporated into the general hospital disaster plan.

Physical Facilities

A well-equipped emergency department provides an efficient patient flow system to manage emergent, urgent, and nonurgent conditions of patients. The design should include an ambulance entrance separate from the ambulatory entrance. A triage nurse at the intake point makes an initial assessment of the patient's priority needs for care. This triage nurse then directs the patient to the appropriate area for treatment or directs the patient to wait for treatment.

Triage has become an integral part of emergency nursing care and emergency department function, especially when many patients request care simultaneously. The triage activity initiates the care and ensures that emergent or urgent patient care is not delayed. Registration clerks and secretaries are also usually available in the emergency department entrance area to manage the registration and business functions of the department. A triage system is a necessity for an emergency department, and triage is assigned to a specific care area.

Treatment areas may be divided into major trauma or arrest rooms, minor suture rooms, gynecologic examination room, psychiatric rooms, family room, and general examination rooms. Some departments have an observation or holding room, an isolation area, a decontamination facility, a cast room, an eye, ear, nose, and throat treatment area, radiographic equipment, and a small laboratory. Administrative offices and offices for pastoral care or social services may also be within the physical setting of the department.

Regardless of its design or size the emergency department is available 24 hours a day and staffed to deal with one or many victims of illness or injury who need either minimal or resuscitative care.

TRENDS IN EMERGENCY CARE

Many advances in technology and treatment are occurring in the field of emergency care, particularly in the area of prehospital care. However, advances in technology will be overshadowed by an increasing demand for emergency care services, particularly for critically ill patients. Most advances in technology in the emergency department come from a growing need for high-technology equipment that once was reserved for intensive care units. The education demands on emergency care providers are increasing at the same time that hospitals are finding it difficult to ensure that emergency departments remain solvent. Emergency administrators, in order to retain or achieve profitability, must assess hospital emergency care systems and increase the sophistication of methods used to classify patients to better assess charges and the collection process.

The aging of the population in the United States has

spurred research in cardiac treatments and technology. Cardiac care accounts for the bulk of the advances in the technology of emergency care. The development of automatic defibrillators has permitted an expansion of accurate, successful prehospital defibrillation. The introduction of thrombolytic drugs that destroy blood clots causing acute myocardial infarctions has been shown to significantly improve patient survival rates. An increasing number of hospitals are administering these drugs in the emergency departments. Preventive medicine has also become prohibitively expensive for the indigent and the elderly. Patients arriving at the emergency department are sicker and stay longer. The introduction of diagnostic related groups has exacerbated the problem. Patients are often being discharged early, resulting in increased visits to the emergency department because the patient is still sick and there is a lack of care and resources in the community.

As a result of the increased demand for critical care skills in the emergency department, providers of emergency care must have additional expertise. This demand for critical and specialized care is likely to continue. Patients with acute conditions frequently have to wait for an intensive care unit bed to become available, and emergency department staff must contend with critically ill patients who remain in the emergency department from hours to days. A recent development in emergency care that has alleviated some of the stress on emergency care personnel has been the designation of "fast track" care areas. Fast track units use triage to distinguish critically ill patients from patients with minor injuries and illnesses. Patients with minor injuries and illnesses can be seen in "fast track," allowing sicker patients to be seen in the emergency department.

Many challenges face nursing, emergency nursing, and the entire health care system in the United States. These challenges can readily be seen as threats. However, as nursing increases its financial and political savvy and, most important, as it becomes more united and speaks with a single voice, these challenges are proving to be brilliant opportunities.

One of the opportunities concerns financial issues in health care. Historically nurses have been given little information about the fiscal aspects of emergency care. Because of the nursing shortage that followed a major fiscal crisis in health care, nurse managers have become more involved in money matters and have shown others how to run a cost-effective department. A nurse manager's accountability now encompasses such areas as unit management, staffing patterns, high-quality patient care, and total responsibility for everyday budget operations.

The nursing shortage and widespread budgetary constraints are forcing managers to demonstrate that nurses provide responsible, cost-effective patient care and that the delivery and coordination of that care are well worth the cost.

Many health care issues confront our nation today: fiscal constraints in health care, the nursing shortage, acquired immunodeficiency syndrome, the ever-increasing elderly population, increasing patient acuity and longer waiting periods in the emergency department, care for the indigent, the cost of care, and access to care. These and many other issues will continue to have effects on nursing; they will change the profession and how it is perceived. In light of these issues nurses must join together with a new energy, come up with fresh ideas, and create a new presence for emergency nursing and emergency care.

REFERENCES

1. Emergency Nurses Association: Annual list of emergency nursing graduate programs, *JEN* 16(5):28A, 1990.
2. Emergency Nurses Association: *Code of ethics,* Chicago, 1989, The Association.
3. Emergency Nurses Association: *Core curriculum,* Philadelphia, 1987, WB Saunders.
4. Emergency Nurses Association: *Position paper: role of the clinical nurse specialist,* Chicago, 1989, The Association.
5. Emergency Nurses Association: *Pre-hospital core curriculum,* Chicago, 1991, The Association.
6. Emergency Nurses Association: Scope of practice statement, *JEN* 15(4):361, 1989.
7. Emergency Nurses Association: *Standards of emergency nursing practice,* St Louis, 1990, Mosby–Year Book.
8. Emergency Nurses Association: *Trauma nursing core course,* ed 2, Chicago, 1991, The Association.

SUGGESTED READINGS

Gelot D, Alongi S, and Edlich RF: Emergency nurse practitioner: an answer to the emergency care crisis in rural hospitals, *JACEP* 6(8):355, 1977.
Health Care Advisory Board: *Trends in emergency care: summary of findings,* Washington, DC, 1989, The Board.
Rockwood CA Jr: History of emergency medical services in the United States, *J Trauma* 16(4):299, 1976.

Prehospital Care

Kathleen S. Robinson

Most people are keenly aware of the health care trends affecting our population. Diagnostic related groups and other pressures from the cost reimbursement industry send more patients home who are sicker and less prepared to deal with the problems of home care than ever before. Each year more than 150,000 Americans die of traumatic injuries, and one person in three has a nonfatal injury; nonfatal injuries disable 10 to 17 million persons a year. Technologic advances in equipment and increased emphasis on training enhance patient survival and decrease morbidity. Prehospital care is a simple concept: Take the expertise of specially trained persons and equipment to the victim at the emergency scene and maintain that level of care during transport to an emergency care facility.

HISTORY OF PREHOSPITAL CARE

Emergency care in the field is not a new concept. In the late 1700s, rudimentary emergency medical service (EMS) systems provided the capability for immediate wound dressing on the battlefield and transport of sick and injured soldiers in covered carts. Military needs also provided the impetus for aeromedical evacuation operations during the Prussian siege of Paris in 1870, when hot air balloons were used to transport 160 wounded infantry soldiers. Professional level emergency care in the field was first provided by a nurse, Clara Barton, during the American Civil War. At the same time, the first organized ambulance corps had their origins in the military, although ambulances did not find application to civilian use until nearly half a century later. Dr. Frank Pantridge is credited with the development of modern EMS systems through his work in Belfast, Northern Ireland, in the late 1960s.

Several legislative initiatives focused federal attention on the problems of prehospital care. In 1966 the National Research Council of the National Academy of Sciences published *Accidental Death and Disability: The Neglected Disease of Modern Society,* which outlined severe deficiencies in trauma care. In the same year, Congress enacted the National Highway Safety Act, the first legislation to address and fund emergency services improvement. Two years later,

personnel training standards were identified and the first U.S. mobile coronary care unit with trained paramedics was established as a pilot project in Dade County, Florida, closely followed by projects in New York, Seattle, and Los Angeles. The Emergency Medical Services Act of 1973 (PL 73-154) defined mandated system components and addressed the need to reduce the number of emergency-related injuries and illnesses resulting in death and disability. However, the National Planning and Resources Development Act of 1974 shifted the focus of the federal government to the planning of activities and services aimed at helping states develop their own EMS systems.

The 1980s witnessed gradual withdrawal of federal funding at a time when EMS systems were expanding to meet the needs of a growing population. Advanced life support (ALS) systems are now available in every major city and are proliferating in many rural areas as well. These systems are equipped with the latest in technology and staffed by persons specially trained in the rigors of prehospital care.

TYPES OF PROVIDERS AND LEVELS OF TRAINING

Most health-related professional organizations consider education basic to their mission. The American College of Surgeons has been developing prehospital training programs since its inception, as have the American Academy of Orthopaedic Surgeons, the American College of Emergency Physicians, the American Heart Association, and the American Red Cross. If there is an official agency designated to develop training standards for prehospital providers, perhaps the National Highway Safety Act charged that responsibility to the Department of Transportation (DOT). Prescribed programs maintained by the DOT are intended to be *minimum* standards for training (first responders, emergency medical technicians [EMTs], and EMT-paramedics); newer courses advocated by professional organizations greatly enhance the knowledge and skill of prehospital providers at every level. Much of the responsibility and jurisdiction defined in early federal legislation, including the training and accreditation of these professionals, has since been relegated to state and local EMS authorities. It is essential that all prehospital providers recognize, understand, and function within these individual hierarchies.

Citizen

The average citizen is frequently overlooked as the true first responder. Most people are relatively uneducated concerning control of bleeding or splinting an extremity, yet more than 70 million people receive hospital emergency care each year. This estimate includes 1000 prehospital sudden deaths per day in the United States and 1.5 million myocardial infarction victims annually. The recommendations and specific standards for both basic and advanced cardiac life support were published as a supplement to the *Journal of the American Medical Association* in 1974. More than 5 million copies in a number of different languages were distributed worldwide. Materials for teaching cardiopulmonary resuscitation (CPR) to laypersons and medical professionals, developed primarily by the American Heart Association and the American Red Cross, were widely distributed. As a result, 12 million Americans had been trained in CPR by 1977 and an estimated 60 to 80 million persons planned to be trained. In 1983 an estimated two thirds of the U.S. population indicated an interest in being trained in CPR. According to a Gallup poll, the proportion of those adults who knew about CPR increased from 66% in 1977 to 87% in 1983. Since 60% to 70% of sudden deaths caused by cardiac arrest occur before hospitalization, it has been suggested that the community has the potential for being the ultimate coronary care unit.

First Responder

Studies clearly demonstrate the benefits of rapid access to emergency care on patient outcomes. Response times of ambulances or other vehicles used to transport more extensively trained persons to the scene can be affected by many geographic and environmental factors such as unfamiliarity with location, traffic, road conditions, and weather. First responders can be law enforcement officers, members of fire and ambulance units, educators, industrial safety officers, or other individuals who are willing and reasonably available to respond to calls for help until an ambulance arrives. The scope of training of the first responder includes lessons in basic access to the patient while using minimal equipment, and moving and lifting if necessary. Basic emergency care provided by the first responder includes recognition and treatment of life-threatening emergencies: airway care, CPR, control of bleeding, prevention of shock, care of soft tissue injuries, internal injuries, fractures, and a variety of illnesses and medical conditions.

Emergency Medical Technician

The emergency medical technician (EMT) is a vital link to the EMS system. Many times the EMT is the first trained person to assess and provide immediate care to the sick and injured. The basic level of training for the EMT consists of 33 lessons involving 100 hours of classroom and field training and 10 hours of in-hospital observation. States may increase program requirements to ensure individual competency. Enhancement of skill levels may include training in the administration of a limited number of drugs, the use of advanced airway skills, and cardiac defibrillation. Individuals with advanced certification and credentials are usually identified by the following titles: EMT-intermediate, EMT I to EMT VI, cardiac rescue technician, EMT-advanced, EMT-defibrillator, critical care technician, EMT-cardiac, and others.

EMT-Paramedic

The military's need to attend to urgent multicasualty situations defined a role for a level of health care provider beyond that of traditional basic life support. In the era of the conflicts in Korea and Vietnam medical corpsmen became physician-extenders and performed even some minor surgical procedures under the direct supervision of the physician. As these conflicts drew to a close, the natural transition of these highly skilled providers to the realm of prehospital care served as part of the force behind the proliferation of advanced life support services through the country. The Department of Transportation curriculum mandates a minimum of 212 hours of didactic time, although it is common for training institutes to nearly double this time when testing and practical laboratory sessions are added. Another 200 hours or more of hospital-based clinical rotations and field internships is required. State certification or licensure is awarded to the paramedic candidate after successful completion of written and practical examinations and is typically valid for a period of 2 to 4 years. However, some EMS agencies require annual reverification of skills through documentation of completed skills, retesting that includes skill demonstration, continuing education, or any combination of these.

Registered Nurse

Many roles for nurses are recognized in the prehospital setting: research, education, management, consultation, patient advocacy, and, of course, clinical practice, which is discussed in the following paragraphs.

Prehospital care is not an entry-level practice specialty. The environment is unlike that of any other area of nursing: extrinsic factors are sometimes difficult to control, and the environment is often unpredictable and at times dangerous. It challenges the nurse to be keenly aware of her surroundings, extremely flexible, and able to identify and use every available resource.

Although nurses have long been functioning in the prehospital environment, standards of practice and training specifically for nurses have been virtually nonexistent. This contradiction has forced many nurses to either turn to practice and training standards intended for other types of providers or refrain from prehospital care. A 1988 position paper cosponsored by the Emergency Nurses Association (ENA) and the National Flight Nurses Association and revised in 1990 discusses these issues more thoroughly. In response to intraorganizational pressure for prehospital training standards, the ENA developed the *National Standard Guidelines for Prehospital Nursing Curricula* in 1991, which are intended to integrate the nurse's prior education and clinical experience with the knowledge and skills needed by the prehospital nurse in basic and advanced life support roles.

Physician

High-quality physician leadership is the cornerstone of every successful EMS system across the United States. With nearly 40,000 active ALS providers, the need for on-line and off-line medical control is more crucial than ever. Supervision and participation in prehospital training programs, accreditation of providers, establishment of standing orders and protocols, direct and indirect communication (medical command or control) with field personnel, research, quality assurance activities, and direct patient care are some of the primary roles assumed by the EMS physician. The American College of Emergency Physicians has described qualifications of the EMS medical director, which include the following:

1. Familiarity with the design and operation of prehospital EMS systems
2. Experience in prehospital emergency care of the acutely ill or injured patient
3. Routine participation in base station radio control of prehospital emergency units
4. Experience in emergency department management of the acutely ill or injured patient
5. Routine, active participation in emergency department management of the acutely ill or injured patient
6. Active involvement in the training of basic life support (BLS) and ALS personnel
7. Active involvement in the medical audit, review, and critique of BLS and ALS prehospital personnel
8. Participation in the administrative and legislative process affecting the regional and state prehospital EMS systems

The demonstrated ability of physicians to improve care will dramatically increase their ability to lead others in the system. The more understanding physicians have of the constraints and problems faced by others in the system, the more likely it will be that physician proposals will fit into the system and be judged acceptable.

Air-Medical Crew

Throughout the 1980s the number of air-medical services grew from less than 50 to nearly 200. Until recently flight programs have relied on military training models and suggestions from the pioneers in civilian air-medical transport for training standards. Crew mixes are variable, blending the expertise of EMTs, paramedics, nurses, physicians, respiratory therapists, and others to provide prehospital and interfacility care. In 1988 the Association of Air Medical Services (then known as the American Society for Hospital-Based Emergency Air-Medical Services) entered into a contract with the Department of Transportation and Samaritan Air Evac in Phoenix, Arizona, to develop a national standard curriculum for air-medical crew members.[1] Air-medical crew members provide prehospital emergency care and interfacility patient transport by fixed-wing aircraft and helicopter according to certification level or licensure. Five levels of competencies are recognized: flight EMT-basic, flight EMT-I, flight paramedic, flight nurse, and flight physician. In addition to meeting training standards previously described, these individuals are educated in the application of basic and advanced principles of altitude physiology as it pertains to specific diseases or conditions and patient care during air transport, patient assessment and care in the airborne environment, patient preparation for air-medical transport, oxygen therapy in the air-medical environment, aircraft safety and orientation, aviation communication, survival, and other pertinent topics. Although didactic, clinical, and supervised flight experience are components of the program, the course emphasizes student competence and recognizes prior clinical experience; hence no mandated, standardized testing or certification has been established.

COMMUNICATIONS

Several elements compose an effective EMS communications system. Some of the more commonly used terms are described in the box on p. 12. However, the technical aspects of radio communication are beyond the scope of this text.

Components

An effective communications system is the glue that holds the whole EMS system together. Each one of the components is essential and depends on the others. Until 911 systems (or enhanced 911 systems, which provide a digital display of the caller's telephone number and the address of the phone to the dispatcher, prevent disconnection, and provide immediate callback) are uniformly available, continued public education programs about accessing the EMS system are essential.

When a call is placed to an emergency operations center, the dispatcher is responsible for notifying units to respond. This notification is usually accomplished by transmission of sequential tones and voice command to radios and personal alerting devices. Responders in turn establish radio communication with the emergency operations center and other responders via preassigned frequencies. Depending on case severity (and protocols) the mobile unit can be directly linked to the medical command center or base station at the

---

TERMS COMMONLY USED IN RADIO COMMUNICATIONS

Base station A transmitter and receiver in a fixed location

Channel For EMS systems, a pair of radio frequencies, one for transmission and one for reception

Communications center A regional center that usually coordinates radio traffic, including dispatch, for fire, police, and ambulance services throughout a geographic area

Federal Communications Commission The federal agency charged by statute to develop the efficient use of nongovernment radio frequencies, including AM, FM, TV, and mobile aircraft, marine, and land frequencies

Hertz Radio frequencies measured in cycles per second

Interference Unwanted signals from other radio transmitters or from electromagnetic radiation

Land line Telephone line between geographically separated points

Medical control terminal Base station usually located in an emergency department for medical control of an EMS system

Phone patch Ability to interface radio reception with telephone lines; allows an individual in a mobile system to communicate with someone in another location via land line

Repeater Ability to relay a radio signal from a transmitter of lower output and transmit it at a higher frequency

Skip Signals bounding off the atmosphere or buildings, which causes an abnormal signal projection that may carry for a great distance and interfere with radio communications

Squelch Receiver circuitry for suppressing unwanted radio signals or noise

Tone and tone code Selective signal used to activate a specific receiver that is designated to recognize the tone

Transceiver Radio capable of transmitting and receiving radio signals

UHF Ultra-high frequencies; in the 300 to 3000 megahertz band

VHF Very high frequencies: in the 30 to 300 megahertz band

VHF high band Frequencies in the 150 to 174 megahertz band

VHF low band Frequencies in the 32 to 50 megahertz band

---

hospital by telephone or radio patches. The BLS or ALS provider can then provide pertinent information, including the transmission of electrocardiogram (ECG) strips, and receive specific commands for intervention. In other circumstances, basic information can be relayed from the scene by the emergency operations center to avoid prolonged or unnecessary mobilization of medical channels or inefficient use of command personnel.

Role of the Dispatcher

The dispatcher is instrumental in the success of the effective communications system. The role of the dispatcher includes receiving as much information as possible about the emergency, directing appropriate vehicles and personnel to the scene, providing instruction as necessary to the caller for life-threatening conditions, and monitoring and coordinating field activity (including that of fire fighters and police officers, in many systems). In the past, emergency dispatchers were not required to have much EMS training, which resulted in poor communications, misunderstanding of priorities, lack of prearrival intervention, and the undermining of the total EMS structure. Although a training course for dispatchers was developed by the Department of Transportation, the course was based on the assumption of a successful diagnosis of the problem; this assumption created a real problem if the dispatcher was not an EMT. An updated approach to training developed by Dr. Jeff Clawson and the Utah Bureau of Emergency Medical Services[2] is gaining wide acclaim and acceptance. The Emergency Medical Dispatch Care Protocol System is the core of a 25-hour training course for the certification of emergency medical dispatchers (EMDs). Using protocols printed on cards, the EMD is able to identify dispatch priorities and provide accurate prearrival instructions to the caller using symptom-based or incident-type guidelines.

Applicable Codes

Signal codes were originally developed and used in the military to disguise top secret information and prevent eavesdropping by the enemy. The Federal Communications Commission developed the Aural Brevity Code (the "10" codes) in an attempt to promote efficient use of air time: number representations were substituted for commonly used words and expressions (for example, "10-4" for "OK"). Early ambulance services adopted the "10" codes but found them to be cumbersome, confusing, and impractical and abandoned their use, opting for clear language. The "10" codes continue to be effective in some areas, however, and many police departments still use them. Other established codes usually serve regional needs. Emergency service personnel are encouraged to contact local EMS authorities for a copy of applicable codes for their area.

Transmission of Medical Information

Society's quest for information enables any person to purchase a mobile scanner or radio that is capable of intercepting nongovernmental frequencies for personal use. Good sense and common courtesy provide the best guidelines for transmission of information over these air waves.

When using biomedical equipment, speak clearly, slowly, and in simple terms. Be familiar with any local codes. Never break into a transmission unless it is an absolute emergency. When giving a report on a patient, be as brief as possible without sacrificing important patient information. Always be sure that the message has been received. If you are not sure that it has been received, ask the receiver to repeat the message. Never use profanity; always be professional. Be sure to identify yourself during each transmission, especially in dual-run situations. Be sure to address the party to whom you are speaking by call-code name, and always sign off at the end of the total transmission. Even if you do not have a comment to make, acknowledge each transmission. Be sure to call each medication order by name, dosage, and route of administration; if receiving an order, make sure to repeat it back to the sender for verification before administration. Whether the medication should be titrated or given rapidly or slowly should also be specified. Be familiar with policies related to dual-run situations. Sending a continuous ECG strip may monopolize the frequency. Send only enough strip for the rhythm to be identified or verified. Be sure that each ECG strip is identified by both the sender and the receiver.

Every effort should be made to protect patient confidentiality; therefore the use of patient names or other identifying factors is discouraged. A standard reporting format is provided in the box at right. Last but perhaps most important, be familiar with your system: the personnel, capabilities and limitations, equipment, and other available resources.

Medical Control

The organization of medical control varies from system to system. On-line medical control is the direct communication between field personnel and the physician (or the physician-surrogate) via radio or telephone for the purpose of providing orders for patient care. Off-line medical control includes those administrative functions that are necessary to ensure the quality of EMS care, such as quality assurance and policy development.

Each state has a division or bureau of EMS, typically within the organization of the health department. A state medical director (physician) is responsible for the development and implementation of rules and regulations pertaining to EMS and for notifying regional or local medical directors of revisions and changes in state policy. Regional medical directors may be responsible for specific geographical regions, cities or municipalities, or one or more counties, depending on population, number of services, or need. It is the responsibility of regional medical directors to iden-

---

REPORTING FORMAT* FOR MOBILE INTENSIVE CARE UNIT

Call code
Base station name _____

Mobile unit
Your number designation _____

Location
Describe where (in general) _____

Age and weight
Estimate _____

Sex
_____

Problem severity
Mild, moderate, or severe _____

Chief complaint (or problem)
_____

History and medications
Determine and describe _____
_____

      Any previous similar problem? _____
      Any serious or chronic illness at present?

Initial vital signs
    General appearance (describe) _____
    Level of consciousness (patient's response to stimulus)

_____
_____

    Skin color and temperature _____
    Pulse (rate and rhythm) _____
    Respiration (rate and rhythm) _____
    Pupils (if appropriate, size, reactivity to light, equality)

_____
_____

Blood pressure _____

* Format developed by R.D. Stewart, Center for Emergency Medicine, University Health Center of Pittsburgh, Pittsburgh, Pa.

---

tify protocols that define specific treatment plans, including standing orders, patient triage and transport guidelines, and other special policies and procedures.

In some areas of the country, particularly in California, on-line medical control is a function of specially trained mobile intensive care unit nurses. These nurses act as a liaison between the field provider and the emergency physician. They do not function independently and are bound to strict, prewritten protocols. The certification process for mobile intensive care unit nurses is extensive, and evidence of continuing education in prehospital care and periodic field experience is also required, to maintain certification.

EMS Documentation

A written, standardized trip report form must be used in most EMS areas to document specific call information for insurance, quality assurance, and liability purposes. This documentation also provides pertinent patient information to the emergency department staff and provides other basic data that are used to establish call demographics and evaluate the use of personnel and equipment. Multiple copies of these forms are usually completed, and the form may or may not become part of the patient's permanent medical record. The standard trip report form is a legal document and should be completed thoroughly and accurately as soon as the call is finished. The general format for such reports includes the date and time of the call, ambulance or other services involved, the location and type of incident, essential patient information, pertinent patient history and assessment information, care provided and equipment used, where the patient was taken, and names and training levels of the providers.

Completion of the form and analysis of data can be time consuming; therefore many states are implementing computerized scan sheets with minimal narratives.

SCENE MANAGEMENT AND RESCUER SAFETY
Rescue and Extrication

Patient access can be one of the most complex problems facing the prehospital provider. From a simple situation such as evacuation through dark, narrow hallways and stairs to vehicle entrapment or high-angle rescue, the ability of the rescuers is critical to the success of an EMS operation. Proper training and experience are essential for personnel and victim safety. Equipment *must* be inspected daily if not more frequently to ensure availability, correct working order, and effective maintenance.

Vehicle rescue involves a series of well-planned, well-executed steps that includes the following:

Preparation	Gaining access
Response	Emergency care of the patient
Assessment	Disentanglement
Hazard control	Removal and transfer of the
Support operations	patient

If emergency service personnel are to perform competently at an accident scene, they must understand the theories and techniques of each phase in this series of steps. Patient care providers are an integral part of the rescue team; practice drills are one way for care providers to maintain familiarity with specialized vehicles, hand tools and powered tools, and the roles of various participants.

Safety

Nothing is more distressing in EMS than a needless injury or death in the line of duty. It is imperative that individual rescuers develop a positive attitude and a strict policy toward personal safety. Wearing head-to-toe protection may not be a practical precaution at every call; therefore, recognition of potential hazards may alert the provider to the need to consider the risk and take appropriate precautions. The key to adequate protection is anticipation.

Personal Safety

In any vehicular accident, rescuers may be exposed to many hazards, including fire, smoke, toxic fumes, dangerous chemicals, radioactive materials, glass shards, sharp metal edges, flying particles of glass, metal, and paint, ice, and extreme temperature variations, not to mention traffic hazards and downed trees, utility poles, or wires. In accident situations that involve certain hazardous materials, fire fighters, police officers, and rescue personnel may be required to evacuate residents and spectators from areas both around and downwind of the scene. Before 1973 there were few guides that emergency service personnel could use to determine initial action in a hazardous materials incident. In that year the Department of Transportation printed and distributed its *Emergency Services Guide to Selected Hazardous Materials*. The guide, revised in 1987, contains basic information about potential fire, explosion, and health hazards. It suggests certain immediate actions to be taken when there is a fire, spill, or leak and also includes suggestions for first aid.

The Occupational Safety and Health Administration's Hazardous Waste Operations and Emergency Response regulation became effective for all emergency service responders in 1990. The regulation imposes standards for training, organization, and operations on all emergency services that will respond to a release of hazardous materials from a stationary facility or incidental to transportation. Specific information about this regulation and available training can be obtained through local, state, or federal emergency management agencies. Additional information about hazardous spills can be obtained through the Chemical Transportation Emergency Center at 1-800-424-9300, or at 1-202-887-1255, a nonemergency number.

The Occupational Safety and Health Administration standards also regulate minimal requirements for the use of protective clothing. Ideal body protection is provided by approved helmets, safety goggles, turnout coat and pants, reinforced boots, and leather gloves. Turnout clothing may not provide adequate protection from poisonous vapors or liquids encountered during incidents involving hazardous materials.

Currently the prehospital care provider encounters a new and potentially lethal threat; the increasing use of common firearms and high-powered weapons in the escalating drug war. Some metropolitan areas have had to resort to the provision of body armor and weapons of defense for ambulance personnel. Although most areas of the country are not yet confronted with this modern menace, emergency personnel both in and out of the hospital must be careful when dealing with violent situations.

3 Communicating with Patients

Susan Budassi Sheehy

Although an almost daily trip to the emergency department is commonplace for most emergency nurses, to the patient and family or friends, this experience may produce any level of anxiety. In addition to pain, difficulty breathing, or other clinical signs and symptoms, the patient and his or her family are confronted with unfamiliar faces, a foreign environment, bleeps and blinks of equipment, usually noisy surroundings, and perhaps even a language (medical terminology) that may be unfamiliar. Patients may also have fear of the unknown and even fear of the known. There may be long waits and long silences from medical and nursing staffs. Some patients may be badly injured; some may have recently died or be close to death.

Privacy is usually at a premium, since we ask personal (and necessary) questions and ask patients to undress and be punctured and probed by complete strangers. We ask patients to trust us and sometimes to literally place their lives in our hands.

We ask family and friends to leave the treatment room or sit in the waiting area while we examine or even resuscitate their loved ones. Minutes seem like hours and hours seem like days. The patient and the patient's family and friends may feel alone and helpless. All these factors and many more would undoubtedly produce stress in most human beings.

As emergency nurses we must be astutely aware of the psychologic and psychosocial factors that are a part of the patient's entry into the emergency care system. How the patient and his or her family perceive the nurse and the system may affect their levels of anxiety and may even affect the situation's outcome. If the emergency nurse is aware of these psychologic and psychosocial factors and is able to understand the anxiety of the patient and the patient's family, the nurse may be able to make a difference in their anxiety level.

However, there are times, despite all our efforts, when anxiety levels run high and may even reach crisis proportions. Identification of this is crucial, if interventions are to be successful.

The main theme in all the interventions used to prevent severe anxiety levels or to deal with the patient or family in crisis is *communication*. Communication is not only the sending of the message but also the receiving and understanding of the message. Communication can be verbal or nonverbal. It is the process through which the patient-caregiver relationship develops. The patient may base his or her perception on the level of the nurse's competence and on what the patient sees as the level of communication and interpersonal skills the nurse has demonstrated. Usually, the better the communication and the patient's perception of that communication, the more smoothly the therapeutic process goes.

The emergency nurse must be acutely aware of the following facts:

Regardless of the method, there is some form of communication in any relationship, even if it is nonverbal or does not involve physical contact.

Communication can be formal or informal.

All behaviors by the nurse, the patient, and the patient's family are forms of communication.

It is impossible *not* to communicate.

What you say may not necessarily be what the patient hears.

Remember that each person perceives the world in his or her own way. How a person perceives a situation can be seen in behaviors, language, and actions. Language is the personal attribute that reflects a person's values, beliefs, and life-style. Awareness of language can provide a useful reference point from which a meaningful communication with the patient can occur. Be sure to talk with the patient at his or her level of understanding. Listen to what the patient has to say: take time to listen. A patient must feel as though he or she is being heard for effective communication to take place. Therapeutic communication skills take training, practice, and learning from mistakes.

Be careful not to confuse *empathy* with *sympathy*. *Sympathy* is subjective. When you are sympathizing with a patient, you are actually sharing the emotion with the patient. Sympathy uses great energy, energy you must have to help patients cope with their problems. You should strive to be *empathetic*. *Empathy* is an objective skill. It allows you to be with patients during their feelings but not be joined with the patients. You can and should demonstrate respect and concern for what the patient is experiencing, but you should ensure a separateness that allows a therapeutic relationship.

ACCEPTANCE OF THE PATIENT'S FEELINGS

It is important for patients to feel that their feelings are noticed and recognized as legitimate by emergency care givers. The nurse should not berate or criticize patients' expressed feelings or those of their families or friends. Convey the attitude that you are willing to assist the patient in recognizing and trying to understand his or her feelings. If you can help the patient to recognize his or her own emotions, you may assist in decreasing the patient's fear of the experience so that the patient's anxiety is reduced to a manageable level. Making a statement such as, "It's OK to be somewhat anxious about what has just happened," can greatly reduce a patient's anxiety level. Accept the patient's feelings as legitimate, and work with the patient. Communicate an attitude of acceptance that encourages problem-solving and promotes health.

Try not to interpret the patient's feelings, since they often cannot be interpreted. You can observe behaviors and make inferences about why the behaviors are occurring, but your inferences may not always be accurate. For example, you may see a patient in the waiting area who has tears in her eyes and on her face. You may assume that she is upset about something. In reality she may have tearing because her new contact lenses have caused her eyes to become extremely photosensitive.

Sometimes a patient expresses his or her feelings as behaviors. It is useful in these cases to encourage the patient to verbally communicate his or her feelings. This approach is preferable to trying to interpret a patient's behaviors.

You must also focus on your own feelings and identify how they affect your therapeutic communications with patients. Always work toward the level of mutual trust and respect between the caregiver and the patient. To establish this level of communication, you must have knowledge of the process, patience, caring, and skill. Learn to accept patients without placing value judgments on them. Recognize each patient as an individual human being with unique needs.

Whenever a person enters the emergency care system, whether it be in the prehospital care phase or the emergency department phase, the first encounter the patient has with a care provider will probably set the tone for his or her attitude toward the entire emergency care experience. Regardless of how urgent the need to perform a procedure, always explain, however briefly, what you are going to do to the patient. You must gain the patient's confidence and respect. Be sure to tell the patient not only what you are doing but also whether what you will be doing will cause any pain or

discomfort. Remember to do this even if the patient appears to be unresponsive.

THERAPEUTIC COMMUNICATION TECHNIQUES

There are many techniques that can be used in therapeutic communications. No technique works well in all situations; the ability to choose the appropriate technique takes practice and patience.

Supportive Technique

If a patient is anxious, the supportive technique is a good way to help the patient regain or maintain self-control. You can be supportive by doing the following:

Verbalizing your support

Acknowledging that the patient is an individual with individual needs

Being a good listener when the patient needs to talk and taking the time to listen

Trying to stay with the patient who is lonely, feels isolated, or is afraid

Accepting the patient's feelings as legitimate feelings, whether or not you agree with what the patient is expressing

Letting the patient know you are trying to understand what it must be like for him or her

Closely observing and carefully commenting on behaviors or actions by the patient that may be clues to his or her true feelings

Providing some therapeutic touch — on an arm, a hand, a shoulder — if it is comfortable for the patient and for you

Showing respect and compassion

Keeping your personal attitudes to yourself

Silence

Although not often thought of as such, silence as an expressive, nonverbal response can be a useful tool in therapeutic communication. Remember, silence is the absence of words but *not* the absence of activity. It may be a natural conclusion of verbally transmitted thoughts. Silence may be useful in the following ways:

Silence allows time to think.

It may be helpful in finding solutions to problems and answers to questions.

It *is* a way to convey your feelings without words.

It may promote acceptance or indicate anxiety in either you or the patient.

When carefully employed, silence can be used to pace, time, alienate, resist, or relax.

Listening

Listening is one way to hear the concerns of our patients. Having the patient talk while you listen may relieve the patient's anxieties and facilitate information collection. Whenever possible, allow the patient to take the conver-

TYPES OF QUESTIONS

Leading question

"Don't you know better than to not wear your seatbelt?"

This type of question restricts the respondent.

It implies the asker's judgment.

It elicits nonverbal clues.

It contains a suggested answer.

Question that provides no choice

"I'm going to give you this injection, OK?"

This type of question can be interpreted as a command and may be interpreted as authoritarian.

Closed-ended question

"How long have you had this pain?"

When you ask this type of question, you elicit a specific response.

"Yes or no" question

"Do you have any pain now?"

Since this question usually requests a "yes or no" response, it can be responded to verbally with little self-disclosure.

Limited choice question

"Do you want a plaster or fiberglass cast?"

This type of question gives the responder two choices. It also implies compliance or agreement with at least one of the two choices.

Double question

"Are you thirsty? Would you like some water?"

This type of questioning actually contains two or more questions, which are asked in sequence, without a pause.

This type of question can confuse both the responder and the asker.

The responder has to choose which question to answer.

Open-ended question

"How did you feel right after you fell?"

This type of question usually begins with "how" or "what" or "tell me more about . . ."

The answer usually conveys feelings and perceptions as well as thoughts.

This type of question encourages the patient to describe, elaborate, and compare.

It allows a free response.

It helps the nurse assess the patient's reliability.

Indirect question

"Tell me about the accident."

This type of question doesn't really seem like a question. (It has no question mark at the end.)

It exhibits the nurse's interest in the patient.

It allows the patient to carry the conversational lead.

---

sational lead. Listening is an active, physically visible process. Being able to listen is a learned skill, acquired through practice. Acknowledge the patient's verbalizations with active listening and comments such as, "Yes, go on," or "Tell me some more about this problem," or "I see," or "This must be really important to you."

Questions

Although questions are necessary to gather information, they do little to develop therapeutic communications. Choose your questions carefully, keeping in mind the following guidelines:

Don't ask "why" questions, since they tend to cast a sense of blame.

Don't ask too many questions.

The use of "your" or "who" at the beginning of a question may be interpreted as accusatory.

Keep questions simple. Compound or double questions may cause confusion.

Unless you are seeking very specific information, don't ask closed or direct questions.

Types of questions nurses ask patients are listed in the box above.

COMMUNICATING WITH FAMILIES AND FRIENDS OF PATIENTS WHO DIE

Care of the patient almost always extends beyond the patient to the psychosocial care of the patient's family and friends. This is especially true when a patient dies. Emergency nurses must provide empathy, support, and direction and act as resource persons. If the patient's death is sudden and unexpected, the first reactions the nurse can expect from family members or friends are shock and disbelief. As the reality of the death of a loved one begins to set in, the feelings of family members and friends may change to guilt, anger, or sorrow. In time, most people will come to understand and accept their feelings of loss and come to some sort of resolve so that they can return to their normal activities in life. This final stage of the grief process is rarely seen in the emergency care setting, and emergency nurses are often faced with families and friends who are in great emotional need. As emergency caregivers, we are directly involved with patients' families and friends who are in the stages of shock, disbelief, guilt, anger, and sorrow that are part of the grief process. Our honesty, sensitivity, and sincere concern will do much for these families and friends when they begin the therapeutic road to resolve. Help them to perceive the event realistically. Assure them that persons such as chaplains, social workers, or other family members or friends are available to provide emotional support. If possible, find a private place for them, a place where they can cry or scream, make phone calls, or sit in silence. Assess the situation to determine what kind of support system is available. Help them contact other family members or friends.

Communication During the Resuscitation Attempts

During the resuscitation attempts, when it becomes apparent that the patient is in extremely critical condition or will soon die, make contact with the family, if contact has not yet been made. Make sure that someone stays with the family during the resuscitation period or if this is not possible, provide the family with frequent updates of the patient's condition. Take some time to listen to what the family is saying, since they may need to verbalize their guilt or anger, sorrow or memories. Be honest: do not give false hope. There is a fine line between being honest and being too blunt. Compassion and concern will usually guide you in deciding how much information to offer and when to give it.

Help the family members make phone calls, and offer to speak with the person they are calling, if they are unable to do so themselves. Gestures such as offering something to drink or your hand to hold may go much further than you think in helping the family through the grief process. Allow the family the right to grieve. Realize that the family may be angry and that anger is a normal part of the grief process. Do not, however, allow that anger to be directed at you. Be aware of differences in normal grief responses in various ethnic groups. Ask for help if you feel that the situation is beyond your understanding or control.

Communication When Death Has Been Declared

You or someone who has been working with the family, along with the attending physician, should speak with the family when death has been declared. Traditionally the physician has been the person to inform the family that the patient has died. Realistically the physician may not be available, or another member of the health care team may be in a more appropriate position to inform the family. In either case the person who tells the family that the patient is dead should do so compassionately yet directly. Allow the family members time to react to the news. If possible, stay with them. As they are absorbing and reacting to this news, you may ask them if they wish to see the patient: most will say yes, some will say no. Viewing the patient is important to grief recovery, but do not force anyone who does not wish to do so.

If the family wishes to see the patient, make sure that the resuscitation room is in good order and that the patient has been prepared for viewing. Remove or cover all bloody sheets or pillows and emesis. Make the patient as presentable as circumstances permit. Dim the lights if possible, and cover open carts or duty equipment. Whenever possible, place a chair by the bedside for a family member, and don't rush the family. Remember that at this moment the family members become your "patients"; they need time to absorb and react to all that has happened.

Usually after the family views the patient, family members return to the family counseling room (if the emergency department has one). Usually at this time necessary questions are asked, such as whether the family requests an autopsy. (In some states the family may be told that an autopsy is mandatory in cases of sudden death.) Give the family instructions, both verbal and written, concerning what must be done next. Often a family will need to return home, contact other family members, and make funeral arrangements. Tell the family whom to call when these arrangements have been made, and give family members a phone number of someone at the hospital to call in case they have additional questions. Ensure that they have transportation and that they have family members, friends, or neighbors they can call, should they need to do so.

Communication After the Family Has Left the Hospital

To send a card or to call the family a few days after the patient's death, although not necessary, is a compassionate gesture. If the patient was a child or a victim of violence or in some other category for which a support group is available to the family, be sure to refer the family to that support group.

SUMMARY

Communication is essential in any therapeutic relationship. Open, honest communication, with sensitivity and compassion, is always best. Allow the patient the opportunity to talk and to express his or her feelings. Assist the patient to identify inappropriate feelings or actions, and provide therapeutic alternatives.

SUGGESTED READINGS

Braulin J and others: Families in crisis: the impact of trauma, *Crit Care Q* 5(3):38, 1982.

Caldwell E: The psychological impact of trauma, *Nurs Clin North Am* 13(2):247, 1978.

Caplan VG: Mastery of stress: psychological aspects, *Am J Psychiatry* 138(4):413, 1981.

Maddison D: Coping with crisis, *Aust Nurses J* 7(8):31, 1978.

Robin PL, Hussain G: Crisis intervention in an emergency setting, *Ann Emerg Med* 12(5):300, 1983.

Swigonski ME, Nagy MB: A team approach to patient death and staff grieving, *J Am Assoc Nephrol Nurs Tech* 8(2):38, 1981.

Legal Issues

Patricia Southard

This chapter explores the legal issues that apply to the emergency department (ED). In addition to being concerned about providing a level of care that falls within the standard of care, ED personnel are affected by evolving federal laws and other court decisions. Health care professionals must have a basic knowledge of the potential legal hazards that can occur in practice. It is equally important that medical and nursing practice be performed within the prescribed professional standards. This type of practice coupled with good documentation skills is the best protection from legal liability. This chapter addresses the sources of law, negligence and other torts, documentation issues, the Consolidated Omnibus Budget Reconciliation Act (COBRA), death and dying, consent, and other topics. Risk management in the ED is also discussed.

SOURCES OF LAW

The United States Constitution is the supreme law of the land. No other constitution, state statute, ordinance, administrative regulation, or case law can be in conflict with the principles defined in the Constitution. Every constitution can be amended using prescribed procedures. The United States Constitution has been amended 26 times. The first 10 amendments are known as the Bill of Rights.

The Constitution provides the framework for the division of government services among the executive, legislative, and judicial branches. This division creates a system of checks and balances, which ensures that each branch is accountable to the others.

The Bill of Rights delineates the rights guaranteed to each individual. These rights include freedom of religion, press, and speech; freedom from unreasonable search and seizure; prohibition of cruel and unusual punishment and excessive bail; right to a speedy trial with the assistance of an attorney; and guarantees of due process before the federal government can deprive an individual of life, liberty, or property. In recent years the Bill of Rights has been the area of contention for many issues related to health care.

There are two different opinions concerning the way in which the nation's founders intended the Bill of Rights to be applied. One opinion is that the Bill of Rights must be read strictly, that is, no interpretation of intent is allowed. The other opinion is that the Bill of Rights was intended to be interpreted in light of current technology and problems. Seldom have these two opinions come into such conflict as in the questions dealing with medical rights. Examples of issues affected by this conflict range from the use of artificial birth control to abortion to the right to die. The question asked in these cases is whether a right to privacy is guaranteed by the Constitution. This difficult question is discussed more fully later in this chapter.

Federal and state statutes are another source of law. The number of statutes that directly affect health care professionals is increasing rapidly.[15] The Medicare laws, along with the section concerning COBRA, are examples of federal statutes. Laws addressing consent for medical care, licensing of health care professionals, child abuse, and reporting communicable diseases are examples of state statutes.

Administrative agencies such as the Internal Revenue Service or state health departments have the authority via legislatures to promulgate regulations. To be valid, the regulations must have been adopted through a clearly defined process that generally requires some type of public comment. Once the regulations are determined to be valid, they have the force of law.

A final source of law is the common law, which comes from the written decisions made by judges after hearing or reviewing a case. Judges who are in the position of making common law are bound by the principle of *stare decisis*. The Latin term, *stare decisis,* means "to abide by or adhere to decided cases."[4] This doctrine ensures that once a principle of law is applied to a certain set of facts, that same principle will apply to all future cases that have the same facts. The doctrine of *stare decisis* ensures consistency and predictability within the common law. Common law provides the source of laws that health care professionals are involved with most frequently.

TORTS

Lawsuits filed for medical negligence (medical malpractice) fall into the legal category known as torts. A tort is a civil wrong committed against a person or property for which the court will provide a remedy of money to be paid to the plaintiff.[4] Torts are divided into intentional and nonintentional torts. Intentional torts require that the person who commits the tort intends to do that which the law forbids. Examples of intentional torts are assault, battery, trespass, false imprisonment, and intentional infliction of mental distress.

Nonintentional torts occur when an individual fails to use the care a reasonable and prudent person would use in similar circumstances.[4] Medical negligence, or medical malpractice, is a nonintentional tort. In legal actions for medical negligence the plaintiff does not have to prove intent but must prove that the care delivered was substandard.

Assault is an intentional threat to inflict injury on another person coupled with the apparent ability to immediately carry out the threat.[4] If a nurse threatens to hit a patient and raises his or her hand as the threat is being expressed, the nurse would probably be liable for assault. An exception occurs when the nurse is responding in self-defense to a threat from the patient. Health care providers have the right to protect themselves from harmful contact.

Battery is the nonconsensual touching of another person that results in harmful contact. If a surgeon operates on a patient without the patient's consent, a battery is committed. In the ED there is always concern regarding battery because patients are cared for according to the theory of implied consent rather than actual or express consent. If life or limb is at risk, it is always safe to assume that treatment will not be considered battery. Nonemergent procedures should only be performed with the express consent of the patient.

A common problem in EDs is the issue of determining blood alcohol levels at the request of the police department. Many if not all states have specific laws that address the issue of police request for blood alcohols. It is essential for ED personnel to know well the specific state law regarding this issue. Oregon's state law, for example, addresses the request to determine a blood alcohol level or to perform other tests in furtherance of a criminal investigation. The statute confers immunity from civil liability to a physician or person acting under the direction of a physician who performs medical tests to gather evidence in a criminal investigation. The procedures must be performed in a medically acceptable manner for the immunity to apply, and the peace officer can only request, not require, the physician to comply.[18]

Another area in tort law deals with property owners and the duty they owe to members of the public who are legally on the property of the owner. By law, property owners must keep their premises safe and free from hazards. If a visitor to a hospital slips and falls on water in the hallway or ice on the walkway to the ED, the hospital will probably be liable.

Negligence is the most common tort involving health care professionals. For a lawsuit to be successful in a negligence

---

ELEMENTS TO BE PROVED BY PLAINTIFF

1. A duty was owed to the patient.
2. That duty was breached by the defendant.
3. The breach of duty was the proximate cause of the patient's injury.
4. The patient sustained actual injuries as a result of the breach in standard of care.

---

action, four elements must be proved by the plaintiff. These elements are listed in the box above.

Duty is the legal concept that defines the responsibilities of conduct in certain relationships such as that of physician or nurse to patient. The law requires that due care or reasonable care be the conduct extended to patient care. In a lawsuit for medical negligence the determination of whether the duty was breached is by testimony from expert witnesses and the review of written professional standards. Sources of material that could be used to determine whether the care in question fell below standards includes the manual of the Joint Commission on Accreditation of Healthcare Organizations, a hospital's policy and procedures manual, and the standards or guidelines from professional associations.

The third element that must be proved is that the plaintiff's injury was a result of the defendant's negligence. This cause-and-effect relationship, termed proximate cause, is the most difficult element to prove. The plaintiff must prove that the injuries would not have occurred in the absence of negligence of the health care provider.

The final element necessary to a successful negligence lawsuit is that the patient sustained damage. The injuries may be physical or psychologic. The amount of money awarded to the successful plaintiff is determined in relation to the extent of injury.

Patients who come to the ED are there to have emergency conditions diagnosed and treated. Therefore one of the major areas for litigation is failure to diagnose a condition in the ED. All ED personnel should know which medical conditions have a high potential for misdiagnosis. These conditions include myocardial infarction, ectopic pregnancies, fractures, appendicitis, ruptured organs following trauma, and others.[12]

Analysis of Case Study

Do the facts in the case study presented in the box on p. 25 suggest that the plaintiff-patient will be successful in litigation? To answer this question, a step-by-step analysis of the elements necessary to prove negligence as they apply to the facts in this case study is provided in the following paragraphs.

The element of duty is the easiest one to establish for the plaintiff-patient. On arrival at the ED the patient was owed

CASE STUDY 4-1

Misdiagnosis Resulting in Lawsuit for Negligence

A 20-year-old man was transported via ambulance to the ED following a motor vehicle collision. He was a restrained passenger in a vehicle involved in a high-speed, head-on collision. The driver of this same vehicle was killed. The trauma patient was awake, somewhat disoriented, and complaining of severe abdominal and shoulder pain. On arrival at the ED, his vital signs were blood pressure, 70 mm Hg, pulse, 134 beats/min, respiratory rate, 36 breaths/min, and Glasow coma score, 11. The trauma surgeon performs a rapid assessment of the patient. She thinks the patient has intraabdominal bleeding and a hemopneumothorax. A radiograph of the chest confirms the presence of a hemopneumothorax, and a chest tube is inserted. A peritoneal lavage returns grossly bloody fluid. A radiograph of the lateral cervical spine demonstrates no fracture to cord level C6. The patient then becomes severely hypotensive with no palpable blood pressure and is taken immediately to the operating room (OR) for exploratory surgery.

The ED nurse who accompanied the patient to the OR gives a report to the nurse who will be circulating during the surgery. The ED nurse reports that the cervical spine was "cleared" in the ED after results of a radiograph of the cervical spine were negative. The anesthesiologist has some difficulty intubating the patient because the patient has a "bull" neck and prominent front teeth. The anesthesiologist wants to remove the cervical collar to achieve better visualization. The circulating nurse passes on the information that the cervical spine was "cleared in the ED." The collar is removed, and the patient is intubated successfully.

After the patient has awakened in the postanesthesia care unit, he is found to have profound neurologic deficits. A second radiograph of the cervical spine is made, and this radiograph shows a fracture-dislocation of the cervical and thoracic vertebrae (C7-T1) with severe cord compromise. The patient is returned to the OR for immediate intervention, but the patient has permanent neurologic deficits. The OR circulating nurse files an incident report with the hospital attorney. The incident report describes the report given to her by the ED nurse regarding the status of the cervical spine. The patient files a lawsuit for negligence against the hospital, the trauma surgeon, and the anesthesiologist. The suit against the hospital alleges negligence by the ED staff nurses and OR nurses for failure to maintain cervical spine immobilization.

thoracic vertebrae, cord level C7-T1, before precautions related to spinal injury are abandoned. The defendant would also have an expert witness, who would testify that this patient's life was at stake, which negated the possibility of maintaining precautions related to the spine. The jury would then decide whether the element of duty was breached, by deciding which of the expert witnesses was more credible. In trauma cases the manual of the Advanced Trauma Life Support Program would be used by the plaintiff to prove care delivery below national standards.

To prove proximate cause, the plaintiff's attorney must show that some action or omission on the defendant's part was the cause of the injury incurred by the patient. If the documentation indicates that the patient did not have neurologic deficits before anesthesia was administered, it seems likely that the element of proximate cause will be found to apply.

Concerning the element of injury, there is no question that this patient has sustained a serious injury. If the jury is convinced that the injury is directly related to the miscommunication regarding the cervical spine, the amount of damages awarded to this patient will be significant, probably in the millions of dollars.

One common concern of nurses is whether they will be personally sued in actions for professional negligence. Generally the employing hospital has a "blanket" insurance policy that includes coverage for the negligent acts of its employees. By law an employer is responsible for the negligent acts of employees who are acting within the scope of their employment.[22] This legal responsibility is termed vicarious liability. Since litigation is expensive and the potential award for damages in this situation is substantial, the plaintiff's attorney will look to the party who has the "deep pockets," therefore the best ability to pay an award. Hospitals are considered to have "deep pockets" because of extensive insurance coverage and are commonly named as defendants in professional negligence actions involving hospital employees.

Another aspect of the case study that is relevant to the concerns of ED personnel is the filing of an incident report on the miscommunication. Incident reports must be filed only with the hospital attorney or the administrative representative for legal matters. There should be no documentation in the chart to indicate that an incident report was made or filed. During the discovery phase of the litigation, the plaintiff's attorney will ask the hospital to submit all relevant records for this patient, including peer review records, incident reports, and other information, in addition to the medical record. Most states have laws that provide protection from discovery for documents related to quality assurance activities or related to the needs of the hospital attorney to perform his or her job. Incident reports are usually among the documents protected from discovery; however, each state's laws must be reviewed to determine whether protection is accorded.

a duty of reasonable care by the physicians and hospital staff involved in his care. He had the right to expect that all reasonable precautions would be observed so that no further harm would come to him.

Breach of duty is proved by demonstrating that the care given to the patient fell below acceptable standards. An expert witness for the plaintiff would testify that it is standard practice to visualize by radiography the cervical and

DUTY TO WARN

The obligation to safeguard patient confidences is subject to certain exceptions that are ethically and legally justified because of overriding social considerations. When a patient threatens to inflict serious bodily harm to another person and there is a reasonable probability that the patient may carry out the threat, the physician should take reasonable precautions for the protection of the intended victim, including notification of law enforcement authorities. Communicable diseases and gunshot and knife wounds should also be reported, as required by applicable statutes or ordinances.[9]

One of the most serious dilemmas faced by ED personnel occurs when a patient who was seen for treatment in the ED poses a threat to the public when discharged. This situation occurs in the case of an intoxicated person who plans to drive home from the hospital, a psychiatric patient who threatens to kill or injure another person after discharge, or a patient with an onset of seizure disorder who drives a commercial truck for a living. When can the ED personnel breach the patient's confidentiality to protect the public? The Tarasoff case gives the best example of the law's exceptions for breaching patient confidentiality.[28,29]

In the Tarasoff case a University of California student sought psychiatric help at the University of California Student Health Service. During the interview with the psychologist, the student related a pathologic attachment to a woman named Tatiana Tarasoff. The student revealed that he had thoughts about inflicting harm on this woman. The psychologist notified the campus police about the intentions expressed by the student, but nothing was done to stop the student or protect Ms. Tarasoff. Shortly after the interview with the psychologist the student had the opportunity to be with Ms. Tarasoff, and he murdered her.

Ms. Tarasoff's family instituted a lawsuit against the university, the psychologist, and the campus police. Their legal claim was based on the theory that the therapist had a duty to warn Ms. Tarasoff or her family of the impending danger. The final decision of the court contained a phrase that has now become famous when these questions are considered: "The protective privilege ends where the public peril begins."[9] The Tarasoff family won their lawsuit, and new rules were established regarding the degree of confidentiality patients could expect in their conversations with medical personnel.

Again, each state's laws must be read to determine if there is specific law that addresses the question of patient confidentiality. In the absence of state law, it is likely that the finding in the Tarasoff case would apply in these types of cases.

DOCUMENTATION

The hospital medical record is the complete document reflecting the events of a patient's hospitalization. Thorough, accurate documentation in the medical record is one of the best defenses against lawsuits for medical negligence. Increasingly the medical record is being used by insurance companies and peer review organizations to substantiate charges and study the quality of care delivery.

When a plaintiff seeks the counsel of an attorney regarding the possibility of a legal action against a medical professional, the attorney immediately requests copies of the medical record. The attorney reviews the contents of the medical record to determine whether a basis for a lawsuit exists. Since it is common for a lawsuit to be instituted several years after the incident has occurred, the medical record provides the only written account of the events of that time. Rules for accurate documentation in the medical record are listed in the box below.

In addition to the specific guidelines for documentation,

RULES FOR DOCUMENTATION IN MEDICAL RECORD

1. Always write legibly, using correct spelling and acceptable medical abbreviations.
2. Leave no lines blank between charting. Blank lines create the impression of an intent to return to the record to do fill-in charting.
3. All medical personnel who participate in the care of the patient must be identified in the medical record by legible signatures and titles.
4. Draw a line through errors in charting, and initial the errors. Never use correction fluid (White-Out) to cover errors. A notation such as "incorrect entry" or "void" should be made above the lined out area.
5. All documentation should be recorded in chronologic order and as contemporaneously as possible.
6. If procedures have been performed in response to verbal orders from physicians, the physician must sign the ED record. His or her signature verifies that the orders were accurate and carried out at the direction of the physician.
7. Late entries should be noted as such on the medical record. Late entries should be made only to complete the documentation, *never* in contemplation of litigation. Experts in documentation analysis have the ability to analyze the document and determine the date when the entry was actually written and who made the entry.[13] The science of documentation analysis evolved after an estimated 10% of medical records in malpractice cases were found to be fraudulently altered.[1]

there are other guidelines expressly related to documentation in the ED setting, which are discussed in the following paragraphs.

All ED charting must be performed in compliance with standards of the Joint Commission on Accreditation of Healthcare Organizations for the region. These standards require the recording of a physical assessment, allergies, patient history, and condition on discharge, among other items.[2] All charting also must be performed in compliance with the specific hospital policies, and the accepted medical abbreviations for that facility must be used.

Every woman of childbearing age (between the ages of 9 and 60) should be asked the date of her last menstrual period. The answer should be recorded on the chart in a prominent place. This information is important when radiographic examinations may be performed and when antibiotics or other drugs may be ordered.

Any patient who has previously been a patient at the hospital should have his or her previous medical record(s) sent to the ED for review, and the obtaining and review of the medical records should be noted on the current record. This procedure is particularly important for patients who are having shoulder or arm pain because of the frequency of missing a diagnosis of myocardial infarction. A previous electrocardiogram or previous enzyme studies can be especially helpful in making the appropriate diagnosis.

Extreme care should be taken when recording comments made by people other than the patient. If the ambulance personnel state that the patient was "probably" unrestrained in the vehicle, it would be prudent to note that restraint use was unknown. Some states decrease the amount of money that can be awarded to a victim in a motor vehicle collision, if the victim was not wearing a safety belt at the time of the collision. Patients can lose money because of incorrect information in the medical record.

The discharge instructions given to the patient represent one of the most critical areas of potential litigation in the ED. A written assurance must be made that the patient has been given the instructions in a written format and in language that was easily understood. If the patient speaks a foreign language, documentation of the accommodation made must be provided to ensure that the patient comprehends the discharge instructions. All discharge instructions should contain a statement that encourages the patient to either return to the ED or contact his or her personal physicians for medical attention to unresolved problems or exacerbation of their physical problems.

The discharge instructions provide the opportunity to ensure that the patient knows what possible complications he or she must be looking for during recovery. The instructions also provide information regarding the possible drug reactions the patient might have with the drugs they received. Additional warnings can be included, such as the warning not to drive a vehicle when an eyepatch is in place[14] or when certain drugs have been given. These instructions furnish the final chance to give the patient all the information needed to continue the prescribed medical care at home, including a comprehensive list of potential problems that must be monitored.

Adequate discharge instructions are one of the best safeguards against litigation from the patient who was discharged and sent home from the ED. A copy of the instructions given to the patient should become part of the permanent medical record.

CONSOLIDATED OMNIBUS BUDGET RECONCILIATION ACT

In the late 1970s and the early 1980s, publicity was focused on the practice in some hospitals of refusing to accept emergency patients or attempting to transfer patients to county hospitals once it was determined that the patients were uninsured. In response to this practice, Congress passed what has been termed the federal "antidumping" law. This law, part of a Social Security act, is known as the Consolidated Omnibus Budget Reconciliation Act (COBRA).[7] This act applied to all hospitals that provided some type of emergency service. The passage of this act placed severe restrictions on the transfer of emergency patients, and the threat of substantial penalties was imposed on hospitals and physicians.[5]

On December 19, 1989, President Bush signed into law amendments that make the previous COBRA restrictions even more stringent. The amendments went into effect on July 1, 1990.[7] These amendments have increased the scope of COBRA's effect so that it now applies to any hospital that has a Medicare provider agreement.[31]

The term "responsible physician" was deleted from the act, and the provisions were made to apply to "any physician who is responsible for the examination, treatment, or transfer of an individual in a participating hospital, including a physician on-call for the care of such individual."[32] Essentially, any physician who practices in the hospital falls under the COBRA provisions. The major provisions of the amendments to COBRA that became effective in 1990 are listed in the box on p. 28.

The financial penalties have remained unchanged; the hospital and the physician face $50,000 fines for violations of the law. The patient maintains the option of filing a civil lawsuit for damages he or she believes were incurred because of hospital or physician violations.

The new amendments also address responsibilities of certain hospitals to accept transfer patients. Regional referral centers and hospitals with specialized capabilities such as trauma centers, tertiary neonatal centers, and burn units are obligated to accept all *appropriate* transfers of patients who require the care provided by these specialty centers, as long as they have the capacity to treat the individual.

It is clear that the amendments to COBRA have far-reaching effects on most U.S. hospitals. Every affected hospital must obtain thorough knowledge of the require-

---

MAJOR PROVISIONS OF AMENDMENTS MADE TO COBRA* IN 1989

1. The word "patient" has been deleted and the term "individual" is in its place. This terminology indicates that the act applies to any person who seeks care at the ED. The individual does not have to be an official patient of the hospital. This provision was probably placed because some hospitals attempted to divert individuals before they registered as patients.[5]
2. The requirement for a routine medical screening examination in the ED is now expanded to include the capabilities of the ancillary services available to the ED.
3. The provisions now apply to any pregnant woman who is having contractions, not only to the woman in active labor.
4. All medicare-participating hospitals must maintain records of patient transfers to and from the hospital. Hospitals must also maintain a call list of physicians who are available to provide the necessary stabilizing treatment following the initial screening examination.
5. Hospitals are prohibited from delaying the screening examination until insurance coverage or the patient's ability to pay is determined.
6. When an individual seeks care at a hospital, the hospital is required to provide informed consent of the risks and benefits of the care that the hospital offers. If the patient refuses the preferred treatment, the hospital must take all reasonable steps to obtain *written informed consent* of the refusal. If a transfer of the patient is contemplated, the hospital is obligated to obtain the patient's informed consent regarding the proposed transfer.
7. When patients are going to be transferred, the hospital

must comply with one of the following requirements:
   a. After informing the patient of the hospital's obligations under the federal law and describing the risks and benefits associated with the transfer, the hospital must obtain the patient's written request for a transfer, or
   b. A physician must sign a certificate confirming that the benefits of transfer outweigh the risks, based on the information available to the physician at the time of transfer, not on information from the initial examination, or
   c. If a physician is not available in the ED a *qualified medical person* must sign the certificate described in "b." A physician must countersign the certificate within a reasonable period (should not exceed 24 hours).
8. When a patient is transferred to another facility, it is the obligation of the transferring hospital to send to the receiving facility all medical records or copies of medical records pertaining to the emergency condition of the patient. This requirement should be understood to include all the medical records generated at the hospital where the patient was first seen.
9. If the transfer was ordered by the ED physician because of his or her belief that the patient required care by an on-call specialist who refused to see the patient, the following information applies: the *name and address of any on-call physician who has refused or failed to appear within a reasonable time to provide necessary stabilizing treatment to the patient* (emphasis added) must be included with other transfer documents.

*Consolidated Omnibus Budget Reconciliation Act (COBRA). Amended Dec 19, 1989, Pub L. No. 101-239, §6211 HR 3299, 140-44 (effective July 1, 1990).

---

ments and develop the appropriate rules and regulations, forms, and on-call policies, to ensure compliance with this federal law. The list of provisions given in the box above is not comprehensive but is reflective of the major changes that were effective July 1, 1990. Hospital attorneys should be consulted to determine the applicability of the federal "anti-dumping" law to the individual hospitals and medical staffs.

CONSENT ISSUES

It is well established in law that a patient must give consent before medical treatment can be initiated. This legal doctrine was eloquently described by Justice Cardozo while he was sitting on the New York Court of Appeals: "Every human being of adult years and sound mind has a right to determine what shall be done with his own body; and a surgeon who performs an operation without his patient's consent commits an assault, for which he is liable in damages."[26]

The presence of either an express consent or an implied consent of the patient for care delivery is a valid defense by the defendant to a legal action in the case of battery. Express consent is an oral or written confirmation of the agreement to receive medical treatment. Implied consent is understood to be given when the patient's conduct suggests agreement, for example, the competent patient who voluntarily submits to the treatment. Implied consent would also be given when the patient arrives unconscious with life or limb at risk. It is understood that if this patient were able to communicate, he or she would consent to lifesaving therapy. If procedures are performed according to the implied consent theory, the documentation should reflect the critical importance of proceeding with treatment before being able to obtain express consent. If at all possible, it would be helpful to have a second documented opinion regarding the need for rapid interventions.

Commonly in the ED a minor requests emergency medical care. The laws addressing the age of consent vary from state to state and often have multiple variations. For example, the law may describe a certain age for consenting to medical treatment[17] and include exceptions for children seeking information about birth control, abortion, or venereal disease.[16] State laws also dictate the financial responsibilities of parents when their children seek medical care.

In the previous discussion on battery, it was mentioned that a patient who was touched in an offensive manner without the patient's consent would probably have a legal suit against the defendant for battery. If the offensive contact was performed without the patient's informed consent, the legal action would be for negligence, not battery.[25] Many states have made the requirements for informed consent a state law. Under Oregon law, for example, informed consent must meet the following criteria:

1. The procedure or treatment must be explained to the patient in general, understandable terms.
2. Any alternatives to the proposed procedure must be explored.
3. An explanation of the risks associated with the procedure or treatment must be given.[19]

In addition to the law concerning the requirements for informed consent, other statutes that required the designated person to provide informed consent were passed for two reasons. First, the physician possesses the technical expertise necessary to answer questions posed by the patient about the procedure and the risks. Second, physicians have a special relationship of trust with patients, which requires that the physician provide the information.[15]

Another statute that is becoming more common throughout the United States applies to patients involved in motor vehicle collisions. The provisions of this statute allow the police to administer a breath test to determine the alcoholic content of the blood of a person who is arrested for driving under the influence of intoxicants. This law deems that if the person operated a motor vehicle on any premises open to the public or on state highways, the patient gave implied consent for the test. If the arrested person refuses to take the test after hearing an explanation of rights, the police are given the authority to suspend the person's driving privileges.[20]

In conjunction with the preceding statute, more states are adopting laws that give police officers the legal authority to obtain blood from patients who are suspected of driving under the influence of intoxicants.[21] This statute may put a burden on ED personnel because of the potential conflict between being a patient advocate and gathering criminal evidence from a patient. It is imperative that every health care professional who works in the ED have complete understanding of the state law in the area of blood alcohol testing.

Any discussion of consent would be incomplete without comments on the right of patients to refuse offered treatment. In a recent Supreme Court opinion, Justice Brennan wrote eloquently on this topic: "The right to be free from unwanted medical attention is a right to evaluate the potential benefit of treatment and its possible consequences according to one's own values and to make a personal decision whether to subject oneself to the intrusion."[8]

All too often medical personnel believe that patients are obligated to accept even those offered medical interventions that have only the remotest possibility of extending life.[15] The current controversies regarding the privacy rights associated with refusal of consent are discussed in the following section. In the ED, one of the most common cases of patient refusal to consent is the Jehovah's Witness patient who refuses to consent to blood transfusions. The refusal by these patients is grounded in their belief that the First Amendment allows the religious right of self-determination.

Hospitals frequently resort to the legal system in attempts to override the refusal of consent for these patients. If after reviewing the facts the court finds that the patient who is refusing the transfusion is an adult who will leave no minor children should death occur as a result of the refusal, the court generally allows the patient's wishes to stand.[10] However, if the patient is a minor or has minor children, the court often orders the transfusion(s) to be given.[3]

The objection Jehovah's Witnesses have to blood transfusion extends to the reinfusion of their own blood via cell savers or autotransfusion units.[30] However, in an emergency situation when the patient's life is threatened by hypovolemia, the blood transfusion should be administered immediately.[11]

During the orientation of new nursing and physician staff in the ED, it would be prudent to include a section on the relevant state laws concerning the issues surrounding consent. A section in the department policy and procedure manual should also be dedicated to this important topic.

THE RIGHT TO PRIVACY

As modern medicine has extended its ability to maintain life at both ends of the life cycle, concerns about the questions related to when life begins and ends are ever increasing. This section focuses on the recently litigated issue of whether patients have a "right to die."

In the 1970s a New Jersey court heard and decided the case of Karen Ann Quinlan. Ms. Quinlan had been to a party where she accidentally overdosed on alcohol and a prescription drug. When the prehospital providers arrived on the scene, she was pulseless and apneic, and CPR was initiated. There was a return of vital signs, and Ms. Quinlan was transported to a local hospital. After a few days, the neurologists advised the Quinlan family that Karen was in a persistent vegetative state.

The Quinlans then asked the hospital to disconnect the ventilator because they believed that Karen would not want to continue to exist in this permanently unconscious state. The hospital refused their request because Ms. Quinlan did not have brain death. The Quinlans then resorted to the legal system to obtain permission to disconnect their daughter from the ventilator. A lengthy court battle ensued before the Quinlans were given the right to disconnect their daughter from the ventilator.[24] After Ms. Quinlan was disconnected, she began spontaneous respirations and lived for several more years in a nursing home.

The decision of the court in the Quinlan case was easily accepted by the medical profession. During the next several years additional cases that were brought before the courts had slightly different facts than those of the Quinlan case. The courts frequently agreed with family members that the patient should not be forced to endure medical care that was palliative only. The concept of termination of life-support systems was expanded to include the termination of tube feeding by surrogate decision makers acting in the patient's best interest.[33]

Until 1989, all the legal cases addressing the "right to die" were decided by state courts or federal appeals courts; the Supreme Court had never agreed to hear a "right to die" case. However, during the 1989-1990 session, the Supreme Court heard the arguments in the Missouri case of Nancy Cruzan.[8]

Ms. Cruzan was involved in a motor vehicle accident (a single-car rollover) in January 1983, in Joplin County, Missouri. When the police arrived on the scene, she was pulseless and apneic and was lying face down in a ditch. The prehospital personnel arrived and initiated CPR. Ms. Cruzan's vital signs returned after the institution of CPR. She was transported to a local hospital and taken to the OR for an exploratory laparotomy. After surgery Ms. Cruzan appeared to be progressing, and the hospital personnel attempted without success to give her fluids from a cup. Her physicians thought that she would recuperate more rapidly with the insertion of a feeding tube. Ms. Cruzan's husband (they were later divorced) agreed to the insertion of the tube.

Soon after the procedure was performed, Ms. Cruzan's condition stabilized and did not further progress. It was determined that she was in a persistent vegetative state. When it became clear that Ms. Cruzan had no chance of recovering her previous mental status, her parents approached the hospital officials and requested the termination of the tube feedings. The hospital refused the parents' request and told the parents that for the hospital to comply with their wishes, a court order would have to be obtained.

The Cruzans then applied to the state trial court for the order requested by the hospital. The state trial court agreed with the Cruzans and issued the order. This order was immediately appealed by the Missouri Department of Health to the Missouri Supreme Court. This court denied the petition of the parents. Ms. Cruzan's parents then appealed to the U.S. Supreme Court, and the Court agreed to hear the case.

In June 1990 the Supreme Court issued its opinion in the Cruzan case. It is important to understand exactly what the Court did and did not say in that opinion. The question the Supreme Court answered was, "Did Missouri have the right to demand clear and convincing evidence of the incompetent patient's wishes regarding termination of life support?" The answer to that question was yes.

The Supreme Court held that Missouri had a strong interest in the preservation of the lives of its citizens. In the exercise of that interest, Missouri had the right to require evidence that it thought expressed with certainty the desires of the incompetent patient. Since the Cruzans did not have evidence that fit the Missouri standard, the termination of tube feedings was not allowed.

If Ms. Cruzan had filled out a durable power of attorney form for health care decisions before the accident, the form probably would have met the standard set by Missouri for clear and convincing evidence. It is clear from the Supreme Court decision that the state court of Missouri will always decide in favor of preserving life when there is any doubt about what the patient would have wanted in the particular circumstances.

The Cruzan decision should alert all health care professionals to the need for education of the public regarding "living wills" and durable power of attorney forms for health care decisions. The proper execution of these documents provides the best reassurance that one's wishes regarding prolongation of life will be honored.

In the late fall of 1990 the Cruzans returned to the Missouri trial court to seek reconsideration of their request for termination of the feeding tube. Additional witnesses came forward who had discussed in detail with Nancy her preference on the issue of prolongation of life-sustaining treatment for patients in vegetative states. These witnesses confirmed the earlier testimony of the Cruzans that if Nancy were in a vegetative state, she would have wanted not to receive life-sustaining treatment.

The Missouri trial court agreed that the new testimony provided the clear and convincing evidence required for termination of tube feeding. The trial court issued the order for termination, and the hospital complied. Nancy Beth Cruzan died 12 days after the feeding tube was removed, on December 26, 1990.

EMERGENCY DEPARTMENT RISK MANAGEMENT

Risk management is the identification and minimization of risks, with the primary focus on reducing liability exposure and financial loss.[15] How do ED personnel identify the greatest risks to their department? Risk identification comes primarily from the monitoring activities associated with the quality assurance review process.

The ongoing ED quality assurance monitoring activities process pinpoints the activities that increase liability exposure. To be effective, the quality assurance process should systematically monitor high-risk and high-volume activities and comprehensively review problems identified through other sources. Once a serious risk factor has been identified, it is crucial that the ED manager or physician director develop a policy or procedure to address the risk. New policies and procedures should not necessarily be developed in response to every identified occurrence but should be developed in response to those events posing the greatest exposure to liability.

The most important factor in reducing liability exposure is comprehensive documentation. The well-written ED flow chart can be used for defense in several types of legal actions frequently filed against ED personnel. As discussed previously, inclusive discharge instructions are also critically important in the management of risk.

The following are examples of problems that have a high potential for associated liability, accompanied by methods of risk management:

Risk

ED radiographs made between 8 PM and 7 AM are not read by a radiologist until 8 AM.

Risk management

1. The discharge instructions specify that the patient must call the ED to get the final reading of the films or must leave a telephone number where he or she can be reached in case of a different radiologic diagnosis.
2. A log that lists the following is maintained in the ED: the names of patients who received incorrect interpretations of radiographs, the time and date when each patient is notified, and instructions given to each patient.

Risk

Women of childbearing age receive radiographic examinations or antibiotics when they could possibly be in the first trimester of pregnancy.

Risk management

1. During the history that is taken for all women of childbearing age, the patient is asked when her last normal menstrual period occurred, and the response is noted on the chart. When the response indicates the possibility of an early pregnancy, a special notation is attached to the chart.

Risk

A patient admitted to the ED in critical condition requires care that is not available at the admitting hospital, and the ED physician plans to transfer the patient to another hospital more equipped to care for this patient.

Risk management

1. A standardized form that details all the COBRA requirements must be available, and the physician must complete this form before the transfer.
2. A nursing checklist for the COBRA requirements is also available.

The preceding examples reflect one approach to incorporating risk management with ED care. Many of the potential risks are identified in applicable state and federal laws such as COBRA and consent laws. Peer review of documentation is another method of risk management that not only ensures medical record review but also provides an educational process for the staff involved in the review process.

The foundation of quality health care is built on this interrelationship of quality assurance and risk management. The ED with a credible risk management program will be rewarded with a decrease in liability exposure and an increase in patient safety and satisfaction. Risk management is further discussed in Chapter 16.

SUMMARY

The essence of liability prevention in all areas of medical and nursing practice is providing and documenting care within accepted standards. ED nurses should practice not in fear of litigation but according to sound medical and nursing principles. Every ED manager should ensure that department personnel have received education regarding consent principles, standard of care, transfer restrictions, and other important medical-legal issues. Additionally, comprehensive written procedures should be available to all staff, and current forms regarding such issues as blood alcohol testing, transfer of patients, and refusal to consent should also be available. All personnel should also be made aware of mandated reporting requirements concerning child abuse, infectious diseases, and injury incurred as a result of criminal activity. Nurses must know the limits of the state's Nurse Practice Act. The prudent ED manager supports continuing education for staff members: the acquisition of knowledge and skills ensures the competence of practitioners. A comprehensive quality management process is a key ingredient in the provision of a safe environment for the ED patient. All the preceding elements combine to provide ED patients with high-quality care that meets acceptable medical and legal standards of care.

REFERENCES

1. American College of Legal Medicine: *Legal medicine: legal dynamics of medical encounters,* St Louis, 1988, Mosby–Year Book.
2. *AMH Accreditation Manual for Hospitals,* Chicago, 1989, Joint Commission on Accreditation of Healthcare Organizations.
3. Application of the President and Directors of Georgetown College, Inc, 331 F 2d 1000 (D.C. Dir. 1964).
4. Black HC: *Black's law dictionary,* ed 5, St Paul, 1979, West Publishing.
5. Brown LC: Patient dumping after COBRA 1989: new problems for hospitals and physicians alike, *Health Lawyer* 4:2, 1990.
6. Reference deleted in proofs.
7. Consolidated Omnibus Budget Reconciliation Act (COBRA). Amended Dec 19, 1989, Pub L. No. 101-239, §6211 HR 3299, 140-44 (effective July 1, 1990).
8. *Cruzan v. Director,* Missouri Department of Health, 58 LW 4916, 4928 (June 25, 1990).
9. Current Opinions of the Council on Ethical and Judicial Affairs of the American Medical Association. Opinion 5.05 (1986).
10. In re Estate of Brooks, 205 N.E. 2d 435 (1965).
11. Gibbs RF: Blood transfusions for Jehovah's Witnesses. In American College of Legal Medicine: *Legal medicine: legal dynamics of medical encounters,* St Louis, 1988, Mosby–Year Book.
12. Goldman B, ed: Curbing the threat of litigation in the emergency

department: a risk management approach, *Emerg Med Reports* 2:2, 1990.

13. Hirsch, HL: Tampering with medical records, *Med Trials Technique Q* 24:450, 1978.

14. *Joy v. Eastern Maine Medical Center,* 529 A 2d 1364 (Maine, 1987).

15. Macdonald MG, Meyer KC, and Essig B: *Health care law: a practical guide,* New York, 1988, Matthew Bender.

16. Oregon Revised Statute 109.610 (1977).

17. Oregon Revised Statute 109.640 (1971).

18. Oregon Revised Statute 133.621 (1989).

19. Oregon Revised Statute 677.097 (1983).

20. Oregon Revised Statute 813.100 (1985).

21. Oregon Revised Statute 813-140 (1985).

22. Prosser WL: *Handbook of the law of torts,* ed 4, St Paul, 1971, West Publishing.

23. Reference deleted in proofs.

24. In re Quinlan, 355 a-2d, 647 (New Jersey, 1976).

25. *Salgo v. Leland Stanford, Jr,* University Board of Trustees, 154 Cal App 2d 560, 317 p 2d 170 (Palo Alto, Calif, 1957).

26. *Schloendorff v. Society of New York Hospital,* 211 New York, 125, 129-30, 105 N.E. 92,93 (1914).

27. Southard P and Frankel P: Trauma care documentation: a comprehensive guide, *JEN* 15:393, 1989.

28. *Tarasoff v. Regents of the University of California,* 13 Cal 3d 177, 119 Cap Rptr 129, 529, P2d, 553 (1974) (Tarasoff I), affirmed on rehearing 17 Cal 3d 425, 131 Cap Rptr 14, 551 P2s 334 (1976) (Tarasoff II).

29. *Tarasoff v. Regents of the University of California,* 17 Cal 3d at 442, 131 Cal Rptr at 27, 551 P2d at 347 1976.

30. Thurkauf GE: Understanding the beliefs of Jehovah's Witnesses, *Focus Crit Care* 16:199, 1989.

31. 42 U.S.C.A. 1395 dd (d) and (e) (3) (1982 and Supp. IV 1986) (amended 1989).

32. 42 U.S.C.A. 1395 dd (d) (2) (b) (Supp. 1990).

33. 42 U.S.C.A. 1395 dd (Supp. 1990).

Emergency Department Management

Barbara Weldon Tone*

Emergency department (ED) management is one of the most exciting, challenging fields in health care today. Emergency medicine is a relatively new, dynamic, and rapidly changing specialty. Many areas of controversy remain, and many areas have yet to be researched. Opening a chest in the ED was unheard of 20 years ago, and 30 years ago almost no one had heard of prehospital care.

The people who work in EDs are unique and challenging to manage. Most emergency personnel do not like routine; they enjoy bringing order out of chaos; they are motivated, aggressive, and not content in a static environment. Keeping up with an ever-changing field and with people who are easily bored is not an easy task, but it can be rewarding.

This chapter does not present new scientific studies in management. It does present some basic, practical, and easily understood ideas about people and systems. In a single chapter it is not possible to explore in depth all the aspects of management. Entire books have been written about motivation, goal setting, performance reviews, and other management topics.

As you read about management, it is important to remember that there are as many management styles as there are managers. Although it is hoped that the ideas presented here are sound and useful, unfortunately no absolutes exist in management. What works in one system or with one person may not be appropriate in every system or with every person. Part of the chapter discusses the importance of common sense and perspective in the manager. If absolutes existed in management, common sense and perspective would not be needed.

The first section of this chapter addresses a few of the "systems" parts of management: goal setting, problem solving, and dealing with structure and change. The second section deals with the management of people. The emphasis in this chapter is more on the people aspect of management for two reasons. First, I tend to be more "people oriented" (sometimes an asset, sometimes a liability) than "systems

oriented"; second, people everywhere are much the same (in a collective sense), but systems vary widely.

Many of the sections overlap and repeat ideas from other sections. Management is an integrated process, and one cannot isolate one component from another, either on paper or in practice.

From these discussions, I would like the reader to remember mainly the ideas, not the formulas. No magic formulas exist. Management is primarily an art, not a science.

MANAGEMENT OF THE SYSTEM

According to Webster, a system is "an established way of doing something." Having a collection of the most talented, motivated people in the world is a good start, but if no systems are in place for guiding their efforts, confusion and chaos result, and the overall output is significantly decreased. To illustrate, suppose you did not have a system for scheduling and simply called around every day looking for people to work. Most of your available administrative time would be spent on the phone. Imagine also a patient's chart that did not have specific areas labeled to indicate what should be recorded. Much time would be spent trying to locate the patient's name, address, and orders on the chart. The same principles apply to less obvious areas, including goal setting and problem solving.

The first part of this chapter discusses a few areas of systems management: goal setting, problem solving, project management, and structure and change. My intent is to convey that systems are essential to smooth operation. This section provides some examples of systems for managing certain areas, but more importantly, the manager must understand the *need* for a defined method of operating. It is easy to understand the need in scheduling and in chart design, but one must also have a systematic process for setting goals and resolving performance problems. For example, suppose a staff member comes to you and says that nobody is restocking the rooms anymore. If you do not understand the need for a defined method of approaching this problem, your response might be to simply *demand* at the next staff meeting that everyone stock his or her room. If you have a

---

*With revisions by Vicky Bradley.

defined approach, the investigation might reveal that someone moved all the supplies and nobody can find anything to restock.

Systems are essential. Develop your own, use somebody else's, or do both, but do not assume that you can successfully manage without them.

Setting Goals and Objectives

If you don't know where you are going,
you will end up somewhere else.
L. Peter

In emergency care the only predictable thing is change, usually rapid and often dramatic. Medical care changes, health care systems change, prehospital care changes— nothing seems to stabilize for more than a few days at a time. One in the midst of all this can easily become caught up in daily "fire fighting" and lose sight of long-term goals.

"Fire fighting" (dealing with the 1001 problems that crop up every day) can be a full-time job if you allow it to be. The only way to avoid this fire-fighting syndrome (or "management by crisis," as it is sometimes called) is to be zealous in your commitment to goal setting and goal achievement.

The importance of goal setting cannot be overemphasized. Conscious attention to where you are versus where you want to be is imperative if you expect to establish and maintain a progressive ED service. Although no one goal-setting method is right for every environment, the following guidelines may be useful in establishing a goal-setting process.

Goal-setting activities should be a cooperative effort between nurses, physicians, and hospital administration. If goals are established independently, it is likely that too many different projects will be activated simultaneously, resulting in staff frustration, stress, and confusion. It is also important that all members of the team understand the objectives, which is difficult to achieve if goals are not mutually agreed on beforehand.

The medical director and nursing manager may be the only ones directly involved in the goal-setting process, or all the administrative staff may be involved. Representatives may be selected from the department staff to participate in the process, or written input may be solicited from all staff members.

The first step in this goal-setting process is to define the *strategic goals* for the department. Two types of strategic goals exist. The first represents the department's overall philosophy. Some examples of overall strategic goals are "provide optimal emergency care"; "meet the needs of all client groups" (that is, patients, physicians, community); and "provide opportunities for professional advancement."

Overall strategic goals should be few in number, no more than five, and they do not change. These philosophic "goals" essentially represent the department's reason for existence, and they provide the basis for all other goal setting. Outlining these philosophies is therefore a very important part of the goal-setting process.

The second type of strategic goals is established annually. Every department should, formally and *in writing*, define the departmental goals for the year. Each of these annual goals should relate to one or more of the philosophic goals. For example, "Ensure appropriate initial patient screening" is an annual goal and relates directly to the overall goal of providing optimal medical care. "Minimize patient processing time" is a goal that relates to meeting the needs of the patient/client group. Annual strategic goals represent *where you want to be* and therefore require that you first know where you are.

Emergency department status survey. The ED status survey on p. 35 is an assessment tool developed by Fulcher[2] for use in the goal-setting process. This survey is an outline of those areas of ED operation that should be assessed annually to provide a clear picture of *where you are*. The outline lists several key areas of operation and subcategorizes each one. Use of this assessment tool is invaluable when establishing annual goals.

The status survey must be done in writing. Each subcategory should be honestly reviewed. All categories should be assessed based on their relationship to what would be "perfection." Clearly, perfection in all areas at all times is not a realistic goal, but aiming for less than 100% only lowers the ultimate result.

Ideally a mixture of objective and subjective data sources should be used to complete the status survey. The more objective data available, the more valid the status survey will be. Gathering data by hand is time-consuming but frequently is the only option available. Using staff downtime or assigning a clerk are temporary options. Strategizing with information management specialists, management engineers, and quality assurance managers to develop computerized information systems is essential to provide today's manager with a clearer picture of how the ED is functioning and changing.

Subjective data can be obtained by two or three key administrative people independently and then compared. It is most interesting to look at different perceptions of the same areas. For even more diverse views, ask two or three staff members to complete the survey.

After the survey has been completed and compiled, the people responsible for annual goal setting should meet to review this assessment and set goals for the year. Annual goal setting requires three "Cs": commitment, compromise, and common sense.

The people involved in goal setting must have a *commitment* to the process and an understanding of its importance. They must also be mature enough to be committed to the achievement of the final goals even if some of the goals decided on are not the ones they would have chosen.

Goal setters must be willing to look at all perceptions and *compromise* when necessary. A spirit of cooperation and mutual respect should exist among the individuals involved.

Finally, goal setting calls for *common sense*. The worse the shape the department is in, the easier it is to set goals;

EMERGENCY DEPARTMENT STATUS SURVEY*

I. Facility and equipment
   A. Size and design
   B. Emergency equipment
   C. Stocking and control procedures
   D. Equipment checking procedures

II. Charts and records
   A. Design
   B. Chart procedures
   C. Storage and retrieval
   D. Statistics

III. Administration/management
   A. Personnel
   B. Policy/procedure manual
   C. Communications
   D. Administrative procedures
   E. Budget

IV. Personnel
   A. Staffing
   B. Back-up procedures
   C. Morale
   D. Evaluation
   E. Orientation
   F. Recruitment standards

V. Logistics of patient care
   A. Triage
   B. Admission procedures
   C. Discharge procedures
   D. Hospital admission
   E. "Processing" paperwork
   F. Telephone communications
   G. Billing/collection

VI. Ancillary services
   A. Radiology
   B. Laboratory
   C. Pulmonary
   D. Electrocardiography
   E. Social services
   F. Other

VII. Attending staff relationships
   A. Private physicians
   B. Back-up physicians
   C. Emergency committee

VIII. Interhospital relationships
   A. Administration
   B. Medical staff office
   C. Business office
   D. Nursing administration

IX. Extrahospital relationships
   A. Police department(s)
   B. Fire department
   C. Others

X. Paramedic/ambulance services

XI. Quality monitoring
   A. Chart review
   B. Standards/protocols

XII. Education
   A. CPR training
   B. Continuing education
   C. Reference materials

Examples of assessment

EXAMPLE 1: Section I, Part A

Size and design

Assessment data

1. Number of annual visits: 30,000
2. Projected trend of visits: annual increase of 7% over the last 5 years
3. Percentage of emergent (critical) patients: 12%; 4% increase last year
4. Percentage of "fast track" (convenience care) patients: 34%; 7% increase last year
5. Percentage of urgent patients: 54%
6. Trends in patient demographics: 20% pediatric patients, 80% adults; 25% of patients admitted to hospital (20% last year); 5% increase in gynecologic patients; 2% increase in major trauma patients
7. Average length of stay: 4 hours
8. Patient complaints related to size or design: 30 complaints related to long length of stay; majority were "fast track" patients

Analysis: The major problem appears to be an increase in critical patients who are using more staff, laboratory, and radiology resources. This is causing a delay in providing rapid care to the "fast track" population. The ED radiology suite is frequently tied up with major trauma patients, eliminating the ability to provide x-ray films of minor injuries expeditiously. This problem warrants further study.

EXAMPLE 2: Section V, Part A

Triage

Assessment data

1. Number of annual visits: 30,000
2. Length of time between initial presentation and beginning of triage: 90% within 15 minutes in patients classified as nonurgent and urgent; 10% longer than the 15-minute standard; all emergent patients immediately triaged
3. Patient complaints: two complaints related to other patients being treated before them (both triage classifications correct)
4. Number of triage misclassifications: audit incomplete

Analysis: The 10% outside the 15-minute standard are typically nonurgent patients who arrive between noon and 10 PM, with higher frequency on Friday and Saturday evenings. This problem warrants further study to investigate whether a second triage is needed on Friday and Saturday evenings.

*Developed by James K. Fulcher.

major deficiencies are then much more obvious. As a department becomes more finely tuned, the lines become much grayer, and deficiencies are not so glaring. Common sense is essential in establishing priorities for departmental improvement. "Thorough knowledge of renal pathophysiology" is probably unrealistic if no one in the department is certified in basic cardiopulmonary resuscitation (CPR). This may be an exaggerated example, but it is not unusual to see lofty goals set when the basics are not yet covered. Therefore, assuming that all the goal setters have the three "Cs," you should be able to determine annual goals without great difficulty.

Before we move to objectives, there is one final goal-setting warning, especially to those who are new to the goal-setting process: *be realistic*. Tackling laboratory and radiology delays, the collection system, medical record problems, new emergency department charts, a facility redesign, and the care of multiple trauma patients all in 1 year only results in frustration and discouragement at year's end. Only two or three major goals should be set for a year. Some minor "cleanup" goals also may be set, but attempting to resolve four or more major deficiencies in 12 months is unrealistic.

Tactical objectives. Once the annual goals have been decided on, each goal should be broken down into *tactical objectives*. Writing objectives helps determine the cause of the deficiency and work toward resolution. "Ensure thorough documentation of all cardiac arrests" is an excellent goal, but the statement is an insufficient basis for action. Going to the emergency department staff and saying "improve your CPR documentation" will not be well received or productive. Possible tactical objectives for this goal follow:

1. Establish criteria for CPR documentation.
2. Review 20 CPR charts and compare with criteria.
3. Assess cause of deficiency.
4. Implement staff education, charting format, and so on to correct deficiency.
5. Review results (reaudit).

A final step in the process is the task outline. A *task outline* is a listing of specific activities necessary to meet each *objective*. Each objective should have a task outline (see the section on project management).

At this point, some readers may be wondering when one has the time to resolve deficiencies after spending all of this effort outlining the deficiencies and the mechanisms for resolution. Responses to this question include the following:

1. With practice, the time involved to set goals and objectives becomes less and less.
2. All these activities already occur mentally if you do any type of goal setting.
3. Knowing the steps beforehand helps diminish confusion and delay later.
4. Although goal setting should be a formal activity with

meetings and the involvement of all key people, the objectives and responsibility for achievement may be parceled out to individuals.

5. Tasks outlines (discussed later) are not necessarily formal, typed, and submitted to a committee. Task outlines can be jotted down and kept for reference so that as one step is completed, you can move rapidly to the next.

Summary. Goal setting is essential. No one can keep up with changes, new regulations, and requirements and maintain systems already in progress unless an organized system for doing so exists. If you doubt this, check with managers who have a well-run, progressive department and find out how they have achieved that state. The department is probably not run by "crisis management."

In summary, the goal-setting process involves:

1. Establishing *philosophic goals* (no more than five)
2. Completing *emergency department status survey* (annually)
3. Establishing *annual strategic goals* (based on status survey; no more than four major goals)
4. Writing *objectives* for each strategic goal
5. Completing *task outlines* for each objective

Problem Solving (Goal Barriers)

There is always an easy solution to every human problem—neat, plausible and wrong.
H.L. Mencken

This section is purposely mistitled for two reasons.

First, although the title is *problem solving*, the discussion relates primarily to problem identification. I believe that identification is more difficult than resolution. Once the real reasons for a deficiency have been determined, correcting that deficiency, although sometimes tedious and time-consuming, is usually the easier of the two tasks. If your car periodically stalls, the difficult part for the mechanic is finding out *why*. Fixing it may be expensive and take a long time, but once the reason is known, the greater challenge has been met.

Second, this section is titled *problem solving* because that is a familiar term to most of us. The word *problem*, however, carries some negative connotation and already sounds discouraging. I prefer the term *goal barrier* simply because it presents a different mental picture, and because all problems are really barriers to a goal. A semantics game? Yes, but at times it is psychologically helpful to choose the words that most accurately represent what we mean. "X-ray is really a problem!" sounds different from "there is a barrier to speedy processing of our patients."

Reading this section is not likely to change established, familiar terminology, but attitude is important in resolving goal barriers. The more positive the approach, the better. A familiar axiom illustrates this concept: "There are no problems, only *opportunities*."

Many opportunities exist in ED management. Goal barriers abound and proliferate, and much effort is directed toward resolving them. Inadequately trained staff may be a barrier to appropriate patient triage; medicines in unlockable cabinets may be a barrier to Joint Commission on Accreditation of Health Care Organizations (JCAHO) approval; and personnel conflicts are barriers to teamwork. Each goal barrier represents an opportunity to use skill and creativity.

Before a goal barrier can be resolved, it is important to identify the difference between *symptoms* and *diseases* and between *people* barriers and *system* barriers. To clarify this discussion, the differences between symptoms and diseases and between people barriers and system barriers are separated. Often, however, when one is differentiating goal barriers, the *symptoms* appear as *people barriers* when the *disease* is the *system*.

Symptoms versus diseases. "We have a morale problem" is not an accurate statement. Low morale is a symptom of a disease and not the disease itself. High staff attrition rates are often symptoms of the job satisfaction disease (barrier); similarly, a decrease in thorough charting with an increased patient census may be a symptom of inadequate staffing.

When approaching goal barriers, one must deal with the "disease" and not the symptom. Weekly requests for better charting will not produce results if there are simply not enough people to care for the patients and thoroughly document that care at the same time.

For those who are new to resolving goal barriers, it is a good idea to practice identifying "diseases" every time a goal barrier is identified. Working on symptoms alone does not produce long-term results and is a waste of valuable time.

People barriers versus system barriers. Much is blamed on people when the system is at fault. Saying that Mike does not care about doing proper chest compression is unfair if Mike has never had a CPR class or has not practiced for a couple of years. Criticizing staff members for not reporting deficiencies when they have never seen results of their reporting is also unfair. "Adequate" documentation can be expected only if "adequate" documentation has been concretely outlined. Many complaints about inadequate performance can be traced to inadequate education, poor feedback, or poorly designed systems, rather than to laziness or apathy.

Any time a significant decrease occurs in overall output, efficiency, or effectiveness in a department, it is unlikely that suddenly all the staff members quit caring. Even isolated, person-specific deficiencies often result from poor orientation or lack of positive feedback. If we assume that the manager has hired reasonably intelligent, well-intentioned people, probably 90% of all barriers are system related.

A simple mechanism exists for differentiating between symptom and disease and identifying people barriers and system barriers: all statements about goal barriers should be followed by *because.* For example:

The morale is low *because* . . .

Patients are leaving without a medical examination *because* . . .

Theresa was rude *because* . . .

Charting is inadequate *because* . . .

The use of *because* starts the thought process on the path to identifying the true barrier. The *because* technique should be taken to its conclusion. For instance, the morale is low *because* there has not been enough feedback *because* the head nurse has not had the time *because* there were too many simultaneous projects *because* of poor planning. Only when taken to its final stage can the real barrier be determined.

If you are seriously looking for real barriers, you will only rarely arrive at *becauses* that end with laziness, apathy, or bad attitude. Even when you do, personal problems (family, school, money) usually have caused the behavior in a particular individual.

Once the barriers have been identified, you can proceed to resolution decisions. Goal barriers come in many sizes, as do solutions. Solutions to barriers may range from 3-minute chats to 12-month projects, and some barriers warrant "waiting it out."

When resolving goal barriers, one must also be careful not to overtreat or undertreat the disease. When caring for patients, the same type of decisions must be made. It is costly and time-consuming to order a complete blood count, urinalysis, tests to measure levels of blood sugar, blood gases, and electrolytes, radiographs, and lung scan on an emotionally upset patient with rapid respirations, numbness, and tingling that were relieved by paper-bag breathing. It is also overtreatment to call a 12-person conference for an isolated abrupt exchange between staff members.

Conversely, a young patient who has sudden onset of severe headache and no prior history of headaches should not be sent home without a neurologic examination and only with instructions to take aspirin every 4 hours. Similarly, an incident of a staff member going berserk in the middle of a cardiac arrest should not be written off as a "bad day."

Resolving deficiencies calls for common sense and good judgment, and no one is always right in that decision-making process. Keep in mind, however, that the treatment should fit the disease.

In summary, the system for identifying goal barriers and the need for resolution asks:

1. Is this a symptom or disease?
2. Is this a people barrier or a system barrier?
3. Have I taken the "because" to its conclusion?
4. What is the magnitude of the problem?
5. What will happen if I do nothing?
6. Does this barrier constitute a real hindrance to a goal, and if so, *what is the goal*?

Once you have identified the goal and the barrier, you have the basis for a project.

Project Management

Project in this context is used to mean any activity undertaken to resolve a barrier to a goal. Remember that nearly 100% of our work is directed toward achieving a goal that is important to the care of patients and the smooth operation of the ED.

A variety of approaches and terminologies are used in the goal-setting process. Many people, when setting goals, use opening words such as "improve," "increase," or "decrease." Some people argue that "improving CPR documentation" is really an *objective* for the *goal* of "ensuring optimal care of the cardiac arrest patient." However, the important concept is to use terminology that is understood by all. It is also helpful to use the same language approach throughout a project outline. The project outline here uses a pure goal-setting format, but if *improve* is more understandable to the reader than *ensure*, use *improve*. Whatever works is a good tool.

If you have a clear understanding of the goal-setting and goal-barrier concepts, outlining objectives, solutions, and tasks is not difficult. An example of goal setting through goal achievement in outline form is shown in the box below. This outline is detailed to provide a clear picture of the process. It is not necessarily recommended that one go through this entire written outline for every barrier that arises. It *is* recommended, however, that the objective/task outline be used for annual goals. (For the reader's information the goal outline identifies the "philosophic" [strategic] goal to which the activity relates. However, it is not usually necessary to include philosophic goals in the project outline.)

PROJECT OUTLINE

Project chairperson: M. Smith
Project name: Triage
Philosophic (strategic) goal: Provide optimal emergency care*
PART I: Goal/objectives
  A. Goal: Ensure appropriate patient triage
  B. Objectives
    1. Develop triage criteria/coding system
    2. Provide staff education regarding triage coding
    3. Audit coding system for accuracy
    4. Reinforce if indicated
    5. Reaudit
PART II: Task outline
  Objective 1: Develop triage criteria/coding system

Task	Assigned to	Deadline	Report to
1. Select three staff members to assist with task	M. Smith	1/15	D. Jones
2. Collect data from three area hospitals about triage systems	J. Rogers	2/1	M. Smith
3. Establish criteria for priority of patients	All	2/28	M. Smith
4. Develop coding system	All	3/15	D. Jones

  Objective 2: Provide staff education regarding triage coding

Task	Assigned to	Deadline	Report to
1. Prepare written guideline for coding system	J. Rogers	3/20	M. Smith
2. Schedule staff meetings	J. Rogers	3/30	M. Smith

  Objective 3: Audit coding system for accuracy

Task	Assigned to	Deadline	Report to
1. Select 30 patient records	S. Brown	6/1	J. Rogers
2. Audit for triage accuracy	J. Rogers	6/15	M. Smith
3. Report to staff	J. Rogers		M. Smith/ D. Jones

---

*For reader information only.

Ideally, each *task outline* should be on a separate page and should be given to the persons involved in completing the task.

As you can see, much of the material contained in these outlines represents the step-by-step process that usually goes on in one's mind. Sitting down in advance to outline the necessary tasks, objectives, and responsible parties helps prevent delays and eliminate overlooking essential steps in the project.

Creativity in project management. Within each project lies the opportunity to meet the challenge of management creatively. Many management mistakes are made because of the tendency to see only what is known or has been experienced. When working toward a goal, do not confine yourself to tradition, and do not put up barriers that do not exist. During the initial brainstorming process, do not limit suggestions and ideas. In a true brainstorming session, the individuals think out loud without regard to feasibility of an idea. Each brainstormer states every idea that pops into mind, and the other people are not permitted, at that point, to make judgments such as "that won't work" or "that's too expensive." Once all ideas have surfaced, the group then begins to eliminate ideas that are truly unfeasible, but the reasons must be stated before an idea is eliminated.

If you are unhappy with the hospital review format, do not assume that the personnel office will not accept an "emergency department addendum" that is specific to your area. If you think a full-time collection person would be helpful, ask for such a 3-month or 6-month trial program. If the hospital has a one-to-one restock system that is inefficient for your area, request a trial program there as well. Visiting other EDs is another good way to open up your "tunnel vision." After 2 or 3 years at one facility we all tend to see it only as it is and not as it could be. If efficiency problems exist, see if some physical redesign might be helpful.

Projects are also a golden opportunity for staff involvement. Those people in the "trenches" have many good ideas that will surface if they are asked. Some of the best improvements come from those who have to face the inefficiency and frustration daily. For example, the ED in which I work has *separate* ambulance and walk-in entrances. Unfortunately, the ambulance entrance is the most visible as you approach the ED. The ambulance entrance doors are automatic and operated by press-plates on the walls, both inside and outside. Many of our patients, upset and in a hurry, did not see the walk-in entrance. We put up more signs, with no improvement. People complained daily about the problem, and the ED staff were constantly frustrated when patients and family members suddenly appeared through the ambulance doors. This went on for 18 months until finally one of the clerks meekly asked, "Is there any reason why we couldn't take the outside handles off the ambulance entrance doors?" It worked!

Administrative Structure and Change

Structure. Finding the administrative structure that meets the department's needs is one of the greatest challenges faced by the department manager. Administrative structure refers to the assignment of responsibilities for people and functions. Administrative structure is that entity on which organizational charts are based; a traditional administrative structure follows:

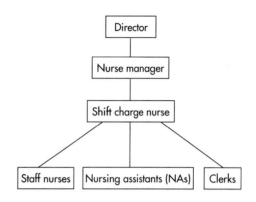

Each of these categories of staff member has some defined area(s) of responsibility. Unfortunately, no one structure works in every environment, and it may take several attempts to find the best method of operation.

Because no one structure works in every ED, it would not be appropriate here to recommend a particular structure for administrative activity. However, one can follow three consistent guidelines in the process of developing an appropriate (*workable*) method for operating a department:

1. Define your needs.
2. Be creative.
3. Match people and functions.

Defining needs. Much defining of needs in administrative structure is instinctive. You have a "feeling" that certain activities are inefficient, not thorough, or inadequate. Also, you may feel pressured for time, indicating either poor time organization, the need for additional administrative help, or the need to redistribute some duties.

If you are setting up a new department or have the previous feelings about a department you are already managing, you can use several approaches when attempting to define the needs. Only one approach is presented here. The important concept is to view the problem in its entirety and not just as a "slice." In the approach that follows, you can take several steps to define the needs:

1. Make a list of all the functions that are not direct "hands-on" patient care or a direct registration/discharge activity. The list should include all the usual administrative duties, such as interviewing, orientation, education, ordering, and restocking. Also, include those factors that are related to patient care but may not be built into the current system, such as triage,

the expediting of patient flow, social service, and the checking of equipment.

2. After the list is made, take each item and categorize it as specialized or nonspecialized. A *specialized* function requires special knowledge or training; nursing education, for instance, cannot be done by the departmental secretary. Ordering medical supplies also requires some knowledge of emergency medicine. Recording departmental statistics, however, can be done by anyone with minimal training.

3. After categorization, indicate those items on the list that are currently not being done and the reasons *why* they are not done. Reasons might include inadequate time available, no system set up, inadequate monitoring, or no trained person available.

When you have completed these activities, you should have a clear picture of what needs to be done and by whom, and you should be ready to move on to creativity.

Creativity. One of the most common errors made when developing a management system is the tendency to see what is and not what could be. Tradition says that an official charge nurse is on each shift, that supervisors do the ordering, and that only social workers can do social service functions. Many managers are unable to clear out the "tradition cobwebs" and look at alternatives without preconceived ideas about the structure.

After you have listed your needs, categorized the activities, and compared what is done with what you feel is desirable, you can begin to develop alternatives for correction of the management deficiencies. This is the time to bring the department's creative thinkers together and have a true brainstorming session, one that opens up the mind so new ideas and concepts are not automatically blocked out.

Many administrative activities can be distributed to people in the ED who traditionally do not have the responsibilities. It is difficult to teach creativity on paper, but the following are examples of some structural resolutions to management problems.

Problem	Solution
Students in the ED are receiving fragmented education.	Staff nurse "preceptors" have been assigned (volunteered, actually); the students work that staff nurse's regular shift and work only with the *one* preceptor.
New staff members are not receiving individual attention during orientation.	"Big brothers and sisters" have volunteered to help orient, answer questions, and encourage the new person for the first 4 weeks in the department (1 to 2 weeks past orientation).
Much staff shift rotation is making it difficult for shift charge nurses to do staff reviews.	Charge nurses assigned to specific shifts have been deleted. Reviews have been reassigned to the nurse manager. Review input is obtained from charge nurses and from co-workers, who are selected *by the staff members being reviewed.*

Problem	Solution
Dual problem: 1. No social worker is available. 2. Patients are not receiving appropriate attention at time of registration; they are being greeted with a business tone.	A new position of patient representative has been created. Patient representatives do initial patient registration (the usual clerical work) and are also responsible for the social service aspects of ED operation: they help with placement problems and perform ED death/crisis counseling. Since "social service" types of people are recruited for the position, patients receive more appropriate initial attention.
Another dual problem: 1. Administrative time available is insufficient to do quality audits. 2. Staff involvement/concern with quality assurance is low.	Departmental audit committee has been created, chaired by, and composed of ED staff.

This list could go on and on, but the general idea should be clear by now. Also, you should not overlook your secretarial talent. Most secretaries are good organizers and do an excellent job of setting up systems.

Brainstorming to develop alternatives works well whether you are changing an entire structure or merely working on one particular area. After you have developed the ideas for new administrative structure, you should begin the process of matching people and responsibilities.

Matching process. Some controversy exists over whether one should define job responsibilities and look for someone who can fulfill those responsibilities or whether one should use available resources and match people to responsibilities. In the real world a combination of both these approaches probably is appropriate.

Matching people and functions is a challenge that often results in an odd distribution of duties. The concept of matching is simple: each of us has areas of talent, and each of us has areas in which we do not excel. Compulsive superorganizers are often not outstanding in interpersonal relationships, and vice versa. Also, some people are very good teachers but cannot develop a budget. The goals of matching are to (1) combine the right people with the right job and (2) balance the talent areas in the department as a whole. With this second goal the department has people who excel in interpersonal relations and people with organizational ability.

There is one caution concerning the matching process. Although no law says individuals have to supervise functions *and* supervise the people doing those functions, it is very difficult to monitor functions unless you also have responsibility for the people who do those tasks. To clarify, suppose you assign a nursing assistant (NA) to oversee all restocking activity. If that NA does not have authority over the people doing the restocking, it can be very frustrating. This system may work, but it requires a special combination of people. Such a system also requires that the person supervising the function and the persons responsible for the people work very closely.

Change. Much has been written about change, especially people's response to it and how to cope with it. There are even "stress points" assigned for certain changes in one's life: a job change, divorce, moving, vacation, and so on.

ED personnel have the same responses to change as most people. In general, however, people attracted to a field as diverse and chaotic as emergency care are usually aggressive and motivated and do not tolerate *stagnation* any better than they tolerate change. Therefore, although they may resist change, they also find it difficult to work in an environment that maintains the status quo for long periods. If the status quo continues too long, ED workers often have many ideas for improvements that involve change.

Implementing changes in work procedures and policies is often difficult. The following guidelines may be helpful in preventing some of the resistance from personnel.

1. Do *not* make more than one major change every 3 months, preferably no more often than every 6 months. Many persons find it very difficult to adjust to major changes in structure and ways of operating. Also, if you have an option, do not terminate people at intervals shorter than every 3 months. Even if everyone understands why, they tend to become nervous.
2. Obtain as much input as possible before making major or minor changes. If preparation and discussion have occurred, the "change resistance quotient" is lowered. In addition, you often receive input you have not considered, which prevents mistakes in system design.
3. When introducing a change, *be sure* everyone understands that if it does not work, they will *not* be stuck with it forever. For internal changes in procedures, staff members should be assured that the goal is to find a *workable* method.
4. *Always* explain the reason for any change. Having a new procedure "dumped" on them without explanation is frustrating to staff, which significantly elevates the resistance quotient.

Summary. Structuring and making changes in an ED can be very difficult. The ED manager faces many challenges, such as external competition with other hospital EDs and free-standing urgent centers and internal competition among departments for capital and human resources. Also, the ED manager must successfully create efficient and productive systems.

One last note about structure and change: something that worked well a year ago does not necessarily work well forever. Needs change, people change, census increases, census decreases, and health care changes. Always be on the lookout for outdated methods of operating. If you do, you will probably not fall into the "tradition trap," and you will be better equipped to maintain a progressive and dynamic ED.

MANAGEMENT OF PEOPLE

The best systems developed are worthless if you do not know how to manage the people. People run the system; the right people run it better. If you place the right people in a good system and manage them well, you have the makings of an outstanding department.

People are complex. Much of what motivates them and causes them to respond so differently is not well understood. Being responsible for a group of people, therefore, is sometimes frustrating. However, it is an incredible challenge and one of the most exciting parts of the management task.

This section explores people: how to find them, motivate them, schedule them, review them, select their leaders, resolve their conflicts, and promote teamwork among them.

The information presented here is primarily a philosophy of management, although some "how-to" advice is included. If you are currently a manager or are thinking about becoming one, the first aspect you should explore is your philosophy about people. The intent here is to convey *concepts*. People and leadership styles differ, and it is the manager's responsibility to develop his or her own specific techniques for dealing with other people. It is hoped that this section will help in developing a philosophic approach conducive to a well-run department and reasonably satisfied staff members.

Selection of Staff Members

Finding a person to fill a particular position can be difficult. Finding the *right* person can be very difficult. The selection process is one of the most important tasks that the manager faces. The responsibility for selecting permanent members of the team should not be taken lightly. Selection of staff is a four-step process:

1. Defining needs
2. Recruiting
3. Interviewing
4. Making the decision

NOTE: This section is concerned primarily with selecting staff for *nonadministrative* positions. Selection of leadership staff is discussed later in the chapter.

Step 1: defining needs. Several selection needs should be considered before you start the recruiting process: the basics, the need for experience, and the ED's personality needs.

Basic needs. Some needs are easily identifiable. If you are filling a registered nurse (RN) position, you should interview only RNs. Can your nonlicensed personnel be staff aides and orderlies, or do you require NA certification? Do you require that people have billing experience before becoming admitting clerks? Most of these questions are easily answered.

Experienced or inexperienced? Before you start recruiting, you must decide whether you need someone with experience or prefer to train someone. This decision should be based on (1) the position and its requirements and (2) the ED census.

Position. If you are looking for a full-time triage nurse or one who will be the only RN on the 11-to-7 shift, you cannot take someone fresh from state board examinations, give her 3 weeks of orientation, and put her in charge. The hazards to patients and to the individual are obvious. If you are looking for a clerical person to type charts, files, and answer phones, you can train a person without jeopardizing patient care. You must decide beforehand what you need and not waste time on people who do not meet the criteria. Occasionally you will miss the one in 100 who could do the job without experience, but the alternative is to interview the 99 others.

Census. If your monthly ED census is 800, you probably have the time and the environment in which to train someone. If your monthly census is 3000, you need somebody who knows the basics: which patients can wait and, more important, which ones cannot. Many gradations exist between 800 and 3000, as well as many other "busy-ness" factors, such as having resident staff or full-time emergency physicians. You must examine your department and determine its special needs.

Personality. The third and final step in determining needs is to look at what "personality" would benefit the ED. This area, unfortunately, is rarely considered when looking for a new staff member, probably because it is viewed as a luxury.

What is meant by "personality"? Most applicants can be divided into two categories: job seekers and career seekers. Before we define these terms, it should be made clear that the terminology is not intended to divide applicants into desirable and undesirable. They are merely different, not better or worse.

Job seekers are usually looking for a position to provide them with an enjoyable means of support while they pursue other interests, such as school, family, or even skiing. Some are undecided about their career, about how much of their lives to commit to a career, or about what specific area to pursue. They may do their work well but usually do not have a high level of involvement.

Career seekers are aggressive, highly committed, full of ideas, and willing to devote the time and energy required for growth and change.

On the surface it would appear that, given a choice, you would want only career seekers. However, do you really want, for example, 30 people with strong convictions about where the copying machine should be placed? What you do want is a balance. If your department is full of job seekers, start looking for some career people. If you already have enough leaders, look for followers. Both are required to accomplish the goals.

Step 2: recruiting. Recruiting is the next logical and probably most difficult step. The ability to recruit depends

on many factors: the geographic location, time of year, and what you have to offer. Having a vacancy at Christmas and knowing that you pay less than anyone in the city can be a problem.

Applicants are obtained primarily by means of three mechanisms: referral, drop-ins, and advertising.

Referrals. Of the three ways to obtain new staff, referral is the most preferable. If someone whose judgment you trust has worked with or knows an applicant, you already have access to much valuable information that cannot be obtained any other way. The applicant's strengths as well as potential problem areas are already identified. The hazard in referral is that the person doing the referring may have poor judgment.

In any case, put the word out. Tell the department staff, and call professional friends and acquaintances. Somewhere the right person is looking for a new opportunity.

Drop-ins. These persons call or stop by, but not in response to an ad. They are usually (1) new in the area, (2) aggressive and intelligent enough to know how to bypass human resources, (3) unaware that there is a personnel office, or (4) 17 years old and looking for their first job. The chances of finding a successful applicant with a drop-in are about the same as when you actively advertise.

Advertising. Advertising is an art, and people do it for a living. Those who have written their first ad usually wish they had taken a journalism elective. It is very difficult, especially when paying by the word, to say everything you want in an ad. A few hints about advertising follow:

1. Do *not* write a narrative ("Hospital was founded in 1920 . . . ").
2. Title it "EMERGENCY NURSES" in large letters.
3. Make the criteria known; it will prevent unnecessary telephone calls.
4. Include incentives that will attract the type of applicant you are seeking, for example, "excellent medical care," "full-time emergency physicians," and "progressive educational program."
5. Have other people review the ad to tell you if it sounds attractive.

Once the ad is written, you must decide where to place it. With professional journals you need to know about the vacancy well in advance, since it is usually 6 weeks before the ad appears. Try local and metropolitan newspapers. You can also place ads in out-of-town or out-of-state papers.

Other possibilities include the newsletter for your professional organization (usually less lead time than a journal), placement centers at colleges and universities, and your own hospital's placement bulletin.

Recruiting "blind," that is, by means of advertisements and drop-ins, is always more risky than the referral method. You have to rely solely on references and your judgment, which is why interviewing is so critical to the selection process.

Step 3: interviewing

There is something that is much more scarce,
something finer far, something rarer than ability.
It is the ability to recognize ability.
E. Hubbard

If a foolproof method existed for weeding out undesirable applicants during the interview process, we would do less documenting of reasons for terminating those people who impressed us at the interview. This section discusses some typical interview techniques, their advantages and disadvantages, and the interviewer's responsibility.

Interview techniques

Panel method. The panel method consists of bringing various representatives from the staff (the interview committee) together to conduct the interview. The representatives usually include the manager, a charge nurse, staff nurses, and the medical director. The structure is generally formal. The advantages are that there is more input, the burden for decision making is shared, the staff feels more involved, and a group perspective may be better than an individual one. The disadvantages are that it is difficult to schedule all people, administrative cost is increased, the applicant tends to be uncomfortable, and a decision is sometimes difficult to reach.

One-to-one method. Only one person does the interviewing, usually the manager. The interview tends to be informal. The advantages are that it is easy to schedule, administrative costs are decreased, decisions are less time consuming, and the applicant is usually more comfortable. If the manager's judgment is poor (or viable), the disadvantages can be disastrous. The staff feels less involved, the burden on the interviewer is increased, and there is no input into the "can't-decide-between-the-two-candidates" situation.

One-to-one series method. The applicant interviews on a one-to-one basis with several selected interviewers. This method is usually used when hiring leadership staff. The advantages are that it is easier to schedule than a panel, there is more input into decisions, and it is more comfortable for the applicant than with the panel. The two disadvantages are that the applicant must make several appointments, which increases administrative costs, and more time is needed to collect information from all the interviewers to make a decision.

One-to-two method. The applicant interviews with (usually) the manager and one other representative of the staff. The advantages are that it decreases the burden on one individual, it is easier to schedule than a panel or a series, there is more input than in the one-to-one method, and the staff is involved. The disadvantages are that it is somewhat more difficult to schedule and administrative costs are slightly increased.

Summary. Is any one method preferable to the other? Except for the panel method, the answer is probably no.

Each of the other techniques may be favored in any given situation. My preference is a one-to-one series for leadership positions and one-to-one or (preferably) one-to-two for staff positions. The panel method is cumbersome, costly, rigid, and tends to promote the asking of questions such as, "What is your nursing philosophy?"

The important thing in deciding interview techniques is to allow flexibility. No one method is perfect for every situation, and the freedom to choose the most desirable can save the department much time and energy.

Interviewer responsibilities. Selecting the right people is one of the keys to success in any program. Most deciding factors in selection come from the interview. Therefore, knowing how to conduct an interview and learning how to obtain the information you need are critical to the selection process. There are as many interview styles as interviewers. Each individual must develop a style that is personally comfortable. However, certain responsibilities should not be ignored.

Be sure you know the basic needs. Do not interview inexperienced people if you know that the job requires experience. Evaluate the entire department, and decide whether you need job seekers or career seekers.

Have a clear picture of your environment. ED environments differ widely. Universities, private hospitals, and public hospitals all offer different challenges and require different types of people. A critical care nurse who really enjoys one-to-one or two-to-one patient care would probably not be happy as a full-time triage nurse. If your environment is flexible, calling for much teamwork and mutual give and take, a person with a militaristic view might have difficulty adjusting. Be sure you understand what your environment needs.

Be sure you are "up" for it. I have, on occasion, postponed interviews because I was not up for them. Interviewing is exhausting, especially if you receive a one-word reply to every question and are basically doing a monologue. You should be rested and fully enthusiastic about your department. Do not forget that the applicants may be interviewing elsewhere. Do not risk losing a good candidate because you are tired and cranky, and do not schedule more than two interviews in a day. By the time you say, for the fifth time in a day, "We have a wonderful education program," you will sound like a recording.

Put the applicant at ease. It is difficult enough to find out what you need to know about the applicant; do not complicate it by increasing his or her anxiety level. If applicants are relaxed, they are more likely to reveal who they really are. Offer a cup of coffee, ask if they had any trouble finding the hospital, or talk about a patient you just had. Do not begin by asking, "What are your career goals?"

Initially providing a brief overview of the department's strengths and weaknesses gives applicants information to help them decide whether this job is right for them. For example, explaining predominant patient populations, staffing patterns, scheduling, orientation, and educational opportunities illustrates employee life in the department. The description also conveys what you expect from your employees. You may also want to review benefits and provide a salary quote unless this is covered by human resources.

Ask questions that have answers, and be direct. Avoid ridiculous interview questions, such as "What is your nursing philosophy?" "How would you compare 2-, 3-, and 4-year graduates?" and "Where do you plan to be in 15 years?" You can find out more by asking applicants which patients they enjoy caring for the most, which ones are they least comfortable with, and why. Often I directly ask such questions as "Are you comfortable with patients who have dysrhythmias?" and "What are your strengths in nursing care?" Most applicants are honest when approached directly and know bluffing is a short-term escape.

Ask if the applicant has any questions, and listen. Beware if the applicant's first question is "How long before I'm eligible for vacation?" or "How many Medicaid patients do you see?" You learn much about what is important to applicants by listening to their questions and answers.

Review the interview. Initially, the review should be done in writing. List the things you liked and your negative observations or any questionable areas. If you have interviewed with other staff members, review your list with them. See if your impressions are the same. Ask yourself if you would want to work side by side with this person 40 hours a week, and pay attention to your instinct. If you cannot pinpoint some quality about the applicant, be cautious. Remember, the best résumés in the world are still only résumés.

Always check references. Obtaining a thorough reference is becoming increasingly difficult. In most states the only information that can be given is hire date, termination date, and eligibility for rehire. Some clues for checking references follow:

1. Determine the name of the applicant's previous supervisor, and call him or her directly. Do not call human resources.
2. If the supervisor hedges, be cautious. If the applicant was a model employee, the supervisor's tone of voice is usually different than if the applicant was not.
3. If the applicant is not eligible for rehire, he or she is usually someone you would not want.
4. If you had negative observations or questionable areas in the interview, ask the supervisor about those specific points.

Once you have decided your department's needs, recruited, and interviewed, the final step is to make the decision.

Step 4: making the decision. Do not panic. If all the applicants were unacceptable, *do not hire anyone*, no matter what your schedule demands. Keep searching. Hiring and then terminating someone 3 months later only doubles your work. Remember number 3 of Murphy's law: "It is easier to make a commitment or to get involved in something than to get out of it."

If you have interviewed other people, review all the candidates when you are finished. (During a 2-year period in my career, I interviewed jointly with one other person. We hired only those applicants about whom we were both enthusiastic. If either of us had reservations about someone, he or she was disqualified. Our success rate was unusually high.)

Finally, do not make a decision immediately. Put recruiting, interviews, and your tight schedules out of your mind for 2 or 3 days. You will find your perspective is different and your mind clearer to make the final decision.

Motivation

Everybody talks about motivation. For example, "How can I motivate this person? He's bright and has so much to offer, but he's just not motivated." Much research has been done to enable us to better understand human behavior. The following is a brief review of some of the better-known theories of motivation.

Motivational theories

Hierarchy of needs. Maslow[4] was among the first to propose a motivational theory. Even though it has been the source of controversy, a brief summary may still provide the ED manager with insight.

Maslow identified five needs that serve as motivators (Fig. 5-1). To understand the hierarchy, one must know the two basic assumptions.

1. A need emerges only when the lower level need has been met. (One would have little concern for self-actualization if one were having severe difficulty breathing.)
2. More than one need may be operating at once, but only one dominates.

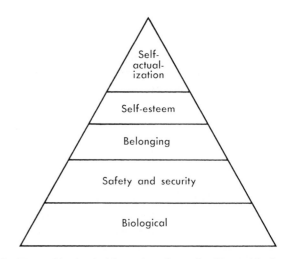

Fig. 5-1 Maslow's hierarchy of needs. (From Maslow A: Toward a psychology of being, New York, 1962, D Van Nostrand.)

Most managers are concerned primarily with the top two or three needs in the hierarchy. Physiologic and safety needs are generally adequate in the work environment, so our attention must be directed toward the higher motivational levels.

N Ach theory. McClelland[5] discusses what divides people in the world into two broad groups: "There is that minority which is challenged by opportunity and willing to work hard to achieve something and the majority which really does not care all that much." This minority, those with a high *need* for *ach*ievement (n Ach) are still a puzzle to psychologic researchers. According to McClelland, the need for achievement is "a distinct human motive, distinguishable from others."[5] People who score high in n Ach testing share several characteristics:

1. They set moderately high, but not unachievable, goals for themselves.
2. They respond only if they can influence the outcome by doing the work themselves.
3. They show strong preferences for situations in which the results of their effort are readily visible.
4. They consistently look for ways to "do things better."

No concrete answers can yet explain why certain people seem to have a higher level of n Ach than others. However, "the evidence suggests it is not because they are born that way, but because of special training they get in the home from parents who set moderately high achievement goals, but who are warm, encouraging and nonauthoritarian in helping their children reach these goals."[6] Can n Ach be increased in a given individual? McClelland's research suggests that it is possible to change an individual's thinking process and increase his or her need for achievement.

Expectancy theory. Developed by Vroom,[7] the expectancy theory states that workers' motivation depends primarily on what they perceive as the result of a given behavior and the value they place on these results. For instance, if a staff nurse highly values a promotion to charge nurse and believes that demonstrating commitment (that is, schedule flexibility and educational participation) will produce the desired promotion, she or he will probably be motivated to work extra shifts and attend lectures. A staff nurse who is content as a staff nurse and has no desire for promotion will probably have less motivation (or at least different motives) to put in additional time and energy. Vroom's theory therefore suggests that employees can be motivated by changing how they perceive the *value* of the outcome of their behavior.

Motivation-hygiene theory. The motivation-hygiene theory, developed by Herzberg,[3] divides worker motivation into two distinct categories: *satisfiers* (motivators) and *dissatisfiers* (hygiene or maintenance factors). When hygiene factors (dissatisfiers) are inadequate or absent, the results are worker dissatisfaction. Dissatisfiers are factors such as working conditions (lighting, space, and so on), salaries, relationships with management and co-workers, and com-

pany policies. If these factors or conditions are inadequate, the employee will be dissatisfied. Adequacy in all hygiene factors does *not*, however, produce motivated employees. Even if the salary is adequate, co-worker and management relationships are good, working conditions acceptable, and company policies reasonable, the employee is not *necessarily* motivated to achieve or contribute.

Satisfiers (motivators) are such factors as achievement, responsibility, recognition, the work itself, and promotion. If these factors are available in the environment, the results are employee satisfaction and motivation.

Motivation methods. Managers do not study motivation theory solely to understand why people *do not* produce. Clearly the goal is to find motivation methods that encourage greater efficiency and productivity. Before you start trying to motivate others, you must first address three questions:

1. What do you personally think about people and what it takes to motivate them? Are you of the school that believes people are basically lazy and stupid, or do you believe that, given the opportunity, most people are eager to contribute something to their jobs and capable of doing so? This is an important question. If you *really* believe that people are inherently lazy, you will probably find it difficult to interact in ways that have a positive effect on another's productivity.
2. What is your usual way of interacting with other people? Do you tend to avoid confrontation? Would you rather "do it yourself" than teaching or even asking someone else to help? Do you give orders or request assistance? Do you ask what happened or accuse others of mistakes before you have all the facts? Evaluate your usual behavior; you may be surprised.
3. Does your usual style of interacting correspond with your answer to question number 1? If not, you have a conflict that needs to be resolved. If you do believe people are willing to contribute but you accuse, dictate, and "do it yourself," something is amiss.

Motivation is *not* a single interaction with another person, a yearly performance review, or a once-a-week pat on the back. Motivation should be an integral part of your style as a manager. Motivation can be very difficult if you have to remember consciously to do it. If it is a natural outgrowth of what you think about people, motivation is much easier. The following section on communication outlines four key components in the motivational process.

Communication. We are naturally social creatures, and communication, both verbal and nonverbal, is an integral part of our daily lives. Communication is vital to motivation.

Later in the chapter the section on leadership addresses the issue of personal communication styles. The discussion here is limited to the areas of communication that should be routine in your motivational system.

Expectations. If you want complete vital signs on every patient but do not tell anyone, you should not criticize staff members for not doing them. This example may be simplistic, but if you begin to question the staff in your department, you will probably be amazed at how many gray areas exist. Do you expect all staff to rotate shifts cheerfully every 3 months or only occasionally? Does everyone in your department really understand their roles in a disaster? Are your patient records supposed to be signed with the beginning of treatment or at the end? Who is supposed to call the blood bank for uncrossmatched blood for trauma patients? Can staff wear tennis shoes? How many lectures a year are considered "educational enthusiasm"?

Employees need to know what criteria are being used to make judgments about their performance. The key here is for the manager to ensure the expectations are clearly understood *without* creating a dictatorial atmosphere.

Feedback. If you have ever made a suggestion to your manager for improving your department and never received a response, you may already understand the importance of feedback. Any question or suggestion deserves a prompt response, even saying you cannot deal with the problem now. When a staff member takes the time (and possibly has the good sense) to question a procedure or recommend an improvement, it is essential that you reply as soon as possible. Write a note to yourself, put it on your calendar, or "to do" list, but do not forget it. Even the worse suggestions warrant discussion and an explanation of why they would not work.

Another feedback area is *constructive criticism.* When a staff member makes an error, do not write it down and present it at a performance review 6 months later. All of us make mistakes, and timely discussion has the most benefit. Three rules for constructive criticism should never be broken:

1. *Never* criticize or reprimand an employee in the presence of others.
2. *Always* ask for the person's version of the story. Often a logical explanation exists for what you observed or heard from others.
3. *Always* explain why the action was an error. People remember a correction if they understand its rationale.

Recognition

A pat on the back is only a few vertebrae removed from a kick in the pants, but it is miles ahead in results.
V. Wilcox

The third communication practice that should be an integral part of your motivational style is recognition. When was the last time you complimented someone on her or his handling of a difficult patient? When did you last express appreciation to a nurse, technician, or clerk who *always* does the assigned duties? We all need recognition for our accomplishments, whether large or small. You can easily become so wrapped up in problems that you do not even see the good. *Take* the time to notice and communicate.

Managers also frequently do not give credit where credit is due. If someone makes a suggestion or an unusual con-tribution, be sure that you publicly recognize his or her effort. Taking someone's suggestion and presenting it as you own ensures that the person involved will never make another suggestion.

Goals. The last communication practice in motivation, the communication of goals, is often ignored. If you expect to receive support from the staff, they must know the goal. Communicating goals includes *all* goals—from the overall departmental goals for the year to the reason for instituting a new procedure. Again, people cooperate if the rationale is clear. If you are talking about departmental goals, explain the mechanisms that will be used to accomplish the goal. For instance, if a goal for the year is to improve clerical efficiency, explain that you are planning to preprint the patient's number on the charts and add an imprint maker, rather than making the clerks work harder.

Staff involvement. The second component of the motivational system is staff involvement. To involve staff members in the growth and progress of the department effectively, the manager should understand the why and how.

Why should the staff be involved? The first reason is based on Herzberg's theory,[3] which states that satisfiers (motivators) are recognition, responsibility, and the work itself. Most of us are more enthusiastic about a project into which we have had direct input. Involving the staff in goal setting and decision making also gives them some control over their work environment. Very few people respond positively to dictatorial leadership.

The second reason that the staff should be involved is that managers are not all-knowing. Unfortunately, no magic answers go with a promotion. Experience, usually by trial and error, may have taught managers how *not* to do things, but they are not the only ones with good ideas. Effective managers find good people and determine how best to utilize their talents.

How should the staff be involved? Every staff member is, at some level, "involved" in the progress of a department. One is either (1) a hindrance to progress or (2) a help to progress. The adage "if you are not part of the solution, you are part of the problem" is true. Rarely is anyone a neutral force. Every time someone "complains," he or she is involved in identifying barriers to a goal. Although the barrier may be of one's own making, it is still a barrier. Allowing individuals to be an asset to progress requires managerial skill and patience, but the benefits far outweigh the disadvantages.

The use of the word "allowing" is not accidental. It is important to remember that managers do not "get" people involved. Managers allow the individual to express a natural inclination, and they establish the mechanisms that encourage the expression of that inclination.

Any staff member, manager or otherwise, is involved in only two activities: goal setting and goal achievement. Here is a simple example. Objective: "correct volume depletion" (more often stated as "start an IV"); to achieve: "take IV bottle from shelf, remove cap," and so on. *Everything* we do is directed toward achieving a goal. Therefore, when we discuss staff involvement, the real questions are (1) What are the goals of the staff member? (2) What are the department's goals? and (3) Are they compatible?

What are the goals of the staff member? Before you read further, choose one member of your department's staff and write down what you think he or she wants from the 8 hours a day spent at work. Having done this exercise, you have a list of the goals for the staff member. If you read things such as "get paid for 8 hours of doing nothing" or "make everyone's life miserable," you need to do some extensive reading about human behavior or seriously assess your interview/hiring abilities. More likely, however, you have written staff goals related to learning, being recognized for achievement, or simply enjoying their workday experience.

What are the department's goals? Every member of the ED team should be able to list the department goals—both the ongoing, permanent goals and the specific objectives for the year. One of the keys to establishing a successful mechanism for staff involvement is ensuring that everyone knows the goals. When new staff members are oriented, they should be given a clear picture of the overall philosophy of the department. When specific yearly, monthly, or weekly objectives are established, they should be shared with all members of the team.

Are the staff member's goals and departmental goals compatible? Everyone who sought employment in your department probably had a reason for choosing that specific area. A critical care nurse may have wanted to broaden his or her base of experience. A nursing student may have wanted more clinical exposure, and a clerk may have wanted exposure to health care to assist in future career decisions. Some of the staff may have been looking for an exciting way to support their ski habit.

The manager's responsibility is to combine (1) the goals of the staff member that are specific to emergency care; (2) the personal goals of *all* individuals: recognition, achievement, and responsibility; and (3) the departmental goals. The manager must combine these goals in such a way that all can be fulfilled. This is no easy task but is not as difficult as it may sound. Meeting all these objectives simultaneously offers the manager another creative opportunity.

Many methods can be established to promote the involvement of staff members. Involvement may range from helping establish annual objectives to deciding how to remove blood from the wall before the next trauma patient arrives. The opportunities for input and assistance are endless, and the mechanism varies from department to department, from year to year, and from individual to individual. The manager is responsible for creating the methods best suited for the environment.

Annual goal setting. Having all staff members agree on annual goals would probably be unwise. However, you can select representatives to assist in the process or ask each category of personnel (nurses, NAs, clerks) to establish one or two group goals. You could also solicit input from staff, formally or informally, concerning their perceptions of the "improvement needed" areas.

Preestablished projects. After objectives have been established, they are, ideally, achieved by one method or another. Solicit assistance. Tell everyone what you are trying to achieve and see who is interested. You may define the overall objective and let the team members break it down into tasks. You may define the tasks and ask for assistance in a specific area. There are long-term projects, short-term projects, ongoing tasks, and one-shot projects. You may want the chairman of a group, a group member, or individual to complete a specific activity. Someone can chair the audit committee; another can take responsibility for all CPR education; someone else may want to oversee follow-up phone contact with patients who were sexually assaulted. Everyone has some talent and an area of special interest.

Personnel problems. If you are having difficulty with a new staff member, ask one of his or her colleagues to be a big brother or sister for a while. Working out performance problems with a peer is often less threatening and more successful than "supervisory counseling."

Orientation. Your full-time employees know what their new colleague *really* needs to know, and many of them are good at sharing that knowledge. Capitalize on that talent by requesting staff input to develop a formalized orientation. Promoting development of staff as preceptors enhances their ability to individualize orientation to meet the needs of each new employee.

Complaints. As stated before, complaints are the identification of a barrier to achieving a particular goal. If someone has identified a barrier, ask if he or she is interested in helping find a solution.

New ideas. Everyone who has a new idea for improving patient care, efficiency, interpersonal relations, or other aspects should be encouraged and praised. Lock into that interest and channel it.

Interviewing. Create a rotating interviewer position, or simply allow those who are interested to sit in on interviews.

Recruiting. If you are looking for a new staff member, ask the staff to help recruit. Be sure to thank anyone who refers an applicant. If you did not hire the applicant, be sure to explain why.

Scheduling. Anyone who expresses an interest in scheduling should be encouraged to help with it.

Hazards in staff involvement. Any system comes with potential hazards, which must be identified to be prevented.

Suppose you are trying to improve your relationship with hospital administration, and the least tactful nurse in your department volunteers to be the liaison. You may want to channel that enthusiasm into another area or at least spend some time discussing the art of diplomacy. If the clerical staff unilaterally decides to increase collections by 200%, you should investigate what methods they intend to use.

These are extreme examples, but we all occasionally tend to get carried away by our enthusiasm. The manager is responsible for ensuring that projects and new ideas are carried out in a manner consistent with departmental philosophy.

Another potential hazard is allowing too many projects to be going on at one time. Change is difficult for everyone, and a barrage of new procedures may create chaos and fatigue among the staff.

Also, remember that all good ideas do not warrant implementation solely because they are good ideas. Calling every ED patient 24 hours after treatment may be a very good idea, but it is probably impractical. The institution of a new policy or procedure should be consistent with current departmental needs.

A final hazard warning involves priority setting. Advanced cardiac life support certification for ED staff is an excellent idea but should follow a well-organized, basic cardiac life support certification system. Offering a 12-week advanced dysrhythmia course is also a good idea, but not if only one nurse is ready to study advanced dysrhythmias. Again, the available time, effort, and energy should be used to meet objectives that are consistent with needs.

Before proceeding to the next section, we should address two questions that many readers may be asking at this point.

1. Staff involvement may work fine for someone else, but what about a department such as *mine*, in which everyone is apathetic?

Lots of folks confuse bad management with destiny.
E. Hubbard

This problem is discussed directly when we discuss the third component of the motivational system: leadership and its effect on motivation. This issue is also addressed indirectly in the section that discusses leadership as a single issue. For now, this summary is sufficient: if you have a department filled with apparently apathetic, unenthusiastic, unmotivated people, the problem is probably not with the staff members.

2. What do I do about the people who aren't motivated?

Dealing with this issue is a relatively simple, two-step process: (a) ascertain the reason(s) and (b) correct the barriers, *if possible*. People choose to be uninvolved for various reasons. They may not have received enough recognition and therefore think they have "nothing to offer." They may not understand that they can be involved without devoting 100% of their life energy to work. They may be insecure enough personally that they believe everyone else has better ideas. They may be temporarily hostile about the administration. They may not yet have seen a project that interests them. Finally, they may simply be one of those people who have chosen not to devote additional energy to their job.

In all but the last example, most of the barriers can be corrected, and your efforts should be directed toward dealing with the real problems and not the symptoms. In the last example, do nothing. As long as the individual is fulfilling the job responsibilities and not creating a negative atmosphere, do not waste valuable time trying to alter someone's view of the world. Nobody receives 100% participation, and expending energy on the 1% or 2% who have chosen not to be involved only diminishes the energy available to the other 98%. Also, keep in mind that in these circumstances nothing is inherently wrong with someone who has actively decided to direct extra efforts to activities outside of work. Remember, you do not "get" people involved, you "allow" them to express a natural inclination.

If these individuals are not fulfilling their responsibilities and are creating a negative atmosphere, you are dealing with a motivation problem. You are confronting either an isolated personnel problem or, in the Herzberg terminology, an unresolved "dissatisfier" factor.

Leadership: its effect on motivation. The third and final component of any motivational system is its leadership. Whether they are titled managers, supervisors, administrators, directors, coordinators, or chiefs, these leaders have been given the responsibility of guiding others' efforts to achieve a defined set of objectives.

Anyone who has ever worked under an incompetent manager knows the effect that incompetence has on motivation. Eventually the best, most motivated people give up trying to make suggestions or improvements. *Incompetent* managers are those who are always right or cannot take criticism, do not listen, appear unconcerned with people's problems, dictate without explanation, do not know what they are doing, always take sides, never delegate, or are power happy. They also seem to keep their jobs forever.

Incompetence, however, is different from inexperience. *Inexperienced* managers, as distinguished from incompetent managers, learn from mistakes and make a genuine effort to correct their deficiencies. No one knows everything about how to lead, but good managers listen, try to learn, make changes if indicated, and enjoy their work.

Trying to maintain enthusiasm when you work for someone you do not respect as a professional or as a person is very difficult. Note the use of the word "respect," as opposed to "like." It is highly improbable that even the best of managers are liked by everyone. If the manager is respected as a reasonable, capable person, being liked is not essential.

Many "motivation" problems could be easily resolved by a change in leadership. This does not mean firing the manager whenever motivation deteriorates. If many team members exhibit chronic apathy and discontent, however, someone should at least examine the quality of leadership.

The other side of this issue is the positive motivating effects of good leadership. When the manager is respected and is enthusiastic about his or her work, that enthusiasm filters to all staff members. Genuine enthusiasm is contagious. Think about the differences in working on a project with someone really excited about it and with a leader who presented the project as drudgery.

Summary. Motivation is complex, and no one approach works in every environment. Each manager must tailor his or her motivational system to fit the milieu. In any system, however, the three components remain the same. Your motivational system should include the following:

1. *Communication.* This addresses expectations, feedback, recognition, and goals.
2. *Self-involvement.* This must be *allowed*, and mechanisms must be established to encourage involvement.
3. *Leadership.* Managers, directors, and charge nurses should be respected and should be enthusiastic.

Scheduling

Emergency care is stressful—mentally, physically, and emotionally—and is a 24-hour-a-day operation. Scheduling for 24 hours a day, 365 days a year is not an easy task. When staff members are vacationing or ill, EDs do not have the luxury of working "short." When trying to fill every position every day, one understandably tends to create many rules and to become insensitive to individual needs and differences.

The nursing profession is currently experiencing great unrest. Since much of the unhappiness is directly related to scheduling, it seems appropriate to discuss scheduling as a single issue.

The manager attempts to meet the following objectives when he or she sits down to make a schedule:

1. Provide staffing that is adequate to ensure that patient care is not jeopardized.
2. Meet individual needs and preferences.
3. Be fair.
4. Be consistent.

These are difficult objectives, particularly because they must be met simultaneously.

The most frequent complaints you hear from disgruntled staff members involve their schedule. "They put me on night shift and didn't even tell me. I had plans for that evening." When making a schedule, you must remember that you are scheduling people's *lives.* Indiscriminate use of that power can rapidly create a morale crisis and subsequently a high attrition rate.

There are no easy answers to the problems of scheduling, but the following guidelines are offered.

1. Have as *few* rules as possible. If a nurse wants an extra weekend off, and he or she can find appropriate coverage, no logical reason exists to deny that request. The same holds true if someone wants to trade a shift. Do not create rules dictating that people can never leave early, arrive late, or work only 1 day a week. Scheduling policies *are* necessary, but only when there is solid justification for them. Solid justification is *not*

manager stress, "hospital policy" (hospital policies *can* be changed and exceptions granted), or abuse of the system by an isolated staff member.

2. Try to have extra help available. Call them *per diem, casual,* or *subject-to-call* personnel, but try to keep enough help available that you are able to ensure some flexibility. On the surface this sounds costly, but if you weigh the cost of per diem help against the cost of the "quit-recruit-interview-orient" cycle, you will probably find that you come out ahead.
3. *Do not* make schedule commitments that you cannot keep, and once you have made them, do not renege. If you have hired someone for 4 days a week in the ED, give her 4 days a week *in the emergency department.* Do not ship her off to the coronary care unit. If you promised 3 to 11 hours, do not schedule her for 11 to 7 without permission.
4. Have an employment agreement. Employment agreements should spell out, at the minimum:
   a. Category—full-time, part-time, per diem, exempt
   b. Number of hours a week commitment
   c. Wages

   Employment aggreements are "clarity" tools for both the employee and the staff member. Be sure to obtain a new agreement if an employee's status changes.
5. Communicate. If you need coverage for the 11 to 7 shift and want to use someone who ordinarily does not work 11 to 7, ask that person if he or she is willing. *Never* put employees into an unusual slot or change their rotation without speaking with them first.
6. Grant all schedule requests. This is not always possible, but it should always be your goal. If you are absolutely unable to grant these requests, explain why.
7. Deal directly with abuses. Making rules that affect everyone in the department solely to resolve one or two offenders is unwise. It is better to be rid of one or two offenders than everyone in the department.
8. Be creative. Two strategies that increase staff satisfaction with scheduling are (1) increasing the variety of positions offered and (2) practicing self-scheduling. Offering more than straight days, evenings, and nights not only provides more options for staff, but also meets departmental needs with census and acuity fluctuations. At 7 AM five nurses may be too many, but at noon five may be very busy. Also, EDs tend to need more RNs on weekends than during the week. Examples of positions are described next.

Option	Description
a. Weekend plan	1 full-time employee (FTE)
	Works two 12-hour shifts every weekend
	Paid 36 hours for days
	Paid 40 hours for nights
	No benefits

Option	Description
b. Weekend plan plus	1.4 FTE Same as weekend plan Full-time benefits included If needed, must work additional 16 hours per week to cover shortages
c. 0.9 plus	1 FTE Works three 12½-hour shifts per week 11 AM to 11:30 PM Saturday, Sunday, and Monday or Friday, Saturday, and Sunday Benefits included
d. 4-day week	1 FTE Works two 8-hour and two 12-hour shifts per week Works every third weekend, 12-hour shifts Benefits included
e. 5-day week	1 FTE Works five 8-hour nights Monday through Friday, no weekends Benefits included
f. Variety of start times	7 AM, 11 AM, 3 PM, 7 PM, 11 PM
g. Variety of shifts	Day/evening rotation Day/night rotation Evening/night rotation Nights, no weekends
h. Bonuses	(1) Quarterly bonus check for a specified number of undesirable shifts, such as evenings or nights (2) 5% bonus after employed for 18 months; 2% at 36 months, 5 years, and 10 years

The idea is to create positions and schedules that meet unit needs and staff needs. These positions and schedules in turn will help decrease the cost of turnover and will increase staff satisfaction and retention.

Self-scheduling has appeared as an option to increase staff control over their day-to-day schedules. Ultimate control and responsibility still remains with the nurse manager. A 6-week schedule is posted for 2 weeks, during which full-time and part-time staff pencil in their desired schedule. Each staff member has their own set of rules to follow based on the position for which that person was hired. For example, staff nurse A may work a 4-day, 50-50 day/evening rotation and work every third weekend. Staff nurse B may work a 50-50 evening/night rotation and work every third weekend. Staff nurse C may work on the weekend plan and alternate every weekend, with 7 AM and 7 PM shift starts. After 2 weeks the per diem/on-call nurses may sign up to fill gaps in the schedule. After another week the nurse manager or designee reviews the schedules to ensure that everyone is fulfilling their commitment. Then the manager negotiates with staff to cover the remaining gaps with overtime, switches, and so on. Self-scheduling is not a perfect answer to scheduling dilemmas, but it is an option that increases the staff nurse's autonomy and thus is worth pursuing.

Despite all the previous guidelines perhaps sounding (1) unworkable and (2) like an administrative nightmare, it is usually well worth the effort. In general, if people are treated with consideration, they will be willing to help out when you are in a bind. Also, your attrition rate will reflect that consideration.

Performance Review Systems

A performance review, if done appropriately, can be a positive, motivating experience for both the staff member and the reviewer. If not done appropriately, a review can be a frightening, negative experience for the staff member and an energy drain for the reviewer.

This section outlines the two types of performance reviews and the objectives of each, lists the responsibilities of the staff member and the reviewer, and briefly discusses review format.

Performance review: formal. When we combine Webster's definitions of *performance, review,* and *formal,* we arrive at an understanding of this process.

Term	Meaning
Performance	The act of performing . . . accomplishment, fulfillment . . . operation or functioning, usually with regard to effectiveness
Review	A look at . . . a general survey, report or account
Formal	Of external form or structure . . . of or according to fixed customs, rules . . . done or made in an orderly, regular fashion . . .

A formal performance review is a structured method of looking at accomplishments and effective function. Probably the most common mistake made in interpreting this definition is assuming that the review process is a one-sided monologue. Good reviews are dialogues. Before a formal review is conducted or a review system is designed, the following questions should be answered:

- What are the objectives of the formal review?
- What are the responsibilities of the staff member?
- What are the responsibilities of the reviewer?

Formal review objectives

1. To establish rapport, particularly with new staff members. Scheduling an uninterrupted hour or more to talk with a staff member provides a rare opportunity for the individuals involved to become better acquainted. This time should be used to open or reopen lines of communication.
2. To provide an opportunity to discuss staff member goals, methods of achievement, and deadlines (Fig. 5-2). Many staff members, especially those who have not previously been involved in personal goal setting, may need to explore that process with a "guide." Outlining work-related goals does not come easily to everyone. Staff members who list such things as "finish school" and "enroll in scuba diving class" as personal goals probably do not yet have a clear enough picture of goal setting in a work environment. Those who do understand goal setting may need education in methods of achievement. For instance, someone

---

EMERGENCY DEPARTMENT

Name _____ Date: _____

Staff performance objectives

Please list below your goals for professional growth in the coming 6 months or year in the first column. In the second column outline your proposed methods for achieving those objectives. In the third column please indicate your projected deadlines for achievement.

Performance objectives may be of an individual or group nature, personal or departmental, and may include such items as clinical expertise, attitude changes, departmental restructure, and so on. If your goals incorporate group or departmental objectives, please indicate what your personal contribution would be toward achieving these objectives.

Goals	Methods	Deadline

Fig. 5-2   Form for review of staff member's goals and methods to achieve them.

might list "improve my attitude about nonemergent patients" as a goal and write "try harder" as a method. This person could probably benefit from suggestions to read about the health care system, talk with colleagues about nonemergent patients, or spend more time with these patients to ascertain why they came to the emergency department. Finally, many people set unrealistic deadlines for themselves. Any nurse who sets a 3-week deadline for "understanding 12-lead ECGs" is either unrealistic or a genius.

When a review is conducted, the staff member and reviewer should look over the goals, methods, and deadlines from the previous review and ask the following questions:

a. Was the staff member able to meet his or her goals? If not, why not?

b. Did the methods work, or did they have to be altered?

c. Were the deadlines realistic?

3. To provide an opportunity for feedback to the staff member regarding performance. This is, traditionally, the primary focus of the review—and probably should not be. Some managers still keep a little black book with all the "bad" things a staff member has done, and at review time this list is dutifully read to the offending party. Inappropriate behavior, in attitude or clinical performance, should be discussed at the time of the incident and not weeks or months later. Reviews should be a general survey of strengths and "improvement-needed" areas. This survey should be conducted primarily by the staff member and only secondarily by the reviewer.

4. To provide an opportunity for education of the staff member. This refers not to clinical education but to education about the changing world of health care, the reasons for internal procedural changes, or the reason why the hospital or ED administration has selected certain goals for the year. The reviewer has a captive audience and an opportunity to answer questions about health care systems, prehospital care systems, and hospital and ED methods of operating—even if the questions are not directly asked.

5. To provide an opportunity for feedback *to the reviewer* regarding departmental problems and administrative performance. *This* should probably be the primary focus of the review or, at the very least, should receive equal time with number 3. The people who take care of the patients, fill out the forms, answer the phone, and interact with other agencies, department heads, and patients' families every day know the real prob-

lems. They also know who works and who does not. Do not pass up this chance to discover what they think and what you are doing (or not doing) that makes their lives more difficult.

6. To document the items just described. Documentation serves two purposes: protection of the staff member and protection of the employer. Lengthy discussion of the importance of documentation is unnecessary, but one thing deserves attention: *nothing* should go into a staff member's personnel file unless he or she has signed it.* People have a right to know what could be released to a future employer.

Although hospital administration requires an annual performance appraisal, once a year is not enough. You should schedule appointments quarterly to review the material from the objectives just listed. Goals are sometimes quickly forgotten, or they may be achieved and new ones may be set. If you wait until the end of the year to learn what a staff member's perceptions are of the unit or yourself, you will be too late. Regular feedback is needed by all staff members as well as by the manager to prevent misperceptions and misunderstandings and, most importantly, to promote growth in the department.

Performance review: informal. Adapting from the definition of formal review, we can define the informal performance review as a casual or unceremonious method of looking at effective function. More specifically, informal reviews are the discussion of single incidents or transient attitudes. The formal review section briefly mentioned the manager who keeps a black book in preparation for formal review. Informal reviews have made these books obsolete and, more to the point, ridiculous. If a problem exists with an individual's clinical performance, attitude, or behavior, it should be discussed at the time it occurs or very soon thereafter. Nobody remembers why he or she went to lunch early 6 months after the fact.

Informal reviews take on many forms. They may be anecdotal records or casual queries such as "I heard there was a problem with the lab last night—what happened?" Informal reviews are conducted daily, even though we may not identify them as such. They are not restricted to discussing problems and negative behaviors. Informal reviews should be balanced with compliments and pats on the back.

Informal review objectives
1. To collect data. Frequently the story you heard initially is the end result of the gossip chain and bears little or no resemblance to the actual incident. Remember the saying, "There are three sides to every story—your side, my side, and the truth."

2. To correct misunderstandings. Maybe the laboratory did not really hang up on the offended party; perhaps the switchboard disconnected the call at the most inopportune moment. Perhaps the charge nurse was conducting two conversations. When she said "yes," it was in answer to the person who asked if Mrs. Smith was still here and not in answer to the staff nurse who asked to go to lunch now.

3. To correct for the future. Some of the best teaching/learning tools are "What would you do differently next time?" and "What can we do to ensure that this doesn't happen again?"

4. To maintain contact. Much of our daily contact with staff members is in the form of reviewing specific situations. If we keep black books instead of handling problems at the time they occur, we could easily and rapidly become isolated from events that are important in the daily lives of the staff.

Performance review responsibilities. This segment applies primarily to the formal review process, although some of the principles are readily adaptable to the informal process as well.

Usually, two primary parties are involved in the formal review. Each of those individuals has responsibilities in the review process. For clarity, the person who is celebrating a 3-month, 6-month, or annual anniversary in the department is called the "staff member," and the person to whom he or she is directly responsible is called the "reviewer."

Staff member responsibilities. The following is an excerpt from a memo that I give to ED staff members in preparation for review.

MEMO
Do I have to do anything for the review?
Yes.
You will be notified when a review is near. You are then responsible for the following:
1. Contact the reviewer to set up a mutually convenient time for the review.
2. Prepare a staff performance objectives sheet *before* the review. If you have never set professional goals, talk with the reviewer ahead of time to discuss your questions.
3. Be prepared to discuss the following:
   a. Your strengths (what you think you are good at)
   b. Your "improvement-needed" areas (what you want to learn and attitudes you want to change)
   c. What you like about the emergency department
   d. Areas of deficiency or inefficiency in the emergency department
   e. What you like about the "administration" (charge nurses, assistant director, medical director, and so on)
   f. What you would like to see changed about the administration
4. If you are eligible for a merit increase and believe you should have one, write out and bring with you a list of the reasons why you feel an increase is warranted.

Responsibilities of reviewer. Some of the reviewer's re-

---

*If obtaining a signature is inappropriate, the documentation should go into a confidential departmental file and *not* into the individual file. The confidential file should be flagged to indicate that the information is used only after consultation with the hospital attorney. Any documentation placed in the confidential file should be signed by at least two people.

sponsibilities are concrete, obvious, and relatively simple to fulfill. Other responsibilities are intangible and sometimes difficult to achieve or measure.

1. Notify the staff member at least 1 week, and preferably 2 to 6 weeks, before the anniversary date that a review should be scheduled.
2. Provide the staff member with written information about the review process. The written material should include information concerning when reviews are done, why they are done, a list of the staff member's responsibilities, a goals sheet, the format to be used in the review, and an outline of procedure in the event of disagreement with the reviewer.
3. Provide adequate time for the review. Fifteen minutes is not enough. Usually the review takes an hour or more.
4. Provide uninterrupted time. Phone calls and drop-in visits should not be permitted during the allotted review time. It is rude and may break the train of thought of the staff member and the reviewer.
5. Prepare for the review. Write down the points you wish to cover, spend time thinking about the staff member's overall performance in the preceding months, talk with his or her direct co-workers, and review the previous goals list.
6. Be honest. You must be able to confront problem areas directly, without beating around the bush.
7. Be fair. Make sure your information is accurate and reflects the opinion of more than one person.
8. Do not attack. Reviews should *not* be structured as criticism. They should be an honest appraisal of the staff member's strengths and areas where further growth and improvement are indicated.
9. Be receptive. If you are going to ask for sincere feedback, you must be prepared to look at your own performance and analyze its strengths and weaknesses. Staff members are a valuable source of input about how others perceive you, and if that input is met with immediate defense or attack, you may lose a source of information that is helpful to your growth as a manager. This does not mean that you must accept all input as a 100% accurate reflection of your abilities, but do listen and ponder.

Learning to conduct true dialogue reviews takes time and practice. Nobody is so completely secure, fair, honest, and receptive that every review goes smoothly and results in enthusiastic, motivated, and happy staff members. If you think the review is not going well, discuss it before you continue; for example, "I feel some tension here. Did I say something that bothered you?" or "I need to clarify something you just said that is bothering me." Do not expect to develop rapport and totally honest dialogue overnight. Also, remember that some people are not able to be open and direct in communicating, no matter how they are approached.

Review formats. A review format is the written document on which the formal review is based. Hundreds of different formats are probably in use, and most hospitals have some type of standardized, required format. Do not feel confined by that. If the hospital standard form does not meet your needs, request the use of an addendum specific to your area.

Formats range from the 10-question review of quality of work, quantity of work, and job knowledge to a totally new, start-with-a-blank-page appraisal.

The start-with-a-blank-page appraisal, when based on a key responsibilities format, is an excellent review tool.[6] It works best, however, when you have no more than five people a year to review. It is time-consuming to write a review with no specific format, and that alone usually means long delays in producing the written document.

The 10-question, quality/quantity, job knowledge format may meet the needs of the human resources office, but beyond that serves little useful function.

The best formats are those specifically designed to review areas that you and the staff consider important in your environment. "Relates well with house staff" is appropriate in teaching institutions only. "Completes restocking assignments thoroughly" is appropriate unless there is a full-time restock person. Design a format that addresses the special needs and philosophies of your ED.

Leadership

In the ED context the discussion of leadership is concerned with the people who have a title: supervisor, charge nurse, head nurse, manager, coordinator. These people have been selected to assume a level of responsibility that is beyond what is expected of a regular staff member.

Essential qualities for leader selection. There is a longstanding tradition in many professions that leaders are selected on the basis of years of service. It is a puzzling tradition that brings to mind a story.

According to legend, the Roman emperor Hadrian once found himself in an analogous position. One of his generals, the story goes, felt overdue for promotion. He took his case to the emperor and cited his long service as justification. "I am entitled to a more important command," he declared. "After all, I'm very experienced—I've been in ten battles."

Hadrian, a shrewd judge of men and their abilities, did not consider the man qualified for higher rank. He waved a casual hand at some army donkeys tethered nearby. "My dear general," Hadrian said dryly, "take a good look at those donkeys. Each of them has been in at least *twenty* battles—yet all of them are still donkeys."[1]

Another quotation also comes to mind: "You can have either 20 years of experience or 1 year of experience 20 times."

The nursing profession has another very puzzling practice. The profession has somehow come to the conclusion that clinical excellence automatically equals management excellence. How all this came to pass is a mystery. The effects of these traditions, however, are not very mysterious and have probably been experienced by all readers. The importance of having respected leaders and the results of incompetent leadership have been discussed. This section outlines the qualities that should be looked at in the selection of a manager, not necessarily in order of priority.

"Natural" leadership. If you put 15 people in a room and give them 10 minutes to resolve a problem, one or two will "naturally" lead the discussion. Title or no title, they are the people in your department to whom everyone automatically goes when a question arises. It appears to be true that certain people are "born leaders." Deciding whether or not they are actually *born* with this talent will be left to the heredity-versus-environment researchers; the practical effect is the same. A percentage of the population seems to have an abstract leadership quality that separates them from the rest of the population.

The importance of this quality deserves an illustration. Picture that person in your department who is capable, does the work thoroughly, but is always quiet, rarely enters into discussion, and does not socialize much. Then picture that same person in charge of a project that represents a major change for the department, or imagine this person recruiting and interviewing. The value of natural leadership is readily apparent. It is essential to reiterate, however, that these qualities do not divide people into desirable or undesirable categories. They are simply different, *not* better or worse.

Competence. Whoever you are asking to serve as a leader should have the skills to do so. No one person can excel in all areas, but he or she should be competent in the specified area of responsibility. For instance, a nurse who does not know a paramedic from a fireman should not be selected as paramedic liaison nurse. The weakest clinical nurse should not be asked to be responsible for the overall departmental in-service training. The least tactful person in the department should not be assigned all performance reviews. A supply technician should know the difference between 4×4s and 2×2s.

Staff members do not respect or follow the guidance of someone who is incompetent in his or her area of responsibility. Leaders should be skilled in their area. Whether the area is interpersonal skills, organizational skills, educational skills, or clinical skills, a leader should be the most competent person you can find. The comic strip in Fig. 5-3 demonstrates a popular misconception about leadership skills.

High level of commitment. Commitment is very difficult to quantify, but everyone knows who the committed people are. Their career development is important to them; they take the time and effort to look for answers; they help resolve problems; they take the time to leave a note if something needs repair; they attend classes; and they demonstrate in word and deed that they do not take responsibility lightly.

Committed people do *not* routinely goof off at work, call in sick when they are not, refuse to help out in scheduling, hang out in the lounge, leave their mess for the next shifts, or refuse to pitch in because "it's not my job."

Enthusiasm. Enthusiasm may resemble commitment. You do not usually find enthusiasm without commitment, but in relation to leadership, subtle but important differences exist. An emergency nurse, NA, or clerk may be highly committed to emergency care and career progress but may not have any enthusiasm for the responsibilities associated with management. Good leaders *genuinely* enjoy the type of work they do. The good leaders are those who accepted the position because of *the work itself* and not because they wanted a title, more money, weekends off, or power.

This quality cannot be overemphasized. The people selected as leaders must receive true enjoyment out of the work itself. Taking a leadership position for *any* other reason will have disastrous effects. Besides, if a leader does not enjoy the work, nothing else makes it worth the hassle. A leader who does not like the job can destroy a department.

Ego strength. No one is 100% secure. Everyone comes equipped with a full complement of assets and liabilities. Ego strength in leadership refers to various qualities, as listed next.

Self-confidence. A good leader should have enough self-

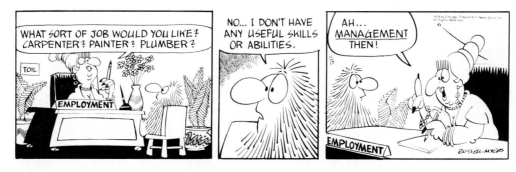

Fig. 5-3 Despite what this comic strip suggests, skills and competence are essential to the ED manager. (Reprinted by permission: Tribune Media Services, Inc.)

assurance that he or she does not hesitate to voice opinions, make decisions, or speak with some degree of authority.

Interpersonal skills. Interacting with others in a genuinely caring way requires some degree of self-love. People whose personal esteem is very low often have difficulty expressing concern and appreciation to others. This difficulty may be demonstrated by abruptness with others, an inability to say "thank you," or a need to "put people down." Frequently these people take sides and do not make an effort to help staff members support each other and "see the other side."

Confrontation skills. A good leader must be able to confront both people and problems. If one's opinion of oneself is regulated solely by external factors, other people's approval carries such impact that confrontation becomes very difficult. Good leaders confront without attack, never accuse, and interact in ways that promote trust in their objectivity and fairness.

Leaders must also confront problem areas and not be afraid to pursue resolutions. They should possess confidence in their ability to solve problems.

Self-assessment. People who are reasonably secure are not afraid to examine their own behaviors and motivations. They are not afraid to admit error. They are not defensive and hostile when criticized, and they do not always need to be right. They solicit feedback from colleagues and make a sincere effort to improve their areas of deficiency.

Good managers know their strengths *and* their weaknesses and are not afraid to surround themselves with talented people. They are able to delegate when appropriate and are not concerned when other people have skills that they do not possess. They also know when stresses are interfering with their judgment and are willing to admit it.

"Realness." People who like themselves are willing to be themselves. They can admit anger, fear, frustration, and "bad days." No one is "in control" all the time. This does not mean that good leaders routinely shout, throw things, or cry a lot. Occasionally, however, everyone reaches a stress limit. Staff members find the manager more believable as a person if he or she is not reluctant to express the feelings we all experience.

Recruiting: "inside" or "outside." The leadership selection topic would not be complete without addressing the inside promotion versus outside recruitment issue. To begin, when a management position is available, the ED staff members should have a realistic picture of what is required to fulfill responsibilities. If previous leaders have had the qualities just described, staff members probably already have a reasonable understanding of the effort and energy necessary to meet the department's needs. If the leadership has previously been too low-key, the people responsible for recruiting have an obligation to explain to all internal candidates that the former level of output was not sufficient and that greater commitment, time, and energy is required. A clear picture of the job will eliminate many applicants.

The next step is to open interviews to anyone in the department who is interested. Those who wait to be asked and do not show the initiative to seek the position actively can be eliminated from the running.

The third step is to evaluate all candidates by the criteria outlined previously. If the recruiters (there should be more than one) honestly believe that none of the candidates is capable, it is necessary to look outside. Leadership recruiting is that simple.

Now you have made an honest assessment and decided to look outside, but you are concerned about resentment from other staff members. You might try asking those staff members who did not apply if they think anyone in the department is capable of doing the job. If your assessment is accurate, they will ponder a bit and concur that there is not. When employees are presented with the possibility of working under someone who is not right for the position, much of their resentment rapidly fades away.

The applicants themselves should be directly, kindly, and honestly informed of the reasons why they were not selected. If the recruiters believe the applicants could be developed, their areas of deficiency should be identified and a program begun to develop them for future positions. If the applicants are mature and the denial is based on reasonable assessment, they will have some understandable adjusting to do, but it should be short-term.

When internal candidates are reviewed, another possible situation may arise. A candidate may be a questionable choice; he or she may be good in some areas but deficient in others. If sufficient reason exists to consider that person for the position, he or she should be offered the leadership position. However, the areas in question should be discussed with the candidate, who must have a clear understanding of what is expected. If the person is, in time, able to fulfill the responsibilities, all is well; if not, *do not leave him or her in the position.* The probationary period should not exceed 3 months. Also, it should be documented that the person understood the requirements and concerns. If possible, some measurable criteria should be established. Weekly conferences to discuss performances and establish direction for the following week should not be necessary; self-assessment and initiative are the responsibilities of a leader. The person's performance and abilities should stand (or fall) on their own merit. A conference at 6 weeks is probably indicated to prevent the "I didn't know I wasn't doing well" allegation, but constant counseling should not be necessary for people in a position to lead others.

This is not intended to be interpreted as a harsh, insensitive approach to managing people. Some people are not yet ready for leadership positions, are wrong for the ED environment, or are not leadership material at all. The effects of leaving these people in management positions are devastating and serve to demoralize the nursing profession.

If such a situation occurs, the person involved should be given every consideration, be provided supportive alternatives, and be commended for willingness to try. Occasionally, the person even may be kept in the same department. Not working out in a "titled" position should not be viewed as a social disgrace. The individual should be reminded of her or his talents and encouraged to pursue areas in which those talents can be used.

One of the great fallacies in nursing is that those who do not "move up" are somehow "failures" or "lacking in commitment." Patients have lost some of the best clinical care available because good nurses felt pressured into "moving up." Good clinical nursing should be recognized and encouraged and should never be second to titles.

Responsibilities of a leader

Role modeling. The leader described earlier is understandably expected to serve as a role model to other staff members in attitude and perspective. No one is a model of perfection, but the departmental leaders should exemplify maturity and professionalism.

Enthusiasm. The leaders should be expected to serve as a positive motivating force in the ED. If a member of the leadership staff is consistently cranky, depressed, and short-tempered and appears to hate coming to work, the effects are predictable.

Support and perspective. The leadership staff should serve as a support system to the department. Support and perspective translate into many behaviors. Department leaders should have the most thorough knowledge of procedures and policies so that they can be looked to for answers. They should also have a level of understanding of departmental philosophies and objectives that enables them to support changes. They should serve as a sounding board for other staff members and should help resolve minor problems before they become major problems. Leaders should be expected to handle their own complaints maturely without creating morale crises by inappropriate "behind-the-back" complaining. They should have a realistic perspective of the department and its relationship to other departments and to outside agencies. Ideally, leaders serve as public relations officers for the hospital and the department.

Problem solving. Good leaders should be able to reason through a problem even when there is no "policy" and come to a logical resolution. They should be able to think clearly, weighing advantages and disadvantages, and not jump to hasty conclusions without knowledge of all the facts. They should also know when it is appropriate to refer a problem to the hospital administrator or the medical director. When unfamiliar situations arise, leaders should find out how to deal with such events the next time.

Communication. Good leaders are skilled in communication. They know that one questions, not accuses. They know that part of their responsibility is to teach perspective, understanding, and a "let's look at it from their side" approach. They also know how to confront their colleagues when differences arise.

Leaders know the importance of communicating to their superior when a problem has occurred. If the state governor was a patient on Friday night and not happy with the care received, a good leader knows it is wise to advise the department director and hospital administrator.

Initiative. Leaders are expected to possess some initiative. Good leaders do not "dump" problems that they could easily resolve themselves. Good leaders also know what is going on in the department. If a sound of breaking glass comes from a treatment room, the charge nurse does not wait for someone to file a report before investigating whether or not the security guard should be called.

Effective leaders take initiative in helping resolve long-term problems as well. If a department-wide deficiency seems to exist in documenting the care of patients with chest pain, leaders help devise education, audit new forms, or whatever it takes to resolve the problem.

Decision making. It has been said that "good managers make decisions—if it is the right decision, so much the better." Although this may be a slight exaggeration, when leaders (particularly those with overall responsibility) are afraid to risk being wrong, they may immobilize the department's growth. A weekend charge nurse who is afraid to call the copier repair people before Monday may risk an uprising if the staff has to run three flights of stairs to have copies made over the weekend.

Clinical time. The final behavior that should be expected, even demanded, of nursing leaders is that they spend some portion of their time working in actual patient care. Several advantages exist to adopting this practice:

1. The nurse leader is able to maintain some percentage of his or her clinical skill.
2. Patient care maintains the leader's perspective about the real purpose of the job. It is too easy to drown in papers and rapidly forget that the reason for being a nurse is the care of patients.
3. This practice is good for mental health. Caring for patients is very rewarding, and the feedback is more immediate than the feedback in management. The nurse leader can, at least for a time, forget about meetings, phone calls, and administrative hassles and do something with rapid, visible results.
4. Patient care diminishes "Monday morning quarter-backing." If you were not there at 2 AM Saturday, it is easy to second-guess and say, "This is what I would have done." You do not know the situation unless you do occasionally perform patient care.

Leadership styles—or how to put together a management team. Teams are two or more people working together to achieve a goal (or goals). When putting a management team together, you should attempt to do the job with the least number of people with titles. Having 30% of the department staff in charge of a project creates confusion and hassle.

No matter what the size of the team, there are three essential ingredients: people skill, clinical skill, and organizational skill.

People skill involves the ability to interact in a genuinely caring, nonthreatening manner, and to confront, counsel, and see the good qualities in others. Persons with this skill remember to ask how your weekend was and really do care if it was rotten.

Clinical skill includes clinical expertise, educational enthusiasm, and commitment to learning and teaching. These nurses are excited when a new, sophisticated procedure is introduced and actually understand how it works.

Organizational skill is the ability to define systems that improve efficiency, to identify inefficiencies, to think logically, and to organize projects. These persons cannot tolerate disorganization and are able to design a workable system for resolving the problem.

Ideally we would be able to find a leader with an equal balance of all these skills. Unfortunately, few people possess *all* these skills.

The key to putting together a management team is to assess what the staff's current skills are and add these skills to work areas found to be deficient. A team project does not work out well if all the leaders are people oriented but do not care that the proper supplies are lacking. The project also does not work well if many supplies are made available but no pats on the back are given for obtaining the materials.

Most leaders have some amount of each skill but are generally weighted more heavily in one area. If possible, you do not want people who have only one skill. If you have an organizer who has no time for people, you still need someone to relate to the staff. If you have a 100% people-oriented leader, no supplies may be available. If you have a 100% clinician, everyone will know how to do the new procedure, but the right equipment will not always be available.

When filling (or creating) a position, assess the current leadership and write a summary of what abilities are needed to resolve the problem areas. Many leaders make the mistake of choosing people similar to themselves in hopes of making life easier. However, a happy, well-organized, and clinically excellent department is not made of people who are all alike. Always agreeing may create a peaceful working environment, but growth, change, and progress come only with new perspectives, some opinion differences, and varied ways of viewing the world.

Should you be a leader? This last part of the leadership section addresses current leaders and persons considering leadership.

Management requires a different set of skills than does patient care. Anyone who has organized even a small project understands that fact. Management is not for everyone, just as emergency care, geriatric nursing, oncology nursing, and surgical nursing are not for everyone.

Discovering that management is not for you should not be perceived as failure or disgrace. People do not criticize nurses who choose oncology over critical care, and they should not criticize nurses who choose direct patient care to management. Nurses try many areas before they find the position best for them, and management is only one of many possibilities.

Should you be a leader? The answer asks two more questions: Do you enjoy management work? Are you good at management? Usually contentment and competence go hand-in-hand, but unfortunately some leaders enjoy the title and prestige and do not have the skills.

The following self-quiz is designed to help you arrive at the answer to these two questions.

Do you enjoy management work?

1. What has been the happiest, most rewarding period in your career? If your answer is "when I was a staff nurse," perhaps you should reevaluate your career.
2. Do you look forward (at least 90% of the time) to going to work? If not, why not?
3. Do you find yourself longing to take care of patients and avoid management hassles?
4. What is your assessment of your mental health? Do you smile often and go home feeling as if you have accomplished something, or do you find yourself grumpy, withdrawn, and always tired and depressed?
5. Do you look forward to new changes and problem-solving challenges with enthusiasm? Or do you find yourself procrastinating and avoiding new projects?
6. What do you think about your colleagues? Do you believe that they are basically a good group with whom you feel comfortable, or do you find you are consistently angry with them, routinely cranky, and critical of their behavior? Colleagues include all department staff—physicians, nurses, technicians, and clerks, as well as nursing and hospital administration.
7. Are you physicially healthy most of the time? If your sick days have dramatically increased, this may be an indication of stress.
8. What do your loved ones think about your job? If your family and friends have expressed concern about your job's effect on your outlook, you may need to look carefully at your career choices.
9. What was your original reason for accepting the position?
10. Do you often think that it is not worth the hassle?

Are you good at management?

1. What is the status of the overall morale in your department?
2. What is the attrition rate?
3. Have you noticed an increase in sick calls?
4. Do staff members come and talk with you regularly in a relaxed and comfortable way?
5. Have you accomplished the goals you set out to accomplish?
6. Do your colleagues feel free to offer advice, input, and suggestions for improvement?
7. Are people in the department actively involved in helping to make changes and improvements in the department?
8. Are there many people in the department whose talents exceed yours in certain areas?
9. Are you ever complimented by your superiors or the staff for the job you are doing?

10. Is there chronic tension and friction between nurses, physicians, technicians, and clerks? Are they consistently critical of one another?
11. Do you regularly have to intervene in resolving petty personnel conflicts?
12. Do the people in the department enjoy coming to work, and do they treat patients with empathy and respect?

This self-assessment should give you a fairly accurate picture of whether this is the right career choice for you.

If you are really unsure and are willing to risk the outcome, go to your immediate superior and tell him or her that you are questioning whether you are effective in management. If the person says, "You're doing an excellent job," you probably are. If you receive a reply such as "Not everyone is cut out for management," or "Do you have other options in mind?" you may want to consider a change.

Making a change is simply that. It is deciding that other options would provide you with a happier, more rewarding career. It is not failure. Your colleagues will respect and appreciate your willingness to assess yourself and admit that you are not happy in that position. Your superiors will probably do everything possible to help you find a position that will meet your needs. Chronic frustration and unhappiness are not healthy for you or for the department.

Teamwork and Personnel Conflicts

No member of a crew is praised for the individuality
of his rowing.
Ralph Waldo Emerson

Emergency care offers unique opportunities and challenges in the area of teamwork. It is the only area in health care in which physicians, nurses, technicians, and clerks work side-by-side on a 24-hour basis. It is also a stressful area, and emergency personnel have a relatively short time in which to meet a variety of goals. First, the patient's medical needs must be met; then the patient's emotional needs and those of the family must be met. Emergency personnel must deal with forms, requisitions, reporting laws, and legal problems. All this must be done and done right, and ED staff members have anywhere from 10 minutes to a few hours to accomplish these varied objectives.

To expect, in such an environment, that staff members will always interact in a calm, quiet, and reasonable manner and never irritate each other is unrealistic. However, if an atmosphere of professionalism and mutual respect is established throughout the department, peer conflicts and related problems can be minimized.

Establishing and maintaining this atmosphere presents a genuine challenge. People attracted to emergency care are generally not low keyed. They have definite ideas and opinions and usually are not at all reluctant to share their perceptions of things. This individualism is, overall, an asset. Dealing with immediate threats to life and limb requires some assertiveness, and it is much easier to tone down assertiveness than to gear up apathy. However, these qual-

ities can also create many injured egos and, if not properly handled, some obstacles on the road to teamwork.

Providing an atmosphere of professionalism and respect is a two-part task. The atmosphere must first be established, and then it must be maintained.

Establishing the atmosphere. Establishing a teamwork milieu is primarily the responsibility of the leadership staff.

Medical and nursing director relationship. If the top leadership people in a department are not able to interact in a mutually supportive manner, the groundwork is already laid for trouble. The physician director and the nursing director should be the role model for teamwork. The planning for a department's growth and progress should be a joint effort between physician and nursing leadership to ensure that goals are agreed on, understood, and supported by both parties. When the top leadership is pulling together, departmental teamwork is a natural result.

Leaders will disagree on occasion, but these disagreements should not be the topic of general discussion throughout the department. The leadership staff should be mature enough that they do not slander the others and solicit allegiance, directly or indirectly, for their side. The goal should always be to arrive at a mutually agreeable method of operating. If the medical and nursing directors are unable to work together, one or both of them should leave.

Selection of staff. (See also earlier section on staff selection.) Selecting staff members who are mature and professional in their outlook prevents personnel conflicts. Staff members whose entire life is focused on work and whose friends are all work friends tend to develop a skewed perspective of the work environment. Also, "chronic complainers" are committed to perpetuating problems and not in resolving them. These are the people who say *nothing* directly, whose complaints are always heard thirdhand, and who never actively work toward resolution of a problem. Do not let one of them be transferred to your department.

Laying the groundwork. When new staff members are hired, their orientation should explain to them how complaints and problems are handled. It must be communicated from the outset that the goal is problem resolution, not problem continuance and magnification. New staff members should understand that, when problems arise, they should confront only the person they have conflict with or the immediate supervisor. Magnifying problems by grumbling to many people should not be tolerated. If this message is delivered early in employment, it may help prevent serious morale problems in the future.

Roles and teamwork. If the leadership staff emphasizes that no one job category is more important than another—that it takes the cooperative effort of all to meet the goals—the hierarchy problems can be minimized. Although good physicians may be more difficult to acquire than good clerks, an ED cannot function adequately without good clerks—or nurses or technicians. No one category can effectively operative without cooperation and expertise in the other categories. The entire staff should understand that all personnel will be treated with respect.

Another factor that ensures a smoothly running department is teamwork. Nurses should not be sitting in groups of two and three while NAs clean suture sets. Clerks should not be idle while nurses are flooded with requisitions. The "whose job is it?" problem can be difficult. For efficiency there must be defined sets of responsibilities, but 5 minutes after duties lists are distributed, someone will invariably say, "That's not my job." Overcoming this mind-set takes time and patience. People are naturally inclined to be relieved when their duties list is completed and are apt to ignore the five other people working diligently without break for the past 8 hours.

During orientation, management should communicate that, although management-defined responsibilities exist, each person is also *expected* to help out if his or her colleagues are overloaded.

Semantics. Our primary method of communication is words, and the words we use should be carefully chosen. Part of laying the groundwork for genuine teamwork is being selective in our terminology. For instance, "The 3 to 11 charge nurse hates the new doctor" has a different sound from "The 3 to 11 charge nurse came to talk to me about the new doctor." "She's really stupid when it comes to dysrhythmias" sounds different from "I think she needs some dysrhythmia education."

The word "employee" immediately says that there is an "employer" or "boss." However, *everyone* is really a *staff member,* and there should be *personnel* manuals, not *employee* manuals.

Finally, do not call the people in the department *my* nurses or technicians or clerks. Staff members do not belong to anyone. They are the nurses in the ED, or she is the department secretary—but not "my" anything or anybody. The ED is *our* department, not *my* department.

It may be difficult to change years of terminology habits, but try listening to yourself and assessing the psychologic impact of your word choices. Whenever possible, use words that are not "loaded."

Maintaining cooperation. The responsibility for maintaining a cooperative atmosphere lies primarily with the leadership staff and secondarily with all members of the team. A mutually supportive, understanding environment requires empathy, the recognition of conflict and differences, and conflict resolution.

Empathy. Encouraging empathy among staff members is an excellent way to promote teamwork. When a new physician working a first shift seems slow and uncertain, staff members should be reminded that they all had a "first day." Slowness complaints seem to be related to physicians more often than to any other job category. People expect that a physician should be able to drop into any environment, not knowing the procedures and ways of working, and function at top speed.

One of the ways to promote empathy is to arrange a "shadow" program. An RN can spend the day "shadowing" a clerk at the registration desk or a clerk can spend the day following a physician caring for patients. This is also helpful between departments, such as the ED and intensive care unit. From a cost standpoint, routine shadowing is not often feasible. If the opportunity is available, however, it should not be passed up. Shadowing is a valuable tool for increasing understanding about the various important roles each team member plays.

Complaints about other staff members should be met with some dialogue about the possible reasons for the person's suspect behavior. These dialogues should also reflect some of the good points about that person. "Yes, I know he can be a little short-tempered occasionally, but there isn't a better nurse in the department, and he really is concerned that the patient gets the best care available."

Department personnel should also be reminded that everyone has idiosyncrasies: some people cannot get to work on time, others hate checking the equipment, some are occasionally grumpy, others are slow, and still others are too compulsive. Each person has some faulty and some redeeming qualities.

However, not all personnel conflicts should be handled by playing the "glad game." Investigating reasons for the conflictive behavior and evaluating that person's overall patterns of performance may reduce the intensity of the complaint.

Conflict recognition. Recognizing conflicts is an important part of maintaining a teamwork environment. Differentiating minor, transient problems from conflicts that interfere with good working relationships is sometimes difficult. Although personal conflicts should not be ignored, they should also not receive more time and attention than they warrant. Calling an eight-person group therapy conference every time an impolite exchange occurs only adds to the problem. Most adults realize that life is full of annoyances, many of which are not worth much emotional energy. Overemphasizing minor situational problems is counterproductive, costly, and time-consuming.

However, all personnel conflicts should be *recognized* and dealt with in some way. Dealing with a conflict may occasionally mean ignoring it or watching for awhile to see if it resolves itself; many times maturity wins out, and the conflict disappears on its own. If some intervention is indicated, it should be done as soon as possible. Allowing problems to brew for weeks may ultimately double the work involved in resolution. Emergency care is stressful enough without expending the energy necessary to remember not to speak to someone.

Differentiating between minor and major problems is a skill that is learned only with time. No magic formulas or graphs guide that decision. The best monitoring device is your own sensing and your knowledge of the people involved and prior events. If you know that the people involved are inclined to bear grudges, or if this minor complaint has surfaced often, it is necessary to address it directly and immediately.

Conflict resolution. This discussion of conflicts is related to those performance problems and personality-related issues that inevitably crop up in any working environment: "Laura is too abrupt," "Sharon doesn't restock her room," "Jeff is lazy," "Bill left early," "Elaine let 14 people stay in the trauma room, and there was so much confusion," "The night shift doesn't . . . ," "The day shift always . . . ," and so on. This discussion is not related to major problems. Staff members who hit patients, steal narcotics, or make gross clinical errors should be dealt with directly and rapidly.

There are many approaches to dealing with personnel conflicts and much controversy over what constitutes the best approach. All people have to decide for themselves what methods work best, but the suggestions that follow may be helpful. New conflicts become known by one of three mechanisms: (1) someone comes into the office to complain directly, (2) some gossip occurs about the incident or person, or (3) someone senses a possible conflict. In each of these situations, decisions have to be made about how much attention the incident warrants. For the purposes of this discussion, however, it is assumed that the decision to investigate is made. A list of helpful hints follows.

Do not overemphasize the problem. Comments such as "How could she be so stupid?" or "He is such a jerk" do not help the situation. Comments such as "Does this happen often?" "Can you give me more specifics?" or "I'm surprised. That's really out of character for him" may add some perspective. If you have not been directly approached but are trying to investigate, it is better to start with "I heard there was a problem Saturday night" than with "Jeff really blew again, huh?" Try to remain neutral and objective and add some perspective rather than taking sides.

Clarify the issues. When discussing the conflict, be sure the *real* problems are identified. What appears to be laziness may be a lack of understanding of what the duties are. What seems to be a lack of caring may be a momentary preoccupation with personal problems or a previous patient. Failure to restock a room could be the result of an unusually busy shift. Abruptness may result from adjusting to a new role and the stresses involved. Review the issues carefully before deciding about intervention.

Leave the resolution decision where it belongs. Once a problem has been identified, ask the *people who identified it* what they think should be done. Are they simply in your office to blow off steam (perfectly appropriate, if *not* spread throughout the department), or do they feel some intervention is indicated? The answer to the "What do you think should be done?" question is often surprising. When the decision is presented to them, often they think that discus-

sion is sufficient and wish to leave it at that or wait to see if the problem recurs. Most people are not anxious to hang their colleagues.

Encourage confrontation. Once it has been decided that intervention is indicated, ask how the complaining party wants to handle it. Staff members are not children. Most of them are capable of dealing directly with the problem themselves. Although uncomfortable and difficult at first, having to say "you" and "I" deescalates the subjective nature of the "he did, she said" conversations. Confronting someone directly forces one to see the other as a real person with assets, liabilities, and feelings.

Clearly, leaders must become involved at times. Chronic problems and performance conflicts that may result in discipline problems should be handled by the appropriate manager. However, most conflicts are best resolved on a one-to-one basis.

Summary. Establishing and maintaining a teamwork atmosphere is not easy. It requires diligence and commitment to the goal, but the benefits are obvious. If a teamwork problem exists, direct, emphatic confrontation with a goal of *resolution* is the recommended approach.

REFERENCES

1. Gellerman S: *Motivation and productivity,* New York, 1963, AMACOM, a division of American Management Associations.
2. Fulcher JK: Personal communications, 1976-1980.
3. Herzberg F: Dual-factor theory of job satisfaction, *Personnel Psychol,* Winter 1967.
4. Maslow AH: *Motivation and personality,* New York, 1954, Harper & Row.
5. McClelland D: That urge to achieve. *Think Magazine,* 1966.
6. Smith HP, Brouwer PJ: *Performance appraisal and human development,* Reading, Mass, Addison-Wesley.
7. Vroom V: *Work and motivation,* New York, 1964, John Wiley & Sons.

SUGGESTED READINGS

Barnum BS, Mallard CO: *Essentials of nursing management: concepts and context of practice,* Rockville, Md, 1989, Aspen.
Buschiazzo L: *The handbook of emergency nursing management,* Rockville, Md, 1987, Aspen.
Drucker PF: *The best of Peter Drucker on management,* New York, 1977, Harper's College Press.
Frank IC: *Managing emergency nursing services,* Rockville, Md, 1989, Aspen.
Glassman AM: *The challenge of management,* New York, 1978, John Wiley & Sons.
Hampton, DR: Behavioral concepts in management, Encino, Calif, 1972, Dickenson.
Mager RF: *Goal analysis,* Belmont, Calif, 1972, Fearon.
Mager RF, Pipe P: *Analyzing performance problems,* Belmont, Calif, 1970, Fearon.
Peters T: *Thriving on chaos: handbook for a management revolution,* New York, 1987, Harper & Row.
Winston S: *The organized executive,* New York, 1983, Warner Communications.

Designing An Emergency Department

Lynne Gagnon

L ittle in nursing school prepares a person for the role of assisting with design of an emergency department (ED). Yet, as a nurse manager you may be required to oversee a multimillion dollar renovation and construction project at your ED. You must be a vocal member of the architecture and construction team. Resources for this role are scarce. This chapter gives the reader an overview of the planning and construction process.

PREPLANNING

The preplanning phase begins long before construction. Because of state and federal mandates to control health care costs, many states have implemented a "certificate of need" process. In that process hospitals must justify the need to renovate or construct new facilities. If that is the case in your state, you should be involved in that process with the hospital planning department or the consultant hired for that purpose. Planning specialists conduct an environmental analysis of the community. They look at population demographics (predicted population increases or decreases), the economic environment (new industries or expansion of existing ones), and competitive services offered in the area. These planning specialists must be familiar with your ED's long-range strategic plan.

The planning specialists need to be educated about the predicated impacts of new services and the forecast of the ED needs. To do this forecasting, identify your ED customers: (1) the percent of adults and children, (2) the types of cases seen (medical, surgical, obstetric, pediatric, and acute versus nonacute cases), and (3) the prehospital providers, police, and allied health professionals such as counselors, organ procurement personnel, clergy, and the like.

Consider special functions that your department will provide, such as regional Emergency Medical Services communication and medical control, a poison information center, organ and tissue procurement, trauma care, a flight program, a hospital-based ambulance, a hazardous substance decontamination unit, psychiatric consultation and care, walk-in care or other "fast-track" services, dictation areas for private physicians, medical records storage, phy-

sician and staff call rooms, storage systems—the list can seem endless. Be sure to consider as many possibilities as you can in your planning. Most construction renovation projects are designed to meet projected needs for 7 to 10 years after completion. In architectural terms, this process is called *functional programming*.

You must look at health care trends that will or may affect the services of the ED, including the following:
1. Who your competition is and what they offer
2. Increasing number of outpatient services
3. Overcrowding, ambulance diversions, unavailable intensive care unit beds, and the nursing shortage
4. Reimbursement issues such as health maintenance organizations, preferred provider organizations, self-payers, ambulatory visit groupings, the underinsured, and the uninsured
5. Technologic advances
6. Exposure to and management of hazardous substances
7. Access issues affected by increasing violence within EDs (for example, the need for security staff or metal detectors or both)

The success and usefulness of your new department will directly correlate to the amount of effort put into forecasting needs and services. Do not expect, however, that you will think of everything—because you cannot.

DESIGN TEAM

After the commitment has been made to build or renovate, the hospital engineers, planners, and administration begin the process of selecting an architect or design firm or both.

You may or may not be involved in choosing the architect or design firm. Regardless of the degree of your involvement, request a firm that has had previous experience in designing EDs. Involve the staff from the beginning; involving the staff helps gain support for the project from the staff. Form a department planning committee made up of staff nurses from each shift, secretarial staff, physicians, and other support staff who provide services within your department.

The committee should choose a spokesperson to represent

them on the hospital's design team. The hospital's design team should have a representative from each discipline that functions within your department, for example, the housekeeping, laboratory, radiology, pharmacology, risk management, and registration departments. The team should also include a representative from the hospital's engineering staff. It would also be wise to invite a lay person to attend some of the design meetings. Those of us who work in the environment every day tend to see things differently or overlook some things that later become apparent when patients or customers begin using the facility. For example, a lay person would be helpful, when the placement of direction signs is being determined. Staff members know how to find their way around the department, so we may not think to put up *enough* clear and accurate signs for those who are not there every day. A lay person on the design team can help identify such issues.

After the design team is formed, establish regular meetings with the hospital engineers and the architect. In the initial meetings the nurse manager and physician director should share the department's strategic plans and long-range goals, including expansion of existing services and new services that are being planned. When you look at the architect's design proposals, review them from all perspectives: the added services, patient flow, communication within the department, and how personnel from outside the department will function within the department.

Examine the exterior aspects of the construction project. How will patients access your department? Will there be separate entrances for ambulatory patients and patients who arrive in ambulances? If you separate the acute care area from the nonacute care area, where will the ambulance entrance be in relation to the acute care area? Will sidewalks be adequately graded for wheelchair access? How many parking spaces are being allocated solely for ED patients, and how close are the spaces to the ED entrance? How will

traffic flow? Is there enough room for the ambulance traffic? Are patient walking areas away from the ambulance area? These and similar questions should be asked.

After the initial plans are formed, the architect and engineer should provide you with blueprints of the area. Do not be concerned with the technical figures on the blueprint. The things you should pay special attention to are the location of doors and windows and planned locations for wall-mounted equipment, radiograph view boxes, electrical connections, medical gases, suction equipment, and restrooms. If you find that there are certain areas in your proposed department that generate staff discussion and disagreement, it would be helpful to have the hospital carpentry shop or the architect produce a model of that area, which allows staff to "walk through" the design and "feel it out." A model was made of a proposed triage area, for example, and those involved were able to foresee problems that the planned space would cause. If the construction project includes renovating existing space, you may have to accept limitations in design and function. For example, one project included renovation of an already existing area that was formerly used as an outpatient clinic. In efforts to keep costs down, the examination rooms that were used as clinic rooms were left "as is," with the exception of new paint and new floor covering. When stretchers were moved into these rooms, it was discovered that they could only fit in the rooms next to a certain wall and that physicians would have to perform patient examinations from one side of the stretcher instead of the other. This may seem a minor detail, but the design could not be altered and became a source of frustration for many physicians (who are also customers of the hospital).

THE CONSTRUCTION PHASE

When the actual construction or renovation process begins, the construction supervisor establishes frequent communication meetings with the hospital engineer overseeing

Product type _____

Product name _____

Unit cost (indicate if approximate) _____

Supplier name _____

Supplier address _____ Home _____

Contact person _____

Trial period _____

Product features _____

User comments _____

Fig. 6-1   Example of equipment trial record.

the project. The ED medical director and nurse manager should participate in as many of these meetings as possible. Participation establishes a communication link between the construction supervisor and the people who will actually be using the new facility.

After the new services are determined and the construction begins, establish lists of new equipment you will need to purchase. The list will be extensive, and necessary equipment ranges from oxygen gauges to cardiac monitors. Most hospital purchasing departments can facilitate the purchasing process by initiating contact with sales representatives from companies whose products you wish to consider. Try as many products as possible before making the decision to purchase. Let the staff use the equipment as it will be used in the new department. Users are the best testers of the durability and functionality of the equipment. Negotiate with sales representatives to allow you to try their products for specified periods.

Because you will be trying so much equipment during a short time, create a product comment sheet (Fig. 6-1). This sheet becomes a "tickler" file of comments about the products that staff members like and dislike and includes the reasons for their preferences.

When equipment cannot be tried, (1) identify the product needed, (2) obtain the manufacturer's product literature through sales representatives or through the hospital's purchasing department, (3) request a current user's list and contact some of those users to determine their level of satisfaction with the product, and (4) consult the hospital's engineering department to review the product standards with you (for example, electrical requirements, product safety, applicability to your need). The biomedical engineering department should also participate in product trials, especially if department staff will be required to maintain or repair the product once it is purchased.

Nurse managers should spend time with product sales representatives. Involve sales representatives in the planning process: they can be instrumental in acquiring the right product for the intended use.

After the decision has been made to purchase equipment, be sure to negotiate delivery time of the product. The last thing you need is either 15 new stretchers arriving in the department without a place to put them *or* a new facility ready to open and no stretchers.

After a comprehensive list of equipment necessary to operate the new facility has been developed, a work sheet used to track the stages of trial, bid, and purchase is also developed. This status sheet is updated monthly.

When you are looking at new products or systems for the department (for example, communication systems or storage systems) ask the sales representatives what kinds of service they can provide toward analyzing your needs. For example, one of the objectives we hoped to accomplish in the construction of a new facility was the conversion from an exchange cart system to a "par-level," that is, a predetermined

inventory level, storage system. When we began to look at storage devices and systems, one company provided us with the consulting services of a nurse specialist. She spent a day inspecting the current storage system and the problems it presented; then she gave us a written recommendation of how many and what types of storage carts we would need to convert from an exchange system to a "par-level" system. These types of resources are invaluable, but often you must ask whether they are available.

As construction progresses, the nursing director and medical director should walk through the site frequently. It is much easier to make changes during the building process. When you walk through the site, visualize caring for a patient in the specific areas. Where should electrical outlets and oxygen be? Where should the cardiac monitors be? Should they be mounted on the wall or suspended on a boom? If it is your option, encourage the placement of extra wiring. If you are not currently using computers but may use them within the next 5 to 10 years, plan for computers now. Visualize how you would move additional equipment such as a portable radiograph unit into the room. Evaluate access to utility areas for clean and soiled equipment and supplies from the patient care areas. Will your medication area or pharmacy station be nearest the area where you will care for the most critically ill patients? Where will you locate code carts? Will you have a separate waiting area for families in crisis? Ask these types of questions.

A whole book could be devoted to interior design and furnishings. Remember that hospitals do not have to be white. Color and lighting elicit both physiologic and emotional responses. Consult with the interior designer (usually associated with the architectural firm) when choosing colors. If you have plans to use color-coded directions for wayfinding, include those plans in your color scheme. The primary objective of using colors in your new department is to create an uplifting, aesthetically pleasing, soothing environment for patients, their families, and staff. Make every effort to incorporate natural lighting along with institutional lighting.

The topic of furnishings should be discussed in detail with the interior designer. If you will be purchasing new chairs, whether for staff or for patient waiting areas, be sure to have accurate information about how to clean them, the durability of fabrics to be used, and the reliability of pneumatics in chairs. Consultation with the housekeeping department concerning furnishings can be helpful. Obtain samples of suggested fabrics so that housekeeping staff can test them by soiling and cleaning them. It is also useful to seek the input of the housekeeping department when selecting floor coverings. The housekeeping staff are the experts when it comes to evaluating floors for durability, ease of cleaning, and appearance. One architect suggested the use of quarry tile in an ED foyer. By his report, quarry tile was durable, aesthetically pleasing, and easy to maintain. His recommendation was accepted; the housekeeping staff and other users were not consulted, and the tile was installed in the main patient entrance. After the tile was installed, it was found to be difficult to clean. It always appears dirty, and because it is a natural tile, it has an uneven surface, which causes jarring of patients in wheelchairs or on stretchers. The quarry tile is slippery when wet and not an appropriate flooring choice in a state where there is snow a large part of the year.

Other general design issues you should consider include the following: acoustics, play areas for young children, security within your department (consider number of entrances and exits, need for security staff space, and need for metal detectors), communication systems within the department (intercom, light boards, buzzers, phones, and patient alarms), as well as backup emergency phone systems and intradepartmental communication. Will you have a pneumatic tube station? Are you considering an ED laboratory? Department planning committees have generated such suggestions as placing ceramic tile on the walls of a critical care room used when treating overdose patients so that the unavoidable messiness of charcoal administration can be easily cleaned up, and installing a beautician sink in one examination room at stretcher height, where it can be used for eye irrigations, hair washing, and similar procedures.

As the construction progresses, you will discover that requirements of many state building regulations and codes, as well as Occupational Safety and Health Administration requirements for employee safety, must be met. Your hospital engineer should be the one to see to it that those standards are being met.

For example, if you are incorporating a decontamination area, there must be a mechanism for collection of the water used for decontamination and a process for disposing of the water. Fire regulations, electrical and plumbing codes, and radiation codes governing the installation of a radiology unit must also be followed.

PLANNING FOR IMPLEMENTATION

Be prepared for construction delays, which occur for numerous reasons. As the project nears completion, begin planning for the move. The amount of time spent planning for the move directly correlates to the smoothness with which the transition occurs. Issues that must be resolved before the actual move include in-service training for users of new equipment and relocation of existing equipment from the old department to the new one (for example, computers, furnishings, and monitors). Stocking of the new area should be completed before the move. Stocking is a time-consuming project, especially if you are converting from one type of storage system to another. One of the best ways to determine whether your new facility is ready for operation is to walk through the facility as though you were taking a patient through it. Is everything that will be necessary to provide care for the patient in place at each phase of the patient's visit? Take the imaginary patient through triage and the ED registration processes. Where does the patient go from there? How does the primary nurse access the patient? How and to whom will laboratory and radiograph orders be communicated? What happens to the patient and the patient's chart while diagnostic studies are pending? Where will radiographs be viewed? Where will chart work and dictation be done? How will the patient be discharged? For each of these steps specific tools and supplies will be needed.

After the actual building and installations are completed and rooms are set up and stocked, the housekeeping department will need time to do a major cleaning of the area. Give them as much time as possible. Staff of departments such as pharmacy, radiology, operating room, registration, and nursing will need to know of your move date and time. Patients, prehospital providers, and private physicians will also need to know this information.

The actual move is best implemented at your department's least busy time, which is usually between midnight and 5 AM. Extra staff should be scheduled to make the move. The actual move should occur on one shift, but know that the transition will take much longer. Expect that there will be problems you did not anticipate and things that will have to be changed. Remember that there will always be a few people who "liked it better the other way." Change is difficult, but with patience both you and the staff will not only survive but also appreciate the new facility.

SUMMARY

Designing or renovating an ED is a challenging opportunity, a time-consuming project during which you will experience many emotional peaks and valleys. You must be the advocate for the consumer and the user. No doubt there will be compromises; there will be many discussions with the architect concerning functionality versus "architectural integrity."

Remember that you are planning and designing not only for now but also for 5 years from now. Build in flexibility. Expect that revisions and changes will be necessary after the move. (We found it necessary to redesign the triage area one month after a move.) Glitches that you could not foresee will occur. For instance, radiant heat panels were installed in the ceiling over each bed in a trauma room so that staff would not have to work around portable heating units. What was not planned was that these heating units activate the air conditioning unit: the room actually became quite cold, despite the radiant heat panels.

Planning efforts directly correlate to the overall success of the new facility. Get involved early, stay involved, and do not hesitate to participate in the construction update meetings. Conduct frequent walk-throughs and speak up if something doesn't "feel right." This process can be an invaluable and enriching experience from which you reap the rewards of success for years to come.

SUGGESTED READINGS

ED Layout and Physical Design. In *Emergency department forms, checklists and guidelines,* Rockville, Md, 1987, Aspen.

Friend P, Shiver J: *Freestanding emergency centers: a guide to planning, organization, and management,* Rockville, Md, 1985, Aspen.

Guidelines to functional programming, equipping and designing hospital outpatient and emergency services, Pub No HRA 77-4002, US Department of Health and Human Resources (Bureau of Health Planning and Resources Development, Division of Facilities Development), Washington, DC.

Triage

Marilyn Rice and **Cynthia Abel**

Triage is the process that places the emergency patient in the right place at the right time to receive the right level of care. In many emergency departments (EDs) a nurse in the triage role has become the "gatekeeper" to medical care. The triage nurse is responsible for the efficient and effective allocation of ED resources.

HISTORICAL PERSPECTIVE

The word *triage* is derived from the French verb *trier*, which means "to pick or to sort."[14] Triage dates back to the French military, who used the word to designate a "clearing hospital" for the battlefield wounded. U.S. military triage first described a sorting station from which battlefield injured were distributed to hospitals. After World Wars I and II, triage became the process that identified the injured who were most likely to return to battle after medical intervention and concentrated medical resources on them. Further battlefield experience with the triage process in Korea and Vietnam was based on the principle of accomplishing the "greatest good for the greatest number of wounded and injured men."[17]

Disaster triage is similar to military triage in its goal to ensure the greatest good for the maximum number of injured. The primary difference is that disaster triage is field oriented and delays initial transport of some victims to prevent ED overloading.[15] Table 7-1 compares priority categories of military and disaster triage.

ED use of triage systems began in the early 1960s, when the demand for emergency services began to outpace available emergency resources. ED space, equipment, and personnel were not adequate to handle the explosive increase in the number of emergency visits.[14] The number of ED visits has more than tripled since 1958. The nation's hospitals reported 18 million ED visits in 1958.[14] By 1968 this figure had increased to 44 million. The American Hospital Association predicted 90 million visits for 1990.[2]

Based on recent trends, estimates are that between 50% and 85% of these 90 million visits are for nonurgent problems. Nonurgent reasons for use of the ED include speed of service, proximity, expediency, 24-hour availability, and cost.[7,13,15]

An estimated 38 million people in this country are either underinsured or uninsured. Many of these people seek their primary health care in the ED.[20]

Increases in ED use, shortages of nurses and intensive care unit beds, and backlogs of emergency admissions have contributed to ED overcrowding and prolonged waiting times. The triage process evolved as an effective method to separate those requiring immediate medical attention from those who can wait.

THE TRIAGE SYSTEM

The primary goals of an effective triage system are (1) to quickly identify those patients with urgent, life-threatening conditions; (2) to regulate the flow of patients through the ED; and (3) to avoid unnecessary congestion in emergency treatment areas.[14]

An efficient and effective triage system may also shorten the length of patients' stays and decrease patient waiting times by combining immediate assessment and intervention. Use of a triage system has been found to increase patient satisfaction with the ED and enhance public relations.[11] An effective triage system should also ensure efficient use of space and all resources.[14,15]

Other functions of the triage system should include reassessment of waiting patients, identification of health care learning needs, screening of individuals who require information, assignment of the appropriate care provider, and evaluation of the system.[14,15]

The extent to which a triage system may encompass all of these functions depends on (1) number of daily patient visits; (2) available staff; (3) presence or absence of walk-in or same-day clinics; (4) type and availability of health care providers; (5) availability of specialty treatment areas; and (6) environmental, legal, and administrative constraints.[14,15]

Triage systems vary widely among EDs. In 1982, Thompson and Dains identified the three most common systems and the differences among them. These systems are type I (traffic director), type II (spot check), and type III (comprehensive). The three systems differ in their urgency categories, staffing patterns, documentation requirements, pa-

Table 7-1   Comparison of military and disaster priority categories

Priority	Military	Disaster
1	**IMMEDIATE CARE** Shock, airway problems, chest injury, crushing injury, amputation, open facture	**CLASS I (EMERGENT)** Critical; life-threatening: compromised airway, shock, hemorrhage
2	**MINIMAL CARE** Little or no treatment needed	**CLASS II (URGENT)** Major illness or injury; requires treatment within 20 minutes to 2 hours: open fracture, chest wound
3	**DELAYED CARE** Treatment may be postponed without loss of life; noncritical: simple fracture, nonbleeding laceration	**CLASS III (NONURGENT)** Care may be delayed 2 hours or more; minor injuries; walking wounded: closed fracture, sprain, strain
4	**EXPECTANT CARE** No treatment until immediate and delayed priority patients have been cared for; requires considerable time, effort, and supplies	**CLASS IV (EXPECTANT)** Dead or expected to die: massive head injury, extensive full-thickness burns

Adapted from Thompson JD, Dains J: *Comprehensive triage: a manual for developing and implementing a nursing care system,* Reston, Va, 1982, Reston.

tient assessment and reassessment, and initiation of diagnostic procedures (Table 7-2).

Type III, or comprehensive, triage is the most advanced system. Assessment is performed by either a registered nurse or a physician and focuses on selected patient data. Urgency categories range from I to IV. Specific diagnostic procedures may be initiated, and patients are reassessed at designated intervals. Documentation is systematic and ongoing. Educational health needs and primary health needs are also addressed.[15] Type III urgency categories are shown in Table 7-3.

Table 7-2   Comparison of triage systems

Elements	Type I: traffic director	Type II: spot check	Type III: comprehensive
ASSESSMENT			
Personnel	Nonprofessional	Registered nurse or physician	Registered nurse
Data	Chief complaint	Chief complaint: limited subjective and objective	Through assessment: complete, subjective and objective; education needs; primary health needs
ANALYSIS			
Urgency category	2 categories: emergent; nonurgent	3 categories: emergent; urgent; delayed	4 categories: I-IV; larger data base
Nursing diagnoses	None	None	Present
PLAN			
Alternatives	Treatment room; waiting room	Treatment room; waiting area; treat and discharge from triage; inconsistent diagnostic procedures	Treatment room; waiting area with planned assessement; diagnostic procedure by protocol
Documentation	Little; inconsistent	Variable	Systematic
EVALUATION			
Client	None	None planned; at patient request	Planned; systematic
System	Difficult	Variable	Systematic

Adapted from Thompson JD, Dains J: *Comprehensive triage: a manual for developing and implementing a nursing care system,* Reston, Va, 1982, Reston.

Table 7-3   Comprehensive triage: four urgency categories

CLASS	I	II	III	IV
Descriptor	Immediate; life threatening	Stable; ASAP	Stable; no distress	Stable; no distress
Reassessment	Continuous	q15 min	q30 min	q60 min
Examples	Cardiac arrest, seizures, major trauma, respiratory distress, major burn	Open fracture, pain, minor burn, surgical abdomen, sickle cell, child, and fever	Closed fracture, laceration without bleeding, drug ingestion over 3 hr with no signs or symptoms	rash, constipation, impetigo, abrasion, nerves

Adapted from Thompson JD, Dains J: *Comprehensive triage: a manual for developing and implementing a nursing care system*, Reston, Va, 1982, Reston.

Urgency Categories

Urgency categories developed for the triage process refer to the system of rating patient acuity. Rating systems vary depending on patient census and available resources. Generally, rating systems have two or more categories for patient classification. Each category is delineated by predetermined criteria. Urgency rating is determined by the following elements: (1) degree to which the problem is lifethreatening, (2) risk of short-term complications, (3) salvageability, (4) clinical assessment of the patient, (5) availability of treatment, (6) algorithms, and (7) department protocols.[14]

Thompson and Dains' four urgency categories[15] for comprehensive triage are shown in Table 7-3. An expanded, five-category urgency rating system is illustrated in Table 7-4. A five-category system allows for better discrimination of the urgent and nonurgent patient and also allows for direct referral. The rating system used should accommodate the needs of the particular ED.[8]

Triage Staffing

Receptionists, ward clerks, nurse aids, emergency medical technicians, licensed practical nurses, registered nurses, physicians, and a variety of other personnel have all been used to perform triage. Recent legislation requires immediate medical screening before inquiries may be made about finances and ability to pay.[1,6] This medical screening must be performed by "qualified" individuals.[1,6] The Joint Commission on Accreditation of Healthcare Organizations requires that prioritization for medical treatment be performed by "specially trained personnel . . . using established guidelines."[9] Use of a specially trained registered nurse in the triage role for the purpose of medical screening and prioritization has proved efficient and cost effective.[21,22]

Nurses may be rotated through this position on a shift-by-shift or partial-shift basis. In some systems the designated triage nurse may not rotate to other treatment areas. However, most nurses find the triage position stressful and demanding as a full-time assignment.

Triage Nurse Qualifications

The hallmarks of the successful triage nurse are experience and skill in rapid patient assessment and correct determination of patient urgency. The ability to recognize who is "sick" and who is not is critical to success. This ability depends on experience, skill, and expert clinical judgment.

An effective triage nurse must have well-developed organizational skills and the ability to function in chaos. The triage nurse sets the pace for the department and is responsible for maintaining an efficient patient flow. Timing of patient disposition from the triage desk can have a significant impact on the department treatment areas and staff.

The triage position involves high visibility and great stress. Ringing telephones, waiting ambulance stretchers, walk-in patients, visitors with inquiries, and miscellaneous interruptions, as well as the need to assess and make rapid decisions, test the endurance of the most experienced emergency nurse.

Triage often takes place in the lobby in full view of patients and visitors. Whether answering the telephone, interviewing a patient, splinting an ankle, or choosing the next patient for an open treatment room, the triage nurse is under constant public scrutiny and pressure to perform well.

Table 7-4   Expanded urgency categories: five-category system

Urgency category	Acuity	Wait time	Examples
Class V	Life threatening	See immediately	Cardiac arrest, shock
Class IV	Urgent	May wait 30-60 min	Fractured hip, severe laceration, asthma, dyspnea
Class III	Semiurgent	May wait up to 2 hr	Cystitis, otitis
Class II	Nonurgent	Indefinite	Rash, cold signs and symptoms
Class I	Referred	Indefinite	Routine physical, minor bruises

Adapted from Hammond B, Lee G: *Quick reference to emergency nursing*, Philadelphia, 1984, JB Lippincott.

The triage nurse is usually the first person encountered by the emergency patient and family. This nurse represents the hospital and may set the tone for the patient's entire visit. Hospital surveys have shown that patient satisfaction with the department and care received can be affected by the triage nurse's actions and demeanor.[11]

The triage nurse must be comfortable with this public role, must be able to establish and maintain good public relations, even under stressful circumstances, and must be able to relate to a variety of patients, regardless of age, culture, or level of intelligence. It is essential that the triage nurse be able to demonstrate understanding, tact, patience, and discretion when dealing with emergency patients, visitors, family members, police, prehospital personnel, other hospital staff, and the media. The triage nurse may also be called on to enforce visiting regulations or perform "crowd control" in the waiting area.[12]

Triage Nurse Orientation

Criteria regarding readiness for the triage role vary with each individual nurse. The decision depends on the institution, the sophistication of the triage system in use, the individual nurse's competence in assessment, clinical judgment, and decision making, and the quality of the triage orientation process. Current legislation and legal implications that affect this role must be considered when designating new triage personnel. A risk-management approach for the ED identifies strategies for preventing litigation. Callahan[3] recommends that the triage nurse be an experienced emergency nurse. The triage position is considered a high-risk position because of the necessity for quick assessment and prioritization of urgent patient conditions.

A formal triage orientation program tends to enhance the effectiveness of personnel in this position.[15] A new triage nurse should complete a triage orientation that includes didactic material, standards and protocols for decision making, and an internship or preceptorship that provides time for work with an experienced and successful triage nurse.

Triage Environment and Space

The ED is often described as a window to the hospital. In communities where more than one hospital ED exists, there is usually competition to capture a greater share of the emergency patient market. An aesthetically pleasing physical environment, in addition to excellent service, may draw more of the market share.[5,18]

Because the triage area is generally the first area a patient views, it can make a lasting positive or negative impression. Consideration should be given to comfort, privacy, and a pleasing atmosphere. Demographic information about the population that is served may be helpful. For example, a large geriatric population, as compared with a large pediatric population, may require structural differences in interview space and waiting room facilities for patients and visitors.[5]

A number of other features are helpful to the efficient operation of the triage area. The area should be designed to promote easy access and observation of patients yet provide privacy for interviews and assessment. Traffic flow should not impede the triage process, but the triage nurse should have easy access to the arriving patient. Entrances and doors should easily accommodate stretchers and wheelchairs. Separate ambulatory and ambulance triage areas and entrances may be necessary. Sinks and other equipment needed to support the use of universal precautions are critically important. Space is needed for supplies, first aid materials, stretchers, and wheelchairs. Space for a computer, radios, or poison control equipment may be necessary.

Equipment for communication is a necessity at the triage desk. Receiving information about incoming patients and communicating with other areas of the ED or with referral services are essential. The telephone, however, has been identified as one of the greatest nurse stressors at the triage desk. All possible effort should be made to route calls about patient location, directions, and advice or information to a separate area. The triage telephone number should not be the main ED number listed in the telephone directory or advertisements. Clerical support for telephone calls can be a helpful addition for staff. Clerks can answer simple questions about the location of and directions to the ED, and route medical and advice calls to the appropriate personnel.

Provision for security in the triage area is critical. Recent events in ED have highlighted the vulnerability of the department and the triage position in particular. Security may be maintained by communication, the physical presence of an armed guard or law enforcement officer, or controlled-access doors.

The waiting area should have ample seating for patients and visitors to help prevent overflow into the working triage area and to promote patient comfort. Restrooms that are nearby and accessible to individuals with handicaps are essential. Pay telephones and vending machines for visitors may also be helpful. A separate waiting area for pediatric patients may be beneficial, if the department has a high volume of pediatric visits.

THE TRIAGE PROCESS

An effective triage system provides quality health care for patients waiting for medical treatment, as well as for those already in the treatment areas. The triage nurse is expected to ensure prompt evaluation of all patients entering the department within 2 to 5 minutes of their arrival. An interview in progress may be interrupted to assess a newly arriving client with an urgent problem. All senses must be used to gather data for analysis and decision making. Analysis of thorough assessment data enhances the triage decision-making process regarding (1) patient acuity, (2) patient priority, (3) appropriate health care provider, (4) appropriate treatment area, (5) initiation of interventions, (6) initiation of diagnostic procedures, and (7) selection of referral services.

IDEAL TRIAGE INTERVIEW

1. Chief complaint
2. History of current complaint
3. Name, age, gender, and mode of arrival
4. Allergies
5. Medications and past medical history
6. Date of last menstrual period for women of childbearing years, including gravida, para, and abortion history
7. Last tetanus immunization
8. Assessment data, including vital signs and weight

The triage process begins when the patient enters the ED. The patient may be ambulatory or on a stretcher. Triage personnel may be called on to assist arriving patients from vehicles on the receiving dock. Emergency equipment such as an Ambu-bag should be readily available for unexpected emergencies. After the patient has entered the department, the triage nurse should introduce herself or himself and begin the interview and assessment. Assessment may be as brief as a quick look at the patient on the stretcher and a terse prehospital report given while the triage nurse directs the crew to the appropriate resuscitation area. The ideal triage interview should provide the information in the box above.

Documentation at triage should include all information elicited and (1) nursing interventions, (2) diagnostic procedures, (3) disposition to appropriate treatment area, (4) reassessment while waiting for treatment, and (5) urgency rating.

The triage nurse may place an identification bracelet on the patient before moving the patient to the treatment area or initiating diagnostic procedures. In addition, color coding by bracelet[15] or colored dots on the patient record may be used to identify urgency category or referral service.

Other triage nurse responsibilities include (1) evaluation of the need for additional wheelchairs or stretchers for incoming patients, (2) initiation of the emergency record by handwriting or computer generation, (3) initiation of diagnostic tests or nursing interventions when appropriate, (4) direction of patients to the treatment area, (5) provision of a nursing report to the treatment area nurse and physician, and (6) communication with the physician and charge nurse about patient conditions and expected arrivals.

The Nursing Process in Triage

The nursing process is an organized manner of determining the patient's health status, identifying problems, planning solutions, initiating and implementing a plan, and evaluating the effectiveness of the plan. The steps of the nursing process are assessment, nursing diagnosis, planning, implementation, and evaluation.

Assessment. Assessment is the collection of objective and subjective data. The triage interview and assessment must be completed in 2 to 5 minutes; triage assessment is not the same as the complete head-to-toe or in-depth assessment performed by the treatment nurse. Triage assessment provides enough information to determine patient acuity and any immediate physiologic, psychosocial, or educational needs. Triage assessment can also provide the data base for initial treatment or diagnostic tests.

Nursing diagnosis. As stated, assessment data are used to determine immediate physiologic, psychosocial, or educational needs. Nursing diagnoses may be identified and patient acuity or urgency categorized based on predetermined criteria. Urgency categories depend on the type of triage system used.

Planning. The triage nurse may be responsible for planning nursing interventions and medical or diagnostic procedures, based on protocols, that can be initiated in the triage area. Examples include splinting, applying ice, or ordering radiographic examinations of extremities.

Implementation. The triage nurse is responsible for assigning patients to an appropriate treatment area and health care provider. The triage nurse may also be responsible for ordering preliminary treatments and diagnostic procedures based on established protocol or physician's order.

Evaluation. Patients should be reassessed based on predetermined criteria for each urgency category. Each waiting patient should be reassessed at least every 60 minutes. Patients with conditions categorized as emergency or urgent conditions may be reassessed as often as every 15 minutes. Recategorization, or retriage, should be performed whenever new information arrives or a change in patient status occurs. Patient follow-up by the triage nurse is an excellent evaluation tool that is used to confirm or refute clinical impressions and decisions.

The Triage Interview

The triage interview is the basis for clinical judgments and decisions made regarding the emergency patient's acuity and need for intervention. The triage interview generally begins with the patient's chief complaint and should include both subjective and objective information. Although the interview usually focuses on the chief complaint, the nurse must elicit associated complaints and significant past medical history that may affect the patient's health or the current complaint.

The triage nurse must be skilled in asking the right questions or pursuing small details to elicit information necessary for determining urgency and the appropriate treatment area. Guidelines, protocols, decision trees, and algorithms may all aid in this process. Algorithms are particularly helpful to the novice triage nurse who needs a guide to the interview and triage process.[15,19]

The interview process is a communication process that includes the giving and receiving of information, both verbally and nonverbally. Language barriers, cultural differences, age, developmental levels, and health status may be barriers to the interview process. Children and parents must be interviewed differently than older patients. For example, the nurse may need to play with the child to gain his or her confidence. Older adults may have hearing losses and may process questions more slowly. A patient with acute pain or anxiety will not tolerate a lengthy interview. Questions should be short and to the point and should be asked in a caring manner. The most time-consuming aspects of the triage process are often relieving patient and family anxiety, establishing rapport, and conveying general concern.

Questioning is a valuable interview technique. Open-ended questions help elicit feelings and perceptions along with information. Closed questions (with yes or no answers) are useful for obtaining facts. Both types of questions are useful, and the triage nurse must balance the number of open-ended or closed questions.

In general, initial questions should be open-ended, whereas closed questions can be used to validate information. Other techniques useful in the interview process include (1) reflecting or restating what the client has said, (2) using silence, (3) displaying acceptance, (4) showing recognition, (5) using broad openings, (6) providing general leads, (7) verbalizing observations, (8) giving information, (9) seeking information, and (10) summarizing. The active triage nurse develops interview techniques that suit his or her communication style, the clientele, and the environment.

Physical assessment accompanies the triage interview. Assessment may begin with the observation that the patient can speak and therefore has a patent airway. Physical assessment must be rapid, concise, and focused. Gathered data should include such objective measures as vital signs, Glasgow coma score, trauma score, or burn percentage if appropriate.

Effective triage requires the use of the senses, sight, hearing, smell, and touch. The patient provides nonverbal clues: facial grimaces, cyanosis, or fear. Listen to what the patient is saying, as well as to what he or she will not say. Listen for a cough, hoarseness, or shortness of breath. Touch the patient: assess heart rate and skin temperature and moisture. Notice odors such as the smell of ketones, alcohol, or infection.

Thorough evaluation of a symptom can be accomplished by using the *PQRST* mnemonic, which is shown in the box below, left.

Remember that the purpose of the triage interview is to gather enough information to make a clinical judgment for disposition, not medical diagnosis.

Attitude and empathy are important aspects of the triage nurse's demeanor. Remaining consistent and nonjudgmental toward all patients is important. Difficult patients such as those who are intoxicated or combative require special care. Try not to prejudge patients based on appearance or attitude.

Triage Documentation

The triage process is not complete until the patient encounter is documented. Triage documentation may be done on the ED record, on a separate form, or as part of the nurses' notes. It is probably best to initiate a clearly separate triage note. The Joint Commission on Accreditation of Healthcare Organizations requires documentation of any patient reassessment performed during extended waiting times that precede medical evaluation. It is helpful to document

---

PQRST MNEMONIC

P (*p*rovokes)
   What provokes the symptom?
Q (*quality*)
   What makes it (the symptom) better? What makes it worse?
Q (*quality*)
   What does it (the symptom) feel like?
R (*r*adiation)
   Where is it (the symptom)? Where does it go? Is it in one spot or more than one spot?
S (*severity*)
   If we gave it (the symptom) a number from 1 to 10, with 1 being the least and 10 being the worst you can imagine, what number would you give this?
T (*t*ime)
   How long have you had this symptom? When did it start? When did it end? How long did it last?

SOAPIE MNEMONIC

S (*subjective data*)
These are the patient's complaints or the reason given for seeking emergency care. This correlates with "chief complaint."
O (*objective data*)
These are the things that the nurse can see, hear, feel, and smell. These are observable, measurable data.
A (*analysis of data*)
Nursing diagnoses and urgency categorization are evidence of data analysis.
P (*plan*)
The triage nurse decides which treatment or diagnostic procedures may be implemented based on protocol or by seeking a physician's order.
I (*implementation*)
The triage nurse may implement treatment or diagnostic procedures based on established protocol.
E (*evaluation*)
Evaluation may include patient reassessment and patient follow-up to determine accuracy of clinical decision-making for acuity and patient categorization.

Triage	Date:	Time:	Arrival mode:	□Walk □W/C □Carried □Ambulances: □PVt. □H.F.D. □Other Unit #								
Chief complaint:				Current medications:								
History of present illness:												
				Private medical doctor:								
Past medical history				Notified: □Yes □ No □ Attempted —Time:								
				E.C. to treat: □ Yes □ No								
Allergies:				**VS** Time	T.	P.	R.	B.P.		Triage		
LMP:	GRAV:	PARA:	AB:							1	2	3 4
Tetanus status:		Weight:								1	2	3 4
Triage nurse signature:				Time to treatment area:			Bed #:					

Fig. 7-1 Example of SOAPIE triage note.

the reason for extended waiting times along with the appropriate reassessment information.

SOAPIE, as shown in the box on p. 72, is the mnemonic for a problem-oriented method of assessment and documentation that is adaptable to triage because patient situations in the ED are problem oriented.[40]

Fig. 7-1 shows an ED record designed to permit use of the SOAPIE format for triage documentation.

SPECIAL TRIAGE CONSIDERATIONS
Multiple Patients

Emergency patients rarely arrive one at a time, or so it seems. The triage nurse must be prepared to evaluate several patients simultaneously. Generally, alert observation of new arrivals and a few carefully chosen questions can be used to screen new arrivals. The nurse may have to interrupt one interview to assess a new patient who has a condition of greater urgency. It may be necessary to "walk the line," or speak briefly with several new arrivals, to determine whether immediate attention is needed. If several acutely ill patients arrive simultaneously, a backup system may be activated, in which nurses from the various treatment areas come to assist until the situation is under control.

Telephone Triage

Management of telephone triage, or advice calls, is a controversial topic. Formal policy and procedures for handling these calls are difficult to find. Most of the literature advises two things: do not give advice, and leave the decision to come to the ED up to the caller. Giving advice or suggesting alternatives for action is difficult without the physical presence of the caller. Callers may be vague and inarticulate when they describe the problem or give a history over the telephone.

Giving generic advice such as suggestions to "call 911" or "come to the ED" may be appropriate but inadequate.

At times, advice about interim measures might make a difference in outcome. For example, cardiopulmonary resuscitation instructions or childbirth instructions may be needed before emergency medical services arrive.

Formal policy and procedure with protocols for specific situations may be a proactive method of handling this dif-

---

TRIAGE "PEARLS"

1. Always validate what you think you heard. Patients sometimes tell you what they think you want to hear.
2. What is visible is usually not the whole story. Patients must be questioned thoroughly; attention must be given to verbal and nonverbal cues.
3. Do not assume that the accident caused the present problem. The opposite is possible.
4. Most psychoneurotic patients ultimately die from organic disease. Even "repeaters" require careful assessment and evaluation.
5. When a patient says he or she has an emergency, the burden of proof is not the patient's.[16] Look for the worst possible cause of his or her symptoms, and plan to intervene.
6. When a woman of childbearing age says there is no possibility of pregnancy, believe her, and perform a pregnancy test anyway.
7. If a patient looks "sick," he or she probably is. Do not assume, just because a patient does not look "sick," that he or she is not sick.
8. Cues to the triage nurse to assign a high-priority category include (1) severe pain, (2) active bleeding, (3) stupor or drowsiness, (4) disorientation, (5) emotional disturbances, (6) dyspnea at rest, (7) cyanosis, (8) extreme diaphoresis, and (9) measurements of vital signs that are outside the normal limits.[19]

CASE STUDY 7-1

Fracture

An 80-year-old woman arrives via basic life support ambulance.

Subjective assessment

The emergency medical technician states that "she fell and broke her hip." Your patient says, "My hip hurts." She denies having syncope, palpitations, chest pain, or dizziness before the fall.

Objective assessment

You note that she is conscious and has a patent airway and no overt bleeding. The left leg is shortened and rotated outward with an external splint that was applied in the field. Pedal pulse rates are present bilaterally, and readings of vital signs are within normal limits. Pain is evidenced by her grimace and muscle tightness when the stretcher is moved.

Analysis

Categorize condition as class II because of age, pain, and large bone fracture.

Plan

If cardiac problems are suspected, transport the patient to medical department for cardiac monitoring. If pulse rates are absent or diminished, transport the patient to the surgery department for evaluation. If the patient's condition is stable, arrange for a radiographic examination of the extremity according to protocol.

Implementation

Implement treatment or diagnostic procedures based on established department protocol and triage plan.

Evaluation

Reassess patient every 15 to 30 minutes if she cannot be placed in the treatment area immediately. Follow up on the patient in the treatment area to determine accuracy of triage decisions.

CASE STUDY 7-2

Fall During Grand Mal Seizure

A 23-year-old woman is brought to the ED via advanced life support ambulance.

Subjective assessment

Paramedics state that she fell during a grand mal seizure, which they witnessed.

Objective assessment

The patient is unresponsive but restless and is breathing on her own. She has a large, heavily bleeding occipital laceration, to which pressure is being applied by one of the paramedics.

Analysis

Categorize condition as class I for maintenance of airway and control of bleeding.

Plan

Arrange for immediate evaluation and control of bleeding. Transport the patient to the resuscitation area for observation of the airway and potential seizure activity. This patient may also require an evaluation of cervical spine integrity.

Implementation

Maintain the airway and control bleeding en route to the treatment area.

Evaluation

Monitor patient changes en route to the treatment area. Follow-up for evaluation of triage decisions.

---

ficult situation. Policy and procedure set a standard, and protocols could be used to guide the interviewer.[10]

If telephone advice is given, calls should be logged with the caller's name, location, callback number, concern, and advice given. It is important to realize that callers may be noncompliant. Documentation, although time consuming, may protect the nurse and institution from liability.

A suicide call or any crisis call requires special attention. Nurses should be trained in crisis intervention techniques before handling such calls. Generally the caller should be kept on the line as long as possible, while authorities attempt to trace the call. The nurse should obtain as much information as possible from the caller and assume that the caller's judgment is impaired.[12]

TRIAGE EVALUATION

Evaluation of the triage process includes three elements, structure, process, and outcome. Structural evaluation includes such things as space, equipment, physical layout, policy, procedure, protocols, staffing, staff qualifications, and urgency categories.

Process evaluation reviews the steps involved in the triage process. Items that may be evaluated include triage time, waiting times, traffic patterns, patient flow, accuracy and completeness of documentation, and adherence to written procedure, policies, and protocols.

Outcome evaluation may review patient assessment, accuracy of triage decisions, referrals, and patient satisfaction.

The Emergency Nurses Association has published the *Standards for Emergency Nursing Practice*. Comprehensive practice standard I addresses comprehensive triage and includes both competence and excellence as outcome criteria. These criteria could be used as a tool for evaluation of triage.[4] The box on p. 73 offers some triage "pearls."

CASE STUDY 7-3

Abdominal Pain

A 19-year-old man with a chief complaint of abdominal pain is brought by a friend to the ED.

Subjective assessment

The patient complains of acute abdominal pain, which began as generalized pain "last night" and is now located in the right lower quadrant. He states that he has vomited, is nauseated, and feels "warm."

Objective assessment

You observe a young man who is doubled over and holding his abdomen. He walks up to the triage desk carefully and you see a grimace of pain on his face. Vital signs include blood pressure of 120/70, heart rate of 120 beats/min, respiration rate of 28 breaths/min, and a temperature reading of 102° F. The patient's skin is pale and warm.

Analysis

Categorize the condition as class II because of pain and potential for emergency abdominal surgery.

Plan

Transport the patient to the surgical area because he has had the pain for less than 48 hours.

Implementation

Move the patient to the treatment area as soon as space is available. Initiate diagnostic tests for abdominal pain as dictated by department protocol. Alert the emergency physician to the patient's presence and complaints.

Evaluation

Monitor this patient for changes in pain or vital signs at least every 15 minutes, until treatment space is available. Follow-up to evaluate triage decisions.

CASE STUDY 7-4

Multiple Simultaneous Admissions

Four patients arrive at the ED at the same time.

Subjective and objective assessment

PATIENT 1
S/O = 60-year-old construction worker with complaints of acute lower back pain; the patient is bent over, holding his back, unable to straighten.

PATIENT 2
S/O = 16-year-old boy complains of ankle pain. He arrives with the aid of friends, hopping on one foot. His ankle is swollen and discolored. He has intact neurovascular status.

PATIENT 3
S/O = 27-year-old male jogger arrives in respiratory arrest via advanced life support vehicle. Paramedics are ventilating the patient via endotracheal tube. The monitor shows sinus tachycardia with palpable pulse rates and a heart rate of 144 beats/min. The neck veins are distended.

PATIENT 4
S/O = A 76-year-old woman complains of vomiting blood. She says she fainted. She is pale and has the following vital signs: blood pressure is 80/palp, heart rate is 130 beats/min, and respiration rate is 24 breaths/min.

Assessment

PATIENT 3
Class I: Immediate, life-threatening condition.

PATIENT 4
Class II: Urgent condition; may become life threatening. You must assume that she is bleeding.

PATIENT 1
Class II: Stable condition but in a great deal of pain.

PATIENT 2
Class III: Stable condition with no neurovascular deficits.

Plan

PATIENT 3
Transport the patient to the resuscitation area immediately. Notify the treatment team.

PATIENT 4
Transport the patient to the treatment area for immediate medical evaluation and monitoring.

PATIENT 1
Transport the patient to the treatment area for evaluation of back pain, as soon as space is available. Implement diagnostic procedures from triage area according to protocol.

PATIENT 2
Nursing interventions include application of ice, elevation of ankle, splint, and radiographic x-ray examination per protocol. Assign the patient to the treatment area as space permits.

Implementation

Move the patients as planned. Initiate diagnostic and nursing measures as allowed by department protocol.

Evaluation

Reassess patients 1 and 2 until they are moved to the treatment area. Follow up to evaluate triage decisions for all patients.

SUMMARY

The basic responsibility of any ED is to provide quality care and optimal patient outcomes. The triage nurse is the first point of contact between the patient and the ED. This contact may be a primary determinant in the final outcome. Currently a wide variety of triage systems exists. Although systems vary, the common element in successful triage systems is a skilled, efficient triage nurse.

REFERENCES

1. American College of Emergency Physicians: New patient transfer laws take effect: experts question impact, *ACEP News* 9:6, 1990.
2. American Hospital Association: Ambulatory care growth continues upward trend, *Outreach* 11:1, 1990.
3. Callahan F: Emergency department nursing risk management, *J Ambulatory Care Management* 12(2):31, 1989.
4. Emergency Nurses Association: *Standards of emergency nursing practice,* ed 2, St Louis, 1990, Mosby–Year Book.
5. Frank IC: *Managing emergency nursing services,* Rockville, Md, 1989, Aspen.
6. Function and transfer of patients with emergency medical conditions affected by revisions made by OBRA '89. In *Health law outlook,* Spring 1990, Wood, Lucksinger, and Epstein.
7. Habenstreit B: Health care patterns of non-urgent patients in an inner city emergency room, *New York State J Med* 10:517, 1986.
8. Hammond BB, Lee G: *Quick reference to emergency nursing,* Philadelphia, 1984, JB Lippincott.
9. Joint Commission on Accreditation of Healthcare Organizations: *Accreditation manual for hospitals: emergency services,* Chicago, 1989, JCAHO.
10. Lyle NA, Clingerman E: *Comprehensive triage: personalized system of instruction.* Unpublished manual.
11. McMillan JR et al: Satisfaction with hospital emergency department as a function of patient triage, *Health Care Manage Rev* 3:21, 1986.
12. Nelson D: The emergency department nurse: changing role? In Findeiss JC: *Emergency medical care,* New York, 1974, Intercontinental Medical Book.
13. Powers MJ, Reichelt PA, Jalowiec A: Use of emergency department by patients with non-urgent conditions, *JEN* 9(3):145, 1983.
14. Rund DA, Rausch TS: *Triage,* St Louis, 1981, Mosby–Year Book.
15. Thompson J, Dains J: *Comprehensive triage: a manual for developing and implementing a nursing care system,* Reston, Va, 1982, Reston.
16. Turner SR: Golden rules for accurate triage, *JEN* 7(4):153, 1981.
17. United States Department of Defense: *Emergency war surgery,* Washington, DC, 1975, US Government Printing Office.
18. van de Lew JH: *Managing emergency nursing services,* Rockville, Md, 1987, Aspen.
19. Vickery DM: *Triage: problem oriented sorting of patients,* Bowie, Md, 1975, Robert J Brady.
20. White SK: President's message. Access to care: the issue of the 90s, *Heart Lung* 19:1, 1990.
21. Willis D: A study of nursing triage, *JEN* 5:8, 1979.
22. Zwicke DL, Bobzient WF, Wagner EH: Triage decisions: a prospective study, *JEN* 8(3):132, 1982.

SUGGESTED READINGS

American College of Emergency Physicians: Emergency care guidelines (revised), *Ann Emerg Med* 15(4):486, 1986.

Broome ME: Telephone protocols for pediatric assessment and advice, *JEN* 12(3):142, 1986.

Emergency Nurses Association: *Emergency nursing core curriculum,* ed 3, Philadelphia, 1987, WB Saunders.

Emergency Nurses Association: *Emergency nursing scope of practice,* Chicago, 1988, ENA Board of Directors.

Estrada EG: Triage systems. In *Nurs Clin North Am: symposium on emergency nursing* 16(1):13, 1981.

Parker JG: Triage: concept and format. In Parker, JG, ed: *Emergency nursing: a guide to comprehensive care,* New York, 1984, John Wiley & Sons.

Ramler C: Triage. In Kitt S, Kaiser J: Emergency nursing: a physiologic and clinical perspective, Philadelphia, 1990, WB Saunders.

Rozovsky LE, Rozovsky FA: Triage and the law, *Can Crit Care Nurs J* 6(3):16, 1989.

Southard PA: COBRA legislation: complying with ED provisions, *JEN* 15(1):23, 1989.

Wheeler SQ: ED telephone triage: lessons learned from unusual calls, *JEN* 15(6):481, 1989.

Wilson MT: Setting up an effective ED triage system, *Nursing* 18(12):55, 1988.

Joe E. Taylor and Janet Taylor

The purpose of this chapter is to acquaint the reader with the concept of nursing diagnosis by providing a brief history, exploring definitions of the term, and presenting related issues and trends. Recommendations concerning how to implement nursing diagnoses are explored, along with methods of validation and research involving diagnosis in the emergency department (ED). Finally, two brief case examples illustrate the use of nursing diagnosis in the ED.

HISTORICAL EVOLUTION

Gordon[17] states that the term *nursing diagnosis* was first discussed in the year 1950. The nursing diagnosis focused on patient problems or conditions, sometimes expressed concretely as lists of strengths and liabilities. Gordon thinks that a list of diagnostic categories could have been synthesized even at that time. Carpenito,[10] however, states that nursing diagnosis was introduced in 1953 and was used to describe the steps necessary in the development of a nursing care plan. This plan included a section resembling a nursing diagnosis. Experts in the area of nursing diagnosis disagree even about the origin of the term.

In the 1960s, some theorists made proposals to move nursing education away from the traditional foundation of medical diagnosis. They suggested that nursing education should be based on nursing problems or patient needs.[10] Henderson's nursing problems[21] included the areas of breathing, eating and drinking, elimination, movement and posture, sleep and rest, clothing, body temperature, cleaning and grooming, avoidance of environmental danger and injury, communication, worship, work, play and recreation, and learning and discovery. Abdellah[1] thought that although the goals of nursing and medicine were similar, the central goals and functions of nursing required specific nursing knowledge. At this point, nursing theory started to separate from medicine and focus on patient problems that nurses could treat.

In 1967 Yura and Walsh published the first edition of *The Nursing Process,* which included the phases of assessment, planning, implementing, and evaluation. The four phases of the process formed a conceptual framework for

the explanation of what nurses did in practice. After 1973, when the American Nurses' Association (ANA) published their *Standards of Nursing Practice,* Yura and Walsh[33] added nursing diagnosis as an integral part of the nursing process in their third edition. The ANA formally brought nursing diagnosis into nursing practice by stating that "nursing diagnoses are derived from health status data" and that "the plan of nursing care includes goals derived from the nursing diagnoses."[2]

The ANA *Standards* formed the foundation of the National Conferences on the Classification of Nursing Diagnoses. The goal was to "initiate the process of preparing an organized, logical, comprehensive system for classifying those health problems or health states diagnosed by nurses and treated by means of nursing interventions."[7] The seven conferences since 1973 have resulted in the following:

1. Development and revision of specific diagnoses with etiologies and defining characteristics
2. Formation of regional and state conference groups that provide for continuous work on diagnostic labeling
3. Establishment of a speaker's bureau and a list of diagnostic experts
4. Publication of conference proceedings

The later conferences emphasized refinement and review of approved diagnoses, use of nursing diagnoses in clinical practice, education and research, and examination of proposed theoretic frameworks for the nursing diagnosis as a part of the nursing process.

The seventh conference in 1986 focused on (1) classification systems; (2) issues related to the development of a taxonomy; (3) diagnostic review criteria to critique proposed diagnoses; (4) examination of studies related to the development, validation, and refinement of nursing diagnoses; (5) exploration of issues related to etiology, research methods, and computerization; and (6) formation of a stronger network of nurses interested in nursing diagnosis. A major consideration for the seventh conference was a proposed conceptual framework for a nursing diagnosis taxonomy.[29] The concept of nursing diagnosis is becoming more refined and validated with each conference.

DEFINITIONS

Since its first mention as a concept, many definitions have been formulated to describe nursing diagnosis. Gordon[16] provided the most widely accepted definition: "Nursing diagnosis, or clinical diagnosis made by professional nurses, describe actual or potential health problems which nurses, by virtue of their education and experience, are capable and licensed to treat."

Guzzetta and Dossey[19] stated that "the purpose of nursing diagnosis is to identify human responses to stressors or other factors that adversely affect attainment of optimal health. Treatment is directed toward causes of the response or factors influencing it. A nursing diagnosis excludes . . . health problems that are treated with prescribed drugs, surgery, radiation, or other modalities legally defined by the practice of medicine."

Bircher[7] described the nursing diagnosis as a "tool which helps to identify a basic difficulty, as a means to judge the worth of importance of a concern, and as a process of measurement which is used to assess the presence, absence, or quality of certain objects, characteristics, functions or events."

Each of these definitions reflects what the individual author thinks nursing diagnosis is, but essentially each definition has the same or a related meaning.

RELATED ISSUES

After the initial introduction of the concept of nursing diagnosis, some authors identified possible flaws in the process. Aspinall[4] pointed out that many gaps in the nursing diagnosis literature led to confusion and lack of a firm knowledge base. She also was concerned that only 25% of nurses surveyed in a small exploratory study labeled patients as having anything other than physiologic problems. Aspinall also implied that nurses might not be educated enough or have enough experience to make sound nursing diagnoses. Finally, she stated that most of the nurses in the study lacked both the theoretic knowledge and the strategy that would enable them to make pertinent nursing diagnoses.

Hagey and McDonough[20] suggested that the term *diagnosis* conveys the erroneous message that nurses are primarily concerned with deviate or pathologic problems instead of with promoting health and the client's potential, which might conflict with the medical diagnosis. They also thought that nursing diagnoses may simplify and even obliterate the client's experience or the importance of the client in a nurse's care. For example, the authors were concerned that nurses might associate the client with the diagnosis instead of with the client's holistic nature.

Other authors, such as Bircher,[7] weighed the negative points associated with nursing diagnosis against positive aspects. Negative factors included lack of agreement about nursing diagnosis between clinicians, lack of appropriate labeling, lack of uniformity, vagueness of definitions, misuse of diagnosis, premature labeling, and stereotyping of clients. On the positive side, Bircher stated that the nursing diagnosis is a convenient shorthand system, a guide for the nurse to plan, easily remembered, and a ready point of reference for the clinician in daily interaction with the patient and family. Overall, Bircher's pros outweighed the cons.

Some confusion probably still surrounds the difference between medical and nursing diagnoses. Bockrath[8] differentiated between the two by stating that unlike the medical diagnosis, the nursing diagnosis does not focus on a disease process but rather on a physical response to the problem. Unlike medical diagnoses, most nursing diagnoses change continually as the patient progresses through various stages of illness to health. Also, unlike the medical diagnosis, the nursing diagnosis might identify potential health problems. Bockrath argued that the nursing diagnosis documents what nursing is and does and distinguishes nursing from any other profession.

Lash[26] also advocated the process by stating that the nursing diagnosis is a route to accountability. Nurses have long been concerned about accountability, and recording nursing diagnoses should overcome the anonymity that has been a major obstacle to accountability. Lash also wrote that nursing started as a basically dependent profession, but eventually autonomy and independent decision making became major issues. She thought that the nursing diagnosis facilitates autonomy and independent decision making by providing deliberate analysis of functions, developing knowledge unique to nursing practice, and changing the nursing educational system to perpetuate autonomy.

Another issue affecting nursing diagnosis is the legal implications of making diagnoses. Fortin and Rabinow[14] cited two legal problems that could arise from the process. The first is the failure to diagnose. The case cited involved a nurse who failed to recognize cancerous skin changes in a postinjury patient. The court ruled that the nurse should have been able to recognize and diagnose such a problem. The second major legal problem is misdiagnosis. The case cited involved nurses who diagnosed a young patient as merely being feverish. The child later died of congestive heart failure following an attack of rheumatic fever. The court ruled that the nurses should have identified the symptoms and signs correctly. Both rulings found in favor of the plaintiff. The authors' summary stated that "nurses do not diagnose because the law demands it; they diagnose because their professional responsibilities cannot be met by doing anything less."[14]

Bruce and Snyder[9] stated that nurses have the legal right and responsibility to diagnose. They wrote that the process of nursing diagnosis has become a standard, especially with the legitimate position of nursing diagnosis in the ANA standards. Therefore the process is part of the care duties the nurse owes the patient. Failure to diagnose adequately and intervene appropriately constitutes a breach of duty of care. The authors listed some diagnostic errors as (1) *premature closure,* in which the diagnosis is based on inadequate data; (2) *lack of closure,* in which adequate data are collected but diagnosis is not made; and (3) *invalid data clustering,* in which diagnostic errors occur because of the assumed relationship of unrelated data. Bruce and Snyder's thoughts on legal issues of nursing diagnosis are similar to those of Fortin and Rabinow.[14] From any viewpoint, nursing diagnosis is supported legally and has become a standard within the nursing process.

IMPLEMENTATION

After nursing diagnoses had been developed and refined, the problem of implementation was addressed. Field[13] introduced an implementation plan using the theory of change. The plan involves two or three change agents with the goal of implementing the nursing diagnosis. The application of the principles of change consists of four steps or phases: (1) assessing preimplementation status, (2) planning for implementation, (3) coping productively with resistance, and (4) developing an ongoing support system. Implementation includes educational activities that attempt to create change in the affective, cognitive, and psychomotor domains. Nursing diagnoses are also incorporated into the implementation process. Field stated that the "use of the taxonomy can both enhance and expedite professional communication. It helps to elucidate the focus of nursing's concern much more readily.[13]

Kieffer[22] recommended implementing nursing diagnosis by having nurses on the unit use a four-step method. Step one is to gather information by observing general problems in day-to-day patient interactions. Step two is to label the problems by using the approved wording when possible. Step three is to "make sure you're right" by asking the patient whether the diagnosis is accurate. Finally, step four is to "clarify your role" by making sure the problem is treatable by the nurse. Although the steps are well conceived, the author mentioned no results.

Two research studies have implications for the implementation of nursing diagnoses. The first, by Meade and Kim,[27] described the effect of teaching on documentation of nursing diagnosis. A group of 16 nurses were given a case study and asked to document nursing diagnoses for that case. Then they received a 5-hour instruction on diagnosis. After this, they were given another case for documentation of nursing diagnoses. A significant difference was found between preteaching and postteaching documentation of nursing diagnosis. From these data it appears that formal instruction on nursing diagnosis might facilitate its implementation.

In the other research study, Carstens[11] examined the effects of an in-service program on nurses' abilities to identify valid nursing diagnoses. Her sample included 24 nurses divided into experimental and control groups. The 12 nurses in the experimental group were given 5 hours of in-service classes using case studies to identify valid diagnoses. The control group was not given any instructions. One week after the in-service program, both groups were tested on their ability to identify valid diagnoses. Results indicated that the classes did not have any statistically significant effect on the ability to identify valid nursing diagnoses. However, the experimental group scored consistently higher than the control group. This supports that in-service programs have an impact on the implementation of nursing diagnoses.

The literature sparsely mentions problems encountered after implementation of nursing diagnosis. In one study, nursing diagnoses were implemented systematically in the emergency department of a 200-bed urban community hospital.[12] Three major concerns emerged. The first involved the appropriateness and usefulness of the taxonomy. For example, "laceration" was considered more concise than "alteration in skin integrity." The second concern was the legality of nursing diagnoses and how they legally affected the treatment given. The third concern involved physician acceptance of nursing diagnoses. This was handled carefully by formal orientation of the physicians to the process. Although some skepticism existed, no real problems occurred. Overall, the implementation was effective, and the value of nursing diagnosis had been proved.

Toth and others[32] also implemented nursing diagnosis in an emergency setting, in this case a shock trauma center. The results indicated that the nurses believed the nursing diagnosis more clearly identified the trauma patient's needs and delineated more specifically what a nurse can treat independently. Another advantage cited was that the nursing diagnosis provided documentation of the steps the nurse had taken to prevent complications formerly unnoticed.

The next logical step in the progression of nursing diagnosis implementation is the incorporation of nursing diagnosis into current computerized record keeping systems.[17] In one study a 541-bed research hospital implemented nursing diagnosis into its existing medical information system (MIS) computer.[31] Before implementation the nurses charted manually using the problem-oriented charting method known as the SOAP method (see box on p. 111) on card flip-files. In this computer system, nursing assessments were broken down into 30 major needs categories, then further subdivided. Those subdivisions were related to the nursing diagnoses and formed a system of charting totally on the computer using the nursing process. As a result of this project, the nursing staff shifted from a medical focus to a nursing perspective. The system served as a form of programmed instruction to make the nursing process more visible.

VALIDATION

Even though five distinct methods exist to validate nursing diagnoses, most of the studies done in this area have used bits and pieces or alterations of these original methods.[5,6,24,28] Only a few validation studies have been done, but more are now under way or are in the planning stages. Only through repeated studies can nursing diagnoses be considered valid for clinical use.

Two validation methods reported in the literature use expert panels of nurse clinicians instead of a clinically based patient population. The first, the *retrospective model,*[18] allows a large group of clinicians to concentrate on a general problem area to identify special concerns within it. Diagnostic categories are constructed using the problem–etiology–signs-symptoms (PES) approach (see later discussion). A vote is then taken to identify diagnostic labels the group has agreed on. A second vote is taken to derive diagnostic categories from the defining characteristics already identified. The advantages of the retrospective model include the possibility of obtaining a large nurse sample as opposed to a patient sample. The disadvantages include heterogeneity of the sample members.

The second expert validation approach, the *Q-sort method,* was modified and adapted by Lackey.[25] A group of nurse experts choose a diagnostic label to work with, then list the defining characteristics on note cards. The cards are individually ranked, and the list is narrowed to a predetermined percentage of the total number of cards. Rank ordering and reducing the number of cards occur once or twice again until the critical behaviors are identified. This method provides for the acceptance or rejection of preidentified defining characteristics.

Two established models are based on validating nursing diagnosis by using a clinical patient sample.[18] The first is the *nurse validation model,* which has two variations. Both variations start by identifying a specific diagnosis. Then a sample of patients exhibiting that diagnosis is systematically assessed by one or two nurses. In the first variation, one nurse assesses the sample and the data are reviewed by two specialists. In the second variation, both the assessments and the reviews are done by the two nurses. Both variations entail identifying defining characteristics in the sample with a subsequent tabulation of defining characteristics. Then a decision is made as to whether sufficient cases are present to validate the nursing diagnosis.

The final model, the *clinical validation model,* starts with a sample of patients who have a particular health problem.[18] Signs and symptoms are observed and tabulated systematically. Additional signs and symptoms may or may not be added to the list of the approved defining characteristics. After the tabulation is completed, the defining characteristics are arranged to determine whether critical clusters are present or not. If critical clusters are present, a second decision is made to determine if sufficient cases exist for a valid nursing diagnosis.

All these models need more testing so that the feedback from research can improve the validation process for nursing diagnoses.

USE IN THE CLINICAL SETTING

The benefits of establishing a unified taxonomy for nursing affect all areas of the profession. Use of nursing diagnoses in the clinical setting can enhance and streamline patient care planning. Patient acuity levels can be more readily evaluated when diagnoses are written for each patient. Also, the use of nursing diagnoses helps the nursing service "parcel out" what is uniquely nursing. This can assist in establishing the "costing out" of nursing services. Finally, a unified taxonomy can aid in computerized documentation of nursing services, which in turn can assist in the implementation of the other services previously described. Nursing diagnosis is the wave of the future; however, its use in the clinical setting must become uniform and second nature to the nurse clinician. This section provides clinical considerations for the use of nursing diagnoses.

As previously mentioned, nursing diagnosis is now seen as a part of the nursing process. However, a more careful examination of the relationship between the nursing process and nursing diagnosis reveals that much of the diagnostic processes have been performed by the clinician in the daily planning of care. The nursing process can be seen as a spiral that is continually changing and evolving. This spiral can be divided into three phases: (1) the preprocess phase, (2) the process phase, and (3) the postprocess phase. All three phases are equally important when identifying possible diagnoses for the patient.

The *preprocess phase* establishes the nurse-patient relationship. The primary goals of this phase include:

1. Establishment of a degree of trust between the client and the nurse
2. Definition of the roles the nurse and the client will play in the client's care
3. Voicing of the client's initial fears and questions
4. Creation of a positive environment in which to implement the nursing process

The *process phase* is implementation of the nursing process, during which the following actions occur:

1. Assessment: begins with the nursing history and the performance of a health assessment; ends with verification of the wellness or illness states; a precursor to diagnosis
2. Diagnosis: a determination or conclusion reached by the nurse based on assessment data; follows the PES format (see following discussion)
3. Planning: determination of a plan of action to assist the client toward the goal of optimal wellness; involves priority setting and yields a written plan of care
4. Implementing: initiation and completion of actions necessary to accomplish the defined goal of optimal fulfillment of human needs
5. Evaluating: appraisal of the changes experienced by the client in relation to goal achievement as a result of the nurse's actions

The *postprocess phase* involves reevaluation and termination of the nurse-patient relationship. The tasks performed during this phase include reassessment, updated diagnoses and care planning, and reevaluation of all phases described.

PES FORMAT FOR NURSING DIAGNOSES

1. Problem (patient problem)
   a. This is usually a diagnosis accepted by the North American Nursing Diagnosis Association (NANDA).
   b. This behavior can be improved through nursing assistance and intervention.
   c. This statement may have qualifying or quantifying adjectives to identify stages, phases, or level of a problem (for example, acute, chronic, mild, severe).
   d. An anatomic site may also be specified.
   e. The problem represents a *state of the patient*, not a nursing activity; for example, "ineffective airway clearance," not "needs suctioning."
2. Etiology
   a. This consists of physiologic, situational, and maturational factors that can cause the problem or influence its development.
   b. Etiology of the patient problem influences the nursing action.
   c. This is preceded by the phrase "related to" in a diagnostic statement.
3. Signs and symptoms (defining characteristics)
   a. Signs are objective.
   b. Symptoms are subjective.
   c. These are used in a diagnostic statement to clarify and justify.
   d. These may or may not be incorporated into the statement.

Table 8-1 Examples of the three domains of nursing practice

Independent domain	Interdependent domain	Dependent domain
NURSING DIAGNOSIS	CLINICAL NURSING PROBLEM	MEDICAL PROBLEM OR DIAGNOSIS
Range of motion	Levine tube	Swan-Ganz catheter
Maintenance of skin integrity	Egg-crate mattress	Fetal monitoring
Psychosocial intervention	Oxygen therapy	Medications
	Diet therapy	

NURSE	PHYSICIAN

Although all phases must be worked through, the most important time related to the development of the diagnostic statement is the diagnosis part of the process phase. A major consideration when developing the diagnostic statement is to be consistent. All diagnoses should be written uniformly for clarity and continuity. One such format is called *PES*; the components are the *problem, etiology,* and *signs* and *symptoms* (defining characteristics). Parts of the PES statement are defined in the box above.

Although nursing diagnosis is a statement of a patient response to the treatment regimens, errors may be made in the diagnostic statements. Basically, three dependency domains exist in nursing. Those domains are located on a continuum and are identified in Table 8-1.

Frequently, statement errors are made because the nurse tries to address problems located in the interdependent or dependent domains. These areas require intervention from someone other than the nurse, and nursing diagnoses cannot be made. Nursing diagnoses are not the following:

1. Medical diagnoses (for example, diabetes mellitus)
2. Medical pathology (for example, decreased cerebral tissue oxygenation)
3. Treatments or equipment (for example, hyperalimentation, Levine tube)

4. Diagnostic studies (for example, cardiac function tests, catheterization)
5. Goals (for example, "Client should perform own colostomy care")
6. Client needs (for example, "Client needs to walk every shift")
7. Nursing needs (for example, change dressing)

Also, when making a diagnostic statement, it is important to avoid judgmental statements or statements that could have legal ramifications. Avoid legally inadvisable or judgmental statements such as the following:

1. Fear related to frequent beatings by her husband
2. Ineffective family coping related to mother-in-law's continual harassment of daughter-in-law
3. Potential altered parenting related to low IQ of mother
4. Noncompliance related to failure to return for follow-up visits

With a good understanding of the information presented in this section, the nurse is now prepared to make diagnostic statements for patients in the real world. The following case examples briefly show how the process described can be applied to the clinical setting.

Case Examples

A 76-year-old male is admitted to your unit with a history of chronic congestive heart failure and a medical diagnosis of acute onset of congestive heart failure, moderate to severe. Your initial assessment reveals that the patient has rales and rhonchi bilaterally, tachypnea, cough with frothy sputum, slight cyanosis, dyspnea, anxiety, confusion, restlessness, coated tongue, and oral plaque.

With the following approved diagnoses, appropriate diagnostic statements might include the following:

1. Ineffective airway clearance related to increased pulmonary secretions
2. Anxiety related to potential cardiac arrest

3. Ineffective breathing pattern related to increased pulmonary secretions
4. Impaired gas exchange related to increased pulmonary secretions
5. Altered oral mucous membrane related to the administration of oxygen by nasal cannula

A 15-year-old female is brought into your unit after being raped within the last hour. You note that she is apprehensive, fearful, and shaken. She has poor eye contact and has extraneous movements in her extremities. She has a guarding behavior and a facial mask of pain. Her parents are not able to meet her emotional needs. Furthermore, she engages in self-blame and seems to be humiliated.

Appropriate diagnoses for this patient could be the following:

1. Anxiety related to fear of further injury
2. Pain related to physical injury sustained during the attack
3. Altered family processes related to withdrawal and social isolation
4. Rape-trauma syndrome related to the rape event

SUMMARY

Nursing diagnosis is a valuable clinical tool for the nurse. Diagnoses assist nurses to provide uniform, consistent, and efficient care because the language is understood by all nurses. From the first mention of nursing diagnosis in the 1950s to the establishment of nursing diagnosis as the second step in the nursing process by 1980, nursing diagnosis has been met with much controversy. However, with clinical validation mechanisms, nursing diagnosis has become more widely accepted. The consistent use of nursing diagnoses is necessary for the further development of nursing as a profession with its own unique body of knowledge.

REFERENCES

1. Abdellah F: The nature of nursing science, *Nurs Res* 18(5):388, 1969.
2. American Nurses' Association: *Standards of nursing practice,* Kansas City, 1973, The Association.
3. American Nurses' Association: *Standards of nursing practice,* Kansas City, 1980, The Association.
4. Aspinall M: Nursing diagnosis: the weak link, *Nurs Outlook* 24(7):433, 1976.
5. Baer C, Delorey M, Fitzmaurice J: A study to evaluate the validity of the rating system for self-care deficit. In Kim M, McFarland G, McLane A, eds: *The classification of nursing diagnoses: proceedings from the fifth conference,* St Louis, 1984, Mosby–Year Book.
6. Balisterieri T, Jiricka M: Validation of nursing diagnosis: role disturbance. In Kim M, McFarland G, McLane A, eds: *The classification of nursing diagnoses: proceedings from the fifth conference,* St Louis, 1984, Mosby–Year Book.
7. Bircher A: On the development and classification of nursing diagnosis, *Nurs Forum* 14(1):10, 1975.
8. Bockrath M: Your patient needs two diagnoses: medical and nursing, *Nurs Life* 2(2):29, 1982.
9. Bruce J, Snyder M: The right and responsibility to diagnose, *Am J Nurs* 82(4):645, 1982.
10. Carpenito L: *Nursing diagnosis: application to clinical practice,* Philadelphia, 1983, JB Lippincott.
11. Carstens J: The effect of an inservice program on nurses' ability to identify valid nursing diagnoses. In Kim M, McFarland G, McLane A, eds: *The classification of nursing diagnoses: proceedings from the fifth conference,* St Louis, 1984, Mosby—Year Book.
12. Dinsdale V: Implementation of nursing diagnosis in one emergency department, *JEN* 11(3):140, 1985.
13. Field L: The implementation of nursing diagnosis in clinical practice *Nurs Clin North Am* 14(3):495, 1979.
14. Fortin J, Rabinow J: Legal implications of nursing diagnosis, *Nurs Clin North Am* 14(3):553, 1979.
15. Gebbie K, Lavin M, eds: *Classification of nursing diagnosis: proceedings of the fifth national conference,* St Louis, 1975, Mosby–Year Book.
16. Gordon M: Nursing diagnosis and the diagnostic process, *Am J Nurs* 76(8):1298, 1976.
17. Gordon M: The concept of nursing diagnosis, *Nurs Clin North Am* 14(3):487, 1979.
18. Gordon M, Sweeney M: Methodological problems and issues in identifying and standardizing nursing diagnosis, *Adv Nurs Sci* 2(1):1, 1979.
19. Guzzetta C, Dossey B: Nursing diagnosis, *Heart Lung* 12(3):282, 1983.
20. Hagey R, McDonough P: The problem of professional labeling, *Nurs Outlook* 32(3):151, 1984.
21. Henderson V: *The nature of nursing,* New York, 1966, Macmillan.
22. Kieffer J: Nursing diagnosis can make a critical difference, *Nurs Life* 84(3):18, 1984.
23. Kim M, McFarland G, McLane A: *Classification of nursing diagnoses: proceedings of the fifth conference,* St Louis, 1987, Mosby–Year Book.
24. Kim M et al: Clinical validation of cardiovascular nursing. In Kim M, McFarland G, McLane A, eds: *The classification of nursing diagnoses: proceedings from the fifth conference,* St Louis, 1984, Mosby–Year Book.
25. Lackey N: *Use of the Q methodology in validating defining characteristics of specified nursing diagnoses,* unpublished manuscript, University of Kansas, Kansas City, Kan, 1984.
26. Lash A: A re-examination of nursing diagnosis, *Nurs Forum* 17(4):333, 1978.
27. Meade C, Kim M: The effect of teaching on documentation of nursing diagnosis. In Kim M, McFarland G, McLane A, eds: *The classification of nursing diagnoses: proceedings from the fifth conference,* St Louis, 1984, Mosby–Year Book.
28. Miller J: Development and validation of a diagnostic label: powerlessness. In Kim M, McFarland G, McLane A, eds: *The classification of nursing diagnoses: proceedings from the fifth conference,* St Louis, 1984, Mosby–Year Book.
29. North American Nursing Diagnosis Association: *Nursing diagnosis: gateway to scientific practice* (Pamphlet), St Louis, 1985, The Association.
30. Perry A: Nursing diagnosis research, *J Neurosurg Nurs* 14(2):108, 1982.
31. Simmons S, Ryan L: The implementation of nursing diagnosis using a computerized information system. In Kim M, McFarland G, McLane A, eds: *The classification of nursing diagnoses: proceedings from the fifth conference,* St Louis, 1984, Mosby–Year Book.
32. Toth L et al: *Implementation of nursing diagnosis in the trauma setting,* unpublished manuscript, Maryland Institute for Emergency Medical Services Systems.
33. Yura H, Walsh M: *The nursing process: assessing, planning, implementing, and evaluating,* ed 3, Norwalk, Conn, 1978, Appleton-Century-Crofts.
34. Yura H, Walsh M: *The nursing process: assessing, planning, implementing, and evaluating,* ed 4, Norwalk, Conn, 1983, Appleton-Century-Crofts.

Patricia Lenaghan

The practice of nursing produces a never-ending stream of challenges to determine the best way to solve problems. Often, nurses can find solutions through logical reasoning, experience, trial and error, or even tradition. Although these methods are legitimate in some situations, the nurse must often search for the best way to solve problems. Research is any activity designed to find a valid answer to a question; it is a way to determine how we know something to be accurate.

In clinical settings, nurses have relied on problem-solving ability they have acquired through experience. An experienced nurse may transfer the knowledge gained from past experiences to other patients and situations. However, the knowledge may have become outdated and stagnant in the ever-changing clinical environment. The traditional practice may have developed haphazardly as a result of unsystematic methods, and other methods may be more useful. Furthermore, this knowledge is often undocumented and thus inaccessible to others.

Clinical problem solving is another method that nurses use. With this method, nurses use intelligence, experience, and formal systems of thought to arrive at a solution for the problem of a particular patient: the nursing process is based on this method. Often this method is not a formal method to evaluate the approach to the problem; thus we may not know if the solution was found in the best possible manner.

Research, then, is the method used to determine the truth as it best can be defined. It is not always possible to determine whether method A is better than method B, C, or D for solving problem X, but the nurse can determine that method A produces more satisfied patients, less pain, and quicker recoveries. The goal of nursing research is to facilitate the development of clinical nursing interventions that improve health outcomes and contribute to the optimal delivery of health care. According to the American Nurses' Association, nursing research "develops knowledge about health and the promotion of health over a full life span, care of persons with health problems and disabilities and nursing actions to enhance the ability of individuals to respond effectively to actual or potential health problems."[1]

The purpose of research is to provide new knowledge by finding valid answers to questions that have been raised or valid solutions to problems that have been identified. Unlike problem solving, research is related to the care of patients in general, and the results benefit many patients.

STEPS IN THE RESEARCH PROCESS

A researcher usually goes through a series of well-defined, logical steps to organize a project. These steps are discussed in this chapter and listed in the box on p. 84.

Ways to seek funding sources, information on protection of human subjects and informed consent, ways to critique a research report, and ways to apply research to nursing practice are also discussed in this chapter.

Identifying a Problem

Research always begins with a question or a "researchable problem." This problem may concern patient care, nursing education, nursing administration, or any issue of interest. Patient care (or nursing practice) problems generally address a difference between how nurses practice and what is ideal or desirable.

Deciding on a specific research question may be difficult for the beginning researcher. Nurses are particularly skilled at explaining things to other nurses and patients; however, envisioning how scientific inquiry can shed light on an old problem is more difficult.

One of the best sources for researchable problems in nursing is personal experience. Many times an observation can be turned into a question such as one of the following:

1. I wonder whether seeing the dying family member before death helps the family during their bereavement?
2. I wonder whether using protocols for laboratory and radiographic examinations can expedite care in the emergency department?
3. I wonder if drawing blood below and above IV sites has any bearing on the laboratory values?

The more you know about one particular problem or area, the easier it will be to decide how to proceed.

Another source of problems to be researched is the nursing literature. Most research studies make recommendations for

---

STEPS IN THE RESEARCH PROCESS

1. Identifying a problem
2. Reviewing the literature
3. Developing a theoretic framework
4. Formulating a question or hypothesis
5. Following nursing research approaches and designs
6. Collecting data
7. Measuring and sampling
8. Performing data analysis
9. Determining results, conclusions, and recommendations
10. Communicating the results

---

future studies. Nursing practice is changed not by one study but by an accumulation of scientific results that indicates the best solution to a problem. Start by reading literature in an area of interest to outline common themes and patterns that you may wish to investigate.

Several nursing and federal organizations have published recommendations for research study. The Emergency Nurses Association, American Association of Critical Care Nurses, and American Nurses' Association all have research priorities for clinical nursing.[12,16] The National Institutes of Health also publishes their priorities in the area of nursing research.

Literature Review

Purpose. The purpose of the literature review is to explore the work conducted in a particular area of interest, thus helping to formulate or clarify the research problem. After critiquing previous research in a particular area, the researcher is more knowledgeable about what has been studied, more skilled in deciding how his or her study would best contribute to science, and more able to assess the feasibility of his or her study. Related research articles may contain relevant theory and research strategies that may be useful in future research. For example, Rebenson-Piano and others used previous studies of blood pressure measurement to help design their study, which evaluated two indirect methods of blood pressure measurement.[36]

Sources and scope. Librarians are excellent resources for the researcher who is conducting a literature review: they are familiar with the literature, literature retrieval, and library services. In addition, they are familiar with the National Library of Medicine and community, state, and regional libraries that make up the Health Science Library Network.

The search for published articles about a specific problem usually begins with either indexes to the literature or computerized data bases. The most commonly used indexes in nursing research are *International Nursing Index, Cumulative Index to Nursing and Allied Health Literature, Nursing Studies Index,* and *Index Medicus.* Abstract journals summarize articles that have appeared in other journals. *Nursing Research* and *Psychological Abstract* both provide useful abstracts of nursing studies.

Computer searches provide the reviewer with complete bibliographic information, thereby saving time and energy. A computer search may be obtained either by requesting one from a librarian or by conducting the search yourself. End-user systems are designed to allow reviewers to conduct their own computer searches in the library or at other locations.[43] The cost of a computer search depends on the type and extent of the search, as well as the data base used. Most libraries have request forms to be completed, and the fees for computer searches are usually posted. Before requesting a computer search, the researcher should know what subject matter and how many years of research are to be included in the search. Many options are available. Literature in foreign languages can be searched, or searches of literature in English only can be conducted; nursing literature only can be searched, or a comprehensive search of all the medical literature can be conducted.

When you receive the final search, you may see many or only a few pertinent articles. Articles that you receive may have rich bibliographies. Books, too, are useful; most books contain references to other sources of information at the end of each chapter.

Writing the literature review. After you have selected those articles that in some way contribute information about your research question, the next step is to critique those studies and summarize them to see how they do or do not fit into the scope of your study. A good review reinforces the need for the study in light of what has already been discovered. What is accepted to be true from other studies is the groundwork on which new studies are based. The written literature review should also include summaries of articles that differ from the proposed point of view; this aspect of the review indicates that the author has conducted an exhaustive review of the available knowledge.

A primary source of information is the description of an investigation that is written by the person who conducted it. A secondary source is a description of a study that is prepared by someone other than the original researcher. Both sources can be helpful, but written literature reviews should be based on primary sources whenever possible.[34] Nonresearch articles, which contribute to ideas or theories about the problem, may be included, but it is best to focus on primary research articles. LoBiondo-Wood and Haber, as well as and Polit and Hungler, have provided guidelines for critiquing and writing literature reviews.[22,34]

Theoretic Framework

One body organ does not function in isolation, nor does one bit of research. Theoretic frameworks are a "set of interrelated constructs [concepts], definitions, and propositions that present a systematic view of phenomena by specifying relations among variables, with the purpose of explaining and predicting the phenomena."[20] The purpose of the theoretic framework in research is to provide a systematic way to organize the information about a particular thing. The theoretic framework is a way to organize the rules or beliefs about what we observe.

Examples of theories used in nursing are psychoanalytic theory, theory of relativity, theory of evolution, theory of gravity, learning theory, systems theory, and theory of homeostasis. Campbell used the theoretic models of grief and learned helplessness to help explain women's responses to battering.[7]

The power of theories is to explain the relationship of variables and the nature of this relationship. Theories then help stimulate research by giving direction and providing impetus. Questions and ideas are formulated about what will occur in specific situations (hypotheses). Then the hypotheses are tested in research to determine whether the information fits into the theory. A theory is not only a necessary way to organize work; it also serves as a springboard for scientific advances.

Characteristics of theories. The two components of a theory are the concepts and a statement of propositions. Concepts, the building blocks of a theory, are abstract characteristics, categories, or labels of things, persons, or events. Examples of nursing concepts are health, stress, adaptation, caring, and pain. Propositions are statements that define the relationships among concepts: a set of propositions may state that one concept is associated with another or is contingent upon another.

Conceptual frameworks represent a less formal, less well-developed system for organizing phenomena. Conceptual frameworks contain concepts that represent a common theme but lack the deductive system of propositions, which give the relationship among concepts. Most research in nursing practice provides conceptual frameworks rather than theories.[34] These conceptual frameworks often lay the groundwork for more formal theories and serve as springboards for the generation of hypotheses and testing.

A conceptual model for nursing practice is a systematically constructed, scientifically based, and logically related set of concepts that identify the essential components of nursing practice. The model is a mental image of the realm of nursing and how it is put together and works. Fawcett named four central concepts of the nursing discipline: person, environment, health, and nursing.[13]

The past few decades has produced several conceptual models of nursing practice: Peplau's Developmental Model for Nursing Practice, Newman's Health Care Systems Model, Orem's Model of Self-Care, King's Open System Model, Johnson's Behavioral Systems Model, Levine's Conservation Model, Rogers' Model of the Unitary Person, and Roy's Adaption Model.[37] You may wish to use a nursing model in your study or review relevant literature that may give direction for a systematic way (theoretic framework) to determine how your research problem fits into what is already known. A research example of the application of a nursing theory used Orem's Model of Self-Care to determine the effects of assertion training and first aid instruction on children's autonomy and self-care.[26]

Formulating Questions or Hypotheses

Before a problem can be researched, it must be narrowed, refined, and made feasible for study. The research interest can be stated as a question or a hypothesis. The research question should identify the key variables under investigation. For example, the research question might be "What effect does the presence of the parent in the child's room have on the child's experience of pain during fracture reduction?" The dependent variable is the child's pain experience, and the independent variable is the presence of the parent in the room. The dependent variable is explained through its relationship with the independent variable. Often research questions begin like the following: "What causes . . . ?"; "Is there a relationship between . . . ?"; and "How effective is . . .?" Both research variables must be specific. The goal is to determine whether a relationship exists between the two variables.

The independent variable is what is assumed to cause or thought to be associated with the dependent variable. Changes in the dependent variable are presumed to depend on the independent variable's effects. The dependent variable is what you want to explain or understand. Be specific about what you want to study in your research. If you try to measure too much, clearly analyzing the data at the end of your project may be difficult. For example, it is known that many factors affect a child's perception of pain, but only one independent variable (parent's presence) would be measured in this study. The researcher can measure several variables if the study is well designed.

Often the dependent variable can have multiple causes. A study may be designed to examine several factors and their influence on a phenomenon. For example, you may want to know whether experience with triage or an educational program concerning triage influences ability to accurately perform triage. Both independent variables (education and experience) can influence triage performance ability (dependent variable).

Several dependent variables can also be designated as measures of treatment effectiveness. Another question may be whether a comprehensive triage system has an influence on length of stay in the emergency department (ED), patient satisfaction, and patient outcome. Length of stay, patient satisfaction, and patient outcome are all dependent variables by which triage effectiveness is measured.

A hypothesis is a tentative prediction or explanation of the relationship between two or more variables. This prediction of expected outcomes is the basis of the research process. Hypotheses, which often stem from theories, are possible solutions or answers to the research problems. The hypothesis is a prediction of the nature of the relationship between several variables. For example, one hypothesis might be that pediatric patients who are promised a reward at the end of a suturing procedure will cooperate and be more compliant than pediatric patients who are not promised a reward. In this example, the researcher is not only questioning whether a relationship between rewards and behavior exists but is also predicting outcomes from this relationship. The null hypothesis is a statement that no relationship exists between the independent and the dependent variable. The null hypothesis is often generated for statistical purposes, data analysis, and discussion.

Nursing Research Approaches and Designs

Experimental and quasi-experimental studies. Experimental studies differ from nonexperimental studies in that the researcher who conducts an experimental study actively participates in the research; he or she does not simply observe a phenomenon. To qualify as an experiment, the research design must possess the following characteristics:

1. Manipulation. The researcher must do something to at least some of the participants in the study.
2. Control. The researcher manipulates the independent variable by giving one group an experimental treatment. The control (comparison) group receives normal treatment, that is, the control group does not receive the experimental treatment.
3. Randomization. Subjects are randomly assigned to either the experimental group or the control group. Each subject has an equal chance of being assigned to either group. This randomization assures the researcher that both groups are exactly alike and that the effect of the treatment or experiment will be caused by the independent variable, not by individual differences. Neff and others used the experimental method to test the effects of respiratory rate and depth and open versus closed mouth breathing on sublingual temperatures.[28]

Quasi-experimental design is similar to experimental design in that it provides manipulation; however, quasi-experimental design lacks either the feature of randomization or the feature of control. When randomization is lacking (usually because the researcher cannot assign subjects to groups) no guarantee exists that both the experimental group and the control (comparison) groups are similar. This design is called a nonequivalent control group design. Osguthorpe, Roper, and Saunders used a quasi-experimental method to study the effects of teaching on the subjects' knowledge related to medications.[31] The researchers compared pretest and posttest scores after subjects participated in an intervention involving either a drug information sheet or a videotape.

A time-series design is often used in nursing research. This method is used when researchers are not able either to randomize or to have a control group. Because only one group is available for study, the phenomenon of interest is studied over a longer period of time and the experimental treatment is introduced during the course of the study. A time-series design was used by Tilden and Shepherd to develop and test an ED interview protocol focused on identification of physically abused women.[45]

Nonexperimental research. When experimentation or quasi-experimentation is possible, these two approaches are the best methods for testing hypotheses. A number of research problems (especially those involving human subjects) do not lend themselves to experimentation because the independent variables (for example, diseases, widowhood, and injury), which are often naturally occurring, cannot be manipulated. The two broad classes of nonexperimental research are ex post facto (or correlational) research and descriptive research. The translation from Latin of *ex post facto* is "after the fact." This term indicates that research is conducted by the use of variations of the independent variable in the natural course of events. Ex post facto studies are also known as explanatory studies,[22] descriptive studies,[46] causal-comparative studies,[46] or comparative surveys.[14] In conducting ex post facto research, the investigator does not have control of the independent variables because they have already occurred. A retrospective study of ex post facto design looks at an existing phenomenon and tries to link it to others from the past. Epidemiologic studies are often of ex post facto design. Many cancer research studies attempt to link past behaviors with current cancerous conditions. Prospective studies start with presumed natural causes and compare groups who have and do not have those independent variables.

The purpose of descriptive (nonexperimental) research is to observe, describe, and investigate aspects of a phenomenon. For example, an investigator may wish to determine the percentage of ED patients who do not have a regular source of health care.

Several other research methods are used to view and interpret phenomena in the practice of nursing. These methods are used to evaluate the past, examine units in depth, develop tools, evaluate programs, and study the principles of nursing.

Historical research provides an account of past events. The investigator systematically collects information relating to past occurrences and also critiques the data. Generally, historical research is performed to test hypotheses or answer questions about causes, effects, or trends relating to past events that shed light on present behaviors or practices.[34] A researcher may wish to know the historical perspective of the nurse's role in prehospital care, including group transport and aeromedical transport. This information would help in the identification of trends and, possibly, in the prediction of future needs.

Survey research is designed to obtain information about distribution prevalence and interrelationships among variables. When this nonexperimental approach is used, intervention is not performed by the investigator but rather explained by the collection of data. A researcher may survey ED nurses to understand how retention may be affected by the increase in ED census, the occurrence of violence, and the spread of infectious diseases. Surveys may be personal interviews, telephone interviews, or questionnaires. Political opinion polls are examples of survey research.

Field research is an investigation of a certain situation in the natural setting. This qualitative research is aimed at describing and exploring the phenomenon. The results of field research define behaviors, beliefs, and practices of individuals or groups in real situations. Anthropologists are probably the most widely recognized field researchers. Nurses conduct field studies in home environments and hospitals to determine what aspects of the patient and environment contribute to the well-being of patients.

Case study designs provide an in-depth analysis of an individual, a small group, a family, a place, or an organization. Natural conditions are usually studied, and variables related to history, current characteristics, interactions, or problems are examined. Case studies usually focus on why the subject feels, thinks, or behaves in a particular way. Meier and Pugh think that case studies are well suited to the study of clinical nursing problems, since case studies focus holistically on individuals.[24]

Evaluative research is the use of scientific research methods and procedures to evaluate a program, treatment practice, or policy; therefore this type of research uses analytic means to document the worth of an activity.[22] Experimental, nonexperimental, or quasi-experimental approaches can be used. Program goals or objectives should be the focus of the evaluation.

Methodologic research is a controlled investigation of the ways of obtaining, organizing, and analyzing data.[34] This type of research addresses the development, validation, and evaluation of research tools or techniques. For example, an investigator may want to develop or perfect a tool for measuring anxiety in the hospitalized cardiac patient. Measuring the level of anxiety in the patient is not the goal of this type of research; the goal is to determine the degree of accuracy with which the tool measures anxiety in all patients.

Data Collection Methods

When you know what you want to study and whom you plan to use in your research, you may use various techniques for collecting the needed information. The key to success in data collection is choosing or developing appropriate methods that will accurately describe the variables you wish to study. Operationalization is the process of translating the concepts of interest into observable and measurable phenomena.

There are five types of data collection methods: physiologic and biophysical, observational, interviews and questionnaires, scales and psychologic measures, and records or available data.

Physiologic measurements fall into several major groups.

Physical measurements are those used to measure characteristics such as temperature, weight, height, cardiac output, muscle strength, and electrical activity of organs. Parsons, Peard, and Page measured physiologic responses of heart rate and cerebral perfusion pressure of patients with head injuries during nursing interventions.[32] Measurements of chemistry include hemoglobin levels, hematocrit percentages, blood sugar and potassium levels, and the like. Microbiologic measurements provide counts and identifications of bacteria. Radiographic studies, biopsies, computerized axial tomography, and magnetic resonance imaging are examples of anatomic or cytologic measurements. One advantage of physiologic measurements is objectivity: the data collected are not influenced by the person performing the study. Physiologic measurements are relatively precise and sensitive.

Certain types of research problems are more amenable to direct observation methods; the researcher actually observes what he or she intends to study. For example, you may want to observe the response of parents to casting or suturing procedures performed on their children. The observation method is most useful for entities that are difficult to measure, such as interactions, nursing process, changes in behavior, or group processes.

Interviews and questionnaires are used to allow subjects to report data for or about themselves. The purpose of questioning participants is to seek direct data (such as age, religion, or marital status) or indirect data (such as level of intelligence, anxiety, and pain). An instrument used or developed for interviews or questionnaires must measure the intended data. Newly developed instruments are often pilot tested. Pilot testing is performed on a small sample of people to evaluate the research tool or method.

Instruments with scales are often used to make distinctions among subjects concerning the degree to which they possess a certain trait, attitude, or emotion. Scales are measuring instruments that permit interindividual comparisons in dimensions of interest.[34] For example, a researcher interested in knowing whether a nerve block or a local injection of anesthetic is more effective for relieving pain during fracture reduction would use a pain scale to measure pain.

Many scales and psychologic measures have already been developed by researchers. To find the appropriate scale or instrument, review the literature related to what you are researching. Research texts discuss measurement methods at the end of most chapters on data collection methods.[34] Some texts provide nothing but instruments for measuring health and nursing care.[15,23]

Measurement and Sampling

The definition of population is not restricted to human subjects. A population can consist of records, blood samples, actions, words, organizations, numbers, or animals. Whatever the unit, a population is always made up of specific elements of interest.

A population can be defined to include thousands of individuals or narrowed to only a few hundred. The population is defined in a study by set criteria. For example, when studying emergency department nurses, the researcher may choose nurses who have 1, 5, or 10 years of experience. The researcher sets the criteria for inclusion in the study, and the criteria define the population.

Because it is nearly impossible (and expensive) to include large populations, the researcher samples only a part of a large group. Samples represent a portion of the entire population to be studied. In Figure 9-1, all ED nurses represent the entire population; the sampling unit consists of ED nurses from City A, and the sample is selected from those ED nurses in City A.

The important factor in sampling is the researcher's ability to verify that the sample represents the entire population (representativeness). The researcher usually verifies representativeness by using probability and nonprobability sampling plans.

Probability sampling is the use of some form of random selection in choosing the sample units. Every element in the population has a known, nonzero probability of being included in the sample. The goal of probability sampling is to ensure that the study population is represented.

The majority of human samples in most types of research (including nursing) are based on nonprobability.[34] There are three types of nonprobability sampling. Accidental samples are based on convenience, such as surveying the first 100 patients in the ED on a particular day. Quota samples are used when the researcher knows an element of the population and bases the sample on that element. A researcher may know that 25% of ED nurses are men; the researcher then makes sure that 25% of the sample consists of men, thus increasing the representativeness of the population. Purposive sampling occurs when the researcher handpicks the cases to be included in the sample. Usually the researcher uses purposive sampling to ensure a wide variety of responses or because the choices are judged to be typical of the population. Remember that the extent to which you can generalize your results depends on the method by which you chose the samples. If you can randomly pick the samples, you will have more widely applicable results.

Sample size. No one simple equation is used for determining sample size, although the largest possible sample should be used. The larger the sample is, the more representative it is of the population. A procedure known as power analysis is often used by advanced researchers to estimate sample size.[11] Sample sizes should be determined according to population and the statistical procedures to be run on the data.

Instrument validity. Validity is the "degree to which an instrument measures what it is intended to measure."[34] Although an instrument may appear to measure some aspect of a construct (or element), the instrument must be evaluated to determine whether it really does provide such measurement. There are three kinds of validity, content, construct, and criterion-related.

Content validity is the degree to which an instrument

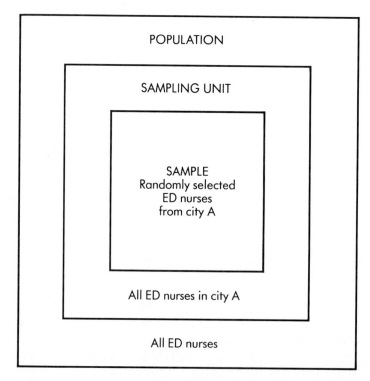

Fig. 9-1   Sample represents portion of population to be studied.

measures the universe of content that it is said to represent or measure. Content validity is often determined by a panel of experts in the field to be evaluated. If you wanted to measure bereavement behaviors in the ED, you might ask social workers and members of the clergy, as well as ED nurses, to review your instrument for measuring content related to grief.

Construct validity is the degree to which a tool measures the construct in the study. A construct is an abstraction that is developed for a scientific purpose. Construct validity is usually determined over time after data from research studies either support the construct to a greater degree or question it further.[49] For example, you may want to determine the sense of hope (a construct) in trauma patients' families. The researcher's instrument must discriminate between families who posssess hope and families who do not possess hope (construct validity.)

Criterion-related validity consists of two types, predictive validity and concurrent validity. In each type, the subject's performance on one measure is used to infer the likely response on another measure (criterion).[4] Predictive validity is a measure used to predict future performance. (For example, a nurses's score on a content knowledge test in emergency nursing predicts how well a nurse will perform with patients.) Concurrent validity is the degree to which an instrument can distinguish subjects who differ on a certain criterion measured at the same time.

Reliability. Reliability of an instrument refers to its ability to consistently and accurately measure a criterion. The reliability of an instrument is the degree of consistency with which it measures something. A test of reliability is whether the tool produces the same measurement when a measurement is repeated several times. The less an instrument varies in repeated measurements, the greater the reliability of the instrument. A thermometer that measures an oral temperature at 98.6° F one moment and 102° F the next is unreliable.

Data Analysis

After completing data collection, the researcher summarizes the data through a statistical procedure. The purpose of analysis is to answer the research questions. The preliminary steps for data analysis include sorting, coding, or entering data into a computer. Researchers who use quantitative methods for data collection should plan for analysis before the research data are collected.

Statistical techniques give meaning to quantitative data; the techniques reduce, summarize, organize, evaluate, interpret, and communicate numeric data.[34]

Statistics are either descriptive or inferential. Descriptive statistics are used to describe and summarize data. Examples of descriptive statistics are mode, median, mean, average, percentage, and frequency.

Inferential statistics are used to draw conclusions about a large population based on a sample from a study, to make judgments, and to generalize information. Inferential statistics are then used to test the hypotheses to determine whether they are correct. Two categories of inferential statistics are parametric and nonparametric.

Most statistical tests are parametric tests, which have the following characteristics: (1) They focus on population parameters, (2) they require measurements on at least one interval or ratio scale, and (3) they make assumptions about the distribution of the variables.[34] Nonparametric tests are used most often when measured variables are either nominal or ordinal; these tests do not make assumptions about the distribution of variables.

Variability refers to the spread or dispersion of data such as range and standard deviation. The range is the spread between the highest and lowest scores. Standard deviation is the most commonly used variability test. The standard deviation is determined by first calculating deviation scores, or the degree to which a score deviated from the mean. The standard deviation indicates how far scores generally deviate from the mean.

Frequently used statistical tests. A *t*-test is a parametric test that determines whether a difference exists between the means of two groups.

Analysis of variance (ANOVA) is also a parametric test used to determine the significance of differences between the means of two or more groups. The purpose then is to determine whether the variability is due to the independent variable or due to other differences such as human or measurement error. Osguthorpe and others used ANOVA to test hypotheses about medication teaching interventions.[31]

The chi-square test is a nonparametric test used when two sets of data can fall into various categories. A contingency table is used to test the significance of different proportions. The table is used to determine total frequencies for each category. The chi-square value is then computed to determine the actual observed frequency and to determine what would be expected if no relationship existed between the variables.

Correlation coefficients are most frequently used to describe a relationship between two measures. When two variables are totally unrelated, the correlation coefficient is 0. If two items always were positively related the correlation coefficient approaches 1.00 (for example, temperature elevation usually correlates with white blood cell count elevation). A negative correlation occurs when one factor or variable increases while the other decreases. For example, increasing intracranial pressure has a negative correlation with level of consciousness. This correlation is called an inverse, or negative, relationship.

More sophisticated tests are being used in research because of the advancing skill of researchers and the rigorous attention to design of studies. Tests used to analyze three or more variables, termed multivariate statistical analyses, include multiple correlation, or multiple regression, analysis of covariance and factor analysis.

Computers. Computers are available at most universities and hospitals for statistical procedures. Computers are widely used to calculate and report results. A wide variety of software packages is available for performing all the necessary statistical procedures. Examples of prepacked statistical programs are Statistical Analysis Systems, Statistical Package for the Social Sciences, and Biomedical Statistical Software. You will probably need assistance in the use of these programs. A computer file must be made for your data entry. Your data must be entered into a file; then the computer is told how to read your data and what procedures to perform. If you need assistance in creating the data file and in telling the computer how to process the data, ask someone who is familiar with both the computer system and statistical procedures. Woods and Catanzaro describe computer software programs, including cost, functions, and program sources.[50]

Results, Conclusions, and Recommendations

Results are often reported in the form of tables and graphs. Van Hoozer, Warner, and Felton describe the use of the MS-DOS computer operating system (any system compatible with International Business Machines [IBM] personal computers) for creating graphics of research.[47] Data summarized in the form of graphs and tables can be more easily interpreted and compared with the research questions or hypotheses and theoretic framework. For example, in a study to test the minimum discard sample required for accurate blood samples drawn from an indwelling arterial catheter, Preusser and others displayed their data to show with a 2 ml discard sample that the results of the analysis did not significantly change.[35] The visual image of their data helps to show the reader the results simply and clearly.

Interpretation of the findings is an extremely important aspect of conducting a study. Results are either positive, negative, serendipitous, or mixed.

Positive findings confirm what the researcher expected. The results are consistent with the logic and theoretic framework of the study. The null hypothesis (no relationship or difference between variables) is rejected. The hypotheses are accepted.

Negative findings mean that nonsignificant results were discovered. The null hypothesis is accepted. The researcher then must evaluate alternative explanations for the negative results.[50] The negative results could be attributed to sampling bias, measurement error, or design or measurement methods.

Serendipitous findings are those that were unexpected. These findings are usually not discussed in the problem statement because the factor or variable was not thought to be part of the conceptual or theoretic framework.

Mixed results contain some results that support the research questions and hypotheses and some that do not. Mixed results may lead the investigator to rethink the theory or to improve methods for study.

Conservative judgment should be used when considering the conclusions drawn from a study. Conclusions should be supported with facts, data, and results, not viewpoints or subjective judgments. Remember that correlation does not prove causation: because two things are associated does not necessarily mean that one causes the other. Alternative explanations for the results should always be considered.

Recommendations stem from changes that the researcher would make in sample, design, or analysis, if the study were repeated. Recommendations may also be based on negative, mixed, or serendipitous findings. Other explanations for results should also be discussed so that progress can be made in future studies of the research problem. Implications of research, for example, how the findings could be used to improve nursing or how best to advance knowledge through additional research, should also be provided.

Communicating the Results

Once the research data are analyzed and conclusions are drawn, you have an obligation to yourself and to the profession to share this knowledge. The results have the potential to influence nursing care, and by reporting the results, nurses add to the available body of knowledge. Because the future of the profession depends on the advancement of this knowledge, nurses must communicate with each other about what has been discovered.

To communicate your research results, you can either write about them or give an oral presentation. Written reports are usually in the form of a thesis, a dissertation, or a journal article. Paper and poster presentations are opportunities to discuss your study with an audience.

Journal articles are the most useful means to reach a large group of professionals. Leading nursing journals that primarily publish nursing research articles include the following: *Nursing Research, Research in Nursing and Health, Western Journal of Nursing Research, Journal of Advanced Nursing, International Journal of Nursing Studies,* and *Advances in Nursing Science.* Clinical research is also published in other nursing and nonnursing journals. Specialty journals such as *Journal of Emergency Nursing* and *Heart and Lung* also publish research. The journal you select depends on the readership you want to reach.[44]

Because your manuscript must compete with those of other researchers, you may want to write a letter of inquiry (a query letter) to determine whether the editor is interested in your manuscript. A positive response increases the likelihood that your article will be published. You can send query letters to as many journals as you wish. You may not, however, submit your full manuscript to more than one journal. It is an unwritten ethical code between editors and authors that you may have your manuscript reviewed by only one journal at a time. This code prevents several journal editors from going through the time and work of reviewing an article, only to discover that the article is being published in another journal. It is not ethical to submit exactly the same manuscript to two different journals, but you can report different information from your research in separate articles.

If your manuscript is not accepted for publication, you may submit it to another journal. Many researchers submit several manuscripts before they abandon hope of getting their results published. Many editors include "information for authors" at the beginning of their journals; following these guidelines improves your chance of acceptance. You may also ask colleagues and friends to read your manuscript for clarity and correctness.

Theses and dissertations are written mainly to partially fulfill the requirements for a master's or doctoral degree. A thesis or dissertation has a limited audience and is the method least often used for dissemination of research results. These manuscripts are generally thorough and scholarly but too lengthy for most readers.

A paper presentation is an oral summary of your research results; it is usually read at scientific or professional meetings where members of the same field gather to share knowledge. Organizations request abstracts 6 to 9 months before the meeting date. Calls for abstracts are published in journals. The call usually lists any requirements that your abstract must fulfill, such as length and format, and includes the deadline for submission and any requirements regarding membership in that particular organization.

You will be allowed 15 to 30 minutes for your oral presentation of introduction, methodology, results, discussion, and time to answer questions. Practice your presentation so that you stay within the time frame; there will be a strict time limit. You may wish to include slides or other audiovisual aids in your presentation.

Sometimes professional organizations give researchers the option of a poster presentation; again the organization will issue a call for abstracts or papers. A poster presentation combines a visual poster of your research and the opportunity to discuss your findings informally with interested persons. Usually a poster session is set up at a specific site at the meeting to allow participants to walk among the researchers and their posters and to ask questions. Following the guidelines for poster presentations will help you give your poster a professional appearance. Instructions regarding the size and number of poster boards are usually provided after the paper is accepted. You may wish to check with your hospital graphic arts department or biomedical department for help in preparing your poster.[27,40]

Writing an abstract. An abstract is a brief summary of the research study; it is located at the beginning of a journal article. An abstract is also located at the beginning of a bound copy of a thesis or dissertation. Some journals publish abstracts of articles that have appeared in other journals or that have been presented orally or as poster presentations at conferences.

Abstracts can be 250 to 1000 words long, depending on the space available. An abstract generally contains a statement about the research purpose of hypotheses, a description of the sample, a brief explanation of the data collection and analysis procedures, and a summary of important findings.

FUNDING

When seeking money to fund research, the researcher must follow formal guidelines. Most funding agencies release the guidelines and standards for review to the public. When requesting grant funds, you should consider both the agency most appropriate for the project and the level of sophistication of the researcher.

The thousands of funding sources for research include federal, state, and local government agencies, private foundations, business and industry, university or hospital funds, private donors, and professional and scientific organizations. In some of the health areas, certain foundations and private businesses are providing more research funding than the federal government is.[19] Public libraries and most university research departments have listings and current information regarding government and foundation sources.

Many universities and hospitals have research funds for staff members. In many cases, these funds are more quickly accessible and require less formal proposal preparation than other sources do. Agencies that are likely to fund clinical researchers and junior investigators include Sigma Theta Tau International, The American Nurses' Foundation (ANF), the National Science Foundation, and the National Institutes of Health (NIH). In terms of dollars, the NIH is the primary source for nursing research funding.

Both Sigma Theta Tau (National Honor Society of Nursing) and the ANF offer small grant programs that have deadlines once each year. The maximum amount awarded by Sigma Theta Tau is $3000, and the application is due by March 1.[48] The ANF awards as much as $2700; the application is due by June 1.[30] These two agencies also offer a joint clinical research grant once each year: this grant must be applied for by June 1 and awards a selected chemically oriented researcher as much as $6000. Application forms and comprehensive guidelines are available from the executive office of each agency.

Many specialty organizations also offer grants for research. The Emergency Nurses Association budgets $1500 to be awarded each year. The maximum individual award is $500, and the deadline for submission of the grant proposal is December 31. Grant application guidelines are available from the national office of the association.[21]

The NIH has 12 freestanding institutes, as well as the National Center for Nursing Research. Other divisions in the NIH that have funded nursing research include the National Institute on Aging, the National Cancer Institute, and the National Institute of Child Health and Human Development. Fundable research proposals submitted to the National Center for Nursing Research should be related to one of three programs: health promotion or disease prevention, acute and chronic illness, or nursing systems. Information about each program can be obtained from the center.

Submitting a Proposal

The first step in submitting a proposal is to obtain specific guidelines from the funding agencies. Agency deadlines, any restrictions, and investigator qualifications are all important components. Be sure to give consideration to any specific directions for preparation of your proposal. You may seek funding from more than one agency but you must meet the specific requirements of each.

After writing a proposal, submit it to several of your peers for review. Select someone who has good knowledge of the content that you are proposing to study. A second person who is not familiar with the content can review it for style, clarity, and logical flow. Mistakes in grammar, spelling, and punctuation may cause the reviewers to question your ability to perform scholarly research.

When a grant application is reviewed, one of the first things reviewers look for is the purpose of the study. The purpose must be stated clearly near the beginning of the proposal. The reviewers ask the following questions: Why is the study important? Who will benefit from the study? Is the study feasible? Are all ethical standards met? How well does this study contribute to what we already know?

Your grant proposal is evaluated by experienced researchers who first determine whether you followed the guidelines for submission. Be sure that you read and follow these guidelines carefully. Remember that deadlines are not usually flexible.

There are many more good research questions than there is money to fund them. If your proposal does not get funded, consider it a learning experience. The guidelines assisted you in clarifying your question and forced you to look closely at important components of your research. Consider the reviewer's comments as free expert advice, and use the advice to improve your proposal. Only 51% of all published research studies were funded in the early 1980s, but this percentage is increasing.[25]

PROTECTION OF HUMAN SUBJECTS

The first federal guidelines requiring that grant applications for research involving human subjects be reviewed by an Institutional Review Board (IRB) were published in 1966 by the United States Public Health Service.[17] The purposes of these guidelines were to safeguard subjects' rights and welfare, to ensure appropriate procedures for informed consent, and to allow subjects to make independent decisions about risks and benefits. Any research activities supported by the Department of Health, Education and Welfare (now the Department of Health and Human Services) were regulated by Congress in 1974.

In 1974 Congress established a National Commission for Protection of Human Subjects of Biomedical and Behavioral Research. This commission recommends legislative and regulatory action to govern agencies issuing research grants.

The National Research Act (P.L. 93-348) was passed on July 12, 1974, and regulated the ethics guidance programs

---

> # INSTITUTIONAL REVIEW BOARD REQUIREMENTS
>
> 1. Risks to subjects are minimized.
> 2. Risks to subjects are reasonable in relation to anticipated benefits, if any, to the subjects and in relation to the importance of the knowledge that may be expected to result.
> 3. Selection of subjects is equitable.
> 4. Informed consent will be sought from each prospective subject or legally authorized representative.
> 5. Informed consent is appropriately documented.
> 6. The research plan makes provision for monitoring data collection to ensure subjects' safety (as needed).
> 7. When appropriate, provisions are made to protect subjects' privacy and confidentiality of data.
> 8. Additional safeguards are included if some or all subjects are likely to be vulnerable to coercion or undue influence.

---

of IRBs. This act requires that any institution applying for a grant or contract for any project involving a human subject in biomedical or behavioral research must show proof in the application that it has established in IRB. Agencies that receive no federal grants usually have a review mechanism similar to an IRB, sometimes referred to as a human rights committee or a research committee.

The box above lists the requirements that an IRB must guarantee before approving a research study.[10]

Expedited Review and Exemption

When risk to subjects is minimal, most IRBs include a process called expedited review, which usually shortens the length of the review process.[10] A list of research categories eligible for expedited review is available from any IRB office. Keep in mind that IRBs usually have set meeting times during the year and that they may have many proposals to review. The IRB ensures protection of subjects; if you are anticipating a starting date for your study, begin the IRB process early (several months in advance is *not* unrealistic). Every researcher should obtain the most up-to-date requirements for review from the institution's IRB office.

Usually exempt from the strict IRB requirements are studies that use existing data, documents, records, or pathologic and diagnostic specimens, if these sources are available to the public or if the information is recorded so that the subjects cannot be identified.[10]

Some institutions require progress reports. All institutions require final reports of the study, including the number of participants, study findings, and how these findings are to be communicated.[29] The IRB usually requests a copy of your publication or presentation, to ensure that proper credit is given to the institution.

INFORMED CONSENT

The federal government has mandated that the following elements of information be included when informed consent is obtained[10]:

1. A statement that the study involves research, an explanation of purposes of the research, a delineation of the expected duration of the subject's participation, a description of the procedures to be followed, and an identification of any procedures that are experimental
2. A description of any reasonably foreseeable risks or discomforts to the subject
3. A description of any benefits to the subject or to others that may reasonably be expected from the research
4. A disclosure of appropriate alternative procedures or courses of treatment, if any, that may be advantageous to the subject
5. A statement describing to what extent, if any, the confidentiality of the records identifying the subject will be maintained
6. For research involving more than minimal risk, an explanation as to whether any medical treatments are available if injury occurs and if so, what they consist of, or where further information may be obtained
7. An explanation of whom to contact for answers to pertinent questions about the research and research subject's rights and whom to contact in the event of a research-related injury to the subject
8. A statement that participation is voluntary, that refusal to participate will not involve any penalty or loss of benefits to which the subject is otherwise entitled, and that the subject may discontinue participation at any time without any penalty or loss of otherwise entitled benefits

The language of the consent form must be understandable. The subject cannot be asked to waive rights or to release the researcher or institution from liability for negligence.[10]

The date, the time, and the signatures of the subject, researcher, and witness must be included on the form. In addition, the researcher should include a phone number where he or she can be contacted about concerns.

Ethical Considerations

In 1985 the ANA issued their *Human Rights Guidelines for Nurses in Clinical and Other Research*[3] and their updated version of *Code for Nurses with Interpretive Statements*.[2] This code states that any proposed nursing research study should meet the following conditions:

1. The study design is approved by an appropriate body.
2. The individual has the right to freedom from intrinsic risks of injury.
3. The individual has rights to privacy and dignity.
4. All people have the right to choose to participate, to

have full information, and to terminate participation without penalty.

CRITIQUES

A research critique is a critical appraisal of a research study that is performed systematically by someone who has knowledge of both research and the content area. The goal is to determine how the new knowledge fits into what is already known. A decision concerning scientific merit is made so that readers can determine whether to incorporate the results into practice. A careful appraisal is made of the study's strengths and weaknesses. The information in a paper that has been accepted for publication will not necessarily be adopted into practice. Usually several strong, similar research results are needed to change practice; therefore, research is often replicated and refined. Each element of the research report is critiqued.

For adequate evaluation of research, expertise is required in the areas of study design, methods, sampling data analysis, and the content area under study. You may want to ask a nurse researcher in a local institution, school of nursing, or college for help in critiquing research. Beck presents a 10-step process for critiquing all dimensions of a research report.[5]

Phillips has devoted an entire text to the critiquing and utilization of nursing research.[33] This text serves as an excellent resource. Shelley summarizes that research critiques should provide answers to the following questions[41]:

1. What new knowledge, if any, has been generated?
2. How does this new knowledge relate to existing knowledge?
3. What are the implications, if any, for practice?
4. How might this research be extended or improved?

APPLICATION TO NURSING PRACTICE

The final step of the research process is to use the results to change nursing practice. Even if your findings have been disseminated in journals, at conferences, or in a paper, your useful data will not necessarily be put into practice. You must be the one to make research-based changes in practice. Often a group of research findings, called innovations, are used to change practice. Rogers has provided a theoretic model of innovation diffusion.[39] She defines innovations as things, ideas, knowledge, or practices that are perceived as new by an individual. Whether you are a researcher or a clinical nurse, you can identify these innovations and put them into practice.

Horsley has presented a seven-step process for producing a research-based practice change,[18] which serves as an excellent resource for any nurse wanting to implement changes. The steps of the process are the following:

1. Systematically identify patient care problems.
2. Identify and assess research-based knowledge, to solve identified care problems.
3. Adapt and design the nursing practice innovation.

4. Conduct a clinical trial and evaluation of the innovation.

5. Decide whether to adopt, alter, or reject the innovation.

6. Develop the means to extend (or diffuse) the new practice beyond the trial unit.

7. Develop mechanisms to maintain the innovation over time.

Brett studied organizational methods for integrating research into practice.[6] She found that hospitals are having difficulty adopting innovations by nurses. Many organizations are now supporting the inclusion of research committees and nurse researchers on the organizational charts. Nursing research is often rewarded through clinical and career ladders. Joint appointments between academic and clinical settings are made to promote research. Reading research-based literature and attending conferences that include research presentations contribute to the nurse's awareness of research findings and understanding of how this supports practice.

Brett found that conducting and publishing research did have a positive impact on the adoption of findings into practice.[6] Collaboration is one method for accomplishing research and changing practice. Smejkal formed a research committee among her critical care nurses, to give their group opportunities to use the resources of several hospitals and to accomplish research goals.[42] Rogers states that collaboration allows joint discussion about problems, combines expertise, provides opportunities to develop and expand research skills, and provides an avenue for dissemination of findings into practice.[38] Chenger lists economic and resource utilization benefits from collaborative studies.[8]

SUMMARY

Nursing research begins, for each nurse, with a "first" research project. Research is a set of logical steps that ensure meaningful and useful results. Start with a small project, and find the resources that help you. Contact nurses in your hospital who have advanced degrees and who have done research. Faculty members of a nearby college or university may be looking for someone with clinical expertise to collaborate with on projects. Finally, look for research results when you are solving clinical problems. If you think there must be a better way to perform a particular aspect of nursing care, there probably is one. Review the literature to see if you can find an answer; if you cannot find one, you have the beginnings of a useful research study.

REFERENCES

1. American Nurses' Association: *Research priorities for the 1980's: generating a scientific basis for nursing practice*, Pub No D-68, Kansas City, Mo, 1981, The Association.

2. American Nurses' Association: *Code for nurses with interpretive statements*, Kansas City, Mo, 1985, The Association.

3. American Nurses' Association: Commission on Nursing Research: *human rights guidelines for nurses in clinical and other research*, Kansas City, Mo, 1985, The Association.

4. American Psychological Association: *Standards for educational and psychological tests*, Washington, DC, 1974, The Association.

5. Beck CT: The research critique: general criteria for evaluating a research report, *J Obstet Gynecol Neonatal News* 19(1):18, 1990.

6. Brett JL: Organizational integrative mechanisms and adoption of innovations by nurses, *Nurs Res* 38(2):105, 1989.

7. Campbell J: A test of two explanatory models of women's responses to battering, *Nurs Res* 38(1):18, 1989.

8. Chenger PL: Collaborative nursing research: advantages and obstacles, *Int J Nurs Stud* 25(4):295, 1988.

9. Clochesy JM: Computer use and nursing research: statistical packages for microcomputers, *West J Nurs Res* 9(1):138, 1987.

10. Code of Federal Regulations: Protection of human subjects, Office of Protection from Research Risks, Reports: Sec 46.111, 46.101(b), 46.110, and 46.116(a), 1985, US Department of Health and Human Services.

11. Cohen J: *Statistical power analyses for the behavioral sciences*, rev ed, New York, 1977, Academic Press.

12. Emergency Nurses Association: *Research priorities*, Chicago, 1987, The Association.

13. Fawcett J: *Analyses and evaluation of conceptual models of nursing*, Philadelphia, 1984, FA Davis.

14. Fox DJ: *Fundamentals of research in nursing*, ed 4, East Norwalk, Conn, 1982, Appleton-Century-Crofts.

15. Frank-Stromborg M: *Instruments for clinical nursing research*, Norwalk, Conn, 1988, Appleton & Lange.

16. Funk M: Research priorities in critical care nursing, *Focus Crit Care* 16(2):135, 1989.

17. Gortner SR, Heath E, and Sanders P: The institutional review board: a case study of no-risk decisions in health-related research, *Nurs Res* 30(1):21, 1981.

18. Horsley JA: *Using research to improve nursing practice: a guide*, New York, 1983, Grune & Stratton.

19. Kehrer BH et al: The research program and priorities of the Robert Wood Johnson Foundation, *Health Serv Res* 19:439, 1984.

20. Kerlinger F: *Foundations of behavioral sciences research*, New York, 1973, Holt, Rinehart & Winston.

21. Lieber S, Executive Director, Emergency Nurses Association: Personal communication, July 10, 1990.

22. LoBiondo-Wood G and Haber J: *Nursing research: methods, critical appraisal, and utilization*, ed 2, St Louis, 1990, Mosby–Year Book.

23. McDowell J and Newell C: *Measuring health: a guide to rating scales and questionnaires*, New York, 1987, Oxford University Press.

24. Meier P and Pugh EJ: The case study: a viable approach to clinical research, *Res Nurs Health* 9:195, 1986.

25. Moody LE et al: Analysis of a decade of nursing practice research: 1977-1986, *Nurs Res* 37(6):374, 1988.

26. Moore JB: Effects of assertion training and first aid instructions on children's autonomy and self-care agency, *Res Nurs Health* 10:101, 1987.

27. Morra ME: How to plan and carry out your poster session, *Oncol Nurs Forum* 11(2):52, 1984.

28. Neff J et al: Effect of respiratory rate, respiratory depth, and open versus closed mouth breathing on sublingual temperature, *Res Nurs Health* 12:195, 1989.

29. Reference deleted in proofs.

30. Nordvig OK: Personal communication, July 13, 1990.

31. Osguthorpe N, Roper J, and Saunders J: The effect of teaching on medication knowledge, *West J Nurs Res* 5(3):205, 1983.

32. Parsons LC, Peard AL, and Page MC: The effects of hygiene interventions on the cerebrovascular status of severe closed head injured persons. *Res Nurs Health* 8:173, 1985.

33. Phillips LR: *A clinician's guide to the critique and utilization of nursing research*, Norwalk, Conn, 1986, Appleton-Century-Crofts.

34. Polit DF and Hungler BP: *Essentials of nursing research,* ed 2, Philadelphia, 1989, JB Lippincott.

35. Preusser BA et al: Quantifying with minimum discard sample required for accurate arterial blood gases, *Nurs Res* 38(5):276, 1989.

36. Rebenson-Piano M et al: An evaluation of two indirect methods of blood pressure measurement in ill patients, *Nurs Res* 38(1):42, 1989.

37. Riehl J and Roy C: *Conceptual models for nursing practice,* ed 2, New York, 1980, Appleton-Century-Crofts.

38. Rogers B: Research and practice: collaborating for improved nursing care, *AAOHN* 36(10):432, 1988.

39. Rogers E: *Diffusions of innovations,* ed 3, New York, 1983, The Free Press.

40. Sexton DL: Presentation of research findings: the poster session, *Nurs Res* 33(6):374, 1984.

41. Shelley SI: *Research methods in nursing health,* Boston, 1985, Little, Brown.

42. Smejkal CW: Research: running with a winning team, *Focus Crit Care* 16(2):147, 1989.

43. Smith LW: Microcomputer-based bibliographic searching, *Nurs Outlook* 37(2):125, 1988.

44. Swanson E and McCloskey J: Publishing opportunities for nurses, *Nurs Outlook* 34(5):227, 1986.

45. Tilden VP and Shepherd P: Increasing the rate of identification of battered women in an emergency department: use of a nursing protocol, *Res Nurs Health* 10:209, 1987.

46. Van Dalen DB: *Understanding educational research: an introduction,* New York, 1979, McGraw-Hill.

47. Van Hoozer H, Warner S, and Felton G: Creating presentation graphics with MS-DOS computer technology, *Comput Nurs* 7(4):161, 1989.

48. Watts N, Executive Director, Sigma Theta Tau (National Honor Society of Nursing): Personal communication, July 18, 1990.

49. Wilson HS: *Nursing Research,* ed 2, Redwood City, Calif, 1989, Addison-Wesley.

50. Woods NF and Catanzaro M: *Nursing research: theory and practice,* St Louis, 1988, Mosby–Year Book.

SUGGESTED READINGS

Baines EM: Winning funds for nursing research, *Nurs Connections* 2(2):5, 1989.

Brower HT and Crist, MA: Research priorities in gerontological nursing for long-term care, *Image J Nurs Sch* 17(1):22, 1985.

Cassidy VR and Oddi LF: Legal and ethical aspects of informed consent: a nursing research perspective, *J Prof Nurs* 2:343, 1986.

Crane J: Using research in practice, *West J Nurs Res* 7(2):261, 1985.

Davis AJ: Ethical issues in nursing research, *West J Nurs Res* 7:249, May 1985.

Fleming JW: Selecting a clinical nursing problem for research, *Image J Nurs Sch* 16:62, 1984.

Funkhouser SW and Grant MM: 1988 ONS survey of research priorities, *Oncol Nurs Forum* 16(3):413, 1989.

Guido GW: *Legal issues in nursing,* Norwalk, Conn, 1988, Appleton & Lange.

Hodgson C: Tips on writing successful grant proposals, *Nurs Pract* 14(2):44, 1989.

Holm K and Llewellyn JG: *Nursing research for nursing practice,* Philadelphia, 1986, WB Saunders.

Horsley JA and Crane J: Factors associated with innovation in nursing practice, *Fam Community Health* 9(1):1, 1986.

Jennings BM and Rogers S: Using research to change nursing practice, *Crit Care Nurse* 9(5):76, 1989.

Johnson SH: Selecting a journal, *Nurs Health Care* 3(5):258, 1982.

Lambert CE and Lambert VA: Clinical nursing research: its meaning to the practicing nurse, *Appl Nurs Res* 1(2):54, 1988.

Leininger MM: *Qualitative research methods in nursing,* Orlando, Fla, 1985, Grune & Stratton.

Lewandowski LA and Kositsky AM: Research priorities for critical care nursing: a study by the American Association of Critical Care Nurses, *Heart Lung* 12:35, 1983.

Lindeman CA: Research in practice: the role of the staff nurse, *Appl Nurs Res* 1(1):5, 1988.

Loomis ME: Knowledge utilization and research utilization in nursing, *Image J Nurs Sch* 17(2):35, 1985.

McClosky JC and Swanson E: Publishing opportunities for nurses: a comparison of 100 journals, *Image J Nurs Sch* 14(2):50, 1982.

Miller P et al: Strategies to promote valid and reliable nursing interventions in research, *West J Nurs Res* 11(3):373, 1989.

Morris JM: Funding strategies for qualitative research. In Morris P, ed: *Qualitative nursing research: a contemporary dialogue,* Rockville, Md, 1989, Aspen Publishers.

Nieswiadomy RM: *Foundations of nursing research,* Norwalk, Conn, 1987, Appleton & Lange.

Nokes K: Exploring the institutional review board process, *J NY State Nurses Assoc* 20(3):7, 1989.

Orsolits M: Reorganizing nursing for the future: nursing commission recommendations and research implications, *Appl Nurs Res* 2(2):64, 1989.

Polit DF and Hungler BP: *Nursing research: principles and methods,* ed 3, Philadelphia, 1987, JB Lippincott.

Rogers M: *An introduction to the theoretical basis of nursing,* Philadelphia, 1970, FA Davis.

Sexton DL: Developing skills in grant writing, *Nurs Outlook* 30(1):31, 1982.

Shapek, RA: Do's and dont's in proposal writing: how to increase your probability of obtaining federal funding, *Grants Magazine* 7(1):51, 1984.

Taunton RL: Replication: a key to research application, *Dimens Crit Care Nurs* 8(3):156, 1989.

Topf M: Response sets in questionnaire research, *Nurs Res* 35(2):119, 1986.

Tornquist EM: Strategies for publishing research, *Nurs Outlook* 31(3):180, 1983.

Tornquist EM: *From proposal to publication: an informal guide to writing about nursing research,* Menlo Park, Calif, 1986, Addison-Wesley.

Veatch RM: The National Commission on IRB: an evolutionary approach, *Hastings Center Report* 9(1):22, 1979.

Ward MJ and Fetler ME: What guidelines should be followed in critically evaluating research reports? *Nurs Res* 27:120, 1978.

Ward MJ and Lindeman CA, eds: *Instruments for measuring nursing practice and other health variables,* Washington, DC, 1978, Government Printing Office.

Waltz CF, Strickland OL, and Lenz ER: Measurement in nursing research, Philadelphia, 1984, FA Davis.

Werby HH and Fitzpatrick JJ: *Annual review of nursing research,* New York, 1985, Springer Publishing.

Western Institute of Nursing: *Communicating nursing research: choices within challenges,* Boulder, Colo, 1989, Western Institute of Nursing.

Western Institute of Nursing: *Communicating nursing research: nursing research: transcending the 20th century,* Boulder, Colo, 1990, Western Institute of Nursing.

Anne Manton

The opportunity for certification in a nursing specialty dates back to 1945, when a certification process was first initiated by the American Association of Nurse Anesthetists. Most certifications in nursing, however, were established in the last two decades. The increase in the number of nursing specialty organizations has been a major factor in the proliferation of nursing certifications. More than 40 certifications are available. Although most specialty organizations offer only 1 certification, the American Nurses' Association (ANA) offers at least 17 certifications.

PURPOSE

What is the purpose of certification? Why do nurses participate in this process? The primary purpose of certification, whether in nursing or another discipline, is to assure the public that an individual has acquired a specific body of knowledge.

In addition to providing information to the public, certification in a nursing specialty benefits the nurse who attains certification; it provides a mechanism by which the nurse can demonstrate mastery of a specific body of knowledge. Achieving certification may also result in greater esteem from employers and colleagues, salary increases, and— perhaps most important, greater self-esteem.

Employers and potential employers also benefit from nursing certification. Certification provides an objective measure of the knowledge base of employees, as well as valuable information about prospective employees. Certification thus benefits both the individual nurse and the employer and serves the public interest.

The nursing profession also benefits from the possibilities for certification. Because of the certification process, bodies of specialty nursing knowledge are defined and examined; certification demonstrates to members of other health care disciplines that nurses are able to articulate their defined body of knowledge and establish levels of specialty competence based on that knowledge.

Another way in which certification benefits the profession of nursing is that, because the certification process requires testing (at least initially), nurses usually study the body of knowledge of the specialty thoroughly in preparation for the examination. In most instances nurses are certified for a specified period of time. Although various methods for renewal of certification exist among the nurse certification agencies, the intent of recertification is to encourage the practicing nurse to remain well informed in all aspects of specialty nursing practice.

APPROACHES TO CERTIFICATION

A nurse can obtain certification in three ways. One way is to be certified by a state or government agency. State certification resembles a legal endorsement of a nurse's ability to function in certain expanded nursing roles. This process is different from that by which a nurse becomes registered. Certification by a state usually refers to a specific aspect of nursing practice that is considered beyond the level addressed in a state board examination (National Council Licensure Examination) for registration. State certification is often based on prior certification by a nurse certification body, completion of an education program, or both. In some instances a certifying examination is administered by a state agency. Requirements for state certification vary from state to state; therefore certification by one state may not be recognized by another state.

State certification has both advantages and disadvantages. Among the advantages are public recognition of specialty nursing and expanded roles in nursing practice. Perhaps most important, state certification allows the state to exercise control over those who perform in specialty or expanded roles. In this way the public may be better protected from persons not competent to practice in specialty roles.

The disadvantages of state certification include the additional responsibilities placed on state boards of nursing, which are usually already overburdened. The cost, in terms of other aspects of a board's responsibilities being neglected or delayed, must be carefully considered. Another possible disadvantage is that regulations may be so narrowly interpreted that they restrict dimensions of usual nursing practice. Perhaps the most obvious and ominous disadvantage is that when practice issues are placed in so public a domain, the door is opened for powerful lobbying groups (for example, third-party payers, medical societies, and other care providers) to influence nursing practice.

Another way in which certification can occur is via an institution. The institution may be a health care facility or an educational system. This type of certification is usually based on successful completion of an educational offering, which may be of varying length and characteristics. Most often the state or the profession does not control content or requisites for such certification. This type of certification has limited appeal outside the particular certifying institution, because consumers and professionals alike seem to more highly value academic degrees or certifications based on national standards. Some local triage, trauma nursing, or mobile intensive care nursing certifications are examples of this type of certification.

The usual way to obtain certification in a nursing specialty area is through a professional organization. Many types of certifications are offered by the ANA; most nursing practice specialty organizations, too, have developed or are in the process of developing a certification process in their specialty. This endeavor is testimony to the belief that knowledge beyond the level of safe basic nursing practice is required for specialty nursing practice.

Although mechanisms for certification vary from one specialty to another, certification granted by a specialty organization has the advantage of being nationally and internationally recognized. Certification associated with specialty nursing organizations is also more relevant to that specialty's nursing practice and defined body of knowledge.

MECHANISMS FOR SPECIALTY CERTIFICATION

The many nursing organizations that offer certification processes have developed various requirements for certification and renewal of certification. Requirements for nursing specialty certification can be placed in the following categories: education, practice, demonstration of knowledge, and renewal mechanisms.

All nursing specialty certification organizations require that candidates be registered nurses. This requirement assumes successful completion of the state board examination. Some specialties either require or are considering requiring a minimum of a bachelor's degree for certification eligibility. The completion of a master's degree is a requirement for eligibility for some ANA certification examinations. The ANA and other certifying organizations also require specific courses and clinical experiences for some certifications (for example, nurse practitioner and nurse midwife certifications).

Some certifications have practice requirements in addition to educational requirements; that is, to be eligible to take the certification examination, the nurse must have spent a certain number of hours in specialty practice. Often, however, the practice component of the certification process is a strong recommendation, not an absolute requirement. It has been demonstrated that nurses with at least 2 years of practice in a specialty are more likely to achieve a passing score on the certification examination than those with less practice time in the specialty.

All nursing specialty certifications require that the applicant for certification demonstrate mastery of the body of specialty nursing knowledge. This mastery is demonstrated by written examination. Certification examinations vary in length and format, but all are sufficient, according to the experts within the specialty, to broadly examine the applicant's knowledge base in the specialty. Written examinations provide the most objective measure of mastery of the core knowledge of the specialty. Although practical or psychomotor examinations would also measure attainment of the requisite knowledge, most certifying agencies find these examinations too cumbersome to conduct with the consistency, objectivity, and integrity necessary for the examination process.

The final component of the certification process that all nursing specialty certification agencies have in common is the renewal of certification. In almost all instances, certification is granted for a limited period of time, most often 4 or 5 years. This requirement is based on the recognition that nursing knowledge is dynamic, always changing and evolving. Thus the certified nurse's continued mastery of the knowledge base of the specialty must be verified at regular intervals. The mechanism by which certification is renewed varies with the certifying body. Many have opted for mandatory continuing education hours, although continuing education's image has been tarnished by several kinds of abuses. Weisfeld and Falk stated that "with the half-life of medical knowledge usually estimated at 5 years, and the pace of obsolescence even faster in some allied occupations, little justification can be found for requiring a demonstration of initial competence, while ignoring the need for continuing competence."[3]

EMERGENCY NURSING CERTIFICATION

The first emergency nursing certification examination was administered in July 1980. The examination has been offered each July and February since that time. Originally, answers to all 250 questions of the examination were calculated into the score, and the number of correct answers necessary for a passing score and certification was consistent at 175. Since 1980 the certification examination has evolved into a much more sophisticated measure of emergency nursing knowledge. All question-and-answer sets are now pretested for accuracy, clarity, and reliability before being included among those questions that determine the passing score. Each examination contains both pretest items (50) and items that are scored (200).

Because the degree of difficulty for each question can be determined in advance through pretesting, each new version of the examination is weighted accordingly; thus the number of correct answers necessary for a passing score and certification varies with each new examination. Because of this weighting procedure, there is no advantage in taking one examination instead of another.

Examination Content for Certification in Emergency Nursing

To ensure that the certification examination reflects current emergency nursing practice, a role delineation study was undertaken by the Board of Certification in Emergency Nursing in 1990.[2] Preliminary scrutiny of the study findings indicates considerable compatibility between current emergency nursing practice and the content of the examination. Changes have been made recently in the Certification in Emergency Nursing (CEN) examination to reflect the findings of the role delineation study. These changes have resulted in a blueprint for the examination beginning in 1992 (Table 10-1).

Because the blueprint for the CEN examination also gives attention to the components of the nursing process, this dimension is also considered in the development and design of each examination. The percentages of the nursing process components of the examination have remained the same since 1988 (Table 10-2).

The number of items for each content area can be calculated based on the 200 items that determine the score for

each examination. Each percentage point translates to 2 items (questions); for example, the content area that includes abdominal emergencies has the assigned weight of 6%. Thus each examination will include 12 items concerned with abdominal emergencies. In addition, the overall examination will have 64 assessment items based on the assigned weight of 32% established in the blueprint design.

Renewal of Certification

Certification in emergency nursing is granted for a period of 4 years after successful completion of the certification examination. Renewal of certification in emergency nursing is by written examination. The decision to require written examination for renewal of certification is rooted in the following beliefs:

1. The primary purpose of certification is to assure the public that the certified person has mastered a specific knowledge base.
2. Emergency nursing knowledge is dynamic, always changing and evolving.
3. The most effective way to determine mastery of a knowledge base is by written examination.

At the request of members of the Emergency Nurses Association and other certified emergency nurses, the possibility of using other mechanisms for renewal of certification has been investigated. No other mechanism has yet been deemed adequate for assuring the public that a nurse has the knowledge necessary for the designation, certified emergency nurse (CEN).

CONTINUING ISSUES REGARDING CERTIFICATION

Because certification is a relatively new process in nursing, many issues concerning certification remain unresolved. Some of the issues that must be addressed concern not only emergency nursing but more broadly, all certifications related to specialty nursing practice. These issues include but are not limited to educational requirements, practice requirements, the length of time for which certification is valid, renewal mechanisms, advanced levels of certification, cost of certification (from many perspectives), validity and reliability of the examination, liability con-

Table 10-1   Content weights for the CEN examination

Content area	Assigned weight
SECTION I CLINICAL PRACTICE (96% OF THE EXAMINATION)	
Abdominal emergencies	6%
Cardiovascular emergencies	9%
Disaster management	2%
Environmental emergencies	3%
Maxillofacial emergencies	4%
General medical emergencies	5%
Genitourinary and gynecologic emergencies	4%
Neurologic emergencies	8%
Obstetric emergencies	2%
Ocular emergencies	3%
Orthopedic emergencies	7%
Mental health emergencies	5%
Patient care management	8%
Respiratory emergencies	8%
Shock and multisystem trauma	8%
Substance abuse and toxicologic emergencies	5%
Surface trauma emergencies	5%
Stabilization and transfer	2%
Patient and community education	2%
SECTION II PROFESSIONAL ISSUES (4% OF THE EXAMINATION)	
Legal	2%
Organizational issues and quality assurance	2%

Table 10-2   Nursing process content weights for the CEN examination*

Content area	Assigned weight
Assessment	32%
Analysis and nursing diagnosis	16%
Planning and intervention	32%
Evaluation	16%

*Only in the Clinical Practice section of the examination are items (questions) also selected by nursing process category when each examination is constructed.

cerns, and recognition by professional colleagues and the public. The need for a national board of specialty certifications has also been discussed recently. The Emergency Nurses Association has been a participant in these discussions.

Certification in nursing specialties is here to stay. What remains to be seen is how the issues mentioned are resolved and what effects such resolutions will have on the emergency nursing certification process.

TESTING

The situation of being tested provokes anxiety in virtually everyone. It is impressive, then, that to become certified, so many nurses choose to place themselves in this situation. The number of certified nurses is a testament to the confidence nurses have in their mastery of the specialty knowledge base and to their high level of professionalism. Not surprisingly, however, many nurses resist the requirement of being tested once again to renew their certification.

Anxiety in the testing situation is *normal*. Uneasiness and anxiety occur because of the significance we (and others) attach to our success or failure on examinations. Although a certain amount of test anxiety is normal and may even be helpful, such anxiety must be kept under control. Uncontrolled test anxiety can interfere with the ability to think clearly and demonstrate knowledge effectively. The following are strategies that may help nurses reduce that uncomfortable feeling of anxiety.

Foremost among strategies to reduce anxiety is to be prepared for the examination by studying well. Confidence in your knowledge base and your ability to respond correctly to a broad variety of questions is essential.

Developing a Study Plan

To study well, you must first undertake a self-assessment to determine your strengths and weaknesses in the context of the material to be tested. You must recognize that everyone has weaknesses. If you can identify your particular weaknesses, you can rectify them.

In preparing for the CEN examination, the next step is to review the content outline for the examination as described in the *Certification Examination for Emergency Nurses Handbook for Candidates*.[1] With the content outline in mind, focus on identification of your specific areas of strength and weakness. Review the *Emergency Nursing Core Curriculum* or another comprehensive emergency nursing text. As you survey each chapter, ask yourself whether you could answer questions related to that content area. Be honest in your self-assessment. Armed with your self-assessment knowledge, look once again at the CEN examination content outline. Your studying priorities should be a combination of your relative strength or weakness in the content area and its importance (that is, percentage of questions) in the examination.

Creating a list of priorities with time lines for your study

plan may be helpful. Areas of your greatest perceived weakness that are also of high importance in the examination should be studied first. Areas of increasing strength of knowledge or areas of decreasing importance in the examination (or a combination of these) should then be studied. The last content areas to be studied should be those in which your knowledge base is strong or those in which content importance in the examination is slight.

When designing a successful study plan, two components should be considered. The first consideration is that studying should be carried out over a period of months, not weeks or days. *Cramming does not lead to success.* The other component is that some time should be left at the conclusion of your study of the content for a review. If you have followed the study plan and prepared well, the review may not be necessary; however, reviewing during the week before the examination may increase your self-confidence, an important element of success in most endeavors.

Remember that developing a study plan is vital to your success in testing. Failing to plan may mean planning to fail.

Study Techniques

Studying from a book is different from reading a novel: just as the purpose is different, so too is the method. The professional literature includes advice on successful strategies for studying; among all the strategies, common suggestions emerge. One common suggestion is to conduct a preliminary survey of the section to be studied. This survey includes a brief preview of the introductory paragraph, headings, definitions, rules, and summary paragraph. The purpose of the preliminary survey is to identify core ideas.

Another common suggestion in the many books and articles about successful studying is to develop questions related to the material being studied. Some experts suggest reading the material for ideas and questions after conducting the survey. Others suggest that, once the core ideas have been identified during the preliminary survey, the learner should construct questions appropriate to the content area and proceed with reading to answer the questions. Whether you read first and then formulate questions to be answered in a self-review or first generate questions to be answered in subsequent reading of the content, the formulation of questions is essential to studying. Although generating questions may seem to take up valuable time at first, it is through asking and answering questions that the content becomes meaningful and therefore, is retained. When studying for the CEN examination, try to relate those questions to the nursing process, because 96% of the examination, beginning in 1992, is nursing-process based. The following are examples of questions that might be formulated:

"How is _____ related to _____ ?"

"What would I look for in assessment of _____ ?"

"What information would lead me to conclude that the problem was _____ ?"

"If I saw _____ in the presence of _____ , what would that tell me?"

"What would be the most appropriate treatment for _____ ? Why?"

"How would I know that the situation was improving? or deteriorating?"

As you read each section, concentrate on the content, giving attention to ideas and concepts rather than to words by themselves. It is important to conceptualize rather than attempt to memorize. Know and understand basic principles, and reflect on their application as you study various sections. Many principles (for example, ensuring adequate airway, breathing, and circulation [ABCs], hormonal responses, and cellular responses) apply in a variety of instances. Keeping such principles in mind as you study each section makes answering those questions about the nursing process, which you have generated for yourself, easier. In this way the significance of an assessment finding or the value of a particular intervention becomes evident as a point of logic, not as something to be recalled from memory alone.

After your in-depth, concentrated reading of each section, attempt to answer questions about that section. This self-questioning reveals areas for further review. Reread those sections until understanding and recollection are achieved.

Additional hints for effective use of texts or other study aids include the following:
- Look for clues that suggest a "larger" meaning, that is, a principle.
- Give particular attention to diagrams, graphs, tables, and illustrations; these often summarize an important concept or idea.
- Note any sentences that are in boldface or italic type and all sequences of numbered items.
- Look for patterns of relationships, that is, look not only for the trees but also for the forest.
- Reduce the subject matter to easily remembered divisions. For the purposes of studying for certification, those divisions may be the nursing process components used in the design of the CEN examination: assessment, analysis and nursing diagnosis, intervention, and evaluation.

Organizing and implementing a study plan is a matter of individual study style. Some people prefer to study alone at an individual pace. Others find that studying in groups is more beneficial because discussion of information can be helpful in generating and answering questions, in identifying larger issues and principles, and in gaining understanding. To make a study group successful, however, some guidelines should be considered. It is important to develop a plan and structure to which all group members can agree. Each member of the group should have a role, or responsibility, in the presentation and discussion of topics. The group should allow time for socialization, preferably at the conclusion of each planned topical discussion. (If socializing is not planned, members often use study time for this purpose.) Be selective about group membership and about the size of the group. Remember that study groups can be an effective way to prepare for the certification examination or they can be a waste of valuable time.

Test-Taking Strategies

Perhaps the most influential factor in successful test taking is *attitude*. It is possible to thoroughly know the test material and yet fail an examination because of a poor attitude. Fear conditions the mind for failure. Fear and anxiety, as mentioned previously, can result in tension and an inability to think clearly. Fear can so overwhelm the thought processes that what was known only a few moments before can no longer be recalled. The ability to think logically, to solve problems, and to determine relationships or associations can be greatly reduced because of fear. Fear can cause careless mistakes. It is imperative to address fear and determine strategies to manage it before taking a test. Test taking involves skill. The test taker must develop a positive attitude toward his or her ability to master this skill.

The person with a successful attitude anticipates the examination as an opportunity to demonstrate what he or she knows, not as a negative situation with the potential for failure. The attitude of challenge rather than defeat leads to constructive preparation, which in turn leads to increased self-confidence and a positive attitude toward the anticipated outcome of the examination.

Because even the most well-prepared test takers experience some anxiety, well-internalized test-taking strategies can be most helpful. It may be beneficial, especially for those considered (by themselves or others) poor test takers, to practice these skills on sample test questions. The CEN handbook for candidates includes a number of such practice questions, as does the computer software and review manual available from the Emergency Nurses Association.

Strategies for enhancing test-taking skills include the following:
1. Pay attention to instructions and follow them. This strategy may seem obvious, but extreme fear and anxiety can influence even the most basic test activities. Conversely, following instructions correctly can allow the test taker time to overcome the initial nervousness and may represent a degree of control that allows a positive attitude to prevail.
2. Read the stem of each item (question) carefully. Observe all qualifying terms such as the following: always, never, most, usually, not, except, first, initial, primary, next, best, most important, highest, lowest, least, and contraindicated. These words tell you what the question is really asking. Failure to notice these words may lead to a misinterpretation of the question and thus to an incorrect answer.
3. After reading the stem of the item carefully, for-

mulate an answer before looking at the answer choices given. (This strategy is effective only when you know the content.) Once you have arrived at what you think the answer is, look to see whether that is one of the answer choices. If it is, select that answer. If your answer is not a choice, reread the stem. Did you misinterpret what was asked? Is there an answer choice that is similar to yours but with different terminology? If you are still not sure of the answer, do you know enough about the content area to rule out some of the answers? Ruling out incorrect answers often leads to the correct answer.

4. When the content is unfamiliar, try to select the best option. Can you rule out any answer choices? Think about any general principles (for example, ABCs) that may assist you in choosing an answer or eliminating choices. Think, too, of answers with content that would be therapeutic, ensure patient safety, promote comfort, demonstrate respect, and communicate acceptance. Look for terminology in the stem of the question that may be compatible with or suggestive of one particular answer choice.

5. When the content is familiar but none of the answers listed is the one you consider correct, do not become flustered. The overriding rule of test taking is to select the *best* answer from those presented. Reread the stem to make sure you have correctly interpreted what the question is asking; then select the *best* choice available, even if it is not the answer you would prefer.

6. Answer first the questions you know. Do not skip freely through the examination, but if you have followed all the suggestions previously listed and are not able to decide on an answer, leave that question and go on to the next one. You may find that information in a later question jogs your memory or that turning your attention to a different question may allow an attitude change, which may permit a new view of the unanswered question later. Remember to leave a space on the answer sheet for the missing answer. (You may want to mark the place lightly in the margin of the answer sheet.)

7. Do not read too much into the question. Assumptions frequently cause knowledgeable individuals to answer incorrectly. Do not make assumptions about information that is not given; use only the information that is included in the stem of the question. Any information that is important to your ability to select the correct answer is included in the stem. Think in terms of the *usual, not the unusual.*

8. If an answer choice includes a totally unfamiliar term, try to decipher the term by considering its roots. If the word remains a mystery, the response is probably not the correct one. The certification examination attempts to test important aspects of emer-

gency nursing; a term that is totally unfamiliar is unlikely to be part of the idea that is being tested. Consider the unfamiliar term a distractor: do not be tricked.

9. There is no penalty on the CEN examination for incorrect responses; your computed score is based only on the number of correct responses. Therefore you should *answer every question on the examination,* even if you have to guess.

10. Once you have decided on an answer, do not change it without good reason. Your first response is likely to be the correct one. Often the temptation to change an answer is the result of reading too much into the question or thinking of the unusual rather than the usual.

11. Although the time allowed for the CEN examination is considered sufficient, it is important to manage time effectively during the examination. There are 250 questions to be answered in approximately 4 hours. To allow ample time for review at the completion of testing, you should answer between 65 and 70 questions per hour. Check periodically to ensure that you are within these guidelines. Some individuals proceed through the examination at a considerably faster pace than others. Do not allow yourself to be distracted from the test by others who are finished. Speed is not an indicator of performance on the examination. Take the time you need to read the questions carefully and answer them correctly.

12. After every 15 to 20 questions, check to make sure that the number on the answer sheet corresponds to the question number on the examination. Mistakes can easily be made in placement of answers on the answer sheet. If this happens, you do not want to discover the error when the examination is completed.

13. After completing the test, check the answer sheet one more time. Make sure that each space on the answer sheet has been filled with an answer selection. If any questions had been deferred, make sure that these have been answered.

14. Throughout the examination, control your fear and anxiety. Remember that to pass the test, you do not have to answer every question correctly. Remember, too, that every examination contains items that are being pretested; these items do not affect your score. Perhaps the questions that are difficult for you are pretest items.

15. Believe in yourself and your ability to successfully pass the CEN examination or any other examination.

REFERENCES

1. Board of Certification in Emergency Nursing: *Certification examination for emergency nurses handbook for candidates 1990 examinations,* Chicago, 1991, Emergency Nurses Association.

2. Certification Review Board: Blueprint for 1992 CEN examination, *CEN Newsletter* 4(2):8, 1990.
3. Weisfeld N, Falk D: Chasing elusive competence, *Hospitals* 57(5):68, 1983.

SUGGESTED READINGS

Carlson ME: Certification in nephrology: credentialing issues, *ANNA* 17(3):264, 1990.
Collins HL: Certification: is the payoff worth the price? *RN* 50(7):36, 1987.
Dickenson-Hazard N: The importance of recertification, *Pediatr Nurs* 14(2):137, 1988.
Knapp JE: Assuring continuing competency: a snapshot of current practice, *Spec Nurs Forum* 2(3):1, 1990.
Kortbawi PA: Test taking skills: giving yourself an edge, *Nurs '90* 20(6): 95, 1990.
Sides MB and Cailles NB: *Nurses guide to successful test-taking*, Philadelphia, 1989, JB Lippincott.
Waherman CE: *Credentialing in nursing: contemporary development and trends. The 1979 study of credentialing in nursing recommendations: where are we now?* Kansas City, Mo, 1986, American Nurses' Association.

Physical Assessment

Joan Kelley Simoneau

The key to all aspects of patient care is a good assessment. A thorough understanding of patient assessment provides insight into the various findings that assist implementation of the steps of the nursing process. A concise yet comprehensive patient assessment allows for proper diagnosis of the patient's problems and application of the appropriate therapeutic interventions.

The spectrum of events that constitutes an emergency varies considerably with each individual patient. In recent years the number of patients seen in the emergency department (ED) has increased markedly, and in this hectic environment it becomes crucial that there be a continuous effort to identify patients with critical or potentially critical conditions. Often the responsibility of the initial evaluation falls to the emergency nurse, who is frequently the first professional to encounter the patient.

Although the degree of assessment and intervention differs for each patient, the process is a dynamic one; it is often of singular importance to establishing management priorities. Development of accurate decisions for action depends largely on whether the nurse employs an organized and systematic approach to the assessment process. Although tools are helpful in the physical examination, the initial observations that serve to focus the assessment require no equipment. During this period the most important tools are the senses of sight, touch, smell, and hearing—in other words, common sense. Much depends on the skill of the observer to interpret what significance the information collected has in the clinical situation.

The potential for deterioration exists for any patient in the department. If subtle changes are overlooked or ignored, this deterioration is not only possible but may rapidly become irreversible, even if recognized and treated vigorously later. If, for instance, we were to place each patient at an arbitrary point of relative wellness or equilibrium (point A), we can plot out a path based on timeliness of intervention. If we recognize the patient's physiologic and emotional

needs at that point and move to provide intervention, we will either maintain this equilibrium or improve the patient's condition. If, however, intervention is delayed or absent, the patient will move down the path to point B. Point B is that place on the curve at which a great deal of effort and skill must be expended to halt and reverse the descent. If the patient does not receive appropriate intervention at point B, he or she will progress further down to point C, or death.

In essence, all our efforts must be directed toward the arrest of any downhill descent at whatever point we receive the patient, whether the patient is sitting up and comfortable with only ankle pain or obtunded and gravely ill. The primary purpose of nursing assessment is to use the scientific method of collecting patient information and implementing a nursing plan and interventions based on a reasonable interpretation of signs and symptoms, thus preventing deterioration and death, as well as evaluating the results.

The focus of this chapter is to identify the practical aspects of nursing assessment. Specific disease assessments are avoided in favor of presenting them within the individual chapters that deal with each system. Rather an overview is provided that serves as a helpful guideline for the emergency nurse to use in the day-to-day situation. Potential barriers to assessments by nurses are also presented to build a respect for the obstacles that may hamper or destroy efforts to assess patients. Equipment and steps of physical assessment are covered in detail. With this information, more nurses may become involved with one of the most important and satisfying functions that the emergency nurse can perform: nursing assessment of the emergency patient. Nursing diagnosis is discussed in Chapter 8.

BARRIERS TO PATIENT ASSESSMENT

If assessment of the emergency patient is such a vital aspect of emergency management, why is it that nursing assessment is not routinely performed in every department? The reason is that there are barriers to effective and consistent assessment. If these barriers can be recognized and reduced or avoided, they may have less impact on the process. The most common barriers can be categorized into

This chapter was originally written for the first edition of the book. Because of its timeless nature and thoroughness, it has been retained for this edition.

three groups: professional, institutional, and patient-related. These same groups are discussed in more detail in this chapter.

Professional Barriers to Assessment

Traditionally many have thought that patient assessment and management were solely the physician's responsibility. Evaluating signs and symptoms, interpreting collected physical data, developing a working diagnosis of the cause of the discovered abnormalities, and initiating treatment were all considered to fall within the physician's purview; nurses were not expected to become involved with this process. Even today *diagnosis* is considered a medical term, and many physicians and traditional nurses are alarmed by the growing use of this word in the nursing vocabulary.

As emergency medicine and critical care became more sophisticated and as greater numbers of patients were seeking care within the ED, there were not sufficient numbers of physicians in each unit to provide timely evaluation for every patient. The on-duty physician began to rely on those nurses who had integrated knowledge with judgment for information about the status of patients within the department. These nurses became adept at aiding in the establishment of management priorities. Within recent years a growing awareness has been developing: many nurses are actively assessing patients and developing a nursing diagnosis through which they are providing initial stabilization and intervention; this function is an important element in meeting the immediate needs of many patients. Particularly within the larger facilities, a healthy respect now exists for the ability of nursing professionals within the ED to ensure that optimal treatment can be made available for each patient.

Unfortunately, many facilities continue to expound the traditional philosophy; in these hospitals the terms *nursing assessment*, *physical assessment*, and *nursing diagnosis* are not acceptable. The concept that a physician is able to rely on nurses for valid information on patient condition and for appropriate intervention in emergencies is a new one. Attitudes that relegate emergency nurses to a position of active involvement in undressing patients and obtaining their vital signs but inactive involvement in assessing their signs and symptoms are frustrating to nurses who have been educated to perform more than simple patient hygiene duties. Moreover, such conditions fail to effectively use the health care team in the department. On the other hand, to develop confidence in their abilities, emergency nurses must use their skills and knowledge wisely and not consider themselves surrogate physicians. Attitudes steeped in tradition retard the development of a solid team within the ED, particularly in environments where there is a failure to perceive that assessment of patients is a necessary function of the emergency nurse. If assessment is not considered part of the nursing obligation, evaluation of patients will be inconsistent and most likely performed only by those nurses who

have a strong sense of identity and have received the necessary education to perform assessments correctly.

Many states have begun to enhance progressive attitudes by establishing nursing practice acts, which allow for the performance of expanded role functions. However, until nurses themselves become more comfortable with the responsibility for performing nursing assessments and initiating appropriate therapy, and until they assertively seek support from the medical community for the development of such skills, this barrier will continue to exist and undermine assessment efforts.

Institutional Barriers to Assessment

Multiple nurse contact. Contact of several nurses with one patient may be a significant barrier to effective assessment and intervention. In departments where nursing personnel frequently work without benefit of specific patient assignments, the confusion and lack of communication regarding patient status, particularly in busy times, can result in inconsistent or delayed intervention. Consider what may happen if one nurse performs triage, another prepares the patient for examination and takes vital signs, another enters the cubicle to complete the assessment process, another carries out treatment orders, and still another discharges the patient. Either perfect or consistent communication must take place, or significant gaps or errors may occur in management of the patient throughout the emergency department visit.

The only way to reduce this barrier to effective assessment and intervention is to implement a system of staff assignment, specific not only to areas of the department but also to treatment beds. Such assignments help establish responsibility and accountability for nursing assessments and nursing management. When a nurse is assigned to a particular bed or area, that nurse is the primary nursing clinician for that patient(s). No other nurse should intervene in the patient care plan thus established unless appropriate communication is carried out between the two nurses.

Float nurse staffing. Using nurses from other areas to help staff the ED may become a significant barrier if a nurse in question serves infrequently as an ED nurse or has never received training in assessment in the emergency setting. Others working in the unit may erroneously assume that the nurse in question is providing equivalent evaluation when this may not be the case.

Superiors in each facility must determine, using input from the nurses in the ED, whether the benefits outweigh the risks of using float or registry nurses in their department. The qualifications and capabilities of such personnel, if they are used, must be clearly identified to the regular department staff, including the physician on duty, to prevent misconception and potential patient compromise. In addition, it is recommended that all float and registry nurses receive an orientation to the department before they are expected to perform without supervision.

Imbalance of staff versus patient volume. If the number of nurses does not allow sufficient time and contact with each patient, a barrier may develop. Nursing staff-to-patient ratios should be calculated based on known and anticipated volume and on the percentage of critically ill patients anticipated within that volume, as determined by past experience and distribution studies. Identification of peak load through study and evaluation may be time consuming, but it can be of tremendous value in setting realistic staffing equivalents and patterns.

Particularly in busy departments, insufficient staffing may promote a dangerous situation in which priorities are not established consistently and symptoms that require prompt intervention might be overlooked or patient flow into treatment areas may be disrupted. The additional danger of insufficient staffing is that although minimal coverage may allow for the assessment process to be carried out under normal circumstances, unexpected volume peaks or depletion of existing staff because of illness or break times may contribute to the same end results as already noted. These factors are uncontrollable, but the institution must allow for sufficient staff to handle potential volume through careful evaluation of peak load trends.

Obviously there are times, such as in a disaster situation, when even careful planning and normally sufficient staff will not be adequate to meet the need. During these times assessments must necessarily be limited to the essentials, but assessments are no less important; each nurse must make effective decisions regarding the extent of evaluation that is appropriate under the circumstances. It is of tantamount importance, however, that during these situations frequent assessments be performed to prevent or to recognize and treat life-threatening conditions.

One of the most devastating effects of inadequate staffing is the eventual burnout that occurs with the nurses who continue to provide effective assessment even though the department is shorthanded and the number of patients is increasing. Continuation of such efforts requires a motivation that often wears out unless administrators address the problems caused by lack of sufficient nursing staff per patient volume.

Lack of appropriate staff resources for assessment. A lack of language interpreters, multisystem laboratory facilities, social service or psychiatric support personnel, and radiologic services can significantly affect nursing assessment, as well as physician assessment and management. Both categories of personnel are affected when the resources necessary to perform thorough examination are not available.

One of the most underrated resources is the language interpreter. It is extremely difficult to adequately assess a patient who cannot speak or understand the same language as the health professional. If a language interpreter is not available, the entire patient history may be unattainable. Although behavioral clues may be interpreted and integrated into the assessment, vital subjective information is lost. This loss of information may contribute to misinterpreting or missing physical symptoms that otherwise might have helped establish a cause of the patient's condition. Moreover, it is sometimes difficult even to establish a primary patient complaint on which to base the assessment.

Accessible laboratory and radiologic services greatly affect the quality of the physical assessment. A major element of the physical data base is lacking or delayed if the laboratory and radiologic services are located far from the emergency department, if they are closed during peak load hours, or if they are not available at all.

Environmental barriers. Within the institution, environmental barriers include poor lighting, excessive ambient noise levels, and lack of patient privacy. Poor area lighting interferes with critical observations such as skin color and wound status. High ambient noise levels interfere with the interpretation of auscultated sounds, if they can be heard at all. Lack of privacy may prevent adequate physical evaluation and collection of personal information, which the patient may be embarrassed to give without adequate privacy. Consider the gynecologic examining table so placed that when the door of the examining room is opened, the patient and examining physician are exposed to a full view of everyone in the vicinity.

The most effective way to reduce the impact of environmental barriers is to recognize them and take appropriate steps to improve the situation. Provide extra lighting if necessary, using focus lighting for the evaluation of wounds and skin color and for illuminating an area before any procedure. Take steps to reduce the noise level in the treatment areas by encouraging only appropriate and necessary conversation. If possible, acoustic tile should be affixed to the ceiling and padded linoleum applied to the floors. Reduced traffic flow of unnecessary personnel and visitors through the treatment areas increases privacy during examination and treatment.

Institutional barriers are not usually insurmountable, yet they tend not to be addressed because, if significant changes are necessary to reduce or alleviate them, money is often required. Hospital administration, aided by the objective input from nurses working in the unit, can do a great deal to effect change. If there are difficulties in explaining existing problems to personnel not exposed to the situation, rational and organized evaluations of the problems with alternatives for change may help those in authority to set appropriate priorities.

Patient-Related Barriers

Patient-related barriers to assessment are unpredictable and present the greatest challenge. It is difficult to present a straightforward listing of all these, since overlapping often occurs.

Language barriers. The language barriers mentioned earlier do not apply only to the non-English-speaking patient; the deaf, deaf-mute, and mentally disabled patient also may not receive adequate assessment because of a language barrier. When there is a significant difference between the medical jargon used and the patient's level of understanding, the assessment process may also be affected, but in a more subtle manner. For example, Mr. Jones, who is obviously alert and oriented, enters the department complaining of pains in his abdomen. Mr. Jones is asked about his past medical history, what medications he is currently taking, and who his private physician is, along with many other questions. Should he manage to understand what is being asked of him and give the appropriate answers, he is taken into a treatment room and asked to undress and put on a gown, climb onto a gurney, and wait to have his vital signs taken. If he is not yet totally bewildered by this alien environment, he will have further opportunity to become bewildered, because he will be expected to have the language tools to describe his symptoms and the ability to interpret what he is expected to do when he is asked to go into the restroom to collect a clean-catch urine specimen.

This example identifies important points. It is extremely difficult to know when a patient understands what is being said. The best-dressed, most sophisticated, most alert patient might be the one patient who has not the slightest idea what "radiation of pain" or any other technical jargon means. It is folly to assume that any patient will be able to integrate what most nurses consider logical and comprehensive. Nor should we assume that the myriad tests or methodologies of assessment will not cause apprehension that will interfere with the patient's ability to make sense of his or her situation.

To prevent the exchange of inaccurate or misleading information, watch the patient's face and behavior carefully to identify whether he or she is able to synthesize what is happening, what you are saying, and what is expected. Although the patient may not understand the events, he or she wants to give the information you are seeking because the patient hopes to receive the correct treatment; for the same reason the patient may not tell you that he or she is confused. Use simple and direct language, but try not to sound patronizing. Lack of understanding medical jargon is widespread but unpredictable: occasionally a patient may be insulted by a patronizing tone or expression.

Interference by family members. In the process of history taking or examination, family interference may become disruptive to the flow of information between patient and nurse. Such intrusion usually occurs when a family member insists on answering questions for the patient even though the patient may be quite capable of doing so. An example is the overprotective mother who does not allow her 20-year-old son to describe his symptoms or who insists on being present during examination so that she can make absolutely certain that her son "doesn't forget anything." More tolerable but certainly just as disruptive is the elderly husband and wife team. After hours of arguing, Mrs. Smith finally talks her husband into coming into the department for treatment of his indigestion. Then she proceeds to interfere with the triage process by giving information that she believes her husband is forgetting or by arguing with him when she thinks his story is incorrect.

Whenever possible, obtain the history directly from the patient. Use language that the patient can understand, and question the patient when anything he or she says does not make sense to you. State clearly what assistance you wish from any family members who might be present, where you wish them to be during the examination process, and what behavior you will not tolerate. To avoid embarrassment of the patient and potential conflict or irritation between staff and family, family members should not be present during the physical examination portion of the assessment if the patient is capable of cooperating and answering questions.

Emergency staff attitudes. Attitudes of the emergency staff are extremely important. The attitude of the nurse performing the assessment may significantly affect the quality of the relations thus established and may subsequently interfere with patient compliance throughout and beyond this visit. If your attitude is one of haste, indifference, or irritation, even if such attitude is not directly related to the current situation, the patient will sense it and respond either accordingly or by becoming agitated. He or she may be afraid of answering questions "incorrectly" or afraid to antagonize you further and so may forget important elements or may even falsify the situation to smooth the interaction. The patient may even react with hostile behavior, beginning a cycle of resistance and counterresistance that is harmful to the assessment process. Remember that each patient who enters the department is extremely sensitive to being placed completely in the hands of strangers and may find it difficult to feel comfortable in trusting them with his or her life or health. If the patient senses that he or she is a burden, is made to feel stupid, or is treated with disrespect, the situation may result in anxiety, fear, panic, or uncooperative behavior.

Prejudgment of the patient. Prejudging may be manifest in a variety of ways, all of which somehow adversely affect the assessment process. The use of "why" questions when taking a patient's history or when performing triage after the patient's arrival at the triage desk is sure to produce defensiveness. Questions such as, "Why did you wait 6 months to come in if you have been having back pain for that long?" imply that the patient is misusing the department or is too stupid to take appropriate care of himself or herself. Other questions that are counterproductive to the interveiw are those directed at why the patient did or did not do something. "Why did you stop taking your seizure medicine?" or "Why did you leave the bleach out where Johnny could get hold of it?" are examples of questions that surely make the patient feel defensive and interfere with the smooth exchange of information. Such questions can be asked much more gently and supportively, and tone and expression play a significant role in how the patient may perceive the questions. When you ask a patient the reasons for not taking prescribed medication, for example, using an accepting expression and a gentle tone can turn a potentially hostile situation into a productive exchange of information.

A much more disturbing type of prejudgment is the premature determination that the patient's condition is nonemergent based on inadequate or faulty data. The tendency to prejudge the patient is often influenced by the patient's attitude ("She doesn't act as if she has just been raped"), the number of visits that the patient has made to the department ("This is the third time this week that James has come in with the same complaint, and there is never anything wrong"), the presentation of history or symptoms that on casual observation do not seem to correlate with the clinical picture, and a variety of other factors. The unfortunate result of prejudgment by health professionals is that the patient ultimately bears the burden of proving that he or she has an emergency. In addition, prejudgment may result in collection of only that information which supports the prejudgment, thus causing errors in assessment or intervention.

It is extremely important to listen to the patient describe his or her history and symptoms no matter what the circumstances may be. As the patient is describing his or her situation, compare the patient's appearance with his or her report and history. Make every attempt not to form conclusions or force the interview in the direction that you think correct. Above all, do not stop collecting information when you have only that which supports your subjective analysis of the patient's status. If you feel judgmental, try to determine why this has happened. Verify your conclusions with someone else before taking action, or more important, before *not* taking action. Finally, recognize that prejudging a patient may lead you into unnecessary error unless you are willing to concentrate on information contrary to your initial diagnosis.

Patient attitude and appearance. The attitude and appearance of the patient may influence the assessment process. If the manner in which a patient responds to questions and directions is derogatory, the attitude of those around the patient may be adversely affected. It is difficult to be kind and gentle with everyone who comes into the department, especially on a busy shift during which you are barely able to maintain a sympathetic attitude. The tenuous hold on your composure may be threatened by an unruly, overbearing patient, especially if you find it hard to tolerate such behavior even on your good days. Resistance to directions, hostility that appears to have no legitimate basis, and mental confusion, particularly when caused by substance abuse, may alienate the staff and reduce effective interaction and assessment. It is most helpful to avoid personalizing antagonistic behavior, which often is an attempt on the part of the patient to cope with feelings of helplessness. Keep in mind that the most positive action that can be taken is to reassure the patient through empathetic and professional

behavior and to let him or her know that assistance will be given. When you think that you cannot cope with the situation, get someone else on staff to take over for you. Most important is to recognize that you can help the patient regain control of his or her behavior only when you refuse to take it personally; when the patient regains control, the inappropriate behavior should subside.

The more difficult patient for the nurses is the dirty, foul-smelling, unkempt one wearing layers of insect-infested clothing. The patient with poor personal hygiene may be subjected to delays in assessment while the staff determines who is willing to touch him or her. In these situations it is likely that the patient will receive only hasty or incomplete evaluation and may never even be completely undressed. Some facilities have showers that can accommodate a stretcher, and the patient can be wheeled into the stall fully clothed and may be washed down while being undressed. Whatever the method used to deal with the situation, this patient should receive the same meticulous and systematic assessment given to any other patient.

Patient age. The age of the patient may present unexpected problems. It is difficult to conduct an assessment on the young or the old patient who cannot describe symptoms or express discomfort appropriately. Elderly patients do not sense pain as acutely as younger patients do and elderly patients also are often confused and forgetful. Even the mother of the pediatric patient may not be able to accurately describe the events relative to the child's illness or injury.

Neurologic, cardiac, and respiratory parameters in the pediatric and geriatric patient differ from normal ranges, and it takes time and practice to develop the skills necessary to identify subtle signs and correlate them into a meaningful picture. With a basic understanding of common pediatric and geriatric disease and trauma, and with practice under the supervision of someone skilled in pediatric and geriatric assessment, the job of evaluating patients in these age ranges becomes easier. Remember that these patients are different from the young and middle-aged adult, and realize that care must be taken to evaluate them carefully to avoid error.

Summary. All the barriers to patient assessment exist in one form or another in health care departments all over the United States. These barriers hamper and retard some professional emergency nurses; others resolve the problems and work around the barriers. The only way to lessen their potential impact on daily operation and their interference with effective patient assessment is to be familiar with their many aspects, to recognize that they exist, and to make every effort to provide optimal evaluation for each patient despite the barriers. Determining how best to reduce barriers will lessen their effect on nursing performance.

DOCUMENTATION OF NURSING ASSESSMENT AND INTERVENTION

Information collected through the assessment process and action taken during the intervention phase must be documented in such a manner that others who are concerned with the care of the patient will be aware of the events that have taken place. Recorded information is not only valuable for continuity of care but it also serves as a helpful tool for auditing and teaching purposes.

Many facilities use separate nursing records in the emergency department, whereas others use the face sheet of the patient's ED record for nurses' notes. Often, however, the face sheet does not contain enough space for the documentation of serial nursing assessments. The form used for nursing documentation depends on the individual facility, but the method of documentation must be clearly understood by everyone involved in the management of cases and should not vary significantly within the department. If several different methods are used in one department, information cannot be abstracted from the record quickly, and fragmentation of care, duplication of effort, and deletions in assessment are more likely to occur.

It is as vital for nurses to chart their findings as it is for physicians to document theirs. An organized method of charting facilitates case management and contributes to the development of an individualized plan of action. Problem-oriented charting is one of the most effective modes; it is based on the problem-oriented medical record (POMR) format, which was developed by a physician who wanted a tool that would aid in the organized management of all known and potential patient problems. The system includes the elements listed in the box below. This method of documenting information provides for a "closed loop," in which one step leads into another until each of the problems has been addressed and resolved. If an action has not been effective in resolving a problem, evaluation of the action naturally returns to the first step, where additional data can assist in the development of further action.

A most effective method of documenting patient management over a long-term (inpatient) period, the POMR is being used more frequently in the ED for charting of a single patient problem that might have numerous associated smaller problems. When the POMR is used, none of the problems can be overlooked, even though some may appear to be inconsequential relative to the entire case. For instance, suppose the plan of action for a victim of a head injury is to discharge him home. If the original problem list that is naturally developed from the history, physical examination, and diagnostic tests reveals that the patient lives alone, is elderly, and has difficulty with physical coordination, the patient cannot be discharged with instructions for head injury care before arrangements are made to have a friend or relative remain with him overnight. If no one is available to do so, then the problem must be resolved differently, perhaps by admitting the patient overnight for head injury observation, even though under other circumstances such action might not have been necessary. If the POMR was not used in this case, personnel in a busy department might have overlooked a potentially dangerous situation fraught with legal liability.

The SOAP process, which is used in problem-oriented charting, is a simple and valuable framework for documentation in the emergency department: the mnemonic SOAP is an abbreviation for the successive recording of *s*ubjective information, or the information that the patient provides in answer to questions; *o*bjective information, or that which is elicited through examination and diagnostic tests; *a*ssessment of the information that has been gathered through the history and physical examination (working diagnosis); and a *p*lan of action to resolve the problem. The SOAP process can be used effectively for documentation of the nursing assessment on nursing flow sheets. Properly completed, the SOAP system can be an extremely effective tool for recording the patient assessment process and intervention performed by nurses or physicians. Such a system emphasizes recorded data rather than memory and reflects an orderly thought process. The system also lends itself to progressive audit; faulty documentation or thinking is readily evident to the reviewer. Even if the evaluation of the patient is abbreviated because of the urgency of the situation, the examiner is not likely to forget anything if the SOAP process of recording is used from the outset. An example of SOAP charting is presented in the box on the next page.

Whatever method of recording is used must be reasonably straightforward and clearly understood and should be used by all the nurses and physicians. Many nurses complain that their charting is never read by anyone other than themselves. It is certainly more likely that this will be the case if they continue to use narrative styles of recording that reflect disorderly thought processes, or if they chart nothing of more significance than "Mr. Jones is complaining of pain."

Memory, verbal reporting, and cryptic notes recorded in small areas of the face sheet of the patient's record or on the bed linen are not acceptable for documenting patient care. The qualitative recording of the history and physical findings is necessary to a systematic thought process and is becoming more important than ever before in legal reviews

---

PROBLEM-ORIENTED MEDICAL RECORD CHARTING

Data base Records the history, physical findings, and diagnostic test results

Problem list Enumerates the problems that can be identified, as well as those that can conceivably be anticipated, and separates them all into active and inactive (resolved) categories

Plan Identifies a written plan for addressing each of the active problems on the list

Action Provides a record of the plans that are to be implemented, those that have been implemented, and an evaluation of their effectiveness

---

EXAMPLE OF SOAP CHARTING

S: 31 y/o cauc female c/o S.O.B. × 2 hrs. States dyspnea onset while brushing teeth. Onset associated c̄ sharp pain (L) midscapular line radiating through to anterior chest. Now "hurts to take a deep breath." Pain now intermittent, on inspiration, and of moderate severity with no relief on position change.

O: Alert, oriented × 4. Appears anxious. Skin moist, cool, pale. Although pain is intermittent, unable to find comfortable position when experienced. Neck veins flat @ 30° elevation. Respirations 30, regular, shallow, symmetric chest rise. Breath sounds diminished (L) apex anteriorly, otherwise vesicular c I > E @ posterior bases. 0 abnormal lung sounds. Peripheral pulses equal bilat., reg. rate & rhythm. Monitor → SVT @ 130. BP 120/80. Heart sounds reg. Abd. nontender, flat. No calf tenderness.

A: Respiratory distress, moderate. SVT per monitor.

P: O₂ @ 5l/cannula. Cardiac monitor continuous Lead 2. Blood specimens drawn, sent for CBC, lytes, hold for further tests. 1000 cc N/S via #18 angiocath and reg. tubing started in dorsum R hand. ABGs drawn from L radial artery before O₂ therapy. Allen's test positive for ulnar circ.

---

of patient records. Documentation must be legible, accurate, and complete to be of most value. Problem-oriented charting that includes the SOAP process readily reveals the thoroughness or sloppiness of the person recording the information. Both systems also depend on the judicious use of abbreviations, which, if not universally understood, may prove more a detriment than an aid to patient care.

SETTING PRIORITIES FOR ASSESSMENT

Often during discussions of nursing assessment, someone protests that not every patient who comes to the department requires the thorough assessment promoted in many textbooks. Some hospitals filter clinic cases through the ED when clinics are not available. Others have such a tremendous volume of cases that serial assessments seem ideal at best. No hard and fast rules can be made either for assessment of each patient or for how assessments must be performed when time permits. However, when the patient volume is heavy, skilled nurses adopt effective methods of assessment if motivation, education, and support are present; therefore heavy volumes are no excuse to neglect the process in most cases. Also, in facilities that have a light emergency department caseload and therefore may not have a physician on duty at all times, it is vital that nurses perform assessments to identify and treat life-threatening conditions.

The individual nurse in each department must determine what extent of assessment is appropriate to each patient situation. Unfortunately, those who are labeled "clinic patients" are almost automatically considered nonemergency patients and are rarely beneficiaries of even the most cursory assessment. This practice is dangerous; it is nearly always appropriate to perform at least a general overview and primary survey and to collect a history and subjective information from the patient to set reasonable priorities for care. Even though the patient is labeled a clinic patient because he or she brought a clinic card or mentioned belonging to a clinic, it cannot be assumed that the patient has no significant health emergency until an objective evaluation is made of the patient's current situation.

It is precisely when patient volumes are heavy, when a department repeater comes in, or when a clinic patient arrives that the assessment process can establish unanticipated and potentially crucial problems and avert a major catastrophe. Nursing assessment should not be reserved for the critically ill patient. If intelligent judgments are made regarding the extent of assessment warranted by each patient, nursing assessment can be performed for everyone who comes to the department for care.

STEPS IN ASSESSMENT

Following organized steps maximizes effectiveness of the assessment, even when some of the steps must be delayed to allow for intervention. Although the steps presented in this section are in flow format, the sequence of steps varies depending on the individual circumstances; therefore the format described is intended as a guide to the vital elements of the assessment process. The environment within the ED often dictates that the process be adapted to the situation at hand, and probably the most important concept for nurses to understand is that they must develop and consistently use the approach that is most meaningful to the individuals using it. Flexibility can be developed if nurses are thoroughly familiar with the steps of assessment and meticulous in follow-through. Proficiency is maintained by constantly practicing assessment skills.

Primary Assessment

The priorities of nursing assessment are always the respiratory and cardiovascular systems. During initial contact with the patient, the nurse must determine the status of the airway and respond to priorities for intervention. Visually observe for patency of the airway and adequacy of ventilation based on skin color, respiratory effort, tidal volume, and use of accessory muscles in breathing. Determine the level of consciousness in terms of whether the patient is able to respond. Simultaneously check the pulse and observe for ventilation.

The primary assessment is mandatory for every patient with whom you come in contact, regardless of presenting status. Also referred to as the *primary survey*, this observation should be completed within 30 seconds. If a patient does not have a patent airway, has inadequate ventilations, or is pulseless, intervention in these life-threatening instances supersedes further assessment. The same holds true if there are variables that also may be life threatening, such as cardiac dysrhythmias that are first noted when checking the pulse and appear to be hemodynamically significant. Under such circumstances, such elements of the assessment process as history are delayed or conducted simultaneously as intervention is implemented.

General Survey

The general survey proceeds beyond the fundamental considerations of airway, breathing, and circulation to a more systematic observation of the patient, which should include observation of the following:

- Affect and mood, including thought organization
- Quality of speech (normal, slurred, silent, unable to speak)
- General appearance (manner of dress, hygiene, color of skin, facial expression)
- Posture and motor activity (upright posture should be observed if possible; motor activity should be observed while the patient walks, sits, undresses, and so on)
- Odors (breath, skin)
- Evaluation of degree of distress, based on all the observations preceding this determination

The general survey can be conducted simultaneously with the primary survey. Combining the two becomes easier with practice. Often both the primary and the general survey can be combined with the patient history interview; the determining factor is the patient's condition at the time. If immediate or unanticipated problems arise, the interview may be delayed and completed either during the physical examination or after the patient's condition has been stabilized.

History

The patient history interview in the ED focuses on the chief complaint, and the questions, although open ended, should be directed by that complaint. The key to obtaining information about the chief complaint–the reason why the patient came to the department—is to listen to what the patients says as he or she tries to tell you what is wrong. What the patient tells you is by definition subjective and therefore demands an objective assessment. The chief complaint should not be recorded as a diagnosis (possible fractured left arm) but exactly as the patient describes the problem (fell from stepladder, now pain and swelling in left arm).

If the patient initially comes to the triage area and is physically able to proceed though the triage process, the history can be completed there. If, however, the patient enters the department by ambulance or other vehicle and cannot be processed through the triage area, it is generally the responsibility of the nurse managing the patient in the

---

EMERGENCY HISTORY DATA

History of the present illness or injury
    How and when the injury or illness first occurred
        Influencing factors
        Symptom chronology and duration
        Related symptoms
        Location of pain or discomfort
        What, if anything, the patient has done about the
          symptoms
Pertinent past medical history
    Has this problem ever occurred before?
        If so, was a medical diagnosis made, and what
          was it?
    Has the patient ever had surgery? If so, for what
        reason, and what was the result?
    Is there any familial medical history that may
        influence the patient's present complaint?
    Does the patient have a private physician? (Obtain
        full name if possible.)
Current medication (prescribed and unprescribed)
Allergies
Age and weight
Tetanus immunization history if an injury is involved
Date of last menstrual period, if the patient is female

---

treatment area to obtain the history and whatever information the prehospital personnel may have regarding status or treatment before the patient's arrival at the department. If the patient can respond to questions, any history obtained from others should be validated with him or her. Often, when the anxiety of the transport into the department diminishes, the patient remembers information that he or she had not been able to recall previously. Whoever obtains the history should tell the patient who he or she is, and should attempt to prevent the patient from having to retell the story several times to different people.

There are times when a patient cannot describe his or her symptoms and reason for coming into the department. When this occurs, attempts should be made to reach someone who can relate the history of the present complaint. If the patient is unresponsive and no one is available to provide the history, treating the patient becomes a much more difficult, time-consuming process, yet treatment must not be delayed until a history is available.

When you are obtaining information from the patient, the elements listed in the box above should be addressed.

In recent years the mnemonic PQRST, which is presented in the box on p. 113, has been used to great advantage in assessing complaints of pain or dyspnea. The PQRST helps define the complaint by focusing on essential elements of provoking factors, quality, location, and radiation, severity, and the timing in terms of onset and duration.

Based on the history shown in the case study on p. 113,

PQRST ELEMENTS

P *(Provoking factors)*
Ask the patient what, if anything, provokes the pain or discomfort. Is there anything that makes it worse or relieves it? What was the patient doing when it began?

Q *(Quality of the pain)*
Ask the patient to describe the pain in his or her own words. It is particularly important to avoid "feeding" descriptive terms to the patient; instead use open-ended questions to allow a personal description. (Can you tell me how your pain feels to you?)

R *(Region or radiation)*
Ask the patient to point to the area of the pain or discomfort, if possible. Ask if it travels anywhere or if there is pain any place else. Ask if the pain has moved from the region of onset. There are times when a patient may not be able to isolate a single area of pain, particularly if the pain is visceral as opposed to cutaneous. In this case ask if the patient can identify the general area for you. Do not touch the patient while he or she shows you where the discomfort is; this may obscure the answers and provide you with incorrect information.

S *(Severity)*
Ask the patient to describe the severity of the pain. It is sometimes helpful to use the scale of 1 to 10. On this scale, 1 is equivalent to no pain at all, whereas 10 is the most severe pain the patient has ever experienced. Ask if the pain has affected normal activity, and if so, how it has affected the activities of daily living. Watch while the patient moves or undresses, and assess the degree to which the pain compromises activities.

T *(Time)*
The time of onset and constancy or duration of symptoms are assessed. It is also helpful to ask if the patient has ever had the symptoms before, what they were related to, and how they were treated.

CASE STUDY 11-1

PQRST Case History

A 32-year-old woman arrives at the department with abdominal pain. Using the PQRST, the nurse obtains and records the following information:

32 y/o ♀c̄ gradual onset RUQ pain that "comes and goes," increases p̄ meals but tolerable remainder of day. Does not awaken her @ noc. Pain has increased past 2 days and remains colicky. θ vomiting or diarrhea/constipation, but nauseated when pain is at its peak. Position changes not helpful, also do not provoke. θ radiation. Pt. has noted increase in skin temperature in past day, did not take temperature. No past hx of this or similar problems. LMP 7/9, θ abnormality noted, Gravida VI para VI, last child now 2 y. No recent weight gain or loss, current wt. 160#.

---

a reasonably reliable working hypothesis can be formulated, particularly in determining the relative urgency of this patient's problem. Without the history, however, such a hypothesis would be necessarily delayed until the physical examination and extensive laboratory and radiographic studies could be employed to determine the possible cause of the pain.

Although the circumstances of the department may dictate compression of the interview into a few pertinent questions, the most important ones should be asked. Those that are most important depend on the individual patient. Regardless of the time frame in which the history is obtained, every attempt should be made to collect as much history as is available and in some cases to track down that which is not immediately available when the patient arrives. There are adjuncts to the history that are sometimes available, such as an identifying (Medic-Alert) bracelet, personal medical information written on papers kept in a wallet, or the Vial-of-Life. The Vial-of-Life is a small vial into which a pre-printed questionnaire, answered by the patient and containing vital medical history, is placed. The vial is then placed in the patient's refrigerator at home (simply because it is less likely to become lost in that location), and a small seal is placed on the refrigerator door that the vial is inside. Paramedics have been advised to look on the refrigerator door when responding at the home of a patient, particularly if the patient is elderly, infirm, or unconscious.

PHYSICAL EXAMINATION

It has been said that 80% of the time a good history will be enough information to establish a diagnosis, but the physical examination remains important to the adequate evaluation of the emergency patient, particularly when not much else is known about him or her. Physical examination is often abbreviated to the situation; skill and judgment are necessary to determine what physical information is vital and appropriate and what need not be evaluated under the circumstances. The routine health examination that we have all experienced is not appropriate to the ED, but some routines do exist that are considered in courtroom deliberations to be the appropriate standard of evaluation. For instance, the minimal acceptable evaluation for a patient with a head injury is mental status and level of consciousness; assessment of posture and motor movements, including reflexes; evaluation of eye movements, including reflexes; evaluation of eye movements and pupil status; and evaluation of gross focal neurologic deficit. The physical examination is then supported by special diagnostic aids as appropriate: radiographic studies of the skull and cervical spine, electroencephalogram (EEG), and computed tomography or magnetic resonance imaging studies. Depending on the cause of the head injury, other body systems might be examined as well, but the evaluator must determine further examination as appropriate unless specific audit guidelines specify which examinations must be performed in every case of head injury.

Nurses can and should perform physical examinations of patients under their charge. However, the main purpose of the examination in an ED with physicians on site is to recognize and treat life-threatening emergencies and to collect enough data to enable the nurse to establish priorities of care within a busy environment. Generally the nursing examination is performed briefly and rapidly; therefore the nurse must be well versed in normal findings to be able to interpret abnormal ones quickly and accurately. This art can be developed by being persistent in performing examinations and by using adequate clinical supervision while learning to integrate your findings.

Probably the most important aspect of the examination is the establishment of a therapeutic and professional rapport with the patient. Here also is the potential for abruptness or prejudgment that could disrupt the process and adversely affect the nurse-patient relationship. Remember to provide privacy and to use touch before the start of the examination to establish contact with the patient. If the patient is unconscious, relating to him or her before evaluation may not be possible, but explaining what you are doing before doing it is considered appropriate even under these circumstances.

Being organized is also a significant aspect of performing a patient examination. Anticipate what tools you will need before beginning so that you do not have to leave the bedside for any reason. You may not use the full gamut of tools for each examination; however, it is helpful to be aware of what you may need so that you can select appropriately.

Tools for Examination

The tools used in the nursing examination of a patient in the ED are not as numerous as those used in the health screening examination in a well-adult clinic or for specialized tests in neurology or cardiology. The major items used in the ED are described here, and a short listing of other tools follows.

Stethoscope. The most common stethoscope is the binaural acoustic instrument that has both a bell and a diaphragm. Ideally the stethoscope should be lightweight, have two large-lumen tubings that are approximately 12 to 14 inches long, have metal sidepieces and flexible earpieces, and have a rubber or plastic rim around the bell and the diaphragm to reduce ambient noise interference. Not all stethoscopes sound alike, and individuals differ regarding the type of instrument they prefer. Try to select one that not only is well constructed but also fits comfortably, particularly in the external ear, and has the features necessary to the situations in which you will be functioning.

Problems commonly encountered with stethoscopes include cracking of the diaphragm, tubing, or earpieces; lack of a bell piece, resulting in an inability to evaluate low-pitched sounds; and poor transmission of sounds because of excessively long tubing between the head of the instrument and the earpieces.

Care of the stethoscope prolongs the life of this vital piece of equipment. Cleanse the earpieces after each use, particularly if someone else has used it. It is preferable that you own your own stethoscope, one that fits your unique ear canal angle. If you lend your stethoscope to someone, protect yourself against cross-contamination by cleansing the eartips with alcohol before you use it. Check the tubing routinely along with the diaphragm, bell, and earpieces to detect cracks. These parts can be cleansed with a mild soap solution but must be dried completely with a soft, clean cloth. Folding the tubing predisposes it to cracking, particularly if you fold it tightly. A well-fitted, well-designed, and well-constructed stethoscope assists you in auscultating breath, heart, and bowel sounds. It does not amplify sounds but transmits them to your ears effectively by eliminating most ambient noises.

Otoscope and ophthalmoscope. Skills in diagnosing eye, ear, nose, and throat disorders are not necessary for the emergency nurse; however, it is appropriate that you know how to use these instruments to evaluate, when necessary, loss of vision, nasal occlusion or bleeding, and presence of foreign bodies.

The otoscope is designed with a handle that is either portable and battery-operated or portable and recharged between use by a counter- or wall-mounted charger base. The instrument has an otoscope head attachment and usually can also accommodate an ophthalmoscope head when the other head is removed.

The otoscope head attaches with a clockwise twist and a snap-on motion. The head has a round ring for the attachment of an aural or nasal speculum and also has a small ring magnifier that can be lined up with the distal opening of the speculum. There is also a light to illuminate the inspection site. When using the otoscope in examining the ear, hold the scope handle firmly between the thumb and fingers of one hand and tilt the patient's head away from you. Grasp the auricle and pull it upward and backward in the adult or downard and back in the child. This maneuver straightens the canal, and if tenderness is elicited with such an action, the tenderness should be noted. The fingers of the hand that is extending the ear canal should also steady the patient's head. Once this position is obtained, turn the scope light on and guide the speculum gently into the canal, visually inspecting the walls as you enter. If difficulty is encountered while advancing the speculum, pull slightly on the auricle to further straighten the canal, or increase the tilt angle of the patient's head.

The ophthalmoscope is used most commonly in the ED by nurses to check pupils or to identify corneal or conjuctival foreign bodies. Few nurses have the time or skill necessary to conduct a more complete eye evaluation. Yet the ophthalmoscope can prove helpful in examining external eye structures, evaluating pupillary response and accommodation, and evaluating the anterior chamber. As you become more familiar with the instrument and more comfortable with its use, practice identifying internal ocular structures such as the retinal wall, vessels, macula, and optic disc. Until you establish skill, it is more expedient to practice viewing normal structures than to view abnormal ones.

The ophthalmoscope head is a simple instrument that has a small aperture through which you view the eye. It also projects a narrow beam of light and has a set of at least 22 lenses, depending on the model being used. These lenses can be rotated into the aperture by turning a lens wheel located on one side of the head. The lenses are used to focus on different structures within the eye, but they can also be adjusted to accommodate myopia or loss of accommodation in either the examiner or the patient. When you turn the lens wheel, a clockwise turn provides lenses with a shorter focus (these lenses are referred to as *plus diopters*), and a counterclockwise turn provides lenses that have a longer focus (these are referred to as *minus diopters*). A diopter is a unit that measures the capacity of a lens to converge or diverge light rays on an object.

The light beam can be adjusted from wide to narrow; generally the wide setting is easiest to use. Also, the light setting can be changed to a narrow slit or to a red-free filter. Passing the light beam through the refractory structures to the retina allows you to evaluate the clarity of these normally transparent structures when the beam of light bounces back into your eye. The light also illuminates the fundus.

When using the ophthalmoscope to examine the eye, seat yourself directly in front of the patient. If either of you has a history of astigmatism, that person should wear corrective lenses during the examination if they are available. The room can be dimly lit; there is no need for it to be completely dark. Ask the patient to focus on an object directly above and at some distance behind your head; this focusing enlarges and steadies the pupil. Holding the ophthalmoscope handle firmly, place the head of the instrument against your cheek and your eye directly behind the aperture. Place your index finger on the lens wheel and set the scope at 0 diopters, a setting that neither converges nor diverges light rays. Using your right eye, examine the patient's right eye while holding the scope in your right hand. Use your left eye and hand when examining the patient's left eye. During the examination keep your thumb on the patient's brow and your palm and fingers on the patient's head to steady it and prevent movement.

The eye examination should begin with the scope held approximately 12 inches away from the patient and approximately 15 degrees lateral to the patient's field of vision.

In this position identify the red reflex of the eye, which is the reflection of the light bouncing off the retinal wall. Following this reflection, move forward until the hand holding the scope nearly touches the patient's cheek. Keep your eye relaxed and identify the retinal wall by its pinkish color. Look for the optic disc, which is a pale pink with variations located to the nasal side. If you cannot locate it initially, find a blood vessel and follow its pathway centrally until you see the disc itself. Arteries appear light red, whereas veins appear dark red in the fundus of the eye. (The arteries pulsate; the veins do not.) By turning the lens wheel, you should be able to bring the disc into sharp focus to evaluate its margins and depth. Look next for the macula, which is located about 1.5 disc diameters from the disc toward the temporal side and is slightly darker than the retina (the retina ranges in color from pinkish yellow in fair-skinned people to brown in darker-skinned individuals). The sequence of examination recommended by most experts follows:

1. Assess pupil equality, size, shape, and reaction to light.
2. Identify the red reflex.
3. Evaluate the disc.
4. Evaluate the vessels.
5. Evaluate the retinal wall.
6. Evaluate the macula.

The otoscope and ophthalmoscope can also be used for nasal inspection by attaching the otoscopic head and a short, wide speculum to the round ring. Place the patient's head in a neutral position and first visualize the inferior nares bilaterally. Then tilt the patient's head backward and visualize the superior nares. Also evaluate the nasal mucosa, septum, turbinates, and middle meatus between the turbinates.

Reflex hammer. The reflex hammer is a triangular-shaped rubber tip attached to a metal handle, which is narrow at the neck and the distal end and wide in the middle. The reflex hammer is used to evaluate the muscular contraction that results when a tendon is stretched suddenly by the force of the reflex hammer striking it. The hammer should be held between the thumb and fingers of one hand at the handle base. Position the patient's limb to produce a slight stretch of the muscle to be evaluated. Strike the tendon with a brisk but light tap of the hammer, controlling the movement of the hammer yet allowing it to move in an arc with your wrist as a fulcrum. The muscles most frequently evaluated in this manner are the biceps, triceps, brachioradialis, and quadriceps. Hyperreflexia and hyporeflexia are evaluated in context with the patient's norm and considered according to the clinical situation; most commonly reflexes are recorded on the following scale of 0 to 4:

4+ Brisk; hyperactive
3+ Brisker than normal but not necessarily pathologic
2+ Normal
1+ Hypoactive
0+ Absent

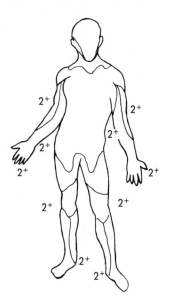

The handle of the reflex hammer is used to evaluate plantar reflexes and abdominal and cremasteric reflexes.

Additional items. Other tools used in patient examination are self-explanatory and include the following:

1. Flashlight
2. Thermometer
3. Sphygmomanometer
4. Watch with a second hand
5. Tongue depressors
6. Safety pins or cotton swabs, to evaluate nervous sensation
7. Flexible tape measure, to compare the size of extremities, skin lesions, and masses, and to measure the circumference of an infant's head

All items necessary for examination should be collected and kept close at hand before you begin the examination so that you do not have to interrupt the process.

Techniques of Physical Examination

There are four essential techniques involved in the physical examination of any patient. The pattern of use may vary depending on the system being evaluated, but the sequence and organization of the approach chosen should be directed at minimizing patient movement and efficiently using time with the patient.

Inspection. Inspection is perhaps the most vital of all of the examination techniques because the observations obtained from the visual inspection of the patient as a whole and each system in particular help integrate what the patient says with what the physical appearance manifests. Inspection must always precede any of the other techniques, and although the technique may be difficult to master at first, continual practice eases your discomfort in simply *looking* at the patient. Keep in mind what you are looking for so that your observations have purpose and organization.

Evaluate the patient's general appearance. Is the patient unkempt, malnourished, well groomed, or overweight? Does the patient appear to take good care of himself or herself or does he or she appear to have poor hygiene? These observations help you to view the patient as a person and to relate the general appearance to the illness. These observations need not be documented in the ED, although often the physician records the patient's nutritional status. Look at the condition of the mucous membranes for information about oxygenation and hydration. Observing body movement and posture provides information about pain, mental status, and mood, as well as clues to degree of debilitation. After this general "quick look," your observations should become specific based on the presenting complaint and the specific system that you are evaluating first. Respiratory excursion and chest symmetry of expansion, apical thrust, and comparison of extremities for size and shape are all examples of routine observations.

Palpation. Your hands become important tools when used to palpate skin temperature, skin texture, vibrations and pulsations, masses or lesions, muscle tenseness or rigidity, and deformities. Different aspects of the hand are better equipped to feel different sensations. The dorsum of the hand is more sensitive to temperature changes, whereas the palm is more sensitive to vibratory sensations. The fingers are sensitive to touch, but because this sensation can be diminished by increasing the pressure on the fingertips, light palpation is generally preferred to deep palpation. However, pressure changes are used to palpate and distinguish one organ from another or to define the borders of the organs. During examination of the abdomen, light palpation is generally followed by deep palpation in the process of identifying abdominal contents.

The preferred method of light palpation is to use the fingertips of one hand to distinguish hard from soft, rough from smooth, and muscle tone. The preferred method of deep palpation is to place the fingertips of one hand over and slightly forward of the fingertips of the other hand, which is placed over the area to be palpated. Both hands are then used to press firmly and deeply over the area. Palpation with both hands can also be employed to fix an organ in place with one hand while palpating its borders with the other, or by using one hand to entrap the organ between the fingertips.

Ballottement is a form of palpation in which the fingertips are lightly bounced along the surface of the skin. A sense of tenseness or resistance in abdominal organs or an increase in pressure within an organ or cavity may be appreciated with the use of ballottement. Ballottement employs light palpation in conjunction with rapid increases and decreases in pressure against the examiner's fingertips, which increases their sensitivity to touch.

When used properly, palpation helps confirm information obtained through observation. The technique is helpful in identifying areas of pain or tenderness and in evaluating where the point of maximal pain or tenderness is located.

Percussion. Percussion is the technique of eliciting vibrations that can be heard and felt when a portion of the body is struck with the examiner's hand or fingers. The extent of the vibration varies depending on the density, position, and size of the tissue underlying the area being percussed. This technique is helpful in outlining the borders of an organ, identifying pain and tenderness within an area of the body, identifying fluid within an organ or cavity, and evaluating lung fields for the presence of consolidation, fluid, or air.

Percussion notes are difficult to describe, because the discrimination of sounds is relative to the amount of practice the examiner has had and to the patient as an individual when areas of the body are compared with one another. Generally sounds are described in terms of pitch, duration, intensity, and quality. The pitch is determined by the speed with which vibrations travel through the body, strike an organ, and bounce back to the examiner's fingers. When the organ is close to the skin surface, the pitch is *high* (not to be confused with *loud*) and is a result of the vibrations being returned rapidly to the examiner. The sound heard is dull, for example, the sound made if you were to strike your thigh, which is fairly dense and does not transmit vibrations at all. The duration is the time the vibration lasts and is dictated by the distance of the organ from the skin surface and thus the amount of time available for the vibration to exist. A fairly solid tissue transmits a sound of short duration, whereas a hollow organ transmits a sound of reasonably long duration. The intensity of the sound is relative to the loudness or softness of the sound heard when an area is percussed. A solid organ transmits a soft sound when percussed because the vibrations are traveling little if at all. The quality of the sound defines what type of organ is making the sound; in other words, the quality of sound that a musical instrument makes gives the listener a clue as to what the instrument is. For example, when the chest is percussed, a certain sound is heard if the lungs are normal and the alveoli are inflated with air. This sound is called *resonant* and has a different quality than would be heard if, for instance, the hemithorax were filled with bowel instead of normal aerated lung.

The art of putting the different characteristics of vibratory sound together to determine abnormal pathologic conditions makes the technique of percussion valuable. Percussion is not at all a harmful technique if the nurse cannot interpret the findings; it becomes a futile exercise unless the sounds are translated into meaningful terms. Most nurses are uncomfortable with percussion because they are unable to interpret their findings. You will never learn to interpret findings, however, unless you percuss normal tissue and abnormal tissue and areas of the body having different density to learn the different sounds. No amount of didactic lecture can provide you with that information.

Percussion notes are obtained through either *direct* means (striking the patient's skin with the fingers of only one hand) or *indirect* means (using fingers of both hands). The indirect method is most often employed, and it is performed by placing the middle finger of the left hand firmly against the patient's skin and striking the distal phalange with the tip of the middle finger of the other hand. The finger placed directly on the patient is called the pleximeter finger, and the striking finger is called the plexor finger. The pleximeter must be placed firmly to avoid damping the sound. No other part of the hand must come in contact with the skin because of the muffling or distorting effect that the other fingers or parts of the hand may cause. Sounds are produced most effectively by striking the pleximeter finger with short, brisk taps, exerted through the motion of the plexor wrist. The lightest percussion force that produces a sound should be used, although there are times when any striking force is uncomfortable for the patient.

Because bone produces a flat percussion note, percussion is not usually carried out in areas where bone overlies cavities or organs. In addition, the deeper the organ lies beneath the surface, the more the tissue lying above it, rather than the organ you are trying to evaluate, transmits the sound. Therefore, it is generally not helpful to try, for instance, to evaluate a kidney using the anterior approach to percussion. An organ that lies more than 5 cm below the surface is generally not detectable by percussion.

Finally, always compare the patient's body from side to side when eliciting percussion notes. Comparison makes it much easier to recognize normal sounds for each patient, and it helps you distinguish changes in quality from organ to organ. Particularly if sounds are subtle, moving from side to side helps you distinguish and differentiate what you are hearing.

Auscultation. Auscultation is the method of transmitting sound from an organ or area of the body to the examiner's ear either by placing the ear directly on the body or by using a stethoscope. The presence or absence of sounds or the deviation from normal sounds heard assist in the development of a diagnosis. Remember that the stethoscope does not amplify sounds; instead it transmits sounds to your ear while reducing external noise interference. The diaphragm is useful when auscultating high-pitched sounds, and the bell is useful when auscultating low-pitched sounds. However, the bell may be converted into a diaphragm if too much pressure is exerted against it and the skin is drawn taut under the bell piece.

As with percussion sounds, auscultation sounds are described in terms of their pitch, intensity, duration, and quality. The systems routinely auscultated during examination are the respiratory, cardiovascular, and gastrointestinal systems.

Auscultating lung sounds. Lung sounds should be auscultated for their relationship to the inspiratory and expiratory (I/E) cycle, as well as for the four elements already listed. There are three basic types of normal sounds that, depending on their location, may indicate a pathologic condition.

Vesicular sounds. Normally heard in the lung periphery, vesicular sounds indicate normal distension of alveoli with air. Their intensity is soft and their pitch is low; many liken the sound to rustling leaves. Their relationship to the I/E cycle is 1.5:1, since the last half of the normal, passive expiratory phase cannot generally be heard in the healthy adult. When the chest is *observed*, however, the expiratory phase should appear to be about one and a half times longer than the inspiratory phase; the extra half is the postexpiratory pause, during which the pressures within the alveoli have fallen and the diaphragm is completely relaxed.

Bronchovesicular sounds. Bronchovesicular sounds are the result of normal air flow in the larger airways other than the trachea and are normally heard only over the mainstem, just inferior to the clavicles anteriorly and between the scapulas posteriorly. As indicated by the name, these sounds are the result of two components: the movement of air through the mainstem bronchi and the inflation of alveoli. In addition, these sounds are associated with a fairly equal I/E cycle that has a slight pause between inspiration and expiration. When heard in the chest periphery, bronchovesicular sounds indicate early pulmonary consolidation or compression.

Bronchial sounds. If you place your stethoscope directly over the trachea, you hear loud, high-pitched, raspy sounds, which are the result of air moving through the trachea and are referred to as *bronchial* or *tubular* breath sounds. The expiratory time is longer than the inspiratory time, generally in a 1:2 ratio. If these sounds are heard anywhere on the chest other than directly over the trachea, pulmonary consolidation or compression such as may be caused by pneumonia, edema, or tumor is indicated.

Breath sounds may change dramatically, depending on the degree of involvement of pulmonary tissues and the time span within which a pathologic condition has existed. The size of the chest may dampen sounds; an obese or muscular chest may exhibit reduced lung sounds. When listening for the normal sounds already described, determine whether or not normal sounds are reduced, distant, or absent, and whether abnormal sounds are present.

Adventitious sounds. Adventitious sounds include two categories of sounds, rales and rhonchi. The use of different descriptive names for these sounds is somewhat controversial; many dictionaries group all adventitious sounds under the heading "rales." Sometimes adventitious sounds are characterized as "crackles and wheezes." To facilitate your understanding, however, adventitious sounds are described in this text as rales and rhonchi.

Rales result from fluid collection in the tracheobronchial tree, generally starting in the alveolar sacs because of gravitational forces on the fluid; when air moves through this fluid, a sound is produced. The following are types of rales:

1. Fine rales are heard as soft clusters of sounds with varying intensity and pitch. They are discontinuous and correlate most often with end-inspiration, since this is the point at which air has moved through the larger airways and entered the alveoli.

2. Medium rales are slightly louder than fine rales but have more of a crackling sound, much like the fizz of a carbonated beverage. They are the result of fluid collection affecting the bronchioles and therefore can be heard in midinspiration, since this is the point at which air moves past the small bronchioles toward the alveoli. The sound extends through the end-inspiration because the alveoli are also involved; therefore the true distinction of whether the rales are fine or medium is based on the point in the cycle at which the sound is heard. Usually the distinction of fine or medium is not nearly as important as describing where in the phase you hear the sound.

3. Coarse rales are often referred to as rhonchi, primarily because the fluid collection has now extended to the large airways. The sound is continuous, not discontinuous as the other types of rales were; the sound of the coarse rales is also rattling, bubbling, or gurgling and can be appreciated throughout the I/E cycle. Another name for this sound is "death rattle," since it is frequently heard in the moribund patient who is unable to clear the airway.

Rhonchi are sounds produced as a result of air passing through mucus or narrowed passages in the larger airways. Their pitch is medium to low, and they are louder than rales. In addition, rhonchi are generally heard on expiration. The following are types of rhonchi:

1. Coarse rhonchi have been described in the preceding paragraph.

2. Sibilant rhonchi are also called "wheezes" and have a musical, whistling, or hissing quality. This sound results from the passage of air through narrowed bronchioles and is heard during expiration. Sibilant rhonchi are of medium pitch and intensity; they are the musical, continuous noise heard in the asthmatic patient.

The *pleural friction rub* is also classified as an adventitious sound. This interrupted, coarse, grating sound develops over an inflamed pleura or over an area where there has been a loss of lubricating fluid within the pleural space. The key to identifying this abnormal sound is that it is usually unilateral and localized, whereas rales and rhonchi are usually not. The rubbing sound may be exaggerated if the patient is positioned toward the involved area, because this positioning brings the involved area closer to the stethoscope. Friction rub is a difficult sound to distinguish without a great deal of practice in auscultating lung sounds.

Adventitious sounds are often associated with changes in the I/E ratio simply because, as in the cases of rales and rhonchi, a pathologic condition exists that disrupts the normal movement of air through the tracheobronchial tree. The phase during which the normal decrease in intraluminal diameter of the airways during expiration is accentuated is prolonged; in emphysematous patients the I/E ratio may be 1:3, 1:4, or even 1:5 in severe cases.

Auscultation of breath sounds takes practice; a few hints are provided to help you become more inclined to develop your skill in this technique. When listening to breath sounds, listen for the normal sounds and for changes in the normal sounds before attempting to identify extra sounds. Begin anteriorly, preferably with the patient in a sitting position and breathing quietly through the mouth. Nose breathing tends to produce more turbulence, which may prove confusing; deep breathing through the mouth tends to produce a bronchovesicular or even bronchial sound, since it increases the velocity of airflow through the airways and mimics the sound heard over the trachea if the breathing is deep enough.

Whenever possible, examine the lungs in a quiet environment and have the chest completely exposed so that you can observe, as well as listen. If the patient cannot sit up, use a semi-Fowler's position to listen to the anterior chest, and roll the patient from side to side to listen to the lateral and posterior walls. Under these circumstances it is difficult and impractical to attempt a side-to-side auscultation as you move down the posterior chest. If help is available, have someone assist the patient to sit forward while you listen to the posterior wall.

Always attempt to auscultate from side to side so that you can compare what you are hearing, and use the interspaces, where sounds are more easily discernible. Anteriorly you should begin at the apex of the lungs and auscultate from side to side and down the chest. Because of the lung topography, the upper lobes can be auscultated anteriorly, whereas the right middle lobe can be auscultated anterolaterally. Listen also on the lateral chest walls for sound in the lower lobes. Proceed to the posterior chest and, again starting at the apices of the lungs, auscultate side to side and downward, ending at the lung bases. It is important to specifically listen for rales with the patient in a sitting position; often these sounds cannot be distinguished unless gravity facilitates collection of the fluid in the alveoli of the lower lobes. In addition, fine rales may be heard only posteriorly because in this area the lower lobes are more closely approximated to the chest wall.

Auscultating heart sounds. Although somewhat more difficult to analyze than lung sounds, heart sounds are nevertheless an important element in the chest examination and can provide information about the integrity of the heart valves, the ventricular and atrial muscles, and the conduction system. Because many of the cardiac sounds have a low pitch, having a bell available is helpful. The goal of listening to heart sounds should be to identify changes in intensity of the normal sounds, changes in timing of the normal sounds, and the presence of extra sounds or murmurs and their relationship to the cardiac cycle.

The sequence of events that occur in the cardiac cycle is presented in the following steps:

1. Blood flows into the atria during diastole; pressure within the atria begins to slightly exceed that within the ventricles.
2. The atrioventricular valves open, allowing access of blood to the ventricular chambers and resulting in ventricular filling.
3. Ventricular contraction begins, and the pressure within the chambers exceeds that within the atria; the atrioventricular valves close.
4. As ventricular pressure continues to rise, it exceeds the pressure in the aorta and pulmonary artery, forcing the aortic and pulmonic valves open.
5. As the ventricles eject the blood, the level of intraventricular pressure again begins to fall; once the level of ventricular pressure falls below the level of pressure within the aorta and pulmonary artery, the aortic and pulmonic valves close.
6. The atria again begin to fill with blood, and the cycle begins again.
7. This entire sequence takes just 1 second at 60 beats per minute.

Heart sounds are the result of vibratory energy that is produced by these changes. While the valves are growing taut, while the ventricular chambers are filling, and while blood is being ejected into the great vessels, sounds occur that can be related to the cardiac cycle and even superimposed onto a phonocardiogram to show their relationship to electric events. Normally each cardiac cycle produces two sounds, the first and second heart sounds.

The *first heart sound* (S_1) is caused by several events but is generally attributed to mitral and tricuspid (atrioventricular valve) closure after ventricular filling has been completed. The first sound signals the onset of systole and is approximately synchronous with the onset of the apical thrust and the carotid impulse. It is heard most loudly at the mitral and tricuspid auscultatory areas.

The *second heart sound* (S_2) is referred to as the closure of the aortic and pulmonic valves but also consists of sounds made by late atrial filling and early ejection of blood into the ventricles through the atrioventricular valves. The pitch of this sound is slightly higher than that of the first sound, and the second sound has a snappier quality. It is heard most loudly at the pulmonic and aortic auscultatory areas at the base of the heart. This sound begins the diastolic phase of the cardiac cycle.

The period between S_1 and S_2 is cardiac systole; this period is shorter than the time between S_2 and S_1, or diastole. Systole must be distinguished from diastole so that extra sounds can be differentiated from normal sounds and murmurs. (The third and fourth heart sounds, S_3 and S_4, are *diastolic* sounds.) The diastolic phase is affected by tachydysrhythmias and is difficult to discern unless the cardiac thrust is used to identify systole and is correlated with the heart sound heard at the same time.

Abnormalities of S_1 are confined primarily to changes in intensity as a result of mitral stenosis or conduction defects. Remember, S_1 should be louder than S_2 over the *apex* of the heart.

Abnormalities of S_2 are confined primarily to abnormal splitting or changes in intensity of S_2 between the aortic and pulmonic auscultory areas. Splitting of heart sound is not always abnormal, however; it may normally be appreciated because of the difference in timing between closure of the aortic valve and closure of the pulmonic valve. Normally the aortic valve closes slightly earlier because pressures within the aorta are greater than pressures within the pulmonary artery; it is these pressures after ventricular contraction that close the aortic and pulmonic valves at the onset of diastole. A splitting sound can best be described as the difference in sound between the word "spit" and the word "split." When "spit" is spoken three times in succession and then "split" is spoken three times in succession, you will be able to appreciate the quality of a splitting sound. The abnormalities of S_2 splitting include a reversal of closure of the valves, resulting in a soft and then slightly louder sound; a prolonged delay in the closure of the pulmonic valve, resulting in a wide split; and a fixed time interval between closure of the two valves, resulting in a fixed split. In the physiologic splitting of the aortic and pulmonic valves, the two sounds usually coincide during the expiration but are separate during inspiration as a result of changes in intrathoracic pressure. For a more in-depth review of splitting, ejection clicks, and opening snaps, the reader is referred to a textbook of cardiac physiology and cardiac examination. These phenomena are difficult to evaluate and are not generally of isolated concern within the ED.

The *third heart sound (S_3)* is a diastolic sound that may be normal in young children and women in the third trimester of pregnancy and pathologic in other adults. The mechanism for both normal and abnormal instances is essentially the same: a low-frequency sound that results from vibrations in the ventricle as the outward motion suddenly stops during early diastolic filling. Also called a *ventricular gallop,* S_3 may occur in cardiac failure, increased preload, and abnormally slow rates.

The *fourth heart sound (S_4)* is a diastolic sound that actually falls before systole and is caused by poor distensibility of the ventricles when the atria contract and force blood into them. S_4 is often referred to as an *atrial gallop.* If both S_3 and S_4 are heard in the diastolic phase, the sound is called a *summation gallop* and is clearly an abnormal finding that must be further evaluated and treated, in context of the clinical setting, as soon as possible.

Murmurs. Murmurs are sounds produced by the following mechanisms:

1. Turbulent flows across a partial obstruction such as a stenotic valve
2. Turbulent flow across a valvular irregularity but without obstruction
3. Turbulent flow into a dilated chamber
4. Turbulent flow out of a high-pressure chamber through an abnormal passage
5. Increased flow through normal passages
6. Regurgitant flow across an incompetent valve or defect

The sounds that result in murmurs can be described either as raspy or harsh or as sounds with a blowing or musical quality. Raspy sound is most often heard over a stenotic valve, and a blowing sound is most often heard over regurgitant valves or dilated chambers and is similar to the bruit heard over a dilated aortic aneurysm. Murmurs are divided into systolic and diastolic, and although there may be innocent or benign systolic murmurs, diastolic murmurs almost without exception indicate some disorder.

The scale commonly used to describe the intensity of a murmur is the Levine Scale, which is shown in the box below. It is necessary to record murmurs according to the scale used to measure their intensity, for example, grade 5 or grade 6.

Some cardiac sounds have both a systolic and diastolic component, such as those heard with *pericardial friction rubs* and *venous hums.* Identifying these sounds can become somewhat confusing if they overlie other extra sounds in the cycle. Probably the most important to learn is the pericardial friction rub that may develop because of inflammation of the pericardial sac and may herald tamponade. The elements of this sound are related to cardiac movement, most notably atrial contraction, ventricular systole, and ventricular diastole. Therefore the sound has a short component that falls between S_1 and S_2, another that falls directly after S_2, and yet another that occurs immediately before S_1. The sound of a friction rub should increase in intensity if the

---

LEVINE SCALE

Grade 1
Very faint: may not be heard in all positions

Grade 2
Quiet but heard immediately on stethoscope contact with the chest wall

Grade 3
Moderately loud but not associated with a thrill; tactile sensation associated with the sound

Grade 4
Loud; usually associated with a thrill

Grade 5
Very loud; may be heard without placing the stethoscope completely on the chest

Grade 6
Extremely loud; may be heard without placing the stethoscope on the chest at all

patient sits forward and you listen during expiration, the quieter of the two respiratory phases. The sound of the pericardial friction rub can best be described as scratchy and high pitched.

Evaluation of heart sounds is difficult for the new practitioner; however, with practice you can successfully recognize normal and abnormal findings. The following techniques of examination will help you develop skill:

1. Use a quiet environment, with the patient's chest exposed.
2. Approach the patient's right side and identify the auscultatory areas.
3. Count the cardiac rate, and identify the rhythm.
4. Place your stethoscope over the aortic and pulmonic areas, and concentrate on S_2. Note the sound's intensity, and listen for splitting.
5. Move your stethoscope to the mitral and tricuspid auscultatory areas, and concentrate on S_1. Note the sound's intensity, and listen for splitting. Splitting of S_1 is not generally appreciated because of its soft intensity.
6. Now concentrate on the interval between S_1 and S_2; note any extra sounds in terms of timing, intensity, and pitch.
7. Listen to the diastolic phase; remember that it will be longer in duration than systole. Note any extra sounds in terms of timing, intensity, and pitch.
8. Listen for systolic murmurs, and identify early, middle, or late systolic murmurs, the location of the sound on the chest, radiation, if any, intensity as measured by the Levine Scale, pitch, and quality.
9. Listen for diastolic murmurs, and identify the characteristics as described for systolic murmurs.
10. Listen for murmurs or other cardiovascular sounds that have both a systolic and diastolic component, such as pericardial friction rubs.

VITAL SIGNS AS AN ASSESSMENT FACTOR

Vital signs are an important element of the assessment process and deserve much more than the casual attention they usually receive. The pulse rate, respiratory rate, blood pressure values, and body temperature can provide valuable information that, when combined with the remainder of the physical examination findings, can greatly affect the nursing diagnosis. In addition, when signs and symptoms conflict with one another or with values of the vital signs, it is imperative to pay meticulous attention to all elements of the physical examination to determine the cause of the conflict. In the hospital the ED is the only unit where there is no prior exposure to each patient and therefore no opportunity to evaluate the present condition in terms of yesterday's laboratory tests or physical findings.

Vital signs are indicators of the patient's present condition and must be obtained serially if they are to have any impact on the identification of trends or developments in the clinical situation. Because the vital signs reflect the activities of compensatory mechanisms within the body, they also provide information regarding the failure of these mechanisms. Variations from normal values and from the patient's own normal values must be explained on clinical examination. Subsequent readings should be considered in light of the therapeutic interventions initiated.

Temperature

Several types of thermometers—tympanic, electronic, and paper—are currently available with which to obtain a measurement of a patient's temperature. In addition, rectal and esophageal probes may be used to measure temperature. The glass thermometer is of no particular advantage over these newer tools. When measuring oral temperatures, place the tip of the thermometer in the pocket of tissue at the base of the tongue against the sublingual artery. Temperatures across the buccal cavity change significantly depending on the distance from this artery. The sublingual site is not only easily accessible in most patients but also easily replicable, as opposed to the rectal and axillary sites, where it is difficult to obtain measurements of temperatures from the same place each time.

The rectal route has been proclaimed to be the only effective route for obtaining accurate temperature readings in the patient who is mouth breathing because of pain or dyspnea. The rectal route does not necessarily provide accurate measurement of temperatures in all cases, however, for the following reasons:

1. The rectum is not known to have thermoreceptive elements and is distant from the central nervous system.
2. The rectum does not reflect early changes in temperature as rapidly as does the sublingual site.
3. The presence of stool may impair accurate readings; if the stool is hard, the thermometer may not reach the suggested 3-inch depth; if stool is soft, the tip of the thermometer may become imbedded in the stool and never touch the rectal wall.
4. The rectal site is not easily accessible, and the procedure may be embarrassing to adults and older children.
5. It is not easy to repeat placement of the thermometer at the same site, and rectal temperatures may vary with placement of the thermometer tip at different sites.

The axillary site is used more frequently in neonatal units where airflow and ambient temperature are carefully controlled. This site is safe and accurate when the proper precautions are taken to avoid environmental influence. These precautions include leaving the thermometer in place for at least 10 minutes, ensuring that the thermometer is resting against the axillary artery, and maintaining contact by keeping the arm tightly enfolded over the thermometer for the entire time the instrument is in place.

When core temperature is desired, readings may be obtained by using a probe, which is placed against the tympanic membrane, by measuring the urine temperature, or by measuring the temperature in the nasal turbinates.

Pulse

In this world of electronic sophistication a habit has developed that is occurring with alarming frequency: the reluctance of paramedics, nurses, and physicians to palpate all peripheral pulses as part of their assessment of the patient's status. When emergency nurses are given pulse rates from the field in a prehospital situation, it is likely that only the mechanically monitored rate is being reported. This information gives no indication of the quality and characteristics of the pulse. Equally important, rhythm disturbances may not be identified unless these changes are seen on the portable monitor. Irregularities of rhythm can be missed on a portable scope if they derive from premature beats or are irregularly irregular. Yet premature beats can be felt on palpation as either missing beats or beats with less amplitude than those preceding them, and irregularly irregular rhythms, even if they tend to be subtle, can be felt as a chaotic rhythm.

In addition to describing the rate and rhythm of the pulse, the nurse should also describe the quality as bounding, normal, weak and thready, or absent. If the pulse rate is parodoxic such as in the sensation under your fingertips of a rising and falling amplitude in concert with aspirations, this finding should be recorded. An unusually snappy and full pulse rate, such as a "water-hammer" pulse, should be recorded. Other characteristic pulse qualities should also be solicited during the cardiovascular assessment of patients by the actual palpation of all peripheral pulses.

In context with other physical findings, the pulse is an important indicator of cardiac function. Often changes in the pulse rate are the first sign that compensatory mechanisms are being invoked to maintain homeostasis. Frequently in early volume depletion a healthy individual with an intact autonomic nervous system may retain normal pressures with only one subtle change: a slight increase in the pulse rate and amplitude. Any deviation from the normal range for the patient's age that cannot be related to psychologic or environmental factors should be considered an indication of a pathologic condition until proved otherwise.

Respirations

Performing a thorough respiratory assessment is not a time-consuming process. In most cases this entire system can be assessed, to the extent necessary in the ED, within 1 or 2 minutes. The objective of assessing respirations as a part of evaluation of the patient's vital signs is to identify impairment of ventilatory function, attempt to isolate the cause, and provide timely intervention. When collecting vital signs, the nurse should not simply count the respiratory rate without completing respiratory evaluation. This practice should hold true for all emergency patients, not only the critically ill ones. The other factors besides respiratory rate and rhythm that should be assessed are discussed in the following paragraphs.

Oxygen saturation. Oxygen saturation measurements are being used commonly in the emergency care setting. Compact, portable equipment and wall-mounted monitors are available. Oxygen saturation values are usually obtained via a finger probe or an ear probe.

Signs of respiratory effort. Signs of respiratory effort include tracheal tugging, nasal flaring, use of accessory muscles, and retractions. Generally a healthy individual does not make extra efforts to breathe; there is no airway noise, the trachea is fixed in midline, the nasal cartilage is quiet, and there is no use of the sternocleidomastoid or intercostal muscles to help lift the chest cage. In addition, there is no suprasternal, intercostal, or substernal indrawing on inspiration to indicate an increase in the work of breathing.

Chest contour. An increase in anteroposterior diameter can generally be seen on casual observation and indicates chronic alveolar distension. Other changes in chest contour are those that are seen in cases of funnel chest, pigeon chest, kyphosis, and kyphoscoliosis. These particular anatomic changes in contour may interfere with normal lung inflation and may complicate or exacerbate the effects of respiratory conditions.

Symmetry of chest expansion. When the healthy individual inspires, the chest expands symmetrically on both sides. When pulmonary or chest wall conditions exist, the chest may rise asymmetrically during ventilation; this asymmetry can often be observed with the chest exposed. The asymmetry can also be palpated during inspiration.

Depth of ventilation. The patient's tidal volume can be estimated by observing the rise and fall of the chest during ventilation or by standing behind the patient and placing your hands around the chest cage with your thumbs placed parasternally. When you palpate in this manner, your thumbs are displaced laterally during inspiration and then move back toward each other during expiration. The depth of ventilations is described as shallow, normal, or deep. A normal adult moves 300 to 500 cc of air at rest and moves as much as 2000 cc during exercise, with a corresponding increase in rate. When evaluating depth, remember that a fast rate is not necessarily moving increased volume, nor is a slow rate necessarily moving less volume.

Breath sounds and inspiratory/expiratory ratio. Simply counting the respiratory rate is not measurement enough; all elements listed here must be evaluated when assessing respiration as a vital sign. The days of rapidly calculating a 15-second rate are long over for the critical care nurse in an intensive care unit or ED.

Blood Pressure

Because the blood pressure varies with numerous factors, including patient condition, age, and gender, blood pressure is not the most reliable indicator of physiologic changes. It is, however, vital information when considered with the pulse and respiration rates and in light of the clinical situation. The systolic pressure is a measurement of pump integrity, and the diastolic pressure is a measurement of vascular status. Normal pressures measured in the ED are not necessarily an indication that all is well. As mentioned previously, a healthy person may not exhibit signs of low circulating volume until all compensatory mechanisms have been exhausted. The patient may have only to change position to cause a precipitous drop in pressure. Thus anyone suspected of having volume depletion, which may be revealed by history or clinical findings, should be evaluated for *postural vital sign* changes.

Also known as *orthostatic vital signs* or the *tilt test*, postural vital sign evaluation should be performed for patients who have had syncopal events, those who appear dehydrated, and those who have a history of volume loss such as in prolonged vomiting, diarrhea, sweating, diuretic therapy, gastrointestinal bleeding, burns, or obvious blood loss. Contrary to the method for the neurologic tilt test, which is used to test the integrity of the autonomic nervous system, a 5-minute period after a change in position is not provided when obtaining postural vital signs. The purpose of the test is to establish whether a significant loss of volume has occurred that has necessitated the use of compensatory mechanisms, including severe peripheral vascular constriction. Therefore immediately after obtaining a pulse rate and blood pressure measurement and writing them down while the patient is lying flat, elevate the patient to a full sitting position and remeasure the pulse rate and the blood pressure level. Significant changes include the following:

1. A subjective feeling of dizziness or blurring of vision
2. Decrease in blood pressure level of 20 mm Hg or more
3. Increase in pulse rate of 20 beats per minute or more

If significant findings occur during a change to the sitting position, the test is considered positive for significant blood loss, and fluid replacement must begin with volume expanders such as Ringer's lactate solution, normal saline solution, or another solution appropriate for the situation. In addition and most important, the site of bleeding must be sought and the bleeding controlled. If the sitting portion of the postural vital sign examination is positive, the standing portion may be deferred, since it will not yield important information in such cases and may prove detrimental to the patient. If there are equivocal changes from the lying to the sitting position or no changes at all, the patient should be moved to a standing position unless this change is contraindicated (for example, in the case of a fractured leg), and the pulse rate and blood pressure level should be remeasured and recorded. Positive findings are the same as those described for the sitting position.

Whenever evaluating the blood pressure values, consider your findings in relationship to the patient's history; if the patient is undergoing antihypertensive therapy, the values obtained during the ED visit may represent a significant deviation relative to the patient's "normal" pressure. Consider also the pulse pressure (the difference between the systolic and the diastolic pressures), which represents the approximate stroke volume when all other variables are constant. Peripheral vascular resistance and elasticity of the vessel walls are also critical determinants of the pulse pressure, and therefore approximating the stroke volume by measuring the pulse pressure is more qualitative than accurate; however, the pulse pressure provides information about the status of the pump and peripheral vessels and indicates otherwise subtle hemodynamic changes.

Blood pressure recordings can be obtained on the arm, using the brachial artery; the thigh, using the popliteal artery; or the calf, using the *flush method*. The flush method is performed on neonates or infants to obtain the mean arterial pressure. The patient's foot is elevated above the heart and the blood is massaged out of the limb. An infant cuff is applied around the calf and pumped to a pressure of approximately 130 mm Hg. The foot is then lowered and the pressure in the cuff released in 5 mm increments until the foot flushes with blood; the pressure at which the foot flushes is the mean arterial pressure.

Both the auscultated method and the palpated method can be used, depending on the patient's condition and the environment, but the palpated method does not provide information about the diastolic, thus the peripheral vascular system, pressure. Be certain to communicate which method has been used so that others who obtain the pressure use the same method or correlate findings from another method. A single blood pressure recording yields little or no information; serial pressures must be measured to monitor the hemodynamic status. All the vital signs must be taken and evaluated serially; the patient's condition in the department is a dynamic continuum that can be assessed only through constant monitoring. Whenever therapy is instituted, all the vital signs should be evaluated to assess the efficacy of the treatment. Also, the vital signs should be measured once more before a decision is made about the disposition of the patient from the department, whether the patient is to be discharged, admitted, or transferred to another facility.

Level of Consciousness

Level of consciousness is one of the most essential of all vital signs because it is an indication of the status of cerebral perfusion and function. One of the more specific ways to describe the level of consciousness is to use the stimulation-response method, stating exactly how the patient responds to a specific stimulus. The stimulation-response method requires judgment, interpretation, and specific documentation to communicate the information to others who may also be evaluating the level of consciousness.

Assessing consciousness in the order in which it may deteriorate is helpful. When the cerebral hemispheres are intact, well oxygenated, and functioning normally, the patient is able to respond with purpose to your normal speaking voice; the patient is able to answer questions readily and remains awake during the interview and examination. In short, he or she is fully conscious. If the patient is conscious, evaluate the degree of orientation, beginning with the one thing the patient is least likely to forget—his or her name. Progressively the patient should be asked where he or she is, what day or time it is, and what has happened. Allowing for possible patient confusion resulting from the stress of the situation or even from the patient not having been told what hospital he or she was being taken to, assess the patient's answers to evaluate whether he or she is oriented to person, place, time, and situation (orientation times 4). These four areas of orientation are lost in a progressive order, beginning with disorientation to the situation, or amnesia for the situation. As a patient becomes less responsive, he or she often becomes less oriented also.

When the cerebral hemispheres become dysfunctional for any reason, the level of consciousness and degree of orientation begin to deteriorate, but the changes may be extremely subtle at first. Unless the same situation is given, these changes may be overlooked until they become obvious. The following list of progressive changes in a particular patient demonstrates how these changes can be identified without the use of confusing labels such as "lethargic," "semiconscious," or "obtunded."

1. Mr. Jones is awake, responds to my voice by turning to look at me, and is oriented times 4.
2. Mr. Jones is sleepy but becomes awake and alert when I call his name. He follows all directions, answers questions appropriately when aroused, and is oriented times 4.
3. Mr. Jones is drowsy but arouses when I shake his shoulder; he is oriented times 3. When stimulation is removed, he drifts to sleep again.
4. Mr. Jones is sleeping most of the time, arouses sluggishly when his shoulder is shaken firmly, cannot follow more than one direction at a time, and drifts back to sleep readily.
5. Mr. Jones is sleeping most of the time; he arouses only to trapezius pinch and pushes my hand away. He is inarticulate when aroused and drifts back to sleep immediately.
6. Mr. Jones responds only to firm trapezius squeeze and evidences decorticate posturing without arousing.
7. Mr. Jones responds to firm trapezius squeeze with decerebrate posturing.
8. Mr. Jones responds to firm sternal rub with increase in pulse and respiration rates only. He does not respond to any other stimulation.
9. Mr. Jones has no physical response to deep, painful stimulation.

Placed in context with other neurologic assessments, including eye changes, respiratory changes, and motor movement and posturing, this stimulation-response method is

---

> ## TYPES OF PAINFUL STIMULATION
>
> **Supraorbital compression**
> Pressure over the supraorbital rim just medial to the midline of the eye traps the nerve against the bony skull prominence and causes pain. This compression is useful in two ways: (1) it should provoke a reaction in all but the most deeply comatose patient, and (2) it may help to demonstrate a motor deficit on one side of the body or the other.
>
> **Sternal compression (rub)**
> "Knuckle rub" causes pain but can leave bruises, especially in elderly persons. Remember to describe the painful stimuli, for example, "The patient responds to sternal compression with purposeful movement."
>
> **Interdigital compression**
> Trapping the digital nerves against a pencil—for example, placed between the fingers or toes—is useful for determining whether the patient will withdraw the limb; this type of stimulation is used when hemiparesis is suspected.
>
> **Trapezius pinch**
> This pinch is painful and can bruise.
>
> **Calf pressure**
> This pressure is quite painful.

---

very informative. The painful stimulations used to assess the level of consciousness need not be barbaric. Types of painful stimulations are presented in the box above. Stimulation should begin with light pain such as pressure on the nailbeds, supraorbital nerve pressure, and interdigital pressure applied with a pencil. Deep pain can be applied by a firm pinch or squeeze of the trapezius muscle, the inner aspect of the thigh, or the inner aspect of the upper arm. Deep pain can also be applied with a firm sternal rub with your knuckles, although this method may result in bruising of the sternal skin. The patient either responds or does not respond to deep pain; there is no need to sadistically apply more severe stimulation. If the patient is unarousable to anything other than deep pain, however, the objective of applying the painful stimulation is not to keep the patient awake. If there is a significant intracranial condition, nothing will keep the patient awake, until the condition is treated. Therefore apply the noxious stimulation briefly and at intervals, rather than constantly.

If the level of consciousness begins to deteriorate, follow through with an assessment of the pupils, respiratory rate and pattern, and muscle reflexes and tone. The Glasgow coma scale (see p. 277) is used to score neurologic function.

Skin Vital Signs

Because the skin is the largest organ in the body and is external, it is an excellent mirror of physiologic changes occurring within the body. The dermis is well supplied by an extensive capillary system that is sensitive to changes in the autonomic nervous system. Sympathetic overactivity results in the release of endogenous catecholamines into the circulation, with a resultant increase in heart rate and blood pressure. The skin reflects these changes by becoming cool, moist, and pale. This sympathetic overactivity is frequently a response to pain, stress, or reduction in cardiac output. Parasympathetic overactivity may be reflected in the skin by ruddiness resulting from relaxation of peripheral vasculature, increased temperature, and dry skin. Changes in skin color, moisture, and temperature are vital signs that can be assessed.

Skin color. Changes in skin color (Table 11-1) depend on many factors, including the size of surface vessels, the content and depth of melanin and carotene, the amount of oxyhemoglobin or reduced hemoglobin, and the lighting of the environment coupled with the skill of the evaluator. Inspection of the skin for color changes should follow an organized pattern. Note whether any changes seen are localized or generalized; then inspect for changes in areas that

characteristically have the least amount of pigmentation that could obscure or confuse findings. These areas are the buccal mucosa, lips, nailbeds, earlobes, palms, and soles. Inspect the palms and soles while the patient is lying flat to prevent gravity-induced changes. In addition, the sclera and conjunctiva may reflect changes when pallor or jaundice exist; they take on a grayish hue in cases of pallor and a yellowish hue in cases of jaundice. The critical color changes to be evaluated are cyanosis and pallor, because rapid intervention is required in both cases to reverse the cause. Cyanosis is not always evident in poorly ventilated patients or in those who have less than 5 g circulating reduced hemoglobin. It is also difficult to see cyanotic changes in highly pigmented skin. If you are unsure whether the cyanosis is central or peripheral, massage a small area of skin with your finger. Peripheral cyanosis disappears on massage, whereas central cyanosis does not. If skin color suggests blood loss or cardiovascular dysfunction, perform a capillary blanching maneuver to help substantiate your suspicion; a decrease in filling is seen after pressure is applied and released suddenly if your suspicion is correct. Patients who have a decrease in hemoglobin content caused by anemia also appear pale, but the vasomotor tone is still good, and the capillary filling test result is normal.

Table 11-1   Color changes in the skin

Color	Cause	Location
Brown	Generic	Generalized
	Sunlight	Exposed areas
	Pregnancy	Localized (exposed areas, palmar creases)
	Addison's disease and some pituitary tumors	Localized (exposed areas, palmar creases) or generalized
Gray brown or bronze	Hematochromatosis	Exposed areas, genitalia, scars; may also be generalized
Reddish	Polycythemia	Face, conjunctiva, mouth, hands, feet
	Excessive heat	Generalized
	Sunburn, thermal burn	Exposed areas
	Increased visibility of normal oxyhemoglobin caused by vasodilation as a result of fever, blushing, alcohol, inflammation	Localized
	Decreased oxygen use in skin, as in cold exposure	Exposed areas
Yellow	Increased bilirubinemia caused by liver disease, red cell hemolysis	Sclera in initial stages, then generalized
	Carotenemia caused by increased carotene pigment as a result of myxedema, hypopituitarism, diabetes	Exposed areas although may be generalized; not seen in sclera or mucous membranes
	Chronic uremia	Exposed areas although may be generalized; not seen in sclera or mucous membranes
Blue	Hypoxemia	Central (lips, tongue, nailbeds)
	Decreased flow to skin because of anxiety, cold	Localized, peripheral
	Abnormal hemoglobin as a result of combination with methylene or sulfa drugs	Central
Pale or white	Obstructive, hemorrhagic, distributive, or cardiogenic shock	Generalized
	Renal failure	Generalized
	Fear or pain	Generalized and self-limiting

Skin moisture. Moisture of the skin should be evaluated by palpating the texture and turgor of the skin. Grasp a small section between your thumb and forefinger and evaluate whether the skin is thin and dry, inelastic or elastic, or thick and mushy, as in the patient with myxedema. If the water content of the skin feels excessive, check to see if pitting is present and where it is located. Remember that a patient who has been confined to bed may not exhibit dependent edema of the lower extremities; instead, check the sacral area for pitting edema. Finally check to see if the skin is dry, damp, or wet. Overactivity of the sympathetic nervous system may produce diaphoresis that may range from light to excessive.

Skin temperature. An increase of blood flow through the capillaries under the skin results in radiation of heat from the surface of the skin, whereas a decrease in flow is manifested by coolness to touch. Evaluate the skin temperature by palpating the skin surface with the dorsum of your hand, which is most sensitive to temperature changes. Identify whether temperature changes are localized or generalized. Skin temperature is also affected by changes in the diameter of capillaries under the skin; dilated vessels produce heat at the skin surface, whereas constricted vessels produce cool skin. All the skin vital signs should be evaluated in concert with one another. If the findings do not correlate with one another, investigate for causes.

EVALUATION OF PAIN

Whenever a patient states that he or she is having pain, the nurse must believe the claim. Pain is an extremely subjective sensation, and although an illness or injury may initially trigger the sensation, the manner in which each patient perceives the pain and thus behaves is unique. Cultural influences, past experiences with pain, individual coping mechanisms, and the gravity of the current situation all contribute to a patient's individual reactions to pain.

A patient's response to pain is also affected by the nature of the pain itself; chronic pain is more difficult to deal with than an acute episode. Whereas acute pain tends to generate anxiety, chronic pain tends to generate depression and the feeling that nothing can be done to relieve it. The patient with acute pain is much more likely to cooperate with treatment procedures and the inevitable delays in treatment. The chronic sufferer is not, even though he or she desperately wants relief.

In the evaluation of pain, use open-ended questions that allow the patient to describe just what sensation he or she is having in terms that are most meaningful to the patient. Watch the patient's face as he or she expresses how the pain feels, and watch the behavior as the patient attempts to deal with the situation and with the anxiety of the ED setting. Often this setting aggravates discomfort and fear, and often pain relief may be engendered by your empathy and support. Depending on the particular pathologic cause, the patient's age, and his or her ability to cope, pain may be described

in many different ways; elderly patients often have diminished pain sensation and may not use the term *pain* at all in their description. It is helpful to have the patient rank the pain on a scale of 1 to 10; a ranking of 1 refers to a complete absence of pain, whereas a ranking of 10 refers to excruciating, unremitting pain. When using this scale, ask the patient to rank this episode of pain in comparison with other painful experiences in his or her life. Find out what experience the patient is using to compare with this situation. Have the patient point to the painful area or place of maximal discomfort if possible. Visceral pain, as opposed to superficial or cutaneous pain, often radiates to other areas of the body because it follows different dermatomes, or tracks of nerves. Thus visceral pain is diffuse and more difficult for the patient to pinpoint. However, the patient can identify areas that are *not* painful or indicate the general area of the pain.

The PQRST mnemonic is helpful in identifying the character, location, and intensity of the pain. Depending on the presenting complaint, physical maneuvers or palpation of the area of discomfort can help identify specific painful areas and pain intensity. Before palpating an area, however, inspect the site. In the case of abdominal pain, auscultate for bowel sounds before palpating the belly, since palpation may change the nature of bowel action. In the case of post-traumatic spinal injury, do not move the spine to identify pain or tenderness before spinal films are taken. Palpation may be performed for paraspinal muscle spasm before films are taken, but motion is strictly prohibited so that cord damage is prevented.

Do not rely on sympathetic nervous changes to substantiate a patient's report of pain. Reflex parasympathetic activity may interrupt common sympathetic findings of cool, clammy, and pale skin, which often is found in cases of severe pain. Continue to assess the patient's subjective description of the level of the pain, and allow the patient to react in his or her own way without making judgments about whether pain is present or whether it is incapacitating. In most cases some type of medication can be given; this medication might be a mild sedative to relieve anxiety and enable the patient to regain effective coping behavior. In some cases medication given for pain has other beneficial effects, as is often the case with morphine sulfate in cases of acute pulmonary edema. Although a patient may use complaints of pain to manipulate others for the purpose of obtaining drugs, this situation rarely occurs and can usually be identified by the careful use of the PQRST mnemonic in combination with a physical examination.

LABORATORY ANALYSIS

The laboratory data base is an essential ingredient in the assessment of patients in the ED. Laboratory tests should not be ordered indiscriminately but should be ordered based on an interview and examination process that indicates the appropriate testing requirements for each patient.

Table 11-2   Tubes for drawing blood

Tube	Preservative or anticoagulant	Test
Red top	None	Serologic studies, chemistry panels, routine chemistry studies
Lavender top	Ethylenediamine tetraacetate	Hematologic studies, lipoprotein electrophoresis, acid phosphatase studies
Blue top	Sodium citrate (0.5 g)	Coagulation studies
Gray top	Sodium fluoride	Blood glucose levels, blood alcohol content, drug screens, and tests with delayed evaluation
Green top	Sodium heparin	Special procedures

A number of laboratory tests are frequently used within the emergency setting. In some departments it is a nursing responsibility to order routine tests when the need is established, whereas in other departments such orders are carried out by the physician on duty. In either case a working knowledge of the commonly ordered tests and the types of containers used to collect specimens for them is necessary for the nurse involved (Table 11-2).

Specific Tests

Complete blood count. A complete blood cell count is a routine hematologic screening test performed on serum; it includes hemoglobin content, hematocrit, total red blood cell count, white blood cell count and differential, mean corpuscular cell volume, mean cell hemoglobin concentration, and mean corpuscular hemoglobin concentration. Elements of this test may on occasion be ordered separately, which saves the patient money. Five milliliters of venous blood is generally required.

Urinalysis. A urinalysis should always be performed on a clean-catch or catheter specimen collected in a sterile, dry container and examined within 2 hours. The standard examination includes analysis of appearance, pH, specific gravity, glucose and ketone values, protein semiquantitation, and microscopic examination of the sediment for casts, crystals, red blood cells, and bacteria.

Blood glucose. Venous blood used for testing glucose levels should be obtained as a clot specimen for patients in whom abnormalities in glucose metabolism are suspected. Collect the specimen before starting intravenous solution infusions or administering dextrose. Two to 3 ml of venous blood is necessary to perform the test. Record the conditions under which the blood was drawn, for example, whether the patient was fasting and the approximate time of the patient's last meal.

Blood urea nitrogen. The blood urea nitrogen test measures the amount of circulating urea in the blood; urea is the end product of protein metabolism and is normally excreted in the urine. An elevation of the blood urea nitrogen level may indicate renal failure, renal hypoperfusion, obstructive uropathy. One milliliter of venous blood is required.

Serum electrolytes. The specimen should be withdrawn from a vein and collected in a specimen container with as atraumatic a procedure as possible to avoid hemolysis, which results in a false elevation of the level of serum potassium. The test for serum electrolytes includes measures of potassium, chloride, and carbon dioxide content. Although each of these elements can be tested individually, the implications of the results may change depending on the values of the other electrolytes.

Serum creatinine. The serum creatinine test evaluates renal function by measuring the level of creatinine, a waste product of creatine metabolism that is found in skeletal muscle and is usually filtered by the renal glomerulus. The serum creatinine level may be elevated in cases of acute renal failure. Three milliliters of venous blood is required.

Cardiac enzymes. Tests of cardiac enzymes include tests that measure the levels of creatine phosphokinase, lactic dehydrogenase, and serum glutamic-oxaloacetic transaminase. Levels may be elevated with cardiac muscle infarction, as well as in patients with acute muscle injury or multiple injections. therefore cardiac isoenzymes are usually evaluated also, specifically those that are known to be elevated with cardiac muscle infarction (lactic dehydrogenase fraction 1 and creatine phosphokinase containing M and B units). Five milliliters of venous blood is required for this test.

Toxic screen. A toxic screen may be ordered specific to a certain drug or used as a screen for sedatives, hypnotics, narcotics, and so on. This test measures the exact amount of circulating drug per volume of plasma. This is an expensive test and takes a long time to run; most facilities send the specimen out to a bioanalysis laboratory, which delays receipt of the results because of transit time. Five milliliters of venous blood is required.

Serum drug level. A serum drug level test is generally ordered specific to a drug such as digoxin. The test measures the concentration of drug in the blood at the time the level is drawn. Two to 5 ml of venous blood is required.

Serum amylase. Serum amylase is generally evaluated in patients with upper abdominal pain. The test measures the amount of circulating amylase, which is a digestive

ASSESSMENT PROCESS

I. Primary survey
   A. Is the airway patent? If not, clear the airway by suction or positioning, and maintain patency. Any airway noise indicates an airway obstruction that must be found and removed.
   B. Is the patient breathing? Is the patient exchanging an adequate amount of air based on your observation of chest excursion and skin color? Apply supplemental oxygen to any dyspneic patient.
   C. Is the patient perfusing? Feel the patient's feet and fingers and palpate the pulse of a major artery (carotid or femoral). Establish cardiac massage if pulses are absent. If the patient is in shock, venous blood samples should be drawn and an intravenous solution started immediately.
   D. Is there obvious bleeding? Apply direct pressure if the site is accessible. If the bleeding is intraabdominal and therefore inaccessible, consider use of the pneumatic antishock trousers until the patient can be moved to surgery.

II. General survey
   A. Observe the general state of health and nourishment.
   B. Observe the manner of dress and hygiene.
   C. Observe for obvious signs of distress, as manifested by behavior and facial expression.
   D. Observe the patient's level of consciousness, awareness, mood, mannerisms, and behavior.
   E. Observe posture, motor activity, and gait.
   F. Observe speech for clarity.
   G. Observe odors such as alcohol, urine, chemicals, ketones, and drugs.

III. Vital signs
   A. Count the rate of respirations; evaluate the rhythm, depth, and symmetry of chest expansion.
   B. Palpate all peripheral pulses for rate, rhythm, quality, and characteristics. Place the patient on a cardiac monitor if there is any indication of a dysrhythmia.
   C. Evaluate skin moisture, color, temperature, and turgor.
   D. Auscultate the blood pressure. Determine postural vital signs if appropriate.
   E. Take oral, rectal, or axillary reading of temperature.

IV. Head-to-toe examination (performed relative to the patient's chief complaint and clinical status at arrival in the ED)
   A. Head
      1. Inspect.
         a. Is any obvious injury present?
         b. Perform a pupil check for size, equality, and reaction. Perform a visual acuity test if appropriate. Check to see whether both eyes move together in all directions; evaluate whether the patient can raise both eyebrows and open the eyes against resistance.
         c. Is there any discharge from the natural orifices of the head? Perform the target test on any nasal or ear discharge in the posttrauma patient; test the discharge for sugar with a Dextrostix. Perform the test for cerebrospinal fluid on drainage from nose or ears in conjunction with Dextrostix evaluation. Allow drainage to drop directly on paper towel. Blood forms a sound ring; clear fluid, which is less viscous, spreads out away from blood.
         d. Perform a funduscopic and otoscopic examination if appropriate.
         e. Check the oral mucosa for color, hydration, inflammation, and bleeding.
         f. Evaluate the jugular veins for distension.
      2. Palpate
         a. Palpate the scalp for lacerations, contusions, and cranial contour.
         b. Palpate the facial bones and front sinuses for pain and tenderness.
         c. Palpate the neck for tenderness and stiffness and the glands for enlargement or pain.
         d. Palpate the trachea for tenderness, crepitus, and deviation.
      3. Auscultate the carotid arteries for bruits.
   B. Chest
      1. Inspect the following:
         a. Chest contour
         b. Obvious deformities of the chest wall
         c. Obvious injury: contusion, open wounds, abrasions, and discolorations
      2. Palpate the following:
         a. Clavicular, sternal, shoulder, and rib regions for pain, tenderness, or crepitus
         b. Point of maximal impulse; identify ventricular heave (accentuated thrust on systole)
         c. Tactile fremitus in the chest periphery
      3. Auscultate the following:
         a. Breath sounds for increase, decrease, or absence
         b. Adventitious sounds
         c. Heart sounds for change in timing, intensity, pitch, and quality; identify murmurs or extra sounds
      4. Percuss chest periphery for normal resonance
   C. Abdomen
      1. Inspect for the following:
         a. Signs of trauma: discoloration or wounds

ASSESSMENT PROCESS—cont'd

   b. Distension, asymmetry beyond normal range, and increased vascularity

   c. Hernias, masses, rashes, and scars

   d. Pulsations or peristalsis

   e. Bulging flanks

2. Auscultate for the following:

   a. Bowel sounds in all four quadrants for at least 1 minute; are bowel sounds increased, decreased, or absent?

   b. Bruit over the abdominal aorta

3. Palpate.

   a. Beginning away from the site of any identified pain, palpate lightly for pain, tenderness, rebound, and guarding.

   b. Establish point of maximal tenderness.

   c. If hernia was seen on inspection, palpate the mass. Can a thrust be felt as the patient coughs or strains?

   d. Palpate both femoral arteries simultaneously. Are they equal in intensity?

   e. Are both pulses present?

   f. Press on the symphysis pubis gently, and inward on the ischial wings. Is pain elicited by this action? If so, where is the pain felt? Does it radiate?

   g. Place your stethoscope on one of the patient's knees, and auscultate through the diaphragm while tapping firmly on the other knee; can you hear the sound transmitted to your ears? If not, suspect a fractured pelvis.

4. If deep palpation is indicated, answer the following:

   a. Is tenderness or pain elicited in any quadrant?

   b. Can the aorta be palpated in the epigastrium? Try to feel the lateral borders with two fingers of each hand; does the aortic pulsation push your fingers apart laterally or anteriorly? Estimate the approximate size of the aorta. (Normal size is 2 cm in the epigastrium.)

   c. Is the liver firm and smooth, or is it soft and tender? How far below the costal margin does it extend? (Normal extension is 2 cm below the costal margin.)

   d. Can the spleen be felt? Unless it is enlarged more than three times its normal size, it usually cannot be felt.

5. Percuss.

   a. If the flanks were observed to be bulging on inspection, test for fluid motion by placing one hand on one flank and striking the other flank with your other hand with a tapping motion while another person places the ulnar surface of the hand at midline. If the bulging is caused by fluid and not fat, you will see and feel the fluid wave transmitted across the belly.

   b. Percuss from side to side and top to bottom in all quadrants. Note any shifting dullness, location of tympany, and normal dullness over the liver.

D. Extremities

1. Inspect.

   a. Compare for symmetry, edema, discoloration, masses, deformities, and open wounds.

   b. Are needle marks present?

   c. Is clubbing or nicotine stains evident on the fingers?

   d. Do the veins of the hand remain elevated when the extremity is elevated above the heart?

   e. Are ulcers or rashes present?

   f. Can the patient move the fingers and toes without effort?

2. Palpate.

   a. Compare pulse rates and skin temperatures in all extremities. Mark the location of the pulse in an injured extremity.

   b. Evaluate lower extremities for clonus. (Support knee in partially flexed position, dorsiflex foot, and observe for rhythmic oscillations.)

   c. If edema is present, press thumb firmly against the edematous area for 5 seconds; evaluate for pitting.

   d. Compare calves for tenderness, increased firmness, and tension.

   e. Gently palpate any enlarged, tender, or cordlike veins for size and quality.

   f. Evaluate distal sensation on all extremities. Ask the patient to tell you where he or she is being touched. Evaluate the subjective ability to discern sharp from dull.

   g. Ask the patient to squeeze your fingers; evaluate for equal strength.

3. Percuss deep tendon reflexes: biceps, triceps, patellar, Achilles, and plantar.

E. Back

1. Inspect.

   a. Is there any deformity or abnormal curvature?

   b. Are there obvious signs of injury?

   c. Are there masses, rashes, or evidence of sacral edema?

2. Palpate to determine whether there is tenderness or pain along the bony processes or paravertebrally.

3. Percuss by striking the costovertebral angles with the ulnar aspect of your closed hand. Is tenderness or pain elicited?

enzyme for carbohydrates and is elevated most notably in acute pancreatitis. Three milliliters of venous blood is required.

Arterial blood gases. Arterial blood gases are analyzed from arterial specimens collected in heparinized tubes or syringes. Elements measured include serum pH, PCO_2, PO_2, and bicarbonate levels. Results help determine the acid-base status of the internal environment and the degree of oxygenation of the tissues. Most test results include the percentage of oxygen saturation of the red blood cells. Three milliliters is the minimal specimen required, and the specimen is collected under aseptic conditions.

White blood cell count and differential. A white blood cell count and differential may be ordered instead of a complete blood cell count when an infection is suspected. However, the white blood cell count and differential must be ordered and evaluated together, since the white blood cell count may not be elevated even in severe infections, whereas the differential will always be elevated in such cases. Mild to moderate leukocytosis may indicate an infectious process that is bacterial in origin. The differential is an evaluation of the different types of leukocytes that are found in the serum: neutrophils (56% of the total), eosinophils (2.7%), basophils (0.3%), and lymphocytes (34%). Neutrophils are also called "polys," or polymorphonucleocytes, and "segs," or segmented cells. Monocytes are nongranular leukocytes, and small numbers of monocytes may be seen in chronic inflammatory conditions. *Bands* are new neutrophils that are formed in response to overwhelming bacterial invasion that taxes the older neutrophil population. Such a condition is referred to as a *shift to the left*. The specimen for the white blood cell count and differential is collected in a clot tube devoid of preservatives or anticoagulants; 3 to 5 ml of venous blood is required.

Coagulation studies. Various elements of the coagulation series evaluate the different stages of clotting. The studies evaluate prothrombin time, partial thromboplastin time, platelet count, Lee-White clotting time, and prothrombin consumption time.

Prothrombin time. This test identifies defects in stage 3 of coagulation. A calcium-binding anticoagulant is added to the patient's serum, and the time between addition of this element and the formation of a fibrin clot is measured.

Partial thromboplastin time. This test identifies defects in stage 2 of coagulation. The test measures factors XII, XI, X, IX, VIII, V, II, and I; thus it measures the clotting time of plasma when elements of the clotting process are added to calcium-free and platelet-poor plasma in a predetermined sequence.

Prothrombin consumption time. This test measures prothrombin utilization time. The test identifies defects in stages 1 and 2 of coagulation and is also used to evaluate coagulation of blood.

Platelet count. This test identifies the number of platelets

in a peripheral smear and confirms defects in stage 1 of coagulation.

Lee-White clotting time. This test measures the time it takes for a fibrin clot to form in venous blood and identifies defects in stage 4 of coagulation.

Summary. For a complete listing of laboratory tests, the reader is referred to current texts on the subject. This review was intended as a quick guide to those tests commonly used in the ED and with which you will likely come into contact often during your career in that unit. Normal values vary depending on the facility conducting the tests; check with the laboratory at your hospital to determine the values at your location.

PUTTING IT ALL TOGETHER

The goal of nursing assessment in the ED is to assess all pertinent measurements rapidly but thoroughly to establish priority needs and prevent death or decompensation. The process is more a question of emphasis on the patient's chief complaint and subjective symptoms than a question of what specific exclusions are appropriate in each case; therefore the process of assessment changes to meet the needs of each patient.

The outline shown in the box on pp. 128 and 129 presents a workable flow upon which you may base your own assessment process. Whatever your approach, try to keep it practical, concise, and organized.

SUMMARY

This chapter presented the essential elements of nursing assessment within the ED: purpose, barriers, tools, and components of the physical examination. In many departments there are more professional nurses in contact with the patients than there are physicians, and priority setting through knowledgeable assessment and appropriate intervention contributes significantly to decreasing mortality and morbidity. This is particularly true for the early moments of the patient's visit, but it is also valid for the patient's entire stay in the department.

Because of traditional philosophies regarding the nursing role and responsibilities, many emergency nurses have never received proper training and supervision in systematic assessment. Thus it is frequently by empiric judgment that intervention is provided—judgment that often is associated with high error rates. On the other hand, interventions that are implemented based on scientific knowledge and a rational therapeutic framework predispose patients for a much more favorable outcome.

Nursing assessment may be brief and confined to a narrow focus or may be a reasonably rapid and efficient evaluation of all systems that may be affected by the current illness or injury. The extent of the evaluation is the decision of the nurse and is based on the patient's condition at that time, the chief complaint, and environmental factors. We believe

that the information presented here reinforces current practice for those nurses who have been practicing logical and complete assessments. For those nurses who have never been trained to initiate assessment, we hope to have stimulated the desire to obtain appropriate education and direction. For those nurses who have been performing assessments but have fallen prey to undesirable behavior, whether because of existing barriers or other factors, we hope to have stimulated a change in attitude toward this most essential of nursing responsibilities within the ED.

SUGGESTED READINGS

Abels LF: *Mosby's manual of critical care,* St Louis, 1979, Mosby–Year Book.

Bates B: *A guide to physical examination,* ed 2, Philadelphia, 1982, JB Lippincott.

Bookman L, Simoneau J: The early assessment of hypovolemia: postural and vital signs, *JEN* 3:43, 1977.

Gröer ME, Shekelton ME: *Basic pathophysiology: a conceptual approach,* ed 2, St Louis, 1983, Mosby–Year Book.

Sheehy SB, Barber JM: *Mosby's manual of emergency care: practices and procedures,* ed 3, St Louis, 1989, Mosby–Year Book.

Thompson J, Dains J: *Physical assessment,* St Louis, 1980, Mosby–Year Book.

Tilkian SM, Conover MH, Tilkian AG: *Clinical implications of laboratory tests,* ed 4, St Louis, 1987, Mosby–Year Book.

Basic Life Support

Susan Budassi Sheehy

Myocardial infarction is the cause of death in more than 650,000 persons in the United States each year. Of these, more than 350,000 persons die within the first 2 hours after the infarct, usually before they are hospitalized. In an attempt to alter these statistics, many cities and towns in the United States have developed sophisticated prehospital care systems in which early medical care is brought to the scene of the incident. Most prehospital care personnel are trained to administer basic life support, if indicated, and many have been trained to provide advanced life support as well. In addition, citizen cardiopulmonary resuscitation (CPR) is taught extensively in many areas of the country.

The original standards for CPR were drawn from the conference on CPR and emergency cardiac care sponsored by the American Heart Association (AHA) and the National Research Council in 1973.[1]

In 1980 and in several subsequent years, the AHA and the National Research Council have updated these standards in a paper, "Standards and Guidelines for Cardiopulmonary Resuscitation (CPR) and Emergency Cardiac Care (ECC)."[2] In these standards the role of the citizen in administering CPR is emphasized, and changes in standard CPR procedures are described.

Basic life support courses are offered by both the American Red Cross and the AHA to all interested persons. The AHA also offers courses in advanced cardiac life support to medical personnel. For more information regarding these courses, the reader is referred to these agencies.

BASIC LIFE SUPPORT
The ABCs

Basic life support is the first component of advanced life support. In basic life support, the rescuer is taught to recognize unconsciousness, establish a patent airway, ensure adequate breathing, and provide chest compressions if circulation is not occurring. These maneuvers are known as the "ABCs": airway, breathing, and circulation, or as CPR.

Establish airway. The basic airway maneuver for an unconscious patient is the head-tilt–chin-lift maneuver (Fig. 12-1). If cervical spine injury is suspected, the jaw-thrust

maneuver is used: the head is left in a neutral position, and the jaw is thrust forward by the rescuer with the use of his or her thumbs and fingers (Fig. 12-2). Both maneuvers serve to pull the tongue away from the posterior pharynx. The tongue is the greatest cause of an obstructed airway in the unconscious patient. When either of these maneuvers is performed, the action may be just enough to open the airway and allow for spontaneous respirations to begin without further assistance. One must remember, however, that it is essential to maintain an open airway either until the patient is intubated esophageally or endotracheally or until the patient can keep his or her own airway open. The only exception to this rule is when the rescuer is performing one-person CPR and it becomes necessary for him or her to leave the airway to perform chest compression.

Ensure breathing. After an airway has been established, the rescuer must check to see if breathing is present. The rescuer checks breathing by watching for the chest to rise, or by hearing or feeling air movement. If spontaneous

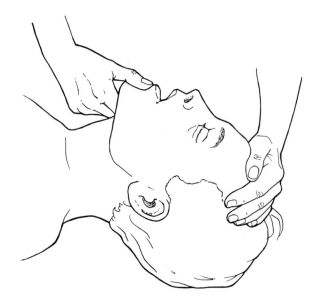

Fig. 12-1 Head-tilt–jaw-thrust maneuver. Pull mandible forward using thumb and forefingers.

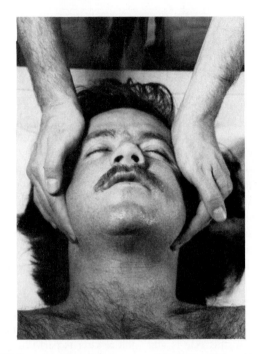

Fig. 12-2 Jaw-thrust maneuver. (Photo by Richard Lazar.)

breathing is present, the rescuer simply continues to maintain an open airway. If spontaneous breathing is *not* present, the rescuer must breathe for the patient. The simplest and most common method is to provide mouth-to-mouth breathing: the victim's nose is pinched shut, and the rescuer places his or her mouth over the victim's mouth and breathes into it (Fig. 12-3). Breathing is initiated by giving four quick breaths in stair-step fashion, without allowing for exhalation. This method permits a "loading dose" of oxygen to be administered before proceeding to the next step in CPR. When breathing into the victim's mouth, the rescuer should see the victim's chest rise (Fig. 12-4). If it does not rise, the rescuer should reposition the airway and try again.

Mouth-to-nose breathing is employed when there is some reason that mouth-to-mouth breathing cannot be used, such as in severe trauma to the mouth. When mouth-to-nose breathing is employed, the rescuer holds the victim's mouth shut with one hand, covers the victim's nose with his or her mouth, and breathes into the victim's nose.

In mouth-to-mouth breathing, the rescuer must remember to remove his or her mouth from around the victim's mouth to allow for passive exhalation. When performing mouth-to-nose breathing, the rescuer must remember to open his or her mouth after each breath into the nose to allow for passive exhalation. The process of breathing for the victim should take place every 5 seconds until spontaneous respiration is resumed or until resuscitation efforts have ceased.

If the victim has a laryngectomy or a tracheostomy, the rescuer should perform mouth-to-stoma breathing by sealing off the nose and mouth and breathing directly into the stoma.

Airway obstruction. Should attempts to ventilate the victim meet with resistance, the rescuer must perform a series of maneuvers to attempt to open the airway. The first maneuver is to reposition the airway. Sometimes in the

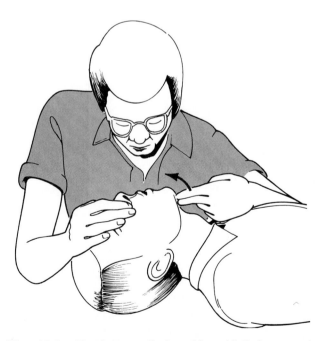

Fig. 12-3 Mouth-to-mouth breathing. Victim's nose is pinched shut, and rescuer places mouth over victim's mouth.

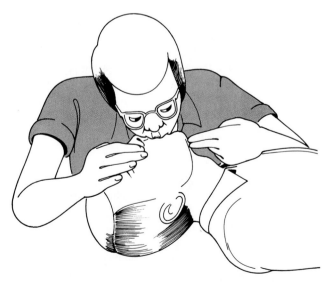

Fig. 12-4 Mouth-to-mouth breathing. Rescuer blows into victim's mouth, observing victim's chest rise.

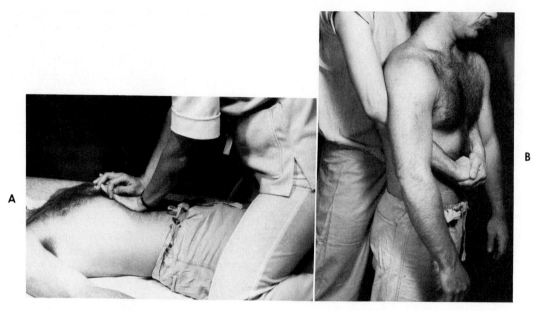

Fig. 12-5 **A,** Heimlich maneuver, lying. **B,** Heimlich maneuver, standing. (Photos by Richard Lazar.)

intensity of the rescue effort, good airway position is lost. Once the victim's head and neck are repositioned, the rescuer should once again attempt to give two quick breaths. If repositioning the victim's head and neck is not successful, the presence of a foreign body is likely.

If a foreign body is present, the rescuer should attempt to dislodge it by employing the subdiaphragmatic abdominal thrust maneuver (also known as the Heimlich maneuver). If the victim is in a prone position, the rescuer should straddle the victim and face the victim's head. The rescuer should place the heel of one hand on the victim's abdomen at the point halfway between the xiphoid process and the umbilicus. The rescuer's other hand should be placed on top of the first hand (Fig. 12-5, *A*). The maneuver is then carried out by administering 6 to 10 quick inward and upward thrusts of the hands in an attempt to increase intrathoracic pressure to dislodge the foreign body. If the airway remains blocked, the rescuer should repeat the procedure for the blocked airway.

The Heimlich maneuver may also be performed with the victim in a standing or sitting position. The rescuer stands behind the victim and places his or her arms around the victim's waist. In this position the rescuer makes a fist, and places the fleshy part of the fist on the abdomen, halfway between the xiphoid process and the umbilicus. The rescuer places his or her other hand on top of the first hand (Fig. 12-5, *B*) and performs a quick inward and upward thrust. This maneuver may be repeated 6 to 10 more times. The entire sequence should be repeated until an open airway is achieved or until advanced life support procedures are available.

Provide circulation. Attempts to assess circulatory status should be performed *only after adequate breathing has been established,* since circulation of unoxygenated blood is essentially a useless procedure. After the airway has been established and artificial breathing is initiated, the rescuer should check for circulation by feeling for the carotid or femoral pulse rate. If a pulse rate is not evident, the rescuer must begin chest compressions to provide artificial circulation. If a pulse rate is evident, the rescuer should be sure to continue to maintain an open airway and adequate breathing status in the victim.

When performing external cardiac compression, also known as cardiac massage, the rescuer should always be extremely cautious about placement of the hands. The rescuer must be sure to locate the xiphoid process and place the heel of one hand 2 finger widths higher, on the lower half of the sternum. The heel of the other hand should be placed on top of the first hand, and the fingers should be "locked" together; no weight should be placed on the chest by the fingers (Fig. 12-6).

The rescuer should be kneeling with the knees slightly separated and up as close to the victim as possible, and the rescuer's elbows should be in a straight, locked position (Fig. 12-7). The rescuer should then begin a smooth, downward compression of the sternum, followed by a smooth, upward decompression. The ratio of downward to upward motion should be in a range of 50% downward and 50% upward. It is important for the rescuer to remember not to administer sharp, quick compressions, since such compressions serve only to contuse the myocardium and do not provide a cardiac output adequate to maintain life.

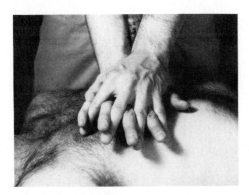

Fig. 12-6 Hand position for chest compression: no weight on fingers. (Photo by Richard Lazar.)

The depth of compression of an adult is approximately 1½ to 2 inches, although compression depth may vary from individual to individual. Chest compression, performed properly, may provide one fourth to one third of the normal cardiac output and may generate a systolic blood pressure of 100 mm Hg, which is compatible with life.

Research has demonstrated that *increased intrathoracic pressure,* not compression of the ventricles between the sternum and the vertebrae, is the force that causes cardiac output in CPR.[5] This research may indicate that chest compressions performed simultaneously with breathing maneuvers produce a better cardiac output. Other theories related to increased intrathoracic pressure and the production of greater cardiac output are being researched, including the use of abdominal compressions and pneumatic counter-pressure devices.

Also, studies have shown that circulation can be maintained during ventricular tachycardia and ventricular fibrillation if the victim is alert enough to cough. A cough increases intrathoracic pressure and provides a small amount of cardiac output.[4]

Chest compressions should be repeated 80 times per minute in a one-person rescue. The individual who is performing one-person rescue should provide 15 chest compressions, followed by two breaths, and then repeat the entire cycle continuously until additional help arrives or until the rescuer is too exhausted to continue.

In a two-rescuer effort, chest compressions should also be repeated 80 to 100 times per minute, and a breath should be interjected during the pause between every fifth compression.

The following points are absolutely essential to remember when performing CPR: (1) Be sure that the victim is on a firm surface when providing chest compression and (2) *always* accompany chest compressions with artificial breathing.

When a rescuer is resuscitating infants and children, the 5:1 ratio of chest compressions to breaths should be maintained. When compressing the chest, the rescuer should use

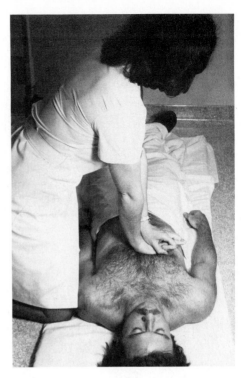

Fig. 12-7 Body position for CPR. Rescuer should be kneeling, with knees slightly separated and elbows in straight, locked position. (Photo by Richard Lazar.)

the index and middle fingers on an infant and the heel of one hand on a larger child. Compression is applied over the center of the sternum at a depth of ½ to 1½ inches, depending on the size of the child. Compression rate should be 80 to 100 times per minute.

It is important to remember that most cardiopulmonary arrests in children are respiratory (airway-related) and that the child will continue to have pulse rates for a while. It is absolutely essential to maintain an open airway and adequate breathing throughout the resuscitation effort.

Cardiopulmonary Resuscitation in Infants

Rescuer procedure. In CPR of an infant, first establish that unresponsiveness is present. Then position the infant on his or her back, supporting the infant's head and neck (Fig. 12-8). Open the airway, using the head-tilt–chin-lift method. Do not hyperextend the neck because hyperextension will cause a posterior airway obstruction. Check for breathing by looking for chest rise, listening for air movement, and feeling the chest rise and feeling air movement against your face. Then check for a pulse rate. Feel for a pulse rate in the upper arm (in the brachial area) for 5 to 10 seconds. If pulse rates are *present,* continue to maintain the airway and breathing at 20 breaths/min. If pulse rates are *absent,* prepare to start chest compressions. Imagine a line between the nipples, and place two fingers 1 finger

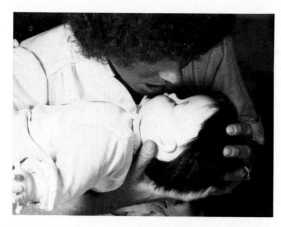

Fig. 12-8 Infant mouth-to-mouth breathing. Place infant's head and neck in a sniffing position. Do not hyperextend infant's neck. (Photo by Richard Lazar.)

width below this imaginary line. Compress the chest ½ to 1 inch in equal compression:relaxation ratio at a rate of 100 times per minute (Fig. 12-9). Compression to ventilation ratio should be 5:1, ensuring a pause for ventilation. Check for the return of a pulse rate after each 10 cycles of respirations and ventilations. If apnea and absence of pulse rate continue, continue CPR.

If the airway is obstructed, reposition the infant's head and attempt to breathe once again. If unsuccessful, place the infant in a head-dependent position, face down, and

administer four blows to the back. Turn the infant to a supine position and administer four chest thrusts in the midsternal region. Perform a jaw lift, and observe for (and remove, if present) any foreign body. Reposition the head and attempt to ventilate the infant. Repeat the entire procedure until the airway is unobstructed.

Resuscitation of Newborns

When CPR is performed on newborns, it is important to suction the mouth first, then the nose (Fig. 12-10).

If a newborn is breathing spontaneously and the heart rate is greater than 110 beats/min, suction the airway and stimulate the infant. Most infants begin to breathe spontaneously at this point. If there is still no breathing, begin mouth-to-mouth or mouth-to-nose breathing by giving two breaths. The newborn will probably begin to breathe. If not, continue breathing for the infant and check for a pulse.

Use supplemental oxygen when breathing for a newborn, and insert an endotracheal tube when possible. Continue to give breaths at a rate of 20 to 30 per minute. If breathing is absent or labored and the pulse rate is less than 110 beats/min, open the airway, suction the airway, and perform mouth-to-mouth or mouth-to-nose breathing. If respirations and heart rate continue to decrease, continue to ventilate the newborn. If a pulse rate cannot be palpated, begin chest compressions at a rate of 100 times per minute. Institute advanced life support measures.

The initial steps in the resuscitation of a newborn are the following:

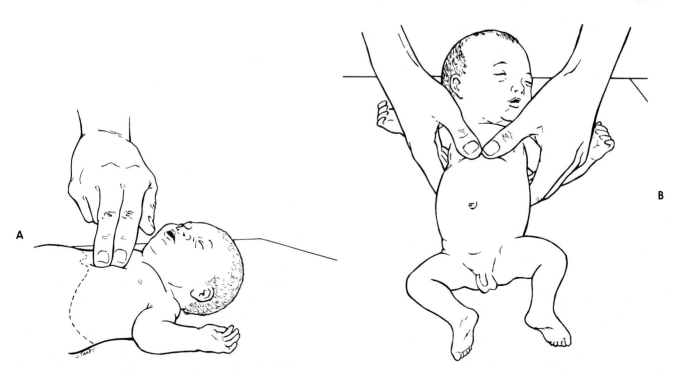

Fig. 12-9 Infant chest compression. **A,** Two-finger technique. **B,** Thumb technique.

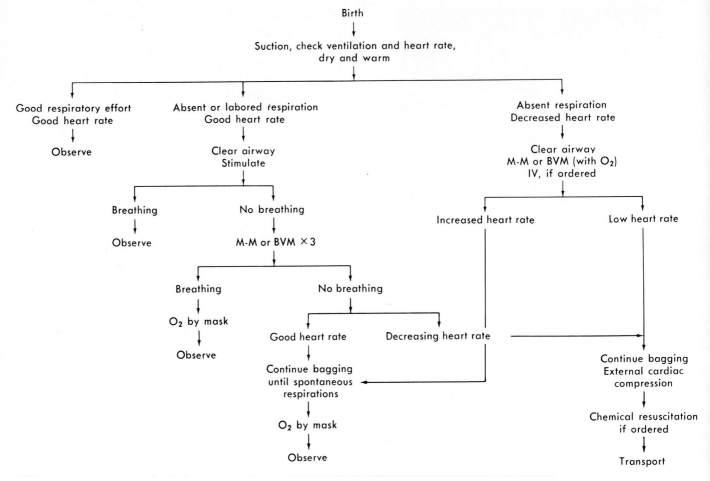

Fig. 12-10 Resuscitation of newborn. (From Melker R: Resuscitation of neonates, infants and children. In Auerback PA, Budassi SA, eds: *Cardiac arrest and CPR,* ed 2, Rockville, Md, 1983, Aspen Systems.)

1. Airway management
2. Breathing with supplemental oxygen
3. Circulation
4. Establishment of an IV line (usually via the umbilical vein)
5. Administration of sodium bicarbonate (2 mEq/kg diluted 1:1) by IV push
6. Administration of epinephrine (0.1 ml/kg of a 1:10,000 solution)

Remember that hypothermia can be detrimental to the resuscitation of newborns, infants, and children; therefore, be sure to keep the patient warm.

Cardiopulmonary Resuscitation in Children

Rescuer procedure. These guidelines are for children under 8 years of age. If the child is 8 years of age or older, use the procedure for CPR in adults.

First, establish that unresponsiveness is present. Position the child on his or her back. Open the airway using the head-tilt–chin-lift method. Assess for breathing by looking for chest rise, listening for air movement, and feeling for chest rise and air movement against your face. If breathing is *present,* maintain an open airway. If breathing is *absent,* make a seal over the child's mouth with your mouth and pinch the nose closed, then administer two slow breaths. Check for a pulse rate in the carotid area. If a pulse rate is *present,* maintain an open airway and artificial breathing. If a pulse rate is *absent,* kneel by the child's shoulders and prepare to administer chest compressions. Place the heel of one hand 2 finger widths above the end of the sternum. Place the second hand on top of the first, and interlock fingers. Compress the chest at a rate of 80 to 100 times per minute; compress 1 to 1½ inches. Ensure that the compression and relaxation phases are equal. The compression:ventilation ratio should be 15:2 in one-rescuer CPR and 5:1 in two-rescuer CPR. In two-rescuer CPR, be sure to allow for a pause in chest compressions while giving the breath.

Reassess the pulse after each 10 cycles of compressions and ventilations. If the airway is obstructed, reposition the child's head and attempt to ventilate again. If unsuccessful, kneel at the child's feet and place the heel of one hand against the child's abdomen just above the umbilicus and well below the xiphoid process. Place the second hand on top of the first hand. Press inward and upward quickly. Repeat this maneuver 6 to 10 times. Check for the presence of a foreign body by performing a jaw-lift maneuver and by attempting to locate the foreign body by visual inspection. If you cannot find a foreign body, reposition the head and attempt to ventilate the child. Repeat the procedure continuously until the airway is unobstructed.

Basic Life Support

Airway management. Airway management should always be the first consideration in an emergency situation. Besides the head-tilt and jaw-thrust maneuvers that are used in basic cardiac life support, several airway adjuncts may be used in advanced cardiac life support.

Oropharyngeal airway adjunct. The simplest airway adjunct is the oropharyngeal airway adjunct (see Fig. 13-2). It is a curved tube that is made of plastic, rubber, or metal. The oropharyngeal airway is inserted into the mouth upside down and rotated 180 degrees until the curve fits comfortably over the tongue with the opening extending into the posterior pharyngeal area. The curved part of the tube prevents the tongue from slipping back into the posterior pharyngeal area. This airway adjunct may also be inserted by moving the tongue to one side with a tongue blade or a similar piece of equipment and placing the airway adjunct with the opening extending into the posterior pharyngeal region (see Fig. 13-3). In infants and children an oropharyngeal airway adjunct should be placed by using the direct visualization–tongue blade technique. Do *not* use the rotation technique in infants and children, since damage may be done to the roofs of their mouths and soft palates. It is essential that the airway adjunct be placed properly: improper placement may actually block the airway. The oropharyngeal airway adjunct cannot be used in a conscious victim, since it may induce vomiting. It is used in those patients who are unconscious. After the airway is in place, continue to maintain the head-tilt or jaw-thrust position to maintain a patent airway. The oropharyngeal airway adjunct may be used in conjunction with a bag-valve-mask device or a demand valve.

Nasopharyngeal airway adjunct. A nasopharyngeal airway adjunct (trumpet tube) may be used in the alert, conscious victim when there is a need for some sort of assistance in maintaining an open airway (see Fig. 13-4). It is particularly useful in patients with soft-tissue facial trauma when edema is anticipated. This airway adjunct is a soft rubber tube that is inserted through a nostril after it has been lubricated with an anesthetic, water-soluble lubricant. The nasopharyngeal airway adjunct extends to the posterior pharyngeal area behind the tongue (see Fig. 13-5). Again, remember to maintain an open airway by using either the

chin-lift or jaw-thrust maneuver in conjunction with use of this airway adjunct.

Esophageal obturator airway adjunct. When a victim is apneic and unconscious, some means of providing positive pressure ventilation is necessary. One method of providing this is via the esophageal obturator airway (EOA) (see Fig. 13-6). This airway adjunct is a piece of equipment that can be inserted by personnel who are untrained in inserting an endotracheal tube. Little technical skill is required to place it, and training takes just a few minutes. The EOA is composed of a mask, which is used to seal off the nose and the mouth, a tube with a blocked distal end and perforations in the area of the posterior pharynx, and a balloon that, when inflated, allows for little or no air passage into the stomach and prevents aspiration of vomitus. Sealing off the nose and the mouth, blowing air into the tube with a blocked distal end, and inflating the balloon ensure that the only other pathway for the air to follow is out of the perforation holes, into the posterior pharyngeal area, and into the trachea (see Fig. 13-7).

To insert the EOA, grasp the lower jaw with one hand and lift it forward (see Fig. 13-8). Advance the lubricated tube into the posterior pharyngeal area with the tip pointing upward. Gently rotate the tube 180 degrees, and advance it carefully behind the tongue, into the posterior pharyngeal area and down into the esophagus. When the mask reaches the face, press it firmly against the face to obtain a tight seal, then blow into the end of the tube. If the tube is in the proper position, the chest should rise. If the chest does not rise, the tube should be removed immediately, since it may have accidentally passed into the trachea.

If after blowing into the tube you see the chest rise, auscultate the chest bilaterally during subsequent ventilatory efforts to ensure that both lungs are being ventilated adequately. Once adequate ventilation is established, inflate the balloon with 35 ml air using a syringe and pushing it through a one-way valve. Continue to ventilate the patient until other means of ventilation are prepared, until the patient resumes spontaneous respiration, or until resuscitation efforts are ceased.

If the patient is unable to maintain his or her own respiratory efforts and a method of long-term ventilation is necessary, he or she should be endotracheally intubated, and the EOA should then be removed.

If the patient begins to breathe spontaneously, the EOA must be removed. It is necessary to follow these instructions carefully for EOA removal: (1) Turn the patient on his or her side (this is not necessary if an endotracheal tube has been placed), (2) deflate the balloon and withdraw the EOA adjunct, and (3) be sure to have suctioning equipment available, since these patients often vomit after the EOA adjunct has been removed.

The advantages of the EOA are that it is easy to use and that training someone to use it is easy. The EOA may be used in those victims who have suspected cervical spine

Table 12-1 Comparison of one-rescuer and two-rescuer CPR

Factor	One-rescuer CPR	Two-rescuer CPR
Initial breaths	2	2
Compression rate	80 to 100/min	80 to 100/min
Compression:breath ratio	15:2	5:1
Other	—	Pause for breath

fractures because it may be placed with the head in a neutral position. Endotracheal tube placement is generally easier to accomplish with the EOA in place. The EOA also prevents aspiration of stomach contents and prevents air from entering the stomach. It allows greater amounts of air to be distributed compared with the bag-valve-mask system, and air intake is equal to that found in endotracheal intubation.

The EOA *cannot* be used in the conscious or semiconscious patient. Because it is available only in adult sizes, it cannot be used in infants and children. The EOA is contraindicated for patients with a history of caustic ingestion or esophageal disease and for patients in whom a foreign body in the trachea made the resuscitation necessary.

The EOA may be passed accidentally into the trachea; this situation is easily correctable if proper attention is paid to the placement procedure and placement verification. A few cases of perforation of the esophagus have been reported, but such cases are rare.

Breathing. Several different devices are available for the delivery of oxygen to a patient. Emergency nurses should be familiar with the various types and should be able to select the proper device for an individual patient's needs (Table 12-1).

Nasal cannula. The nasal cannula is the most commonly used oxygen delivery device. It can be used on a patient who is breathing spontaneously. If the oxygen flow rate is adjusted to 6 L/min, an oxygen concentration of 25% to 40% can be achieved.

Face masks. (See Fig. 13-10.) Face masks are tolerated well by most individuals except those who have severe dyspnea: the face mask may make such individuals feel as though they are suffocating. This device must be used on the spontaneously breathing patient. At a flow rate of 10 L/min an oxygen concentration of 50% to 60% can be achieved.

Oxygen reservoir mask. (See Fig. 13-11.) The oxygen reservoir mask is equipped with a plastic bag reservoir that fills with 100% oxygen when the patient is exhaling. Then, when the patient inhales, with the flow rate set at 10 to 12 L/min, the patient can receive a concentration of about 90% oxygen, provided that the mask has a tight seal. This piece of equipment must be used on the spontaneously breathing patient.

Venturi mask. If a victim gives a history of chronic obstructive lung disease and is currently having respiratory distress, one should consider using the Venturi mask, which allows for delivery of a fixed concentration of oxygen by adjustment of the oxygen flow caps on the device (see Fig. 13-12). With an oxygen flow rate of 4 L/min, one can obtain an oxygen concentration of 24% to 28%. By turning the oxygen flow rate up to 8 L/min and changing the oxygen flow cap, one can obtain an oxygen concentration of 35% to 40%. The proper method for using this device is to initiate the flow rate at the setting for 24% oxygen concentration and observe the patient closely. If respiratory depression is not present, one may elect to increase the oxygen concentration to 28% and repeat the observation, continuing to increase the oxygen concentration as long as the patient tolerates the previous, lower concentration well.

Pocket mask. (See Fig. 13-13.) A pocket mask may be carried by the rescuer and used when other forms of artificial ventilation are not available. The pocket mask allows for mouth-to-mask breathing. The mask fits snugly onto the victim's face, covering the nose and the mouth. The victim's head should be tilted back and the jaw pulled forward, with the victim's mouth slightly open. The rescuer can then blow into the opening in the top of the mask (see Fig. 13-14). One can add supplemental oxygen by attaching an oxygen source to the one-way valve located at the bottom of the mask. If the oxygen flow rate is regulated at 10 L/min, one can achieve a delivered oxygen concentration of about 50%. For pediatric use the mask may be turned upside down, with the wide end placed at the top of the child's head and the narrow end placed just below his or her mouth.

Bag-valve-mask device. A bag-valve-mask device can deliver 21% oxygen (room air) to a victim. By adding an additional oxygen source at a rate of 12 L/min, one can achieve an oxygen concentration of 40%. By adding a plastic cap and a 3-foot corrugated tubing reservoir (see Fig. 13-15) with an open end, one can obtain an oxygen concentration of about 90%.

The mask of the bag-valve-mask unit is applied in the same way as the pocket mask, and a tight seal must be obtained around the nose and the mouth. It is appropriate to use an oropharyngeal or nasopharyngeal airway adjunct in conjunction with the bag-valve-mask device.

Although there are many brands of bag-valve-mask devices on the market, a transparent device is recommended so that one may observe and intervene rapidly should emesis occur.

Oxygen-powered devices. (See Fig. 13-16.) Oxygen-powered devices can deliver 100% oxygen at a rate of 100 L/min to a pocket mask, an attached mask, an EOA adjunct, an endotracheal tube, or a transtracheal catheter insufflation device. Timing and length of oxygen delivery are determined by the operator. This device should *not* be used in children under 12 years of age unless a special pediatric adapter is available.

Circulation. During CPR when a chest compression is being performed, make sure that the victim is lying on a firm surface. Follow the recommendations from the AHA that were presented earlier in this chapter.

REFERENCES

1. American Heart Association and National Research Council: *Conference on standards for cardiopulmonary resuscitation and emergency cardiac care,* Chicago, 1973, The Association and The Council.
2. American Heart Association and National Research Council: Standards and guidelines for cardiopulmonary resuscitation and emergency cardiac care, *JAMA,* 244(suppl):453, 1980.
3. Bennett MA, Pentecost BL: Warning of cardiac arrest due to ventricular fibrillation and tachycardia, *Lancet* 1:1351, 1972.
4. Criley JM, Blaufuss AH, Kissell GL: Cough-induced cardiac compression: self-administered form of cardiopulmonary resuscitation, *JAMA* 256:1246, 1976.
5. Wolf Creek Conference, Maryland Critical Care Medicine, Silver Spring, Md, 1981.

SUGGESTED READING

American Heart Association: *Healthcare provider manual for basic life support, Chicago,* 1988, The Association.

CHAPTER
13 Advanced Life Support

Cynthia L. Stemper

Each year approximately 1.5 million Americans have an acute myocardial infarction (AMI); 540,000 of these people die. AMI occurs when there is inadequate blood supply to an area of the heart, resulting in tissue necrosis. This inadequate blood supply most commonly occurs as a result of severe atherosclerotic narrowing of one or more of the coronary arteries and thrombus formation. Other causes include rupture or hemorrhage of the atherosclerotic plaque and spasm of the artery. Complete myocardial necrosis following occlusion of a vessel may occur within 4 to 6 hours, thus the need for immediate intervention by health care providers.

When cardiac arrest occurs, there is complete cessation of systemic circulation; the patient is unconscious, apneic (or may have gasping agonal respirations), and cyanotic or pale, and pulses are absent in major arteries (for example, the carotid or femoral artery). Palpation of a major artery is necessary because auscultation of heart sounds is an unreliable measure of circulatory status. Unconsciousness usually occurs within 15 seconds after complete cessation of circulation; apnea and pupil dilation begin after 30 to 60 seconds. When there is no cerebral blood flow for 4 to 6 minutes or longer, the chances of recovery without brain damage are slight. Immediate intervention with both basic and advanced life support measures is necessary for survival. A coordinated team effort between prehospital care providers and emergency department staff improves the patient's chances for optimal resuscitation.

Advanced life support measures discussed in this chapter include the assessment and interventions for patients with AMI and cardiac arrest, interpretation of dysrhythmias, pharmacologic and thrombolytic therapy, and resuscitation of newborns, infants, and children.

ASSESSMENT

Establishing a diagnosis of AMI is based on the following components: history, physical examination and assessment, initial and repeat 12-lead electrocardiograms, and cardiac enzyme analysis. Prompt assessment and intervention are important because the incidence of ventricular fibrillation is 15 times more frequent during the first hour after the onset

of symptoms than during the next 12 hours. A person delays seeking assistance for an average of 3 hours. American Heart Association guidelines recommend that individuals with a history of angina seek assistance for chest pain that is unrelieved by 3 nitroglycerin tablets taken for a period of 10 minutes; a person without a previous diagnosis of coronary artery disease should seek assistance when he or she has symptomatic chest pain for more than 2 minutes.

History

Most patients are at rest or engaged in moderate activity at the onset of AMI. Chest pain indicative of AMI is usually severe, lasts longer than 30 minutes, and is usually not relieved by rest or vasodilators such as nitroglycerin. However, chest pain may be absent in as many as 20% of patients or it may not be the patient's main complaint. Classic signs and symptoms of AMI include crushing substernal chest pain, radiation of the pain down the arm(s) or up into the jaw or both, diaphoresis, and a sense of impending doom. Associated symptoms include nausea, vomiting, indigestion, dyspnea, and syncope.

The following PQRST mnemonic is helpful for obtaining from the patient a concise, brief history of the pain:

P (provokes, palliates)
What provoked the pain? What makes it better? What makes it worse?
Q (quality)
What does the pain feel like? Is it burning? Crushing? Tearing? Sharp?
R (radiates)
Does the pain radiate? If so, where?
S (severity)
How severe is the pain? If you were to rate the pain on a scale of 1 to 10, with 1 being the mildest and 10 being the most severe pain you can imagine, what number would you give this pain?
T (time)
When did the pain start? How long did it last? Does it come and go?

In addition to obtaining a history of the pain, the emergency nurse obtains the patient's past medical history. A

Table 13-1 Differential diagnosis of cardiopulmonary arrest*

Causes	Specific cause	Signs and symptoms	Therapeutic intervention	Notes
Metabolic	Hypoglycemia	Physical signs of insulin or oral hypoglycemic agent usage; tachydysrhythmias; seizures; aspiration	Dextrose, 50%	Consider hypoglycemia a strong possibility in patients who have a history of diabetes
	Hyperkalemia	ECG Prolonged Q-T interval; peaked T waves; loss of P waves; wide QRS complexes	Calcium chloride; sodium bicarbonate	Often seen in hemodialysis and renal failure patients; also seen in patients taking Aldactone
Drug-induced	Tricyclic antidepressants (Elavil, Triavil, Tofranil, Etrafon, Sinequan, Vivactil)	Tachydysrhythmias	Sodium bicarbonate (to keep pH at 7.50); physostigmine (however, efficacy has been questioned)	Causes direct cardiac toxicity; often delayed toxicity in adults
	Narcotics	Bradydysrhythmias; heart blocks	Naloxone (Narcan)	There is a question of direct cardiac toxicity
	Propanol	Cardiac Heart blocks; bradydysrhythmias; PVCs Respiratory Bronchospasm Metabolic Hypoglycemia	Isuprel Atropine Aminophyline Dextrose, 50%	PVCs may be caused by slow rate
Pulmonary (any disease causing severe hypoxia)	Asthma	Severe bronchospasm causing hypoxia and respiratory acidosis; ECG Tachydysrhythmias (especially ventricular fibrillation)	Endotracheal intubation and ventilatory support	Abuse of sympathomimetic inhalants
	Pulmonary embolus	Pleuritic chest pain; shortness of breath in high-risk patients (postoperative, those taking birth control pills); syncope (recent study shows 60% have syncope as part of initial complaint); tachydysrhythmias	Good ventilatory support; consider thrombolytic agents	Pathophysiology; acute hypoxia and cor pulmonale leading to tachydysrhythmias
	Tension pneumothorax	Distended neck veins; tracheal deviation; asymmetric chest expansion ECG Often electric mechanical dissociation	Needle thoracotomy; chest tube	Often seen in patients with blunt chest trauma; often occurs during CPR because of chest compressions (especially in patients with COPD)

*Many causes of cardiopulmonary arrest exist in addition to primary cardiac abnormalities. It is important for the nurse or rescuer to be familiar with these causes and to be alert to their signs and symptoms, as identification of these may modify the type of therapeutic intervention given. This table lists some of the conditions that may lead to cardiopulmonary arrest but are not primary cardiac abnormalities. All therapeutic interventions listed are in addition to basic and advanced cardiac life support measures.

SPECIAL NOTE FOR PREHOSPITAL CARE: Consider early transport for young patients in cardiac arrest, since definitive therapeutic intervention will most likely include procedures not performed in the field situation.

Table 13-1   Differential diagnosis of cardiopulmonary arrest—cont'd

Causes	Specific cause	Signs and symptoms	Therapeutic intervention	Notes
Neurogenic	Increased intracranial pressure from any cause (e.g., subarachnoid hemorrhage; subdural hematoma)	Central neurogenic breathing; dilated pupil(s); decerebrate decorticate posturing; ECG Wide range of dysrhythmias, especially heart blocks	Central neurogenic hyperventilation (causes respiratory alkalosis, which results in cerebral vasoconstriction); steroids; diuretic agents; surgery	Damage to brain stem and autonomic centers
Hypovolemic	Anything that causes volume loss such as gastrointestinal bleeding, severe trauma with organ damage, ruptured ectopic pregnancy, dissecting or leaking aneurysm	Tachycardia; decreasing blood pressure; skin cool, clammy, pale; obvious signs of external blood loss	IV fluids; pneumatic antishock garment (PASG); shock position; surgery	A major cause of cardiopulmonary arrest that may be unrecognized
Other cardiac causes	Pericardial tamponade	Distended neck veins; decreasing blood pressure; distant heart sounds ECG Electromechanical dissociation of bradydysrhythmias	IV fluids: PASG; atropine; Isuprel; pericardiocentesis; thoracotomy; widening pulse pressure	Look for it, especially in patients with blunt chest trauma or prolonged CPR efforts

differential diagnosis of cardiopulmonary arrest is given in Table 13-1. Has the patient ever had heart problems? Does he or she have a history of hypertension, diabetes, lung problems, or vascular insufficiency? Ask the patient what medications he or she takes daily. Also ask the patient whether he or she smokes or consumes alcohol regularly. Each of these factors places patients at greater risk for AMI.

The clinician can ascertain the answers to these questions while initiating oxygen therapy, monitoring cardiac function, and obtaining intravenous access.

Physical Assessment

Begin by assessing the patient's vital signs and neurologic status and auscultating the lungs. Signs of a decreasing cardiac output include hypotension, cool, clammy skin, tachycardia, decreasing level of consciousness, distended jugular veins, and crackles in the bases of the lungs. Initially the patient's blood pressure may be hypertensive because of the catecholamine released by the adrenal glands and the sympathetic nervous system in response to the patient's pain and stress.

12-Lead Electrocardiogram

Changes in the electrocardiogram (ECG) provide information about the site of coronary artery occlusion, myo-

cardial ischemia, and the presence of tissue necrosis. Serial ECGs are used in conjunction with the assessment of the patient to confirm the diagnosis of AMI. A single ECG cannot be used exclusively because ECG findings are sensitive to changes only 50% of the time.

Elevation of the portion of the segment between the end of the S wave and the beginning of the T wave (the ST segment), which is indicative of injury, occurs within minutes after occlusion of the artery, and the ST segment may remain elevated for 24 hours. T-wave inversion occurs 6 to 24 hours after occlusion and may persist from months to years; it is the result of ischemia. Pathologic Q waves measure more than 0.04 second both in width and depth and are 25% or more of the overall height of the complex consisting of the Q, R, and S waves (QRS complex). This change in the Q wave usually occurs within 24 hours and indicates irreversible cell death.

Cardiac Enzyme Analysis

Serum glutamate oxaloacetate transaminase, creatine kinase, and lactic dehydrogenase (LDH) are nonspecific cardiac enzymes that become elevated when myocardial damage occurs. The creatine kinase level begins to rise 2 to 4 hours after the infarction and peaks in 24 hours. The LDH level rises and peaks in 12 to 48 hours. Analysis of myocardial-specific isoenzymes (creatine phosphokinase myocardial bands [CPK-MB], LDH_1, and LDH_2) is more helpful in identifying injury. The level of CPK-MB rises within 4 to 8 hours after the infarction and usually peaks after 20 hours. In 8 to 12 hours, the levels of both LDH_1 and LDH_2 rise and peak in 24 to 48 hours. Because even the earliest rise in enzyme levels occurs 2 hours after the AMI, the usefulness of cardiac enzyme analysis is limited primarily to the inpatient critical care setting.

INITIAL MANAGEMENT

While you are obtaining the patient's history and assessing the patient's condition, the steps associated with initial management can be accomplished. It is essential to treat a patient who is having chest pain as though he or she were having an AMI. One of the most important interventions is to communicate with the patient calmly and reassuringly. Let the patient know what you are doing, why you are doing it, and how you are going to carry out procedures. As soon as practical, remember to inform the family about what is occurring.

If a person is thought to be having an AMI but does not have dyspnea, administer oxygen by nasal cannula at 6 L/min. Have the person sit up and attempt to find a position of comfort. Significant hypoxemia may occur even in patients with uncomplicated infarction. If the patient is having any dyspnea, administer oxygen at 12 L/min with a nonrebreathing mask.

After oxygen therapy is initiated, an intravenous (IV) line should be established for the administration of any medications that may be required: a 5% aqueous dextrose solution (D_5W) is usually the fluid of choice. A peripheral site should be chosen, and an 18-gauge catheter, at least, should be used. If thrombolytic therapy is being considered, use a double-lumen catheter and use only compressible veins.

Any patient complaining of chest pain should be monitored for dysrhythmias and treated according to the appropriate protocol. When monitoring for dysrhythmias, use limb lead II (for the strongest wave forms) or lead MCL_1 (for early recognition of bundle branch blocks) (Fig. 13-1). Avoid monitoring on limb lead I because lead I often does not pick up atrial dysrhythmias.

One major problem with myocardial infarction is pain, which can cause anxiety, increased heart rate, increased oxygen consumption, and therefore increased ischemia. Thus one key to treating myocardial ischemia is to provide early pain relief.

One method of providing pain relief is the administration of nitroglycerin. Nitroglycerin may be used in the treatment of both angina and myocardial infarction. Nitroglycerin is a nitrate preparation that dilates the vessels of the peripheral venous circulation, which causes a decreased venous return to the heart. This effect decreases ventricular dilation and filling so that less work is required to empty the heart, resulting in a net decrease in myocardial consumption. An added benefit of nitroglycerin is that it dilates coronary arteries. Nitroglycerin is usually not given unless the systolic blood pressure is at least 100 mm Hg because nitroglycerin may cause a drop in blood pressure. If the patient does become hypotensive, elevate the patient's legs to increase venous return; if this procedure does not improve the patient's hypotensive state, consider a fluid challenge.

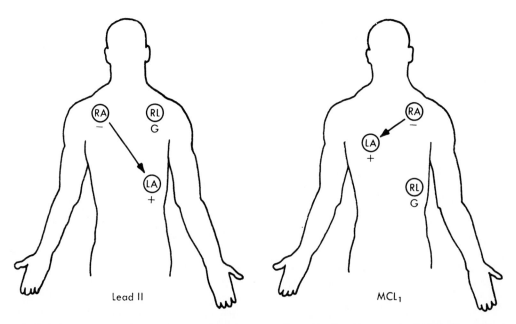

Fig. 13-1   Monitoring on 3-lead ECG monitor. Leads II and MCI_1 are best leads to use for monitoring dysrhythmias.

If the first attempt to relieve the chest pain with nitroglycerin is unsuccessful, the dose may be repeated twice at 5-minute intervals if the systolic blood pressure remains above 100 mm Hg. If the patient tells you that he or she has taken several of his or her own nitroglycerin tablets without obtaining relief, it may be that the patient's medication has become impotent. For this reason it is always better to use the nitroglycerin stocked in the department than to use the patient's own supply.

An alternative to nitroglycerin tablets is transdermal nitroglycerin paste (Nitropaste). It is applied to the chest wall over the left side of the chest in a 1- to 1½-inch strip. Because transdermal nitroglycerin paste is absorbed through the skin, its onset of action is a bit slower than that of sublingual nitroglycerin tablets, but its duration is longer. Nitroglycerin paste can lose its potency over time and with exposure to light. Be sure to check the expiration date on the tube before applying the paste.

If attempts to relieve pain with the various forms of nitroglycerin fail, the next drug of choice is morphine sulfate. This narcotic–analgesic helps to relieve chest pain, decreases preload, decreases myocardial oxygen consumption, and relieves anxiety. If the blood pressure is normal or elevated, administer a dose of 3 to 10 mg IV (slow push) over a period of 2 or more minutes, until pain relief is obtained. If this amount does not relieve the pain, an ad-

ditional dose may be given; the total amount of morphine sulfate given should not exceed 15 mg. Hypotension occurring after morphine administration should be treated in a manner similar to that described for hypotension following nitroglycerin administration. If respiratory depression occurs, naloxone hydrochloride (Narcan) is the antagonist of choice. It should be administered in a bolus of 0.4 to 0.8 mg. A response from naloxone hydrochloride within 4 minutes can be anticipated. It is therefore mandatory that you support the airway and maintain respirations until the naloxone hydrochloride takes effect. If the patient has a history of chronic obstructive pulmonary disease, the use of morphine sulfate is often contraindicated.

A combination of 50% oxygen and 50% nitrous oxide (Nitronox, Entonx) may also be used for relieving chest pain. When the nitrous oxide mixture is administered, it must be given by self-administered mask. As the nitrous oxide mixture takes effect, the patient allows the mask to fall away, which eliminates the danger of over-administration. Nitrous oxide is a rapidly acting gas (3 to 4 minutes) that has been shown to effectively relieve pain without causing hemodynamic deterioration or dysrhythmias.

ADVANCED LIFE SUPPORT MEASURES

Basic life support measures are used to establish an airway, provide oxygenation, and provide minimally adequate

Table 13-2   Cardiac medications for adults

Drug	Category	Actions	Indications	Dose	Comments
Bretylium (Bretylol)	Category III anti-dysrhythmic	Elevates threshold for VF; suppresses reentry dysrhythmias; positive inotrope; transiently positive dromotrope	VF, VT, PVCs refractory to lidocaine	VF: 5 mg/kg rapid IV push; may be repeated twice at 10 mg/kg VT: 500 mg diluted in 50 ml IV solution, given 5 to 10 mg/kg over a period of 10 minutes; repeat every 1 to 2 hours when required Maximum dose is 30 mg/kg IV drip: 1 g/250 ml D$_5$W (4 mg/ml) at 1 to 4 mg/min (15 to 60 μgtts/min)	May cause hypotension, syncope, bradycardia, vertigo, dizziness, nausea, and vomiting; patient should be supine; response is not as rapid with VT as with VF
Dopamine (Intropin)	Sympathomimetic	Dose dependent Dopaminergic effects: 0.5 to 5 μg/kg/min Beta effects: 5 to 10 μg/kg/min Alpha effects: 10 + μg/kg/min	Cardiogenic shock; hypotensive states not caused by volume depletion; congestive heart failure	400 mg/500 ml D$_5$W (800 μg/ml) given at 2 to 10 ug/kg/min; titrate to desired blood pressure	Adverse effects: tachycardia, palpitations, PVCs

Continued.

Table 13-2 Cardiac medications for adults—cont'd

Drug	Category	Actions	Indications	Dose	Comments
Atropine	Parasympatholytic; anticholinergic	Increases rate of SA node firing; increases conduction through AV node; decreases vagal tone	Hemodynamically significant bradycardia; asystole; high-degree AV blocks	Bradycardia and AV blocks: 0.5 mg IV (rapid push) or intratracheally every 5 minutes to maximum dose of 2.0 mg Asystole: 1.0 mg IV (rapid push) or intratracheally; repeat once after 5 minutes Minimum dose is 0.5 mg; maximum dose is 2 mg	May cause paradoxic slowing of heart rate when given slowly or in doses of less than 0.5 mg
Epinephrine (Adrenalin)	Sympathomimetic	Both alpha and beta adrenergic effects; increases mean arterial pressure; decreases fibrillatory threshold; stimulates heart in asystole and idioventricular rhythms	Allergic reactions; cardiac arrest; bronchoconstriction or bronchospasm	Available as 1:10,000 solution (1 mg in 10 ml) Cardiac arrest*: 1.0 mg IV (rapid push) or intratracheally; repeat every 5 minutes when required	Adverse effects: tachycardia, palpitations, PVCs, angina
Propranolol (Inderal)	Category II antidysrhythmic, nonspecific beta-blocker	β_1 and β_2 receptor blockade; beta-adrenergic blocker	Tachycardia, hypertension, after myocardial infarction, to reduce myocardial oxygen consumption secondary to recurrent tachycardias	1 to 3 mg IV (slow push) (<1 mg/min); repeat after 5 to 10 minutes when required Maximum dose is 0.1 mg/kg	May precipitate severe bronchospasm in patients with chronic obstructive pulmonary disease; may precipitate congestive heart failure Side effects: hypotension, bradycardia
Isoproterenol (Isuprel)	Sympathomimetic	Nonspecific beta-adrenergic stimulation	Temporary control of hemodynamically significant bradycardia refractory to atropine	1 mg in 250 ml D_5W (4 μg/ml); 2 to 20 μg/min IV (30 to 300 μgtts/min); titrate to heart rate of 60 to 70 beats/min	Causes an increased workload on the heart; use with extreme caution: exacerbates ischemia and extends infarct size
Furosemide (Lasix)	Loop diuretic	Venodilation, diuresis	Congestive heart failure, pulmonary edema, cerebral edema	20 to 40 mg IV (slow push); repeat every 30 minutes when required Maximum dose is 2 mg/kg If patient is already receiving furosemide orally, begin with an IV dose equal to half the daily oral dose	May cause hypovolemia or hypotension; monitor urine output; insert a Foley catheter; contraindicated for patients with allergy to sulfa drugs

*In some institutions "high-dose" epinephrine (5 mg IV or intratracheally) is given initially, in accordance with local protocols.

Table 13-2 Cardiac medications for adults—cont'd

Drug	Category	Actions	Indications	Dose	Comments
Lidocaine (Xylocaine)	Category IB antidysrhythmic	Decreases automaticity; suppresses ventricular ectopy; depresses conduction through reentrant pathways; elevates VF threshold	PVCs, VT, VF, preintubation for patients with suspected increased intracranial pressure or laryngospasm	1 mg/kg IV (slow push) over a period of 2 minutes, or intratracheally; repeat at 0.5 mg/kg every 8 to 10 minutes when required Maximum dose is 3 mg/kg Preintubation: 1.5 mg/kg IV push, wait 90 seconds, then intubate IV drip: 1 g in 250 ml D$_5$W (4 mg/ml) at 2 to 4 mg/min (30 to 60 μgtts/min)	Adverse effects: central nervous system depression, drowsiness, dizziness, confusion, anxiety Contraindications: bradycardia-related PVCs, bradycardia, idioventricular rhythm; if given too rapidly, may cause seizures
Morphine	Narcotic analgesic (opiate)	Analgesia, venodilation, sedation	Ischemic chest pain, acute cardiogenic pulmonary edema, anxiety, apprehension	2 to 5 mg IV (slow push), repeat every 5 to 30 minutes when required Usual maximum dose is 20 mg	Adverse effects: hypotension, respiratory depression, apnea Have narcotic antagonist (naloxone) available
Procainamide (Pronestyl)	Category IA antidysrhythmic	Suppresses PVCs; suppresses reentry dysrhythmias; may elevate VF threshold; negative chronotrope and dromotrope; mild negative inotrope; potent peripheral vasodilator	PVCs and VT refractory to lidocaine; hemodynamically significant supraventricular tachycardia	100 mg IV (slow push) (20 mg/min), repeat every 5 minutes when required IV infusion: 1 g in 250 ml D$_5$W (4 mg/ml) at 1 to 4 mg/min (15 to 60 μgtts/min)	May cause hypotension, bradycardia Contraindications: third-degree AV block, digoxin toxicity
Sodium bicarbonate	Alkalotic agent	Buffers or neutralizes metabolic acidosis	Suspected acidosis in cases of cardiac arrest	1 mEq/kg IV (slow push); repeat 0.5 mEq/kg every 10 to 15 minutes when required	May inactivate catecholamines when given together in same IV line; when possible, use arterial blood gas levels to guide administration
Verapamil (Calan)	Category IV antidysrhythmic, Ca^{++} channel blocker	Blocks entry of Ca^{++} into cells; negative dromotrope and depresses atrial automaticity; negative chronotrope; negative inotrope; vasodilator	Supraventricular tachycardia	0.075 to 0.15 mg/kg IV (slow push) Elderly patients: 2 mg over a period of 3 to 4 minutes Maximum dose is 10 mg	Hypotension

circulation with chest compressions. For restoration of spontaneous circulation, more complex or invasive measures may be required. These measures frequently include the administration of drugs (Table 13-2) or fluids, cardioversion, and defibrillation.

AIRWAY MANAGEMENT

Airway management should always be the first consideration in any emergency situation. In addition to the head-tilt and jaw-thrust maneuvers used in basic life support, several airway adjuncts may be used in advanced cardiac life support.

Oropharyngeal Airway Adjunct

The simplest airway adjunct to use is the oropharyngeal airway (Fig. 13-2). It is a curved tube, most commonly made of disposable plastic. The tube is inserted upside down into the mouth until the tube just touches the hard palate; the tube is then rotated 180 degrees and advanced until the curve fits over the tongue and the opening of the tube extends into the posterior pharynx. This adjunct prevents the tongue from slipping back and occluding the posterior pharynx. Alternately the tube may be placed by depressing or moving the tongue to one side with a tongue blade and then inserting the airway directly into the pharynx, following the curvature of the tongue (Fig. 13-3). This airway must be placed properly; improper placement may result in pushing the tongue into the posterior pharynx, which blocks the airway. This airway adjunct cannot be used in a conscious patient because it may induce vomiting or laryngospasm. The oropharyngeal airway is used in patients who are unconscious and flaccid, to prevent the tongue from falling back and creating an obstruction. Use of this airway adjunct also helps prevent the patient from biting and occluding an endoctracheal tube. Once the airway adjunct is in place, you must continue to maintain the patient's head-tilt or jaw-thrust position to keep the airway open.

Nasopharyngeal Airway Adjunct

A nasopharyngeal airway adjunct (trumpet tube) may be used in the semiconscious victim when some assistance in maintaining the airway is needed (Fig. 13-4). This adjunct is also useful for patients with soft tissue facial trauma when edema is anticipated or when insertion of an oropharyngeal airway adjunct is difficult. This airway adjunct consists of a soft rubber tube that is inserted through a naris after being lubricated with an anesthetic, water-soluble lubricant. The tube extends to the area of the posterior pharynx behind the tongue (Fig. 13-5). During insertion, remember to direct the tip straight back along the floor of the nose rather than up into the turbinates. Again, remember to maintain an open airway by using either the head-tilt or jaw-thrust maneuver in conjunction with the use of this airway adjunct. Use of the nasopharyngeal airway adjunct may cause vomiting and laryngospasm.

Esophageal Obturator Airway Adjunct

When a victim is apneic and unconscious, a means of providing positive-pressure ventilation is necessary. One method of providing this ventilation is via an esophageal obturator airway adjunct (EOA) (Fig. 13-6). Placing this airway adjunct requires little technical skill and does not

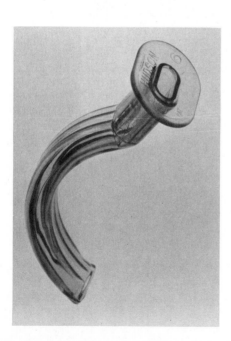

Fig. 13-2 Oropharyngeal airway. (Photo by Richard Lazar.)

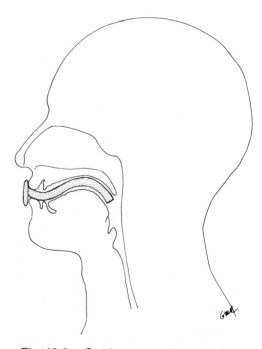

Fig. 13-3 Oropharyngeal airway in place.

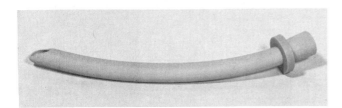

Fig. 13-4 Nasopharyngeal airway. (Photo by Richard Lazar.)

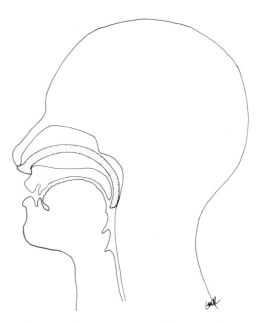

Fig. 13-5 Nasopharyngeal airway in place.

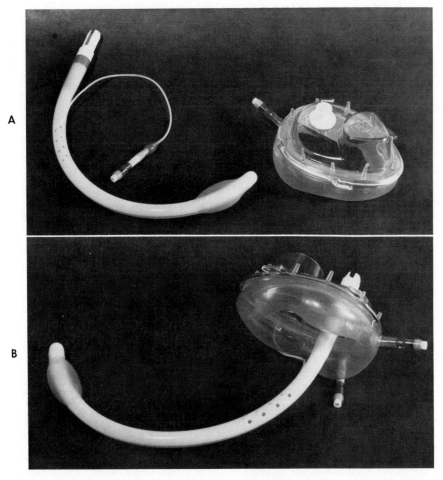

Fig. 13-6 **A,** Esophageal obturator airway and mask, separated. **B,** Esophageal obturator airway and mask, connected. (Photos by Richard Lazar.)

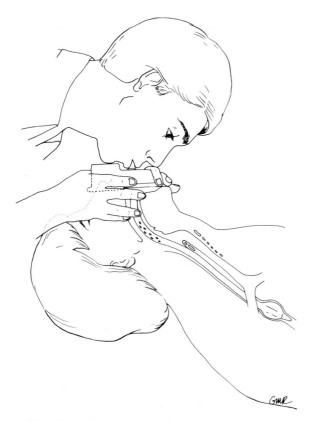

Fig. 13-7   Esophageal obturator airway in place.

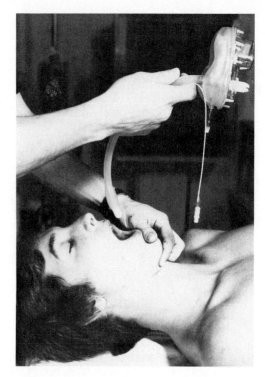

Fig. 13-8   To insert EOA, grasp patient's lower jaw with one hand and lift EOA forward. (Photo by Richard Lazar.)

require hyperextension of the neck. Also, since visualization is not required for insertion, an EOA can be introduced more easily and quickly than can an endotracheal tube.

An EOA is composed of a mask that is used to seal off the nose and mouth; a tube with a blocked distal end and perforations in the area of the posterior pharynx; and a balloon, which, when inflated, allows for little or no air passage into the stomach, preventing aspiration of vomitus. Sealing off the nose and mouth and inflating the esophageal balloon ensure that the only pathway for air to follow is out of the perforated holes, into the posterior pharynx, and into the trachea (Fig. 13-7).

To insert the tube, hold the patient's head to midneutral or slightly flexed position and elevate the tongue and jaw with one hand (Fig. 13-8). With the other hand, insert the tube through the mouth into the esophagus until the tube is advanced fully and the mask is seated on the face. Next, deliver positive-pressure ventilation and watch for the chest to rise. If the chest rises, inflate the cuff with 35 ml of air. If the chest does not rise, the tube should be removed immediately, since it may have passed into the trachea. After inflation of the cuff, confirm breath sounds bilaterally at the midaxillary line. Continue to ventilate the patient until other means of ventilation are prepared, until the victim resumes spontaneous respirations, or until resuscitation efforts are discontinued.

If the victim begins to have spontaneous respirations, the EOA must be removed. To remove the airway adjunct, turn the victim on his or her side (this step is not necessary if an endotracheal tube is in place), deflate the balloon and withdraw the airway, and have suction equipment available, since it is common for these patients to vomit following EOA removal. To minimize esophageal mucosal necrosis, do not leave an EOA in place for more than 2 hours.

While the EOA is still in place, an endotracheal tube should be inserted as soon as possible, to better secure the airway.

The EOA cannot be used for the conscious or semiconscious victim because it may cause laryngospasm, vomiting, aspiration, or a combination of these. It cannot be used for patients less than 5 feet tall (that is, infants and children). It is contraindicated for those with a history of caustic ingestion, esophageal disease (for example, varices), or the presence of a foreign body in the trachea. A few cases of esophageal perforation from various causes have been reported.

Esophageal Gastric Tube Airway Adjunct

An esophageal gastric tube airway adjunct (EGTA) is a new modification of the EOA in which the esophageal tube is open throughout its length to allow passage of a gastric tube for stomach decompression. Since air is not blown into

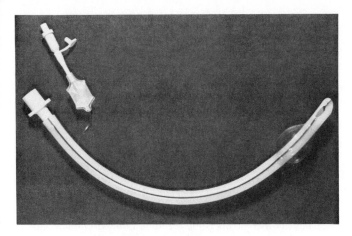

Fig. 13-9 Endotracheal tube.

the esophageal tube of the EGTA, a second port in the mask is provided. The technique for insertion and the complications of the EGTA are the same as those for an EOA.

Endotracheal Intubation

Indications for endotracheal intubation include the inability to ventilate the patient by other means, the inability of the patient to protect his or her own airway, and the need for prolonged ventilation. Intubation should *never* be the first method used to control a patient's airway. Other measures such as mouth-to-mask ventilation or the use of a bag-valve-mask device with supplemental oxygen should be used first.

Efficient, effective intubation begins with careful preparation and organization of equipment. Begin by testing the suctioning equipment and having it close at hand. Select and prepare the correct size of endotracheal (ET) tube. An ET tube has a standard 15 mm adapter that can be used with a bag-valve-mask device or other types of resuscitation and ventilation equipment. An ET tube also has a balloon (cuff) located at the distal end of the tube (Fig. 13-9). For men and women of average size, choose an 8 mm tube and a 7 mm tube, respectively. Insert a malleable stylet until the end is just short of the Murphy eye (side hole), and bend the tube to resemble a hockey stick. If time permits, lubricate the front third of the tube with a water-soluble gel. Test the cuff by inflating it with 7 ml of air and removing the syringe. If the cuff is patent, remove the air and leave the syringe in place. Choose an intubation blade appropriate for the patient. A curved (MacIntosh) blade permits slightly better visualization of the cords than does the straight (Miller) blade; a curved blade is the best choice when the patient has a short neck. The size of the curved blade must be chosen carefully so that the end will fit into the vallecula. The anteroposterior dimension of the curved blade makes scraping the enamel of the upper teeth or prying on (and possibly breaking) the upper teeth more likely with the MacIntosh blade: use of the straight (Miller) blade generally

results in slightly less visualization of the cords but results in less frequent contact with the upper incisors. After choosing an intubation blade, make sure the bulb on the blade is tightly seated and bright. Finally, have available an appropriately sized oropharyngeal airway adjunct to be used as a bite block. Position the patient's head in the "sniffing" position: the neck is slightly hyperextended, with the head forward. A pillow placed under the head helps maintain this position. Monitor the patient's cardiac rhythm, observing for tachydysrhythmias or bradydysrhythmias secondary to the possible hypoxia, vagal stimulation, or increased intracranial pressure that accompanies intubation. These untoward responses can be blunted by administering atropine (0.5 mg IV [rapid push] to block the parasympathetic response) and lidocaine (1.5 mg/kg of body weight IV push to block the sympathetic response). Wait 90 seconds after administering these medications; then attempt to intubate the patient.

Begin by holding the ET tube in your dominant hand. With your other hand, insert the laryngoscope. If you are using a curved blade, insert it into the right side of the mouth and sweep the tongue to the left until the blade is in the midline; then follow the curvature of the anterior surface until the tip of the blade is in the vallecula. If you are using a straight blade, direct it straight down the midline until the blade tip just touches the posterior pharynx; then lift the blade up to move the epiglottis out of view. To lift the tongue and mandible out of the visual line to the vocal cords, push the laryngoscope away from you, directing the force along the axis of the blade handle (toward the corner where the wall opposite you meets the ceiling). Do not bend your wrist or touch the upper teeth with the bottom of the blade. If the laryngoscope is properly placed, you should be able to see the vocal cords. If you are having difficulty seeing the cords, have an assistant perform the Sellick maneuver (posterior cricoid pressure) to bring the cords down into view. Many practitioners insert the straight blade too deeply and see only the esophagus; if the laryngoscope is slowly withdrawn, the glottic opening may drop into view.

When the cords are visible, gently introduce the ET tube from the right corner of the mouth until the cuff has passed completely through the cords; then withdraw the laryngoscope. Do not use the slot in the straight blade as a tube guide; the slot straightens out the tube and makes directing the tube up into the cords more difficult (if not impossible). If you cannot see the cords (or at least the posterior aspect of the arytenoid cartilage), *do not* insert the tube. If more than 15 seconds has elapsed, remove the laryngoscope and reoxygenate the patient for at least 1 minute; then try again.

The tube should be inserted far enough that the cuff does not impinge on the cords but not so far that the end is past the carina and directed into the right mainstem bronchus. For women the tube is usually inserted to a depth of 21 cm at the teeth; for men, 23 cm. Hold the tube against the upper teeth or hard palate with your right hand while removing the stylet with your left. This procedure helps ensure that the tube remains in place. Quickly reconnect the bag-valve-mask device and begin to ventilate the patient. With the stethoscope, listen in at least five places, first over the epigastrium. If you hear gurgling, remove the bag-valve-mask device immediately to prevent gastric distention. Listen over the apices and at the midaxillary line bilaterally. If the tube is properly positioned, inflate the cuff, insert the oropharyngeal airway adjunct, and secure the tube. Check breath sounds and the depth of the tube periodically.

The ET tube may also be placed via the nasotracheal route. This procedure is typically a blind intubation attempt and should be performed only by those who are extremely skilled in this technique. The nasotracheal route is the intubation route of choice for patients who are still breathing and is contraindicated for patients with midfacial fractures.

If the patient has spontaneous respirations in the emergency department and arterial blood gases are at an acceptable level, you may elect to remove the ET tube. Removal is accomplished by, first, suctioning the patient's nose, mouth, and posterior pharyngeal area. The cuff should then be deflated and the tube withdrawn. Never withdraw the airway adjunct without first deflating the cuff. Be prepared to suction the patient in case of vomiting. Also, be sure to monitor the patient for cardiac dysrhythmias.

The advantages of endotracheal intubation are that good control of the airway can be maintained, and the patient can be protected from aspiration. With the tube in place, gastric distention is minimal. The trachea can be suctioned through the ET tube, and the patient can be ventilated with 100% oxygen under positive pressure.

Disadvantages of an ET tube are that the tube can easily be placed in the esophagus during intubation, which results in hypoxia, and that insertion requires skill. Some ventilations must be discontinued while the tube is being inserted; the patient may become hypoxic if insertion is prolonged.

Several medications may be administered via an ET tube, which is especially useful when an IV line has not yet been established. The lungs absorb medications rapidly, so an ET tube is an efficient route of administration. The following medications are readily absorbed via the intratracheal route: lidocaine (Xylocaine), atropine sulfate, naloxone (Narcan), and epinephrine. The following drugs *should not* be given via the intratracheal route: sodium bicarbonate, norepinephrine, calcium chloride, and diazepam (Valium).

Dilute the medication with 5 ml of saline solution to minimize the amount of drug that adheres to the wall of the endotracheal tube. When administering intratracheal medications, place them as far down the endotracheal tube as possible; a long, small-bore catheter (such as a feeding tube) may be used to accomplish this placement. After administration of the medication, instill four or five positive-pressure ventilations to distribute the medication.

Tactile endotracheal intubation. Tactile or digital endotracheal intubation is an alternate method of intubation that may be used when the vocal cords are visually obstructed or when there is a strict need to maintain the head and neck in alignment. Do not use this method unless the patient is deeply comatose.

Prepare the endotracheal tube by inserting a stylet and making an open-ended J at the end of the tube.

Face the patient. Insert the index and middle fingers of the gloved, nondominant hand along the side of the patient's tongue, moving the tongue out of the way as the fingers are advanced to the anterior pharyngeal region. Advance the fingers until the epiglottis or opening of the trachea can be palpated. Grasp the endotracheal tube in the dominant hand and insert it into the patient's mouth. Advance the tube to the posterior pharyngeal area until the tip of the tube can be felt by the fingers of the nondominant hand. Slip the tube into the trachea.

Remove the stylet and force air into the tube, observing for chest rise and listening for breath sounds bilaterally.

Proceed with the remaining steps to secure the tube, as in any other type of intubation procedure.

Lighted stylet. An alternate method of intubation is the use of a lighted (nasal or oral) stylet. The lighted stylet is inserted into the nasal or oral tracheal tube. When the tube is advanced, if it is placed correctly, the light can be visualized through the soft tissue of the anterior neck.

Surgical Techniques and Procedures for Airway Management

If neither the EOA nor the ET tube can be placed, additional methods of obtaining an airway must be attempted, particularly in cases of massive facial trauma or when an occlusive foreign body is present and cannot be removed by the abdominal thrust (Heimlich) maneuver or direct laryngoscopy. Surgical methods for gaining access to the airway are transtracheal catheter ventilation, cricothyrotomy, or tracheostomy. These procedures should be attempted only by specially trained personnel.

BREATHING

A variety of devices are available for the delivery of oxygen to a patient. Emergency nurses should be familiar with the various devices and should be able to select the one that is appropriate for a particular patient (Table 13-3). The basic principle of oxygen delivery is to use a system that provides an adequate concentration of inspired oxygen. If results of an arterial blood gas test are available, a P_{CO_2} of 35 to 45 mm Hg and a P_{O_2} of at least 80 are considered adequate. When blood gas test results are unavailable, observe the patient. Somnolence may be caused by hypercapnia, whereas hypoxemia may be manifested by restlessness, tachycardia, and cyanosis. Remember, though, that the absence of cyanosis does not eliminate from consideration the

Table 13-3   Summary of oxygen assist devices

Type of breathing device	Oxygen flow rate	Oxygen concentrations	Advantages	Disadvantages
Nasal cannula	2-6 L/min	25%-40%	No rebreathing of expired air	Can be used only on patients who are breathing spontaneously
Face mask	10 L/min	50%-60%	Higher oxygen concentration than nasal cannula	Not tolerated well by severely dyspneic patients; can be used only on patients who are breathing spontaneously
Oxygen reservoir mask	10-12 L/min	90%	Higher oxygen concentration than nasal cannula or face mask	Must have tight seal on mask; can be used only on patients who are breathing spontaneously
Venturi mask	4 L/min 8 L/min	24%-28% 35%-40%	Fixed oxygen concentration	Can be used only on patients who are breathing spontaneously
Pocket mask	Expired air to 10 L/min	18%-50%	Avoids direct contact with patient's mouth; may add oxygen source; may be used on apneic patient; may be used on child	Rescuer fatigue
Bag-valve-mask	Room air 12 L/min	21% 40%-90%	Quick; oxygen concentration may be increased; rescuer can sense lung compliance; may be used on both apneic and spontaneously breathing patients	Air in stomach; low tidal volume
Oxygen-powered breathing device	100 L/min	100%	High oxygen flow; positive pressure	Gastric distention; overinflation; standard device cannot be used for children without special adapter

possibility of hypoxemia. Some patients may not have enough hemoglobin to become cyanotic.

A pulse oximeter may be used for assessing the adequacy of oxygenation efforts. This device measures the saturation level of the arterial oxygenation of the blood. The device is easily used by attaching the probe or monitoring device to the patient's finger, ear, or toe. The saturation level is calculated and displayed by the device within a few seconds.

Nasal Cannula

A nasal cannula is the most commonly used oxygen delivery device for patients who are spontaneously breathing. When the oxygen flow rate is adjusted to 6 L/min, the inspired oxygen concentration is approximately 25% to 40%. Increasing the flow rate by 1 L/min, increases the inspired oxygen concentration by approximately 4%.

Simple Face Mask

The simple face mask is used on the spontaneously breathing patient. Face masks (Fig. 13-10) are tolerated well by most individuals but not by those who have severe dyspnea, since the mask may exacerbate the feeling of a patient with

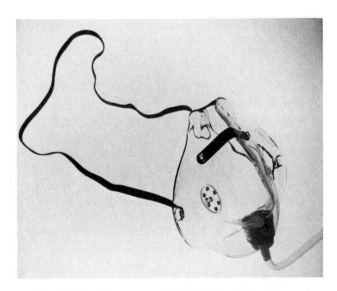

Fig. 13-10   Oxygen mask. (Photo by Richard Lazar.)

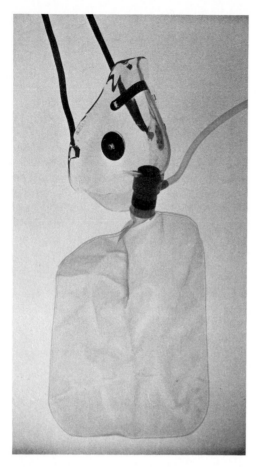

Fig. 13-11 Oxygen reservoir mask. (Photo by Richard Lazar.)

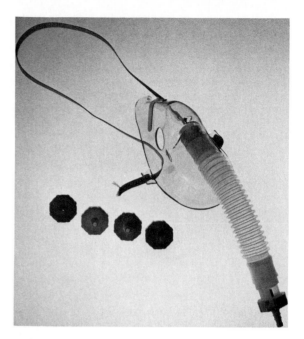

Fig. 13-12 Venturi mask and oxygen regulators. (Photo by Richard Lazar.)

severe dyspnea that he or she is suffocating. At a flow rate of 10 L/min, the inspired oxygen concentration delivered by a face mask is 50% to 60%. The oxygen flow rate should always be higher than 5 L/min, to prevent rebreathing of the exhaled air that may accumulate in the mask.

Oxygen Reservoir Mask (Partial Mask, Nonrebreathing Mask)

An oxygen reservoir mask (Fig. 13-11) is equipped with a plastic reservoir bag that fills with 100% oxygen while the patient is exhaling. During inhalation, with the flow rate at 10 to 12 L/min, the patient may receive a concentration of as much as 90% oxygen, if the mask has a tight seal.

Venturi Mask

If a patient has a history of chronic obstructive pulmonary disease and is currently having respiratory distress, first consider the use of a Venturi mask. This mask allows for delivery of a fixed concentration of oxygen. By adjusting the oxygen flow cap on the device and adjusting the flow rate of oxygen, oxygen delivery can be regulated (Fig. 13-12). For example, with an oxygen flow rate of 4 L/min, a

concentration of 24% or 28% oxygen is delivered. Turning the oxygen flow rate up to 8 L/min and changing the oxygen flow cap results in delivery of an oxygen concentration of 35% or 40%. A low PaO_2 stimulates the respiratory center in patients with chronic obstructive pulmonary disease. Because a sudden increase in PaO_2 may cause respiratory depression, these patients must be observed carefully. The proper method for using a Venturi mask is to set the initial flow rate at 24% oxygen concentration and observe the patient closely. If respiratory depression is not present and the patient remains hypoxemic, increase the oxygen concentration to 28%. Continue to increase the oxygen concentration as long as the patient needs additional oxygen. Never withhold oxygen (even high-flow oxygen) simply because the patient has chronic obstructive pulmonary disease.

Pocket Mask

A pocket mask (Fig. 13-13) may be carried by the health care provider and used when other forms of artificial ventilation are not available. The pocket mask allows for mouth-to-mask breathing. Exhaled air contains 16% to 18% oxygen; this concentration is considered adequate, if the patient's lungs are normal and the rescuer uses about twice the normal tidal volume. The mask fits snugly onto the victim's face, covering the nose and mouth. The victim's head should be tilted back, and the jaw pulled forward, with the victim's mouth slightly open. The rescuer can then blow into the opening in the top of the mask (Fig. 13-14). Supplemental oxygen can be added by attaching an oxygen source to the one-way valve located at the bottom of the

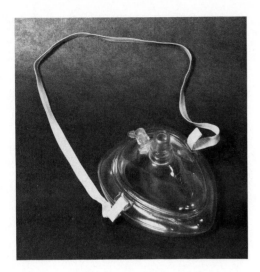

Fig. 13-13   Pocket mask. (Photo by Richard Lazar.)

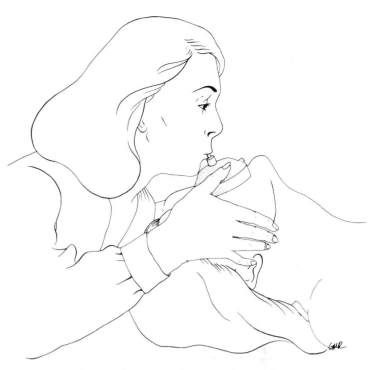

Fig. 13-14   Blowing into pocket mask.

mask. If oxygen is provided at 10 L/min, the delivered oxygen concentration is about 50%. For pediatric use the mask may be turned upside down, with the wide end placed at the bridge of the child's nose and the narrow end tucked under the chin.

Bag-Valve-Mask Device

Using room air, a bag-valve-mask device can deliver 21% oxygen to a victim. By adding oxygen at a rate of 12 L/min, the oxygen concentration is increased to 40%. By adding a reservoir (bag or long, corrugated tubing) (Fig. 13-15), the delivered oxygen concentration is elevated to 90% with the same flow rate.

The mask of the bag-valve-mask unit is applied in the same way that the pocket mask is applied, and a tight seal is obtained around the nose and the mouth. An inadequate seal during ventilation of the patient is the most frequently encountered problem with the bag-valve-mask device. Two individuals should be assigned to ventilate the patient, one to maintain a good seal using both hands and the other to squeeze the bag. The mask should be transparent so that any emesis can be seen and dealt with immediately. Some airway adjunct—an oropharyngeal or nasopharyngeal airway adjunct, an EOA or an EGTA, or an ET tube—must be used at the same time that the bag-valve-mask device is used.

Oxygen-Powered Devices

Oxygen-powered devices (Fig. 13-16) can deliver a concentration of 100% oxygen at a rate of 10 L/min through an attached mask, an ET tube, or a transtracheal catheter. An oxygen-powered system consists of high-pressure tubing connected to a supply of oxygen and a lever or push button. When the valve is opened, oxygen flows into the patient. The timing and length of oxygen delivery, typically 1 second

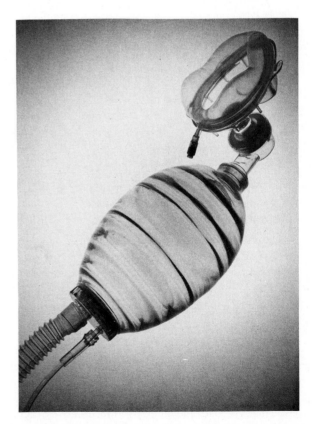

Fig. 13-15   Bag-valve-mask device with oxygen reservoir. (Photo by Richard Lazar.)

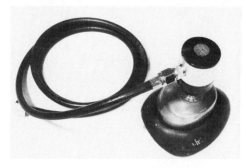

Fig. 13-16   Oxygen-powered breathing device. (Photo by Richard Lazar.)

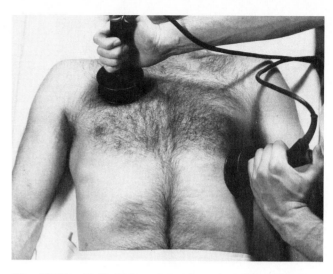

Fig. 13-17   Defibrillation. Anterolateral paddle placement. (Photo by Richard Lazar.)

of inflation (or until the chest rises) and 4 seconds of passive exhalation, are controlled by the operator. The device should not be used for children younger than 12 years of age.

CIRCULATION

Properly performed chest compressions produce about 30% of normal cardiac output, which is enough blood flow through the heart and brain to sustain tissue viability for a short time. Cerebral blood flow must be at least 50% of normal to maintain consciousness.

When performing chest compressions, make sure that the victim is lying on a firm surface to allow for compression of the thoracic cavity, which will result in increased intrathoracic pressure. Chest compressions should be forceful enough to generate a carotid or femoral pulse.

Chest compressions may be performed manually or with the assistance of automatic, gas-powered devices. Although these machines provide more consistent chest compressions than the manual method, they should be used only by trained personnel: internal injuries may result from improper use. The person monitoring use needs to maintain the patient's head tilt and ventilations. These devices are not used for children and infants. The devices are useful during long transports and allow emergency medical personnel to perform tasks other than compressions.

OPEN CHEST MASSAGE (OPEN THORACOTOMY)

Open thoracotomy and cardiac massage may be required in cases of penetrating wounds to the heart, penetrating abdominal trauma with deterioration and arrest, pericardial tamponade, tension pneumothorax, crushing chest injuries, or for patients with chronic lung disease who have a barrel chest when other more conservative measures for chest compression in CPR have failed. Direct cardiac massage provides better hemodynamics than closed chest compressions. This procedure should be performed only by trained physicians and is not recommended for the patient who is having an uncomplicated arrest. This procedure must be performed within 15 minutes of the arrest to be effective.

Defibrillation

Defibrillation is used in the treatment of ventricular fibrillation and pulseless ventricular tachycardia. Defibrillation may also be used when it is unclear whether the rhythm is fine ventricular fibrillation or asystole. In the latter situation, try to verify the rhythm in at least two leads. Defibrillation is generally not used for the patient with asystole unless fine ventricular fibrillation is suspected. Cardiopulmonary resuscitation (CPR) should be started immediately, while the equipment is being prepared, in all cases of pulselessness and nonbreathing. For defibrillation to be effective, an electric current sufficient to depolarize a critical portion of the left ventricle must pass through the heart. Success depends on the metabolic state of the heart and decreasing resistance to the countershock. For the treatment of ventricular fibrillation and pulseless ventricular tachycardia in adults, up to three countershocks should be delivered rapidly, the first at 200 J, the second at 200 to 300 J, and the third at 300 J. Remember to check the pulse and rhythm between shocks. The use of epinephrine and antidysrhythmic agents follows these defibrillation attempts. To improve the chance of success, select paddles and electrodes of appropriate size, defibrillate as quickly as possible, apply 25 pounds of pressure per paddle, and use a conductive gel.

Begin by making sure that the machine has a charged battery or is plugged into an electrical outlet. Turn the machine on and select the "defib" mode. Select the energy level, and prepare the paddles with a small amount of conductive gel. Place the paddles on the patient's chest, choosing one of two positions. Most commonly the anterolateral placement (Fig. 13-17) is used. Place one paddle to the right of the upper sternum just below the right clavicle and the other just to the left of the nipple on the midaxillary line. For placement in the anteroposterior position (Fig. 13-

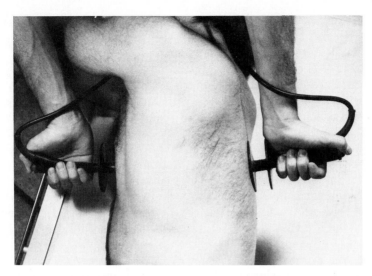

Fig. 13-18   Defibrillation. Anteroposterior paddle placement. (Photo by Richard Lazar.)

18), place one paddle over the precordium, just to the left of the lower sternal border, and place the other paddle posteriorly behind the heart. Reconfirm the rhythm before defibrillating the patient. To defibrillate, apply firm pressure, be sure the area around the patient is clear of personnel and electrical equipment, then discharge the paddles by depressing both discharge buttons simultaneously.

To perform internal defibrillation (during open cardiac massage), use internal paddles and follow the same procedure. Apply sterile saline solution to sterile gauze sponges placed over the internal paddles. The shock energy level is usually between 10 to 50 J for an adult.

Defibrillation may cause, as well as correct, dysrhythmias. Be prepared for potential dysrhythmias with the necessary equipment and medications. The defibrillator should be tested routinely. It should be discharged at full power once a week and discharged daily at the manufacturer's suggested level.

Cardioversion

Synchronized cardioversion is used when the patient becomes hemodynamically unstable or when pharmacologic intervention has been unsuccessful in the management of sustained ventricular tachycardia, paroxysmal supraventricular tachycardia, and atrial fibrillation or atrial flutter or both. In synchronized cardioversion the energy delivered to the heart occurs during the absolute refractory period, a fraction of a second after the occurrence of the QRS complex. Synchronized cardioversion decreases the possibility that the energy delivered may hit on the tail of the T wave, which can cause ventricular fibrillation.

The procedure for cardioversion is the same as that for defibrillation with two exceptions: the machine must be set on the synchronous mode and, if the patient is conscious, sedation may be necessary. For the purpose of sedation, diazepam (Valium) may be administered slowly by IV push in small increments. In preparation for elective cardioversion, explain the procedure to the patient and obtain an informed consent when possible. Check the serum potassium level: hypokalemia predisposes the heart to ventricular fibrillation. Ask the patient to empty his or her bladder and remove dentures. Obtain a 12-lead ECG to establish a baseline measurement. After cardioversion is completed, monitor the patient's vital signs and cardiac rhythm frequently.

Complications of cardioversion include asystole, junctional rhythms, premature ventricular contractions, ventricular tachycardia, embolization, and reversion to atrial fibrillation or atrial flutter.

PACEMAKERS

Temporary pacing is used when a patient's condition deteriorates secondary to tachycardia dysrhythmia or bradycardia dysrhythmia that is unresponsive to other therapy. Indications for the use of pacing include severe bradycardia, high-degree atrioventricular (AV) blocks, atrial tachycardia and flutter, recurrent ventricular tachycardia, transient bradycardia as a complication of myocardial infarction, and hemodynamically significant tachydysrhythmias.

There are three methods for pacing, the transthoracic, transvenous, and external (transcutaneous) methods. The transthoracic approach is usually not used in an emergency setting because the associated risks are high, completing the procedure takes time, and application interferes with chest compressions. The transvenous method involves inserting a catheter electrode percutaneously into the right atrium or ventricle via the subclavian, internal jugular, brachial, or femoral vein. The procedure is guided by changes in the ECG. Atrial pacing is used to suppress atrial tachydysrhythmias. Similarly, ventricular pacing can be used to suppress ventricular ectopy. The more widely used approach in an emergency setting is the external, or transcutaneous, method.

When the external approach is used, a negative electrode is placed posteriorly at the midthoracic level of the spine and a positive electrode is placed anteriorly at the chest lead V_3 position. This position provides a lower pacing threshold and is away from large skeletal muscles, thus decreasing muscle stimulation. Electrode placement should not interfere with placement of defibrillation paddles, which may be needed. If electrical safety guidelines are followed, health care personnel are in no danger of receiving an electrical shock when using the transcutaneous pacer. Because various types of equipment are used, become familiar with the equipment in your department.

The rate of pacing impulses may be fixed (asynchronous, competitive, or nondemand) or placed on the demand mode. The fixed rate delivers an electrical current at regularly set intervals and is usually used when patients are having third-degree heart block. A fixed-rate mode may create competition with the patient's supraventricular beats, causing ventricular fibrillation. Demand pacing is generally used when some degree of electrical conduction is still present. The demand mode senses the patient's own QRS complexes and generates an impulse only if the patient does not have a QRS complex during a certain time period (usually within about 0.08 second). Ventricular tachycardia may occur if the pacing impulse fires on the T wave of the patient's own cardiac cycle.

Successful pacing depends on the condition of the myocardium. Patients with severe bradycardia, heart block, or an idioventricular rhythm who can generate a pulse with each QRS complex usually have a better outcome. Patients with asystole are not likely to respond to pacing.

Factors that may indicate successful capture, that is, a successful electrical stimulation followed by a mechanical response, include a combined pacing artifact and QRS complex of more than 0.14 second in duration, a T wave following the pacing artifact, and resolution of the dysrhythmia being treated. Electrical capture occurs when the heart's conduction system is effectively stimulated by the current from the pacer; electrical capture can be seen on the ECG monitor. Mechanical capture occurs when the heart responds to pacing with effective contractions. Mechanical capture is evaluated by the presence of a pulse consistent with the paced beats. Both types of capture must be present for pacing to be effective. Assess the patient's hemodynamic and neurologic response by palpating the carotid or femoral pulse, obtaining a full set of vital signs, and evaluating the patient's level of consciousness.

Two common reasons for lack of capture are acidosis and hypoxemia. If capture does not occur after correcting these metabolic problems, consider problems with the electrodes. Reposition the posterior electrode to the fifth intercostal space, midaxillary line (V_6 chest lead position). If the gel in the electrodes is dry, replace it. The skin should be clean and dry before the electrodes are applied, and benzoin may be used to improve adherence to the skin.

Automatic Implantable Cardioverter Defibrillator

An automatic implanted cardioverter defibrillator (AICD) provides an approach to treatment that helps reduce the incidence of sudden death from AMI. Approved in 1985, the AICD is a device that monitors the patient's cardiac rhythm and treats ventricular tachycardia and ventricular fibrillation by delivering a countershock directly to the patient's heart. The use of this device is becoming the standard treatment for tachydysrhythmias.[10] Emergency nurses should be aware of its use and should be prepared to manage these patients.

Models available on the market differ in detection criteria and the amount of energy used for defibrillation. Detection criteria include the monitoring of the heart rate and the shape of the QRS complex. The range of measurement for heart rate varies from 120 to 200 beats/min. The unit also monitors the amount of time the ECG is at the isoelectric baseline. In normal sinus rhythm the ECG is predominantly on the baseline; in ventricular tachycardia and ventricular fibrillation there are few intervals during which the ECG is on the baseline. This lack of an isoelectrical interval triggers the device.

An AICD consists of electrodes, which are surgically implanted around the heart, and a pulse generator, which is implanted subcutaneously in the paraumbilical area. Patients are instructed to wear identifying (Medic-Alert) bracelets indicating that they have AICD devices. A surgical scar on the patient's chest and a subcutaneous device may indicate the presence of an AICD. Confirmation can be obtained by making a radiograph of the chest and abdomen; the radiograph visualizes the pulse generator and provides information about the manufacturer, model number, and type of device.

The patient should be managed normally. If defibrillation is necessary, the paddles should be placed in the anteroposterior position. A special magnet must be used to deactivate the AICD. The use of nuclear magnetic resonance imaging is contraindicated because such imaging may cause tissue damage or failure of the device. Computed tomography scanning may be used after the device is deactivated. Ultrasound may be used to evaluate the patient without taking any special precautions.

THROMBOLYTIC THERAPY

The goal of thrombolytic therapy is to dissolve occlusive clots in coronary arteries. Thrombus formation in narrowed coronary arteries containing atheromatous plaques leads to complete occlusion. In some patients coronary vasospasm leads to clot formation because of stasis of blood. Whatever the cause, if occlusion is not reversed, death of myocardial tissue begins after approximately 20 minutes in areas most severely restricted and total necrosis of myocardial tissue occurs within 6 hours of occlusion.

If thrombolytic therapy is initiated within 4 to 6 hours of onset of chest pain, left ventricular function is improved and mortality decreases.[1,3] Other benefits of thrombolytic therapy include the decreased incidence of heart failure and cardiogenic shock.

Pathophysiology of Fibrinolytic System

A review of the physiology of the fibrinolytic system provides the framework for understanding the mechanism of action of the different thrombolytic agents.

Thrombogenesis, or the formation of a thrombus (clot), begins when circulating blood comes into contact with any rough surface such as traumatized tissue (for example, torn vascular walls) or atherosclerotic plaques. The combination of platelet aggregation and activation of the coagulation cascade results in the production of thrombin. Thrombin then stimulates the production of fibrinogen, which leads to the formation of fibrin. Cross-linked fibrin strands trap red blood cells and platelets to form a clot.

Fibrinolysis is the term used to describe the process of clot degradation. Lysis of the clot begins with the activation of plasminogen, which converts to plasmin. Plasmin degrades or breaks down the fibrin in the clot and circulating fibrinogen. Endogenously, plasminogen is activated by the initiation of the coagulation cascade or by the release of tissue activators. Thrombolytic agents are an exogenous source of plasminogen. For example, streptokinase forms a complex with circulating plasminogen. This streptokinase-plasminogen complex leads to conversion of circulating plasminogen to plasmin, which results in degradation of the fibrin clot, circulating fibrinogen, and coagulation factors.

According to the physiology of the fibrinolytic system, the best thrombolytic agent would be clot specific and would not alter circulating fibrinogen or the coagulation cascade. Based on these same physiologic principles, if the thrombolytic agent is not clot specific, hemorrhage is the major complication of thrombolytic therapy. Contraindications to the use of thrombolytic agents include recent major surgery, cerebrovascular disease, intracranial neoplasm, recent trauma (within 10 days), recent gastrointestinal or urinary tract bleeding (within 10 days), previous puncture of noncompressible vessels, persistent uncontrolled hypertension (pressure greater than 180 mm Hg systolic or pressure greater than 110 mm Hg diastolic or both), pregnancy, diabetic hemorrhagic retinopathy, patients who are 75 years of age or older, liver disease, known bleeding diathesis, and acute pericarditis. Thrombolytic therapy is contraindicated in the case of anyone for whom bleeding would constitute a significant hazard or for whom bleeding would be difficult to manage because of its location or the patient's condition.

Indications for the use of thrombolytics are (1) ischemic chest pain lasting longer than 30 minutes and occurring less than 6 hours from the onset of the chest pain, (2) chest pain that is unresponsive to sublingual nitroglycerin, (3) ECG changes indicative of AMI (ST segment elevation greater than 0.1 mV in at least two contiguous leads), and (4) no contraindications.

Thrombolytic Agents

Four different thrombolytic agents are available for use: urokinase, streptokinase, tissue plasminogen activase, and anisoylated plasminogen streptokinase activator complex. Drug selection is based on the patient's history, physician preference, availability, funding, and the mechanism of action. For a comparison of the different drugs, refer to Table 13-4. Sometimes a heparin infusion is used in conjunction with thrombolytic agents. The rationale for its use is that a heparin infusion may help prevent formation of a new clot and reocclusion of the vessel.[5] The heparin is titrated to maintain the partial thromboplastin time at 1½ to 2 times the control levels.

Evaluation

Effectiveness of thrombolytic therapy is best evaluated by cardiac catheterization 90 minutes after the initiation of therapy. However, catheterization is not always practical or desirable. Noninvasive measures of effectiveness are resolution of the chest pain, normalization of the ST segment, and the presence of reperfusion dysrhythmias. The most frequently seen dysrhythmia is an accelerated idioventricular rhythm.

Reocclusion of the vessel usually occurs within 24 to 48 hours after dissolution of the clot. When treatment begins within 3 hours of the onset of new symptoms, the incidence of successful reperfusion is 60% to 70% for all thrombolytic agents.[3]

Nursing Care

Patients should be moved carefully and, in an effort to decrease the incidence of bleeding, a limited number of venipunctures should be performed. Common laboratory tests include a complete blood cell count, measurements of prothrombin time, partial thromboplastin time, cardiac enzymes, and fibrinogen, and a platelet count. Observe the patient carefully for signs of internal and external bleeding. Signs of internal bleeding include a decreasing hematocrit and hemoglobin, hypotension, and tachycardia. If signs of bleeding occur or if the patient is experiencing an allergic reaction, the infusion should be discontinued and a physician should be notified.

RECOGNITION AND MANAGEMENT OF DYSRHYTHMIAS

Premature ventricular contractions (PVCs, also termed ventricular premature beats or premature ventricular beats) are the most commonly occurring dysrhythmia associated with ischemia and AMI. This dysrhythmia occurs in ap-

Table 13-4   Comparison of thrombolytic agents

Agent	Cost	Action	Dose	Comments
Streptokinase	$200	Exogenous plasminogen activator; not clot specific	Usually 1.5 million U IV over a period of 1 hour; intracoronary: 20,000 U IV bolus followed by infusion of 2000 U/min IV for a period of 60 minutes (total dose is 140,000 U)	Half-life in plasma is 18 minutes; has a prolonged effect on coagulation because of depletion of fibrinogen, which persists for 18 to 24 hours; antibodies to the drug may be present in persons who have been exposed to *Streptococcus* infection; allergic reactions (rash, fever, and chills) may occur; patients should not be retreated with streptokinase for a period of 2 weeks to 1 year after initial administration because of secondary resistance to development of antibodies
Urokinase	$1500	Proteolytic enzyme; directly activates plasminogen to plasmin; not clot specific	2 to 3 million U IV bolus or IV over a period of 30 to 60 minutes; intracoronary: 6000 U/min	Half-life in plasma is 10 to 16 minutes
Tissue plasminogen activator	$2200	Proteolytic enzyme; direct activator of plasminogen; high degree of clot specificity	10 mg IV bolus followed by continuous infusion of 50 mg IV over a period of 1 hour, then 20 mg/hr IV over a period of 2 hours (total dose is 100 mg)	Half-life in plasma is 5 to 7 minutes; may cause sudden hypotension; in-line IV filters can remove as much as 47% of the drug
Anisoylated plasminogen streptokinase activator complex (Eminase)	—	—	30 U IV over a period of 2 to 5 minutes; dilute only with 5 ml sterile water	Do not give to patients who are allergic to streptokinase; may not be as effective as usual when administered more than 5 days after the previous dose or after streptokinase therapy or streptococcal infection; discard if not used within 30 minutes after mixing

proximately 85% of patients with myocardial infarction. After the initiation of oxygen therapy, lidocaine is usually the best of the drugs used to abolish PVCs. Lidocaine may also be used prophylactically for patients having a possible myocardial infarction, even without ectopy, because ventricular tachycardia, ventricular fibrillation, and electric-mechanical dissociation may not be preceded by warning dysrhythmias. However, recent studies suggest that prophylactic use of lidocaine in hospitalized patients with AMI may increase mortality.[4] Other causes of PVCs such as hypoxemia, acidosis, alkalosis, electrolyte imbalances,

digoxin toxicity, and bradycardia should be evaluated and corrected.

Lidocaine is given to reduce or prevent ectopy by decreasing ventricular irritability. To maintain therapeutic blood levels, the initial lidocaine bolus should be followed by additional boluses or a lidocaine IV drip. For bolus administration, the dose is 1 to 1.5 mg/kg IV over a period of 1 to 2 minutes. If lidocaine is given too rapidly, seizures may occur. The initial bolus is followed in 2 to 5 minutes by half of the original dose, which may be repeated up to a total dose of 3 mg/kg or until the desired effect occurs.

The second method of administering lidocaine is to give an initial bolus of lidocaine (1 to 2 mg/kg), followed by an IV drip of 2 g lidocaine in 500 ml D_5W solution running at a rate of 2 to 4 mg/min. Do not rely solely on a lidocaine drip: an initial IV loading dose or bolus must be given. If a bolus is given without supplemental boluses or a drip, the therapeutic blood level of lidocaine (2 to 5 μg/ml) diminishes within 5 to 15 minutes. Conversely, if a lidocaine drip is initiated without the benefit of a loading dose, a therapeutic blood level will not be reached in the first half hour of treatment.

Lidocaine should not be given to patients who have a third-degree atrioventricular (AV) block with an escape rhythm or to patients who have bradycardia with PVCs. These PVCs may be contributing to the patient's blood flow; giving lidocaine could effectively reduce this output and cause further decompensation or asystole.

If the patient needs an antidysrhythmic agent but has a history of liver disease, is in shock, or is older than 70 years of age, the dose of lidocaine should be reduced to half, or an alternate antidysrhythmic drug should be considered. Always choose an antidysrhythmic drug of a category different from that of the drug that was not successful. This choice increases the likelihood of controlling or eradicating the ectopy efficiently.

If the use of lidocaine is unsuccessful or the victim is allergic to lidocaine, other antidysrhythmic drugs to consider are procainamide (Pronestyl) and bretylium (Bretylol). Procainamide should be given as a 100 mg IV bolus over a period of 5 minutes to avoid hypertension. The dose may be repeated until the ectopy is resolved, the QRS complex widens by 50% of the original width, hypotension occurs, or the maximum dose of 1000 mg has been given. If the medication is effective, the initial bolus should be followed by a continuous infusion at the rate of 1 to 4 mg/min.

Bretylium is administered as an IV bolus of 5 to 10 mg/kg body weight over a period of 8 to 10 minutes. Dilute the drug in 100 ml of normal saline solution and infuse slowly to avoid severe hypotension, nausea, and vomiting.

The second most commonly occurring dysrhythmia in patients with AMI is bradycardia. Bradycardia is defined as a heart rate of less than 60 beats/min. This dysrhythmia occurs in 65% of patients with AMI, particularly in those sustaining inferior wall infarctions. Treatment of bradycardia is required when the patient becomes symptomatic and has chest pain, dyspnea, syncope, lightheadedness, hypotension, or ventricular ectopy. Atropine sulfate is the drug of choice and is given IV rapid push in increments of 0.5 mg to a maximum dose of 2 mg. Atropine should not be administered slowly or in doses of less than 0.5 mg because it may cause a paradoxic decrease in heart rate.

AV blocks may also occur in patients having AMIs. These rhythms indicate an impairment in the conduction at the AV junction. Four different types of blocks may occur, depending on the area and degree of damage to the conduction system. These are referred to as first-degree, second-degree Mobitz I (Wenckebach), second-degree Mobitz II, and third-degree, or complete, blocks. Blocks in conduction may be caused by infection, degenerative changes in the conduction system, rheumatic heart disease, medications (that is, beta blockers, calcium channel blockers, and cardiac glycosides), or AMI.

First-degree AV block is recognized by prolongation of the interval between the P wave and the QRS complex (PR interval) beyond 0.20 second. This prolongation signifies a delay in conduction from the atria to the ventricles. A first-degree heart block occurs in 10% of patients with AMI, and of these blocks, 75% progress into second- and third-degree blocks when the block is associated with AMI or is drug induced. This dysrhythmia does not usually affect heart rate or cardiac output and does not require treatment. Second-degree Mobitz I block, (Wenckebach), is evidenced by a repeated sequence of a gradually prolonged PR interval that leads to the loss of one QRS complex. This rhythm is associated with a defect in conduction through the atrioventricular (AV) node and is usually both benign and transient. This rhythm is commonly associated with an inferior wall infarction because the right coronary artery supplies this area and the AV node.

Second-degree Mobitz II block occurs when conduction through the bundle branches is impaired. This impairment usually occurs because of blockage of the left coronary artery, which supplies the anterior wall and the bundle branches. This form of second-degree block is more likely than the other form to progress to a third-degree block.

Treatment of second-degree blocks includes careful monitoring of the patient's rhythm and hemodynamic condition. For a Mobitz I block, treatment is usually limited to observation; atropine is needed only if the patient's condition deteriorates. For a Mobitz II block, use of atropine and pacing is determined by the patient's condition. An infusion of isoproterenol (Isuprel) at a rate of 2 to 10 μg/min may also be used but isoproterenol exacerbates ischemia. Isoproterenol should be used only as a temporizing measure while a pacemaker is being prepared.

Other rhythms that commonly occur with myocardial infarction are the supraventricular tachycardias, which may be indicative of myocardial ischemia or an anterior wall infarct. Often associated with chest pain, tachycardias are dangerous because they increase myocardial oxygen consumption and may extend the size of the infarct. Treatment depends on the clinical findings. For unstable patients with supraventricular tachycardia, synchronized cardioversion is the treatment, beginning with countershocks at 75 to 100 J, with subsequent countershocks at 200 J and then at 360 J. If a patient's symptoms are life threatening, defibrillation, rather than cardioversion, may be used, if defibrillation saves time. If possible, an IV should be established before cardioversion, and a sedative should be administered if the patient is awake. If conversion occurs but the supraventricular tachycardia recurs, a second electrical cardioversion is not indicated until pharmacologic therapy has been initiated.

Vagal maneuvers or the administration of verapamil or adenosine or both measures are used for patients who are stable and have supraventricular tachycardia. Verapamil is a calcium channel blocker that slows conduction through the sinoatrial (SA) and AV nodes, decreases myocardial contractility, and dilates peripheral arteries. The initial dose is 0.075 to 0.15 mg/kg (maximum dose, 10 mg) IV over a period of 1 minute. Peak therapeutic effects occur in 3 to 5 minutes. The dose may be repeated in 30 minutes at 0.15 mg/kg (again, not to exceed 10 mg). Bradycardia may occur, if the patient has received previous cardioversion. Verapamil is contraindicated for patients receiving beta blockers because of the synergistic effect. Verapamil should not be used in patients with heart failure or ventricular tachycardia because the drug may induce severe hypotension and may predispose the patient to ventricular fibrillation.

Adenosine acts directly on the AV node to slow electrical conduction, thus interrupting the reentry circuit that perpetuates most causes of supraventricular tachycardia. The initial dose is 6 mg IV over a period of 1 to 2 seconds. If conversion does not occur within 1 to 2 minutes, 12 mg should be given as a rapid IV bolus; repeat this dose once, if needed. The drug has a half-life of 10 seconds. The advantages of using adenosine instead of verapamil include rapid onset of action, transient side effects, lack of associated bradycardia or hypotension, relative specificity for the treatment of reentry dysrhythmias of the atrioventricular node, and safety of use for patients with Wolff-Parkinson-White syndrome.

Vagal Maneuvers

The vagus nerve may be stimulated by a Valsalva maneuver, retching (emesis), stimulation of the face with ice water, or carotid sinus massage. Ocular pressure is no longer recommended. The ice water should be placed in a thin plastic bag, which is then applied to the patient's face. Placing the ice water in a plastic bag minimizes the mess and eliminates the chance of aspiration secondary to a reflexive gasp (especially in children).

Carotid Sinus Massage

Carotid sinus massage is appropriate for young to middle-aged patients who are having supraventricular tachycardia other than atrial flutter and who are refractory to less invasive vagal maneuvers. If the patient is having atrial flutter, this procedure may increase the block already present. During carotid sinus massage, pressure is placed on the carotid bodies, stimulating the baroreceptors and thereby stimulating the parasympathetic branch of the autonomic nervous system. This stimulation sends signals via the vagus nerve and causes a drop in blood pressure and heart rate.

Begin the massage by placing the victim in a supine position and administering oxygen at 4 to 6 L/min by nasal cannula. Initiate an IV line of D_5W solution in a peripheral vein, and monitor the patient closely. Before applying carotid pressure, auscultate the carotid arteries for the presence of bruits. This turbulent flow suggests the presence of an atherosclerotic plaque, which could break off if manipulated, resulting in a stroke. If a bruit is heard over one of the arteries, do not perform the massage at the site of that artery.

Ideally, you should start by massaging the right carotid sinus. In more than 75% of the population, massage of the right carotid body will affect the SA node preferentially and massage of the left side will affect the AV node.[2,6] Even if the SA node is completely shut down, the AV node has a chance to provide pacemaker activity. If you massage the left side first, the massaging may cause a complete block of the AV node and force activation of a very slow (and possibly inadequate) pacemaker in the ventricles. Locate the carotid pulse. Gently press the carotid artery just below the mandible between the fingers and the vertebral transverse processes. Apply pressure in a small, circular motion, rotating your fingers backward and medially. Continue this motion for no more than 5 to 10 seconds; discontinue the motion sooner if a rhythm change occurs. If the first attempt is unsuccessful, you may repeat the procedure.

Even when properly performed, carotid sinus massage may cause asystole for 15 to 30 seconds, followed by a few idioventricular complexes, before a new pacemaker site becomes active. Always be sure to have resuscitation equipment available during the procedure. *Never massage both carotid arteries at once.* If carotid massage is successful, monitor the patient continuously for several hours after the procedure. Complications of the procedure include further dysrhythmias such as ventricular tachycardia, ventricular fibrillation, and asystole, cerebral occlusion, which leads to a cerebrovascular accident, cerebral anoxia, and seizures.

If the diagnosis of a wide-complex tachycardia is unclear, assume that the rhythm is of ventricular origin and react accordingly. However, available data suggest that administration of adenosine for wide QRS-complex tachycardia is not harmful.[7] Cardioversion, digoxin, beta blockers, and pacing may also be used to treat supraventricular tachycardia, if other measures are unsuccessful.

The primary dysrhythmias resulting in cardiopulmonary arrest are ventricular tachycardia, ventricular fibrillation, and asystole. Ventricular fibrillation is the absence of any organized electrical activity. The patient does not have a pulse and loses consciousness within 15 seconds. Remember that pulseless ventricular tachycardia is treated as though it were ventricular fibrillation. Survival from ventricular tachycardia requires *immediate* defibrillation. If equipment for monitoring and defibrillation is immediately available when the arrest occurs, the rhythm should be checked and defibrillation should be performed before CPR is initiated.

Initially, defibrillation is performed three times at increasing energy levels. Begin with 200 J; then increase the levels to 200-300 J and 360 J. Remember to check the patient's pulse rate and rhythm between countershocks. If defibrillation is unsuccessful, begin CPR, establish IV access, and intubate the patient. After the IV access is established or the patient is intubated, administer 1 mg epinephrine 1:10,000, IV push or intratracheally. The administration of epinephrine should be repeated every 5 minutes as needed. Recent studies suggest that high doses of epinephrine (10 to 14 mg IV bolus) may be effective for treating patients who do not respond to currently used protocols.[8]

Epinephrine is an endogenous catecholamine having both alpha-adrenergic and beta-adrenergic properties. Its major actions include increasing the force of the myocardial contraction (inotropism), increasing the heart rate (chronotropism), increasing blood pressure by increasing peripheral vascular resistance, increasing the automaticity and spontaneity of ventricular contractions, and increasing perfusion pressure generated from chest compression. The risks associated with the use of epinephrine are the development of deteriorating tachydysrhythmias, PVCs caused by increased automaticity, and increased myocardial oxygen consumption, which may lead to myocardial ischemia and necrosis resulting from an increased cardiac workload.

After the epinephrine is administered, defibrillation should be performed again at a level of 360 J. At this point during treatment, administration of medications is alternated with defibrillation. Other drugs that are effective for the treatment of ventricular fibrillation include lidocaine (1 mg/kg IV push) and bretylium (5 mg/kg IV push). Both of these medications raise the ventricular tachycardia threshold (the energy required to induce ventricular fibrillation). After medications are administered, give a 50 ml bolus of IV fluid and elevate the arm to enhance delivery of the drug to the central circulation.

The use of sodium bicarbonate should be considered, although its use is no longer generally recommended. The administration of sodium bicarbonate causes a paradoxic worsening of intracellular hypercarbia and acidosis. Other adverse effects include hypernatremia and hyperosmolality. In addition, sodium bicarbonate may cause a left shift in the oxyhemoglobin dissociation curve, which inhibits the release of oxygen to the tissues. Measures such as prompt defibrillation, effective chest compressions, endotracheal intubation, and hyperventilation with 100% oxygen should be instituted and evaluated before considering the use of sodium bicarbonate.

If sodium bicarbonate is given, the initial dose is 1 mEq/kg. Half of this dose may be given 10 minutes later and repeated as necessary. Ideally, administration of sodium bicarbonate should be determined by arterial blood gas values.

Asystole is referred to as cardiac standstill because there is no electrical activity in the ventricles. Asystole may occur as a primary event, or it may follow ventricular fibrillation or electromechanical dissociation. The prognosis is poor because this rhythm may be the result of end-stage cardiac dysfunction or a prolonged arrest. The diagnosis of asystole should be confirmed in two leads because low amplitude VT may resemble asystole; stronger fibrillatory wave forms may be evident in the second lead. If the diagnosis is dubious, the patient should be treated as though the rhythm is ventricular fibrillation. For asystole, CPR should be initiated and followed by the administration of epinephrine (1:10,000, 1 mg IV push) and atropine (1 mg IV push). Both the epinephrine and atropine may be repeated after 5 minutes. The maximum dose for atropine is 2 mg.

When there is an organized electrical impulse (a QRS complex) but no cardiac muscle resulting in a pulse, the patient's condition is known as electromechanical dissociation. The prognosis for this rhythm is poor unless the underlying cause can be quickly identified and corrected. Assessment of the patient's history and condition before the arrest occurred helps to identify the underlying cause. For example, normovolemic patients with cardiac arrest that is not caused by external physical trauma have an elevated venous volume and pressure during CPR. The neck veins should be distended when these patients are in the supine position, and the veins should have a free blood return when a central line is being inserted. Common causes of electromechanical dissociation to be eliminated from consideration are hypovolemia, cardiac tamponade, tension pneumothorax, hypoxemia, acidosis, and profound shock. Others include massive myocardial damage, prolonged ischemia,

---

SYSTEMATIC EVALUATION OF CARDIAC RHYTHMS

Rate
Bradycardia: <60 beats/min
Normal rate: 60 to 100 beats/min
Tachycardia: >100 beats/min

Rhythm
Is the rhythm regular or irregular?

P waves
Are P waves present? Does one P wave appear before each QRS?

QRS complex
Normal duration is 0.06 to 0.12 second. Are the QRS complexes of normal shape and configuration?

P/QRS relationship
Does a QRS complex follow every P wave?

PR interval
Normal duration is 0.12 to 0.2 second. Is the interval prolonged? Is it shortened?

and pulmonary embolism. Initial treatment includes CPR, administration of epinephrine (1:10,000, 1 mg IV push), establishment of IV access, endotracheal intubation, and correction of the underlying cause. A tension pneumothorax is relieved by needle decompression of the chest. Acidosis may be corrected with improved ventilations and possibly with the use of sodium bicarbonate. Improved ventilations and oxygenation should correct hypoxemia. Hypovolemia can be treated with a fluid challenge or the use of the pneu-matic antishock garment. Cardiac tamponade is relieved by pericardiocentesis.

CARDIAC DYSRHYTHMIAS

Dysrhythmias in limb lead II, their significance, and the associated therapeutic interventions for adults are described in this section. When interpreting rhythms, it is helpful to use a systematic approach such as the one provided in the box on p. 165.

Dysrhythmias originating in the sinus node
Normal sinus rhythm

Rate	60 to 100 beats/min
Rhythm	Regular
P waves	Present
QRS complex	Present; normal duration
P/QRS relationship	P wave preceding each QRS Complex
PR interval	Normal

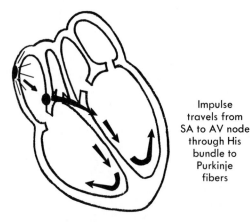

Impulse travels from SA to AV node through His bundle to Purkinje fibers

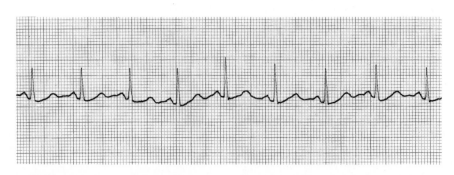

Significance: The sinoatrial (SA) node is the normal pacemaker of the heart; it is influenced by both the parasympathetic and the sympathetic branches of the autonomic nervous system.
Intervention: None required.

Sinus tachycardia

Rate	>100 beats/min; seldom >160 beats/min
Rhythm	Regular
P waves	Normal; present; with rapid rates, the P waves may be buried in the previous T wave.
QRS complex	Present; normal duration
P/QRS relationship	P wave precedes each QRS complex
PR interval	Normal

NOTE: If the patient's rate is exactly 150, consider the possibility that the rhythm is atrial flutter with a 2:1 conduction.

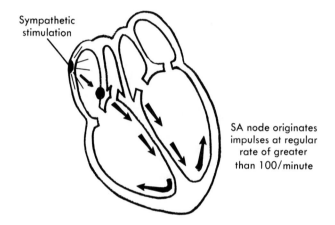

Sympathetic stimulation

SA node originates impulses at regular rate of greater than 100/minute

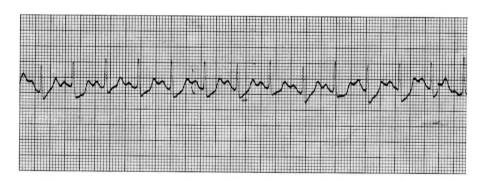

Significance: The normal pacemaker of the heart is firing at an increased rate because of anxiety, fever, pain, exercise, smoking, hyperthyroidism, heart failure, volume loss, specific drugs, or other reasons that may cause increased tissue oxygen demands. This condition may also be caused by decreased vagal tone (parasympathetic stimulation), which allows the sinus node to increase its rate. The cardiac output may decrease with rates greater than 180 beats/min because of inadequate ventricular filling. Very rapid rates during AMI may lead to further ischemia and tissue damage.

Intervention: Treat the underlying cause. No specific drug is given for sinus tachycardia except in the case of congestive heart failure; in that case digitalis is usually the drug of choice.

Sinus bradycardia

Rate	<60 beats/min; seldom <30 beats/min
Rhythm	Regular or slightly irregular
P waves	Present; normal
QRS complex	Present; normal duration
P/QRS relationship	P wave precedes each QRS complex
PR interval	Normal

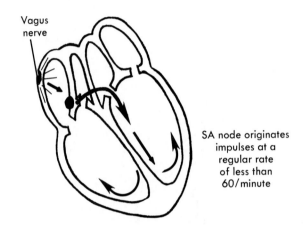

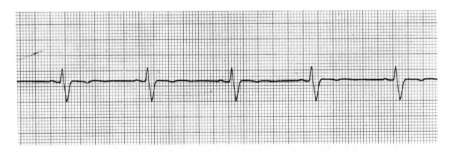

Significance: The normal pacemaker (SA node) is slowed by increased vagal tone (parasympathetic stimulation). Causes include rest, a normal athletic heart, anoxia, hypothyroidism, increased intracranial pressure, acute myocardial infarction, vagal stimulation (such as vomiting, straining at stool, carotid sinus massage, or ocular pressure), and specific drugs.

Intervention: When the heart rate decreases to less than 50 beats/min, the patient's cardiac output, coronary perfusion, and electrical stability may be reduced, causing PVCs to occur. No treatment is needed if the patient is alert, has a normal blood pressure, and has no PVCs. Hypotension and PVCs should be treated. PVCs should be treated with oxygen and atropine, not lidocaine; increasing the heart rate may eradicate the PVCs.

Sinus arrhythmia

Rate	60 to 100 beats/min, but this rate may increase with inspiration and decrease with expiration
Rhythm	Regularly irregular
P waves	Present
QRS complex	Present; normal duration
P/QRS relationship	P wave precedes each QRS complex
PR interval	Normal

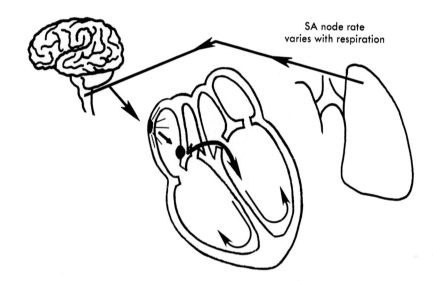

SA node rate
varies with respiration

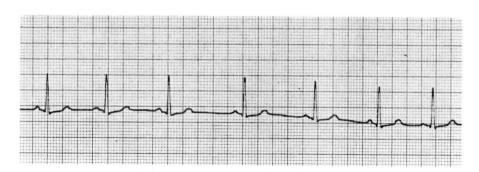

Significance: This arrhythmia is a normal finding in children and young adults in whom there is a variation of vagal tone in response to respirations. As an abnormal finding, it may occur in patients with mitral or aortic valve problems or as a response to intracranial pressure or to specific drugs. For this variance to be considered an arrhythmia, the variation must exceed 0.12 seconds between the longest and shortest cycles.

Intervention: Observe the patient and document findings. If the arrhythmia is not related to respiratory problems, treat the underlying cause.

Dysrhythmias originating in the atria
Premature atrial contractions (extrasystoles)

Rate	Usually 60-100 beats/minute
Rhythm	Usually regularly irregular; may be regular
P waves	Present/but premature P wave may appear different in configuration because it did not originate in the SA node
QRS complex	Present; normal duration
P/QRS relationship	P wave precedes each QRS complex
PR interval	Normal in regular beats, variable in premature atrial contractions (PACs)

NOTE: Always describe the underlying rhythm. For example, document the following: "Sinus tachycardia with approximately 2 PACs per minute."

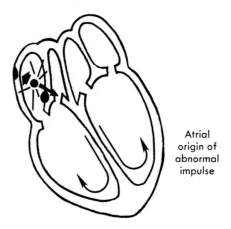

Atrial
origin of
abnormal
impulse

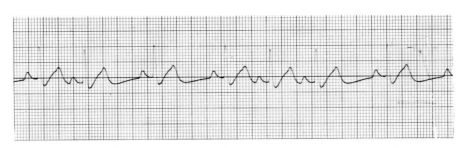

Significance: PACs are the result of an irritable ectopic focus that may be caused by fatigue, alcohol, coffee, smoking, digoxin, congestive heart failure, or ischemia; sometimes the cause is unknown. PACs may be a prelude to atrial fibrillation, atrial flutter, or paroxysmal atrial tachycardia.

Intervention: Treatment is usually unnecessary. If the patient has symptoms the use of tranquilizers, quinidine, procainamide, verapamil, beta-adrenergic blockers, and diltiazem may be tried. Encourage the patient to limit alcohol and coffee consumption and smoking.

Supraventricular tachycardia

Rate	140 to 220 beats/min; atrial rate is usually 160 to 240 beats/min
Rhythm	Atrial rhythm regular; ventricular rhythm usually regular, may be a 2:1 AV block
P waves	Absent or abnormal; may be difficult to identify if P waves are buried in the preceding T wave; differ from normal sinus P waves
QRS complex	Normal or prolonged because of bundle branch block or aberrant conduction
P/QRS relationship	May be a block
PR interval	Normal or prolonged

NOTE: A rhythm that is regular, greater than 150 beats/min, and associated with a narrow QRS complex is considered supraventricular tachycardia. A part of the atria or AV junction, not the SA node, is serving as the pacemaker for the heart. The dysrhythmia may be called paroxysmal supraventricular tachycardia when it abruptly begins and ends.

Significance: In elderly individuals and persons with heart disease, the rapid heart rates may precipitate myocardial ischemia, infarction, or pulmonary edema. This dysrhythmia may also be caused by digoxin overdose.

Intervention: Treatment should be promptly initiated when the patient has chest pain, is hypotensive, has pulmonary edema, or is showing signs of AMI. Determine whether the rhythm is paroxysmal supraventricular tachycardia or ventricular tachycardia. Vagal maneuvers, verapamil, digoxin, overdrive pacing, and synchronized cardioversion are used to treat this rhythm.

Wandering atrial pacemaker

Rate	Usually 60 to 100 beats/min
Rhythm	Irregular
P waves	Present; configuration varies
QRS complex	Present; normal duration
P/QRS relationship	P wave preceding each QRS
PR interval	Normal, although may vary from beat to beat

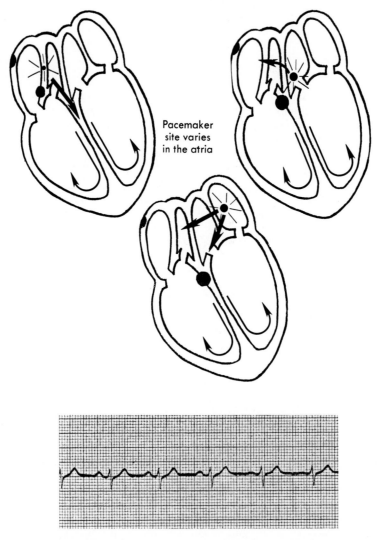

Pacemaker site varies in the atria

Significance: Either the SA node is suppressed or other atrial foci become excited and take over the pacemaker function of the heart. This dysrhythmia may be caused by specific drugs, inflammation, or chronic obstructive pulmonary disease.

Intervention: Treatment is usually unnecessary. If the patient is receiving digitalis, consider withholding it and measuring the serum digoxin level. When treatment is necessary, treat the underlying cause.

Atrial flutter

Rate	Atrial rate of 240 to 360 beats/min
Rhythm	Regular or irregular
P waves	Saw-toothed pattern (F waves, or flutter waves)
QRS complex	Present; normal duration
P/QRS relationship	Because of rapid atrial rate, ventricular response varies; there may be a regular or irregular response
PR interval	Not measurable

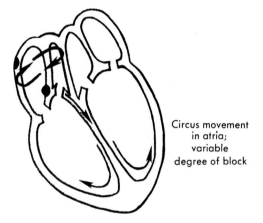

Circus movement
in atria;
variable
degree of block

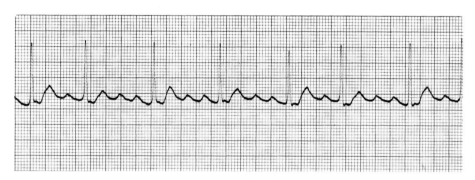

Significance: An irritable focus in the atria is responsible for this dysrhythmia. There is usually a 2:1 AV block with a ventricular rate of approximately 150 beats/min. The ventricular response may be regular or irregular. New-onset atrial flutter is a dangerous dysrhythmia because ineffective atrial contractions may cause mural clots to form in the atria and subsequently break loose, forming pulmonary or cerebral emboli. Atrial flutter may occur with coronary artery disease, rheumatic heart disease, chronic obstructive pulmonary disease, shock, anoxia, electrolyte imbalance, hyperthyroidism, and as a response to various drugs.

Intervention: Synchronized cardioversion is the treatment of choice if the patient has symptoms of atrial flutter. Otherwise the ventricular rate may be slowed with the use of digitalis, verapamil, or beta-blocking agents. If pharmacologic therapy is unsuccessful, cardioversion is indicated. Verapamil and beta blockers may exacerbate bradycradia or congestive heart failure or both.

Atrial fibrillation

Rate	Atrial rate of 350 to 600 beats/min; ventricular rate of 60 to 160 beats/min
Rhythm	Irregularly irregular
P waves	No P waves; F waves (fibrillatory) appear
QRS complex	Irregular rhythm; normal duration
P/QRS relationship	Indistinguishable P waves; irregular ventricular response
PR interval	Indistinguishable

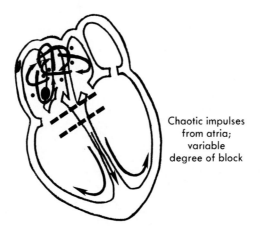

Chaotic impulses
from atria;
variable
degree of block

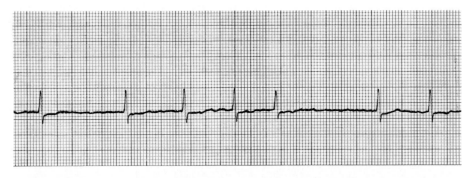

Significance: There is chaotic firing of multiple atrial pacemakers in rapid succession. The atria never firmly contract. The ventricles respond irregularly. Because of poor atrial emptying, there is danger of mural clot formation and embolism. Cardiac output drops because of a lack of "atrial kick" (drops to 15% to 20% of cardiac output). Patients who have chronic atrial fibrillation that is controlled with digitalis and whose ventricular rate is less than 100 beats/min do not need treatment. This dysrhythmia frequently occurs with presence of coronary artery disease, rheumatic heart disease, hyperthyroidism, and, most commonly, with digitalis toxicity.

Intervention: Cardioversion is recommended for patients with ischemic heart disease. For asymptomatic patients, the heart rate may be controlled with the use of digitalis, verapamil, or beta-adrenergic blockers. The use of the latter two drugs in the undigitalized patient may not be effective and may cause congestive heart failure.

Dysrhythmias originating in the AV node

Nodal (junctional) rhythm

Rate	Usually 40 to 60 beats/min
Rhythm	Regular
P waves	May appear inverted before or after the QRS complex, or may not be present
QRS complex	Regular; normal duration
P/QRS relationship	Variable
PR interval	<0.12 second when the P wave precedes the QRS complex

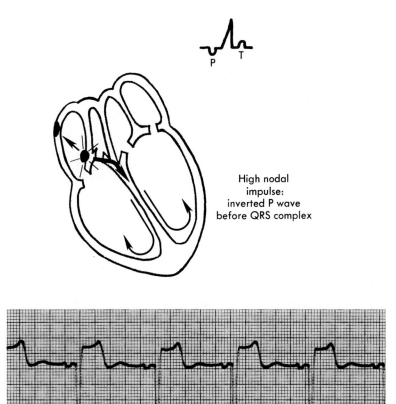

High nodal
impulse:
inverted P wave
before QRS complex

Significance: The AV junction has assumed the pacing function for the heart. There is retrograde depolarization of the atrium, which may or may not result in a detectable P wave.

Intervention: If the patient has been receiving digitalis therapy, withhold the digitalis and obtain a measurement of the serum digoxin level to check for toxicity. There is no specific therapy for this dysrhythmia. If the patient becomes symptomatic from a decreased heart rate, atropine may be administered. If no response to the atropine occurs, pacing and the temporary administration of isoproterenol are indicated.   *Continued.*

Nodal (junctional) rhythm—cont'd

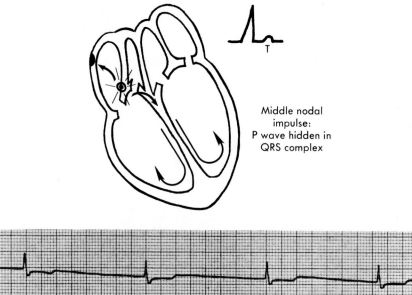

Middle nodal
impulse:
P wave hidden in
QRS complex

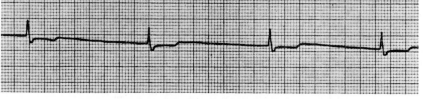

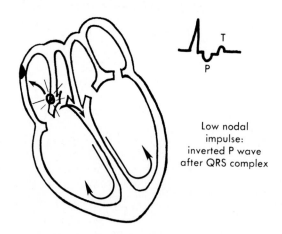

Low nodal
impulse:
inverted P wave
after QRS complex

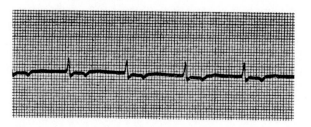

Premature nodal contractions and premature junctional contractions

Rate	Usually normal or bradycardic
Rhythm	Irregularly irregular
P waves	May appear inverted or may not be present
QRS complexes	Regular; normal duration
P/QRS relationship	P waves may appear inverted, may be absent, and may occur before, during, and after the QRS complex
PR interval	<0.12 second when the P wave is seen in a premature beat

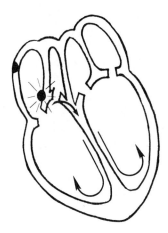

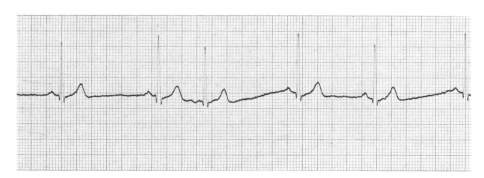

NOTE: See the description of premature atrial contractions.

Significance: The AV junction serves episodically as the pacemaker for the heart. This dysrhythmia is less frequently seen than premature atrial contractions or PVCs; it may precede heart block of the first, second, or third degree.

Intervention: Premature nodal contractions and premature junctional contractions are usually benign. If therapy is indicated, treatment is similar to that for premature atrial contractions.

Nodal tachycardia (junctional tachycardia)

Rate	100 to 800 beats/min
Rhythm	Regular
P waves	May appear inverted or may not be present
QRS complex	Regular; normal duration
P/QRS relationship	P waves may appear inverted before or after the QRS complex or may be absent
PR interval	<0.12 second when the P wave is present

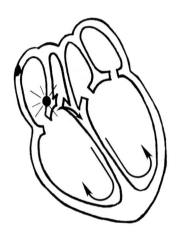

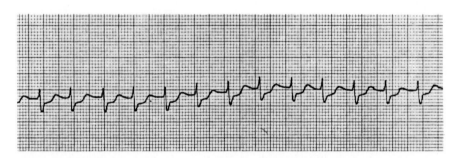

NOTE: An accelerated junctional rhythm is the same as a junctional rhythm but occurs with increased sympathetic stimulation. The rate is 60 to 100 beats/min.

Significance: An irritable focus takes over as the heart's pacemaker. Nodal tachycardia may be caused by heart disease, electrolyte imbalance, chronic obstructive pulmonary disease, anoxia, or specific drugs.

Intervention: This dysrhythmia is generally considered a variant of supraventricular tachycardia and is treated accordingly. In cases of nonparoxysmal episodes caused by digitalis intoxication, the digitalis should be withheld and the serum level checked. A serum potassium level should also be obtained.

First-degree AV block

Rate	Usually 60 to 100 beats/min
Rhythm	Usually regular
P waves	Present; normal configuration
QRS complex	Regular; normal duration
P/QRS relationship	P wave precedes each QRS complex
PR interval	>0.20 second

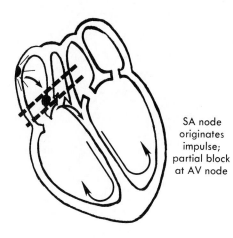

SA node originates impulse; partial block at AV node

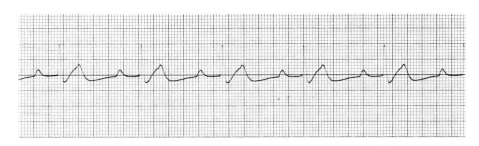

Significance: Conduction of an impulse generated by the SA node is delayed through the atrioventricular node. Causes are varied and include anoxia, ischemia, atrioventricular node malfunction, edema after open-heart surgery, digitalis toxicity, myocarditis, thyrotoxicosis, rheumatic fever, clonidine, and tricyclic antidepressants.

Intervention: Usually no treatment is required. Observe the patient, noting his or her level of consciousness and vital signs. If the patient becomes symptomatic (rarely), atropine is the drug of choice. If the patient is on a regimen of digitalis, withhold it and obtain a measure of serum digitalis and potassium levels.

Second-degree AV block (Mobitz I, Wenckebach)

Rate	Usually normal
Rhythm	Regularly irregular
P waves	One P wave preceding each QRS complex, except during regular dropped ventricular conduction, which occurs at periodic intervals
QRS complex	Cyclic missed conduction; when QRS complex is present, it is of normal duration
P/QRS relationship	P wave before each QRS complex, except during regular dropped ventricular conduction, which occurs at intervals
PR interval	Lengthens with each cycle until one QRS complex is dropped, then repeats

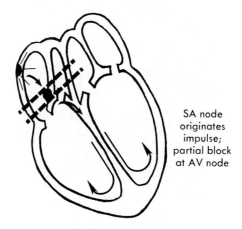

SA node
originates
impulse;
partial block
at AV node

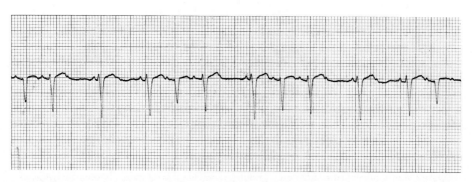

Significance: Each atrial impulse takes longer to travel through the AV node until finally a beat is dropped, and the cycle begins again. This dysrhythmia is the less serious form of second-degree heart block; it is usually transient and reversible. In rare instances this dysrhythmia may progress to complete heart block. This dysrhythmia commonly occurs after an inferior wall infarct.

Intervention: Treatment is needed when the heart rate falls to less than 50 beats/min or if the patient becomes symptomatic. Therapy includes the administration of atropine, temporary pacing, and isoproterenol.

Second-degree AV block (Mobitz II)

Rate	Atrial rate is usually 60 to 100 beats/min; ventricular rate is slower
Rhythm	Usually, regularly irregular
P waves	Two or more P waves for every QRS complex; normal configuration; regular interval
QRS complex	Normal duration, when present
P/QRS relationship	One or more nonconducted impulses appearing as P waves not followed by QRS complexes
PR interval	Normal or delayed on the conducted beat but regular throughout the dysrhythmia

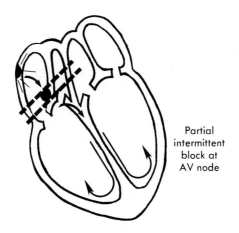

Partial
intermittent
block at
AV node

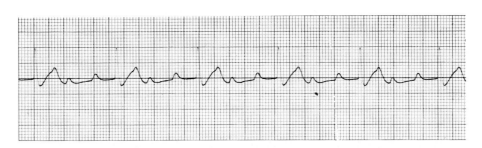

Significance: One or more atrial impulses are not conducted through the AV node to the ventricles. This dysrhythmia may occur in an anterior myocardial infarction and may progress rapidly to complete heart block. Other causes are anoxia, digitalis toxicity, and hyperkalemia.

Intervention: If the patient is asymptomatic, no immediate treatment is required. As with other types of heart block, atropine, isoproterenol, and pacing measures are used. If the patient is taking digitalis, it should be withheld and the serum level should be checked.

Third-degree AV block (complete heart block)

Rate	Atrial rate is 60 to 100 beats/min; ventricular rate is usually <60 beats/min
Rhythm	Usually normal for atria and ventricles when these are examined separately
P waves	Occur regularly
QRS complex	Slow; usually wide (>0.10 second)
P/QRS relationship	Completely independent of each other
PR interval	No PR interval because there is no consistent relationship between the P wave and the QRS complex

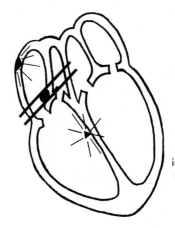

Complete
block at
AV node;
may have
nodal or
ventricular
independent
pacemaker

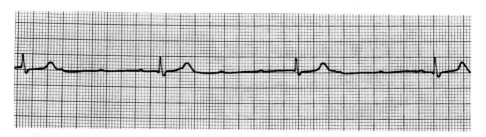

Significance: No conduction of SA impulses through the AV node occurs. The AV node or ventricle initiates its own impulse; the atria and ventricles beat independently of each other. The bradycardia from the block reduces myocardial perfusion and may lead to ventricular tachycardia or ventricular fibrillation.

Intervention: Insertion of a pacemaker is required. Transcutaneous pacing may be used until a transvenous pacer can be placed. Atropine and isoproterenol may be used until the pacing unit is available. Be prepared to perform CPR and advanced life support measures. Do not give lidocaine to a patient with complete heart block, not even when wide, bizarre QRS complexes are present.

Dysrhythmias originating in the ventricles

Premature ventricular contractions (premature ectopic beats, extrasystoles, premature ventricular beats, ventricular premature beats)

Rate	Usually 60 to 100 beats/min
Rhythm	Irregular
P waves	Present with each sinus beat; do not precede premature ventricular contractions (PVCs)
QRS complex	Sinus-initiated QRS complex is normal; QRS complex of PVC is wide and bizarre: >0.10 second; full compensatory pause
P/QRS relationship	P wave before each QRS complex in normal sinus beats; no P wave preceding PVC; compensatory pause following PVC
PR interval	Normal in sinus beat; none in PVC

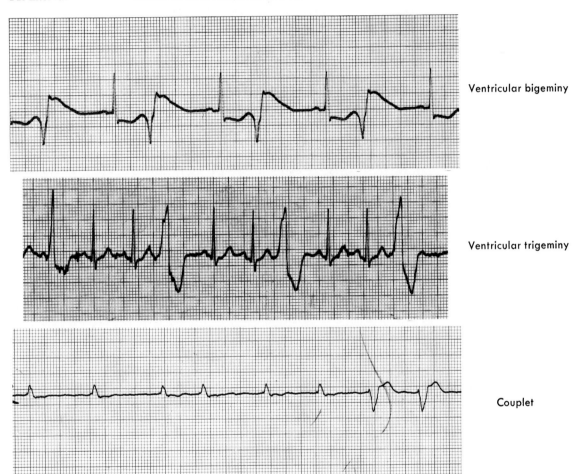

Ventricular bigeminy

Ventricular trigeminy

Couplet

Significance: PVCs indicate ventricular irritability. The impulse is initiated by a ventricular pacemaker cell. PVCs may occur as a result of hypoxia, hypovolemia, ischemia, infarction, hypocalcemia, hyperkalemia, acidosis, or from the use of alcohol, tobacco, coffee, or other stimulants. PVCs may originate from the same focus (unifocal) or from various foci (multifocal). Multifocal PVCs have various morphologies. PVCs may occur in repetitious patterns. If they occur at every other beat, the condition is known as bigeminy; at every third beat, trigeminy. If PVCs occur as in pairs, the pattern is known as a couplet; three contractions occurring together form a triplet. A series of four or more consecutive PVCs is referred to as a short run of ventricular tachycardia.

Intervention: Administer oxygen. If possible, treat the underlying cause. If treating the cause is not possible, pharmacologic therapy is indicated. First try administering lidocaine as a bolus. If this treatment is not successful, procainamide and bretylium may be used. After the ectopy is resolved, an IV drip of the effective antidysrhythmic drug should be instituted. When the PVCs are related to a slow heart rate, atropine is the drug of choice.

Ventricular tachycardia

Rate	150 to 250 beats/min
Rhythm	May be slightly irregular
P waves	Not seen
QRS complex	Wide and bizarre; width is >0.12 second
P/QRS relationship	None
PR interval	None

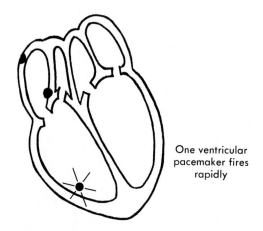

One ventricular
pacemaker fires
rapidly

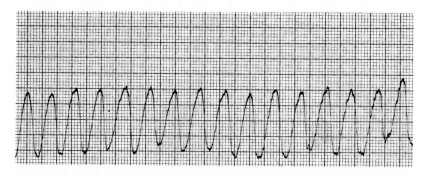

Significance: This rhythm cannot be tolerated for long periods because cardiac output is significantly reduced. If the rhythm persists, it will deteriorate into ventricular fibrillation and asystole.

Intervention: Pulseless ventricular tachycardia should be treated as ventricular fibrillation is treated. If a pulse is present and the patient's condition is stable, the administration of an anti-dysrhythmic agent (lidocaine, procainamide, or bretylium) is indicated. If the patient's condition becomes unstable, the patient should receive cardioversion. Be prepared to begin CPR and initiate advanced life support measures.

Ventricular fibrillation

Rate	Rapid, disorganized
Rhythm	Irregular
P waves	Not seen
QRS complex	Absent; instead, fibrillatory waves of varying size, shape, and duration occur
P/QRS relationship	None
PR interval	None

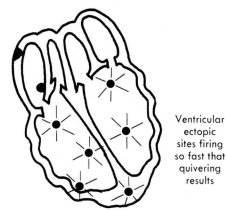

Ventricular ectopic sites firing so fast that quivering results

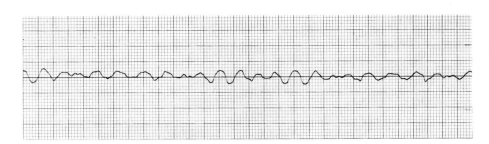

Significance: This dysrhythmia is the most common cause of sudden cardiac death. Ventricular fibrillation produces no cardiac output; cerebral death results when the dysrhythmia is allowed to persist for more than 4 to 6 minutes. Ventricular fibrillation may be preceded by ventricular tachycardia.

Intervention: Begin CPR until a defibrillator is available. Check the rhythm, differentiating between asystole and fine ventricular fibrillation. Defibrillate the patient; start with an energy level of 200 J, continue with 200 to 300 J, and increase the level to as high as 360 J if no response occurs. If no pulse is present, continue CPR while establishing IV access or intubating the patient or both. Next, administer epinephrine (intravenously or endotracheally),* defibrillate up to a level of 360 J, administer lidocaine, defibrillate at 360 J, administer bretylium, and defibrillate again. At this stage, administration of antidysrhythmics is alternated with countershocks. Remember to check the pulse and rhythm between each countershock. If ventricular fibrillation reoccurs after conversion, begin defibrillation at whatever energy level was previously successful.

*Consider the administration of "high-dose" (5 mg) epinephrine IV or intratracheally, in accordance with local protocols.

Idioventricular rhythm

Rate	Usually <40 beats/min
Rhythm	Regular or irregular
P waves	None
QRS complex	Wide and bizarre (>0.10 second)
P/QRS relationship	None
PR interval	None

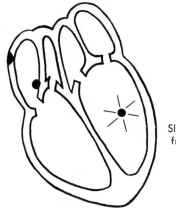

Slow impulses
from ectopic
site in
ventricle

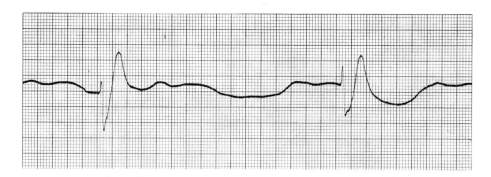

Significance: This rhythm represents an escape rhythm of ventricular origin. Effective cardiac contractions and pulses may or may not be present. This dysrhythmia may be caused by complete heart block, AMI, cardiac tamponade, or exsanguinating hemorrhage. Outcome is usually poor.

Intervention: Administer atropine and isoproterenol; consider pacing. Treat the underlying cause (for example, treat hemorrhage with fluid resuscitation).

Electromechanical dissociation

Rate	Varies
Rhythm	No characteristic pattern
P waves	None
QRS complex	Relatively normal or wide and bizarre
P/QRS relationship	None
PR interval	None

NOTE: By definition a patient is having electromechanical dissociation (EMD) when he or she has a rhythm that should be perfusing but the patient has no pulse. An idioventricular rhythm at a rate of 20 beats/min without a pulse is *not* electromechanical dissociation, but a normal sinus rhythm at a rate of 72 beats/min in a patient who is unconscious, pulseless, and apneic is electromechanical dissociation.

Significance: Electrical complexes are present without mechanical contraction of the heart. The most common causes of this dysrhythmia are tension pneumothorax, acidosis, hypoxemia, hypovolemia, cardiac tamponade, and pulmonary embolism.

Intervention: Perform CPR and treat the underlying cause. Administer epinephrine every 5 minutes as needed.* IV access and intubation should be established.

*Consider the administration of "high-dose" (5 mg) epinephrine IV or intratracheally, in accordance with local protocols.

Asystole (ventricular standstill)

Rate	None
Rhythm	None
P waves	May or may not appear
QRS complex	Absent or rare, with a bizarre configuration
P/QRS relationship	None
PR interval	None

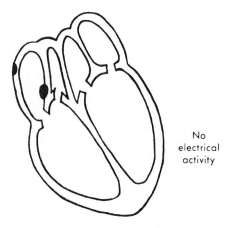

No
electrical
activity

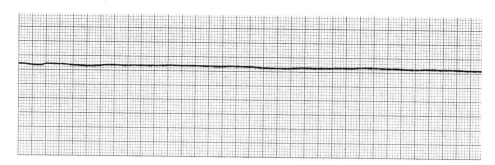

Significance: Mortality is greater than 95%. Asystole often implies that the patient's heart has been in arrest for a prolonged period. Confirm the presence of asystole in two limb leads.

Intervention: Begin CPR. Differentiate between asystole and ventricular fibrillation. Establish IV access and intubate the patient. Administer epinephrine; repeat the dose every 5 minutes as needed. Next, give atropine (repeat once in 5 minutes). If these measures are unsuccessful, pacing may be considered, but it is rarely effective.

CARDIOPULMONARY ARREST IN INFANTS AND CHILDREN

Cardiac arrest in children and infants usually results from hypoxia rather than from primary cardiac disease or dysrhythmias. Causes include airway obstruction, near-drowning, trauma, burns, smoke inhalation, poisoning, upper airway infections, and sudden infant death syndrome. Asystole occurs more commonly in children with cardiopulmonary arrest than does ventricular fibrillation. Bradycardia deteriorating to asystole is usually reflective of profound hypoxia and acidosis. The principles of advanced life support for infants and children are similar to those for adults. Infants are persons from birth to 1 year of age, and children are persons from age 1 to 8 years. Children older than eight years of age may be treated as adults.

Airway

There are some anatomic differences between the airway of a child and that of an adult. Familiarity with these will improve your success in ventilating and intubating pediatric patients. In children and infants the larynx is higher in the neck (C2 in infants, C3-4 in children, and C5-6 in adolescents and adults); the tongue is proportionately larger; the cricoid ring, not the cords, is the narrowest part of the airway; and the airway is collapsible with flexion or hyperextension of the neck. To open the airway of an infant or child, use the jaw-thrust or the head tilt–chin lift maneuver. Use only the jaw-thrust maneuver when a cervical spine injury is suspected. Suction any obvious vomitus or secretions that could occlude the airway.

Breathing

Assisted ventilation techniques are essential in the arrest situation. Assisted ventilation can usually be managed with an appropriately sized bag-valve-mask device or with the mouth-to-mask technique. The proper mask size should provide an airtight seal on the face. The mask should extend from the bridge of the nose to the cleft of the chin, covering the nose and mouth. If the only mask available is adult sized, turn the mask upside down and place the pointed end under the child's chin and the wide area at the bridge of the nose. Avoid hyperextending the neck; this can collapse the airway. Oxygen concentrations of 60% to 95% can be provided by a reservoir-equipped bag-valve-mask device with an oxygen flow rate of 10 to 15 L/min.

If a mask is unavailable, ventilations may be provided by using the mouth-to-mouth or mouth-to-nose technique. Encircle the mouth and nose with your mouth. For larger children, use mouth-to-mouth breathing, pinching the nose with your hand that is placed on the forehead. When mouth-to-mouth breathing is being performed and supplemental oxygen is available, the rescuer should apply a nasal cannula to his or her own nose, breathe in through the nose, and then give the breath. This procedure provides some supplemental oxygen to the breath given to the child.

Table 13-5   Size of endotracheal tubes for infants and children

Age	Weight (kg)	Tube size (cm) (interior diameter)
Newborn	Less than 1	2.5-3.0
Newborn	More than 1	3.0-4.0
6 months	7	3.5-4.5
1 year	10	4.0-5.0
3 years	15	4.5-5.5
5 years	20	5.0-6.0
6 years	22	5.5-6.5
8 years	25	6.0-6.5
10 years	30	6.5-7.0
12 years	40	6.5-7.0
16 years	50	7.0-7.5

Begin by giving two moderately slow breaths (1 to 2 seconds each), remove your mouth, and let the chest fall. Moderately slow breaths, given just until the chest inflates, help avoid gastric distention. The rate should be 1 breath every 4 seconds or 15 breaths per minute. Ventilations should be given after every fifth chest compression. If the chest does not rise, readjust the position of the head and neck and attempt to ventilate the patient again. If this attempt is unsuccessful, the airway is most likely obstructed. Maneuvers for removal of a foreign body should be performed.

When prolonged ventilation is required, or when adequate ventilations cannot be achieved with a bag-valve-mask device, the child should be intubated. Recommended tube sizes are listed in Table 13-5. To visually estimate the size of tube needed, select a tube that has the same outside diameter as the diameter of the child's little finger. The depth of the ET tube is as important as the proper diameter; the tube should be inserted to a depth of three times its diameter. For example, an ET tube with a diameter of 4.5 cm should measure 13.5 cm at the lips. Immobilize the head and neck to prevent extubation; movement of the head upward or downward may cause the tube to become dislodged. A straight laryngoscope blade (Miller) is usually used in infants and children. Successful placement of the ET tube should be evaluated by observing for symmetric chest movement; by auscultation of bilateral, equal breath sounds; by noting the absence of breath sounds over the stomach; and by observing condensation in the ET tube during expiration. Whenever ventilation is performed via mouth-to-mouth breathing, mouth-to-mask technique, or bag-valve-mask device, an orogastric tube should be placed to relieve gastric distention.

Circulation

For infants, palpate the brachial artery to assess the presence of a pulse. If CPR is needed, the rescuer should place the index and middle fingers of one hand or both thumbs so that the hands encircle the chest 1 finger's breadth below

Table 13-6   Guide to estimating weight by age in children

Age (years)	Weight (kg)	Weight (lb)
Newborn	3-5	6-11
1	10	22
3	15	33
5	20	44
8	25	55
10	30	66
15	50	110

From Melker R: Resuscitation of neonates, infants and children. In Auerbach PA and Budassi SA, eds: *Cardiac arrest and CPR,* ed 2, Rockville, Md, 1983, Aspen Systems.

the intermammary line to compress the sternum to a depth of ½ inch to 1 inch at a rate of at least 100 compressions per minute. For children older than 1 year of age, presence of a pulse should be determined by palpating the carotid or femoral artery. To perform chest compressions, the rescuer should place the heel of one hand in the center of the sternum and compress the sternum to a depth of 1 inch to 1½ inches at a rate of 80 to 100 compressions per minute.

Vascular Access

Initially, establishing vascular access is unnecessary for resuscitation because essential medications can be given endotracheally. For fluid resuscitation, a physiologically balanced solution such as Ringer's lactate can be administered at 20 ml/kg IV push. Central access may be easier to obtain; commonly used vessels are the femoral, internal jugular, external jugular, and subclavian veins. Peripheral sites include the scalp, hand, saphenous veins, external jugular vein, and dorsum of the foot. Small-gauge needles or cannulas may be used; a 21- or 23-gauge butterfly or a 20- or 22-gauge cannula is adequate for administering medications.

If rapid vascular access is not possible, intraosseous cannulation may be used. All resuscitation drugs, as well as intravenous fluids, may be administered via this route. For intraosseous access in infants and children younger than 5 years of age, a bone marrow needle is inserted into the proximal tibia 1 to 2 cm below and medial to the tibial tuberosity on the flat surface or into the distal femur 3 cm above the external condyle. For older children and adults, the distal tibia 2 cm proximal to the medial malleolus is the site of choice. Contraindications for this procedure are recently fractured bones and overlying areas of cellulitis or burns.

Medications

Medication doses are calculated based on the patient's weight in kilograms (Table 13-6). Remember that atropine, epinephrine, lidocaine, and naloxone can be administered through the ET tube (Table 13-7). Do not exceed the stan-

Table 13-7   Medications for pediatric resuscitation

Medication	Dose	Comments
Aminophylline	5 mg/kg IV slowly for a period of 20 to 30 minutes (loading bolus); 0.6 to 0.9 mg/kg/hr IV drip	
Atropine	0.02 mg/kg IV, intratracheally, IO	Minimum dose is 0.1 mg; may repeat every 5 minutes to a total vagolytic dose of 1 mg for children, 2 mg for adolescents
Calcium chloride	20 mg/kg (equals 0.2 ml/kg of 10% solution)	Give slow IV push for a period of 5 minutes; may repeat in 10 minutes
Dopamine	2 to 20 μg/kg/min	Titrate to desired blood pressure
Epinephrine	0.01 mg/kg IV, ET, IO	
Isoproterenol	0.1-1.0 μg/kg/min	Titrate to desired heart rate
Lidocaine	1 mg/kg IV, intratracheally, IO	May repeat half initial dose every 8 to 10 minutes to a total dose of 3 mg/kg
	20 to 50 μg/kg/min IV drip	—
Naloxone (Narcan)	0.1 mg/kg IV, intratracheally, IM, IO	—
Sodium bicarbonate	Newborn: 1 to 2 mEq/kg	Dilute 1:1 with D$_5$W
	Children: 1 mEq/kg	May repeat every 10 minutes with half the initial dose; infuse slowly and only if ventilations are adequate

dard adult doses in pediatric patients. If a dose that is calculated in milligrams per kilograms for a medium-sized child exceeds the adult dose, give the adult dose rather than the calculated dose.

Defibrillation

Ventricular fibrillation is extremely rare in children. To perform defibrillation, use paddles of appropriate diameter: 4.5 cm paddles for infants and small children, 8 cm paddles for older children, and 10 cm paddles for adolescents. If pediatric-sized paddles are not available, you may use adult-sized paddles placed in the anteroposterior position. This placement prevents contact of the two paddles and electrical arcing. The initial dose recommended for infants and small children with ventricular fibrillation and pulseless ventricular tachycardia is 2 watt-seconds per kilogram. If initial attempts are unsuccessful, increase the wattage to 4 J/kg.

For synchronized cardioversion the dose is 0.1 to 1.0 J/kg.

Resuscitation of the Newborn

Immediately after delivery of the infant's head, gently suction the nose and pharynx to clear the airway. If thick meconium is present during delivery, it is essential to clear the oropharynx and nasopharynx before the onset of breathing. To prevent aspiration, suction the airway when the head is delivered but before delivery of the thorax. The goal is to remove as much meconium as possible before the baby's first breath, which will draw meconium into the distal airways.

If the newborn has a pulse rate of more than 110 beats/min and is breathing spontaneously, keep the infant warm and under close observation. Remember that acrocyanosis is normal in newborns. If breathing is labored or absent but heart rate remains above 100 beats/min, attempt to suction the airway, and stimulate the infant by vigorously drying the infant. Most infants then begin to breathe spontaneously. If breathing is still absent, begin ventilation. Open the newborn's airway with a moderate backward tilt of the head with chin support. Use a bag-valve-mask device to ventilate the newborn with supplemental oxygen. If the bag-mask unit has a pressure-limiting pop-off valve (preset at 30 to 35 cm H_2O), tape the valve closed because high pressure may be necessary for initial lung inflation. If the neonate still does not become pink, intubation with a 3.0 to 3.5 mm ET tube is indicated.

Cardiac arrest in the newborn usually occurs secondary to asphyxia or shock from prolonged intrauterine hypoxia. In these cases a prolonged resuscitation almost always re-sults in irreversible brain damage.[9] In the case of a period of only transient pulselessness after a complicated delivery, the use of CPR is usually effective.

Assess for pulselessness by palpating the brachial artery and auscultating the heart. If there is no pulse or if the heart rate is less than 60 beats/min, compressions should be initiated. Draw an imaginary line between the nipples, and compress the chest one finger's width below this line with the index and middle fingers of one hand. Compressions should be performed at a rate of 120 per minute at a depth of ½ inch to 1 inch. Usually ventilation and oxygenation restore a normal heart rate of more than 100 beats/min. Administration of medication is rarely needed. Venous access may be obtained by umbilical vein catheterization.

REFERENCES

1. Belle-Isle C: Patient selection and administration of thrombolytic therapy, *JEN* 16:3, 1989.
2. Evans E: The carotid sinus: its clinical importance, *JAMA* 149:46, 1952.
3. Hammond B: Thrombolytic therapy for acute myocardial infarction: implications for emergency nursing, *JEN* 15:2, 1989.
4. Hine L, Laird N, Hewitt P, Chalmers T: Meta-analytic evidence against prophylactic use of lidocaine in acute myocardial infarction, *Arch Intern Med* 149, 1989.
5. Magee M: Nursing care of the patient receiving thrombolytic therapy, *JEN* 15:2, 1989.
6. Rizzon P, DiBase M: Effect of carotid sinus reflex on cardiac impulse formation and conduction: electrophysiologic study. In Schwartz PJ, Brown AM, Malliani A, Zanchetti A, eds: *Neural mechanisms in cardiac arrhythmias*, New York, 1978, Raven Press.
7. Rothenberg M, ed: Adenosine released to treat supraventricular tachycardia, *ACLS Alert*, June, 1990.
8. Rothenberg M, ed: Further evidence favors use of high dose epinephrine, *ACLS Alert* 3:8, 1990.
9. Safar P, Bircher N: *Cardiopulmonary cerebral resuscitation*, ed 3, London, 1988, WB Saunders.
10. Schuster D: Patients with an implanted cardioverter defibrillator: a new challenge, *JEN* 16:3, 1990.

Intravenous Therapy

Susan R. Cullen

An intravenous (IV) line is initiated to provide a means of administering fluids, medications, blood, blood products, and blood substitutes. In the emergency care setting, an IV line is usually placed because the patient either needs fluids immediately, requires fluids over a short period, or requires administration of emergency medications. In most situations, placement of an IV line in an anatomically acceptable site is important. Use of a preferred anatomic site may lose priority status if a line is urgently needed for a life-threatening problem.

When starting an IV line, be cautious to cause as little pain as possible. Large-bore needles are often necessary in emergency situations for fluid administration and for administration of medications. If a patient is alert, a small bleb of 1% lidocaine may be administered at the insertion site of a large needle before the IV is started. Sterile technique should be as well maintained as possible during the procedure to prevent further complications. Complications that may occur are hematomas at the puncture site, infiltration of fluid, phlebitis, embolism of blood, air, or catheter fragments, infection, cellulitis, and pulmonary edema caused by fluid overload.

INTRAVENOUS INFUSION SITES IN ADULTS

The most commonly chosen IV sites in adults are in the upper extremities, the jugular and subclavian veins, and the greater saphenous veins of the legs (Fig. 14-1). When choosing an IV site, consider the condition of the vein. A tourniquet should be applied proximal to the selected site, to distend the vein for inspection and palpation. If the vein selected already appears distended or is easily palpable, a tourniquet may not be necessary. Elderly patients may have fragile veins that may not withstand the pressure of a tourniquet, or hematomas may develop in these patients as a result of poor tissue integrity. The length of time that the IV will be in place, the size and age of the patient, and the reason for starting the IV line should also be considered.

Veins of the Upper Extremities

The digital veins are located on the dorsal aspect of the fingers. These veins can be cannulated with a scalp vein needle or a small angiocatheter. Because large volumes of fluids cannot be passed through these veins, they should be used only in absolute emergencies.

The metacarpal veins are located on the dorsal aspect of the hands (Fig. 14-2). These veins can be cannulated with any type of catheter. A metacarpal vein is a good site, if long-term therapy is indicated; metacarpal veins are usually good sites in children but should not be used in elderly patients. The skin in this area is usually slightly tougher than that of the antecubital fossa.

The cephalic veins are located at the radial aspect of the dorsal venous network. Cephalic veins are good sites for a large-bore cannula, and their location provides a natural over-board splint. The accessory cephalic vein originates from the union of the dorsal veins and joins the cephalic vein below the elbow. The accessory cephalic vein is a good site for large-bore cannulas and for blood administration. The basilic vein, which has a large capacity but provides poor access, originates from the union of the dorsal veins on the ulnar aspect of the arm. When the arm is flexed at the elbow, the basilic vein can be seen.

Median Veins

The median antebrachial vein, which is sometimes difficult to find, originates from the union of many veins in the palmar aspect of the hands. The median cephalic, or median basilic, vein is found in the antecubital fossa. This vein is frequently used for drawing blood and as an IV site in extreme emergency situations because it is easily accessible and can accommodate large-bore cannulas.

Peripheral Veins of the Lower Extremities

The saphenous vein overlies the ankle. Because of the danger of embolism, this vein should be used only in extreme emergency situations. If an IV line is initiated at this

193

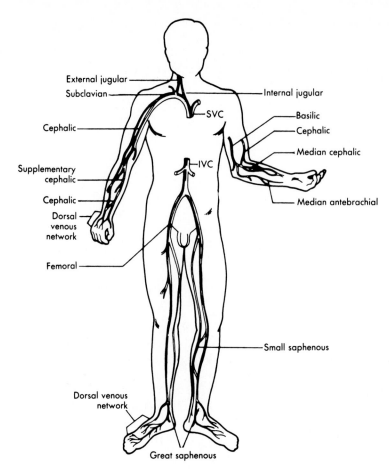

Fig. 14-1   Major veins of body.

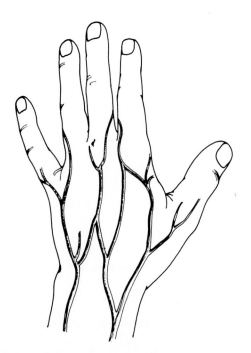

Fig. 14-2   Dorsal and metacarpal venous networks on back of hand.

site, and the pneumatic antishock garment (PASG) is inflated, a pressure cuff must be placed over the IV bag. Be sure that the pressure in the cuff exceeds that of the PASG so that the IV solution can run.

Peripheral Veins of the Neck

Although the site of the external jugular vein is often overlooked, it is large and should be considered, especially in cases of cardiopulmonary arrest and multiple trauma and when large volumes of fluid are required. The external jugular vein can accommodate large-bore cannulas.

NEEDLE AND CANNULA SELECTION

Many types of needles and catheters may be used to cannulate a vein. The decision regarding which device to use depends on the type of therapy to be given and the condition of the patient's veins. In many situations a young person could probably tolerate a large-bore needle; however, an elderly person may have tiny, sclerosed, and tortuous veins, which may necessitate the use of a smaller catheter. If an elderly person is to receive a large volume of fluid, fluid over a short period, or blood or blood products, the larger vein sites should be selected for optimal therapy with an appropriate cannula.

In an emergency situation, when the person's life may depend on the establishment of an IV line to administer medications, look for a vein that is easy to cannulate. Do not waste time looking for a site that is anatomically comfortable for the patient. If the patient's condition stabilizes, the IV site can be changed. Be sure that the vein you select is large enough to hold the cannula. If the purpose of the IV line is to provide large amounts of fluid over a short time, initiate a cannula with the largest possible bore. In cases of cardiopulmonary arrest, the ideal method of administering medications is via the IV route, followed by the endotracheal route. Be sure that all the equipment you require is ready before you initiate the IV line, especially if you are alone. Once the line is established, secure it so that it cannot be inadvertently pulled out.

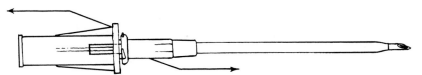

Fig. 14-3 Butterfly infusion set.

Uses

Be sure to use the appropriate cannula for the therapy to be given. When administering blood or blood products, use an 18- to 20-gauge catheter; for the administration of colloids, use a 20-gauge catheter; for the administration of crystalloids, use a 21- to 22-gauge catheter. To administer large volumes of fluids rapidly, use the cannula with the largest bore that can be initiated at that time.

Types

A *butterfly cannula* (Fig. 14-3) is also known as a scalp vein needle or winged needle. The butterfly cannula is made of steel and has plastic, winglike projections that are used for easy placement.

An *indwelling* catheter, a plastic cannula designed for long-term use, may be used when a cutdown is performed by the physician.

A *catheter-over-needle* (Fig. 14-4) is a tapered catheter fitted over a needle. The needle is used to puncture the skin and the vein; then the catheter is advanced into the vein while the needle is simultaneously withdrawn.

A *catheter-inside-needle* (Fig. 14-5) is a sharp, hollow needle with a catheter inside. The needle is used to perforate the skin and the vein; the catheter is then advanced through the needle, and the needle is withdrawn from the patient. Usually the needle remains outside the patient and over the end of the catheter, which is secured with a plastic clip; the clip ensures that the catheter cannot accidentally be cut. This type of catheter is often used for a subclavian line.

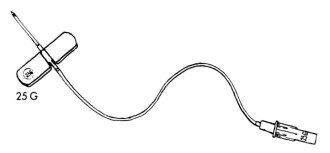

Fig. 14-4 Catheter-over-needle.

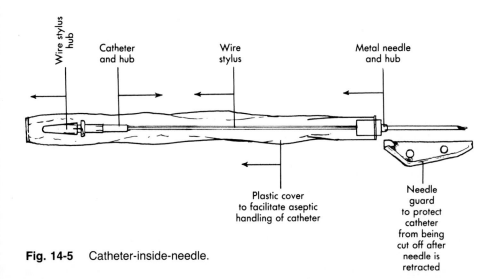

Fig. 14-5 Catheter-inside-needle.

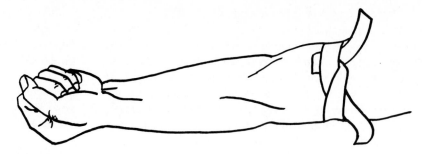

Fig. 14-6   Tourniquet proximal to puncture site.

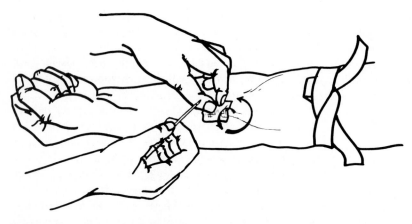

Fig. 14-7   Just before venipuncture, antiseptic solution is applied to area of needle insertion.

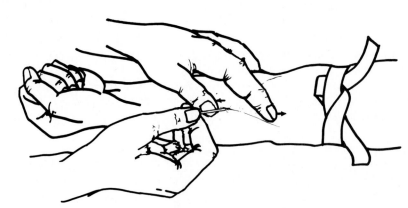

Fig. 14-8   Proper handling and alignment of needle with axis of vein contributes to successful venipuncture.

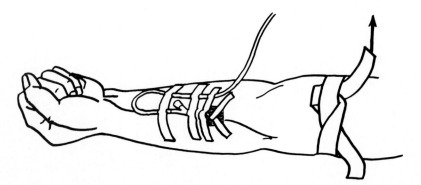

Fig. 14-9   Needle is immobilized and tourniquet is removed.

Preparing the Site of Intravenous Cannulation

Before attempting to cannulate a vein that is in an extremity, apply a tourniquet proximally (Fig. 14-6). In many elderly patients veins may be more prominent, and a tourniquet may not be necessary. Sometimes in these patients the pressure in the veins caused by the tourniquet may rupture the vein before catheter insertion. Care must be taken to assess the need for a tourniquet in the elderly patient.

Do not leave the tourniquet in place for more than 5 minutes. When the tourniquet is tightened, tap or briskly rub the vein to allow it to dilate. Holding the limb in a dependent position, if possible, is also helpful. Before catheter insertion you may ask the patient to take several deep breaths and open and close his or her hand a few times to dilate the vein. If these measures fail, apply a hot pack or a warm towel over the vein to be cannulated and wait for about 5 minutes. Prepare the area for cannulation by cleansing it with a surgical preparatory solution such as povidone-iodine (Betadine) solution (Fig. 14-7). Be sure that the patient is not allergic to povidone-iodine. Next, wipe the area with an alcohol wipe and then with a sterile 2- by 2-inch gauze. If time permits and the catheter is large bore, a 1% solution of lidocaine without epinephrine may be injected subcutaneously, according to hospital policy or standard. Also, when a large-bore needle is to be used, a scalpel may be used to make a small skin incision through which a large-bore catheter can be passed.

After the site is prepared, stabilize the vein with the thumb of the nondominant hand distal to the puncture site. Keeping the bevel of the needle up, puncture the skin using the smallest angle possible between the cannula and the skin. (Fig. 14-8). The vein may be entered either from above or from the side. Advance the catheter slowly, and check for a flashback, or blood return. Once this flashback occurs, advance the catheter either over or through the needle, depending on the type of catheter-needle device used. Remove the tourniquet, and connect the IV tubing to the hub of the catheter. If resistance is met while advancing a catheter into a vein, connecting the tubing and flushing the vein with fluid may facilitate cannulation. Place a dressing over the IV site. Hospital procedures related to dressings may vary. An Op-Site or Bioclusive dressing or a sterile 2- by 2-inch gauze dressing may be used. IV lines should be taped securely (Fig. 14-9), and the site should be marked with the date, time, and needle size and the initials of the person starting the IV line. Hospital policies dictate when the catheter should be replaced or when the IV dressings should be changed. The container of IV solution should also be marked with the date and time when it was hung, as well as with the names of any medications it may contain. The bag or bottle should be marked with the time the bag was hung and with the rate at which the IV is to be infused.

Heparin or saline lock. A heparin lock or a saline lock is a cannula that is not connected to IV tubing. Instead, a rubber adaptor is attached to the end of the IV catheter, and this adaptor is flushed with either a heparin solution or a saline solution; the type and amount of solution are dictated by hospital policy. Medications may be administered through the cap, or if a solution is to be infused, the cap may be removed and the tubing may be connected directly to the catheter. This device is ideal for the purpose of intermittent IV access or emergency IV access.

INTRAVENOUS INFUSION SITES IN INFANTS AND CHILDREN

There are preferred sites for intravenous infusions in infants and children. In neonates and small infants, those sites may be the dorsal surfaces of the hands or feet, antecubital veins, scalp veins, or, in newborns, the umbilical vessels. The use of hypertonic solutions or hyperalimentation for infusion in the peripheral veins is contraindicated. If an infant has been receiving long-term IV therapy and the peripheral accesses have been exhausted, a cutdown may be necessary. A cutdown is a surgical procedure that is usually performed on the saphenous vein or the basilic vein just above the joint of the elbow: a small incision is made, to expose the vein; then the vein is cannulated. The cannula is then secured to the vein with a suture, and the wound is closed and dressed.

One or two commonly used IV sites in children are on the arms and feet; four to eight sites are on the scalp. Because there is so little subcutaneous tissue in the scalp, vein visualization is easier. Also, scalp veins have no valves, so they can be infused in either direction. These veins are frequently used in infants younger than 9 months of age. Shaving hair from the scalp may be necessary so that the vein may be better visualized and so that tape will adhere. As little hair as possible should be removed and parents should be made aware of the necessity of the procedure, since shaving the baby's head may be upsetting to them.

Infants and children usually have a large amount of subcutaneous fat, which may make visualization of an IV site difficult. Warm compresses applied to the preferred site may enhance visualization. Placing the extremity in a dependent position may help to distend the vein. Applying a tourniquet may sometimes be helpful, but because a child's veins may be thin walled or fragile, the back pressure may cause the vessel to rupture. Gentle tapping against the wall of the vein may aid in distention.

Types of Catheters

Scalp vein needles or butterfly needles for children are usually from gauge 21 to gauge 25 in size. These needles have winged tabs that can be easily secured to the skin with tape. These needles are used for short-term therapy. For longer term therapy, 22- to 24-gauge over-the-needle catheters are available. A 26-gauge over-the-needle cather can be used in small veins and is usually used for the neonate. In the newborn, the umbilical vessels, which contain two veins and one artery, are present for use. Special umbilical catheters are available in gauge sizes 3, 5, and 8 for cannulation of these vessels. Hospital policies dictate who places these catheters. Placement is performed according to sterile procedure, and special attention is given to the measurement of the vessel and the length of the catheter that is introduced. Chest and abdominal radiographic examinations are necessary to confirm proper placement. The catheter is then secured with a suture to the stump of the umbilicus, and proper taping is performed. Because umbilical lines are considered central lines, intravenous fluids may be infused in these lines and blood samples may be obtained from these lines according to hospital policies.

Intraosseous Infusion

When other types of venous access are not obtainable, intraosseous infusion is used in children 3 years of age or younger as a method of venous access for temporary infusion of fluids and medications. Any solution that can be given IV can be given by the intraosseous method into the bone marrow. The preferred site for this method is the flat medial surface of the proximal tibia, 1 to 2 finger breadths below the tibial tuberosity, below the growth plate of that bone (Fig. 14-10). The marrow cavity is large, and there are no adjacent nerves in the area. A 15- to 18-gauge bone marrow needle (Fig. 14-11) or an 18- to 20-gauge short spinal needle can be used because these needles are not easily plugged off. The needle should be inserted perpendicular or at a 60-degree angle to the skin with a rotary motion and moderately applied pressure. A popping sensation and loss of resistance indicate entry into the marrow. A 5 cc syringe of saline is then attached; when flushing occurs easily with no extravasation into the surrounding tissues, the line is properly placed. Any reattempts for insertion should be made in the other leg. IV tubing can be plugged directly into the needle hub. The needle is stable, and little taping is necessary; supporting the needle with gauze pads should be sufficient. Infusions may run more slowly than ordinary IVs that are run with a needle of the same gauge. Pressure bags may be necessary to achieve higher rates of infusion.

Intraosseous needles should not be placed in a recently fractured bone.

Preparing the Child

Children are fearful of injection; if time allows, explanation of the procedure should be provided to both the child and the parent. The nurse should perform the procedure in as quiet a setting as possible; privacy decreases the child's anxiety regarding loss of control in front of other people. The assistance of another person during the procedure is

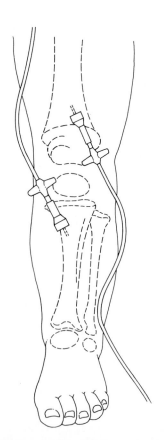

Fig. 14-10 Recommended sites for intraosseous infusion. (From Manley L: *JEN* 14[2]:66, 1977.)

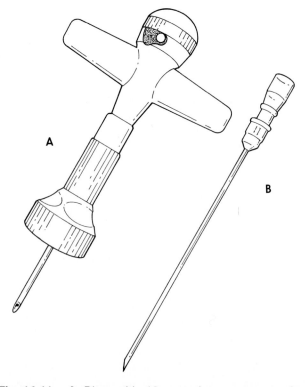

Fig. 14-11 **A,** Disposable 16-gauge bone marrow aspiration needle (Illinois Sternal). **B,** Three-inch, 18-gauge spinal needle (Becton, Dickenson and Co., Rutherford, N.J.). (From Manley L: *JEN* 14[2]:66, 1977.)

preferable, since the child may lose control, but restraint should not be used until necessary. Explanations of each step of the procedure are often helpful in reducing the child's anxieties. The nurse can decide whether the parents should remain in the room during IV insertion. If the parents choose to stay, they should not be asked to help restrain the child; rather, they should be asked to comfort the child after insertion has been completed.

When IVs are begun in children's extremities, limiting the motion of the hand or foot may be necessary. Small armboards may be applied and secured with either tape or elasticized gauze. Care should be taken not to wrap too tightly; circulation must be maintained, and the insertion site should be visible and easily accessible.

Care of the Intravenous Site

When armboards are applied to the extremities of infants and children, care should be taken to keep the hand or foot in an anatomic position as nearly normal as possible. Use gauze pads or rolls for positioning. An armboard should have enough padding to ensure that no tissue damage over bony prominences or impedance of nerves occurs. With active children, restraining the extremity may be necessary. A restraint that is attached to the arm or leg may be secured to the bed. Never attach a restraint to the siderail; this can cause damage to the limb if the rail is inadvertently lowered. For infants the armboard can be pinned to the blankets or to a sandbag for immobilization. Frequent supervised removal of the restraints is necessary so that the child may move around.

IV dressings for infants and children can be applied the same way that adult IV dressings are applied. A clear plastic dressing such as Op-Site or Bioclusive provides ideal visualization of the site.

CANNULATION OF CENTRAL VEINS

The central vein that is most commonly cannulated is the subclavian vein (Fig. 14-12). The box below, left, describes the cannulation procedure. This vein is used for the administration of fluid and to measure central venous pressure. The internal jugular vein can also be cannulated, if a large volume of fluid must be administered over a short period. Cannulation of the internal jugular vein is described in the box below. Because the use of either of

---

SUBCLAVIAN VEIN CANNULATION

This vein is located in the neck between the median and middle thirds of the clavicle and the sternal notch.

1. Place the patient in Trendelenburg's position to increase the size of the vein and decrease the possibility of air embolism.
2. Place a rolled towel between the patient's shoulder blades to provide a better angle.
3. Prepare the neck and upper chest with an antiseptic solution.
4. Anesthetize the area with 1% lidocaine at the inferior edge of the clavicle where the medial and middle thirds join.
5. Insert a 14-gauge or larger cannula (with a syringe on the end to avoid air embolism), aiming toward the suprasternal notch and keeping the cannula just under the clavicle.
6. Aspirate as the needle is advancing; if nonpulsating blood is drawn, the vein has been cannulated.
7. Advance the catheter through the needle; do not pull back on the catheter because it may be sheared off.
8. When the catheter is in place, withdraw the needle.
9. Clip on the catheter guard so that the needle will not shear off the catheter.
10. Suture the catheter and guard in place.
11. Apply antibiotic ointment to the puncture site.
12. Apply a dry sterile dressing.
13. Apply a waterproof dressing.
14. Label the cannulation site.

INTERNAL JUGULAR VEIN CANNULATION

1. Place the patient in Trendelenburg's position to increase the size of the vein and decrease the possibility of air embolism.
2. Place a rolled towel between the shoulder blades to provide a better angle.
3. Prepare the neck and upper chest with an antiseptic solution.
4. Drape the neck and upper chest area.
5. Anesthetize the area with 1% lidocaine at the junction of the middle and lower thirds of the anterior border of the sternocleidomastoid muscle.
6. Insert a 14-gauge or larger cannula (with a syringe on the end to avoid air embolism) close behind the sternocleidomastoid muscle, aimed toward the space formed by the clavicular and sternal heads.
7. Aspirate as the needle is advancing; if nonpulsating blood is drawn, the vein has been cannulated.
8. Advance the catheter through the needle; do not pull back on the catheter because it may be sheared off.
9. When the catheter is in place, withdraw the needle carefully.
10. Clip the catheter guard so that the needle will not shear off the catheter.
11. Suture the catheter and guard in place.
12. Apply antibiotic ointment to the puncture site.
13. Apply a dry sterile dressing.
14. Apply a waterproof dressing.
15. Label the cannulation site.

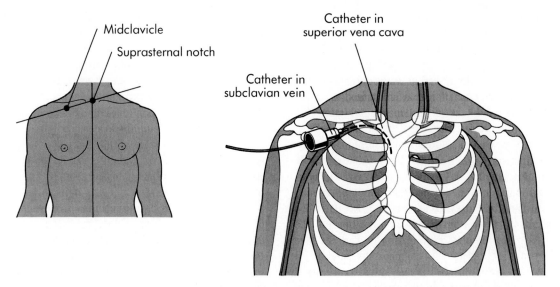

Fig. 14-12 Technique of percutaneous intraclavicular subclavian catheterization. Needle, inserted under midclavicle and aimed in three dimensions at top of posterior aspects of sternal manubrium (indicated by fingertip in suprasternal notch), lies in plane parallel with frontal plane of patient and enters anterior wall of subclavian vein.

these cannulation routes may puncture the lung and cause a tension pneumothorax, these procedures should be performed only when absolutely necessary.

Multilumen central catheters, which usually have three color-coded lumens, the proximal (white), medial (blue), and distal (brown), may be introduced into these central veins. The proximal lumen is 18-gauge and can be used for blood drawing or for general access. The medial lumen is also 18-gauge and is used for general access. The distal lumen is 16-gauge and can be used for drawing blood, for monitoring central venous pressure (CVP), or for general access. If blood must be drawn from these lumens when IV fluids are infusing through them, the fluids must be stopped and an adequate amount of blood drawn off for waste, so

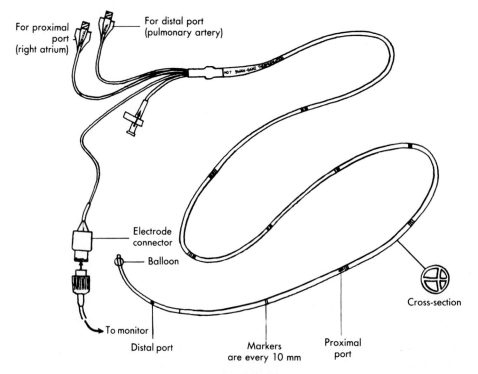

Fig. 14-13 Swan-Ganz catheter.

that the laboratory values are not distorted. The lumens must be flushed after each use and per routine when they are not being infused, according to hospital policies and procedures. The usual solution for flushing is heparin 100 U/ml. The insertion site must be checked frequently for redness, swelling, or drainage, as with any catheter. If any problems are noted, the physician must be notified.

The Swan-Ganz Line, or pulmonary artery catheter (Fig. 14-13), is a multilumen catheter that may be used for drawing blood, measuring pressure within the heart, reading EVPs, and measuring cardiac output, as well as for multiple infusions. This line is placed percutaneously or with a venous cutdown approach.

Single-lumen catheters are also used to provide central venous access for the administration of fluids and medications and for blood drawing. These catheters usually are managed and flushed according to the same protocols as for multilumen catheters, but the hospital's specific policies and procedures should be followed.

CENTRAL VENOUS PRESSURE

The central venous pressure (CVP) is a measurement of the right-sided pressures of the heart, blood volume, effectiveness of the heart as a pump, and vascular tone. The procedure for measuring CVP is given in the box below. The CVP can be obtained from a triple-lumen distal port, a single-lumen catheter, or a Swan-Ganz line. A normal CVP reading is 4 to 10 cm H_2O. A reading of greater than 10 cm H_2O may indicate a pericardial tamponade, right-sided heart failure, fluid overload causing pulmonary edema, tension pneumothorax, or any other condition that causes an increased pressure on the right side of the heart.

PROCEDURE FOR MEASURING CVP USING A SUBCLAVIAN INTRAVENOUS LINE

1. Place the patient in a supine (flat) position.
2. Measure at the midaxillary line (5 cm from the top of the chest) in the fourth intercostal space at the level of the right atrium.
3. Place the manometer zero-reading at this point.
4. Fill the manometer from the attached IV solution (do not let it overflow).
5. Turn the stopcock on the IV line open to the patient and the manometer. The fluid level will fall and fluctuate (decreasing on inspiration and increasing on expiration).
6. When the fluid level appears stable, note the measurement at the top of the fluid column.
7. Record this reading as the CVP.
8. Adjust the stopcock to close the manometer and open the IV line to the patient. (Make sure to readjust the IV solution drip rate.)

A CVP of less than 4 cm H_2O may indicate hypovolemia, vasodilation, dehydration, septic shock, neurogenic shock, anaphylactic shock, drug-induced shock, or any other condition that causes a decreased pressure on the right side of the heart.

PULMONARY ARTERY PRESSURE

The pulmonary artery pressure may be measured with a Swan-Ganz catheter. The proximal port of the catheter site is in the right atrium (Fig. 14-14). The distal port is in the pulmonary artery. Many catheters also have a paceport. Pulmonary artery wedge pressure is a reflection of pressure in the left ventricle. The normal wedge pressure is 6 to 12 cm H_2O. The catheter is advanced into the superior vena cava and floated, with the assistance of the balloon tip, into the right atrium and ventricle, into the pulmonary artery, then into the lung. Once the catheter reaches the lung, the balloon is deflated and advanced a few centimeters until it is located in one of the smaller branches of the pulmonary artery. The balloon is reinflated, occluding this smaller branch of the artery. The tip of the catheter then transmits waves that indicate pressure in the left ventricle of the heart.

To keep these ports patent, the distal port in the pulmonary artery must be connected to a continuously flushing and pressurized solution of normal saline and heparin in all lines, in accordance with hospital policy. The other ports, that is, the venous impedance port, paceport, sideport, and CVP port, should be flushed according to particular hospital policies and procedures.

Laboratory specimens may be drawn from the venous impedance port or the CVP port. The first 5 ml of blood should be discarded; blood is then drawn for the specimen, and a flush of 3 to 5 ml normal saline solution is followed by the heparin flush appropriate for that institution. When these lumens are flushed, pressure should not be forced. If the line does not flush with gentle pressure, notify the patient's physician.

Dressings for the Swan-Ganz, triple-lumen, and single-lumen catheters should be applied using sterile technique. Prepackaged kits that contain all the items necessary for a change are available. A mask and sterile gloves must be worn. The area around the catheter insertion site is swabbed in a circular motion, from the inside to the outside, with three alcohol wipes or swabs. This step is repeated with three povidone-iodine (Betadine) swabs. A small amount of Betadine ointment may be applied to the insertion site based on preference. A 2- by 2-inch gauze pad is placed over the insertion site, and a clear plastic dressing such as Op-Site or Tegaderm is placed over this dressing. Some hospitals may prefer to use a gauze 4- by 4-inch dressing with tape. The plastic dressing provides better visualization of the site. The insertion site should be checked frequently for redness, swelling, or drainage, and the patient's physician should be notified if these occur. Dressings are usually changed every 72 hours.

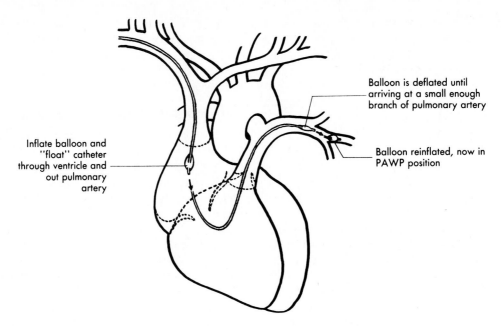

Fig. 14-14   Insertion of Swan-Ganz catheter.

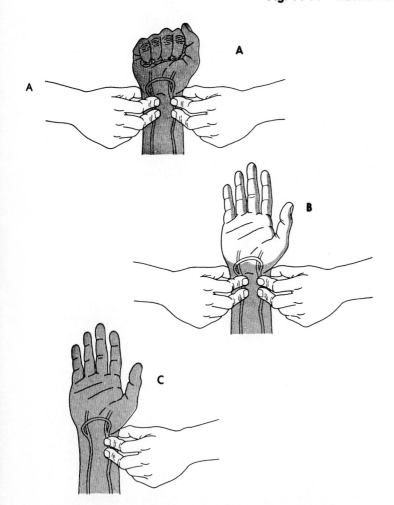

Fig. 14-15   Assessing for Allen's sign. **A,** Occlude both radial and ulnar arteries with firm pressure. **B,** Raise arm to blanch hand. **C,** Release ulnar artery to check for return of color to hand and for patency.

Arterial Line

The arterial line is placed to measure arterial pressures. If the line is to be inserted into the radial artery, you should be certain that the collateral circulation is sufficient to provide circulation to the limb. An Allen test (Fig. 14-15) measures the ability of the ulnar artery to provide circulation to the hand. First, palpate both the radial and ulnar pulses. Then occlude both pulses and raise the arm, causing the hand to blanch. Release the ulnar artery and check to see that color returns to the hand; this return ensures that the ulnar artery is able to provide circulation to the hand. A lack of circulation is considered a negative Allen sign, meaning that the ulnar artery is unable to maintain adequate circulation on its own. If a negative sign is found, an arterial cannula should not be inserted into the radial artery because circulation to the hand is insufficient.

An arterial line should be connected to a pressurized bag containing a normal saline and heparin solution via a special arterial line with a valve (Sorenson) that allows periodic flushing of the line at approximately 3 ml/hr. Blood samples and arterial blood gases may be drawn from a 3-way stopcock; the line can then be flushed with the use of the "pigtail" device attached to the valve. A transducer may be attached to the line and connected to the monitoring system to provide a readout of both systolic and diastolic arterial pressure.

LONG-TERM CENTRAL LINE CATHETERS
Types

There are several types of long-term central line catheters, including the following: Hickman, Groschong, Portacath, and Broviac. These catheters are used for patients who are receiving long-term IV therapy or chemotherapy and whose other venous access sites have been exhausted. Blood drawing for laboratory tests can also be performed from these lines, which are all surgically inserted and removed.

The Hickman and Broviac catheters are similar; they are silastic central venous catheters that are tunneled and have single or multiple lumens. These catheters vary in size from pediatric to adult sizes and are surgically placed through the chest wall and tunneled to the vein, then threaded so that the tip of the catheter lies at the junction of the superior vena cava and the right atrium. A Dacron graft that is placed just under the insertion site eventually adheres to the subcutaneous tissue; as a result the device is more permanently attached and sutures are unnecessary.

The Groschong catheter is similar to the Hickman and Broviac catheters. This Silastic catheter is also implanted, but it has a closed distal end and a slit valve on the side. When the device is not in use, the slit valve stays closed so that blood or air cannot enter the catheter. Because of this feature, heparinization of the catheter may be unnecessary. Only saline flushing may be necessary. Groschong catheters are also available with single or multiple lumens.

Also available for long-term therapy are totally implanted vascular devices. These Silastic catheters are attached to a self-sealing diaphragm surrounded by a stainless steel or plastic case. These devices, some called Portacaths or Groschong Portacaths, are implanted under the subcutaneous tissue; the Silastic tubing is threaded into the vein or artery to be used. These catheters are also available with single or double lumens. These devices have no external feature. To use the Portacath, the Silastic dome underneath the tissue is palpated, and a Huber needle, a needle beveled at a 90-degree angle, is inserted into the center of the dome until the metal resistance is met. If blood is aspirated from the needle, the needle is properly placed. This device can be used for the same purposes as other catheters; it also helps preserve the patient's body image: no dressing over the site is needed if no needle is in place.

Groschong Portacaths have features of both the Portacath and the Groschong catheter. The distal end of the Silastic tubing is the same as that of the Groschong catheter, and heparinization of the line is unnecessary.

Drawing Blood and Care of the Site

When blood is drawn from these central lines, infusions must be stopped and disconnected, 5 to 10 ml of waste must be discarded, the laboratory sample must be drawn, and a 10 ml saline flush must be performed before the tubing is reconnected. Care must be taken to ensure that the catheter is clamped when the tube is being disconnected so that air does not enter the catheter. It is also helpful to ask the patient to perform a Valsalva maneuver during disconnection. Blood should always be drawn from the proximal lumen of multiple-lumen catheters.

When the catheters are not in use, they must be heparinized, with the exception of the Groschong catheters. A heparin solution of 100 U/ml is usually used. Hospital policy dictates how much and how often heparinization is to be performed. Groschong catheters are flushed with 5 to 10 ml of normal saline solution according to hospital policy.

Central line dressings are prepared in much the same way that the dressings for triple-lumen and single-lumen temporary central line catheters are prepared. Using sterile technique, the nurse prepares the skin first with three alcohol wipes, then with three Betadine wipes, always wiping in a circular motion from the inside to the outside. The excess Silastic tubing is conveniently coiled, and a dressing, preferably clear plastic, is placed over the site. The dressing is labeled with the date and time and the initials of the person performing the procedure. Dressings are usually changed twice a week and when required. Dressings are necessary for Portacaths and Groschong Portacaths only when they are in use. Sterile technique must be used, however, when a needle is being introduced into a Portacath.

Central line insertion sites must be inspected frequently for redness, swelling, or exudate because these sites can be a source of a significant infection.

Declotting Central Lines

Central lines may become occluded by a blood clot within the catheter. Urokinase, a thrombolytic agent, may be used to dissolve the clot. A physician's order is always necessary for this procedure. The concentration of urokinase for this procedure is 5000 U/ml. The amount instilled is always equal to the internal volume of the catheter lumen. After the determination is made that the lumen is clotted, urokinase is instilled into the lumen. A prescribed amount of time must pass before attempts may be made to aspirate blood from the catheter. This action may be repeated several times. If blood cannot be aspirated, the urokinase is withdrawn, the line is capped, and the physician is notified. Care must be taken not to instill the urokinase into the patient's blood stream because urokinase is thrombolytic. Policies and procedures may vary and must always be followed.

Intravenous Solutions

There are several types of IV solutions. The type used depends on the reason for use. The most common types of IV solutions and the uses of each are given in the box on p. 204.

BLOOD AND BLOOD COMPONENTS

When a patient is losing blood, all components of blood are being lost. Replacement of lost blood is best provided with fresh whole blood cells. However, large amounts of fresh whole blood are difficult to obtain. Sometimes banked whole blood or blood components must be used (Table 14-1). Properly determining blood type and crossmatching blood takes at least 30 to 45 minutes. Blood other than fully typed and crossmatched whole blood may be used. Type O negative blood may be given when the need for blood is

COMMONLY USED INTRAVENOUS SOLUTIONS

Dextrose (5%) in water (D₅W)

A hypotonic solution of dextrose in water containing 50 g dextrose monohydrate/liter

Use: TKO IV lines and nonelectrolyte fluid replacement; medical lines (emergency and other)

Contraindications: Head injuries; may increase intracranial pressure

Normal saline

A crystalloid, isotonic solution containing the following:

9 g NaCl/liter

145 mEq Na/liter

145 mEq Cl/liter

Use: Restoration of water and salt loss in hypovolemic states; as irrigation solution

Contraindications: Congestive heart failure, pulmonary edema, renal impairment, edematous states with sodium retention

Dextrose (2.5%) and half normal saline

An isotonic solution containing the following:

25 g dextrose monohydrate/liter

4.5 g NaCl/liter

Use: Maintenance fluid

Contraindications: Congestive heart failure, renal impairment, edema with sodium retention

Dextrose (5%) and Ringer's lactate

A hypertonic solution containing the following:

50 g dextrose monohydrate

8.6 g NaCl/liter

300 mg KCl/liter

330 mg CaCl/liter

Use: To replace fluid and electrolyte loss

Contraindications: Congestive heart failure, renal impairment, edema with sodium retention

Ringer's lactate

A crystalloid isotonic polyelectrolyte solution equaling the electrolyte concentration in human plasma and containing the following:

13 mEq Na/liter

4 mg K/liter

109 mEq Cl/liter

2.8 mEq lactate/liter

Use: In hypovolemia for volume replacement

Contraindications: Congestive heart failure, renal impairment, edema with sodium retention, head injury, liver disease, respiratory alkalosis

Dextran 75

A colloid solution containing the following:

6% Gentran in 0.7% NaCl

Should be administered through a blood filter

Use: Treatment of shock, hemorrhage, burns

Contraindications: Bleeding disorders, congestive heart failure, renal impairment

Plasma

A colloid solution and the liquid fraction of unclotted whole blood containing the following:

135 to 150 Na/liter

3.5 to 5 K/liter

98 to 106 Cl/liter

22 to 30 HCl₃/liter

Should be administered through a blood filter

Use: Volume replacement

Contraindications: Congestive heart failure, pulmonary edema

Plasmanate

A colloid and commercial IV solution containing the following:

Human albumin, 88%

Alpha globulin, 7%

Beta globulin, 5%

Polyelectrolyte solution containing the following:

100 mEq Na/liter

50 mEq Cl/liter

Should be administered through a blood filter

Use: Blood volume expansion

Contraindications: Congestive heart failure, pulmonary edema

Salt-poor albumin

A colloid solution containing the following:

Normal human albumin, 25%

Alpha globulin, 7%

Protein, 12.5%

Should be administered through a blood filter

Use: Urgent fluid volume replacement because of trauma or burns; rarely used in trauma management

Contraindications: Congestive heart failure, pulmonary edema

Table 14-1 Blood and blood products

Blood product	Tubing	Solution	Uses	Notes	Blood type	Run time
Red blood cells	#2C2147 Travenol Y type blood administration set	Normal saline	Acute or chronic anemia, aplastic anemia, bone marrow failure, congestive heart failure, chronic renal failure, hepatic coma	Obtain baseline vital signs; run transfusion slowly for first 5 minutes; at this time, transfusion reaction typically occurs	*Must* be ABO compatible	Minimum of 2 hours per unit, unless otherwise ordered by physician; should hang no longer than 4 hours
Whole blood	#2C2147 Travenol Y type blood administration set	Normal saline	Acute massive blood loss, hypovolemic shock	Obtain baseline vital signs; should *not* be stored for prolonged periods; factors deteriorate after 24 hours	*Must* be ABO compatible	Minimum of 2 hours per unit, unless otherwise ordered by physician; should hang no longer than 4 hours
Platelets	Fenwal #4C2196 Y type blood component set (sent from blood bank)	Normal saline	Thrombocytopenia, platelet function abnormality	Do *not* use microaggregate filter	Need *not* be ABO compatible	May be given rapidly, usually 4 to 10 units at a time
Fresh frozen plasma	#2C2147 Travenol Y type blood administration set	Normal saline	Hypovolemia combined with hemorrhage due to deficiencies	Do *not* use microaggregate filter; fresh frozen plasma is rich in clotting factors V, VIII, and XI; if thawed, must be used within 6 hours	*Must* be ABO compatible	May be given rapidly
Cryoprecipitate	Fenwal #4C2196 Y type blood component set (sent from blood bank)	Normal saline	Hemophilia, von Willebrand's disease, hypofibrinogenemia, factor XIII deficiency	Unstable to heat and storage; once thawed, must be used within 6 hours	Need *not* be ABO compatible	May be given rapidly
Albumin	Blood bank sends filtered tubing set	Normal saline	Shock caused by burns; maintains blood volume in patients with hypovolemia; hypoproteinemia	Tubing must have filter; must use vented tubing because albumin is supplied in nonvented bottles	Need *not* be ABO compatible	May be given as rapidly as necessary for shock patients
Leukocyte-poor red blood cells	Microaggregate filter Pall filter #060-00806	Normal saline	Repeated febrile reaction; reaction from leukocyte antibodies and patients who are candidates for organ transplants	Obtain baseline vital signs	*Must* be ABO compatible	Minimum of 2 hours per single unit; should hang no longer than 4 hours, unless otherwise ordered by physician

Courtesy Eastern Maine Medical Center, Bangor, Maine.

Table 14-2 Transfusion reactions

Reaction	Cause	Prevention	Assessment	Intervention
Hemolytic	Blood incompatibility	Type and crossmatch; infuse first 50 ml slowly	Fever, chills, dyspnea, tachypnea, lumbar pain, fever, oliguria, hematuria, tightness in chest; collect blood and urine samples	Discontinue immediately; fatality may occur after 100 ml infused
Allergic	Antibody reaction to allergens	Screen donors for allergy; administer antihistamines before transfusion	Mild: chills, hives, wheezing, vertigo, angioneurotic edema, itching Severe: dyspnea, bronchospasm	Mild: slow infusion; give antihistamine as ordered Severe: stop infusion; epinephrine may be ordered
Pyrogenic	Infusing chilled blood	Screen donors; use aseptic technique in administration	Fever, chills, nausea, lumbar pain	Stop infusion
Hypothermic	Infusing chilled blood	Give at room temperature; use warming coils for rapid infusion	Chills	Slow infusion; cover client
Circulatory overload	Infusion of large amounts of blood, especially to clients with cardiac disease or extremes of age	Infuse slowly; check drip rate frequently	Rales, cough, dyspnea, cyanosis, pulmonary edema, increased CVP	Stop infusion; treat pulmonary edema; apply rotating tourniquets
Air embolism	Entry of air into vein	Use proper infusion technique; avoid giving under pressure; check connections to tubings; avoid Y-tubes; use filter; use plastic containers	Chest pain, dyspnea, hypotension, venous distension	Stop infusion; position on left side; give oxygen; embolectomy may be performed
Hypocalcemic	Precipitate from acid citrate dextrose	Use blood immediately	Numbness, tingling in extremities	Stop infusion; give calcium as ordered
Hyperkalemic	Hemolysis of red blood cells releases potassium	Use blood immediately	Nausea, vomiting, muscle weakness, bradycardia	Stop infusion

From Barber J, Stokes L, Billings D: *Adult and child care: a client approach to nursing,* ed 2, St Louis, 1977, Mosby–Year Book.

immediate. If the patient can wait for about 20 minutes, type-specific (A, B, AB, or O) blood may be used, thus decreasing the risk of a reaction.

Many complications can occur as a result of a blood transfusion. Some of the causes include mismatched blood, hypothermia, hypocalcemia, hyperkalemia (potassium levels in stored blood increase by 1 mEq/L/day), acid-base problems (that occur while the preservative converts to bicarbonate when it enters the liver), and coagulation defects, such as disseminated intravascular coagulation (Table 14-2).

CARE OF THE PATIENT RECEIVING VOLUME REPLACEMENT

The following steps should be followed when caring for the patient receiving volume replacement:
1. Check the airway frequently.
2. Auscultate the lungs.
3. Monitor the ECG.
4. Check urinary output.
5. Check temperature.
6. Check electrolyte values.
7. Check the hematocrit.

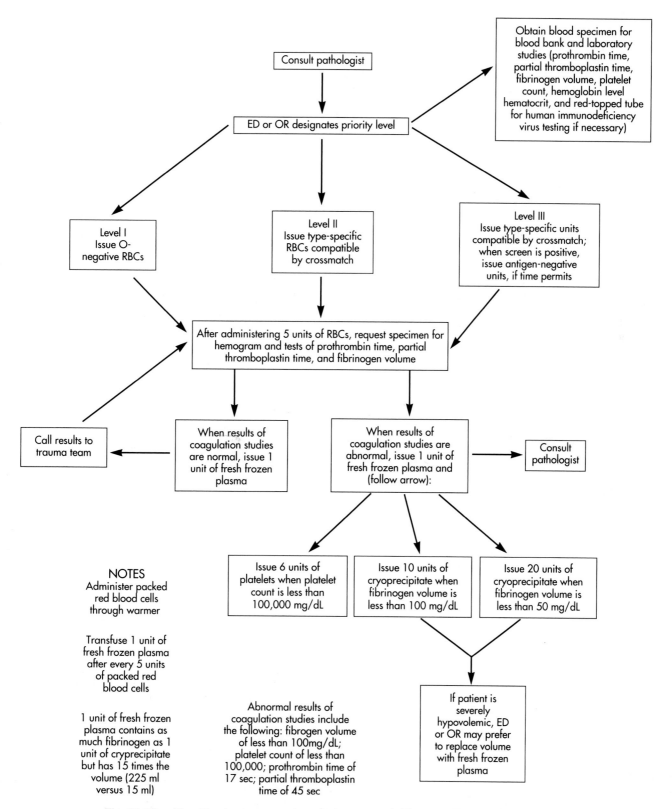

Fig. 14-16 Blood bank emergency transfusion protocol. (Courtesy Eastern Maine Medical Center, Bangor, Me.)

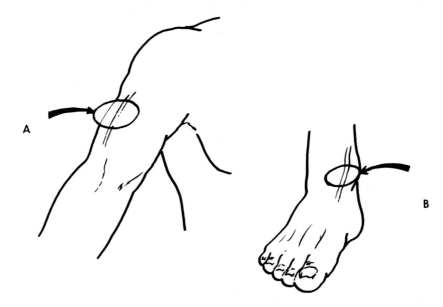

Fig. 14-17 Common sites of venous cutdown. **A,** Cephalic vein. **B,** Saphenous vein.

VENOUS CUTDOWN

Equipment

Surgical gloves
Surgical mask
Scalpel handle and blades (11- or 15-gauge)
Vascular scissors
Suture scissors
Lidocaine (1% or 2%)
Suture material
Forceps
4- by 4-inch gauze squares
Sterile towels

Catheter (may use infant-feeding tube or IV connecting tubing)
Antiseptic solution
Hemostats
Syringe and needle (25-gauge)
Antibiotic ointment
IV setup
Tape
Small vein retractor

Procedure (usually performed by a physician) (Fig. 14-18)
1. Prepare the extremity with antiseptic solution.
2. Drape the limb.
3. Apply a local anesthetic.
4. Make a transverse incision.
5. Dissect the tissue down to the vein.
6. Lift the vein.
7. Nick the vein with a scalpel.
8. Insert the cannula.
9. Secure the cannula with a suture.
10. Suture the wound around the cannula.
11. Apply antibiotic ointment.
12. Tape the cannula in place.
13. Label the IV site (gauge and type of cannula, date, time, caregiver's initials).

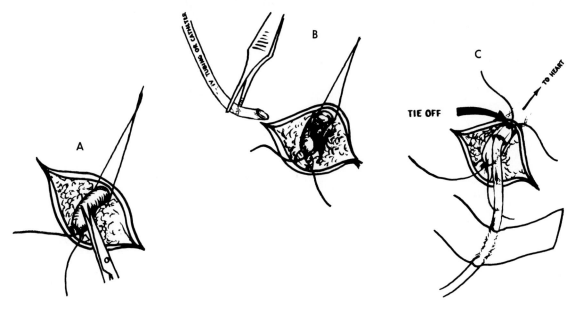

Fig. 14-18 Venous cutdown. **A,** Isolating and cutting vein. **B,** Inserting cannula. **C,** Suturing cannula in place.

MASSIVE TRANSFUSION

If a patient must receive large amounts of blood, a massive transfusion protocol must be instituted so that complications can better be avoided. Figure 14-16 is a sample algorhithmic protocol that is used in cases of major trauma or massive transfusion.

VENOUS CUTDOWN

A venous cutdown is a minor surgical procedure that is used if a peripheral IV site cannot be located or if a large volume of fluid is to be administered over a short period. The procedure is presented in the box on the preceding page. A cutdown is usually performed on the basilic vein (just above the elbow) or the saphenous vein (above the ankle). The saphenous vein is usually chosen when a cutdown is performed on a child (Fig. 14-17).

SUGGESTED READINGS

American Heart Association: *Textbook of advanced cardiac life support,* Dallas, 1987, ANA National Center.

Guhlow L and Kolb: Pediatric IVs: special measures you must take, *RN* 42(3):50, 1979.

Hadaway LC: Evaluation and use of advanced IV technology. I. Central venous access devices, *J IV Nurs* 12(2):73, 1989.

Holder C and Alexander J: A new and improved guide to IV therapy, *Am J Nurs* 90(2):44, 1990.

Insalaco SJ: Massive transfusion, *Lab Med* 15:325, 1984.

Mannucci PM et al: Hemostasis testing during massive blood replacement, *Vox Sang* 42:113, 1982.

Oberman HA et al: Transfusion of plasma components, *Transfusion* 24(4):281, 1984.

Whaley LF and Wong DL: *Nursing care of infants and children,* ed 3, St Louis, 1987, Mosby–Year Book.

Wilson RF et al: Problems with 20 or more blood transfusions in 24 hours, *Am Surg* 53:410, 1987.

Jay Rankin

$\mathbf{I}$n the treatment of disease, few disciplines offer the wide range of information that the modern clinical laboratory is able to provide to the clinical practitioner.

A viable specimen is central to the entire practice of clinical laboratory medicine. The art of obtaining blood specimens is termed *phlebotomy*. Phlebotomy, the letting of blood in the treatment of disease, has been practiced since antiquity.

Specimens obtained in the emergency department (ED) are used both for diagnosis and for determining baselines for treatment. Without a proper specimen, all the instrumentation, the highly trained personnel, and the information regarding patient care may be of little value. Depending on institution policy, emergency personnel may be called on to obtain specimens for laboratory analysis.

Although the techniques for obtaining specimens are not complicated, they do require attention to detail and practice.

SPECIMEN COLLECTION SYSTEMS
Venous Specimen Systems

Evacuated blood collection system

The evacuated blood collection system (EBCS) is the most widely used and recognized specimen collection system. The system allows for the collection of multiple specimens with a single needle puncture. Fig. 15-1 details the components of the system.

Central to the system is an evacuated specimen tube. A vacuum within the tube causes blood to be pulled into the tube after a blood vessel has been cannulated. The tubes have color-coded stoppers, which indicate what each tube is to be used for and what additives are present in the tube (Table 15-1).

The EBCS needles are color-coded by the manufacturer. The color coding refers to both the needle length and the needle diameter. As with IV catheters, the smaller the number is, the larger the needle diameter is.

Nonevacuated systems. Nonevacuated systems, although not used as extensively as the evacuated system, are valuable for blood collection. The ED must provide treatment for a number of compromised patients. In many cases lowered peripheral blood pressure in these patients causes the vein to collapse when the EBCS is applied. The nonevacuated system, in which pressure is applied on the vein

Table 15-1 Commonly used evacuated specimen tubes

Stopper color	Additive	Action; notes
Red	None	—
Red/black	Inert silicon gel	Acts as a separator between red blood cells and serum after centrifuging
Purple	Ethylenediamine tetraacetic acid (EDTA)	Chelates calcium from the blood, thus preventing clotting; the potassium salt of EDTA is usually used
Blue	Sodium citrate	Same action as for EDTA; the anticoagulant of choice for coagulation studies
Black	Sodium citrate	Same action as for EDTA; used for red blood cell sedimentation studies
Gray	Potassium oxalate	Same action as for EDTA; is also a glycolytic inhibitor for glucose determinations
Green	Heparin	Prevents clotting by deactivating thrombin and thromboplastin; both sodium and lithium salts are used

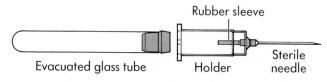

Fig. 15-1 Evacuated blood collection system.

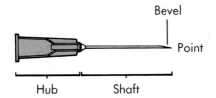

Fig. 15-2 Needle, *above,* may be attached to syringe to form nonevacuated system.

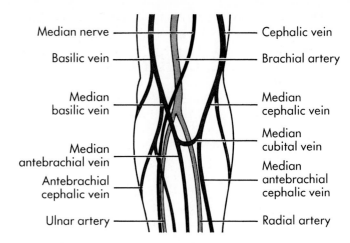

Fig. 15-3 Superficial arteries and nerves in antecubital fossa.

manually, may be used in these cases. The nonevacuated system is also useful for drawing blood from patients whose blood is difficult to draw and for obtaining microbiologic specimens.

A needle attached to a syringe is an example of a nonevacuated system (Fig. 15-2).

Capillary systems. Capillary systems are used primarily for obtaining specimens from infants, small children, or patients such as those with diabetes, from whom multiple blood samples must be taken over a period of time.

A number of microdraw systems, or capillary draw systems, are marketed for a variety of uses. The basic components of a capillary draw system are the lancet, which is used for puncturing the skin either manually or with an automated lancet device, and a container for the specimen. The container may hold a variety of anticoagulants (Table 15-1).

Arterial Specimen Systems

Arterial specimens are obtained by using a nonevacuated collection system; heparin (1000 U/ml) is used as the anticoagulant. Concentrations of heparin that are higher than 1000 U/ml have been shown to alter the measured values.

SPECIMEN COLLECTION
Venous Collection

A patient's venous system is the primary source for obtaining blood specimens used for laboratory testing. Only a few of the many veins in the human body are accessible for venipuncture or intravenous (IV) therapy; therefore, care must be exercised in the use of these veins so that these limited sources are preserved for future specimen collection and therapy.

The proper performance of a venipuncture is mandatory if a viable specimen is to be obtained for testing. Improper venipuncture or careless handling of a specimen may render the specimen useless for laboratory purposes. If laboratory personnel are unaware of improper handling and the specimen is used, inaccurate results may be reported. A proper specimen is the foundation of accurate and useful diagnostic laboratory information.

Equipment. Equipment for venous collection of specimens includes the following:

Disposable gloves
Tourniquet
Isopropyl alcohol wipes or pads
Evacuated tubes, depending on test ordered
Tube holder
Multidraw needle
Dry gauze
Band-Aid or adhesive tape

Procedure. Venous specimens are usually obtained by puncture of veins in the antecubital area of the arm. Fig. 15-3 presents the most commonly used veins in the antecubital area.

Review all requests for tests, to ensure that you have the proper tube for each test ordered. This review helps prevent unnecessary needle sticks to the patient.

Always be courteous to the patient. Knock before entering the patient's room, and when you enter, identify yourself and explain what you will be doing.

Identify the patient. If the patient is conscious and can talk, ask for the patient's full name. The name given should match the name on the test request form or forms. If your institution uses an armband system, also ensure that the name on the armband matches the name on the request form(s). If the patient is unable to identify himself or herself and no armband is available, the patient's primary nurse should identify the patient. Be sure to write this nurse's name on the request form(s), and write that the nurse identified the patient.

Tell the patient what you will be doing. Emphasize that, to help the patient, the physician has ordered the tests. This reassurance is especially important when you are testing apprehensive patients or small children.

Position the patient. If possible, have the patient lie down. If the patient is ambulatory, allow the patient to sit in a chair designed for venipuncture or another chair. Never draw blood from a patient who is standing.

Prepare your equipment. Always wear disposable gloves when working with blood or body fluids. Ensure that everything you may need is at hand, including extra tubes. Generally a 20- or 21-gauge needle is used; smaller gauges tend to cause hemolysis of specimens. For children or patients with small veins, a 22-gauge needle may be necessary.

Select the site to be used. The area should be free of rashes and injuries. *Never* draw from an area proximal to an IV infusion site. (Some institutions have policies that permit venipuncture above an IV site when no other site is available.) *Never* draw from a fistula. Drawing from a hematoma should be avoided if possible.

A tourniquet is applied using a slip knot. Commercially available tourniquets with Velcro, surgical tubing, or Penrose drain tubing may be used.

Wrap the tourniquet around the arm 2 to 3 inches above the area to be used (Fig. 15-4, *A*). Pull one end taut while holding the other in place (Fig. 15-4, *B*). Loop the opposite end under the taut end to form the slip knot (Fig. 15-4, *C*).

Select the vein to be used, visually if possible, and using palpation in all cases. Learn to use the fingers on your nondominant hand to palpate veins. Calluses tend to build up on the fingers of the dominant hand, decreasing sensitivity. Vein visualization will be assisted by having the patient open and close the fist several times and then keep the fist closed. Take your time finding the best possible vein to use. Checking both arms may be necessary.

Never leave the tourniquet in place for more than 2 minutes. The resulting hemoconcentration will affect the test results. Release and reapply the tourniquet before preparing the puncture site.

Using 70% isopropyl alcohol, cleanse the puncture site in a circular manner (Fig. 15-4, *D*). Move from the center to the periphery. Allow the area to dry before performing the puncture.

Remove the needle cover and inspect the needle tip for burrs. Put tension on the skin 1 to 2 inches below the puncture site with your thumb. This tension helps prevent the vein from rolling and the needle from pulling the skin as it goes in. Insert the needle into the skin at a 20- to 30-degree angle to the arm, with the needle bevel up (Fig. 15-4, *E*).

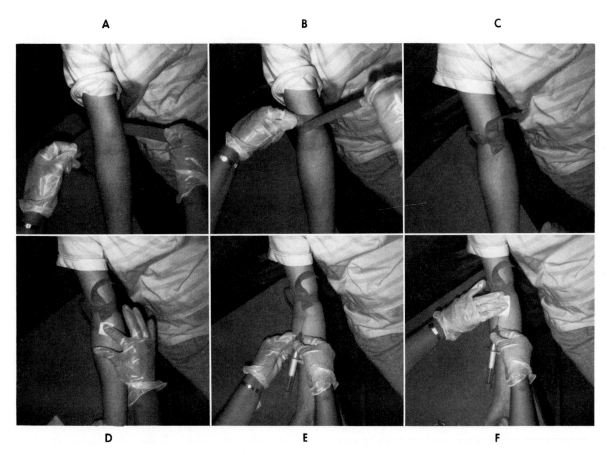

Fig. 15-4   **A,** Wrap tourniquet around arm. **B,** Pull one end taut while holding other in place. **C,** Loop opposite end under taut end to form slip knot. **D,** Cleanse puncture site with 70% isopropyl alcohol, using circular motion. **E,** Insert EBCS needle into skin at 20- to 30-degree angle to arm with needle bevel up. **F,** As you remove needle, place pressure on site.

The puncture should be made in a single smooth motion. As soon as the needle is in place, push the tube as far as it will go into the tube holder. Ensure that the needle does not move as the tube is pushed in.

Tubes containing additives or anticoagulants should be gently inverted and mixed several times as soon as they are taken out of the tube holder. Vigorous mixing may cause hemolysis.

When multiple tubes are to be drawn, the following sequence is recommended:
1. Blood cultures
2. Red-topped clot tubes
3. Blue-topped coagulation tubes
4. Purple-topped hematology tubes

Blood may fail to enter the tube for several reasons, including the following:
1. The vacuum has collapsed the vein. A syringe may then be used.
2. The needle has gone through the vein. Retract the needle slowly until blood enters the tube.
3. The vein has been missed. Try again.
4. The tube has lost its vacuum. Insert another tube.

If you miss the vein, do not attempt any more than a total of two punctures. If you are unable to obtain the specimen, be sure to notify the appropriate person.

Release the tourniquet.

Place dry gauze over the puncture site. As you remove the needle, place pressure on the site (Fig. 15-4, *F*). Pressure should be maintained for at least 5 minutes by the patient. For patients receiving anticoagulant therapy, maintaining pressure for as long as 20 minutes may be necessary. Place pressure tape over the gauze to form a dressing.

Label all the tubes drawn. Minimum labeling includes the following: (1) patient name, last and first; (2) date and time drawn; and (3) collector's initials. The best specimen is of no value, and is potentially dangerous, if it is not correctly labeled.

Properly dispose of your gloves and wash your hands after drawing blood from each patient. Be sure to properly dispose of all equipment before leaving the room.

Thank the patient.

The venipuncture technique for using a nonevacuated system is the same as for the EBCS. When preparing your equipment, be sure the needle is securely attached to the syringe to prevent the needle from being detached. When pulling the syringe plunger back, take care not to put excessive pressure on the vein. Excessive pressure can cause vein collapse and specimen hemolysis.

After the syringe needle is withdrawn, quickly transfer the specimen to the appropriate tubes. Be sure to remove the needle from the syringe and the stoppers from the tubes. Gently depress the plunger and allow the blood to flow down the sides of the tubes, which helps prevent hemolysis of the specimen. Replace stoppers on the tubes, label the specimens, and transfer them to the laboratory.

Remember the following guidelines, during venous collection:
1. Always wear disposable gloves when handling any laboratory specimen.
2. Do not draw from an area proximal to an IV site.
3. Be sure that the tubes are filled correctly. Incompletely filled tubes can affect results. Tubes with liquid additives such as sodium citrate must have the correct amount of blood to maintain the blood : additive ratio around which testing is structured. The blood : additive ratio of 9 : 1 is especially critical in coagulation testing.
4. Always label the tubes *after* drawing from the patient. *Never* prelabel tubes.
5. Check for diet restrictions (for example, should the patient be fasting before the test?).

Capillary Collection

Specimen collection from infants and small children is best performed by a capillary draw. In children younger than 1 year of age, the heel or great toe is generally used. The ring finger of the nondominant hand is preferred for performing capillary draws on children and adults.

Equipment. Equipment for capillary collection includes the following:

Capillary collection system

Lancet (should not allow for a penetration of greater than 2.4 mm, to help prevent puncture of the calcaneus bone)

Disposable gloves

Isopropyl alcohol wipes

Dry gauze pads

Procedure. Select the puncture site. Fig. 15-5 illustrates the foot surfaces that are acceptable for puncture in small children. The use of areas outside those shown in Fig. 15-5 and the use of lancets or surgical blades that allow for a

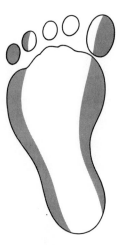

Fig. 15-5 Shaded areas represent areas on infant's foot that are used for obtaining blood specimen.

penetration of greater than 2.4 mm have been reported to cause osteomyelitis and sepsis.

To increase circulation, warm the area for 3 to 5 minutes with a towel or cloth soaked in warm (not hot) water. Clean the area with isopropyl alcohol wipes. Ensure that the area is completely dry before performing the puncture. Avoid using povidone iodine, since it has been shown to affect laboratory test results by falsely elevating potassium, phosphorus, uric acid, and bilirubin levels.

Grasp the heel with a moderately firm grip. Puncture the heel at a slight angle to the surface of skin. The first drop of blood will contain tissue fluids. Wipe this drop away.

Apply moderate pressure. Excessive pressure can cause specimen hemolysis, bruising to the heel, and contamination of the specimen with tissue fluids. Use the capillary collection system to collect the blood.

An adequate puncture produces 0.5 to 1 ml of specimen.

When drawing is completed, apply a dry, clean gauze to the site and maintain pressure until the bleeding has stopped.

The technique for a finger stick is the same as that for the heel stick. Ensure that the stick goes into the pulp of the finger (Fig. 15-6).

Label the specimen containers; then transfer them to the laboratory. Guidelines for capillary specimen collection include the following:

1. Be sure that the area is completely dry before puncturing.
2. Inform laboratory personnel that the specimens are from capillary draws.
3. If a platelet count has been ordered, draw for this test first. Platelets tend to clump, and the count tends to be lower in capillary draws.
4. Take care not to penetrate too deeply when puncturing the fingers of small children. The same problems that may occur with heel punctures may occur with finger punctures.

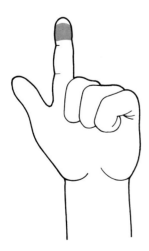

Fig. 15-6   Shaded area represents area commonly used for obtaining blood specimen from fingertip.

Arterial Collection

Arterial blood gas (ABG) values are obtained to assess cardiopulmonary hemostasis. The conditions of many patients received in the ED are such that ED personnel are required to obtain arterial specimens.

Equipment. Equipment used for obtaining arterial specimens includes the following:

5 ml syringe (glass or plastic, specifically designed for obtaining ABG specimens)
21- or 22-gauge needle
Heparin, 1000 U/ml
Isopropyl alcohol wipes
Dry gauze
Pressure dressing
Syringe cap
Disposable gloves
Ice

Procedure. The radial artery is the preferred site for arterial puncture (Fig. 15-7, *A*) because (1) there is collateral blood flow to the hand via the ulnar artery, (2) the vessel is easily accessible for palpation and stabilization, and (3) the surrounding tissues are relatively insensitive.

The second choice of sites for arterial puncture is the brachial artery (Fig. 15-7, *B*). However, this site has no collateral blood flow, the vessel is not as stable as that of the radial artery, and the vessel is in close proximity to the brachial nerve. A third site for arterial puncture is the femoral artery (Fig. 15-7, *C*).

An Allen test is performed to ensure that there is collateral circulation to the hand. Performing an Allen test includes the following steps:

1. Have the patient clench the fist, thereby forcing blood from the area.
2. Place pressure on both arteries, and have the patient open the hand. The opened hand should be blanched.
3. Remove pressure from the ulnar artery: if proper collateral circulation is present, the blanched areas flush within seconds.

The rapid flushing of the hand indicates that the ulnar artery alone is capable of supporting the area's circulatory needs. If the test result is negative (that is, the ulnar artery is not able to support the circulatory needs), an alternate site should be found.

Prepare the equipment by securing the needle to the syringe. Draw up approximately 1 ml of 1000 U/ml heparin to flush the syringe barrel and needle. Expel all excess heparin. The ratio of heparin to blood should be no more than 0.05 to 0.1 ml heparin to 1 ml blood. Excessive heparin alters pH values.

Explain the process of arterial puncture to the patient.

The wrist is hyperextended downward by the patient (Fig. 15-8). This positioning places the artery closer to the surface and stabilizes it.

Palpate the artery to locate the puncture site. Clean the puncture site, using the same technique as for venipuncture.

Amniotic fluid
Pericardial fluid
Peritoneal fluid
Gastric fluid
Spinal fluid

These specimens are usually obtained with a sterile syringe. Specimens to be used for cell counts are placed in tubes containing either EDTA or heparin, which prevents clotting. Fluids for which chemistry testing has been ordered are placed in red-stoppered tubes. Synovial fluid to be used for crystal analysis is placed in tubes containing heparin.

Specimens to be cultured are generally left in the syringe, which is stoppered to ensure anaerobic conditions.

Emesis and gastric specimens are used primarily in toxicologic examinations. When these specimens are submitted, all available information concerning suspected substances should be included with the specimens.

Spinal fluid is submitted for examination in three to five tubes, each tube containing 0.5 to 1 ml of fluid. Tubes are numbered serially as each tube of fluid is obtained. Various facilities and physicians prefer to submit particular tubes for particular tests. In general, tube 1 is used for chemistry analysis, tube 2 for cell counts and differential counts, and tube 3 or 4 for microbiology culture; tube 5 is held for special testing if needed. When difficulty is encountered in obtaining the sample, microbiology testing is generally given priority. Cerebrospinal fluid must always be promptly transported to the laboratory for processing.

Amniotic fluid must be protected from light immediately when the sample is obtained and during transport to the laboratory. This protection from light prevents the breakdown of any bilirubin in the specimen before analysis.

All body fluid specimens should be properly labeled and placed in transport bags, which prevent spillage. Delay in transport to the laboratory results in the deterioration of specimen quality.

Stool Specimens

Fresh, warm stool is preferred for culture. Place a small amount from a bedpan into a dry sterile container, taking care not to contaminate the sample with urine.

Specimens for parasitologic examination should be submitted as soon as possible. Unpreserved specimens must be examined within 1 hour to prevent the death of trophozoites. Therapy should be withheld until specimens have been obtained. Specimens may be preserved for later examination by dividing the specimen into three portions. One is left unpreserved, one is mixed with polyvinyl alcohol (PVA), and the third is mixed with 10% formalin. Generally samples are obtained on 3 consecutive days.

Microbiology Specimens

Specimens for culture are submitted as soon as possible after collection on transport media. Microbiology specimens are divided into aerobic and anaerobic types. Aerobic spec-

imens are obtained when the organism to be identified may be grown in the presence of oxygen. Examples of aerobes are the bacteria *Streptococcus* and *Staphylococcus*. Anaerobic specimens are obtained when the organism to be identified requires a lack of oxygen to grow. Examples of pathogenic anaerobes are the clostridia species, which may cause gangrene or botulism.

Various swabs with transport media are available commercially for both aerobic and anaerobic cultures. Specimens that may contain anaerobic pathogens should be submitted quickly and in the correct transport medium. The swabs should be properly labeled with the patient's name, the date and time of collection, the specimen source, and any antibiotic therapy the patient is receiving at that time.

When rapid monoclonal antibody testing for strep throat is available, two throat swabs should be submitted. One is for confirmatory culture, and the other is for rapid testing.

GUIDE TO SELECTED LABORATORY RESULTS

Laboratory results are assessed using normal values, which represent a range of values for a given test or result. This range is usually plus or minus 2 standard deviations from the mean result for a representative, healthy population. Most health care facilities determine and publish the ranges of normal values for the given area and population they serve. The normal ranges included in this discussion are generally accepted values. The values for a specific facility must be used in the assessment of specific results. When assessing values for pediatric and geriatric patients, be sure to refer to tables of normal values that are specific to these patients.

Arterial Blood Gas Values

The results usually reported in tests of blood gases are a combination of measured values and calculated values. Generally the pH, P_{CO_2}, and the P_{O_2} values are measured, whereas the other values of HCO_3, TCO_2, O_2 saturation, and base excess are calculated. Normal values are given in the box below.

The assessment of ABG test results is usually a two-step process. First, the acid-base status is determined. Second, the oxygen status is determined based on the patient's test results.

Table 15-2 provides useful assessments of ABG test results.

NORMAL ARTERIAL BLOOD GAS VALUES

pH: 7.35 to 7.45
P_{CO_2}: 35 to 45 mm Hg
P_{O_2}: >80 mmHg
HCO_3: 22 to 28 mEq/L

Table 15-2   Assessment of arterial blood gas values

Condition	pH	PCO_2	HCO_3
Acute metabolic acidosis	<7.30	<30	Depressed
Chronic metabolic acidosis	Normal	Depressed	Depressed
Acute respiratory acidosis	<7.30	>50	Normal
Chronic respiratory acidosis	Normal	>50	Elevated
Acute metabolic alkalosis	>7.50	Elevated	Elevated
Chronic metabolic alkalosis	Normal	>50	Elevated
Acute respiratory alkalosis	>7.50	<30	Normal
Chronic respiratory alkalosis	Normal	<30	Depressed

Table 15-3   Normal ranges of electrolyte values

Electrolyte	Serum	Urine
Sodium (Na)	136 to 142 mEq/L	80 to 180 mEq/24 hours
Potassium (K)	3.8 to 5.0 mEq/L	40 to 80 mEq/24 hours
Chloride (Cl)	93 to 105 mEq/L	110 to 250 mEq/24 hours
Carbon dioxide (CO_2)	24 to 30 mM/L	—
Magnesium (Mg)	1.8 to 3.0 mg/100 ml	6.0 to 8.5 mEq/24 hours
Calcium (Ca)	8.5 to 10.5 mg/100 ml	100 to 250 mg/24 hours

Common causes of changes in acid-base status include the following:

Metabolic acidosis

Renal failure

Ketoacidosis (for example, diabetes or starvation)

Lactic acidosis (for example, cardiopulmonary collapse or hepatic disease)

Metabolic alkalosis

Extended IV therapy

Diuretics

Diarrhea

Gastric suction or vomiting

Steroid therapy

Excessive use of $NaHCO_3$ (for example, during or after cardiopulmonary resuscitation [CPR])

Respiratory acidosis

The body's inability to move CO_2 out of the body as quickly as the metabolism produces it. The situation may be either acute or chronic (for example, chronic obstructive pulmonary disease).

Respiratory alkalosis

Central nervous system trauma

Central nervous system infection

Carbon monoxide poisoning

Anemia

Anxiety or psychosis

Pain

Hyperventilation

Electrolytes

Body fluid is composed primarily of water and dissolved substances, usually referred to as electrolytes. Electrolytes may have either a positive charge (cation) or a negative charge (anion). Normally these charges are found in equal, or balanced, concentrations, which are expressed in milliequivalents per liter (mEq/L).

Electrolytes and the normal ranges of laboratory values used to assess electrolyte balance are given in Table 15-3. Causes of electrolyte imbalance and the relative value changes that occur include the following:

Extracellular fluid volume deficit is caused by decreased water intake, diarrhea, vomiting, intestinal obstruction, or infection. Changes include the following:
1. Decreased values
   Electrolytes
   Ca
   Mg
   Proteins
2. Increased values
   Hematocrit
   Hemoglobin
   Red blood cell count

Extracellular fluid volume excess is caused by congestive heart failure, renal disease, or treatment with adrenal cortical hormones. Changes include the following:
1. Decreased values
   Hematocrit
   Hemoglobin
   Red blood cell count
2. Increased values
   Electrolytes
   Ca
   Mg

Sodium deficit (hyponatremia) is caused by excessive sweating or excessive intake of plain water, treatment with diuretics, or adrenal insufficiency. Changes include the following:

Na < 137 mEq/L

Cl < 98 mEq/L

Specific gravity < 1.010

Cl + HCO_3 < 123 mEq/L

Sodium excess (hypernatremia) occurs with diarrhea, decreased water intake, intake of seawater, impaired renal function, febrile illness, or inability to swallow. Changes include the following:

Na > 147 mEq/L

Cl > 106 mEq/L

Specific gravity > 1.030

Potassium deficit (hypokalemia) is caused by diarrhea, vomiting, treatment with diuretics, burns (after 3 days), heat stress, ulcerative colitis, potassium-free IV therapy, or recovery of diabetic ketoacidosis. Changes include the following:

K < 3.5 mEq/L

Potassium excess (hyperkalemia) occurs with renal disease, excessive potassium IV therapy, crushing injuries, early burns, or adrenal insufficiency. Changes include the following:

K > 5.6 mEq/L

Complete Blood Cell Count

The complete blood cell count (CBC) is generally used to determine the hematologic status of a patient. Historically a CBC has been reported in two portions, the cell count and the differential count. With the advent of electronic particle counters, this method of reporting has changed. The relative speed of result determination has been enhanced. Instead of reporting a manual differential count, many cell counters are now able to provide an automated differential count with the cell count.

Only when the automated cell counter indicates an abnormal result is it necessary to perform a manual differential count and examination of the stained blood smear. The determination of what constitutes an abnormal result should be defined at the specific facility.

The basic CBC components are listed in Table 15-4.

The stained blood smear, or differential count, is used for the following purposes:

1. To study red blood cell morphology
2. To evaluate blood parasites such as malaria
3. To determine the percentage distribution of leukocytes in the specimen
4. To study such variations in white blood cell morphology as inclusion bodies and the presence of atypical cells

Urinalysis

Urine is composed of approximately 95% water and 5% solutes. Solutes normally found in the urine include nitrogenous wastes, including creatinine, uric acid, and urea, electrolytes, and pigments, which are derived from bile.

A urinalysis is used to test for the presence of abnormal constituents. In the urinalysis of normal urine the results of tests for these constituents are negative. Abnormal constituents include the following:

1. Protein, primarily albumin, which may indicate the presence of glomerulonephritis
2. Glucose, which indicates the presence of excessive amounts of glucose in the blood, possibly caused by insulin deficiency, severe stress, or renal disease
3. White blood cells, which are evidence of infection
4. Red blood cells, which may be present in cases of inflammation or renal trauma or after catheterization
5. Ketones, which may be present when fats are being incompletely oxidized, such as with starvation or diabetes

The urinalysis further includes tests for pH, specific gravity, color, and appearance, and in some cases includes a microscopic examination of urine sediment. Many of the screening tests available today are reliable enough that when

Table 15-4   Components of complete blood cell count

Component	Normal values	Comments
White blood cell count	5 to 10,000/mm^3	

Red blood cell count	Male
	    4.6 to 6.2 mil/mm^3
	Female
	    4.2 to 5.4 mil/mm^3	

Hemoglobin level	Male
	    14 to 18 g/100 ml
	Female
	    12 to 16 g/100 ml
		A conjugated protein responsible for oxygen and CO_2 transport in the blood

Hematocrit	Male
	    40% to 54%
	Female
	    37% to 47%
		Percentage (volume) of red blood cells in a volume of blood, generally equal to the hemoglobin level × 3 ± 2

Mean corpuscular volume (MCV)	82 to 92 μm^3	Average volume of red blood cells in a sample
Mean corpuscular hemoglobin (MCH) content	27 to 37 μg	Average hemoglobin content of red blood cells in a sample
Mean corpuscular hemoglobin concentration (MCHC)	32% to 36%	Average hemoglobin content in 100 ml of blood
Platelets	150,000 to 400,000/μL	Platelets aid in hemostasis and maintenance of vascular integrity

results of these tests are negative, the microscopic examination of the urine sediment is unnecessary.

The most commonly used form of urine testing is the reagent strip or dipstick. Each strip contains pads that show reactions to specific components in the urine. The strips provide a color reaction that can be compared with standards either visually or through the use of an automated strip reader. The combinations of testing pads on the strips are easy to use. To prevent false readings, always follow the written instructions and heed the stated precautions.

SUGGESTED READINGS

Bauer John: *Clinical laboratory methods,* ed 9, St Louis, 1982, Mosby–Year Book.

Chapman F: Eastern Maine Medical Center Laboratory in-service handout, Bangor, Me, November, 1978.

Davidson I and Henry J, eds: *Todd and Sanford: Clinical diagnosis by laboratory methods,* ed 15, Philadelphia, 1974, WB Saunders.

Memmler R and Wood D: *The human body in health and disease,* ed 6, Philadelphia, 1987, JB Lippincott.

Metheny N and Snively WD: *Nurses' handbook of fluid balance,* ed 2, Philadelphia, 1974, JB Lippincott.

Pendergraph G: *Handbook of phlebotomy,* Philadelphia, 1984, Lea & Febiger Co.

Shapiro B, Harrison R, and Walton J: *Clinical application of blood gases,* ed 2, Chicago, 1977, Mosby–Year Book.

Quality Assurance and Risk Management

Linda C. Carl

The purpose of this chapter is to define the scope of quality assurance data collection as it relates to risk management in the emergency department (ED).

With the advent of the recommendations of the Joint Commission on Accreditation of Health Care Organizations (JCAHO) that nurses be able to demonstrate their impact on patient outcome, quality assurance as it relates to risk management has become one entity comprising the accumulation of data, the analysis of data, and the collection of outcome information. To close the loop on quality assurance, that is, to determine whether or not change is necessary to improve patient outcomes, correlation of risk management outcome data with nursing standards of practice and hospital policies and procedures is also necessary.

Information flows into risk loss prevention programs, which benefit the nurse and hospital by decreasing risk loss potential. Dollars are saved and care is improved.

Through the implementation of selected nursing actions the hospital extends quality assurance beyond the traditional data collection and renders specific outcome information that changes patient care by identifying the potential for problems before they are evident in clinical practice.

There have been major changes in the JCAHO standards for nursing services. Specific quality assurance programs must be operational in order to receive accreditation.

The *Accreditation Manual For Hospitals* offers minimal requirements regarding quality assurance. For example, a copy of the ED record is available to whomever the patient sees for follow-up care. According to Whitcomb and others,[11] radiographs and the results of laboratory tests and electrocardiograms (EKGs), reviewed and including official interpretations, are made available to the follow-up party. Mistaken preliminary interpretations of results are rectified through some mechanism of patient call-back. A daily review of documentation and care given in the ED is assessed based on a representative sample. Particular attention is paid to patients transferred elsewhere such as patients receiving blood or antibiotics in the ED or patients having surgical specimens collected in the ED. Transfer of patients is accomplished safely and in accordance with a written transfer

protocol. The use of blood and antibiotics is open to review by committees that scrutinize modalities of care throughout the hospital. Surgical specimens removed from the patient, except specimens given directly to law enforcement officers for legal reasons, are sent to a pathologist.

Dedication and commitment to a process of identifying deficiencies and taking action based on the results of monitoring is accomplished when the JCAHO standards are used; these are the most basic standards necessary to the practice of safe, appropriate patient care in the emergency milieu.

The Joint Commission indicates that health care providers should monitor, assess, document, and improve patient care.[6] According to Whitcomb and others, monitoring implies the need to create a system of watchful alertness that can capture potential deficiencies.[11] The intent is to identify deficiencies rather than wait until they present themselves. Anticipation of problems through astute data collection and identification is intended to prospectively prevent poor patient outcomes.

For example, telephone follow-ups within 24 hours of discharge from the ED are documented and evaluated in relation to patient outcomes. Patient complaints and feedback are provided by a staff evaluator. Analysis of follow-up care in relation to outcome is based on the JCAHO accredited level of emergency services of the specific institution, as well as the designated level of trauma centers and neonatal and pediatric services.

Tracking by telephone follow-up is one way to demonstrate that nursing care positively affects patient outcomes. Valid nursing patient outcome studies are the modus operandi in the emergency patient care setting for the 1990s.

The JCAHO addresses the application of quality improvement interventions in the hospital such as successfully involving nurses in all aspects of quality assurance.[6] Data management and risk management are imperative components in the delivery of quality assurance and quality care. When monitoring and evaluation are the foundation of an integrated quality assurance program and are coupled with utilization review and sound risk management, data collection promotes establishment and application thresholds for evaluation; these thresholds are a critical component of emergency nursing care. Traditional and nontraditional sources of data collection display data in a meaningful manner; data application becomes an agenda for change in identified clinical indicators.

To maintain a successful quality assurance and risk management program, the hospital must commit dollars and resources: a quality assurance nurse and a risk manager are essential to the task of gathering the data that must be collected in the ED.

As an essential facilitator the nurse manager is actively involved in both quality assurance and risk management; in this way the loop is closed between the two disciplines that are necessary to effect change. The manager is responsible for flowing information from the risk management and quality assurance department back to the clinical staff so that nursing intervention and actions change based on the promulgation of adequate ED policies and procedures and the revision of existing nursing standards of care. The revisions are made based on outcome data derived from each clinical study. After data are collected and compared to patient outcome, problem identification is factored by the pivotal agent for change, the nurse manager.

According to Albaros and others,[1] quality assurance is an issue that all nurse managers must consider so that optimal health care delivery is provided to every patient. A quality assurance program systematically provides data collection, assessment, and evaluation of care based on outcome; the program is accomplished by using a reliable data analysis collection method to evaluate the quality of nursing care.

The assessment of outcome focuses on how the patient responds to the nursing care rendered and on the outcome of care as it relates to the nursing action. Policies, procedures, and nursing standards of care create the platform from which nurses function in the ED setting so that nursing action and intervention can be evaluated. The predetermined criteria are consistent with the goals of the institution and based on the type of care being delivered to a specific patient population in each ED. Criteria statements reflect specific outcomes and represent optimal levels of care that are achieved within a reasonable period. The care rendered is evaluated based on whether confirmation to criteria exists.

Once a deficiency is identified and actions are changed, reevaluation of the process takes place to determine whether outcomes change as predicted. The nurse manager ascertains that observations are factual, accurate, and relevant to the patient care indicator being evaluated. Although in most instances quality assurance and risk management information cannot be obtained by opposing counsel in malpractice litigation, nurses should collect and analyze data and write outcome measures with the guiding assumption in mind that the data will be obtained by opposing counsel. Be certain that what you write is what you mean and that it relates to written nursing standards of care and complies with hospital policy.

According to Marianne Shanahan[9] the processes of care and practitioner performance are evaluated indirectly when patient outcomes at discharge from the hospital are measured retrospectively. In the ED, nursing performance in all areas of care is screened continuously so that performance complies with the standard of care required of the hospital and nurse.

According to Spath and others,[10] from a marketing perspective the image of the ED reaches many potential patients, all of whom offer the possibility of future business should their initial experience prove satisfactory. Annual visits to the ED are made by an estimated one third of the total population of the hospital's market share area. High-quality patient care in the ED points out the need for a comprehensive quality assurance and risk management program. Although a happiness index is not considered valid data in the ED, it is critical to elicit the consumer's perception of the hospital. Assessments of patient satisfaction with care rendered by the health care team are valid indicators of quality of care when combined with patient outcome data.

IDENTIFYING SCOPE OF PRACTICE

The first step in merging quality assurance and risk management is to identify the scope of services rendered in the ED in comparison to patient population.

Spath and others[10] recommend that the ED health care provider develop a scope of services statement that evaluates the health needs of the ED patient; defines the patient population most frequently seen within the institution; differentiates between stable and life-threatening conditions; defines the provision of emergency services; lists the provision for definitive care for patients not requiring emergency care; and evaluates follow-up instructions for patients discharged from the department. An example of an ED quality assurance statement is given in the box on p. 225.

The scope of service becomes the foundation for development of a precise measure of quality indicators. Patients who present a high risk of liability exposure to the institution or patient care management problems are promptly identified. Analysis and staff input will help identify patient outcome data that reflect deficiencies in care.

In 1988 the Emergency Nurses Association Board of Directors approved a definition for the emergency nursing scope of practice that forms the basis for every ED in the United States. The following is an excerpt from the scope of practice definition[4a]:

The scope of emergency nursing practice involves the assessment, diagnosis, treatment and evaluation of perceived, actual or potential, sudden or urgent, physical and psychosocial problems that are primarily episodic or acute and which occur in a variety of settings. These may require minimal care or life-support measures, patient and significant other education, appropriate referral, and knowledge of legal implications.

Emergency patients are people of all ages with diagnosed, un-

EMERGENCY DEPARTMENT QUALITY ASSURANCE STATEMENT

Purpose To evaluate and ensure optimal patient care
Policy
1. Each member of the ED team has his or her own personal copy of a current, updated manual for reference.
2. Data base sheets are evaluated on selected patients, and an evaluation form is sent to each nurse participant and to the quality assurance nurse for data compilation. Data are then sent to the risk manager.
3. There is an annual performance review; information is kept in each nurse's personnel file, and each nurse plans yearly goals and evaluates his or her performance based on patient outcomes.
4. ED cases are presented and reviewed routinely at mortality and morbidity meetings. Nurse attendance is required.
5. Clinical studies are performed by the quality assurance department using a computer data storage and retrieval system. Outcomes are presented to the risk manager, and policy changes are implemented.

diagnosed or misdiagnosed problems of varying complexity. Emergency nurses also interact with and care for families, communities and potential consumers.

Emergency nursing occurs in various health care settings (primary, secondary, tertiary) and exists whenever and wherever an emergency patient and an emergency nurse interact. The practice of Emergency Nursing also includes the delivery of care to consumers through education, research and consultation. Emergency nursing practice can occur in hospital emergency departments; prehospital and military settings; clinics, health maintenance organizations, and ambulatory services; business, educational, industrial, and correctional institutions; and other health care environments. Emergency care is also delivered where the consumer lives, works, plays, and goes to school.

Emergency nursing is multidimensional. The dimensions of Emergency Nursing include the responsibilities, functions, roles, and skills that involve a specific body of knowledge. These dimensions are manifest through emergency nursing characteristics, roles, processes, and behaviors.

Characteristics unique to emergency nursing practice include the following:
1. assessment, diagnosis and treatment of emergent, urgent and non-urgent individuals of all ages, often with a limited patient data base
2. triage and prioritization
3. disaster preparedness
4. stabilization and resuscitation
5. crisis intervention for unique patient populations, such as sexual assault survivors
6. provision of care in uncontrolled or unpredictable environments.

Other characteristics unique to emergency nursing environments include unplanned situations requiring intervention, allocation of limited resources, need for immediate care as perceived by the patient/others, and contextual factors. Contextual factors are the variety of geographic settings, unpredictable numbers of patients, and unknown patient variables which include severity, urgency, and diagnosis.

Nursing roles include those of patient care, research, administration/management, education, consultation and advocacy. The specialty practice of emergency nursing is defined through the implementation of specific role functions which are delineated in documents such as the "Emergency Nursing Core Curriculum", the "Standards of Emergency Nursing Practice" and the Trauma Nursing Core Course.

Emergency nursing practice is systematic in nature and includes nursing process, decision making, analytical and scientific thinking, inquiry, and triage.

Professional behaviors inherent in emergency nursing practice are the acquisition and application of a specialized body of knowledge and skills, accountability and responsibility, communication, autonomy, and collaborative relationships with others. Certification in Emergency Nursing, as recognized by ENA, validates the defined body of knowledge for emergency nursing practice.

The scope of emergency nursing practice is bounded both externally and internally. The external boundaries include legislation/regulation, societal demands for expedient quality emergency care, economic climate, and health care delivery trends. Individual State Nurse Practice Acts which define nursing are an example of legal boundaries used to provide the basis for interpretation of the safe practice of nursing. As well, rules and regulations which evolve from these acts are used as guidelines by state boards of nursing to issue licenses and ensure the public safety.

Examples of the legislative/regulatory factors unique to emergency nursing include the Emergency Medical Services Systems (EMSS) Act, the Joint Commission for Accreditation of Healthcare Organizations (JCAHO) regulations for Emergency Services/Ambulatory Care, and mandated reporting requirements. Health care delivery trends, such as an increase in the number of ambulatory care centers and patient participation in Health Maintenance Organizations (HMOs) and Preferred Provider Organizations (PPOs) influence the demand for emergency nursing services.

The internal boundaries include those forces which fall within the practice of professional nursing. Specific internal boundaries include the ANA guidelines for practice such as the Social Policy Statement, quality assurance monitoring activities, and institutional and departmental policies and procedures.

Boundaries are dynamic rather than static. Changes within the external boundaries may be the driving forces which necessitate changes to the internal boundaries.

Within the internal environment, the "Standards of Emergency Nursing Practice," ENA Position Statements, the "Code of Ethics for Emergency Nurses Core Curriculum" and the Trauma Nursing Core Course define boundaries unique to Emergency Nursing practice.

The practice of Emergency Nursing intersects with a variety of professional and governmental groups outside the domain of nursing such as related health organizations, medicine, allied health, and prehospital care providers. Emergency nursing intersects with other professional groups within the domain of nursing such as the American Nurses Association (ANA), the National Federation of Specialty Nursing Organizations (NFSNO) and other nursing specialties. Intersection is not limited to these groups however, and may occur with any group as appropriate.

At these intersections, emergency nurses participate for the common purpose of improving health care through education; administration; consultation; and collaboration in practice, research and policy decisions. Within these roles, emergency nurses communicate, network and share resources, information, research, technology, and expertise. This is done to address common concerns such as bioethical issues, humanism, bio-psychosocial needs of patients, trends, management of patient care, and alternative care modalities.

While health care professions interact with a common overall mission, the unique knowledge, environment, and focus of Emergency Nursing influences the process and outcomes at the intersections. The emergency nurse is a focal point at the crossroads of primary, secondary, and tertiary care, and on the wellness-illness continuum. Based on the broad range of emergency patients, emergency nursing is involved with other groups in a variety of activities such as disaster planning, organ and tissue procurement, injury prevention campaigns, and prehospital care.

CLINICAL CARE EVALUATION

After the scope of services has been identified, data collection is accomplished in two ways. The simplest way is to collect data retrospectively, that is, to examine patient care forms, logs, and charts that were kept before the date of the study. Tracking patient care back as far as the nurse chooses enables astute analysis of past patient outcomes. This methodology is effective for implementing change after the fact; the drawback is that problem identification occurs after the problem has surfaced.

The preferable methodology in risk management is called the prospective study. Concurrent analysis of patient care identifies the potential for a problem, which allows prevention and improves trends in patient care.

According to Whitcomb and others[11] the distinction is important between the prospective protocol, which directs the actions of the provider, and the retrospective criteria map, which reviews the recorded action. Cases can be reviewed and deficiencies corrected. If quality assessment is to provide meaningful results, it must accurately reflect the nursing care process. As Whitcomb and others[11] suggest, criteria mapping by tracking improves evaluation of care.

Data collection begins by evaluating existing assessment tools (Table 16-1). The patient care record determines whether data are readily gleaned from the ED. The patient assessment sheet addresses head-to-toe assessment in a check-off form so that when data are collected they are easily obtainable. At the same time, a check-off sheet for the ED nurse creates an almost foolproof nursing assessment by reminding the nurse of what needs to be assessed in the patient care evaluation process. A concise emergency patient data base is the framework on which to build an accurate nursing diagnosis (Fig. 16-1).

The record is a data storage and retrieval system. Often the record is inaccurate, incomplete, and unreliable. To decrease risk loss, the record must be accurate. Therefore, nurses must in every way attempt to "idiot-proof" the medical record so that documentation error is prevented and a document replete with information is created. Such documentation is used to assess, evaluate, and improve patient care.

Often in the ED, little time is available for complete documentation of patient assessment. However, this fact does not excuse the nurse from documenting accurately and completely what patient care is rendered. All EDs need triage criteria, an initial assessment protocol sheet, and a neurologic assessment and trauma assessment format, as well as a format for adding narrative notes if necessary. In that way risk management personnel obtain data based on protocol and notes provided from the direct patient care provider, and these data provide a picture of the clinical care rendered.

Alteration of patient records has a significant influence on jurors in malpractice litigation. The Report of the Secretary's Commission on Medical Malpractice stated that 24% of the attorneys surveyed mentioned the impact of record alterations.[8] In the report the following comment appears:

Surprisingly, about one fourth of plaintiff and defense attorneys mention that evidence of record alteration has a significant influence on jurors. What is surprising is not that record alteration influenced jurors, but that it was mentioned with sufficient frequency as to suggest it is not a rare practice among defendants accused of an act of medical malpractice. However, it is not valid to assume from the fact that 24% of lawyers mentioned record alteration as a factor that influences a jury in a medical malpractice case that record alteration occurs 24% of the time.

According to Hershey and others[5] the patient's chart is invariably introduced as evidence at the trial of a malpractice or negligence suit. The attorney for the plaintiff can seize defects in records and develop inferences that are unfavorable to the nurse defendants. Inadequate, misleading, or deficient documents can prevent the successful defense of a legal action.

The absence of data can be just as condemning as the alteration of records. In each patient assessment, normal and abnormal findings based on specific pathologic conditions are documented. Whenever index of suspicion is factored into patient assessment, normal and abnormal findings are documented completely. For example, this type of documentation is mandatory particularly when children seek medical advice because of persistent flu symptoms, which raise an index of suspicion that developing or smoldering meningitis may be present. The chart becomes especially important when the nurse who had been on duty when the patient's condition changed is not available as a witness at trial.

According to Hershey and others, when the chart is devoid

Table 16-1   Guidelines for head-to-toe patient examination

Body region	Assessment	Components of assessment
Entire body	Identify race, sex, age, history, risk factors	
	Observe physical appearance, emotional appearance; document base line	General state of health, facial expression, mood, speech, memory, skin color, body development, nutritional state
	Obtain vital signs; document triage and baseline if normal; repeat every half hour	Respiratory rate, rhythm, chest excursion, heart rate, rhythm, blood pressure (both arms) flat sitting, temperature
	Obtain height and weight; document	
Head	Level of consciousness	Glasgow coma scale
		Repeat every hour
	Examine scalp and face	Symmetry, size, contour of skull, skin color, lesions, periorbital edema, masses, abnormal hair growth, scaliness, lumps, parasites
	Facial sensory response	Light touch; pain and vibration
	Examine eyes	Pupil reaction: equal, round, react to light; accommodation, conjugate gaze, redness or jaundice, visual acuity
	Examine ears	Size, shape, and presence of deformities, lumps, lesions, nodules; drainage or pain on manipulation, tinnitus, hearing balance, equilibrium
	Examine nose	Deformity, symmetry, inflammation, drainage, epistaxis, sneezing, obstruction, absence of nares hair
	Examine lips	Color, hydration, lumps, ulcerations, symmetry of smile, frown
	Examine oral cavity	Color, movement, symmetry, ulcers, dentition
	Reflexes	Gag (swallowing), corneal (blink), sensory, movement
Neck	Inspect	Symmetry, skin conditions
	Palpate	Carotid pulses, thrills, bruits, murmurs, trachea midline, cervical spine tenderness
Chest	Inspect and palpate	Skin color, rashes, lesions, crepitus, tenderness of vertebral spine, tenderness of costovertebral areas, deformities, symmetry
	Observe, percuss, auscultate	Chest excursion, lung fields, breath sounds
	Inspect, palpate, auscultate	Precordial area: apical pulse (compare to radial pulse) rate and rhythm, physiologic splitting, S1-2 abnormal intensity splitting S3-4, murmurs, thrills, rubs, heaves
Back	Log roll, inspect for abnormalities	
Abdomen	Inspect	Color, lesions, scars, rashes, contour, herniation, drainage, distention
	Auscultate	Bowel sounds, bruits, murmurs
	Percuss	Tympany throughout, comparison of solids, fluids, gas
	Palpate	Soft, firm, rebound, tenderness, temperature, masses
Genitalia	Inspect	Size, shape, opening, edema, drainage, masses, hernia, parasites, lesions, drainage
Rectum	Inspect	Lesions, fissures, hemorrhoids, sphincter tone, tenderness
Extremities	Inspect	Deformities, color, lesions, hair patterns, swelling, pulses, turgor, tenderness, texture
	Palpate	Tenderness, motion, turgor, pulses, stiffness, assess motor strength, skeletal configuration

Documentation: The key to determining deteriorating trends is constant documentation of normal and abnormal findings.

of specific information, even when the testimony of the nurse describes the situation, the nurse's testimony may not be given credence by the court if the documentation is absent from the medical record.[5] No absolute rules have been established for distinguishing the data important enough for notation; however, to decrease risk loss potential, a complete head-to-toe assessment of normal and abnormal findings and a complete history of every patient who enters the ED is advisable. The information supports a sound risk management program and serves to refresh the nurse's memory if he or she becomes a party to litigation. The entire process requires documentation and record keeping so that data and

Prehospital report

Patient name _____ Age _____ Patient number _____

Hospital number _____ Incident location _____ Time _____ Date _____

Medic unit _____ Base station _____ Mode of transportation _____

Incident description _____

_____

Mechanism of injury _____

_____

Team	Notified	Responded	Arrived
Trauma surgeon			
Neurosurgeon			
Trauma nurse			
Critical care nurse			
Anesthesia			
Nursing supervisor			
Respiratory therapist			
Other response called			

Patient history _____ Allergies _____

_____

_____

_____ Weight _____

Psychosocial _____ Height _____

Family contact name _____ Phone number _____

Other   Time summary

Family notified _____

Notified by _____ Time and date _____ ED OUT _____

Admit to room _____ Time _____ CT completed _____

Transfer to _____ Time _____ Radiology completed _____

Disposition of valuables or

property to _____ To or time _____

Signature of recipient _____ Subspecialist notified _____

Fig. 16-1 Emergency patient data base.

information are compared to past data. Quality assurance combined with risk management is a way to discover and solve problems that have occurred and problems that could occur in the future, as well as a way to minimize economic loss and decrease mortality and morbidity.

In addition to retrospective and prospective data collection obtained from accurate and precise documentation, the other quality assurance components that must be evaluated are occurrence screening and random case review, according to Murphy and Jacobson.[7] A formal problem identification mechanism is developed; the most important feature of the monitoring system is the physician and nurse involvement at both the management and staff level.

Without a coordinated approach to quality assurance and risk management, the program is scattered at best. The program works effectively only if the physicians, nurses, management staff, and direct patient caregivers participate in the program.

According to Spath and Miller[10] the main activities that are mandatory for a sound quality assurance program are (1) clinical care monitors of important aspects of care or services, (2) occurrence screening (Fig. 16-2), to identify possible problem areas, (3) random care review, to identify possible problem areas and increase the individual nurse

involvement in case review, and (4) education opportunities. The guidelines presented in Table 16-1 assist the nurse in the process of patient evaluation. An initial assessment is performed in the triage area; then a comprehensive examination is completed in the ED. A formal mechanism for obtaining input from the staff to identify possible problem areas is mandatory. The boxes on pp. 230 and 231 provide examples of quality assurance mechanisms.

Hospital risk management programs came into being in the 1970s in response to the escalating malpractice crisis. As a result, one of the internal programs implemented by the hospital to improve patient care and decrease risk liability was incident or occurrence reporting. Incident or occurrence reporting is mandatory to the implementation of an effective quality assurance and risk management program. Although in most instances the report cannot be obtained by opposite counsel in malpractice litigation, the document at times has been obtained. Although the document may not be introduced into court, the information on the document may be used by opposing counsel to discredit emergency nursing care. Therefore, all information is placed in incident or occurrence reports with the knowledge that the document may be read by opposing counsel. Be certain that any information included in the report is also placed

	NO	YES
I. Surgical case indicators	—	—
A. Penetrating wound of abdomen, lower chest, back, perineum		
1. Perforated viscus	—	—
2. History	—	—
a. Gunshot wound		
b. Stab wound with exposure of visvera or leakage of gastrointestinal contents from wound	—	—
c. Stab wound with abdominal tenderness and positive paracentesis or peritoneal lavage of free air	—	—
d. Injury to urinary tract demonstrated by radiologic examination	—	—
B. Blunt trauma of abdomen, lower chest, back, or pelvis	—	—
1. Ruptured viscus	—	—
2. History		
a. Injury with abdominal tenderness and abdominal paracentesis	—	—
b. Lavage of free air determined by radiologic examination	—	—
c. Injury of urinary tract demonstrated by radiologic examination	—	—
C. Massive abdominal bleeding	—	—
1. History of injury with resistant hypotension	—	—
2. Injury of spleen, liver, kidney as demonstrated by radiologic examination	—	—
a. Ruptured viscus	—	—
b. Perforated viscus	—	—
II. Postoperative complications	—	—
A. Intraperitoneal sepsis		
B. Intraperitoneal hemorrhage	—	—
C. Obstruction	—	—
D. Prolonged ileus	—	—
E. Fistula	—	—
F. Pancreatitis	—	—
III. Postoperative validation of diagnosis		
A. Surgeon's reports before and after surgery inconsistent	—	—
B. Pathology report inconsistent	—	—
IV. Discharge status		
A. General criteria not met	—	—

Fig. 16-2   Occurrence screening for case review procedure: abdominal trauma laparotomy.

EMERGENCY NURSING MINIMAL CRITERIA FOR PATIENT TRIAGE

Scope Utilized when patient presents to hospital, to determine entry level into system of care

Purpose To assess the severity of a patient's illness by utilizing anatomic or physiologic considerations as assessment indicators

Policy statement Presence of criteria indicates need to expedite examination by emergency medicine specialist to determine need for referral to subspecialist or tertiary care facility

Text Criteria categories include but are not limited to the following:
1. Abnormal vital signs
2. Extremes of age (0 to 12 or more than 65 years of age)
3. Prolonged extrication
4. Glasgow coma score of 10 or less
5. Champion trauma score of 12 or less
6. Penetrating wounds of the head, neck, chest, abdomen, or groin, no matter what extent they appear
7. Cardiorespiratory abnormalities, even if present by history
8. Infant 2 years of age or less who arrives at the ED with recurrent upper respiratory infection while receiving antibiotics; even absent hyperpyrexia requires septic workup and pediatric referral

MINIMAL CRITERIA FOR NEUROLOGIC PATIENT TRIAGE

Scope All patients with suspected or present neurological deficit (a high index of suspicion should be the rule)

Purpose To define neurosurgical patients and expedite referral to subspecialty

Policy statement The universal Glasgow coma scale will be used to monitor the potential for deteriorating neurological trends indicative of deficit

Text 1. In suspected head and spinal cord trauma the neurosurgeon will be called as part of the team response
   Neurosurgical patients include, but are not limited to, those patients with trauma resulting in:
   — open injury and/or suspected fracture of the skull or spine with or without neurological deficit
   — closed head injury associated with G.C.S. less than 10, posturing or evidence of impaired consciousness or weakness of the extremities
   — open or closed injury to the spinal column associated with or without weakness of the extremities
2. Patients who present with signs and symptoms consistent with cerebral aneurysm in spite of psychiatric history will be treated as a surgical emergency until worked up and seen by a neurosurgeon
3. Age 0-12 presenting with neurological sequelae of any degree or etiology require neurosurgical consultation

Quality assurance monitoring and evaluation activities Year _____					
Date	Monitoring activity	Criteria used	Method for monitoring	Monitored by whom	Frequency

Fig. 16-3 Quality assurance monitor and evaluation activities.

BRAIN DEATH CRITERIA

Brain death criteria An individual with irreversible cessation of all functions of the entire brain, including the brainstem

Policy

1. Cessation is recognized when evaluation discloses the following:
   a. Absent cerebral responsivity and receptivity
   b. Absent brainstem functions
   c. Absent spontaneous respirations, in the face of normal arterial Pco_2 tensions
2. Irreversibility is recognized when evaluation discloses the following:
   a. Cause of coma is established and is sufficient to account for the loss of brain functions
   b. Possibility of recovery of any brain function is excluded
   c. Cessation of all brain function persists for an appropriate period of observation or trial of therapy or both
3. Conditions causing possible unreliability include the following:
   a. Drug intoxication
   b. Metabolic abnormalities
   c. Hypothermia
   d. Shock
   e. Near-drowning
   f. Age of less than 2 months
4. Confirmatory tests include the following:
   a. Isoelectric electroencephalogram, repeated at least every 12 hours (at least after 48 hours if age is less than 2 months, or 24 hours if age less than one year)
   b. Absent cerebral circulation is seen on angiography or isotope blood flow test

somewhere in the medical record. In this way it is less likely that opposing counsel may obtain the report, which is considered strict qualified privilege when the information in the chart is redundant.

Each hospital develops a risk management program that best fits the particular hospital's individual characteristics (Fig. 16-3). The incident report alone does not capture many critical areas that cause medically related incidents. Therefore the report should be expanded to include medically or surgically related patient care modalities. The document is to be nonjudgmental; it serves as a fact report of the occurrence and outcomes. The information is communicated to risk management and quality assurance personnel and is either examined as epidemiologic regarding an entire patient population or type-specific regarding treatment of a subgroup of the patient population seen within an institution. Both examinations provide useful information in trending analysis that demonstrates emerging patterns of unusual numbers of hazards. Integrating information from programs in surrounding hospitals determines whether the standard of care is consistent across geographic boundaries.

CHOOSE A PATIENT POPULATION

Once a clinical evaluation method has been identified, choose a specific patient population to study. Identify patient conditions that are identified by the clinical staff as potentially high-risk and/or high-volume nursing diagnoses. Develop achievable standards of nursing practice, policies, procedures, and protocol for the selected patient population. Define the minimal level of quality expected of the ED nurse; use similar ED within a geographic region as a barometer of expected care. Develop patient management guidelines and treatment protocols, including key information rendering data placed into outcome studies (Fig. 16-4). Arrange criteria into a quality assurance monitoring and multidisciplinary planning plate, and ensure follow-up by selecting the changed nursing action according to the patient's clinical condition. Address the most important aspects of care, and review and assess the outcome with the physicians and staff in a multidisciplinary setting.

When patient care is evaluated in relation to nursing standards of care in the ED, nursing care plans are used as a depository of information. There are many standard and approved care plans for numerous types of emergency patient conditions. The emergency nurse's focus on the minimal standards that have already been developed eliminates any need to "reinvent the wheel" and saves time and effort. Be certain the plan fits the patient.

Preprinted care plans are acceptable, provided that information from the nursing care plan is evaluated retrospectively using data not only from the nursing care plan but also from the emergency room logs, the patient admission sheet, and the medical record. Retrospective evaluation ensures that the plan meets the patient care requirements in your institution. All sources of documentation reflect information consistent with the nursing diagnosis. Certification by the JCAHO no longer requires care plans, provided the plan of care is found somewhere in the nurses' notes. If you choose not to use a format care plan, be sure to include in your notes at least the following: nursing diagnosis, intervention, expected outcomes, and follow-up.

Include the staff nurse in the retrospective review of medical records as part of the continuing educational process. Learning from what is reviewed in the records assists in immediate identification of problem areas. All nurses are held accountable to analyze a portion of cases. Identification of complications and review of patient complaints and abnormal findings are included in the data collection process by the data collector. Data collection and staff education become a cost-effective means of education and problem identification.

Patient _____ Adm/disch date_____

Medical record no. _____ Physician _____

Trauma no. _____

	I. Admission evaluation		3. Leukocytes >500/cu mm
_____	A. Admission criteria	_____	4. Amylase >175 U
_____	1. Physical examination	_____	5. Blood, food, feces, bacteria
_____	2. History	_____	6. All of above
_____	3. Laboratory tests	_____	7. None of above
_____	a. HG, HCT (series of three)	_____	8. More than one
_____	b. Amylase value	_____	C. Surgery
_____	c. Type, crossmatch, screen blood	_____	1. To operating room
_____	d. Alcohol modified	_____	2. Not to operating room
_____	e. ABSAG		IV. Intravenous lines
_____	f. Modified coma panel	_____	A. Two lines initiated PTA
_____	g. Urinalysis	_____	B. One line initiated PTA
_____	4. Radiographs	_____	C. No line initiated PTA
_____	a. Crosstable lateral cervical spine	_____	D. Two lines initiated in ED
_____	b. Anteroposterior CXR	_____	E. One line initiated in ED
_____	5. Two IV lines	_____	F. No line initiated in ED
_____	6. Nasogastric tube	_____	G. Other
_____	7. Foley catheter		V. Computed tomography scan of head
_____	8. Tetanus prophylaxis	_____	A. Indications
_____	9. Antibiotics	_____	1. Low risk
_____	B. Other _____	_____	2. Moderate risk
_____	II. Intubation	_____	3. High risk
_____	A. Indication	_____	4. Extremes of age
_____	1. Extremes of age		VI. Abdominal computerized tomography
_____	2. Cardiopulmonary distress	_____	A. Indications
_____	3. Inability to cooperate	_____	1. Blunt thoracoabdominal trauma
_____	4. Blunt chest trauma	_____	2. Retroperitoneal injury
_____	B. Pavulon use	_____	3. Pelvic fracture
_____	C. None of the above	_____	4. Unreliable response to abdominal examination
_____	III. Peritoneal lavage		
_____	A. Indications	_____	5. Abdominal scarring from previous surgeries
_____	1. History of blunt thoracoabdominal trauma		
_____		_____	6. Pediatric patient
_____	2. Clinical signs of hemorrhage	_____	7. Penetrating injury
_____	3. None of the above	_____	8. Previous DPL (12-24 hours)
_____	4. Repeat lavage		
_____	B. Results		
_____	1. Frank blood aspirated		
_____	2. Erythrocytes >50,000/cu mm		

Quality Assurance Assessment

1. _____ Acceptable for the following: _____

_____

2. _____ Controversial for the following: _____

_____

3. _____ Probably unacceptable for the following: _____

_____

4. _____ Unjustified for the following: _____

_____

Referred to: risk manager   Follow-up: risk manager

Reviewing physician signature: _____

Reviewing nurse signature: _____

Fig. 16-4   Major trauma patient guidelines.

RISK LOSS POTENTIAL

Once the patient population is identified, the risk loss potential is evaluated. The quality assurance process identifies problems, and the risk management process changes actions so that the problems do not occur again (Fig. 16-5). If the staff does not know how frequently a problem occurs, they do not know that it needs correction. It is virtually mandatory that information be given to the clinical staff so that they can be aware of problems and the need for correction. When assessing a problem, evaluate how often the problem occurs and how serious the problem may become; then establish a standard of care or promulgate a new policy or procedure to prevent reoccurrence of the deficiency.

According to Whitcomb and others,[11] unlike generic screening, in which broadly based judgment is applied to randomized diagnoses, standards of care or specific standards apply to a specific diagnosis against which a specific review may be conducted. As each problem is reviewed, an ongoing quality assurance program that systematically reviews problems gradually accumulates standards specific for a particular institution.

In addition, nationwide standards are available for specific problems. The Emergency Nurses Association has a core curriculum and standards of nursing practice that form the basis from which to develop nursing standards of care and policies and procedures specific for each institution and for patient population requirements.

STANDARDS OF EMERGENCY NURSING PRACTICE

The development of standards of care in the ED minimally meets the standards set forth in the Emergency Nurses Association's publication concerning standards of emergency nursing practice. Once the standards have been reviewed, they are streamlined to meet the needs of the patient population seen in each institution.

In addition, the JCAHO *Manual For Hospitals*[6] specifically spells out the minimal standards necessary for ED quality assurance and is used as a map for the development of a program specific to any given institution.[6]

Once standards of practice are complete and the assessment process is refined, the next step is to change behavior based on the results of the study. The plan is complete when monitoring shows that the process has effected change. For example, emergency nursing diagnosis requires observation and evaluation of physical conditions, mental conditions, behavioral changes, symptoms of illness, and reactions to treatment.

According to Dean,[3] a medical negligence lawsuit was filed alleging various acts of negligence on the part of the attending physician and alleging that the hospital's nursing staff failed to insist that the physician personally evaluate the patient during the time his condition deteriorated, which resulted in his condition's ensuing downhill course.[3] The failure to make a nursing diagnosis or to correlate the patient's signs and symptoms and determine whether they represent a deviation from normal resulted in a failure to formulate a plan of nursing care.

If the nursing diagnosis dictates that an emergency evaluation by a physician is necessary, the nurse should follow through and ensure that the patient is seen by a physician immediately. If a physician does not respond, the nurse calls administration, the director of nursing, the director of the emergency services, and the chief executive officer if necessary to obtain a physician evaluation. The independent duty responsibility that the nurse holds to the patient is independent of the physician.

Study title: Orthopedic injuries/infection	Study no: 100	Indicated by: Emergency services Date: 7/91

Data summary
240 patients, out of 517 patients admitted through the Emergency Room Service, had 284 orthopedic injuries. 15% of the orthopedic injuries were compound, and 41 surgical procedures were performed.

Data conclusion
Infection rate is less than 10%; however, the incidence for Hoffman pin sites infection is 1 in 4.

Data recommendation
1. Staff education
2. Antibiotic usage assessment
3. This further validates the need for change in orthopedic culture policy: "all wounds."
4. Continue monitoring and compare current data to data collected one year after policy change to assess outcome.

Fig. 16-5   Patient populations at risk, problems identified, and recommendations.

Anderson's *Legal Boundaries of Florida Nursing Practice*[2] states the following:

Emergency nursing includes the performance of those acts requiring substantial specialized knowledge, judgement and nursing skill. This standard of professional nursing means that we must adhere strictly to the nursing process. Recognition of pathophysiologic conditions on the part of the nurse in making a nursing diagnosis cannot stop here. The nurse will decrease risk loss potential once the nurse devises a workable nursing plan for nursing care.

The process of effected change is consistent with the Emergency Nurses Association *Code of Ethics*[4] for emergency nurses, which is provided in the box on this page.

Necessary components of quality assurance are multidisciplinary committee review, mortality and morbidity review, and ED committee review. It is essential that a representative from the ED nursing staff participate in each one of these committees so that programs to be established have staff nursing input. Within the committee a format for activity, a method of cataloging activity, a method of gathering data, and formalization of the review process all take effect in a multidisciplinary forum.

For example, a staff nurse may identify a problem with prolonged patient waiting and missed triage or mislabeling of specimens. The nurse brings this problem to committee to identify the deficiency and kick the quality assurance study into effect. Tracking outcome is not difficult if the gathering of data renders a workable solution. Outcome is not a happiness index; rather, it is compliance with a standard, which renders a positive physiologic patient outcome that is implemented by adequately educated staff.

For example, neurologic assessment and cervical spine injury assessment are two actions of educated nursing staff that have been examined closely in malpractice lawsuits. Both require nursing standards of care, protocol, and evaluation methods that include tracking of outcomes and follow-up. The boxes on pp. 235 and 236 provide nursing practice standards and protocols that are used in neurologic assessment and cervical spine injury to improve outcome. In addition, the Glasgow coma scale is used to track neurologic trends that correlate with percentage probability of survival. The Glasgow coma scale is a useful clinical tool and an adjunct to sound quality assurance.

The quality assurance nurse develops a monitoring system to determine that assessment matches protocol and to determine the percent probability of survival when available. Information is documented and used for future analysis and comparison. When the method of program description is used, sample selection and outcome assessment render readily identifiable indicators of complications. Based on documentation, changes in practice consistent with study findings are implemented and reevaluated again 6 months after policy change so that the impact of change on patient care can be determined. Studies that demonstrate the ab-

---

EMERGENCY NURSES ASSOCIATION CODE OF ETHICS

The Emergency Nurse provides services with respect for human dignity and the uniqueness of the patient unrestricted by considerations of social or economic status, personal attributes, or the nature of health problems.

The Emergency Nurse safeguards the patient's right to privacy by judiciously protecting information of a confidential nature.

The Emergency Nurse acts to safeguard the patient and the public when health care and safety are affected by the incompetent, unethical or illegal practice of any person.

The Emergency Nurse assumes responsibility and accountability for individual nursing judgements and actions.

The Emergency Nurse maintains competence in nursing.

The Emergency Nurse exercises informed judgement and uses individual competence and qualifications as criteria in seeking consultation, accepting responsibilities, and delegating nursing activities to others.

The Emergency Nurse endeavors to participate in activities that contribute to the ongoing development of the profession's body of knowledge.

The Emergency Nurse endeavors to participate in the profession's efforts to implement and improve standards of nursing.

The Emergency Nurse endeavors to participate in the profession's efforts to establish and maintain conditions of employment conducive to high quality nursing care.

The Emergency Nurse endeavors to participate in the profession's effort to protect the public from misinformation and misrepresentation and to maintain the integrity of nursing.

The Emergency Nurse endeavors to collaborate with members of the health professions and other citizens in promoting community and national efforts to meet the health needs of the public.

From Emergency Nurses Association: Code of ethics, Chicago, 1989, The Association.

---

sence of negative clinical indicators are as acceptable as those that identify and correct deficiencies.

The final step in educating the nursing staff includes the acquisition of minimal body of knowledge set forth in the Emergency Nurses Association *Emergency Nursing Core Curriculum*. Each ED develops a core curriculum preceptor program, complete with clinical evaluation checklist and ongoing evaluation process, and uses the core curriculum to guide program development (Fig. 16-7 and the box on p. 238). The program is revised based on outcome studies, which identify ongoing learning needs.

ASSESSMENT OF THE UNCONSCIOUS PATIENT

Purpose Upon completion of the head-to-toe assessment, the following will be assessed in the unconscious patient.

I. Assess
  A. Mechanism of injury: automobile
    1. Driver or passenger side of patient impact
    2. Seat belt, shoulder harness
    3. Front seat or back seat
    4. Speed of vehicles
    5. Extrication time
    6. Length of skid marks
  B. Mechanism of injury: motorcycle
    1. Helmet or no helmet
    2. Passenger or driver
    3. What did the vehicle hit?
    4. Surface and side of body patient landed on?
    5. Was victim thrown from vehicle and how far?
  C. Pedestrian or automobile, bike, truck, other
    1. What did the patient hit?
    2. What type of surface did patient fall onto and from what height?
    3. What position was patient found in and on what side?
    4. How far from the scene was patient?
    5. Speed of vehicle?
    6. Distance from impact to where patient was found?
    7. Length of skid marks?
  D. History
    1. What had the patient been doing before incident?
    2. Was the patient intoxicated? Document drug screen and blood alcohol level
    3. Identifying (medic-alert) tags or other available information; document

II. Physical assessment
  A. Observe
    1. Areas of bleeding, including ears, nose, and mouth
    2. Look for Battle's sign
    3. Palpate for depressions
    4. Excessive tearing from lacrimal ducts
    5. Scars from prior injuries or surgeries
    6. Pupil size, reaction to light, movement of eyes
    7. If no cervical spine injury, attempt to elicit "doll's eye" reflex
    8. Contusions and hematomas
    9. Position and movement: decerebrate or decorticate or none
  B. Auscultate
    1. Lung sounds (to rule out chest problems and airway complications)
    2. Bowel sounds, to rule out abdominal injury (if present in the chest, suspect rupture of diaphragm)
  C. Palpate
    1. Areas of deformity
    2. Subcutaneous emphysema
  D. Vital signs
    1. Temperature: core
    2. Pulse: character, rate, intensity
      a. If pulse rate is rapid and weak, look elsewhere for bleeding
      b. If pulse rate is slow and weak, could be indicative of neurogenic shock or late anoxic insult
    3. Respirations: character, depth, rate
      a. If respirations are depressed, evaluate for brainstem damage
      b. Assess hyperventilation or hypoventilation by obtaining arterial blood gas levels
      c. Biot's respirations: irregular periods of apnea, respirations of equal depth, indicative of increased intracranial pressure
      d. Cheyne-Stokes respiration: rhythmic waxing and waning of depth of respirations with irregular periods of apnea, indicative of damage to the nervous system
    4. Blood pressure: abnormal blood pressure can indicate severe anoxia or neurologic damage. Be sure to look for all causes. Use systematic Glasgow coma scale.
  E. Motor system
    1. Evaluate muscle strength
    2. Reflex testing: Babinski, Kernig's sign
    3. Does patient respond to stimuli: smell, pain, verbal, noxious stimuli
    4. Never use an ammonia inhalant to arouse an unconscious patient with suspected cervical spine injury
  F. Triage
    1. When in doubt, transfer out
    2. Maintain high index of suspicion and call in nursing supervisor and neurosurgical consultation if uncertain of patient progress

ASSESSMENT OF SUSPECTED CERVICAL SPINE INJURY

Purpose To timely diagnose cervical spine injury and expedite immobilization with referral to subspecialist

I. Mechanism of injury
   A. Type of vehicles involved
   B. Patient's position in vehicle
   C. Seat belt or shoulder harness
   D. Position found
   E. Was patient moved by untrained personnel?
   F. A cross table lateral cervical spine radiograph visualizing C1-7 should be made based on mechanism of injury

II. History
   A. Drug ingestion or alcohol intoxication, which may cloud or mute pain
   B. Mechanism of injury
   C. History

III. Assessment
   A. Observe for
      1. Respiratory compromise
      2. Movement of extremities
      3. Position (Do not alter position of head and neck. Maintain immobilization until neck and spine radiograph rules out injury.)
      4. Deformity
      5. Lacerations, contusions, abrasions
      6. Evidence of paralysis from prior accident or illness (should not alter the index of suspicion until radiographic examination rules out new injury)
      7. Sensorium level
      8. Pallor
      9. Signs of shock
   B. Listen
      1. Airway obstruction
      2. Quality of respirations
   C. Palpate
      1. Crepitus
      2. Subcutaneous emphysema
      3. Deformity
      4. Sensation; check strength of grip (squeeze and release); foot push (plantar and dorsi flexion)
      5. Lacerations and bleeding
   D. Vital signs
      1. Temperature
      2. Pulse rate at bilateral arms; do not permit sitting up until injury to neck and spine are ruled out by radiographic examination.
      3. Respiration rates
      4. Blood pressure (Document every 15 minutes.)
   E. Miscellaneous
      1. Do not leave patient unattended until injury is ruled out by radiographic examination.
      2. Do not leave patient alone; ensure that patient lies flat and that immobilization is maintained.
      3. Do not have patient raise head to sign consents.
      4. Maintain stiff collar and backboard until injury is ruled out. (Radiographic plate is placed under backboard.)
      5. Use restraints if necessary, but do not assume immobilization is intact unless in attendance at all times.

Multidisciplinary planning				
Date _____				
Patient name/DX Admit date	Patient need	Patient goal	Plan/intervention	Evaluation

Fig. 16-6 Multidisciplinary planning form.

Orientee name _____ Date _____

Rating done by preceptor:
    0 = Orientee cannot function independently
    1 = Requires extended orientation
    2 = Qualified to function without preceptor
    4 = Integration sufficient to function at supervisory level

TITLE	RATING				
Role of the ED nurse	0	1	2	3	4
ED policies	0	1	2	3	4
Role of the pharmacist	0	1	2	3	4
Admitting orders	0	1	2	3	4
Admitting laboratory panel and order sets	0	1	2	3	4
Follow-up laboratory work	0	1	2	3	4
Care of the patient in ED	0	1	2	3	4
Head-to-toe survey	0	1	2	3	4
Assessment of unconscious patients	0	1	2	3	4
Asessment of blunt injury	0	1	2	3	4
Assessment of penetrating chest trauma	0	1	2	3	4
Assessment of nonpenetrating chest trauma	0	1	2	3	4
Assessment of the neurotrauma	0	1	2	3	4
Assessment of fractures	0	1	2	3	4
Glasgow coma scale	0	1	2	3	4
Trauma score	0	1	2	3	4
Role of the neurosurgeon	0	1	2	3	4
Neurosurgical drug usage	0	1	2	3	4
Evaluation of abdomen	0	1	2	3	4
Transport cart usage	0	1	2	3	4
Cervical spine injuries	0	1	2	3	4
Gardner Wells tongs	0	1	2	3	4
Halo traction	0	1	2	3	4
Burr holes	0	1	2	3	4
Pneumatic antishock garment	0	1	2	3	4
Administration of warmed fluids	0	1	2	3	4
IV access and procedures	0	1	2	3	4
Blood pump use	0	1	2	3	4
Bard rapid infuser	0	1	2	3	4
Autotransfuser and cell saver	0	1	2	3	4
IV cutdown	0	1	2	3	4
Central line	0	1	2	3	4
Art line insertion	0	1	2	3	4
Chest tube insertion and drainage	0	1	2	3	4
Cricothyrotomy	0	1	2	3	4
Transtracheal ventilation	0	1	2	3	4
Tracheostomy	0	1	2	3	4
Peritoneal lavage	0	1	2	3	4
Pericardiocentesis	0	1	2	3	4
Bladder catheterization	0	1	2	3	4
Endotracheal intubation	0	1	2	3	4
Pediatric assessment	0	1	2	3	4
Triage	0	1	2	3	4
Subspecialty consult	0	1	2	3	4
Obtaining supervisory assistance	0	1	2	3	4

Comments:

Plan:

Preceptor signature _____

Orientee signature _____

Date _____

Fig. 16-7   Emergency nurse skills checklist.

EMERGENCY DEPARTMENT CLINICAL ORIENTATION

Purpose To become familiar with the ED in preparation to function as an independent member of the emergency team

Policy Statement Eight to 16 hours will be allowed for orientation.

Text

1. Locate and check carts, supplies
2. Operate equipment
   - Cardiac monitors
   - Defibrillators
   - Suction units
   - Gurneys
   - Oxygen regulators
   - Blood warmers
   - Blood pump tubing
   - Arterial line monitoring
   - Noninvasive BP monitoring devices
   - Pneumatic antishock garment
   - Central line insertion
   - Chest tube insertion
   - Chest tube drainage setup.
   - Bard rapid infuser
3. Review infection control policy concerning gowning and gloving
4. Locate lead apron and don appropriately
5. Demonstrate a complete understanding of the head-to-toe survey and ongoing assessment protocols
6. Provide direct patient care for ED patients
7. Locate life support equipment in computed tomography and radiology departments
8. Review standing orders for emergency patient stabilization
9. Delineate triage procedures

SUMMARY

The hospital administration's melding of risk management and quality assurance is essential to effect positive patient outcomes in the ED. Risk management is a technique used to reduce financial loss that, when coupled with quality assurance, forms a process for monitoring the quality of care delivered; at the same time, risk loss potential is decreased as a result of targeted improvement in the quality of patient care.

The hospital facilities, operations, and services are evaluated and assessed to determine institutional risk exposure and commitment to improving patient outcomes. Lines of authority for problem resolution are mandatory and match hospital policy, which establishes the chain of command through which the nurse proceeds when a problem is perceived and not resolved at the staff nurse level. The chain of command varies from institution to institution, yet a consistent mechanism is tantamount to a successful risk management program. All incidents are shared with risk management staff for follow-up.

A focused program targets actions while reducing risk, thus playing a vital role in identifying strategies that prevent poor patient outcomes. The nursing staff collaborates with medical staff and administration to develop realistic, documented guidelines and to provide ongoing education. Formation of multidisciplinary committees provides a forum to examine deficiencies while promoting problem resolution. Practicing quality assurance activities that decrease risk loss potential by conducting chart audits and ensuring accurate documentation mandates that the staff nurse play a vital role in preventing claims against emergency nurses while all nurses consider themselves their own risk managers. Being aware of the potential for pitfalls associated with emergency nursing care is an institutional and an individual duty and responsibility that promotes safe, appropriate patient care.

A comprehensive hospital ED has a written plan for quality assurance, which outlines a well-organized, problem-oriented approach to evaluating the quality of patient care and clinical performance. Adequate quality assurance programs stress the integration of risk management and risk loss prevention. Problem identification is prompt, and action taken is effective; such a program provides a safe patient care environment and contains costs associated with high-risk patient care scenarios.

Once problems are identified, whether potential or real, they should be recognized by the clinical staff and management. Analysis of the cause and degree of the problem, which includes corrective action and documentation, results in astute future monitoring practice. Documentation of all data and results is critical to the success of a quality assurance and risk management program. Periodic review and reevaluation of methodology is essential. A recommended 6-month follow-up study demonstrates whether the implemented change is working. Staff conferences and committees, along with monthly review, follow-up care, periodic review of test results, and a multidisciplinary approach to risk management, are necessitated by the urgent patient care needs in the ED.

The overall institutional commitment to the concept of quality assurance and risk management is evidenced by the departmental patient care outcomes and by dollars spent to initiate an effective program. Comparison of the initial plan of action and patient outcomes with those of hospitals that have the same or similar patient populations is necessary; comparisons ensure minimal practicing levels, which are reflected by the standard of care. An efficient program is one that includes careful surveillance, systematic scanning of potential problems in patient care, and the ability to render solutions to those problems before they negatively affect patient outcomes.

A comprehensive program identifies potential problems

and promptly resolves them. ED has its own specific priorities, which necessitate a quality assurance and risk management program separate from that of the rest of the institution. Each department's program will be different from other programs. When problem identification and prevention are taking place and ongoing monitoring of nursing actions and patient outcomes are being reviewed consistently, a successful quality assurance and risk management program is in place.

REFERENCES

1. Albaros RS, McCall V, Thrane M: Computerized nursing documentation, *Nurs Manage* 21(7):64, 1990.
2. Anderson: *Legal boundaries of Florida nursing practice.*
3. Dean K: Legal issues in nursing: duty to the patient, *Focus on Crit Care* 11(5):24, 1984.
4. Emergency Nurses Association: *Code of Ethics*, Chicago, 1989, The Association.
4a. Emergency Nurses Association: *Standards of emergency nursing practice*, ed 2, St Louis, 1991, Mosby–Year Book.
5. Hershey N et al: The influence of charting upon liability determinations, *J Nurs Admin,* March-April, 1976.
6. The Joint Commission on Accreditation of Health Care Organizations: The Joint Commission 1990 AMH accreditation manual for hospitals, Chicago, 1989, The Commission.
7. Murphy JG, Jacobson S: Assessing the quality of emergency care: the medical record versus patient outcome, *Ann Emerg Med* 13(3):158, 1984.
8. Secretary's Commission on Medical Malpractice: *Report*, Appendix, p 112, Table III-39, Factors dealing with facts unique to case that influence jurors, Washington, DC, 1988.
9. Shanahan M: One stage at a time: evaluation of nursing care of the patient with acute myocardial infarction in the emergency room and coronary and post-coronary care units, *QRB* 2(9):17, 28, 1976.
10. Spath PL, Miller MS, Crawford B: Comprehensive quality measurement in the hospital emergency department, *Top Health Rec Manage* 10(3):44, 1990.
11. Whitcomb JE et al: Quality assurance in the emergency department, *Ann Emerg Med* 14(12):1199, 1985.

SUGGESTED READINGS

Albin SL et al: Evaluation of emergency room triage performed by nurses, *Am J Public Health* 65(10):1063, 1975.
American College of Emergency Physicians, Illinois Chapter: *Quality assessment in the emergency department: a practical handbook*, Des Plaines, Illinois, 1984, Quality Assurance Healthcare Handbooks.
Anderson GV et al: A unique approach to evaluation of emergency care, *JACEP* 6(6):254, 1977.
Bailey A, Hallam K, Hurst K: Nursing practice: triage on trial, *Nurs Times* 83(44):65, 1987.
Beers MH, Storrie M, Lee G: Potential adverse drug interactions in the emergency room: an issue in the quality of care, *Ann Intern Med* 112(1):61, 1990.
Bell JW: Why readmissions? Audits can discover the reasons, *QRB* 4(8):16, 1978.
Bernzweig E: Legally speaking: how an emergency can spell trouble, *RN* 49(3):57, 1986.
Boyd CR, Tolson MA, Copes WS: Evaluating trauma care: The TRISS method: trauma score and the injury severity score, *J Trauma* 27(4):370, 1987.
Britton RM, Magen BS: Preventative measures to limit legal liability in pediatric emergencies: an analysis through cases concerning failure to diagnose meningitis, *Pediatr Emerg Care* 2(2):109, 1986.
Brook RH, Stevenson RL Jr: Effectiveness of patient care in an emergency room, *N Engl J Med* 283(17):904, 1970.
Burda D: Dumping laws spurs look at ED, *Risk Management Hospitals* 61(4):34, 1987.
Burke MC, Aghababian RV, Blackbourne B: Use of autopsy results in emergency department quality assurance program, *Ann Emerg Med* 19(4):363, 1990.
Callahan F: Emergency department nursing risk management, *J Ambulator Care Management* 12(2):31, 1989.
Carros DH: Emergency x-ray report system reduces risk of misdiagnosis, *Hospitals* 42(22):78, 1968.
Caszuba A, Gibson G: Hospital emergency department surveillance system: a database for patient care, management, research and teaching, *JACEP* 6(7):304, 1977.
Cecchini RA, Ferraro PJ: The standard of care in emergency room procedure, *Legal Aspects Med Pract* 5(12):45, 1977.
Cohen AG, Tucker E: Department of nursing implementation of JCAH standards: a quality assurance program applied, *Hosp Top* 58(20):38, 1980.
Cohen SW, Leads MP: The moonlighting dilemma balancing education, service, and quality care while limiting risk exposure, *JAMA* 262(4):529, 1989.
Cordell W, Zollman W, Karlson H: A photographic system for the emergency department, *Ann Emerg Med* 9(4):210, 1980.
Creighton H: Law for the nurse-supervisor: liability in the emergency room, *Supervisor Nurse* 3(10):14, 1972.
Creighton H: Failure to adequately supervise PA's, *Nurs Management* 13(12):44, 1982.
Creighton H: The legal aspects of emergency services–part I, *Nurs Management* 19(9):18, 1988.
Cross RE Jr: Transfer of the emergency patient: avoiding legal complications, *Tex Hosp* 35(7):11, 1979.
Cuypers ME: A computerized log and integrated quality assessment program for the small emergency department, *QRB* 15(5):144, 1989.
Davis JL, Kearns S: Trauma registers: planning and developing reports, *JEN* 15(5):436, 1989.
Day SC et al: Evaluation and outcome of emergency room patients with transient loss of consciousness, *Am J Med* 73(1):15, 1982.
DeBard ML: Emergency department staffing by nonspecialists, *J Emerg Med* 1(3):269, 1984.
Derlet RW, and Nishio DA: Refusing care to patients who present to an emergency department, *Ann Emerg Med* 19(3):262, 1990.
Dunn JD: Risk management in emergency medicine, *Emerg Med Clin North Am* 5(1):51, 1987.
Dwyer WA, Jr.: Method for evaluating hospital emergency department treatment, *J Med Soc N J* 82(7):523.
Edwards C: Quality assessment in the emergency room of a small rural hospital, *QRB* 10(4):119, 1984.
Eisner M et al: Efficacy of a standard seizure work-up in the emergency department, *Ann Emerg Med* 15(1):33, 1986.
Emergency department quality assurance: survey, *Nurs Forum* 17(4):9, 1989.
Emergency Nurses Association: *Emergency nursing core curriculum*, Philadelphia, 1987, WB Saunders.
Fahey TM: Update on emergency department staffing requirements, *Hosp Med Staff* 10(5):25, 1981.
Flint LS, Hammett WH, Martens K: Quality assurance in the emergency department, *Ann Emerg Med* 14(2):134, 1985.
Frey CF: Quality assurance in trauma care, *Hospital Physician* 23(5):15, 18, 1987.
Frew SA, Roush WR, LaGreca K: COBRA: implications for emergency medicine, *Ann Emerg Med* 17(8):835, 1988.
George JE: A prescription for avoiding malpractice suits in the ED, *Emerg Nurse Legal Bulletin* 6(1):2, 1980.
George JE, Quattrone MS: Law and the emergency nurse: complications of ED treatment: who is liable?, *JEN* 13(3):175, 1987.

Greenfield S et al: The clinical investigation and management of chest pain in an emergency department: quality assessment criteria mapping, *Med Care* 15(11):898, 1977.

Hansen PJ: A new approach for quality assurance, *Aviat Space Environ Med* 52(10):627, 1981.

Hawkins ML, Treat RC, Mansberger AR, Jr: The trauma score: a simple method to evaluate quality of care, *Am Surg* 54(4):204, 1988.

Heister K, Johnson B, Trimberger L: ED standards and audit criteria, *JEN* 8(2):83, 1982.

Henry DL: One way to teach malpractice: sue a resident on his first day, *Emerg Depart News* 6(7):1, 4, 1984.

Henze HM: Putting together a quality assurance program, consult problems, unite disparate interests, *Emerg Depart News* 6(3):15, 18, 1984.

Hill MB: Preventing malpractice in emergency medicine: identifying the scope of the problem, *QRC Advis* 5(12):1, 1989.

Holbrook J: Computerized audit of 15,009 emergency department records, emergency department quality assurance, *Ann Emerg Med* 19(2):139, 1990.

Holthaus D: Hospital liable for negligence of ED physician, *Hospitals* 62(1):46, 1988.

Horsley JE: When you have to get tough with a doctor, *RN* 50(7):61, 1987.

Hospital Association of Pennsylvania: *Emergency department quality assessment*, Camp Hill, Pennsylvania, 1976, Hospital Association of Pennsylvania.

Illinois hospital reduces ER liability risks, *Hospitals* 59(18):66, 1985.

Isaacman DJ: Pediatric emergency medicine-current standards of care: results of a national survey, *Ann Emerg Med* 19(5):527, 1990.

Jones J et al: Efficacy of a telephone follow-up system in the emergency department, *J Emerg Med* 6(3):249, 1988.

Keith JD et al: Emergency department revisits, *Ann Emerg Med* 18(9):964, 1989.

Kresky B, Cohen A: Considerations for evaluation of patient care in emergency departments, *QRB* 6(12):8, 1980.

Letourneau CU: Emergency room records, *Hosp Manage* 107(1):30, 1969.

Levy R, Goldstein B, Trott A: Approach to quality assurance in an emergency department: a one year review, *Ann Emerg Med* 13(3):166, 1984.

Mandell M: Preventing patient injury: what you don't do can land you in court, *Nurs Life* 7(1):26, 1987.

Maroncelli RD et al: A protocol for risk management, *Vet Hum Toxicol* 27(6):512, 1985.

Mates S, Sidel VW: Quality assessment by process and outcome methods: evaluation of emergency room care of asthmatic adults, *Am J Public Health* 71(7):687, 1981.

Mays ET: Continuing education for emergency department nurses, *Surg Gynecol Obstet* 137(3):480, 1973.

McDermott S: Emergency department organization and management: a checklist of action items, *J Ambulator Care Manage* 9(1):1, 1986.

McLain NB: Risk management in the emergency department, *JEN* 7(6):269, 1981.

Mitchell JH, Hartwick K, Beck B: Telephone follow-up for ER audits: one facility's experience with studies of laceration and head trauma, *QRB* 4(7):6, 1978.

Moore SL: A QA program in a small rural hospital, *QRB* 9(8):233, 1983.

Nakayama DJ et al: Quality assessment in the pediatric trauma care system, *J Pediatr Surg* 24(2):159, 1989.

O'Leary MR et al: Application of clinical indicators in the emergency department, *JAMA* 262(24):3444, 1989.

Peters D: Hospital malpractice: eleven theories of direct liability, *Trial Magazine*, November 1988.

Rea R et al: *Emergency nursing care curriculum*, ed 3, Philadelphia, 1987, WB Saunders.

Regan WA: Poorly equipped ER is factor in infant death, *Hosp Prog* 59(6):80, 1978.

Regan WA: Telephone orders: legally speaking: Regan report, *Nursing Law* 21(7):1, 1980.

Regan WA: Legally speaking: how to force that on-call MD to respond, *RN* 45(2):77, 1982.

Regan WA: Doctor on call, ER nurse sued: case in point: Regan report, *Nursing Law* 24(10):4, 1984.

Reitz JA: Legal issues and risks of ED care, *JEN* 10(2):82, 1984.

Rhee KJ, Donabedian A, Burney RE: Assessing the quality of care in an emergency unit: a framework and its application, *QRB* 13(1):4, 1987.

Roy A, Looney GL, Anderson GV: Prospective versus retrospective data for evaluating emergency care: a research methodology, *JACEP* 8(4):142, 1979.

Rubenstein L, Mates S, Sidel VW: Quality of care assessment by process and outcome scoring: use of weighted algorithmic assessment criteria for evaluation of emergency room care of women with symptoms of urinary tract infection, *Ann Intern Med* 86(5):617, 1977.

Rusnak RA et al: Litigation against the emergency physician: common features in cases of missed myocardial infarction, *Ann Emerg Med* 18(10):1029, 1989.

Ryan M: The phenomenon of the corridor patient, *Br Med J* 281(6253):1483, 1980.

Sateia MJ, Gustafson DH, Johnson SW: Quality assurance for psychiatric emergencies: an analysis of assessment and feedback methodologies, *Psychiatr Clin North Am* 13(1):35, 1990.

Selfridge J: Criteria based performance evaluations using the ENA standards of emergency nursing practice, *JEN* 13(2):91, 1987.

Selfridge J, Nitta D, Saltzer E: Development and design of an ED nursing flow sheet, *JEN* 9(1):30, 1983.

Simchuc CJ: Development of criteria for emergency department nursing audit, *JEN* 3(5):47, 1977.

Simon JE, Smookler S, Guy V: A regionalized approach to pediatric emergency care, *Pediatr Clin North Am* 28(3):677, 1981.

Sklar C: You and the law: good communications a must, even in the ER, *Canadian Nurse* 79(6):51, 53, 1983.

Smeltzer CH, Curtis L: Emergency department care: many perceptions, *Nurs Management* 18(11):96a, 96d–96f, 96h, 1987.

Sniff D: The evolution of a quality assurance program, *QRB* 6(1):26, 1980.

Soreff S: Quality improvement: a collaborative discipline approach, *Psychiatr Clin North Am* 13(1):187, 1990.

Sparger G: JCAH survival guidelines for 1983, *JEN* 9(2):114, 1983.

Spivak HR et al: Patient and provider factors associated with selected measures of quality assurance, *Pediatrics* 65(2):307, 1980.

Stafford VG, Gibson G: The impact of an emergency department nursing audit, *JEN* 21(4):22, 1976.

Stair TO: Quality assurance, *Emerg Med Clin North Am* 5(1):41, 1987.

Taliaferro E: Too stressed-out to care (editorial; comment), *Ann Emerg Med* 18(11):1248, 1989.

Tammelleo AD: Nurses fail to communicate: death results: case in point: Regan report, *Nursing Law* 28(1):4, 1987.

Tammelleo AD: Deficient charting: weak link in evidence: case in point: Regan report, *Nursing Law* 29(12):2, 1989.

Tammelleo AD: Legal case briefs for nurses. GA: incident report altered: punitive damages: Co: concealing death: indictment dismissed: Regan report, *Nursing Law* 29(8):3, 1989.

Tammelleo AD: When a phone call is your liability lifeline, *RN* 52(2):69, 1989.

Tanner JR: Expert reveals tactics to take high risk out of nurses knowledge of legal liability, *JEN* 14(4):225, 1988.

Taylor JE Jr, Taylor JP, Sieh MK: Emergency nurses knowledge of legal liability, *JEN* 14(4):225, 1988.

Trautlein JJ, Lambert RL, Miller J: Malpractice in the emergency department: review of 200 cases, *Ann Emerg Med* 13(9 Pt1):709, 1984.

Travis LW: An audit of otitis media treated in the emergency room, *QRB* 2(9):13, 27, 1976.

Vasey EK: Evaluation of care in the emergency department: a comparison of process and outcome criteria, *QRB* 2(9):12, 27, 1976.

Wachsman L, Singleton AF: Assessing the quality of care provided to pediatric patients by emergency room physicians, *J Natl Med Assoc* 75(1):31, 1983.

Wallas JL: Family practice forum in defense of the emergency room, *J Family Pract* 2(5):389, 1975.

Walters BC, McNeill I: Improving the record of patient assessment in the trauma room, *J Trauma* 30(4):398, 1990.

Walts L, Blair F: Making quality assurance work in the emergency department, *JEN* 9(1):59, 1983.

Waskerwitz S, Unfr SM: Quality assurance in emergency pediatrics, *Pediatr Emerg Care* 3(2):121, 1987.

Weiland DE et al: Trauma malpractice claims related to trauma level designation, *Am J Surg* 158(6):553; Discussion 555, 1989.

Wilbert CC: Timeliness of care in the emergency department, *QRB* 10(4):99, 1984.

Wolcott BW, Ornelas-Wilson LA, Weindorf B: The morning after: daily audit and its effect in emergency divisions at Brooke Army Medical Center, *QRB* 4(7):2, 1978.

Brain death criteria

American Neurological Association: Recommendations from the collaboratory study on cerebral death, 1971–1972, Chicago, The Association.

Ropper A, Kennedy SK, Zervax N: *Neurological and neurosurgical intensive care*, Baltimore, 1983, University Park Press.

Task Force for the Determination of Brain Death in Children: Guidelines for the Determination of Brain Death in Children, *Arch Neurosurg* 44:587, 1987.

Margaret M. Miller

RATIONALE FOR PATIENT TEACHING

During the past 15 years significant changes have affected the emergency nurse's responsibility for patient teaching. First, patient teaching is explicitly incorporated into the role and responsibilities of the professional emergency nurse as stated in the *Standards of Emergency Nursing Practice* and the nurse practice acts of most states, and patient teaching is included in the nursing diagnosis index as "knowledge deficit." Second, documentation of patient teaching is mandated by both quality assurance and accreditation criteria. The following must be documented: date and time, who the learner is, and whether he or she is a patient or family member, content and teaching method used, supplemental learning aids provided, the learner's response, and referrals and signature of the nurse and patient. Third, the variety and sophistication of patient education materials have increased significantly. Two decades ago most patient education materials were "homemade" mimeographed copies of information chosen by interested nurses (Fig. 17-1). Now, however, colorful, humorous, informative booklets and videotapes are published or produced by patient education departments and companies, and educational materials are available from medical supply and pharmaceutical companies. In addition, some learning materials are published in languages other than English and in picture format for patients with limited reading abilities.

Although patient education has traditionally been an accepted component of emergency patient care, the emphasis on the need for patient teaching has increased dramatically. Influential factors include fear of litigation, cost containment, and restriction of patient admissions. In many instances patients formerly admitted to the emergency department (ED) are now treated and sent home. The promulgation of the Patient Bill of Rights by the American Hospital Association in 1972 informed the public of the right of all hospital patients to be informed of procedures used in providing care and self-care methods to be used after dismissal. The Patient Bill of Rights has been widely reprinted in the popular press and in some agencies is distributed to all admitted patients; thus public awareness of the teaching responsibilities of health care professionals has increased. In addition, the increased educational level of the general public and derogatory publicity regarding errors of omission and commission by health care providers have increased the number of malpractice suits. In an effort to contain rising health care costs, patient admissions have been restricted to those persons with illness or injury defined in specific diagnostic related groups. Because of this economic situation, many patients formerly admitted are dismissed from the ED with specific instructions for home care and referral for follow-up care.

Compounding the fear of litigation and restricted admission, the public is focusing on prevention of illness for both personal and financial reasons. We are all aware of the numerous national advertising campaigns focusing on cholesterol control and the prevention of heart and lung disease and occupational and vehicular accidents. Many businesses and industries are subscribing to health maintenance organizations that promote illness prevention and health maintenance.

All these efforts are aimed at containing escalating health care costs by decreasing the use of hospital care. At the same time, the number of patients seen at EDs has increased during the past decade. Whether this increase is due to a lack of personal physicians, the limited office hours of nonemergency services, transportation problems, or financial reasons, many persons perceive the ED to be the only consistently available access to the health care system. Even though the numbers and acuity levels of emergency patients are increasing, staffing restrictions resulting from the nursing shortage have affected the ED as much as they have affected other hospital departments. Despite staffing shortages and increasing numbers of ED patients, effective patient teaching remains one of the top 10 priorities of local, state, and federal government. Patient education is perceived not only as a patient right but also as a means to contain health care costs and prevent expensive litigation.

When these professional, governmental, and economic factors are considered, the need for effective patient teaching by the professional emergency nurse is evident. The re-

HOW TO TAKE A CHILD'S TEMPERATURE

1. Shake the thermometer down.
2. **Oral Thermometer**
   a) Place the long, silver tip of thermometer under child's tongue.
   b) Have child close lips gently, being careful not to bite the thermometer.

Rectal Thermometer
   a) Lubricate silver end of the thermometer.
   b) Spread the buttocks so that rectum can be seen easily.
   c) Insert thermometer gently into the rectum until silver tip can no longer be seen.
3. Hold thermometer in place for 3-5 minutes.
4. Remove the thermometer.
5. Rotate the thermometer until the wide silver line can be seen.
6. Read degree of temperature (exactly where the mercury stops). Read the temperature at the end of the silver line and write down the number.

CU/BMC 6-75

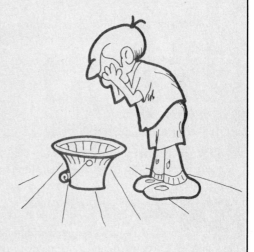

YOUR CHILD IS VOMITING

Saint Joseph Hospital
Emergency Service

YOUR CHILD IS VOMITING

Persistent vomiting — If your child cannot keep down even plain water for more than half a day, contact your physician. Vomiting causes loss of body water resulting in dehydration.

Stop: All feedings
Rest the stomach
No milk
No solid foods
Nothing by mouth for at least an hour

Infants: Start feeding sugar water* or 7-Up in a bottle or with a spoon.

*Sugar water — Add 1 teaspoon of sugar to 4 ounces (½ cup) of boiled cool water.

Older Children: Feed small quantities of cold water or ice chips.

When: The child can keep water or ice chips down, then you may give several sips OR swallows every 15 minutes of:

   a. Weak tea, kool aid, sweetened
   b. 7-Up
   c. Gingerale

When: The child can keep down gingerale, 7-Up, or tea, you can further add other liquids such as:

   a. Clear broth
   b. Fruit juices — apple, pineapple, or orange
   c. Jello — liquid or solid form

Medication: Do not give any medications to stop vomiting, unless ordered by your doctor.

Do Not Give Aspirin: It may increase your child's vomiting.

If your child needs medicine for fever, you may use Tylenol or Tempra in liquid form

If: your child has not vomited for 8-12 hours and feels hungry, you may give the following foods:

First Day
1. Cereal — Rice, oatmeal, cooked cream of wheat
2. Mashed potato, soft cooked rice with butter
3. Dry toast, Soda crackers
4. Apple sauce, Jello
5. Mashed ripe bananas

Second Day
1. May start 2+ or skim milk
2. Lean meat suitable for age: Chicken or Beef
3. Vegetables — Green beans, peas, carrots, spinach cooked tender
4. Vanilla ice cream or puddings, or fruit — jello

Fig. 17-1   "Your Child is Vomiting." (From St. Joseph Hospital Emergency Services.)

sponsibilities of teaching rest with emergency nurses because of the professional and governmental mandates for effective patient teaching; despite the nursing shortage and increasing numbers and acuity levels of patients in the ED, professional emergency nurses are responsible for the design and implementation of effective patient teaching for all patients. Patient teaching in the ED is a special challenge. Constraints and potential impediments to teaching and learning include the varied patient population, the multiplicity of illnesses and accidents, the physician, the psychoemotionally compromised condition of patients, the various age-groups of patients, the typically tense ED environment, and the increased anxiety levels of emergency patients and their families.

To minimize the constraints and to teach effectively, the emergency nurse must be familiar with the teaching and learning process, maintain current knowledge and skills regarding a large variety of health problems affecting all age-groups, and be able to decrease the patient's anxiety level, thus enhancing the learning opportunity. As with the use of any process involving knowledge and skill, familiarity with the sequential steps increases ease and effectiveness. Recall your first attempt at starting an intravenous infusion: initial attempts are awkward. However, with repetition and familiarity with the equipment and process, skill and confidence improve quickly.

Unlike in the specialized units of the hospital such as the orthopedic or coronary units, in the ED the wide variety of health problems and the varying age-groups of patients present a major problem for the emergency nurse and teacher: maintaining the current knowledge and skills necessary to teach self-care to patients of all age-groups and patients with the multiplicity of illnesses and accidents seen in the ED is challenging. The nurse's responsibility to update required knowledge and skills can be met in several ways. Professional continuing education can be acquired during in-service educational programs, by participation in local, regional, or national professional meetings and symposiums, or by independent study courses, which are available in nursing journals or computer-assisted learning programs. Occasionally we fail to take advantage of the knowledge of peers who have specific areas of expertise; these persons could present educational programs to the department, develop teaching protocols that the less experienced nurses could use as references, or serve as preceptors or mentors in their specialized areas. Although moderate anxiety enhances learning, high anxiety inhibits learning. Emergency nurses must be able to ensure effective learning by using various verbal and nonverbal methods to reduce high patient anxiety levels. Most patients have increased stress and anxiety while in the ED. Compounding the health problem that resulted in their emergency visit is the ED environment itself. The numerous unfamiliar stimuli such as bright lights, unfamiliar equipment, strange sounds, unusual sights, and bustling personnel speaking in medical jargon increase the patient's anxiety. Although the total environment cannot be changed, the emergency nurse can explain patient care procedures in nonmedical terms before or during the procedures. Nonverbal communication, including touch, facial expressions, and body language, can be used effectively to reduce anxiety. Other anxiety-reducing approaches include actively listening to what the patient is saying and staying with, or allowing a relative to stay with, frightened patients. Privacy screening or simply dimming the lights can also reduce the patient's anxiety.

Regardless of the constraints of time, number of patients, or nursing shortage, patient teaching is an integral component of professional emergency nursing care. Because patient teaching in the ED is necessarily "telescoped," that is, it focuses on the immediate needs and the patient is provided with referral for concomitant long-term care, familiarity with the process of patient teaching is essential.

TEACHING AND LEARNING PROCESS

To ensure effective use of the teaching and learning process, an analysis of the following sequential components of the process is necessary:

1. Identify the implied and expressed learning needs of the patient or learner.
2. Assess the learner's readiness, capabilities, and motivation.
3. Cooperatively establish realistic learning goals.
4. Select and use the appropriate teaching method based on the identified learning needs, the content to be learned, and the individual characteristics of the learner.
5. Provide time, space, necessary equipment and supplies, and teaching tools such as visual aids, videotapes, or written instructions for home care.
6. Evaluate the effectiveness of teaching.
7. Document the content taught, the method used, the home care instruction sheets provided, the learner's response, and referrals made.

To use this process effectively, the nurse and teacher must have knowledge and skills regarding the content area, astutely assess the learner, establish realistic learning goals, and communicate effectively.

IDENTIFYING LEARNING NEEDS

The initial step in the teaching process, identification of implied and expressed learning needs, is directly related to the patient's problem. For example, if the patient has a fractured arm that must be casted, the implied learning need is for measures that promote healing and prevent complications in the care of the casted arm. However, the patient may request information regarding the advisability of taking previously prescribed medications. Specific questions asked by the patient identify expressed learning needs. If these questions are ignored, the patient's anxiety about medications may block his or her ability to learn the information about cast care that you are sharing.

Categories of home care learning needs are (1) procedures

or techniques and (2) general supportive care. When procedural and technical needs have been identified, the nurse teacher includes the following content: what procedures and techniques are to be performed and why, specifics of how and when to perform them, the anticipated results, a list of necessary supplies or equipment with instructions for care of the equipment, situations in which professional help is necessary, and whom to call for help. For example, a right-handed patient has a laceration on the left thumb, which has been sutured. The physician has prescribed a procedure of twice-daily suture line cleansing, application of antibiotic ointment, and reapplication of sterile dressing. The nurse explains that this procedure is necessary to prevent infection and demonstrates the procedure. To define frequency, the nurse may suggest performing the procedure in the morning and at night or relate timing to the patient's working schedule. A picture and a verbal explanation of a noninfected sutured wound identify the anticipated results. The same method can be used to illustrate an infected suture line that indicates the need for professional help. The nurse either gives the patient a prescription or provides the prescribed ointment and dressings. The patient is also given a referral card, which provides the name and phone number of the health care professional to be contacted if problems arise.

When identifying learning needs related to general supportive care, the nurse teacher selects the appropriate content from an extensive list of potential needs. Included in this broad category are hygiene, rest and nutritional requirements, elimination needs, skin and pressure-point protection, correct body alignment and position changes, oxygenation and ventilation needs, range-of-motion and activity levels, safety factors, and the scheduling of medications nad prescribed therapeutic measures. Obviously the supportive needs list can be long. In the telescoped teaching time available in the ED, the nurse must astutely select the most pertinent content and provide referral for less pressing needs.

Patients being transferred to another unit within the agency or to another health care facility also have urgent learning needs. Specifically, these patients need to know where they are going, how they will get there, and the reason for their transfer. Explaining the reason for the transfer and the logistics of it minimizes the patient's anxiety and reduces the potential for undesirable physiologic stress responses in the patient.

ASSESSING THE LEARNER

After identifying the probable learning needs of the patient, the nurse must assess the learner's readiness to learn, capabilities, and motivation level. Numerous factors influence the patient's readiness to learn self-care measures, including the patient's age, education, culture and primary language, present anxiety level, contact with health care professionals for concomitant or previous health problems, prior experience with self-care, and self-concept. The nurse obtains this information from various sources. The patient's

record indicates the patient's age, family status, nationality, and ability to finance health care. However, much necessary information is obtained from the patient interview and pertinent observation. For example, during the admission process, patients are asked about medications taken at home and current health problems. The patient's method of speaking or answering questions may indicate his or her primary language and educational level.

The patient's record indicates anticipated or completed diagnostic and therapeutic measures. This information is extremely important because the nurse must select a time for patient teaching that does not interfere with or counteract diagnostic and therapeutic measures used in treatment. To illustrate, if a patient has received a central nervous system depressant for treatment of severe pain, the stimulus of initiating patient teaching may counteract the desired effect of the medication. Questions about the previous health care experiences can provide a helpful point of reference for teaching. Using analogies and similes to relate new content to previous experiences increases the meaningfulness of the new content.

Pertinent observations provide additional information. If the patient's basic physiologic needs are not met, his or her readiness to learn is diminished. When a person is dehydrated or has hypoxia, a full bladder, or acute pain, initiating patient teaching is unproductive. These physiologic conditions require prompt remediation. Patient behaviors and appearances that typically indicate a poor self-concept include poor hygiene, lack of eye contact, or muffled voice quality. Generally an inadequate self-concept results in a lack of the self-confidence necessary to learn new self-care behaviors. Because these patients doubt their own capabilities to learn a new behavior, the likelihood that they will attempt to learn or will successfully learn is severely limited.[2] It is equally important to observe the patient for the presence of physical limitations that prohibit the learning of some skills. Physical wholeness and dexterity are prerequisites for learning some psychomotor skills.

In assessing motivation level, look for verbal, nonverbal, and behavioral clues. Verbal clues indicating increased motivation might be specific questions the patient asks or the patient's initiation of a discussion about home self-care measures. A less direct verbal clue is a statement such as "I'm going to have to learn to do that." Nonverbal clues include changes in facial expression that indicate interest in what the nurse is doing: watching rather than turning away can be a clue. Observations of small independent behaviors such as initiating position changes indicate the patient's desire to change from the dependent, sick role to increasing independence. Certain physical behaviors and extensive muscle tenseness can indicate excessive anxiety, which interferes with readiness and motivation to learn. Anxious persons may exhibit either excessive or decreased activity of voluntary muscles. Although some anxious persons exhibit withdrawal behaviors, such as maintaining a fetal position, covering the face, or lowering the eyes, the majority exhibit hyperactive behaviors. For example, these persons may tense the arm, facial, or neck muscles, fidget with bed sheets, smack or purse lips, or have tremors while attempting purposeful movements. Information regarding the patient's age helps the nurse determine the patient's ability to comprehend specific learning content and adhere to self-care measures. For example, a 2-year-old child is incapable of comprehending information about sterile dressings and lacks the physical dexterity necessary to apply a sterile dressing. Therefore the parent or guardian must be taught to complete this procedure at home. Conversely an elderly person may be able to comprehend information about dressing changes but unable to complete the task because of impaired sight and osteoarthritic finger joints.

Because of the cultural and ethnic diversity in the United States, language can present a problem. If the ED staff is unable to converse in the patient's language, a resource person must be obtained. This person can help not only with translation but also with knowledge of cultural factors that may enhance or detract from the patient's adherence to the home care measures being taught. In some instances home care instruction materials and other learning aids are available in the different languages prevalent in the community.

Collecting assessment data is nonsensical unless the data is used. In the teaching and learning situation, nurse teachers must build on assessed strengths and minimize or delete factors that inhibit learning.

ESTABLISHING LEARNING GOALS

The third step in the teaching and learning process is to establish realistic, individualized learning goals. Although health care educators advise designing both short-term and long-term learning goals, the time constraints and the emergency patient's anxiety level preclude addressing long-term teaching needs except through referral. Goals for the emergency patient, based on the learner's assessment data and time constraints, should be realistic. For example, if the patient has a fractured tibia, concomitant diabetes, a hangnail, and a sinus problem, the emergency nurse must determine the paramount learning needs without attempting to meet all the learning needs of this patient. Because of the diverse health problems, the patient would probably be unable to comprehend all the necessary information if the nurse tried to discuss all concerns at once. Realistically the nurse might focus on two of the patient's most pressing needs. The nurse might share the identified learning needs with the patient and ask which are most important to him or her, thereby cooperatively establishing learning goals. The patient's remaining needs can be met by referral to his or her physician, a community health agency, or local groups such as the American Diabetes Association. Local phone companies and public health agencies publish listings of resources available in various communities. These lists are handy reference resources for any ED.

To individualize the teaching and learning process, the nurse must interview the patient regarding his or her work and home situation to discover potential problems the patient might have in adhering to prescribed home care measures. For example, a man is admitted to the ED with acute back pain sustained after 2 hours of sawing, lifting, and stacking logs for his fireplace. After taking vertebral radiographs, the physician diagnoses low back muscle strain and prescribes a muscle relaxant. Proper lifting and bending methods are demonstrated, and a back care instruction sheet is given to the patient for future reference. It is also appropriate to inquire about the man's occupation. If he has a desk job, his return to work the next day would not interfere with his recuperation. However, if his job involves loading trucks, which requires a significant amount of bending and lifting, return to work must be delayed until he has recuperated. For maximum effectiveness, the patient's medication schedule should be correlated with his work schedule. Absorption of medication depends on the metabolic rate; if the patient works from 4 PM to midnight, his schedule for taking the prescribed muscle relaxant will be different from that of a person working from 9 AM to 5 PM. When medications are prescribed, administration scheduling and other pertinent information regarding food and activity restrictions that enhance the effectiveness of the medication should be discussed.

In addition to considering the patient's home and work situation, the nurse can further individualize and adapt the learning experience based on the patient's previous experiences with self-care, potential work-related problems, and family or cultural taboos or expectations. If the patient has had positive experiences with self-care, his or her attitude toward learning is more positive. It is advantageous to use teaching approaches that have been successful previously. For example, if a patient finds it easy to remember to take medications at mealtime or when a specific television program begins, that approach should be used in designing a medication schedule. For others, keeping a record helps to ensure that medications or treatments follow the prescribed timing. When patients admit previous noncompliance, tactfully ask them why they have not adhered to prescribed home care measures. The reason may be lack of finances or failure to comprehend all the components of a procedure. In these instances referral for financial or home health assistance may be the answer. You may also discover that the patient did not learn because of the teaching approach. For example, many young people learn best by using videotaped or computer-assisted instruction, whereas an older person may prefer demonstration and discussion. Occasionally, patients state that they did not follow through with home care measures because they did not understand what was expected of them. Possibly compliance would have been increased if their preferred learning method had been used.

Some occupations, because of either the nature of the work or unusual hours, may cause problems with follow-through in home care measures. Consider, for example, the needs of a long-haul truck driver who is treated for a bladder infection. The physician prescribes 500 mg sulfisoxazole (Gantrisin) to be taken 4 times daily. Recognizing the sulfa base of this medication, the nurse must teach the patient that increased water intake prevents the formation of sulfa salt urinary stones. Because the patient is a truck driver, carrying a thermos of water in the truck may be a logical home care measure. The nurse should also discuss with the patient a list of fluids and foods that produce the desired acid ash.

In some instances the expectations of the patient or family conflict with adherence to prescribed home measures. Consider the compulsive worker who is admitted to the hospital with recurrent angina. Because of his role as family breadwinner, he states that he has to "get right back to work." Obviously the nurse cannot change the patient's culturally based life-style with a single teaching opportunity in the ED. However, the nurse can seize this moment to explain briefly the causes and effects of angina and the anticipated results of the prescribed medications, and the nurse can refer the patient to the support group for persons with heart diseases in the community.

The objective of this step in the teaching and learning process is to elicit data and adapt the teaching approach to realistic, individualized learning goals that will help the patient adhere to prescribed self-care and prevent potential complications.

SELECTING AND USING APPROPRIATE TEACHING METHODS

The fourth step in the teaching process is to select and use the teaching method or methods appropriate to the content to be taught and the assessed capabilities and preference of the learner. Some patients require only a quick review of previously learned information or answers to specific questions. For example, consider the parent of many children, several of whom have had fractures and casts. This parent may need a quick review of cast care and activity restrictions. Other patients, however, require a more structured teaching approach.

Types of Learning

Three types of learning are cognitive, effective, and psychomotor. Cognitive learning involves thinking and reasoning: the focus is on comprehension of content and practical application to real-life situations. Effective learning involves a change in attitude or values. Typically, effective learning requires more time than cognitive or psychomotor learning. In the ED an effective learning goal is often achieved by referring the patient to a community health agency or a support group such as an ostomy or stroke club. Psychomotor learning requires coordination of the brain and extremities to complete a task. After skills are demonstrated, the learner needs practice time before a return demonstration is given.

Principles of Learning

The effectiveness of learning depends on several teaching and learning principles. A major tenet of learning is that active participation by the learner increases the meaningfulness and retention of the content. For this reason two-way discussion and demonstration followed by practice are more effective than a lecture of "do's" and "don'ts." Both verbal and physical incentives motivate learning. Physical incentives such as lollipops, balloons, or a coloring book are effective motivators for children. Adults typically respond positively to verbal reinforcement, especially when the reinforcement is accompanied by appropriate nonverbal behaviors. Successful efforts should be noted because this recognition increases the self-confidence of the learner.

Another principle of learning is that building on past experiences makes learning new content easier and increases retention. This type of learning is enhanced by the teacher's use of analogies and similes. Providing successful experiences by starting with the easiest content and progressing to the more difficult also motivates learners. Recall the old saying, "nothing succeeds like success." Actually, the building-step concept is the basis for our entire educational system.

Although a comfortable atmosphere promotes learning, the mild degree of anxiety prevalent in the emergency setting is not detrimental in most instances. Another principle of learning is that repetition strengthens learning, which is particularly true of psychomotor skills.

Teaching Methods

Teaching methods commonly used include discussion, question and answer, use of visual aids, and the lecture. The advantage of lecturing, or telling information to the patient, is speed, but the major disadvantage outweighs the primary advantage: there is no opportunity to evaluate the patient's comprehension of the content. Lecturing violates the first principle of effective teaching: participation in the process increases retention. Teaching is not complete until the learner has learned.

The advantage of discussion is that it involves two-way responsive communication. The patient and the teacher are free to question and respond to one another. The sequence leads to discussion of "what if" situations, which increase the practicality of learning. The question and answer approach is the most direct because the nurse is responding to the patient's specific learning needs.

Using visual aids as an adjunct method increases the sensory experience of the patient and gives meaning to abstract terms or concepts. For example, showing a patient the radiograph of his or her fractured bone provides a graphic description of the problem. A chart or illustration of the location of body organs aids in describing illness, defining the anticipated effects of prescribed treatments, or explaining the extent of trauma.

Demonstration is the most effective method to teach psychomotor skills. You may spend 30 minutes explaining the technique of figure-eight bandaging, but a 5-minute demonstration is more meaningful. When demonstration is used, the patient must have an opportunity to practice the skill before dismissal. This practice prevents errors in technique and provides the opportunity for active participation and repetition. Recent research has revealed that use of videotapes for skill demonstration provides accurate and consistent information in a cost-effective manner.[3,4] In addition, the visual appeal results in increased retention of the content. Another visual participative teaching technique is computer-assisted learning, which is particularly effective for patients with reading or hearing problems and for many computer-literate patients.[1] However, the use of videotapes and computer-assisted learning programs requires an initial financial investment in hardware and the purchase or development of software and also necessitates dedication of space in or adjacent to the ED. An extensive amount of software is available for purchase, rental, or loan. A number of pharmaceutical and medical supply companies produce and are willing to loan patient teaching videotapes and computer software programs to EDs.

Generally, the content and the learning goal dictate the most appropriate teaching method. In most instances more than one method is used. For example, if the patient needs to learn the technique of sterile dressing change, demonstration is the teaching approach of choice. However, an explanation of the rationale for the procedure and a discussion regarding the list of necessary supplies is also necessary. Potential problems related to bleeding and infection should likewise be discussed. A picture of both properly healing wounds and infected wounds would be helpful. This teaching scenario illustrates that in most patient teaching situations, multiple teaching methods are used to achieve a single learning goal. Planning ahead regarding essential content, necessary equipment and supplies, and potential teaching tools decreases interruptions detrimental to the teaching and learning process.

Effective communication is the one prerequisite common to all teaching methods. Recalling that the goal of communication is mutual understanding, use common, nontechnical words rather than medical jargon. When using health care terms, define words the patient may not comprehend. Avoid using medical abbreviations not generally intelligible. To emphasize the content of your message, match your tone of voice, facial expression, and body language with what you are saying. Consistency of verbal with nonverbal communication prevents the patient from receiving conflicting messages. Because enthusiasm in the learning situation is contagious, be enthusiastic about patient teaching. When the same content is taught repeatedly, sustaining enthusiasm may be difficult. Recall, however, that although this may be your fiftieth presentation of this content, it is the first for the patient. To maintain enthusiasm for teaching specific content, be creative and vary the teaching methods you use. Having a repertoire of teaching approaches benefits the learner, particularly when you are able to adapt your approach to his or her most effective learning style.

After the appropriate teaching method is implemented, provide the time, space, and necessary supplies and learning tools to permit the patient to absorb the content and practice newly learned skills. Learning new content and skills takes time. Rushing the patient's dismissal inhibits effective learning of the content and skills required for home care. Allowing time for the patient to consider practical questions and practice skills enhances retention and compliance with prescribed home care measures.

Occasional visits to the home by the nurse teacher permit the nurse to observe the patient's skill proficiency level and noncomprehension of content or technique and exhibits the teacher's interest in responding to the patient's questions, concerns, or fears. Also, during these visits errors in technique can be corrected before they become habitual. Occasionally a patient may ask a question you are unable to answer. When this occurs, consult another professional; then be sure to provide the answer for the patient.

When the patient obviously does not comprehend the content, try another teaching approach. In some instances, relating your personal experience is beneficial. For example, if you use a date and time calendar to keep track of medications taken, share this approach with the patient. Lack of space in an extremely busy or small ED can present a problem. However, to learn and retain home care measures, the patient needs a place to practice skills and to reflect on potential problems or concerns that may affect the patient's compliance. The use of an adjacent office or conference room for this purpose frees a patient treatment room and provides proximity that allows the nurse teacher to stop by to observe skills and answer questions as they arise.

EVALUATING LEARNING EFFECTIVENESS

Evaluating the effectiveness of learning is the sixth step in the teaching and learning process. The content and teaching method dictate the appropriate evaluation method. To illustrate, discussion has been used to teach home care of a casted lower arm. An appropriate evaluative question may be "To keep the cast dry, is it better to take a shower or tub bath?" If a picture has been used to depict the outcome of figure-eight bandaging that prevents elbow extension, ask the patient to identify the areas on his or her arm that require the thickest part of the bandage. Another valuable evaluation approach is to ask "what if" questions. For example, if an anticonvulsant medication has been prescribed, ask, "What will you do if you have the flu and vomit your morning pill?" Remember that the patient's ability to rephrase and respond correctly to practical questions indicates a higher level of comprehension than his or her ability to simply restate what has been said.

The most valuable method to evaluate skill learning is the return demonstration, whether the patient was taught by personal demonstration or by videotaped instructions. Recall, however, that practice should precede evaluation of skill proficiency. Many computer-assisted learning programs have built-in evaluation. One distinctive feature of computer-assisted learning programs is that the learner progresses only after learning the essential content. Incidental observations indicating incorporation of new learning into the patient's repertoire of behaviors is another valid evaluation method. To illustrate, after teaching active ankle range-of-motion exercises to a patient with dependent edema, you pass the door of his room and observe him doing the exercises without prompting. Likewise, when a patient asks pertinent questions related to self-care measures in his or her work situation, the patient has obviously correlated new learning with his or her real-life situation. Remember that the patient must understand the content before he or she can answer questions regarding how he or she will implement instructions for home care.

In a rushed ED, evaluating attitudinal changes is difficult but possible. For example, a patient with newly diagnosed diabetes says he will attend the local American Diabetes Association meetings, which indicates his interest in self-help. To validate his attendance, you may phone the patient or the association to ascertain whether the referred patient did actually attend. In some instances, when referrals are repeatedly made to a specific agency, a reporting system is designed to inform EDs of follow-through with referred patients.

Other evaluative approaches used by some agencies are analysis of statistical data regarding readmissions for the same problem and patient callbacks, in which patients are asked about their needs for additional information regarding home care measures.

DOCUMENTATION

The final step in the teaching process is documentation. Because of hospital policy regarding discharge instructions

---

SAMPLE PATIENT TEACHING DOCUMENTATION

7/10/92

9:45 AM   Sterile hand bandaging technique demonstrated. Instruction sheet "Sterile Bandage Changing" given to patient's husband, Jerry Howard. Correct return demonstration of sterile bandage change completed. Appointment card for stitch removal on 8/17/92 given to patient.

M. Miller, RN

---

and accreditation criteria and to prevent litigation, accurate documentation of teaching and of the patient's response is essential. As with all other nursing procedures, if the teaching is not documented, it is assumed that the teaching was not done. Complete documentation includes the following information: content taught, method used, patient response, adjunct instructions provided, date, time, and nurse's name and status. If someone other than the patient was taught the self-care measures, his or her name and relationship to the patient should be included. The box below illustrates correct documentation. In some agencies the patient also signs the form to indicate that the information was provided. Because the patient record is a legal document, precise documentation is essential.

HOME CARE REFERENCE SHEETS OR BOOKLETS

Because high anxiety levels decrease retention of newly learned content and skills, it is advisable to provide patients with home care instructional handouts. The diversity of instructional media has increased dramatically in the past decade. Whether you intend to purchase the handouts or design and publish them in-house, statistical data regarding patient admissions should be used as a guide when priorities are set for the purchase or development of these materials.

Sources other than patient care publishing companies and the hospital publication department include many national health care associations, such as the American Lung Association or American Diabetes Association, and state health departments. In some instances these publications are free; sometimes a nominal fee is charged.

If the hospital intends to publish instruction sheets, decisions regarding design, content, and personal responsibility for the project must be made. Within the ED, nurses with specific areas of expertise and interest can develop home care instruction material. Using the staff's special talents such as drawing, writing, and editing can be motivating; because involvement begets commitment, opinions and ideas about the final publication should be solicited from other emergency nurses. Williams and Manske[4] have suggested that when color, humor, and pictures that move or suggest movement are incorporated in the design of instructional media, the result is a more useful product. Successful patient education publishing companies have incorporated these elements in their design of information booklets (Fig. 17-2).

Home care instructions should be brief and clearly stated. They should be written in simple, nontechnical language. For example, if the patient prescription reads, "Bacitracin oint. To suture line, b.i.d.," the patient instructions should read: "After cleaning stitches with peroxide, apply antibiotic ointment to suture line in AM and PM." If dressings are to be reapplied, instruction for reapplication should be included.

THE BENEFITS OF MODERN MEDICINES

Used carefully, today's medicines
can do wonders. They can:

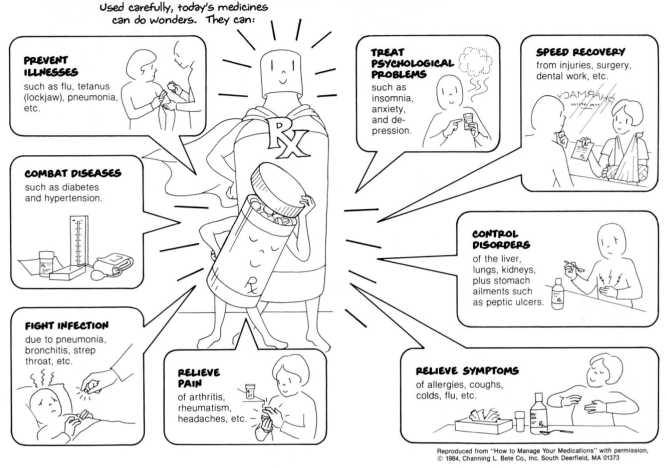

PREVENT ILLNESSES
such as flu, tetanus (lockjaw), pneumonia, etc.

COMBAT DISEASES
such as diabetes and hypertension.

FIGHT INFECTION
due to pneumonia, bronchitis, strep throat, etc.

RELIEVE PAIN
of arthritis, rheumatism, headaches, etc.

TREAT PSYCHOLOGICAL PROBLEMS
such as insomnia, anxiety, and depression.

SPEED RECOVERY
from injuries, surgery, dental work, etc.

CONTROL DISORDERS
of the liver, lungs, kidneys, plus stomach ailments such as peptic ulcers.

RELIEVE SYMPTOMS
of allergies, coughs, colds, flu, etc.

Reproduced from "How to Manage Your Medications" with permission,
© 1984, Channing L. Bete Co., Inc. South Deerfield, MA 01373

Fig. 17-2 "The Benefits of Modern Medicines." (From Channing L: *How to Manage Your Medications,* South Deerfield, Mass, 1984, Bete.)

As illustrated in Fig. 17-3, pictures can provide graphic directions. These pictures are particularly beneficial for patients who do not speak English or for those with low reading proficiencies. A graphic or a listing of objective signs and symptoms that indicate the need to contact a physician or the ED should also be included in a home care instruction sheet. When a language other than English is predominant in a community, providing instruction sheets in that language is beneficial. In some areas of the country all instruction sheets are available in both Spanish and English. In addition, some pharmaceutical companies are now producing patient handouts in languages other than English.

To ensure accuracy of information, institute a trial use period before reproducing large quantities of teaching tools developed in-house. In some instances minor refinements of content placement or wording result in a more practical and accurate teaching tool. Some agencies color-code the various patient instruction sheets to increase visibility. Store the instruction sheets in an easily accessible space.

Development of a teaching plan file benefits the teaching nurses who are newly employed or work as needed, as well as those who may be unfamiliar with the teaching needs of specific types of patients, especially those with rarely seen conditions. Typically contained in a looseleaf notebook or card file, the teaching plan outline should include the following information: patient problem and diagnosis; potential resulting problems; therapeutic, restorative, and preventive home care measures; specific content to be taught, in logical order; list of necessary equipment and supplies; and suggestions for teaching and evaluation methods.

To ensure inclusion of patient teaching as an essential component of patient care, the process of patient teaching and a review of the learning tools available should be included in the orientation of new employees and presented as an annual in-service educational program for experienced staff. In most agencies a policy and procedure for patient teaching is incorporated in the agency and department policy and procedure manuals. Documentation of patient teaching

COPING WITH DIGESTIVE PROBLEMS

If you are one of the millions of people who suffer from acid-related gastrointestinal discomfort, there are things you can do to improve your health and enhance the quality of your life.

1 Avoid spicy, acidic, and tomato-based foods like fruit juices and Mexican and Italian food (eg, pizza).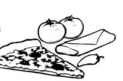

6 Don't exercise too soon after eating.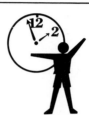

2 Avoid fast-food hamburgers and other fatty foods. Chocolate in any form should also be avoided by people with gastric reflux.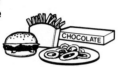

7 Avoid bedtime snacks and eat meals at least 3 to 4 hours before lying down.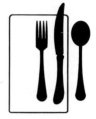

3 Limit your intake of coffee, tea, alcohol, and cola.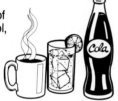

8 Stop (or at least cut down on) smoking.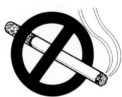

4 Watch your weight. (Being overweight increases pressure in the abdominal area, which can aggravate reflux.)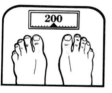

9 Elevate the head of your bed with wooden blocks. (*Don't* elevate your head by using extra pillows; this can increase abdominal pressure.)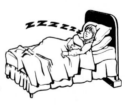

5 Don't gorge yourself at mealtime. Eat moderate amounts of food.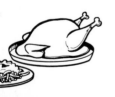

10 See your physician if you are taking antacids three or more times a week.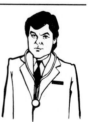

Provided in the interest of good health by: **Glaxo Pharmaceuticals™**
DIVISION OF GLAXO INC.
Research Triangle Park, NC 27709

Fig. 17-3 "Coping with Digestive Problems." (From Glaxo Pharmaceuticals, Inc., Research Triangle Park, N.C.)

is one of the elements listed in quality assurance criteria and in some instances is included in staff performance evaluation criteria.

Even though home care instruction tools have improved significantly in the past decade, they are only an adjunct to the individualized teaching approach selected by the nurse teacher.

SUMMARY

To ensure adherence to prescribed therapeutic, restorative, and preventive measures, the ED nurse is responsible for providing effective, individualized instruction regarding home care measures and the process involved in emergency care. This responsibility necessitates familiarity with the sequential steps in the teaching and learning process. The process includes identifying learning needs, assessing the learner, establishing realistic goals, selecting and using appropriate teaching methods, allowing for learning time, evaluating the results, and documenting the instruction. Application of learning and communication principles are prerequisite to effective teaching. Because all ED nurses must be familiar with the process involved in carrying out their professional role as nurse teacher, content regarding the patient teaching process is included in orientation and in-service educational programs. In addition, patient teaching is a criterion of quality assurance and clinical ladder or performance evaluation.

Home care instruction sheets or booklets are worthwhile teaching tools. These tools can be purchased from patient education publishing companies or designed and published in-house. These tools should be selected based on the typical patients seen in the ED. For inexperienced personnel and for atypical patient conditions, development of a teaching plan file can provide a handy reference.

Because knowledge of home care is a patient's right and also benefits the ED by reducing the number of callbacks and return visits, patient teaching can be considered an integral component of emergency patient care.

REFERENCES

1. Luker K, Caress AL: Rethinking patient education, *J Adv Nurs* 14:711, 1989.
2. Merritt S: Patient self-efficacy: a framework for designing patient education, *Focus Crit Care* 16(1):68, 1989.
3. Taylor JE: Recall and retention of adult patients using videotaped versus written discharge instructions in a hospital emergency department. Presented at 1989 Emergency Nurses Association Scientific Assembly, Washington, DC, Sept 8, 1989.
4. Williams M, Manske P: Efficacy of audiovisual tape versus verbal instructions on crutch walking: a comparison, *JEN* 13(3):156, 1987.

SUGGESTED READINGS

Armstrong M: Orchestrating the process of patient education, *Nurs Clin North Am* 24(3):597, 1989.

Emergency Nurses Association: *Standards of emergency nursing practice,* ed 2, St Louis, 1990, Mosby–Year Book.

Falvo DR: *Effective patient education,* Rockville, Md, Aspen Systems, 1985.

Miller A: When is the time ripe for teaching? *Am J Nurs* 85(7):801, 1985.

Miller M: *The nurse manager in the emergency department,* St Louis, 1983, Mosby–Year Book.

Padberg RM, Padberg LF: Strengthening the effectiveness of patient education: applying principles of adult education, *Oncol Nurs Forum* 17(1):65, 1990.

Pohl ML: *The teaching function of the nurse practitioner,* ed 4, Dubuque, Iowa, 1981, Wm Brown.

Redman B: *The process of patient education,* ed 6, St Louis, 1988, Mosby–Year Book.

Shipes E: Is your patient ready to learn? *Nursing* 17(11):131, 1987.

Tripp-Reimer T: Cross-cultural perspectives on patient teaching, *Nurs Clin North Am* 24(3):613, 1989.

Wound Management

Susan Budassi Sheehy

The two basic principles of wound care are to decrease the likelihood of infection and to promote optimal wound healing. To assess the injury and plan for care, several questions must be asked. Perhaps most important is to determine how the wound was created, what caused the injury, and what the circumstances were in which the injury occurred.

EVALUATION OF THE WOUND

Determine where the wound is. Location may make a difference in cosmetic attention, mobility, and the like. Look closely at the wound and determine the condition of the surrounding tissues. Determine whether the wound is jagged or smooth and how easily the edges of the wound can be approximated.

The patient's age, physical condition, and occupation may play large parts in the wound healing process. If the patient has a significant medical history or is taking any medications, this should be determined, because it may relate to the care given to the wound and to the healing process. Is the patient's skin in good condition and likely to heal well?

Find out when the wound was inflicted. Ask whether any care was given before the patient's arrival at the ED and what the care was. Finally, determine whether there is movement and sensation distal to the wound and whether pulse rates are present, indicating an intact vascular system, distal to the wound.

PROCESS OF WOUND HEALING

To effectively assess and treat a patient with a wound, it is important to understand the process of wound healing. Vasoconstriction occurs immediately when a wound is inflicted. Blood sludges, then vasodilation occurs, which causes the redness and swelling that soon becomes apparent in the subepithelial layer of the skin. Fibrin begins to form within 24 hours, when epithelial cells begin to migrate. This process is known as the proliferative phase of wound healing. Layers of collagen continue to form around the area of the wound that sustains the greatest stress during the sub-

sequent days and for as long as a year. The tensile strength of a wound site is weakest 3 days after injury.

Several factors affect wound healing. Some of these are the presence of preexisting illnesses or infections, the variability of the vascular supply, obesity, altered electrolyte levels, various oxygen levels, nutritional state and age of the patient, stress, and certain medications.

GENERAL PRINCIPLES OF WOUND MANAGEMENT

When a wound is large and obvious, it may be easy to forget that priorities of care should always begin with attention to airway, breathing, and circulation (ABCs). After attention has been given to these lifesaving priorities, direct attention to controlling bleeding and preventing the onset of or treating shock. After bleeding and shock have been treated, the wound itself may be assessed. Check the area distal to the wound for neurovascular and motor status, including skin color, temperature, distal pulse rates, sensation, and movement. Splint a limb if there is the possibility of a fracture or dislocation. If there is a possibility of wound contamination from the wounding object, culture the wound before irrigating it. Before cleansing or scrubbing the wound, anesthetize the wound area. Irrigate the wound with isotonic saline solution or another solution in accordance with local protocols (Table 18-1). The wound should be irrigated, using pressure for at least 5 minutes (longer if the wound is heavily contaminated). Avoid soaking wounds, with the exception of puncture wounds, which should be soaked for 10 to 15 minutes. Be sure to cleanse both the wound and the surrounding tissue. Removal all foreign material and debris. Consider shaving the area in accordance with hospital protocols. In any case, *do not shave the eyebrows,* since they may not grow back.

Before the wound is closed, devitalized tissue should be debrided. The wound can then be closed with suitable closure material such as sutures, staples, or tape strips. Usually the wound is dressed, and a light layer of antibiotic ointment is applied. In most cases, the wound is covered with a nonadherent dressing.

Table 18-1   Suture material for wound closure

Type	Description	Security	Strength	Reaction	Workability	Infection	Comments
NONABSORBABLE							
Silk	Silk	+ + + +	+	+ + + +	+ + + +	+ +	Nice around mouth, nose, or nipples, but too reactive and weak for universal use
Mersiline	Braided synthetic	+ + + +	+ +	+ + +	+ + + +		Good tensile strength; sometimes preferred for fascia repair.
Nylon	Monofilament	+ +	+ + +	+ +	+ +	+ + +	Good strength, decreased infection rate; knots tend to slip, especially the first throw
Prolene Polypropylene	Monofilament	+	+ + + +	+	+	+ + + +	Good resistance to infection; often difficult to work with; requires an extra throw; costly
Ethibond	Braided coated polyester	+ + +	+ + + +	+ + ½	+ + +	+ + +	
Stainless steel wire	Monofilament	+ + + +	+ + + +	+	+	+	Hard to use; painful to patient; sometimes preferred for tendons
ABSORBABLE							
Gut (plain)	From sheep intima	+	+ +	+ + +		+	Loses strength rapidly and is quickly absorbed; rarely used
Chromic (gut)	Plain gut treated with chromic salts	+ +	+ +	+ + +		+	Similar to plain gut; often used to close intraoral lacerations
Dexon	Braided copolymer of glycolic acid	+ + + +	+ + + +	+		+ + + +	Braiding may cause material to "hang up" when knots are tied
Vicryl	Braided polymer of lactide and glycolide	+ + +	+ + + +	+		+ + +	Low reactivity with good strength; therefore, nice for subcutaneous healing; good in mucous membranes
Polydioxanone	Monofilament	+ + + +	+ + + +	+	Excellent	Unavailable	First available monofilament synthetic absorbable suture; appears to be excellent.

From Swanson NA, Tromovitch TA: *Int J Dermatol* 21:373, 1982.

The patient should be given follow-up instructions that include care of the wound, indications of infection, and return visit information. The patient also needs to know about restrictions on his or her activity level and whether bathing or showering is permissible.

TYPES OF WOUNDS

Wounds are categorized into six basic types: abrasions, abscesses, avulsions, contusions, lacerations, and punctures. An abrasion is also known as a "brush burn." Such a wound is caused by the rubbing of skin against a hard surface. This friction removes the epithelial layer of the skin and may also remove the epidermal layer of the skin, leaving deeper layers of skin exposed. An abrasion has the same physiologic effect as does a second-degree burn. A major concern, in addition to risk for infection, is loss of a large surface area of skin layers, which may result in fluid loss.

Therapeutic intervention for an abrasion includes controlling pain, anesthetizing the wound if necessary, cleansing the wound by irrigation, scrubbing, or both, removing any foreign bodies to prevent "tattooing," and applying a topical antibiotic ointment and a nonadherent dressing. Occasionally these wounds are kept open to air. If a dressing is placed, it should be changed daily until an eschar forms. The patient should be instructed to avoid exposing the wound to direct sunlight for at least 6 months.

An abscess is a localized collection of pus. One should not wait for the abscess to "come to a head" before treating it. Therapeutic intervention includes preparation of the area by scrubbing it, anesthetizing the area, and draining the abscess with the use of a needle and syringe while the involved part is in a dependent position. An elliptic area of tissue should be removed with a scalpel. The wound should then be cleansed, packed loosely to allow for drainage, and covered with a loose dressing. The patient should be referred for follow-up care every 2 days until the wound shows good healing progress. If the patient is febrile, administration of antibiotics should be considered.

An avulsion is a full thickness skin loss in which approximation of the wound edge may not be possible. A severe type of avulsion injury is a degloving injury, that is, the full-thickness skin appears to be "peeled away" from a hand or foot or greater extent of the limb. Therapeutic intervention includes consideration of administering local anesthesia either by injection or topical application. If the avulsion is major, consider sedation and pain control. The wound should be thoroughly irrigated, and devitalized tissue should be debrided. Careful attention must be paid to the repair of disrupted tendons or muscles. Occasionally it may be necessary to use a split thickness graft or flap if the area of avulsion is large. The repaired wound should be covered with a bulky dressing.

A contusion is an extravasation of blood into the tissues without disruption of the skin. This type of wound usually results from a blunt mechanism of injury. Therapeutic intervention includes the assessment of neurovascular status, application of cold packs, and administration of analgesic agents if necessary. Covering this type of wound with a dressing is usually unnecessary. The wound must be closely observed if the contusion is large and located on an extremity, since compartment syndrome may develop.

A laceration is an open wound or cut that may range in severity from minor to major. A superficial laceration refers to a laceration that involves only the dermis and epidermis. A deep laceration is one that extends through the tissues below the level of the epidermis. Therapeutic intervention begins with control of bleeding by means of direct pressure. Neurovascular status distal to the wound must be evaluated and documented. The wound should be anesthetized and cleansed by irrigation. Take care to remove any foreign bodies and to excise any necrotic or devitalized tissue. The wound edge should be approximated and the wound should be closed with sutures or tape. The wound may require closure in layers if the cut is deep. Once the wound is closed, a topical antibiotic ointment should be applied, followed by the placement of a nonadherent dressing. Remember that if the laceration is deep and if there is a question of damage to underlying structures, the wound should be explored, either in the ED or during surgery.

A puncture wound results from penetration of the tissues by a sharp object such as a nail or a knife blade. A puncture wound may also result from injection of material from a high-pressure source such as a paint gun or nail gun. With injection injuries, underlying damage may be great, even though the wound at the surface may appear minimal. Be acutely aware of the possibility of gross contamination. Therapeutic intervention for puncture wounds depends on the depth of the penetration and the possibility of underlying damage. Some general guidelines for determining care of a puncture wound follow.

The wound should be soaked twice a day for 2 to 4 days. If the wound is thought to be contaminated, it should be soaked, anesthetized, and inspected carefully. Consider the possibility of the presence of a foreign body. If the foreign body is small, remove it if you are certain that its removal will not cause further damage. If the foreign body is deep and removal may cause further damage, determine whether the object can be left in place or must be removed during surgery. Necrotic tissue should be debrided. A drain can then be placed, and a sterile dressing can be placed over the drain.

If an impaled object is in the wound, the object should be left in place until it can be determined whether removal is safe. Be prepared to handle any complication that may arise as a result of removal of the impaled object. If the object is cumbersome, it may be cut to facilitate patient care and transport. Be sure to secure the impaled object so that it is not accidentally removed.

A gunshot wound is also considered a penetrating wound. The amount of damage inflicted by the bullet or missile depends on the mass of the bullet, its size, the velocity at which it was fired, and the angle of yaw, or entry into the body. If the bullet strikes muscle mass, because of the density of muscle mass, damage is usually severe. If the bullet strikes bone, the direction of the bullet may change and a fragment of the bone may break away and also become a damaging missile.

A small entrance wound and a large exit wound indicate that a high-velocity missile was fired at close range. The energy dissipated by a high-velocity missile is equal to the difference between the energy present when the missile enters the body and the energy left when the missile exits the body. Usually there is a violent expansion of the missile tract, which causes the disruption of arteries, veins, nerves, muscles, and bone. If there is a small entrance wound and no exit wound, this evidence usually indicates that the missile was low in velocity and is retained in the body.

The following considerations related to forensic matters must be considered in the case of a patient with a gunshot wound:

1. All gunshot wounds must be reported to the police, regardless of the circumstances surrounding the incident.

2. Carefully document both the condition of the patient and the appearance of the wound, including powder burns, bleeding, and the like, when the patient arrives at the ED.

3. Before moving the patient, prehospital personnel should make careful note of the environment in which the patient was found, including the position in which the patient was found, his or her relationship to objects, doorways, and so forth.

4. Do as much as possible to preserve the scene, but remember that preservation of evidence does not take priority over patient care. Lifesaving measures take precedence over forensic matters. Do not touch or move weapons or other objects unless moving them is necessary so that patient care can be conducted.

5. Whenever possible, place the patient on a "catch-all" sheet so that any bullets or other items may be found easily.

6. If clothing must be cut, cut it along the seams. Do not begin a cut by using the bullet hole or the stab hole in clothing.

7. Once clothing is removed, handle it carefully. Do not drop it into a pile on the floor. Whenever possible, hang clothing. Allow any blood or other fluid to dry before packaging the patient's clothes. When packaging, place each item of clothing in a separate paper bag. Do not use plastic bags, since they cause condensation to occur and may destroy evidence. Seal and number each bag and attach a patient identification number to each bag. Document the number of bags on the patient's medical record, fill out appropriate forms, and obtain signatures to ensure that the chain of evidence has not been broken.

8. Be sure to keep all clothing as evidence: do not give it to the family unless permitted to do so by the medical examiner, coroner, or law enforcement officers.

9. Avoid scrubbing any powder (gunpowder) from the skin. The area of powder dispersal is a clue to the distance between the patient and the weapon that was fired. If the powder must be removed for medical reasons, carefully document the appearance of the wound and the presence of gunpowder before removal. Whenever possible, take a photograph.

10. If tissue from the wound is debrided, save the tissue for forensic analysis.

11. If a bullet is to be removed, do so with gloved fingers or padded forceps. The teeth on ordinary surgical instruments can make marks on bullets and alter them, making them useless as evidence.

12. If a bullet is removed, mark the base with an identifying letter or number for later identification. Be sure to identify this bullet on the medical record in accordance with the body site from which it was retrieved from the patient and by whom it was retrieved.

13. Place the bullet in a small padded container such as a urine specimen cup. Do not place bullets in bottles or basins, which may cause additional marks to be made on the bullet.

14. When more than one bullet is removed, place each in a separate container that will be sealed and labeled with the patient's name, date, time, exact site of removal, and any other pertinent patient identifier information.

15. If it is not possible to turn the physical evidence over to law enforcement authorities or to the medical examiner's office immediately, place it in a locked box until it can be properly turned over.

16. Always obtain a receipt from the authorities when turning over evidence items.

17. If the wound is a shotgun wound, save any wadding, pellets, and the inner lining of the cartridge, since these may assist in matching the wound to the weapon that was fired. As with bullets, place the material in properly marked containers and follow requirements for preserving the chain of evidence.

18. If the patient dies, do not clean the body. Leave all tubes and other medical equipment that have invaded the body in place. If it is necessary to remove intravenous catheters or the like, circle the needle marks with a pen and label them according to their cause. Also mark any sites at which intravenous catheter placement was attempted but was unsuccessful.

19. Place brown paper bags over the patient's hands to protect potential sources of evidence such as fingernail scrapings, foreign hair, skin, blood, and gunpowder. Do not use plastic bags.

20. Do not probe the wound further after the death of the patient in an attempt to locate the bullet. Unnecessary probing could create false or misleading evidence for forensic reports.

A high-pressure paint gun wound is a form of penetrating injury that requires special attention. The wound may appear to be relatively benign, yet the injury may actually be quite serious. This type of injury usually occurs when a person attempts to clean the tip of the paint gun. The gun injects an aliquot of paint into the fingertip and, perhaps, up into the hand and arm. The result of this type of injury is a large amount of tissue swelling and compromised circulation, leading to ischemia and necrosis.

The patient who has been injured by a paint gun may demonstrate a small puncture wound, usually on the tip of the finger. Swelling of the extremity may be present, and the upper extremity may appear mottled. There may be local tenderness, and the extremity may be cool to touch.

Therapeutic intervention includes obtaining a radiograph of the injured part to check for the presence of paint, which is usually radiopaque. The patient's current tetanus prophylaxis should be ensured, and the patient should also be given tetanus immunoglobulin. Administration of antibiotics should be considered. Surgical debridement is usually performed in the operating room; a fasciotomy may be performed in the ED before surgery. *Do not perform* the following measures: (1) *Do not* soak the wound in warm water and (2) *do not* inject the wound with a local anesthetic agent. These measures may increase edema and ischemia and may induce vasospasm.

ANESTHESIA FOR WOUND MANAGEMENT

The most commonly used agent for local anesthesia and regional anesthesia is lidocaine, with or without epinephrine. Lidocaine is used with epinephrine when bleeding must be controlled in a highly vascular area. Lidocaine is usually preferred to other anesthetic agents because it is more potent than other agents, it is not irritating, and it has a long-lasting anesthetic effect. The disadvantage is that lidocaine is more toxic than the other anesthetic agents. Some other commonly used anesthetic agents are procaine, mepivacaine (Carbocaine), bupivacaine (Marcaine), and tetracaine (Pontocaine).

Regional anesthesia may be selected instead of local anesthesia to provide a greater area of anesthesia. Regional anesthesia is accomplished by applying a tourniquet proximal to the body from the wound and injecting an anesthetic agent distal to the injury. After wound repair is completed, the tourniquet is released and the anesthetic agent is slowly absorbed.

A local nerve block may also be the chosen mode of anesthesia. To accomplish a local nerve block, the anesthetic agent is injected along the course of the nerve; this mode of anesthesia causes the abolition of afferent and efferent impulse conduction for the duration of the anesthesia.

A mixture of 50% nitrous oxide and 50% oxygen may be used as an inhalational anesthetic agent for those procedures that are short but painful, such as debridement of a burn wound. Nitrous oxide is administered by the patient.

If wounds are extensive and wound care will be prolonged, consider the administration of intravenous sedatives or narcotics.

SUTURES AND SUTURE REMOVAL

Suturing is performed to approximate and attach wound edges, which decreases infection, promotes wound healing, and allows for minimal scar formation. The technique used to close the wound and the type of suture chosen depend on the extent of the wound injury. In some cases the choice depends on the preference of the practitioner who is repairing the wound. In certain cases the practitioner may elect to use tape strips or skin staples to repair the wound, again, depending on the extent of the wound and on personal preference.

Some general guidelines are used to determine when sutures should be removed. The variable is the state of healing of the wound. In most cases the following are recommended:

Eyelids	2 days
Face	3 to 5 days (followed by tape strips)
Scalp	7 to 10 days
Trunk	7 to 10 days
Hands and feet	10 to 14 days
Arms and legs	10 to 14 days
Over joints	14 days

TETANUS PROPHYLAXIS

Clostridium tetani is a gram-positive, spore-forming, anaerobic bacillus that causes the condition known as tetanus. Once the bacillus is activated, it is highly resistant to almost anything done to destroy it, including sterilization, because of its remarkable ability to form spores when conditions are adverse for bacillus growth. The incubation period can be anywhere from 2 days to 2 weeks or longer. The organism is present in many common places such as soil, garden moss, and anywhere that animal and human excreta can be found.

C. tetani enters the human circulatory system through an open wound. The bacillus attaches to cells within the central nervous system and causes depression of the respiratory center in the medulla. Signs and symptoms range from mild to severe. Mild tetanus is evidenced by local joint stiffness and mild trismus (the inability to open the jaw). Moderate tetanus is characterized by generalized body stiffness, moderate trismus, difficulty swallowing, and a decreased vital capacity. Severe tetanus causes a patient to demonstrate severe trismus, back pain, penile pain, tachycardia, hypertension, dysrhythmias, hyperpyrexia, opisthotonos, seizures, and mental alertness (at times other than during and after seizures).

Therapeutic intervention for a patient with tetanus includes ensuring the ABCs; administering oxygen at a high flow rate; and providing hyperalimentation, antibiotics, ventilatory support, and a great deal of general supportive nursing care.

Schedule for Tetanus Prophylaxis

The following schedule for tetanus prophylaxis is recommended by the American College of Surgeons Committee on Trauma.

Initial immunization series. In infants and young children give diphtheria, tetanus, and pertussis (DPT) injections as follows:

0.5 ml	At 2 months of age
0.5 ml	At 4 months of age
0.5 ml	At 6 months of age
0.5 ml	At 18 months of age
0.5 ml	At 4 to 6 years of age

For persons 6 years of age and older, give tetanus and diphtheria toxoid (TD) absorbed injections as follows:

0.5 ml	Initially
0.5 ml	4 to 6 weeks later
0.5 ml	6 months to 1 year later
0.5 ml	Booster every 10 years

Wound care. For the patient who is fully immunized (last dose given within 10 years), the schedule is as follows:

Non-tetanus-prone wound	No prophylaxis required
Tetanus-prone wound	If last dose was given more than 5 years ago, administer 0.5 ml absorbed toxoid. This procedure may be omitted if the patient has had many absorbed toxin injections

For the patient who is partially immunized (two or more previous injections, with last dose given more than 10 years ago), the schedule is as follows:

Non-tetanus-prone wound	0.5 ml absorbed toxin
Tetanus-prone wound	0.5 ml absorbed toxoid (passive immunization considered unnecessary)

For the patient who is not adequately immunized (one or no previous injections or if injection history is unknown), the schedule is as follows:

Non-tetanus-prone wound	0.5 ml absorbed toxoid
Tetanus-prone wound	0.5 ml absorbed toxoid plus 250 units (or more) of tetanus antitoxin* (TAT); also consider use of antibiotics

Tetanus-Prone Wounds

Tetanus-prone wounds are the following:
1. Wounds more than 6 hours old
2. Stellate or avulsed wounds
3. Wounds caused by a missile
4. Wounds caused by a crushing mechanism
5. Wounds caused by heat or cold
6. Wounds showing obvious signs of infection
7. Wounds showing signs of devitalized tissue
8. Wounds containing known contaminants

BITES

All bites, regardless of the source, are considered contaminated. In most cases, bites result in puncture wounds, possibly crush injuries, and perhaps, lacerations. When assessing a patient with a bite wound, determine the origin of the bite, the age of the patient, the general physical condition of the patient, the site of the wound, and the severity of the wound, including location, size, depth, and amount of contamination. Also identify the time between the infliction of the bite and the time at which the patient came for medical assistance. Find out what aid if any was given at the scene of the incident, and determine the risk for wound infection.

Infection, abscess, cellulitis, septicemia, osteomyelitis, tenosynovitis, pyarthrosis, rabies, and the loss of an injured body part are all potential complications of bites.

---

*Equine TAT should be given if human tetanus antitoxin is not available and only if the possibility of tetanus outweighs the danger of a reaction to the equine TAT.

Regardless of the origin of the bite, patients should be given similar discharge instructions, which should include keeping the wounded part elevated whenever possible, taking medications as ordered, and returning to private physician, clinic, or ED if a fever, redness, or swelling develops. Patients should also be instructed to return if red streaks appear, if the site becomes hot to touch, if pain at the site increases, if a foul odor develops, or if drainage occurs.

Human Bites

Because of the many organisms that can be found in human saliva, a human bite is one of the most serious bites a person can sustain. Remember that a human bite can be self-inflicted or caused by another person. The most common site for a human bite is the metacarpophalangeal joint on the ring finger. This site can become easily infected. Human saliva contains 10 bacteria per milliliter of saliva.[2] The gram-positive organisms are *Staphylococcus aureus* and streptococci. Gram-negative organisms may be *Proteus* species, *Escherichia coli*, pseudomonads, neisseriaceae, or klebsiellae. More than 3% of these organisms are coagulase-positive, penicillin-resistant *S. aureus*.

Human bites are diagnosed by means of history, teeth marks, and lacerations across the knuckles, which may have been caused by an impact with a tooth or teeth. The patient may be hesitant to tell you that the wound was caused by a human bite. Therapeutic intervention includes evaluation of distal neurovascular status, injection of local anesthesia, culture and Gram stain, irrigation and scrubbing of the wound, debridement of devitalized tissue, administration of broad-spectrum antibiotics, ensuring current tetanus prophylaxis, and giving the patient instructions for strict follow-up care. In general, the wound should not be sutured unless it is a facial wound.

Complications resulting from human bites include abscesses, cellulitis, osteomyelitis, and pyarthrosis.

Dog and Cat Bites

Dogs and cats bite approximately one-half million to 1 million people each year in the United States.[1] The organism that is usually present in the wound is *Pasteurella multocida*.[4] A large dog's teeth and jaws can exert a pressure of up to 400 pounds per square inch.[5] Certain factors increase the risk of infection: if the patient is less than 4 years of age or more than 50 years of age, if much time has elapsed before care is sought, if the location of the wound is in a poorly vascularized area, or if the wound is a puncture wound,[6] the patient is at greater risk for infection.

Dog and cat bites can be diagnosed by means of history, visual inspection of the wound(s), or the presence of infection, pain, swelling, inflammation, regional lymphadenopathy, and a low-grade fever. Therapeutic intervention includes a culture and Gram stain of the wound, possibly the administration of topical or local anesthesia, irrigation and scrubbing, debridement of devitalized tissue, suturing if necessary (although many practitioners prefer not to suture unless the wound is on the face), the administration of antibiotics, ensuring current tetanus prophylaxis, application of a wound dressing (optional), and consideration of rabies prophylaxis.

RABIES AND RABIES PROPHYLAXIS

Rabies is a virus that is found in the saliva of some mammals. The virus is highly neurotoxic. The incubation period is from 10 days to many months long. The patient who seeks medical advice with a history of a mammal bite is at risk for rabies. Find out the type of animal, where (geographically) the bite occurred, and whether or not the animal was provoked. If the patient has a reaction to the rabies virus, he or she may have symptoms that include malaise that has lasted for 2 to 4 days, a fever, headache, granulomatous lymphadenitis, photophobia, muscle spasms, or coma.

Therapeutic intervention includes ensuring the ABCs, performing a culture of the wound tissue, considering the administration of topical or local anesthesia, irrigating and scrubbing the wound, debriding devitalized tissue, considering closure of the wound with sutures (many practitioners omit this intervention), administering antibiotics, ensuring current tetanus prophylaxis, and adhering to the Centers for Disease Control rabies prophylaxis guidelines.[3]

Centers for Disease Control Rabies Prophylaxis Guidelines

Domestic dogs and cats. If the animal is healthy, can be observed for 10 days, and is without signs of rabies, no prophylaxis is required. If the animal shows signs of rabies, the animal must be destroyed and laboratory analysis of the animal must be performed. If the animal cannot be found, the patient must be treated as if he or she were exposed to rabies. Treatment includes administration of human rabies immunoglobulin and human diploid cell rabies vaccine.

Wild animals. Wild animals include wolves, foxes, coyotes, bobcats, skunks, raccoons, bats, and other carnivorous animals. All these animals should be considered rabid unless proven otherwise by laboratory analysis. Patients who have been bitten by wild animals should be treated with human rabies immunoglobulin and human diploid cell rabies vaccine.

Domestic animals, rodents, and rabbits. Animals such as cattle, rodents, rabbits, squirrels, gerbils, hamsters, and guinea pigs are usually considered nonrabid. If a bite occurs, consult the local health authorities for instructions. Usually no intervention is required.

SUMMARY

Regardless of the nature of the wound, patients should be given careful discharge instructions so that complications are minimized. Instructions should include information about keeping the injured part elevated whenever possible, how and when to change the dressing, and immobilization techniques, as well as a list of possible signs of infection such as redness, swelling, red streaks, pain, and local heat. Patients should also be given follow-up instructions concerning whom to see (for example, personal physician, specialist, or follow-up in the ED) and when to see him or her for further care.

REFERENCES

1. Callaham ML: Treatment of common dog bites: infection risk factors, *JACEP* 7:11, 1978.
2. Henrich JJ et al: Human bites, *JEN* 2:21, 1976.
3. Immunization practices advisory committee, *MMWR* 33:399, 1984.
4. Parks B, Hawkins L, Horner P: Bites of the hand, *Rocky Mountain Med J* 71:85, 1974.
5. Scarella J: Management of bites: early definitive care of bite wounds, *Ohio State Med J* 65:25, 1969.
6. Thompson HG and Svitter V: Small animal bites: the role of primary closure, *J Trauma* 13:20, 1973.

PRACTICE

UNIT

II

19 Shock

Susan Budassi Sheehy

"A momentary pause is the act of death."
JC WARREN

Shock occurs when oxygen and nutrients cannot be transported to the cells and waste products cannot be transported away. Shock may be caused by conditions that produce hypoxia or cause poor cellular perfusion. The components of the body that mainly affect the delivery of oxygen and nutrients to the cells are the heart, which functions as a pump, the blood, which transports oxygen and nutrients, and the vascular system, which provides the pipeline through which these substances are delivered.

TYPES OF SHOCK

The three basic types of shock are hypovolemic, cardiogenic, and vasogenic or distributive.

Hypovolemic shock is caused by loss of blood or fluid volume that may result from the following: trauma, hemorrhage resulting from other causes such as gastrointestinal bleeding or a ruptured ectopic pregnancy, severe burns, or dehydration resulting from vomiting, diarrhea, profuse diaphoresis, or nasogastric suctioning. Hypovolemic shock is primarily a fluid problem.

Cardiogenic shock results when the heart becomes inefficient as a pump. The heart can become inefficient as a result of myocardial infarction, pericardial tamponade, pulmonary embolus, or indirectly by tension pneumothorax. Cardiogenic shock is primarily a "pump" problem.

Vasogenic or distributive shock occurs when the vasculature dilates. Septic shock, anaphylactic shock, and neurogenic or spinal shock are three types of vasogenic shock. Sepsis, or septic shock, occurs when a massive infection results in an endotoxin release that causes vasodilation. Anaphylaxis occurs when a severe allergic reaction results in the following: histamine release, increased capillary permeability, and dilation of arterioles and venules. Neurogenic or spinal shock occurs when a spinal cord injury causes a disruption of sympathetic tone and a dilation of arterioles and venules. Vasogenic shock is a vascular or "pipe" problem.

Management of the patient in shock is most successful when therapeutic intervention begins as early as possible. For patients who are in shock, mortality is high. Care of the patient in shock presents one of the most difficult challenges in nursing. Determining the cause of shock is key to applying the appropriate therapeutic intervention so that patient survival is improved. Pay close attention to signs and symptoms: they may offer clues to the type of shock that is occurring. When shock is present, the entire body is affected. Most important is the effect on the vital organs. To function efficiently as a pump, the heart requires good perfusion of the coronary arteries. Coronary artery perfusion is decreased during shock, and the heart functions inefficiently as a pump. Stroke volume and cardiac output decrease, causing a decrease in blood pressure. Brain function begins to diminish as the supply of oxygen and nutrients to the brain decreases. The lungs do not function efficiently because the partial pressure of oxygen decreases as a result of a decrease in blood pressure or blood volume. Adequate oxygen exchange does not occur at the level of alveolar capillary cellular membranes, and the patient becomes hypoxic.

The liver normally detoxifies the blood by filtering out metabolic acids and other waste products. When shock ensues, the stores of liver glycogen are depleted because of an excess of circulating epinephrine. Because glycogen stores are depleted, the liver is no longer able to filter out metabolic acids, and metabolic acidosis results. Perfusion to the kidneys is reduced, metabolic acids accumulate, and renal failure sets in.

PATIENT MONITORING

A patient who has the potential to go into shock or who is already in shock must be closely monitored because the elements that are being monitored may offer early signs or symptoms of improving or deteriorating conditions.

Blood Pressure

Blood pressure is determined by multiplying the measure of cardiac output by the measure of peripheral vascular resistance (BP = CO × PIR). When either cardiac output or peripheral vascular resistance decreases, blood pressure decreases. Cardiac output is determined by preload, afterload, and heart rate. Preload is the length and force of the myocardial contraction. Afterload is the amount of pressure in the left ventricle necessary to cause the muscle to contract. An increased afterload causes stroke volume and cardiac output to decrease. Heart rate is the number of heartbeats per minute (beats/min). During shock the blood pressure is usually decreased, but in the early stages of shock blood pressure may remain relatively normal because of activation of compensatory mechanisms.

Pulse Rate

When the sympathetic nervous system is activated, pulse rate increases to provide a compensatory mechanism for a decreased cardiac output. During neurogenic shock the sympathetic nervous system cannot be activated, and the pulse usually remains normal. Bradycardia in the patient in shock may be a terminal event. The values that indicate the presence of tachycardia vary with age.[1] The box below provides these values.

Temperature

During septic shock, temperature is usually increased. During other types of shock, temperature may remain normal or decrease slightly.

Skin Vital Signs (Color, Temperature, and Moisture)

During all types of shock except vasogenic shock, skin usually becomes pale, cool, and clammy in response to sympathetic nervous system activation and subsequent peripheral vasoconstriction.

CAPILLARY REFILL

Normally capillary refill occurs in less than 2 seconds. When capillary refill is delayed in potential shock situations, the nurse should be aware that the delayed refill may offer a sign of shock or impending shock, and the nurse should observe the patient for other signs and symptoms. Capillary refill may be delayed in patients with hypothermia, Raynaud's syndrome, or other peripheral vascular diseases.

TACHYCARDIA VALUES FOR VARIOUS AGE-GROUPS

Infants: >160 beats/min
Preschool-age children: >140 beats/min
School-age children: >120 beats/min
Adults: >100 beats/min

Pregnant women may have a normal capillary refill response even though they are in shock because of the increased blood volume in pregnant women after the first trimester of pregnancy.

JUGULAR VEINS

Jugular veins may provide a clue to the cause of the shock. Check the patient's jugular vein while the patient is in a supine position. Distended jugular veins may indicate that the cause of the shock is obstructive (usually tension pneumothorax or pericardial tamponade); obstruction causes an increased collection of blood in the jugular veins. Flat jugular veins may indicate hypovolemia, which can be caused by hypovolemic shock or extreme vasodilation such as occurs during distributive shock. Be aware, however, that if hypovolemia is present concurrently with pericardial tamponade or tension pneumothorax, neck veins may be flat.

CARDIAC DYSRHYTHMIAS

In early stages of shock the most commonly seen dysrhythmia is sinus tachycardia that occurs as the result of the activation of sympathetic nervous system response. As the shock worsens and epinephrine stores are depleted, sinus bradycardia, a variety of heart blocks, ventricular fibrillation, or tachycardia may occur.

LEVEL OF CONSCIOUSNESS

During shock the level of consciousness in patients may vary from restlessness and anxiety to unconsciousness resulting from decreased brain tissue perfusion and cerebral hypoxia.

ARTERIAL BLOOD GASES

In early stages of shock, tachypnea usually occurs, CO_2 is blown off, and respiratory alkalosis occurs. While the process of anaerobic metabolism continues, metabolic acidosis ensues. Then, while the patient's respiratory rate decreases, respiratory acidosis occurs.

CENTRAL VENOUS PRESSURE

Central venous pressure (CVP) measurements reflect pressures on the right side of the heart and are indirect measures of blood volume, the effectiveness of the heart as a pump, and vascular tone. Normal CVP measurements range from 4 to 10 cm H_2O pressure. CVP measurements of less than 4 cm H_2O pressure are indicative of hypovolemia or vasodilation. When pressure exceeds 10 cm H_2O, pericardial tamponade, fluid overload, pneumothorax, or pulmonary edema may be present. When the pneumatic antishock garment is used, CVP readings may be falsely high.

PULSE OXIMETRY AND OXYGEN SATURATION

Pulse oximetry is a noninvasive method of measuring arterial hemoglobin saturation, thus, hypoxia. Light is transmitted through tissue, and provided that the other tissues remain constant, the variability of the transmission is determined by pulsated arterial blood flow. A sensor containing two diodes that emit light and a photodiode (light detector) are attached to the patient, usually in a fingertip or an earlobe. One of the light-emitting diodes emits a red light and the other an infrared light. The light absorption abilities of oxyhemoglobin and deoxyhemoglobin have been calculated and programmed into the monitor. A calculation can then be made of the percentage of arterial saturation.

TRANSCUTANEOUS OXYGEN MONITORING

A transcutaneous oxygen monitor can be applied to the skin to measure the tension of oxygen in the skin's surface. This device works by warming the skin and allowing oxygen to reach the electrode. The tension of oxygen is then reduced by contact with another electrode. This contact causes an electrical current to form; the current can be measured and correlates to oxygen tension. This type of oxygenation monitoring does not work well in patients who are obese or hyperthermic, or in those with severe edema. During transcutaneous oxygen monitoring it takes time for the electrode to warm the skin to 40° C, so this type of monitoring may not prove useful in many urgent situations.

ARTERIAL PRESSURE

Intraarterial lines may be placed via percutaneous puncture or surgical incision. Normally, mean arterial pressure is between 70 and 90 mm Hg. Readings of less than 70 mm Hg may be indicative of hypovolemia or vasodilation.

URINARY OUTPUT

During shock, when renal perfusion is decreased, urinary output, which is a function of renal perfusion, decreases. In adults the average hourly urine output is normally 0.5 to 1 ml/kg. A urinary output of less than 35 ml/hr may indicate shock.

PULMONARY ARTERY WEDGE PRESSURE

A measurement of pulmonary artery wedge pressure (PAWP) provides the caregiver with a precise indication of left ventricular function, which contributes to the evaluation of cardiac competence. Measurements of the patient's PAWP during shock provide a guide for fluid administration. Measurements are obtained via a flow-directed balloon-tipped catheter known as a Swan-Ganz catheter (Fig. 19-1). During the insertion procedure, the patient should be placed in Trendelenburg's position if the Swan-Ganz catheter is to be placed via the internal jugular, external jugular, or subclavian vein. Scrub the insertion site with an antiseptic solution such as povidone-iodine, and allow the site to dry. A percutaneous stick procedure or surgical cutdown is then performed to gain access to either the internal or external jugular vein, the supraclavicular or infraclavicular subclavian vein, the brachial vein, the antecubital vein, or the femoral vein. The highest incidence of pneumothorax occurs when the infraclavicular vein is used.

Advance the Swan-Ganz catheter through an appropriate needle or catheter. When the Swan-Ganz catheter is in the vena cava, inflate the balloon tip with room air or carbon dioxide and float the catheter through the right atrium and right ventricle into the pulmonary artery (Fig. 19-2). While the catheter is being floated into the pulmonary artery, monitor the patient closely for dysrhythmias, especially when the catheter is being advanced through the right ventricle.

Advance the catheter smoothly to discourage venospasm. When the catheter can no longer be advanced, deflate the balloon and advance the catheter slightly. Reinflate the balloon (Fig. 19-3). This reinflation should enable you to obtain

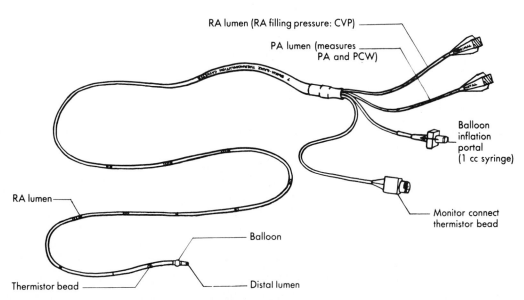

RA lumen (RA filling pressure: CVP)
PA lumen (measures PA and PCW)
Balloon inflation portal (1 cc syringe)
Monitor connect thermistor bead
RA lumen
Balloon
Thermistor bead
Distal lumen

Fig. 19-1 Swan-Ganz thermodilution catheter.

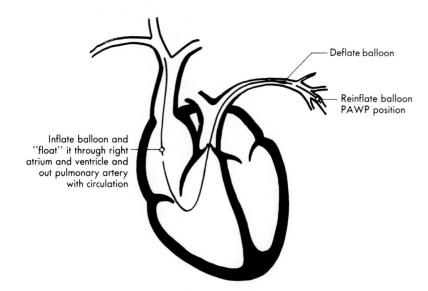

Fig. 19-2 Position of Swan-Ganz catheter in heart and great vessels.

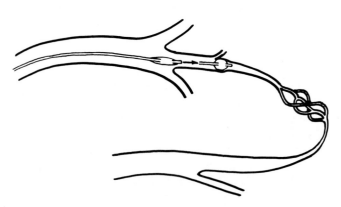

Fig. 19-3 Balloon inflated and floated into wedge position.

a PAWP measurement. To avoid local necrosis and pulmonary infarction, inflate the balloon for only a few minutes at a time. Always remember to deflate the balloon after obtaining the PAWP reading. Secure the catheter with a suture that also closes the small incision. Apply a sterile dressing to the site. Tape the catheter securely to protect both the dressing and the catheter.

COMPLICATIONS OF SHOCK

There are many major complications of shock. Tissue hypoxia, which is caused by chemoreceptor stimulation, results in an increased respiratory rate and increased peripheral vascular resistance. Hypoperfusion and hypoxia result in anerobic metabolism and metabolic acidosis. Respiratory acidosis also occurs when gas exchange is decreased at the alveolocapillary cellular membrane level. Acidosis results in increased coagulation, causing blockage of small vessels and congestion at the postcapillary sphincter. Precapillary sphincters relax, platelets aggregate and disseminate, and intravascular coagulation results. As perfusion to the coronary arteries and renal arteries decreases, myocardial infarction and renal failure may result. Cerebral edema also occurs when cerebral perfusion decreases and carbon dioxide accumulates.

When intestinal mucosa and endothelial cells are damaged because of decreased perfusion, sepsis may result. When intravascular volume, blood pressure, and colloidal osmotic pressure decrease, adult respiratory distress syndrome may occur. The box on p. 269 lists causes of shock.

HYPOVOLEMIC SHOCK (Hemorrhage, Low Blood Volumes)

Hypovolemic shock occurs when a significant deficit in intravascular fluid volume occurs. Normally shock is evident in a previously healthy individual when volume loss exceeds 25%. The degree of shock depends on the following factors:

- Amount of blood lost
- Rate of blood loss
- Age of the patient
- Patient's overall condition
- Patient's ability to mobilize compensatory mechanisms

The adult of average weight (70 kg or 150 lb) contains approximately 5000 ml of blood. A blood loss of 1250 ml results in shock if not corrected. A child contains 80 to 90 ml/kg of blood.[1] The most common cause of hypovolemic shock is trauma; trauma occurs when organs are ruptured or lacerated, vasculature is disrupted, long bones are fractured, or pelvic fractures occur. Hypovolemic shock can also occur in other conditions that result in massive loss of blood volume such as a massive crush injury, a severe burn injury, a gastrointestinal hemorrhage, a ruptured ectopic pregnancy, severe vomiting, severe diarrhea, or severe diaphoresis.

```
        CAUSES OF SHOCK

Hypovolemic
External major bleeding
Hemothorax
Hemoperitoneum
Fractures
Gastrointestinal bleeding
Major vomiting
Major diarrhea
Major diaphoresis
Renal failure
Excessive diuretic use
Fluid loss from diabetes
Burns
Ascites

Cardiogenic
Myocardial infarction
Cardiomyopathy
Cardiac contusion
Dysrhythmias
Diseases of heart valve

Distributive
Sepsis
Anaphylaxis
Spinal cord injury
Overdose
Anoxia

Obstructive
Tension pneumothorax
Pericardial tamponade
Pulmonary embolus
Intracardiac clot
Vena cava clot
Aortic aneurysm
Aortic stenosis
```

The diagnosis of hypovolemic shock is usually made based on close clinical observation, physical examination, laboratory analysis, and hemodynamic monitoring.

The box on p. 270 presents the four classes of hypovolemic shock.

Regardless of the classification of shock, be aggressive, identify the cause, and rapidly apply therapeutic interventions.

COMPENSATORY MECHANISMS IN SHOCK

When a previously healthy person has a traumatic injury with resulting blood loss, the body activates compensatory mechanisms. Four key compensatory mechanisms are activation of the sympathetic nervous system, activation of the renin-angiotensin mechanism, the release of antidiuretic hormone, and intracellular fluid shift.

Activation of Sympathetic Nervous System

Activation of the sympathetic nervous system occurs after trauma with blood loss. Epinephrine is released, and because of beta-adrenergic stimulation, heart rate increases and cardiac output increases. The result of epinephrine's alpha-adrenergic stimulation is peripheral vasoconstriction and a resulting increase in blood pressure. If a patient is in hypovolemic shock and is still conscious, he or she usually feels cold as a result of peripheral vasoconstriction.

Activation of Renin-Angiotensin Mechanism

As renal perfusion decreases, the renin-angiotensin mechanism is activated. When renin is released, it causes the release of angiotensin I, which triggers the release of angiotensin II. The effect of this activity is the release of aldosterone. Aldosterone promotes sodium resorption at the renal tubule level. When sodium is resorbed, water is also resorbed. This resorbed fluid is returned to the venous system in an attempt to maintain intravascular fluid volume, increase blood return to the right side of the heart, and to maintain cardiac output, thereby maintaining blood pressure. This compensatory mechanism also results in a decrease in urinary output.

Release of Antidiuretic Hormone

When hypovolemia ensues, the anterior pituitary gland releases antidiuretic hormone. Antidiuretic hormone promotes the resorption of water at the renal collecting duct. This water is returned to the venous system, where, as with water and sodium returned in the renin-angiotensin mechanism, there is an attempt to maintain intravascular volume so that blood return to the right side of the heart is improved, cardiac output is improved, and blood pressure is maintained. Urinary output decreases as a result of this compensatory mechanism.

Intracellular Fluid Shift

During hypovolemic shock, fluid shifts from intracellular spaces to intravascular spaces in an attempt to maintain vascular volume. Because of the cellular dehydration, if the patient is awake, he or she usually has severe thirst.

PNEUMATIC ANTISHOCK GARMENT

Although it is postulated in some of the literature that application of the pneumatic antishock garment (PASG) may cause an increase in systolic blood pressure, the mechanisms of action of the PASG are not clearly understood and its described actions are sometimes disputed. During the past few years there has been much controversy regarding the efficacy of the PASG; the garment's use has been diminishing because of claims of unchanged outcomes and possible delays in transport while the PASG is being placed.

For patients who are in hypovolemic shock or patients who are at risk for hypovolemic shock,[1] the PASG is intended to be used as an adjunct to other therapies.

CLASSES OF HYPOVOLEMIC SHOCK

Class I: Less than 15% blood loss
SIGNS AND SYMPTOMS
Mild tachycardia
THERAPEUTIC INTERVENTION
Control bleeding
No other action usually required

Class II: 15% to 30% blood loss
SIGNS AND SYMPTOMS
Tachycardia
Mild decrease in blood pressure
Mild increase in diastolic pressure
Mild increase in respiratory rate
Mildly cool skin
THERAPEUTIC INTERVENTION
Manage airway
Administer oxygen
Administer IV fluids
Consider pneumatic antishock garment
Control bleeding if possible
Consider surgery

Class III: 30% to 40% blood loss
SIGNS AND SYMPTOMS
Possible airway difficulties
Tachycardia
Restlessness, anxiety, or decreased level of consciousness
Cool, clammy skin
Cool extremities
Delayed capillary refill
Tachypnea
Hypotension
Decreased urinary output
Decreased central venous pressure and PAWP

THERAPEUTIC INTERVENTION
Manage airway
Administer oxygen
Administer IV fluids (crystalloids and blood products)
  NOTE: Replace blood loss with crystalloids at a rate of 3 L of crystalloids for each liter of blood loss. Consider blood replacement when beginning third liter of crystalloid infusion.
Control bleeding, if possible
Consider pneumatic antishock garment
Prepare patient for diagnostic studies or surgery or both

Class IV: Greater than 40% blood loss
SIGNS AND SYMPTOMS
Decreased level of consciousness
Tachycardia
Hypotension
Tachypnea
Cool, clammy skin
Delayed capillary refill
Narrowing pulse pressure
Decreased urinary output
Central venous pressure of less than 5 mm H_2O
PAWP of less than 4 mm H_2O
THERAPEUTIC INTERVENTION
Manage airway
Administer oxygen
Administer IV fluids (blood products as soon as possible)
Consider pneumatic antishock garment
Control bleeding if possible
Consider emergency thoracotomy

Adapted from American College of Surgeons Committee on Trauma: *Advanced Trauma Life Support*, Chicago, 1988, American College of Surgeons.

BLOOD AND FLUID REPLACEMENT DURING HYPOVOLEMIC SHOCK

After airway management, one of the most important therapeutic interventions for patients in hypovolemic shock is to gain vascular access and infuse fluids and blood products to replace lost fluid volume. For patients with major trauma, initiate at least two large-bore IV lines; use the cannula with the largest gauge and the shortest length possible. For adults, 16-gauge or larger cannulas are recommended.

The peripheral vein access sites used for patients with trauma are the external jugular vein of the neck, the antecubital vein in the antecubital fossa of the arm, and the saphenous vein of the foot. The central veins most commonly cannulated in patients with trauma are the internal jugular vein of the neck and the subclavian vein of the chest.

Often, surgical cutdown sites are cannulated in patients with trauma. The most commonly used surgical cutdown sites are the brachial vein of the arm, the femoral vein in the groin, and the saphenous vein of the foot. Usually a 7.5- or 8-gauge catheter is used.

Standard macrodrip IV tubing or larger "trauma" tubing provides maximum flow rate and should be used. Inline manual pumping devices, pressure cuffs, or commercially available rapid-infusion devices may be used to increase the rate of fluid delivery. Whenever possible, avoid the use of extension tubing, which slows the rate of fluid flow.

Ideally, fluids and blood products administered intravenously should be warmed before infusion: fluids that are room temperature or colder may cause hypothermia. A commercially available warmer may be used to warm fluids and blood. In addition, crystalloids (*not* blood or blood products) may be warmed by placing the IV bags on the defroster unit of an ambulance, by heating the bags in a microwave, by placing chemical heat packs on the IV bags, or by coiling IV tubing through basins of warm water. Regardless of the method chosen, fluid temperatures should not exceed 104° F. Remember, if blood products are cold, viscosity is greater and flow rate is slower.

Crystalloid solutions should be used in the early phases of trauma. Most commonly Ringer's lactate is used because it is similar to plasma in osmolality and electrolyte composition. Although normal saline solution is sometimes used, it should be used with caution because it may cause hyperchloremia, hypernatremia, and acidosis when given in large amounts. Hypertonic saline solution (7%) is being used in some institutions and in prehospital care systems on a trial basis.

The use of colloid solutions such as albumin and plasma substitutes is not recommended in trauma situations because these solutions often cause increased bleeding from raw surfaces, infusion is slower than with crystalloids, and colloid solutions often cause confusion during typing and crossmatching.

When the condition of a patient who has received 3 to 4 L of crystalloid solutions does not improve or when vital signs are indicative of shock, or when both situations are present, blood should be administered. The use of whole blood or packed red blood cells (PRCs) should be considered in major trauma situations. When blood is given, hematocrit should be maintained at 30 to 35 ml/dl, the level at which oxygen can safely be transported without delay in circulation time caused by viscosity increase. Local protocol should dictate the amount of blood ordered for type and crossmatch; type and crossmatch enough blood to provide at least 4 units, and instruct the blood bank always to stay 2 units ahead of the demand.

Blood that is used in trauma situations is usually PRCs. PRCs are whole blood from which plasma has been extracted. Risks of transfusion reactions and transmission of infectious diseases are greatly reduced when plasma has been extracted. Also, there is less citrate, phosphate, free potassium, and debris in PRCs than in whole blood. When large amounts of PRCs are given, bleeding disorders may result because of minimally functional platelets and clotting factors.

O-negative PRCs are given when there is no time to wait for blood to be typed and crossmatched. O-negative blood is known as universal donor blood. When large amounts of O-negative blood have been given, a reaction may occur when type-specific or typed and crossmatched blood is given.

Type-specific, uncrossmatched red blood cells may be given if the administration of blood can be delayed for 15 to 20 minutes while this type of blood is being processed. Type-specific blood is preferable to O-negative blood. Processing of typed and crossmatched red blood cells may take from 30 minutes to 1 hour. Obviously, type-specific blood is preferred, if time for processing is available.

The use of stroma-free hemoglobin is in the experimental phases. Stroma-free hemoglobin is hemoglobin that has been extracted from current or outdated red blood cells. This type of hemoglobin has no incompatibility factors and has great affinity for oxygen; disadvantages include a short half-life (2 to 4 hours) and the tremendous affinity for oxygen. So great is this affinity that it is difficult for stroma-hemaglobin to release oxygen at any level. In addition, stroma-hemoglobin may cause increased coagulation problems.

The use of several synthetic blood products is currently in experimental stages. Of these products, hetastarch and perfluorocarbon appear to be most promising. Hetastarch is a synthetic compound with an indefinite shelf life; it is similar in makeup to albumin and can be used as a volume expander. Perfluorocarbon is being used in a few health care facilities; it has oxygen-carrying ability and has been used in some patients such as Jehovah's Witnesses whose religious beliefs forbid the administration of blood products. To obtain information on how to care for a Jehovah's Witness trauma patient, you can call 1-800-NO BLOOD. This phone number will put you in contact with a group of physicians in California who are experts in the care of patients who cannot or will not accept blood products.

If a trauma patient has received transfusions that replace more than 50% of his or her blood volume during a 3-hour period, the patient should be closely observed for the following conditions.

Hypothermia

A patient who has received many units of unwarmed blood often becomes hypothermic. Hypothermia causes the oxyhemoglobin curve to shift to the left.

Hyperkalemia

When red blood cells hemolyze, potassium is released. Thus the patient's serum potassium levels must be monitored closely. If hyperkalemia does occur, it is usually transient and potassium levels return to normal when the patient stabilizes. If the patient becomes symptomatic or if levels do not return to normal, therapeutic intervention may be necessary.

Hypocalcemia

Banked blood contains citrate. Citrate binds free calcium. When citrated whole blood is administered at a rate greater than 100 ml/min, give 10 ml of a 10% solution of calcium chloride with every 10 units of whole blood.

Acidosis

The pH of banked blood is 7.1. If large amounts of banked blood are transfused, acidosis may become a problem. Mon-

BASELINE LABORATORY TESTS OBTAINED BEFORE AUTOTRANSFUSION

Prothrombin time and partial thromboplastin time
Thrombin time
Plasma fibrinogen level
Split product of fibrinogen
Serum potassium level
Serum calcium level
Arterial blood gas levels
Blood urea nitrogen and creatinine levels
Complete blood cell count
Hemoglobin level
Platelet count
Hematocrit
Urinalysis

itor arterial blood gas levels carefully, and pay particular attention to dysrhythmias that are induced by acidosis.

Alkalosis

Even though acidosis is an immediate problem when a patient is receiving large amounts of banked blood, eventually the citrate contained in the banked blood is converted to bicarbonate in the liver. As with acidotic conditions, arterial blood gas levels in patients with alkalosis should be carefully monitored.

Clotting Problems

Clotting factors are lost in most banked blood. Therefore coagulation times may be prolonged, and clotting disorders become evident. Observe the patient carefully for excessive bleeding. After 10 units of whole blood are transfused, give 1 unit of fresh-frozen plasma.

Debris

Although it is not known whether debris found in banked blood is harmful, a 160-mm micropore filter should be used when banked blood is transfused.[1]

AUTOTRANSFUSION

Autotransfusion is a procedure in which lost blood is collected, filtered, anticoagulated, and retroinfused into the same patient. In emergency situations, when massive blood loss occurs in the thoracic cavity and banked blood may or may not be available, autotransfusion should be considered. Blood from other body cavities, particularly the abdominal cavity, is considered contaminated blood and should not be used for autotransfusion in the emergency setting. Also, autotransfusion should not be used when the patient has a coagulation disorder or cancer.

Autotransfusion may prove useful in cases of hemorrhage because the blood is readily available, there is little delay in obtaining the blood, the patient will not have a transfusion reaction, all clotting factors are viable, red blood cells are available, the blood is warm, and there is no likelihood of disease transmission.

Although autotransfusion may prove to be a lifesaving procedure in many cases, it may not be available because no one who can set up the equipment and perform the procedure is available. A risk of bleeding exists because blood used for autotransfusion must be heparinized to prevent clotting during the procedure. Also, if the procedure operator is not careful when connecting tubing to the collection chamber, the possibility of air embolus exists.

The use of autotransfusion in the emergency setting should be limited to cases of intrathoracic bleeding. Blood from other body cavities should not be used. Autotransfusion is contraindicated in patients with poor liver function.

Baseline laboratory tests should be obtained before autotransfusion, and baseline values should be monitored after the procedure. The box on this page lists baseline laboratory tests that should be obtained before autotransfusion.

During autotransfusion continue other resuscitation measures, take readings of vital signs frequently, and record the amounts of chest drainage and autotransfused blood. Be sure to document the type and amount of anticoagulant used, and observe the patient for excessive bleeding, hypothermia, air embolism, and fat embolism.

CARDIOGENIC SHOCK

Cardiogenic shock occurs when systolic blood pressure drops to less than 90 mm Hg during an acute myocardial infarction, which causes the heart to fail as a pump. When the heart fails as a pump, the myocardial muscle is unable to contract effectively, that is, unable to pump enough blood to meet the body's needs. Cardiogenic shock usually occurs when more than 15% of the left ventricular myocardium has been infarcted. Concurrently, an increase in left ventricular end-diastolic pressure occurs. When cardiac output decreases, perfusion to the tissues decreases. In about 15% of patients having an acute myocardial infarction, cardiogenic shock develops; 85% to 90% of these patients do not survive.

Signs and Symptoms

Signs and symptoms of cardiogenic shock include signs of myocardial infarction, decreased peripheral pulses, increased but shallow respirations, and decreased blood pressure. (If blood pressure elevates, the myocardial oxygen supply is compromised and cardiac output decreases.) In addition, the patient has a lowered level of consciousness preceded by a period of anxiety and restlessness, clammy skin develops, and urinary output is decreased. The patient is also in a state of metabolic acidosis, electrocardiogram changes are evident, cardiac enzyme levels are elevated, and PAWP is greater than 18 mm Hg.

Therapeutic Intervention

Therapeutic interventions include administration of high-flow oxygen, initiation of IV lines, and administration of pharmacologic agents. These agents include inotropic agents, which decrease the left ventricular work load, increase cardiac output, and improve coronary artery perfusion. Appropriate inotropic agents are dopamine (Intropin) and dobutamine (Dobutrex).

Vasodilators are given to decrease left ventricular outflow problems, peripheral vascular resistance, and left ventricular filling pressures and to increase cardiac output. Agents used are sodium nitroprusside (Nipride) and nitroglycerin.

Corticosteroids are used to stabilize lysosomal membranes, increase lactate metabolism, and decrease systemic vascular resistance and the size of the infarct.

The intraaortic balloon pump (intraaortic diastolic assist device) is used to increase cardiac output, oxygen delivery, and blood flow to the coronary arteries. This device also assists in decreasing myocardial oxygen consumption.

VASOGENIC SHOCK

Categories of vasogenic shock include septic, anaphylactic, and neurogenic shock, all of which cause severe vasodilation.

Septic Shock

The most common cause of septic shock is an overwhelming infection that causes vasodilation and decreased tissue perfusion. Septic shock may also be caused by a suppression of the immune system. Blood volume in septic shock is normal—the problem lies with dilated vessels. The infection may result from an indwelling catheter, a massive burn injury, or a postpartum complication, among many other causes. The mortality from septic shock is 30% to 50%. Death from septic shock is more common in young infants and the elderly adults.

The organism that most commonly causes septic shock is a gram-negative enteric bacillus such as *Escherichia coli, Pseudomonas, Staphylococcus, Proteus, Salmonella,* or *Bacteroides.* Occasionally septic shock can be caused by a gram-positive coccus; septic shock is rarely caused by viruses or yeasts. These organisms enter the vascular system and cause the release of endotoxins, which causes fluid to leak into the interstitial spaces, increases vascular permeability and vasodilation, and causes severe hypotension.

Signs and symptoms. Signs and symptoms of septic shock are decreased blood pressure, elevated temperature, and elevated pulse rate. The patient may have chills and tremors, although the skin is warm and dry. The patient may also have nausea and vomiting, a decreased level of consciousness, diarrhea, and an increased cardiac output.

In the initial stages of septic shock, peripheral vascular resistance decreases and the amount of vasodilation is minimal, with an increased cardiac output. This phase is known as warm shock. Later, plasma volume decreases when plasma leaks into interstitial tissues and cardiac output drops because of a decreased preload and a decreased perfusion of the cells. This event causes a stagnation of blood and results in anaerobic metabolism and metabolic acidosis.

Therapeutic intervention. Therapeutic intervention includes administration of high-flow oxygen, IV fluids, and antibiotics. If any draining wounds are present, specimens should be sent to the laboratory for culture. Administration of inotropic agents (dopamine or dobutamine), naloxone (Narcan), and corticosteroids may be considered. In the literature authorities are increasingly advocating the use of naloxone in patients with septic shock. Naloxone blocks the release of endotoxin into the system and may reverse the shock.

Anaphylactic Shock

Anaphylactic shock is an antigen-antibody reaction that occurs when sensitized persons are exposed to an antigen to which they have an allergy. Usually the symptoms have a rapid onset. Antigens to which persons commonly have allergies include Hymenoptera (bee or wasp) stings, monosodium glutamate (a food additive), shellfish, and penicillin preparations. In addition, many antigens present in the environment, in food, and in pharmacologic agents can cause anaphylactic shock. When an antigen-antibody reaction occurs, tissue permeability increases and intravascular fluid leaks into the interstitial spaces, producing a form of relative hypovolemia.

Signs and symptoms. Signs and symptoms include respiratory difficulty, stridor, bronchospasm, wheezing, airway obstruction, or respiratory arrest. Airway obstruction may be caused by laryngeal edema or an edematous tongue. The patient's skin is warm and dry, and he or she may demonstrate urticaria or angioneurotic edema, dysrhythmias, or cardiopulmonary arrest.

Therapeutic intervention. Therapeutic interventions include maintaining airway, breathing, and circulation, administering high-flow oxygen, initiating an IV line, and giving epinephrine, 0.1 to 0.5 ml of a 1:10,000 solution by slow IV push. If profound vasoconstriction occurs, repeat the dose 5 to 15 minutes later. Remember that in true anaphylactic shock, epinephrine should be given intravenously in a solution of 1:10,000, not subcutaneously in a 1:1000 solution. A subcutaneous injection given to a person in shock may not be effective. Keep available a dose of IV propranolol (Inderal), since severe hypertension and tachycardia may develop as a result of epinephrine administration. You may choose to administer aminophylline for bronchospasm, antihistamines such as diphenhydramine (Benadryl), and corticosteroids.

Neurogenic Shock (Spinal Shock)

Neurogenic shock is caused by a decreased sympathetic tone resulting from a disruption of the spinal cord. This loss of sympathetic tone causes the arterioles and venules to dilate, and a relative hypotension results. Neurogenic shock can result from a spinal cord injury, direct damage to the medulla, or spinal anesthesia.

Signs and symptoms. Signs and symptoms include a decreased blood pressure, rapid, shallow respirations, a rapid pulse rate, paraplegia or quadriplegia, and priapism. If the patient has diaphoresis, the diaphoresis occurs only above the level of the cord injury.

Therapeutic intervention. Therapeutic intervention includes maintaining airway, breathing, and circulation, protecting the cervical spine, applying the PASG, and administering fluids intravenously.

Obstructive Shock

Obstructive shock occurs when an obstruction prevents blood from circulating. This type of shock can be caused by tension pneumothorax, a pericardial tamponade, a pulmonary embolus, an aortic aneurysm, a large intracardiac clot, severe aortic stenosis, or a vena cava obstruction.

Signs and symptoms. Signs and symptoms vary, depending on the cause of the obstruction.

Therapeutic intervention. Therapeutic intervention is aimed at removing the obstruction. The reader is referred to the discussions in various sections of this book concerning therapeutic interventions for specific causes.

SUMMARY

Because all cells require oxygen and nutrients to function and depend on waste removal, understanding the components of the all-encompassing term "shock" is important. Perhaps most important is prevention of shock. By understanding the possibility of the onset of shock and its early signs and symptoms, the nurse may help prevent the de-

velopment of a life-threatening condition. By being able to process the findings in patients who are already in shock and by acting rapidly to reverse this condition, the nurse may save lives. Thus the nursing process becomes invaluable: the assessment, the planning, and implementation of care, and the evaluation of that care are keys to preventing or reversing this deadly process.

REFERENCE

1. American College of Surgeons Committee on Trauma: *Advanced Trauma Life Support*, Chicago, 1988, American College of Surgeons.

SUGGESTED READINGS

Cardona V et al: *Trauma nursing*, Philadelphia, 1988, WB Saunders.
Davis JH: *Clinical surgery*, St Louis, 1987, Mosby–Year Book.
Fronaszeb JB: Cardiogenic shock. In Rosen P et al, eds: *Emergency medicine*, ed 2, St Louis, 1988, Mosby–Year Book.
Lawrence P: *Essentials of general surgery*, Baltimore, 1988, Williams & Wilkins.
Lumb PD: Critical care technology. In Gallagher TJ, Shoemaker WC, eds: *Critical care state of the art*, vol 9, Fullerton, Calif, 1988, Society of Critical Care Medicine.
Middleton E Jr: *Allergy: principles and practice*, ed 3, St Louis, 1988, Mosby–Year Book.
Miliken JS et al: Rapid volume replacement for hypovolemic shock: a comparison of techniques and equipment, *J Trauma* 24:428, 1984.
Robin ED: The cult of the Swan-Ganz catheter, *Ann Intern Med* 103:445, 1985.
Saletta JD, Gees WP: Initial assessment in trauma. In Moylen JA, ed: *Trauma surgery*, Philadelphia, 1988, JB Lippincott.

CHAPTER 20

Multiple Trauma

Susan Budassi Sheehy

In the management of multiple trauma injuries, the key to good patient care is a plan that is well conceived, well researched, and well practiced and that involves every member of the trauma team. If any phase of trauma care can be pointed to as most important, perhaps it is the primary assessment phase, when life-threatening injuries or events are identified and therapeutic interventions take place. The ABC4 primary assessment tool was designed for use by those who practice in the first-hour setting. ABC4 is a mnemonic that allows the caregiver to assess the trauma patient and intervene in an organized manner. The following are the components of the ABC4 primary assessment tool:

A (airway)

Ensure that the patient has an open, adequate airway.

B (breathing)

If the patient is not breathing adequately (poor rate, rhythm, or depth), adequate oxygenation and ventilation should be established.

C1 (circulation)

Assess central pulse rates and ensure that adequate circulation is occurring.

C2 (cervical spine)

Establish and maintain cervical spine protection by means of immobilization.

C3 (chest)

Identify the presence of life-threatening chest injuries: flail chest, tension pneumothorax, pericardial tamponade, or massive hemothorax; apply the appropriate rapid therapeutic intervention(s) when necessary and possible.

C4 (consciousness, level of)

Assess the patient's level of consciousness, if it is not already known.

ABC4 PRIMARY ASSESSMENT IN DETAIL
A (Airway)

In any situation, airway is of primary importance. No other therapeutic assessment or intervention should take place before airway management (except in the case of personal safety). The first action of a caregiver who provides assistance to victims of trauma should always be to establish an open airway. In the trauma patient, airway management

should be based on the clinical findings or assumptions of what has occurred. In general, always assume that a cervical spine injury is possible and manage the airway accordingly.

If the patient does not have an open airway, begin with the modified jaw thrust maneuver, in which the cervical spine is maintained in a neutral position. At this point, consider using one of the many airway adjuncts available (see Chapters 12 and 13). These adjuncts include oropharyngeal, nasopharyngeal, and esophageal obturator adjuncts, endotracheal tube, and surgical intervention such as a cricothyrotomy or tracheostomy.

As part of airway management, always ensure that adequate suction is readily available, that the suction cannula is the correct size, that the waste container is of adequate size, and that the energy source is adequate.

B (Breathing)

The goal of breathing and ventilation is to provide oxygenation at the alveolar-capillary cellular membrane level and to remove carbon dioxide and waste from the blood. Once an adequate airway has been established, ensure that appropriate oxygenation is occurring, which can be verified by obtaining measurements of oxygen saturation levels or arterial blood gas levels. All major trauma patients should receive supplemental oxygen, usually at high flow, until sufficient oxygenation can be assured. It may be necessary to provide positive pressure ventilation via mouth-to-mouth, mouth-to-nose, mouth-to-stoma, or mouth-to-mask resuscitation or via bag-valve-mask device or mechanical ventilation.

The need for endotracheal intubation must be assessed, and the appropriate means by which to accomplish intubation must be selected.

C1 (Circulation)

In the patient with multiple trauma injuries, first check for a central pulse rate, for example, in the carotid or femoral area. Peripheral pulse rates may be absent because of a proximal injury, in response to blood loss and peripheral vasoconstriction, or as a result of shock. Assess the quality of the pulse rate, its rhythm and regularity. Obtain a set of

275

vital signs including pulse rate, respiration rate, temperature, blood pressure, and skin vital signs (skin color, temperature, and moisture). Pay particular attention to signs of shock, especially to early signs and symptoms such as tachycardia and cool clammy skin. Be ready to intervene immediately should these signs be evident. The initiation of two large-bore (14- to 16-gauge) intravenous (IV) lines should be accomplished, and crystalloid solutions such as Ringer's lactate should be administered in accordance with hemodynamic findings. Before fluids are given, a blood specimen should be drawn to be used for type and cross-match procedures and other trauma-related laboratory tests.

Shock is a state in which oxygen and nutrients are not transported to the cellular level and waste products cannot be removed (see Chapter 19). In cases of trauma, shock may be due to hypovolemia, vasodilation, or cardiac problems such as those caused by pericardial tamponade or tension pneumothorax. Mild shock may be evident in an adult when there has been a 10% to 20% blood loss. A 20% to 40% blood loss usually causes moderate shock, and a blood loss of greater than 40% would most likely cause severe shock.[1]

Remember that blood pressure may be an unreliable indicator of hypovolemic shock, since activation of compensatory mechanisms (such as the sympathetic nervous system, the renin-angiotensin mechanism, release of antidiuretic hormone, and intracellular fluid shift) may keep the blood pressure within a more normal range for a period of time. Some of the first signs of early shock are restlessness and anxiety, followed closely by cool clammy skin, cool distal extremities, a rapid pulse rate, and a prolonged capillary refill time (longer than 2 seconds). Capillary refill may also be delayed if the patient is hypothermic or has peripheral-vascular disease. If the patient is conscious, he or she may complain of being cold, thirsty, or both. In the pregnant patient, even though she may be severely hypovolemic, capillary refill may remain normal because of the excess blood volume during pregnancy.

Use of the pneumatic antishock garment (PASG) is controversial in the treatment of shock. Refer to local protocols concerning its use.[2]

In addition to replacing volume, control obvious major bleeding whenever possible by using direct pressure, pressure points, or both. Vascular clamps and a tourniquet may be used if extreme measures are necessary to control bleeding.

C2 (Cervical Spine)

All patients who have sustained major trauma should be suspected of having a cervical spine injury until the possibility can be ruled out by radiographic studies. Three views are necessary to provide this information: a cross-table lateral view, an anteroposterior view, and an oblique view. All seven cervical vertebrae and the top of the first thoracic vertebra (T1) should be visualized. If this visualization is not possible, the patient must remain immobilized until a cervical spine injury can be ruled out by further radiographic studies, computed tomographic (CT) scan, or another method.

Meanwhile, the patient should be immobilized from the top of the head to the hips, protecting the thoracic and lumbar spine as well as the cervical spine. In addition to using commercially available immobilization devices, place a 2-inch-wide strip of adhesive tape across the patient's eyebrows and secure each end to the backboard. To remove the tape, cut it between the eyebrows and remove each piece from the center laterally.

C3 (Chest)

In the early minutes after a traumatic injury, several types of chest injuries that may otherwise prove lethal can be readily corrected to avoid catastrophe. Among the more common chest injuries is a tension pneumothorax. A tension pneumothorax may be seen after blunt or penetrating trauma to the chest region. If a patient has a tension pneumothorax, he or she may be dyspneic, anxious, cyanotic, have distended jugular veins, complain of chest pain, and have diminished or absent breath sounds, a deviated trachea, tachycardia, and decreased blood pressure and cardiac output. On a radiograph of the chest, a mediastinal shift may be seen, as well as the darkened area indicating where air has entered the chest cavity.

Immediate therapeutic intervention is to relieve the tension by inserting a needle into the anterior chest wall or by inserting a chest tube (see Chapter 25). There is also the possibility that the patient may require surgery to repair the injured area.

A flail chest is evidenced when two or more ribs are fractured in two or more places or when the sternum is detached. A patient with a flail chest is dyspneic and cyanotic, has tachycardia, and may demonstrate paradoxic movement of the chest wall. Early therapeutic intervention should include endotracheal intubation and positive pressure with the use of 100% oxygen. Fluid administration should be carefully monitored, since pulmonary contusion is usually present and pulmonary edema may be facilitated through this damaged lung tissue.

Pericardial tamponade can occur as the result of a blunt or penetrating injury. Pericardial tamponade is difficult to differentiate from tension pneumothorax because many of the signs and symptoms are the same, such as tachycardia hypotension, distended jugular veins, dyspnea, and cyanosis. In addition, muffled heart sounds may be heard. Therapeutic intervention includes administration of oxygen at high flow, placement of two large-bore IV lines, and pericardiocentesis (see Chapter 25).

A massive hemothorax is evidenced by the appearance, signs, and symptoms of shock. Immediate therapeutic intervention includes administration of high-flow oxygen, initiation of two large-bore IV lines, and preparation of the patient for emergency surgery.

C4 (Consciousness, Level of)

Usually by this time in the primary survey, you are familiar with the neurologic status of your patient. If, however, you have not had time to quickly assess the patient's neurologic status, you should do so. Use the Glasgow coma scale provided in the box below. In addition, use the *DERM* mnemonic provided in the box below to check the patient's level of consciousness, pupils, respiratory status, and motor function.

SECONDARY ASSESSMENT SURVEY

After completing the primary assessment, perform the following thorough, head-to-toe secondary survey:
- Observe the head; check for bleeding or deformity.
- Palpate the head and face (gently) for deformities.
- Check the eyes for pupillary response to light and for accommodation.
- Check the ears and nostrils for the presence of blood or other fluids.
- Check the mouth for foreign bodies, lacerations, or malocclusion of the teeth.
- Palpate the neck for deformities, the presence of pain, subcutaneous emphysema, or a deviated trachea.
- Observe the external jugular veins for distension or flatness.
- Palpate the clavicles.
- Observe the chest wall for bruises, hematomas, symmetry, or defects.
- Palpate the chest wall for the presence of subcutaneous emphysema, pain, or defects.
- Auscultate the chest for heart sounds and breath sounds.
- Observe the abdomen for the presence of bleeding, bruises, hematomas, or lacerations.
- Palpate the abdomen for the presence of pain, tenderness, or guarding.
- Auscultate the abdomen for bowel sounds.
- Perform a hip-rock maneuver or compress the pelvis to elicit a pain response.
- Check the perineum and urinary meatus for the presence of blood or obvious injury.
- Perform a rectal examination.
- Check the back and flank for bruises, lacerations, hematomas, or defects.
- Palpate the thoracic and lumbar vertebrae to elicit a pain response.
- Check the buttocks for obvious trauma.
- Check the lower extremities for the presence of bleeding, bruises, or deformities.
- Palpate the lower extremities for the presence of pain or deformities or both.
- Check for the presence of pedal pulses.
- Check skin temperature, color, and moisture.
- Check motor function and sensation.
- Check the upper extremities for bleeding, bruises, lacerations, or deformities.
- Palpate the upper extremities for the presence of pain or deformities.
- Check skin temperature, color, and moisture.
- Check motor function and sensation.
- Check capillary refill.

Order appropriate diagnostic tests and perform appropriate therapeutic interventions in accordance with local protocols. A rapid and organized systematic approach to the patient with multiple trauma injuries may prove to be lifesaving.

GLASGOW COMA SCALE

Best motor response
Obeys simple commands–6 points
Localizes noxious stimuli–5 points
Flexion withdrawal–4 points
Abnormal flexion–3 points
Abnormal extension–2 points
No motor response–1 point

Best verbal response
Oriented–5 points
Confused–4 points
Verbalization, exclamatory or disorganized–3 points
Moans or groans–2 points
No vocalization–1 point

Eye opening
Spontaneous–4 points
To speech–3 points
To noxious stimuli–2 points
No eye opening–1 point

DERM MNEMONIC

D (*depth of coma*)	Give a stimulus (verbal or painful) and note the response.
E (*eyes*)	Check pupil size and reactivity to light, and check for extraocular movement.
R (*respirations*)	Check rate, rhythm, and depth.
M (*motor movement*)	Check for movement of extremities, including decerebrate or decorticate posturing.

Protocols for use with the patient with multiple trauma injuries should be determined in advance and activated when the patient arrives at the facility. The following are sample protocols for use with the patient who has multiple trauma injuries.

SAMPLE TRAUMA TEAM PROTOCOLS

These are samples of trauma team protocols that employ a minimal number of personnel. Team assignments vary on the basis of the number of available team members. Also, protocols vary slightly in accordance with individual facility requirements.

Priorities in the Treatment of the Patient with Multiple Trauma Injuries

Before the patient's arrival

Incoming patient report taken	Nurse or ED physician
ED physician notified	Charge nurse
Trauma surgeon notified	ED physician or charge nurse
Personnel assignments made	Charge nurse
Trauma room set up	Nurse no. 1 or nurse no. 2
Blood bank and surgery department notified of potential case	Charge nurse
Respiratory therapy department and laboratory notified	Unit secretary

While patient is in the ED

Meet ambulance outside in driveway and assist in transport	Nurses
Scribe notes	Admit clerk
Patient transfer—ambulance gurney to hospital gurney, using cervical spine precautions	Paramedics and emergency medical technicians Nurse no. 1, nurse no. 2
Verbalization of initial priorities	ED physician or trauma surgeon*
Airway management	ED physician and respiratory therapy department
Intubation	ED physician
Suction	Respiratory therapy department
Breathing	
Lung sounds	ED physician
Arterial blood gases	Respiratory therapy department
Respirator or bag-valve-mask device	Respiratory therapy department
Circulation	
Vital signs every 5 to 15 minutes	Nurse no. 2
Chest compression	Nurse no. 2
Correct hypovolemia	Nurse no. 1 or nurse no. 2
IV lines	Nurse no. 1
Central line or arterial line	ED physician
Blood collection (4 clot tests and complete blood count)	Nurse no. 1, ED physician, and laboratory
Laboratory slips	Admitting clerk
Hemorrhage control	ED physician

*From this point on, physician may be either emergency medical physician or trauma surgeon.

Depth of coma (neurologic assessment)	ED physician
Electrocardiogram (that is, monitor leads)	Nurse no. 2
Record rhythm strip	Nurse no. 2
Drugs and defibrillation	Nurse no. 1
Cross-table lateral cervical spine film	Radiology department
Read film	ED physician
Completely undress patient	Nurse no. 1 and nurse no. 2
Examine back	ED physician
Further assessment	ED physician
Order diagnostic tests	ED physician
Consultations	ED physician and admitting clerk
12-lead ECG	Laboratory
Notification of surgery (potential surgery)	Charge nurse
Chest evaluation	ED physician
Chest tube set up	Nurse no. 1
Pleur-Evac (Deknatel Division, Pfizer Hospital Products Group, Inc. Fall River, Mass.)	Nurse no. 2
Instruments and surgical field	Nurse no. 2
Thoracotomy set up (instruments and surgical field)	Nurse no. 1

HEAD INJURY

Consider notification of trauma surgeon at time of radio contact. Anticipate need for CT scan.

1. Airway
   - If possible, maintain with nasopharyngeal airway.
   - If endotracheal intubation is required, perform blind nasotracheal intubation (contraindicated if cribriform plate fracture or severe maxillofacial injury is suspected).
   - Use vasoconstrictor (cocaine 4%) in nose before nasotracheal intubation.
   - Prepare cocaine, cotton balls, bayonette forceps, and nasal speculum.
   - Consider administration of lidocaine bolus 1 mg/kg before nasotracheal intubation to decrease chance of dysrhythmias and to cause a temporary decrease in intracranial pressure.
   - If results of cervical spine radiograph are negative, use nasotracheal route.
   - Consider cricothyroidotomy if unable to maintain airway by other means.
   - Consider use of pancuronium (Pavulon) or other neuromuscular blocking agent for the combative patient, especially if CT scan will be performed.
2. Breathing
   - Obtain ABCs (65% of patients have hypoxia or hypercapnia).
   - Hyperventilate patient with 100% oxygen using bag-valve-mask device to maintain P_{CO_2} at about 28 torr.
   - Have suction equipment ready.
   - Anticipate emesis.
   - Be prepared to ventilate patient.

3. Circulation
   - Ensure carotid, femoral, or radial pulse rates.
   - Apply chest compression if necessary.
   - Control external bleeding.
   - Administer IV fluids:
     Start two large-bore IV lines (14- to 16-gauge), and administer Ringer's lactate or normal saline solution. Run at rate to maintain blood pressure above 100 mm Hg.
   - Use PASG as indicated by local protocols.
   - Have laboratory tests performed before surgery.
   - Type and screen blood for 2 + units packed red blood cells.
4. Protect cervical spine.
   - Immobilize cervical spine completely.
   - Leave as is until results of cervical spine radiographs have been read as negative.
   - Obtain cross-table lateral cervical spine radiograph.
   - Visualize spine to C7-T1 level if possible; may need left lateral swimmer's view.
   - Anteroposterior open-mouth odontoid and oblique views should also be obtained.
5. Undress patient.
   - Examine back (if cervical spine has not been cleared, use caution).
   - Logroll the patient when changing positions.
6. Neurologic assessment
   - Use Glasgow coma scale or DERM mnemonic when the patient is admitted to the ED, 15 minutes after admission to the ED, 1 hour after admission to the ED, every hour after that, and more often as indicated.
   - Include rectal examination to check for anal wink, sphincter tone, or both.
   - Consider administration of diazepam (Valium) to control seizures.
   - Consider use of mannitol, furosemide, or both in cases of head injury with intracranial pressure, to decrease cerebral edema.
7. Check vital signs frequently.
   - Blood pressure
   - Respiration rate
   - Pulse rate
   - Temperature
   - Skin vital signs (color, temperature, and moisture)
8. Notify anesthesia and surgery departments if surgery is possible.
9. Consider performing a CT scan.
10. Ensure tetanus prophylaxis.
11. Consider administration of dextrose 50% and naloxone (Narcan) for the unconscious patient.
12. Prepare intracranial pressure monitoring tray.
13. Maintain good head alignment in patient. Do not allow head to tilt to one side or the other.
14. Check for seizures, agitation, increased intrathoracic pressure, hypoxia, or hypotension, since all increase intracranial pressure.

CERVICAL SPINE INJURY

Consider notification of trauma surgeon at time of radio contact.

1. Airway
   - If necessary and possible, maintain with nasopharyngeal airway adjunct.
   - If endotracheal intubation is required, obtain cross-table lateral cervical spine radiographs before intubation if possible.
   - If cervical spine fracture or dislocation is present, if unable to get cervical spine radiograph, or if intubation is necessary, perform blind nasotracheal intubation. Use vasoconstrictor (cocaine 4%) in nose before nasotracheal intubation. Have ready cocaine, cotton balls, bayonette forceps, and nasal speculum. Consider administration of lidocaine bolus 1 mg/kg before nasotracheal intubation to decrease chance of ventricular dysrhythmias. If bradycardia occurs during intubation (probably as a result of vagal stimulation), consider atrophic administration.
   - Consider cricothyroidotomy.
2. Breathing
   - Assure adequate ventilation.
   - Provide supplemental oxygen via nasal cannula or face mask.
   - If patient has concurrent head injury, hyperventilate patient with 100% oxygen.
   - Have suction equipment ready.
   - Anticipate emesis; prevent aspiration.
3. Circulation
   - Apply chest compression as required.
   - Start IV lines with Ringer's lactate or normal saline solution to maintain blood pressure above 100 mm Hg.
   - Consider PASG according to local protocols.
   - Have laboratory tests performed before surgery.
   - Type and screen patient's blood to always stay 2 units ahead of need.
   - Control external bleeding.
   - Consider use of a vasopressor (dopamine).
4. Stabilize cervical spine.
   - Avoid hyperextension, flexion, or lateral movement.
5. Obtain cross-table lateral cervical spine radiograph (visualize at least to C7-T1 level) as an initial screen. Eventually a full spinal series or scan must be performed before injury can be ruled out.
6. Undress patient; observe back.
   - If there is risk for or presence of cervical spine injury, cut away clothing.
   - Logroll patient.
7. Neurologic assessment
   - Use either Glasgow coma scale or DERM mnemonic when the patient is admitted to the ED, 15 minutes after admission, 1 hour after admission, and every hour thereafter or as required.

- Perform rectal examination to check for anal wink, sphincter tone, or both.
8. Administer high-dose methylprednisolone in accordance with protocols (see Chapter 22).
9. Check vital signs frequently.
    - Blood pressure
    - Pulse rate
    - Temperature
    - Respiration rate
    - Skin vital signs (color, temperature, and moisture)
    - ECG monitor
10. Consider use of nasogastric tube.
    - Place earlier if airway is unprotected (to decompress stomach).
    - Carefully monitor cardiac rhythm, since vagal stimulation may cause severe bradycardia or even asystole.
11. Keep patient in fasting state.
12. Consult with trauma surgeon and neurosurgeon. Notify anesthesia and surgery departments if surgery is considered a possibility.
13. Consider use of traction. Usually Gardner-Wells tongs or Tippi-Wells tongs can be employed with traction.
14. Insert a Foley catheter.
    - Check urine for presence of blood with dipstick.
    - Send specimen to laboratory for urinalysis.
    - Measure hourly urine output.
15. Consider pharmacologic intervention to decrease likelihood of cord edema. Consider administration of diuretics.
16. Collect information regarding time of accident and mechanism of injury.
17. Consider performing blood alcohol or toxicology screen.
18. Carefully assess for other injuries, recognizing that patients with spinal cord injuries may not be aware of injuries to other parts of their bodies.
19. Consider administration of antibiotics.
20. Consider tetanus prophylaxis.
21. Review causes of unconsciousness using the following mnemonic:
    - A = Alcohol (acute or chronic)
    - E = Epilepsy
    - I = Insulin (too much or too little)
    - O = Overdose (or underdose)
    - U = Uremia (or other toxic problems)
    - T = Trauma or tumors
    - I = Infections (usually central nervous system)
    - P = Psychiatric
    - S = Stroke (or other neurologic or other cardiovascular cause)

CHEST TRAUMA

Consider notification of trauma surgeon at time of radio contact.

1. Airway
    - Maintain open airway.
    - Use appropriate airway adjunct.
2. Breathing
    - Give supplemental oxygen; ventilate well.
    - Have suction readily available; anticipate emesis; prevent aspiration.
    - Treat tension pneumothorax using anterior chest needle(s) or chest tube(s).
    - Prepare chest tube and collection device.
    - Prepare patient for autotransfusion.
3. Circulation
    - Check capillary refill (>2 seconds = shock).
    - Check jugular venous distension.
    - Ensure adequate carotid or femoral pulse rates.
        If carotid pulse rate is present, blood pressure is at least 60 mm Hg. If femoral pulse is present, blood pressure is at least 70 mm Hg.
    - Check radial or brachial arteries for equality.
    - If radial pulse rate is present, blood pressure is at least 80 mm Hg.
    - Start 2 large-bore IV lines and administer warmed Ringer's lactate or normal saline solution.
    - Consider use of autotransfusion.
    - Prepare for thoracotomy if cardiopulmonary arrest or suspected penetrating injury to heart with severe cardiovascular deterioration has occurred.
    - Prepare for pericardiocentesis or pericardial window if pericardial tamponade is present.
    - Monitor ECG.
    - Control external bleeding.
    - Check vital signs frequently; check skin vital signs (color, temperature, and moisture) frequently.
    - Obtain routine surgical laboratory tests.
    - Measure hourly urine output.
    - Type and cross-match blood for packed red blood cells.
    - Do *not* remove penetrating objects unless ensured that consequences can be controlled.
4. Consult trauma surgeon.
5. Protect cervical spine and lumbar-sacral spine; obtain cross-table lateral cervical spine radiographs.
6. Undress patient.
    - Keep patient warm by covering him or her with warm blanket.
    - Examine patient's back.
7. Have portable chest radiograph (upright if possible and safe) made.
8. Assess level of consciousness. Use Glasgow coma scale and DERM mnemonic or ATLS mnemonic (A = Alert; V = Verbal stimulus, response to; P = Pain, response to; U = Unresponsive).
9. Monitor 12-lead ECG.
10. Notify anesthesia and surgery nursing staff if surgery is a possibility (if not notified earlier); nurse may wish

to come to the ED to evaluate patient's potential operating room needs; may assist with thoracotomy.

11. Insert Foley catheter.
    - Check urine for presence of blood with dipstick.
    - Send specimen to laboratory for urinalysis.
12. Consider nasogastric intubation as early as possible, since it also assists with identification of anatomic landmarks and helps rule out a ruptured diaphragm, tension pneumothorax, and ruptured aorta.
13. Perform secondary, head-to-toe trauma survey. Be sure to include the following in history:
    - A = Allergies
    - M = Medications
    - P = Past medical history
    - L = Last meal
    - E = Events surrounding the incident*
14. Consider administration of antibiotics.
15. Consider administration of tetanus toxoid.
16. Consider performing blood alcohol or toxicology screen.

ABDOMINAL AND PELVIC TRAUMA

Consider notification of trauma surgeon at time of radio contact.

1. Airway
   - Maintain open airway.
   - Use appropriate airway adjunct.
   - Protect cervical and lumbar-sacral spine.
2. Breathing
   - Ensure adequate oxygenation.
   - Give supplemental oxygen via appropriate delivery system.
   - Have suction equipment readily available.
   - Anticipate emesis; avoid aspiration.
3. Circulation
   - Ensure adequate circulation.
   - Provide chest compression if necessary.
   - Start 2 large-bore IV lines, and administer Ringer's lactate or normal saline solution.
   - Run IV lines wide open if systolic blood pressure is less than 90 mm Hg and there are other associated signs of shock (such as rapid pulse rate or decreased level of consciousness).
   - Consider use of PASG if blood pressure is less than 80 mm Hg.
   - Do *not* remove penetrating objects unless they are life threatening (for instance, blood pressure is extremely low and abdominal section of PASG is absolutely necessary).
   - If patient is pregnant,† or has chronic obstructive

---

*From American College of Surgeons, Advanced Trauma Life Support, 1984.

†Note: If a pregnant patient is hypotensive, the condition may be caused by pressure on the inferior vena cava from the uterus and fetus. Therefore attempt to elevate the right hip, turn the patient on her side if possible, or manually distract the uterus.

pulmonary disease or tension pneumothorax, inflate leg units only, initially.
   - Control external bleeding with direct pressure.
   - Obtain routine surgical laboratory tests.
   - Type and screen blood for 4 to 10 units of blood.
   - Monitor vital signs (including motor movement).
4. Notify anesthesia department and operating room if surgery is a possibility.
5. Undress patient.
6. Check level of consciousness.
7. Insert Foley catheter.
   - If blood at meatus, scrotal hematoma, or high-riding prostate is found during rectal examination, do not perform urethral catheterization until urethrogram is performed and confirms that urethra is intact.
   - Check urine for presence of blood with dipstick.
   - Send specimen to laboratory for urinalysis.
8. Insert nasogastric tube.
9. Consider peritoneal lavage or abdominal CT if patient's condition is stable. If CT will be performed, instill contrast dye in accordance with local protocol.
10. Monitor 12-lead ECG.
11. Perform secondary trauma survey.
12. Perform bimanual rectal examination. Consider pelvic examination for women with direct trauma to lower abdomen or genitals.
13. Consider administration of antibiotics.
14. Consider tetanus prophylaxis.
15. Consider performing blood alcohol or toxicology screen.
16. Consider pregnancy test.
17. Consider "one-shot" intravenous pyelogram to check for renal involvement.

LIMB TRAUMA

Consider notification of trauma surgeon, orthopedic surgeon, or both, at time of radio contact.

1. Airway
   - Ensure open airway.
   - Use adjuncts as indicated.
   - Protect cervical spine.
2. Breathing
   - Administer oxygen as indicated.
   - Have suction equipment readily available.
   - Protect cervical spine.
3. Circulation
   - Ensure adequate carotid or femoral pulse rates.
   - Provide cardiopulmonary resuscitation (CPR) if necessary.
   - Start IV lines in accordance with early assessment of injury.
   - Use PASG if indicated.
   - Have laboratory tests performed before surgery.
   - Type and screen blood for 2 to 4 units of blood.
4. Check chest for tension, flail, tamponade, or massive intrathoracic hemorrhage (life-threatening conditions).

5. Undress patient. Check patient's back.
6. Perform neurologic examination.
   - Use DERM mnemonic or Glasgow coma scale.
7. Control external bleeding.
8. Check distal neurovascular status of involved limb(s), and record status on chart.
9. Pad and splint from joint above and below the joint injury to immobilize limb.
   - Use traction on femur fracture.
   - Apply manual skeletal traction if indicated.
10. Recheck distal neurovascular status and record after splinting has been performed.
11. Apply ice and elevate limb or body part if possible.
12. Obtain radiographs.
13. Consult orthopedic surgeon or trauma surgeon.
14. Notify anesthesia department and operating room if surgery is a possibility.
15. Obtain culture of open wound.
16. Irrigate open wound and dress with povidone iodine (Betadine) dressing.
17. Consider administration of antibiotics.
18. Consider tetanus prophylaxis.
19. Use the following mnemonic, P6, to check for arterial injury:
    P = Pain
    P = Pallor
    P = Pulselessness
    P = Paresthesia
    P = Paralysis
    P = Puffiness (edema)

For amputations, refer to protocol concerning care of the amputated extremity.

THE PATIENT WITH MULTIPLE TRAUMA INJURIES*

Use the ABC4 mnemonic (see p. 277). Consider notification of trauma surgeon at time of radio contact.
1. A = Airway
   - Clear airway.
   - Open airway (observe cervical spine precautions).
   - Use appropriate airway adjuncts.
2. B = Breathing
   - Ensure adequate ventilation.
   - Give supplemental oxygen via appropriate delivery system.
   - If head trauma is possible, hyperventilate with 100% oxygen and positive pressure to maintain $Paco_2$ at 28 torr.
   - Have suction equipment readily available.
   - Anticipate emesis; avoid aspiration.
   - Auscultate lungs.
   - Obtain measurement of arterial blood gas levels.

*See individual injury protocols for more details specific to localized or system injury.

3. C1 = Circulation
   - Ensure adequate circulation.
   - Apply chest compression if necessary.
   - Start at least 2 large-bore IV lines with warmed Ringer's lactate or normal saline solution.
   - Consider use of cutdown, jugular line, or central (subclavian) line.
   - Check vital signs.
   - Consider PASG with blood pressure below 80 mm Hg.
   - Control external bleeding.

If ABCs are not present, prepare for emergency thoracotomy. Mortality is extremely high in cases of massive blunt traumas.
   - Prepare hyperthermia blanket and warm IV solution.
4. C2 = Cross-table lateral cervical spine radiograph (must visualize to C7-T1 level). Also, anteroposterior, open-mouth odontoid and oblique views should be obtained.
5. Undress patient. Check patient's back.
6. C3 = Check patient's chest.
   - For tension pneumothorax or hemothorax: Perform needle thoracotomy or insert chest tube(s).
   - For tamponade, give fluid volume; consider pericardiocentesis, pericardial window, or thoracotomy.
   - For flail chest, intubate endotracheally and administer positive-pressure oxygen.
7. C4 = Consciousness
   - Assess level of consciousness. Use DERM mnemonic or Glasgow coma scale. Perform a rectal examination to check for sphincter tone and prostate position. Consider administration of dexamethasone, mannitol, or both for head trauma.
8. Have laboratory tests performed before surgery.
   - Type and cross-match patient's blood for 4 units of blood *now*, and include instructions to "stay 2 units ahead" at all times.
9. Perform secondary survey (head-to-toe).
   - Head and neck
   - Face
   - Eyes, ears, nose, and throat
   - Chest
   - Abdomen
   - Spine and back
   - Extremities
   - Perineum
   - Buttocks
10. Insert Foley catheter (may be inserted earlier).
11. Insert nasogastric tube and connect to suction (may be performed earlier).
12. Consider peritoneal lavage (may be performed earlier).
13. Consider administration of antibiotics.
14. Consider tetanus prophylaxis.

TRAUMA TEAM ASSIGNMENTS

Nurse No. 1
Set up room.
Meet ambulance.
Apply PASG.
Start IV lines.
Collect blood samples.
Record monitor strip.
Administer drugs and perform defibrillation.
Undress patient.
Set up surgical instruments and field.
Insert Foley catheter (if nurse no. 2 is busy).
Perform limb assessment (neurovascular).
Ensure or administer tetanus prophylaxis.
Write intensive care unit and surgery reports.
Assist with transport to operating room or intensive care
    unit.
Cancel type and cross-match procedure if indicated.
Clean up room.
Take critical care notes.
Provide restock assistance.

Nurse No. 2
Set up room.
Transfer patient from ambulance to ED.
Monitor vital signs every 5 to 15 minutes.
Perform chest compressions.
Remove patient's clothing (anterior clothing).
Apply PASG.
Change monitor leads.
Undress patient completely.
Control bleeding.
Apply dressings.
Set up chest tube collection system.
Set up peritoneal lavage tray.
Splint fractures.
Insert Foley catheter.
Assist with transport.
Clean up room.
Restock room.

Physician (team captain)
Administer overall coordination of team.
Perform patient assessment.
Provide patient care.
Give all orders to nurse no. 1 and nurse no. 2.
Coordinate consultations.
Convey anticipated plans to team.

Order medications.
Determine diagnostic tests.
Perform surgical procedures.
Assist with transport to surgery if indicated.
Speak with family of patient.

Admitting clerk or scribe
Obtain patient name and home telephone number.
Scribe notes.
Provide name band.
Contact consultants and communicate with unit secretary.
Contact surgeons and communicate with unit secretary.
Notify charge nurse of patient admission (that is, change
    to inpatient status).
Provide laboratory slips.
Act as runner outside of trauma room.
Provide death forms.

ED charge nurse
Obtain consents.
Act as family liaison.
Act as police liaison.
Arrange for specimens to get to laboratory.
Arrange for blood to be picked up at blood bank.
Arrange for messengers.
Arrange for admission of patient.
Act as press liaison (if indicated).
Perform all administrative coordination.
Assign personnel.
Monitor crowd control.
Provide initial notification of blood bank and operating
    room.
Forward laboratory reports to trauma room.
Act as resource for organ donation information.

Respiratory therapists
Maintain open airway.
Suction.
Monitor blood gas levels.
Monitor ventilations.
Assist in transport to surgery or intensive care unit.

Pastoral care and social service personnel
Act as family liaison.

Unit secretary
Notify respiratory therapy department.
Notify laboratory.
Make all other phone calls as required.

Table 20-1   Levels of hospital categorization and their essential* or desirable* characteristics

Hospital category	Level I	Level II	Level III
I. HOSPITAL ORGANIZATION			
A. Trauma service	E	E	D
B. Surgery departments, divisions, services, and sections			
1. Cardiothoracic surgery	E	D	—
2. General surgery	E	E	E
3. Neurologic surgery	E	E	—
4. Ophthalmic surgery	E	D	—
5. Oral surgery (dental)	E	D	—
6. Orthopedic surgery	E	E	—
7. Otorhinolaryngologic surgery	E	D	—
8. Plastic and maxillofacial surgery	E	D	—
9. Urologic surgery	E	D	—
C. Emergency department, division, service, and section (see notes)[1]	E	E	E
D. Surgical specialties availability			
1. In house 24 hours a day			
(a) General surgery	E[2]	E[2,17]	—
(b) Neurologic surgery	E[3]	E[3]	—
(c) Orthopedic surgery	E[4]	E[4]	—
2. On call and promptly available from inside or outside hospital (see notes)[5]			
(a) Cardiac surgery	E	D	—
(b) General surgery	—	—	E[6]
(c) Neurologic surgery	—	—	D
(d) Microsurgery capabilities	E	D	—
(e) Hand surgery	E	D	—
(f) Obstetric and gynecologic surgery	E	D	—
(g) Ophthalmic surgery	E	E	D
(h) Oral surgery (dental)	E	D	—
(i) Orthopaedic surgery	—	—	D
(j) Otorhinolaryngologic surgery	E	E	D
(k) Pediatric surgery	E	D	—
(l) Thoracic surgery	E	E	D
(m) Urologic surgery	E	E	D
E. Nonsurgical specialties availability			
1. In house 24 hours a day			
(a) Emergency medicine	E[7]	E[7]	E[10]
(b) Anesthesiology	E[8]	E[8,9]	—
2. On call and promptly available from inside or outside the hospital			
(a) Anesthesiology	—	—	E
(b) Cardiology	E	E	D

*E, essential characteristics; D, desirable characteristics.

From the American College of Surgeons Committee on Trauma: *Optimal Care of the Injured Patient*, Chicago, 1991.

[1] The emergency department staff should ensure immediate and appropriate care for the trauma patient. The emergency department physician should function as a designated member of the trauma team. The relationship between emergency department physicians and other participants of the trauma team must be established on an individual hospital basis, consistent with resources but adhering to established standards that ensure optimal care.

[2] Evaluation and treatment may be started by a team of surgeons that will include, at a minimum, a PGY 4 or senior general surgical resident who is a member of that hospital's surgical residency program. The trauma attending surgeon's participation in major therapeutic decisions and presence at operative procedures are mandatory and must be monitored by the hospital's trauma quality assurance program.

[3] An attending neurosurgeon must be promptly available and dedicated to that hospital's trauma service. The in-house requirements may be fulfilled by an in-house neurosurgeon or surgeon who has special competence, as judged by the chief of neurosurgery, in the care of patients with neural trauma, and who is capable of initiating measures directed toward stabilizing the patient as well as initiating diagnostic procedures.

[4] An attending orthopaedic surgeon must be promptly available and dedicated to that hospital's trauma service. The in-house requirement may be fulfilled by an in-house orthopaedic surgeon or a surgeon who has special competence, as judged by the chief of orthopaedic surgery, in the care of patients with orthopaedic trauma, and who is capable of initiating measures directed toward stabilizing the patient as well as initiating diagnostic procedures.

[5] The staff specialists on call will be immediately advised and will be promptly available. This capability will be continuously monitored by the trauma quality assurance program.

[6] Communication should be such that the general surgeon will be present in the emergency department at the time of arrival of the trauma patient.

Table 20-1 Levels of hospital categorization and their essential* or desirable* characteristics—cont'd

Hospital category	Level I	Level II	Level III
(c) Chest medicine	E	D	—
(d) Family medicine	D[11]	D[11]	D[11]
(e) Gastroenterology	E	D	—
(f) Hematology	E	E	D
(g) Infectious diseases	E	D	—
(h) Internal medicine	E[11]	E[11]	E[11]
(i) Nephrology	E	E	D
(j) Pathology	E	E	D
(k) Pediatrics	E[11,12]	E[11,12]	D[11,12]
(l) Psychiatry	E	D	—
(m) Radiology	E	E	D
II. SPECIAL FACILITIES, RESOURCES, AND CAPABILITIES			
A. Emergency department (ED)			
1. Personnel			
(a) Designated physician director	E	E	E
(b) Physician who has special competence in care of critically injured and who is a designated member of the trauma team and is physically present in the ED 24 hours a day	E	E	E
(c) A sufficient number of RNs, LPNs, and nurses' aides to handle caseload	E	E	E
2. Equipment for resuscitation and to provide life support for the critically or seriously injured shall include but not be limited to			
(a) Airway control and ventilation equipment including laryngoscopes and endotracheal tubes of all sizes, bag-mask resuscitator, pocket masks, oxygen, and mechanical ventilator	E	E	E
(b) Suction devices	E	E	E
(c) Electrocardiograph-oscilloscope-defibrillator	E	E	E
(d) Apparatus to establish central venous pressure monitoring	E	E	E
(e) All standard intravenous fluids and administration devices, including intravenous catheters	E	E	E
(f) Sterile surgical sets for procedures standard for ED (e.g., thoracostomy, venisection, lavage)	E	E	E
(g) Gastric lavage equipment	E	E	E
(h) Drugs and supplies necessary for emergency care	E	E	E
(i) Radiographic capability, 24-hour coverage by in-house technician	E	E	D
(j) Two-way radio linked with vehicles of emergency transport system	E	E	E
(k) Skeletal traction device for cervical injuries	E	E	E
(l) Swan-Ganz catheters	E	D	D
(m) Arterial catheters	E	D	D
(n) Thermal control equipment			
(1) For patient	E	E	E
(2) For blood and fluids	E	E	E

[7] In Level I and Level II institutions, requirements may be fulfilled by emergency medicine chief residents capable of assessing emergency situations in trauma patients and providing any indicated treatment. When chief residents are used to fulfill availability requirements, the staff specialist on call will be advised and be promptly available.

[8] Requirements may be fulfilled by anesthesiology chief residents who are capable of assessing emergent situations in trauma patients and of providing any indicated treatment, including initiation of surgical anesthesia. When anesthesiology chief residents are used to fulfill availability requirements, the staff anesthesiologist on call will be advised and be promptly available.

[9] Requirements may be fulfilled when local conditions assure that the staff anesthesiologist will be in the hospital at the time of or shortly after the patient's arrival. During the interim period, prior to the arrival of the staff anesthesiologist, a certified nurse anesthetist (CRNA) capable of assessing emergent situations in trauma patients and of initiating and providing any indicated treatment will be available.

[10] This requirement may be fulfilled by a physician who is credentialed by the hospital to provide emergency medical services.

[11] The patient's primary care physician should be notified at an appropriate time.

[12] The pediatrician is not required in a system that has a designated pediatric trauma center to which all patients are taken.

Continued.

Table 20-1 Levels of hospital categorization and their essential* or desirable* characteristics—cont'd

Hospital category	Level I	Level II	Level III
B. Operating suite			
1. Personnel: operating room adequately staffed in-house and immediately available 24 hours a day	E	E	D
2. Equipment: special requirements shall include but not be limited to:			
(a) Cardiopulmonary bypass capability	E	D	—
(b) Operating microscope	E	D	—
(c) Thermal control equipment:			
(1) For patient	E	E	E
(2) For blood and fluids	E	E	E
(d) X-ray capability including c-arm image intensifier with technologist available 24 hours a day	E	E	D
(e) Endoscopes, all varieties	E	E	E
(f) Craniotome	E	E	D
(g) Monitoring equipment	E	E	E
C. Postanesthetic recovery room (surgical intensive care unit is acceptable)			
1. Registered nurses and other essential personnel 24 hours a day	E	E	E
2. Appropriate monitoring and resuscitation equipment	E	E	E
D. Intensive care units (ICUs) for trauma patients			
1. Personnel			
(a) Designated surgical director	E	E	E
(b) Surgeon, credentialed in critical care by the trauma director, on duty in ICU 24 hours a day or immediately available in hospital	E	E[17]	D
(c) Minimum nurse-patient ratio of 1:2 on each shift	E	E	E
2. Equipment: appropriate monitoring and resuscitation equipment	E	E	E
3. Support services: immediate access to clinical diagnostic services	E[13]	E[13]	E
E. Acute hemodialysis capability	E	D	D
F. Organized burn care	E	E	E
1. Physician-directed burn center staffed by nursing personnel trained in burn care and equipped properly for care of the patient with extensive burns, or			
2. Transfer agreement with nearby burn center or hospital with a burn unit			
G. Acute spinal cord or head injury management capability	E	E	E
1. In circumstances in which a designated spinal cord injury rehabilitation center exists in the region, early transfer should be considered; transfer agreements should be in effect			
2. In circumstances in which a head injury center exists in the region, transfer should be considered in selected patients; transfer agreements should be in effect			
H. Radiologic special capabilities			
1. Angiography of all types	E	E	D
2. Sonography	E	D	D
3. Nuclear scanning	E	D	D
4. Computed tomography	E	E	D
5. In-house CT technician 24 hours a day	E	D	D
6. Neuroradiology	E	D	—

[13] Blood gas measurements, hematocrit level, and chest x-ray studies should be available within 30 minutes of request. This capability will be continuously monitored by the quality assurance program.

[14] Toxicology screens need not be immediately available but are desirable. If available, results should be included in all quality assurance reviews.

[15] Regular and periodic multidisciplinary trauma conferences that include all members of the trauma team should be held. These conferences will be for the purpose of quality assurance through critiques of individual cases.

[16] Documentation will be made of severity of injury (by trauma score, age, ISS) and outcome (survival, length of stay, ICU length of stay), with monthly review of statistics.

[17] The Committee on Trauma feels that the criteria outlined contribute to the optimal care of the injured patient. It is recognized that in certain Level II Hospitals, because of the size of the community, the surgeons can rapidly be available at the hospital on short notice. Under these circumstances, local criteria may be established that allow the general surgeon to take call from outside of the hospital, but with the clear commitment on the part of the hospital and the surgical staff, that the general surgeon will be present in the emergency department at the time of arrival of the trauma patient and be available to care for trauma patients in the ICU. Communications should be established to provide for advance notice, and the availability of the surgeon and compliance with this requirement must be monitored by the hospital's Quality Assurance Program. In such hospitals, the requirement for initial neurosurgical and orthopaedic in-house coverage may also be fulfilled by the above-mentioned general surgeon.

Table 20-1 Levels of hospital categorization and their essential* or desirable* characteristics—cont'd

Hospital category	Level I	Level II	Level III
I. Rehabilitation medicine			
1. Physician-directed rehabilitation and service staffed by personnel trained in rehabilitation care and equipped properly for care of the critically injured patient, or	E	—	—
2. Transfer agreement when medically feasible to a nearby rehabilitation service	—	E	E
J. Clinical laboratory service (available 24 hours a day)			
1. Standard analyses of blood, urine, and other body fluids	E	E	E
2. Blood typing and cross-matching	E	E	E
3. Coagulation studies	E	E	E
4. Comprehensive blood bank or access to a community central blood bank and adequate hospital storage facilities	E	E	E
5. Blood gas levels and pH determinations	E	E	E
6. Serum and urine osmolality	E	E	D
7. Microbiology	E	E	E
8. Drug and alcohol screening	E	E	D[14]
III. **QUALITY ASSURANCE**			
A. Organized quality assurance programs	E	E	E
B. Special audit for all trauma deaths and other specified cases	E	E	E
C. Morbidity and mortality review	E	E	E
D. Trauma conference, multidisciplinary	E[15]	E[15]	D[15]
E. Medical nursing audit, utilization review, tissue review	E	E	E
F. Trauma registry	E[16]	E[16]	E[16]
G. Review of prehospital and regional systems of trauma care	E	D	D
H. Published on-call schedule must be maintained for surgeons, neurosurgeons, orthopaedic surgeons, and other major specialists	E	E	E
I. Times of and reasons for bypass must be documented and reviewed by quality assurance program	E	E	E
J. Quality assurance personnel dedicated to and specific for the trauma program	E	E	D
IV. **OUTREACH PROGRAM:** Telephone and on-site consultations with physicians of the community and outlying areas	E	D	—
V. **PUBLIC EDUCATION:** Injury prevention in the home and industry and on the highways and athletic fields; standard first-aid; problems confronting the public, medical profession, and hospitals regarding optimal care for the injured	E	E	D
VI. **TRAUMA RESEARCH PROGRAM**	E	D	D
VII. **TRAINING PROGRAM**			
A. Formal programs in continuing education provided by hospital for			
1. Staff physicians	E	E	D
2. Nurses	E	E	E
3. Allied health personnel	E	E	E
4. Community physicians	E	E	D
VIII. **TRAUMA SERVICE SUPPORT PERSONNEL:** trauma coordinator	E	E	D

TRAUMA TEAM ASSIGNMENTS

Trauma team assignments are listed in the box on p. 283. As important as protocols or guidelines are for the assessment and treatment of the traumatized patient, it is equally important to ensure that the patient gets to the right hospital at the right time. To assist with this process, the American College of Surgeons' Committee on Trauma has established three levels of hospital categorization and has identified criteria that are essential or desirable for each of these categorizations (Table 20-1).

SUMMARY

Optimal care of the patient with multiple trauma injuries requires an enormous amount of effort. This effort begins with the planning and preparation phases of system development, in which personnel are educated and trained, equipment is selected, and criteria are met for qualification at the various levels of hospital verification and designation. Protocols or guidelines should be established, and trauma registries and quality assurance programs should be put into place. Guidelines must include all aspects of the patient's care so that nothing is overlooked. The team must be drilled well and prepared to respond at any time of the day or night. The plan must be well conceived, well researched, and well practiced.

REFERENCES

1. American College of Surgeons Committee on Trauma: *Advanced trauma life support, provider course manual*, Chicago, 1988, American College of Surgeons.
2. McSwain N: PASG: state of the art, *Ann Emerg Med* 17:506, 1988.
3. Sheehy SB, Marvin JA, Jimmerson CL: *Manual of clinical trauma care: the first hour*, St Louis, 1989, Mosby–Year Book.

SUGGESTED READINGS

American College of Surgeons Committee on Trauma: *Resources for optimal care of the injured patient*, Chicago, 1990, American College of Surgeons.

Clinical indicators for initial testing. *Agenda for Change*, Joint Commission on Accreditation of Healthcare Organizations, September 1989.

Davis JD et al: The significance of critical errors in causing preventable death in an organized trauma system [Abstract], *J Trauma* 30:918, 1990.

Emergency Nurses Association: ENA to develop joint trauma nursing resource document. *Etcetera* 14:3, 1990.

MacKenzie EJ, Steinwachs DM, Ramzy AI: Evaluating performance of statewide regionalized systems of trauma care. *J Trauma* 30:681, 1990.

Zuspan SJ: Essential trauma nursing knowledge included in level I trauma center orientation and continuing education programs. *JEN* 16:141, 1990.

Head Trauma

Susan Budassi Sheehy

Half of all trauma deaths in the United States each year can be attributed to head injuries, and more than 4000 of those who die as a result of head injury are children.[5] In addition, more than 80,000 persons have head or spinal cord injuries that cause disabilities and more than 2000 of these persons will remain in a vegetative state.[4] The mechanism of injury in 75% of serious head injuries is a high-speed motor-vehicle accident,[7] which causes rotational injuries and severe translational injuries that result in diffuse shearing of brain tissue. In these accidents, the most severe head injuries occur to passengers in the front seat.[8] Seventy-five percent of children who have multiple trauma injuries have head injuries.[9]

After motor vehicle accidents, falls, recreation-related injuries, gunshot (accidental and intentional) and stab wounds account for the majority of head injuries.[9]

BRIEF REVIEW OF ANATOMY (Fig. 21-1)

The hair, scalp, skull, meningeal layers, and cerebrospinal fluid protect the brain. The scalp has five layers of tissue: *s*kin, *c*onnective tissue, *a*poneuroses, *l*igaments, and *peri*osteum. The skull is composed of the frontal, parietal, occipital, and temporal areas. It is divided into two major sections: the calvarium or cranial vault, which houses the brain, and the base, which provides an opening for the spinal cord to enter the cervical area.

The three meningeal layers provide protection for both the brain and spinal cord. The layers of meninges, from the surface of the brain outward, are the *pi*a mater, the *ar*achnoid, and the *d*ura mater. The pia mater is thin and mucuslike and adheres to the cortex of the brain. The arachnoid layer is also thin, and vasculature in the arachnoid area appears spiderlike (thus the name, arachnoid). The tough dura mater adheres to the surface of the skull. The meningeal arteries are between the internal surface of the skull and the dura mater in an area known as the epidural ("above the dura") space.

The ventricles of the brain produce cerebrospinal fluid (CSF) and are found in the subarachnoid space. CSF provides a cushion of fluid for both the brain and the spinal cord.

The brain itself is composed of delicate tissues and contains a lot of water. The main body of the brain is divided into the right and left hemispheres. Each hemisphere is subdivided into the four lobes of the brain—the frontal, parietal, occipital, and temporal lobes.

The functions of the frontal lobe are to conceptualize, to think abstractly, and to form judgments. If this area of the brain is injured, judgment and reasoning may be impaired.

The parietal lobe is the area in which the highest integration and coordination of perception and interpretation of sensory phenomena occur. Injury to this area of the brain causes the patient to have difficulty in receptive communication.

The occipital lobe is the area that is responsible for vision. Injury to this area of the brain may cause blurred vision, double vision, or blindness.

The temporal lobe, which is located on each side of the brain and resembles the thumb of a boxing glove, is frequently damaged in head injury because it is located in a relatively bony chamber. Injury to the temporal lobe may affect memory.

The brain stem contains the reticular activating system and is responsible for consciousness. The medulla, which is the lower part of the brain stem, contains the cardiorespiratory centers.

The cerebellum can be found next to the brain stem, under the cerebrum. The cerebellum is responsible for movement and coordination. The area in which the cerebrum and the midbrain meet is known as the tentorial notch. The tentorial notch has sharp edges, and damage to the brain stem or herniation or both often occur there.

CRANIAL NERVES

There are 12 pairs of cranial nerves. The olfactory nerve (I) is responsible for the sense of smell and can be tested by checking the patient's sense of taste. If this nerve is injured, which is common in head trauma, the patient is able to taste "bitter" and "sweet" but is not able to determine any other taste.

The optic nerve (II) allows the patient to perceive light, count fingers, and blink.

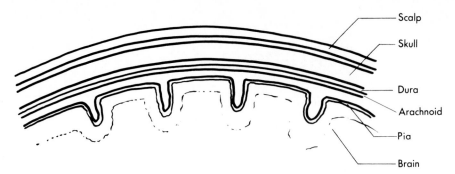

Fig. 21-1   Layers of protection for brain.

The oculomotor (III), trochlear (IV), and abducens (VI) nerves have much to do with the function and movement of the eye. Check the pupil size, shape, and reactivity, and check for the presence of any extraocular movements. The third cranial (oculomotor) nerve passes through the tentorium. Brain-stem herniation puts pressure on this nerve and causes pupil dilation on the ipsilateral (same) side as the herniation. A 1 mm difference in pupil size may be significant. Be sure that flashlight batteries are good and that the light used to test these nerves is bright.

The trigeminal (V) nerve controls facial sensation and jaw movement. These nerves can be tested by checking for facial sensation, strength of mastication muscles, and movement of the jaw.

The facial (VII) nerve controls facial expression and also taste in the anterior two thirds of the tongue. To test this nerve, have the patient raise his or her eyebrows, close his or her eyelids tightly to resistance, show his or her teeth, smile, frown, and puff his or her cheeks. If there is a peripheral ipsilateral injury, both the upper and lower face is involved. If there is a central injury, the brow of the contralateral (opposite) side is spared.

The eighth cranial nerve is divided into two branches— the acoustic branch, which controls balance, and the auditory branch, which controls hearing. The acoustic branch can be tested with the use of a cold calorics examination. The auditory branch can be tested by having the patient respond to a loud voice or clap.

The glossopharyngeal and the vagus nerves, which are the ninth and tenth cranial nerves, are usually evaluated together because of their close anatomic and functional relationships. The glossopharyngeal nerve controls taste in the posterior two thirds of the tongue and sensation in the nostrils and pharynx. The vagus nerve controls the soft palate, the pharynx and larynx muscles, the heart, the lungs, and the stomach. Both of these nerves can be tested by checking for gag and swallow reflexes and by assessing the patient's ability to discriminate between salty and sweet tastes.

The accessory (XI) nerve controls movement of the sternocleidomastoid and trapezius muscles. To test this nerve, ask the patient to turn his or her head against resistance or to shrug his or her shoulders. Before testing this nerve, cervical spine injury must be ruled out.

The hypoglossal (XII) nerve controls movement of the tongue. Ask the patient to stick out his or her tongue. If the tongue is in midline, this nerve is considered intact.

BRIEF NEUROLOGIC EXAMINATION

When evaluating a patient with a head injury, obtain an initial neurologic examination as soon as possible and continue with frequent reexamination as the situation requires. With the use of both the DERM mnemonic for neurologic evaluation (see box below and Table 21-1) and the Glasgow coma scale (see box on p. 291) a brief neurologic examination can be performed in a quick, consistent, and precise manner, by observing clinical findings and changes and by measuring precalculated improvements or deteriorations, which assist in the predictability of outcome.

MNEMONIC FOR NEUROLOGIC EVALUATION

D (depth of coma)

Give a stimulus and note the response. If the stimulus is *voice*, note whether the response is appropriate and state how. If the stimulis is *touch*, record an inappropriate response and state how it was abnormal. Also, observe for any verbalized or nonverbalized signs of *pain* and record findings.

E (eyes)

Note size of pupils, reactivity to light, and accommodation. If the corpus callosum is intact, simultaneous consensual reaction of the unstimulated pupil occurs during light stimulation. Ten percent of the population have unequal but reactive pupils without disease. This condition is known as anisocoria.

R (respirations)

Note rate, rhythm, depth, and regularity of respirations.

M (motor function)

Note whether the patient is able to move extremities; if so, check whether they move bilaterally.

Table 21-1 Use of the DERM mnemonic for assessment of brain stem function

Brain stem	Herniation levels	D = Depth of coma	E = Eyes	R = Respirations	M = Motor function	Posturing
	None	Aware, alert, oriented	Equal and reactive	Eupnea	Normal	None
	Thalamus	Painful stimulus causes nonpurposeful response	Small; react to light	Cheyne-Stokes respirations	Hyperactive deep tendon reflexes	Abnormal flexion (decorticate)
	Midbrain	Painful stimulus causes no response	Midpoint to dilated; fixed; no reaction to light	Central neurogenic breathing	Decreased deep tendon reflexes	Abnormal extension (decerebrate)
	Pons and cerebellum	Painful stimulus causes no response	Pinpoint; fixed; no reaction to light	Biot's respirations	Flaccid	No tone
	Medulla	Painful stimulus causes no response	Midpoint to dilated; fixed; no reaction to light	Ataxia; apneusis	Flaccid	No tone

GLASGOW COMA SCALE

The Glasgow coma scale has been designed to relate consciousness quantitatively to motor responses, verbal responses, and eye opening. Coma is defined as no response and no eye opening. Scores of 7 or less on the Glasgow scale qualify as "coma"; all scores of 9 or more do not qualify as "coma." The examiner determines the best responses the patient can make to a set of standardized stimuli. Higher points are assigned to responses that indicate increasing degrees of arousal.

I. **Best motor response.** (Examiner determines the best response with either arm.)
   A. 6 points. Obeys simple commands. Raises arm on request or holds up specified number of fingers. Releasing a grip (not grasping, which can be reflexive) is also an appropriate test.
   B. 5 points. Localizes noxious stimuli. Fails to obey commands but can move either arm toward a noxious cutaneous stimulus and eventually contacts it with the hand. The stimulus should be maximal and applied in various locations, that is, sternum pressure, or trapezius pinch.
   C. 4 points. Flexion withdrawal. Responds to noxious stimulus with arm flexion but does not localize it with the hand.
   D. 3 points. Abnormal flexion. Adducts shoulder, flexes and pronates arm, flexes wrist, and makes a fist in response to a noxious stimulus (decorticate rigidity).
   E. 2 points. Abnormal extension. Adducts and internally rotates shoulder, extends forearm, flexes wrist, and makes a fist in response to a noxious stimulus (decerebrate rigidity).
   F. 1 point. No motor response. Exclude reasons for no response; for example, insufficient stimulus or spinal cord injury.

II. **Best verbal response.** (Examiner determines the best response after arousal. Noxious stimuli are employed if necessary.) Omit this test if the patient is dysphasic, has oral injuries, or is intubated. Place a check mark after other two test category scores after noting to indicate omission of the verbal response section.
   A. 5 points. Oriented patient. Can converse and relate who he is, where he is, and the year and month.
   B. 4 points. Confused patient. Is not fully oriented or demonstrates confusion.
   C. 3 points. Verbalizes. Does not engage in sustained conversation, but uses intelligible words in an exclamation (curse) or in a disorganized, nonsensical manner.
   D. 2 points. Vocalizes. Makes moaning or groaning sounds that are not recognizable words.
   E. 1 point. No vocalization. Does not make any sound, even in response to noxious stimulus.

III. **Eye opening.** (Examiner determines the minimal stimulus that evokes opening of one or both eyes.) If the patient cannot realistically open the eyes because of bandages or lid edema, write "E" after the total test score to indicate omission of this component.
   A. 4 points. Eyes open spontaneously.
   B. 3 points. Eyes open to speech. Patient opens eyes in response to command or on being called by name.
   C. 2 points. Eyes open to noxious stimuli.
   D. 1 point. No eye opening in response to noxious stimuli.

From Teasdale G, Jennett B: *Lancet* 2:81, 1974.

The examiner should remember that the Glasgow coma scale may be invalid in patients who have used alcohol or other mind-altering drugs, patients with hypoglycemia, patients in shock who have a systolic blood pressure of less than 80 mm Hg, and patients with hypothermia (body temperature of less than 34° C).

OTHER DIAGNOSTIC EXAMINATIONS USED TO EVALUATE PATIENTS WITH HEAD INJURY

Many examinations are useful when assessing and diagnosing head trauma; the most commonly used examinations are presented in the following paragraphs.

Cross-Table Lateral Cervical Spine Radiograph

All seven cervical vertebrae should be visible on a cross-table lateral cervical spine radiograph. To optain this visualization, the examiner must pull the patient's shoulders down. If a good cross-table lateral radiograph of the cervical spine cannot be obtained, obtain a "swimmer's view" of the cervical spine.

The most commonly injured areas are cord levels C5-6 and C6-7. Remember that 10% of patients with significant head trauma have concurrent cervical spine injuries.

Radiographs of the Skull

Radiographs of the skull probably offer the least information, since therapeutic intervention is based on the clinical findings in the patient. If computerized tomography is not available, radiographs of the skull may help confirm a diagnosis.

Computed Tomography

A computed tomography scan (CT scan, computerized axial tomographic [CAT] scan, electromagnetic imagery [EMI] scan) can accurately detect 90% of head trauma. Computed tomography should be performed quickly if the patient has an altered level of consciousness, hemiparesis, or any type of aphasia.

Nuclear Magnetic Resonance Imaging

The atoms of the cells emit transmissions from which images may be created. Nuclear magnetic resonance (NMR) imaging ionizes radiation or sound waves in a noninvasive method to obtain a visual image. Cellular content can also be analyzed with this method to measure the amount of phosphorus emissions. This procedure is not generally used in cases of trauma because the patient must remain absolutely still. Also the patient is inaccessible during the NMR imaging procedure.

Doll's Eye Reflex Examination

Do not perform a doll's eye reflex examination if a cervical spine injury is suspected. A normal doll's eye response occurs when the eyes move in one direction as the head is rotated in the opposite direction (Fig. 21-2, *A* and *B*). An

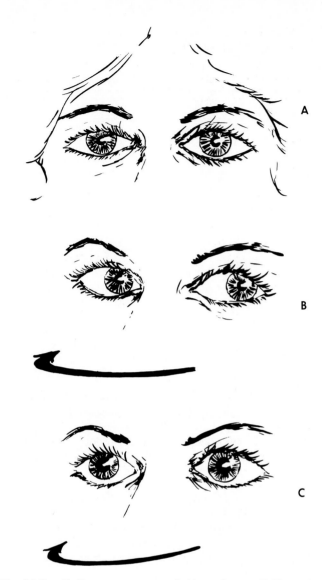

Fig. 21-2 Doll's eye maneuver. **A,** Normal gaze. **B,** Normal reflex. When head is rotated to right, eyes move to left. **C,** Abnormal or absent reflex. When head is turned to right, eyes stay in midline.

abnormal response occurs when the eyes remain fixed in midline position as the head is rotated (Fig. 21-2, *C*).

Cold Calorics (Iced Water Calorics)

Check to see whether the tympanic membranes are intact before performing this procedure. Ice water is squirted into the ear of a comatose patient. A normal response is that the eyes move slowly away from the ice water. A comatose response is that the eyes move toward the ice water. When the brain stem is injured, no response occurs.

Pupils

Normal pupil reaction consists of constriction when eyes are exposed to direct light. Light shined into one pupil causes the other pupil to constrict. If pupils are fixed and pinpoint, this is an abnormal response and usually indicates opiate use or pons involvement. Pupils that are dilated and fixed unilaterally indicate early third cranial nerve involvement. Pupils that are dilated and fixed bilaterally usually indicate complete third cranial nerve involvement. Ptosis may also indicate third cranial nerve involvement.

Reflexes

When the cornea is stimulated, a normal response is to blink; an abnormal reflex will be no response. Gag reflexes are normally intact; loss indicates abnormality. Cranial nerves IX and X are affected. When deep-tendon reflexes are abnormal, hypoactivity or absence of reflexes indicates cerebellar involvement, intricate peripheral nerve disease, or anterior horn cell disease. Hyperactivity indicates pyramidal tract lesions and possibly psychogenic disorders. These reflexes are scored from 0 to 4. Following are the scores:

    0 = Absent
    1 = Decreased
    2 = Normal
    3 = Increased
    4 = Hyperactive

Babinski's sign is a reflex that is elicited by performing a cutaneous stimulation on the plantar surface of the foot. Normally the toes curve downward. An abnormal reflex, also known as a positive Babinski's sign, occurs when the great toe points upward to the head ("to where the problem is").

A posturing reflex *(rigidity)* is elicited by verbal or painful stimuli. Abnormal flexion (decorticate rigidity) occurs when the arms pull "toward the core" and the legs and feet extend; abnormal flexion indicates a lesion above the midbrain (Fig. 21-3). Abnormal extension (decerebrate rigidity) occurs when the arms are extended with wrists flexed and the legs and feet are extended; abnormal extension indicates brain stem compression (Fig. 21-4).

TYPES OF HEAD INJURIES
Scalp Lacerations

Scalp lacerations are probably the type of head injury most frequently seen in the ED. The scalp contains hair, subcutaneous tissue, and glia (the tough fibrous layer), as well as some loose fibrous connective tissue. Scalp lacerations usually bleed profusely because of the great vascular supply. Because of this profuse bleeding, scalp infections are rare. When a person's head hits a car windshield, the scalp absorbs the first 33% of the force.[9] Signs and symptoms are laceration and bleeding.

Therapeutic intervention is the application of direct pressure to control any bleeding. Check the underlying structure with a gloved hand, palpating gently with the fingertips. Be aware that a small puncture wound of the scalp may also indicate a penetrating injury to the brain. Cleanse the area with an antiseptic soap solution, and suture the wound if indicated. Give the patient aftercare instructions about suture and wound care and head injury.

Skull Fracture

A skull fracture does not necessarily indicate a cerebral injury. Observe the patient carefully and perform appropriate therapeutic and diagnostic steps. Basic types of skull fractures include simple, depressed, and basilar fracture.

Simple skull fracture. A simple skull fracture is a linear crack in the surface of the skull; there is no bone displacement.

Therapeutic intervention includes observation of the patient. If there are no obvious neurologic deficits, the patient

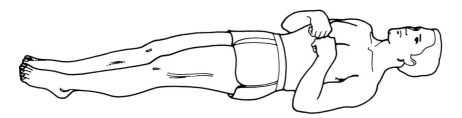

Fig. 21-3   Abnormal flexion (decorticate posturing).

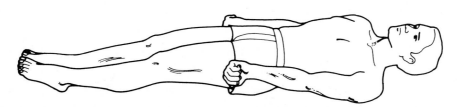

Fig. 21-4   Abnormal extension (decerebrate posturing).

should be released to home and to the close observation of family or friends.

Depressed skull fracture. A depressed skull fracture is a depression in the bony portion of the skull. Surgery is indicated if the depression is deeper than 5 mm. If the depression is overlying the sinuses, profuse bleeding may occur, indicating underlying brain contusion or tears of cerebral tissue. In addition to examining the head, check for cervical spine injury and check the mandible and maxilla.

Therapeutic intervention for a depressed skull fracture includes controlling bleeding, admitting the patient to the hospital for observation, and considering surgical intervention to elevate the depressed fragment, to remove any loose fragments, to debride necrotic tissue, to remove hematomas, and to repair lacerations. Administration of antibiotics should also be considered.

Basilar skull fracture. A basilar skull fracture is a fracture at the base of the skull. Although a basilar skull fracture can be visualized on a radiograph, diagnosis is usually made on the basis of clinical findings. Dangers are associated with this fracture. Most important, a fracture of the middle meningeal artery may cause a scalp hematoma. (Disruption of the middle meningeal artery is the cause of 90% of epidural hemorrhages.) A basilar fracture may also cause intracerebral bleeding.

There are four major signs of basilar skull fracture. Periorbital ecchymoses (raccoon eyes) occur as a result of intraorbital bleeding caused by an intraorbital root fracture. Battle's sign indicates formation of an ecchymosis behind the ears in the area of the mastoid and occurs 12 to 24 hours after injury. Hematotympanum is the presence of blood behind the tympanic membrane caused by a fracture of the temporal bone near the tympanic membrane. A CSF leak from the nose or ear is caused by a fracture of the temporal bone that creates an opening between the cranium and the outside of the skull. The absence of visible CSF does not eliminate from consideration the possibility that the patient may have a basilar skull fracture. If the patient states that he or she has a salty taste in his or her mouth, be suspicious. If CSF leakage is suspected, test the fluid by placing some of it on a piece of filter paper. The formation of two distinct rings is known as a "ring" sign, a "target" sign, or a "halo" sign and may indicate the presence of CSF. If the tympanic membrane is intact, the CSF exits via the eustachian tube and appears as CSF rhinorrhea.

Therapeutic intervention is to obtain a radiograph. However, remember that 25% of basilar skull fractures are not seen on routine skull radiographs. Also, initiate antibiotic therapy if there is a CSF leak, and admit the patient to the hospital for observation. A scar may form at the site of a basilar skull fracture and may dislodge, forming an open fistula into the cranium and causing a CSF leak. Do not attempt to stop a CSF leak. Rather, place a loose, bulky dressing over the opening of the ear or the nose. Be sure to obtain a baseline neurologic examination, and perform frequent neurologic checks.

Concussion

A concussion occurs as a result of a direct blow to the head or is caused by an acceleration or deceleration injury; such an injury occurs when impact does not take place but the brain collides with the inside of the bony skull. After a concussion a brief interruption of the reticular activating system may occur, which causes a brief period of amnesia. The amnesia is usually transient and requires no therapeutic intervention other than observation for the development of further complications. Occasionally, late sequelae develop in patients with concussions, including headache, nausea, memory loss, decreased organizational skills, difficulty in handling more than one task at once, syncopal episodes, loss of coordination, numbness, tinnitus, diplopia, loss of menstrual periods, and abnormal breast secretions. The patient who has had a severe concussion should receive a CT scan; another scan or magnetic resonance imaging should be performed 2 weeks after injury.

Signs and symptoms of a concussion are nausea and vomiting, brief loss of consciousness, brief amnesia, possible skull fracture, headache, and possible brief loss of vision.

Therapeutic intervention includes observation, especially if the loss of consciousness is prolonged (greater than 2 to 3 minutes) or if the skull is fractured. If loss of consciousness continues for more than 6 hours, the injury is considered a cerebral contusion. If there is nausea and vomiting and a possibility of severe dehydration, the patient should be admitted to the hospital, given antiemetic agents, and rehydrated. A nonnarcotic analgesic agent may be administered for the complaint of headache. If it appears that reliable friends or family are present and that the patient has none of the complications that warrant hospitalization, he or she may be discharged to home in the care of family or friends for observation, after complete aftercare instructions have been given.

Postconcussion syndrome occurs when late sequelae of a concussion appear, including headache, memory loss, and syncopal episodes. Therapeutic intervention includes only administration of a nonnarcotic agent for the headache.

Contusion

A contusion is a bruise on the surface of the brain, which causes a structural alteration. Signs and symptoms include an altered level of consciousness for more than 6 hours; nausea and vomiting; visual disturbances; neurologic dysfunctions such as ataxia, weakness, hemiparesis, confusion, and speech problems; and in 5% of patients, seizures. Therapeutic intervention is admission to the hospital for close observation and the administration of an antiemetic agent.

Cerebral Edema and Intracranial Bleeding

Three meningeal layers cover the brain: the pia mater, the arachnoid, and the dura mater. When intracranial bleeding occurs or when there is cerebral edema, the sinuses can accommodate about 75 ml of fluid. When more than this amount of fluid is present, the brain begins to shift downward toward the brain stem. This shifting causes an increase in intracranial pressure (ICP). An increased ICP is the most frequent cause of severe brain damage after a traumatic event. Sustained ICP above 20 mm Hg is associated with significantly increased morbidity and mortality. An increase in ICP causes a decrease in cerebral blood flow and possibly cessation of cerebral blood flow, which leads to cerebral infarct or death. Regional ischemia leads to anaerobic metabolism, accumulation of free radicals, a decrease in adenosine triphosphate, and lactic acidosis.

Cellular swelling (cytotoxic edema) may be caused by the loss of high-energy phosphate bonds, which results in disabled enzyme systems and destruction of intracellular electrolyte concentrations.

The release of free radicals causes capillary endothelial toxicity and results in vasogenic edema. Edema, regardless of the cause, increases ICP.

Intracranial bleeding occurs in 30% to 50% of patients with severe head injuries. Intracranial bleeding results in increased ICP and possible herniation of the medial temporal lobe through the tentorial notch, causing third cranial nerve compression and brain stem compression.

Rapid, early surgical intervention to avoid herniation is imperative. In one study, patients with traumatic intracranial bleeding who had surgery within 2 hours of the accident had 25% mortality; when surgery was delayed for more than 4 hours, mortality was greater than 85%.[6]

Epidural (extradural) hematoma. An epidural hematoma is bleeding between the skull and the dura mater. Epidural hematoma occurs as a result of severe trauma to the head that is caused by a direct blow. There is usually an accompanying skull fracture and possibly a tear in the middle meningeal artery. This torn middle meningeal artery produces an arterial hemorrhage and a rapidly forming hematoma. This type of hemorrhage carries a mortality of 50% and a morbidity of 70%. Half of the patients who have an epidural hematoma have no evidence of a skull fracture.

Signs and symptoms include a short period of unconsciousness followed by a lucid period, followed by another loss of consciousness. It is thought that the initial loss of consciousness results from a concussion and that the second loss of consciousness is caused by the increased ICP. Do not be fooled, however, if there is no initial loss of consciousness or if the patient is brought to the ED unconscious and does not regain consciousness. The patient with an epidural hematoma, if conscious, complains of a severe headache and may demonstrate hemiparesis and an ipsilateral dilated pupil. He or she may also demonstrate bradycardia and increased blood pressure, and positive findings of bleeding result from a CT scan.

Acute subdural hematoma. When an acute subdural hematoma (Fig. 21-5) occurs, there is bleeding between the dura mater and the arachnoid membrane. Acute subdural hematoma is usually the result of severe trauma to the head, such as an acceleration or deceleration injury, in which bleeding occurs from a vein that has been lacerated where it crosses the subdural space. Seventy percent mortality and 90% morbidity are associated with subdural hematomas. If you see evidence of a subdural hematoma in a child less than 1 year of age, suspect that the child was violently shaken during an incident of child abuse. The bleeding that occurs in a child less than 18 years of age is usually caused

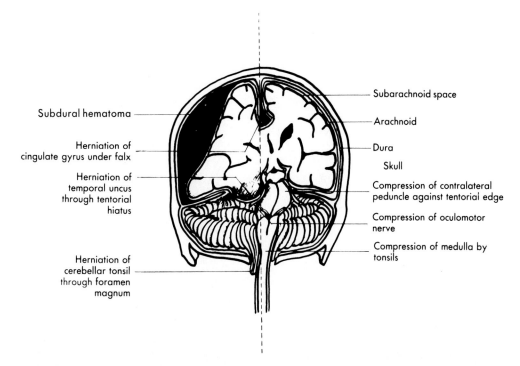

Fig. 21-5   Brain displacement in subdural hematoma. (From Budassi SA, *JEN* 5:45, 1979.)

by a cerebral laceration or a contusion that begins to bleed on the surface of the cortex.

Signs and symptoms include loss of consciousness, fixed dilated pupils, hemiparesis, localized hyperreflexia, and a positive Babinski's sign. A patient with a subdural hematoma also has an elevated temperature and positive findings on CT scan with positive pressure and 100% oxygen. Therapeutic intervention consists of administration of furosemide or mannitol or both and antipyretic agents and possibly surgery. If the patient is an infant with a retinal hemorrhage and decerebrate rigidity, the neurosurgeon may perform a subdural tap in the ED.

Chronic subdural hematoma. A chronic subdural hematoma may occur up to 4 to 8 weeks after a traumatic head injury. At the time of the accident, the patient may have been free of symptoms or may have had an altered level of consciousness that rapidly improved. Chronic subdural hematoma is a condition that may occur without trauma, especially in elderly individuals or patients with chronic alcoholism.

Signs and symptoms include progressively worsening headache, ataxia, and incontinence, decreasing level of con-sciousness, and increasing dementia. It is easy to see how this condition can be confused with senile dementia. Findings of a CT scan are positive.

Subarachnoid hematoma. A subarachnoid hematoma is bleeding between the arachnoid membrane and the pia mater. This hematoma is usually caused by the rupture of a congenital aneurysm known as a berry aneurysm; it may also be caused by severe hypertension or severe head trauma.

Signs and symptoms include a piercing, severe headache, meningism, nausea and vomiting, delirium, blunted responses, syncope, or coma. The patient may also appear to be in a metabolic coma and have respiratory difficulty (eupnea to central neurogenic breathing), dilated pupils, papilledema, and retinal hemorrhage. He or she may also demonstrate focal motor signs, grand mal seizures, and positive findings on CT scan.

INTRACRANIAL PRESSURE MONITORING
(Fig. 21-6, *A* and *B*)

The brain, CSF, and blood are contained in the skull, which allows little space for expansion of these substances. When one of these substances increases in volume, the

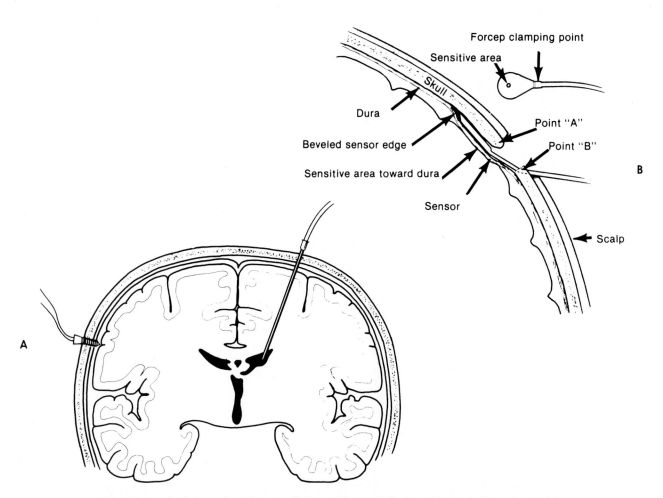

Fig. 21-6   A, Subarachnoid screw *(left)* and intraventricular catheter in lateral ventricle *(right).* **B,** Sensor implantation. (From Budassi SA, *JEN* 5:45, 1979.)

others compensate by decreasing in volume, thereby maintaining a constant ICP. This compensation can occur only when there is a slight increase in volume. If volume increase is excessive, ICP rises.

When ICP increases beyond mean arterial pressure, the brain cells become anoxic because of inadequate perfusion of brain tissue and eventually are irreparably damaged. The brain tissue itself begins to shift, compressing the ventricles and forcing brain tissue into the tentorial notch, which compresses the brain stem and the third cranial nerve.

It is therefore necessary to avoid or at least to moderate activities that cause an increase in ICP in those patients who are already at risk for increased pressure.

Signs and symptoms of supratentorial herniation are the following: coma caused by impairment of the reticular activating system; changes in pupil size and reaction to light, including the dilated fixed pupil; decreased motor responses (decerebrate rigidity if the herniation is at the midbrain level or decorticate rigidity if the herniation is at the thalmic level, and flaccidity if the herniation has reached the level of the lower pons); and Cheyne-Stokes, central neurogenic, or ataxic respirations. ICP monitoring may be indicated when there is suspicion of increased ICP, such as may be found when there has been head trauma that has resulted in cerebral edema, when increased ICP is caused by a tumor or other expanding lesion, and when increased ICP may have occurred as a result of an obstruction in the path of the CSF.

Normal ICP is 5.8 to 13 mm Hg (70 to 190 mm H_2O). Brief elevations in ICP to more than 13 mm Hg during such activities as suctioning, turning, or sneezing are normal. A prolonged ICP of greater than 13 mm Hg, however, is abnormal. If ICP increases to 50 mm Hg or greater for more than 20 minutes, the prognosis is poor.

Cerebral perfusion pressure can be calculated by subtracting ICP from mean arterial pressure. A result of less than 60 mm H_2O indicates cerebral ischemia, and a cerebral perfusion pressure of less than 30 mm H_2O results in death.

Therapeutic intervention for increased ICP includes systemic neuromuscular paralysis and administration of sedatives to prevent increased ICP that results from agitation and patient movement, decreasing the volume of CSF, hypothermia, administration of mannitol or barbiturates, and possibly surgery. Hyperventilation causes a reduction in the partial pressure of carbon dioxide (PCO_2), which reduces vasodilatation, thus decreasing ICP.

Hyperventilation

Hyperventilation is not without controversy. In one study[10] it was found that the condition of patients who were hyperventilated to a PCO_2 of 24 ($\pm$ 2) became significantly worse than did the condition of those whose PCO_2 was kept in the normal range of 35 ($\pm$ 2). It is thought that vasoconstriction as a result of a lowered PCO_2 is accommodated after about a day and that lowered PCO_2 becomes ineffective. A second explanation is that of "inverse steal," that is, in

injured areas of the brain the cerebrovascular vasoconstriction or dilation does not occur.[1] The hyperventilation may, therefore, cause severe vasoconstriction in areas where normal, viable tissue is present. Blood from these "normal" areas moves to the brain-injured area, where there is less resistance; this movement possibly causes ischemia or infarction of normally viable brain tissue, resulting in further cerebral edema and an increased ICP.

Therefore, PCO_2 levels should be kept at 35 ($\pm$ 2) unless acute neurologic deterioration is present or other therapeutic interventions have been unsuccessful.

Mannitol. When mannitol is given, it lowers ICP by causing a significant decrease in blood viscosity, which results in a reduction of cerebral blood volume by decreasing mean transit time of blood through the brain. Fifteen to 20 minutes after mannitol is given, a dose of 0.5 to 1 g/kg should be given IV slowly over a period of 5 to 10 minutes, since rapid infusion may cause a transient increase in ICP. Mannitol should not be used when serum osmolality is greater than 320.

Barbiturate coma. Many studies have demonstrated that use of barbiturate coma has failed to improve outcome for the patient with a severe head injury. It has been found, however, that barbiturate coma may be useful in those patients who have intact vasoresponsivity.[6] Barbiturates cause the cerebral metabolic rate to decrease, and by reducing blood volume they reduce ICP.

Hypothermia. Hypothermia is usually induced only as a last resort to lower cerebral metabolic rate, thus, ICP. A major problem with hypothermia (core temperature less than 90° F) is its association with an increased incidence of infection and myocardial depression.

Corticosteroids. Although corticosteroids were used widely in patients with head injuries in the 1960s, subsequent studies have proven that corticosteroids do not improve outcome. In addition, there is evidence that the use of corticosteroids causes a higher incidence of malnutrition and infections. Thus corticosteroids no longer should be used for patients with head injuries.[2]

Control of free radicals: an experimental idea.[3] It is thought that a catecholamine surge occurs soon after a head injury and results in cerebral vasoconstriction and cerebral ischemia when adenosine triphosphate is depleted and normal levels of intracellular electrolytes can no longer be maintained. When the level of intracellular calcium increases, enzyme systems that cause the release of free radicals are activated. These free radicals are toxic to cerebral cells and may cause cytotoxic and vasogenic edema. In addition, it is thought that free radicals disrupt cerebrovascular autoregulation and vasoresponsiveness to carbon dioxide. Therefore free radicals are thought to be fundamentally responsible for secondary brain injury. In light of this theory the drugs superoxide dismutase with polyethylene glycol (PEG-SOD) and nonglucocorticoid 21-aminosteroids ("lazeroids") are being tested. Results of experiments with PEG-

SOD suggest that this drug, without serious side effects, lowers the levels of free radicals in areas of brain injury after blunt head trauma. In experimental studies the "lazeroids" have been shown to suppress injury-induced lipid peroxidation and improve neurologic function.[9]

THERAPEUTIC INTERVENTION FOR PATIENTS WITH SEVERE HEAD INJURY

- Maintain an open airway.
- Consider endotracheal intubation.
- Ensure adequate breathing.
- Do not routinely perform hyperventilation; hyperventilate the patient only if the patient's neurologic condition is deteriorating.
- Provide adequate oxygen.
- Maintain partial pressure of oxygen at greater than 60 torr.
- Ensure adequate circulation.
- Maintain systolic blood pressure greater than 90 mm Hg.
- Monitor oxygen saturation.
- Frequently assess neurologic status.
- Consider neuromuscular paralysis.
- Administer mannitol (even before the patient reaches the hospital if he or she is normotensive and if transport time is longer than 20 minutes).
- Do not administer corticosteroids.
- Consider other causes of coma such as hypovolemia or metabolic changes.

NURSING DIAGNOSES FOR PATIENTS WITH HEAD INJURIES

Many nursing diagnoses may be applicable for the patient with a head injury. The following are some of the diagnoses most commonly seen.

Breathing Pattern, Ineffective

Injury to the respiratory centers of the brain may cause ventilatory patterns to change and result in ineffective breathing. Commonly seen patterns of breathing in the patient with a head injury are central neurogenic breathing, ataxia, Biot's respiration, and apnea.

Defining characteristics include a pattern of breathing that is irregular, too shallow, or too deep.

One nursing intervention is the administration of oxygen. Hyperventilation is recommended only if the patient's neurologic condition is deteriorating. Pharmacologic intervention should be performed in accordance with physician's orders or protocol. Continue to monitor the patient's vital signs and assess the patient for the presence of additional injuries. Obtain arterial blood gas values. Explain all procedures to the patient, regardless of whether he or she appears conscious.

Evaluation can be made by observing vital signs and arterial blood gas values.

Pain

Pain management for the patient who has a head injury is always a challenge; because the patient may have an altered level of consciousness, assessing the patient for the presence of pain may be difficult. In addition, the nurse should be particularly cautious about administering pain medications, particularly narcotics, since they may decrease the level of consciousness. In most cases, narcotics, especially long-acting ones, are not given. If the management of pain is necessary, short-acting analgesic agents should be considered first.

If the patient appears agitated, this agitation may be due to pain but may also be due to anoxia or hypoxia. Hypoxia can be ruled out by determination of arterial blood gas values. If anoxia is ruled out, the reason for the pain should be sought. Pain may result from a distended bladder or from appliances or devices that may be causing discomfort. If the cause cannot be isolated, chlorpromazine may be the appropriate drug for treatment of agitation.

Thought Processes, Altered: Secondary to Injury

Altered thought processes secondary to injury may be caused by a direct injury to the brain, cerebral edema, or bleeding that results in increased ICP, hypoxia, or brain stem herniation. Assessment can be performed by repeating neurologic examinations. Use the Glasgow coma scale or the DERM mnemonic or both, and carefully assess the cranial nerves.

Nursing interventions include repeated neurologic assessments every 5 to 15 minutes (or as indicated by the patient's condition) and preparation of the patient for surgery, if indicated. The patient's family must be kept informed of the patient's condition and should be supported psychologically. Protect the patient from further injury, particularly if the patient's airway is unstable or if the patient is having seizures. Consider restraining the patient if necessary. Evaluation can be performed by noting changes in the patient's neurologic status.

Infection, Potential for: Secondary to Scalp Laceration or Penetrating Wound into Brain Tissue

Assessment can be made by observing the scalp laceration or the penetrating injury. Nursing interventions are to cleanse and debride the wound with gentle irrigation for a scalp laceration. Protect any exposed tissue with a moist saline (sterile) dressing covered with a dry sterile dressing. Systemic antibiotics should be administered as prescribed, and tetanus prophylaxis should be ensured. that all wounds have been cleansed and dressed appropriately and that the patient's wounds have been protected from further contamination.

REFERENCES

1. Darby JM et al: Local "inverse steal" induced by hyperventilation in head injury, *Neurosurgery* 23:84, 1988.
2. Dearden NM et al: Effect of high-dose dexamethasone on outcome from severe head injuries, *J Neurosurg* 64:81, 1986.
3. Flamm ES et al: Free radicals in cerebral ischemia, *Stroke* 9:445, 1978.
4. Kraus JF: Epidemiology of brain injury. In Cooper PR, ed: *Head injury,* ed 2, Baltimore, 1986, Williams & Wilkins.
5. Kraus JF et al: The incidence of acute brain injury and serious impairment in a defined population, *Am J Epidemiol* 119:186, 1984.
6. Marion D: Head injury. Lecture, International Disaster and Emergency Medicine Conference, Pittsburgh, 1990.
7. Rosen P et al: *Emergency medicine,* ed 2, St Louis, 1988, Mosby–Year Book.
8. Shea J: Lecture, Tacoma Fire Department Trauma Conference, Tacoma, Wash, August, 1986.
9. Shea J: Lecture, Whatcom County EMS Conference, Bellingham, Wash, October, 1988.
10. Ward JD, Choi S, et al: Effect of prophylactic hyperventilation on outcome in patients with severe head injury. In Hoff JT, Bets AL, eds: *Intracranial pressure VII,* Berlin, Heidelberg, 1989, Springer-Verlag.

Susan Budassi Sheehy

More than 12,000 persons have spinal cord injuries each year in the United States.[5] More than half of these persons remain permanently disabled.[5] The most common mechanism of injury is a motorcycle accident. Lack of safety device use and the subsequent ejection from a vehicle result in 1 chance in 13 that the person being ejected will sustain a spinal cord injury.[5] Eighty percent of all spinal cord injuries occur in male victims.[3]

The human body has 7 cervical, 12 throracic, 5 lumbar and 1 sacral (the fusion of four bones) vertebrae (Fig. 22-1). A fracture of the first cervical vertebra (the atlas) at the vertebral arch is known as a *Jefferson fracture,* which is usually due to an axial loading. With this type of fracture, initially there may be no neurologic deficit. This patient requires cervical traction and surgical fixation. A bilateral arch fracture of the second cervical vertebrae (the axis) is known as a *hangman's fracture.* This patient must be maintained in absolute immobilization because excessive head movement may cause spinal cord transection (Table 22-1). The vertebrae, spinal cord, and nerve roots may be injured as a result of fractures, dislocations, or subluxations. Six basic categories of movement that can result in injury to the spinal cord are the following:

1. Hyperextension. When hyperextension occurs, the head is forced back and the vertebrae of the cervical region are placed in an overextended position.
2. Hyperflexion. When hyperflexion occurs, the head is forced forward and the cervical vertebrae are placed in an overflexion position.
3. Axial loading. Axial loading is caused by a severe blow to the top of the head, causing a blunt downward force on the vertebrae and the spinal column.
4. Compression. Compression is caused by forces from above and below the vertebrae.
5. Lateral bend. Lateral bend occurs when the head and neck are bent to one side, beyond normal range of motion.
6. Overrotation and distraction. Overrotation and distraction occur when the head turns to one side and the cervical vertebrae are forced beyond normal limits.

This movement causes the cervical vertebrae to be pulled out of alignment.

The spinal cord is an extremely delicate collection of tissues. So sensitive is the cord that as little as 400 ml of weight (about the weight of a Kennedy half-dollar) dropped onto the cord from a height of about 7 inches will cause a permanent injury and paralysis.[4] In most cases (approximately 93%), problems result from intramedullary bleeding and edema, not from a laceration of the spinal cord.[4]

The spinal cord controls consciousness, regulates body movement and function, and transmits nerve impulses. It is an integral part of the central nervous system. The spinal cord functions both voluntarily and involuntarily; it travels through a canal that extends through the vertebrae.

The spinal cord has anterior and posterior divisions. The anterior division contains motor nerve tracts, and the posterior division contains sensory nerve tracts. Thus, an incomplete lesion is possible. An incomplete lesion occurs when one tract (either the anterior or the posterior tract) is left intact but the other is disrupted, producing sensation without movement or movement without sensation.

The primary function of the spinal cord is to regulate function and movement of the body by transmitting nerve impulses to and from the brain and body. The spinal cord,

Table 22-1   Vertebrae and levels of innervation

Vertebrae	Level of innervation
C2-4	Diaphragm, neck muscles
C5-6	Biceps brachii, deltoid muscle, triceps brachii, wrist extensors
C6-T1	Latissimus dorsi, hand muscles
T2-7	Intercostal muscles
T12-L2	Quadratus lumborum
L1-5	Leg muscles
L2-3	Psoas muscles
L2-4	Quadriceps
L4-5	Tibialis anterior
S1	Bowel, bladder

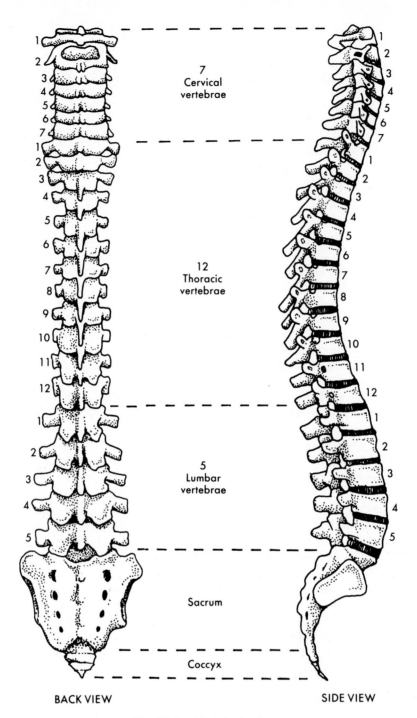

Fig. 22-1 Vertebral column.

much like the brain, is protected by three layers of meninges, the pia, the arachnoid, and the dura. The cord is also protected by the vertebrae and the paravertebral muscles. The round opening in the center of each vertebra forms the canal through which the spinal cord passes. Injury to the spinal cord may result from concussion, contusion, edema, or transection. A concussed cord produces transient changes that usually resolve within minutes to hours. A contused spinal cord may cause a structural defect and a permanent disability. Edema, as a result of trauma, may cause spinal cord compression and transient or permanent damage. Spinal cord transection causes permanent disability and possibly death if the transection is at or above the level of the cord where respiratory function is controlled. In general, a spinal cord injury causes loss of motor and sensory function at and below the level of the injury. An acute transection that causes loss of sympathetic tone may also cause neurogenic shock (see Chapter 19).

The immediate concern with any patient who has or is suspected of having a spinal cord injury is to ensure an adequate airway and ventilations. Cervical vertebrae 3, 4, and 5 (C3-5) contain the area of the spinal cord that controls the phrenic nerve. Injury at or above this area causes loss of control of the diaphragm and loss of respiratory effort. Survival from such an injury is rare; death usually ensues rapidly.

INCOMPLETE SPINAL CORD LESIONS
Central Cord Syndrome

Central cord syndrome (Fig. 22-2) is most frequently caused by hyperextension and is seen most commonly in elderly patients after a fall. This syndrome causes loss of function in the upper extremities. Bowel and bladder function are maintained.

Anterior Cord Syndrome

Anterior cord syndrome (Fig. 22-3) usually results from occlusion of the anterior spinal artery, a herniated nucleus pulposus (ruptured disk), or a transection of the anterior portion of the cord. The patient has hyperesthesia, hypoalgesia, and incomplete or complete paralysis. The patient is able to feel vibrations and has proprioception because of a preserved posterior column.

Brown-Séquard Syndrome

Involvement of the hemisection of the cord in the anteroposterior plane is known as Brown-Séquard syndrome (Fig. 22-4). The most common cause is a penetrating injury such as a gunshot wound or a missile fragment penetration. Brown-Séquard syndrome is characterized by ipsilateral (same side) paresis or hemiplegia and contralateral (opposite side) reduced sensation to pain and changes in temperature. A person with this syndrome can feel one side of the body but not the other and can move one side but not the other.

Nerve Root Injuries

Injuries to nerve roots often occur as a result of spinal cord trauma (Fig. 22-5). Most commonly symptoms include hypoalgesia, pain, or referred pain.

PATIENT ASSESSMENT

Before an assessment begins, the nurse must ensure that the patient has a patent airway and is breathing adequately. Check respiratory rate and rhythm and depth of respirations. Pay particular attention to the use of accessory muscles of respiration, especially the diaphragm (diaphragmatic breathing).

Also ensure that the spine is immobilized completely: the patient must be immobilized from the top of the head to the hips. To accomplish immobilization, the nurse may use one of many commercially available devices; adhesive tape 2

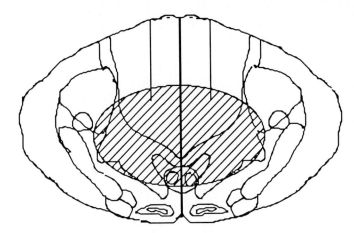

Fig. 22-2   Central cord syndrome.

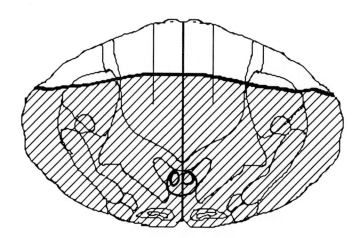

Fig. 22-3   Anterior cord syndrome.

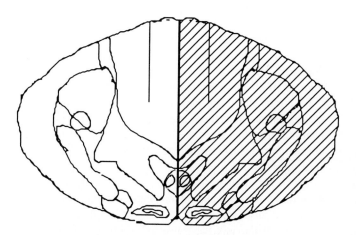

Fig. 22-4   Brown-Séquard syndrome.

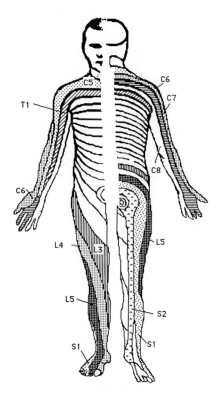

Fig. 22-5 Nerve roots and muscles innervated.

Table 22-2 Cervical spine and spinal cord lesions and resultant physiologic function

Lesion	Resultant function
C3, C4, or above	Respiratory arrest; flaccid paralysis; quadriplegia
C5, C6	Reduced respiratory effort; almost total dependence; flaccid paralysis; quadriplegia
C7	Reduced respiratory effort; almost total dependence; splints necessary for functioning of forearms; quadriplegia
T1	Reduced respiratory effort; partial dependence; paraplegia
T1, T2	Reduced respiratory effort; complete independence; paraplegia
T7	Complete independence; walking with long-leg braces; paraplegia
L4	Complete independence; walking with foot braces; paraplegia

inches wide can also be used. Tape across the patient's eyebrows, and ensure that the patient is fixed to a backboard, along with rolled blankets. The use of sandbags is discouraged, since they often slip and provide little stabilization of the cervical vertebrae.

Evaluate the patient's vital signs, including blood pressure, pulse rate and skin vital signs (skin color, temperature, and moisture). Observe the patient carefully for the presence of a cerebral spinal fluid leak from the nose or ear (or the patient may complain of a salty taste in the mouth). Carefully palpate the spine with your fingertips. Assess for the presence of pain, tenderness, a step-off deformity, edema, or a combination of these.

Assess the patient's motor strength and weakness and document what you find. Also, assess sensory levels and document reaction to touch and pain. Also document any findings of paresthesias and paralysis (Table 22-2).

Carefully check the patient for the presence of ecchymosis, tracheal deviation, and a hematoma in the posterior pharyngeal area. Check the rectum for sphincter tone and check for priapism (a sustained erection indicative of a spinal cord injury).

Check for diaphoresis. Injuries above the thoracic cord level of T4 usually cause sympathetic nervous system disruption. If this disruption occurs, vasodilation occurs below the level of the injury because of the body's inability to

vasoconstrict below the level of the injury. If the patient is diaphoretic, the diaphoresis is evidenced above but not below the level of the injury.

Be sure to check the patient for the presence of other associated injuries, such as a head injury, skull and facial bone fractures, and chest injuries. Twenty-seven percent of patients with spinal cord injuries have concurrent head injuries.[4]

SIGNS AND SYMPTOMS OF SPINAL CORD INJURY

Many signs and symptoms may indicate the presence of a spinal cord injury. Pay particular attention to the presence of neck and cervical tenderness or pain. There may also be weakness of the extremities, numbness, tingling, or paralysis. There may be decreased motor activity distal to the injury. The patient may also have unexplained hypotension with bradycardia, an altered level of consciousness, or a feeling of "electric shock" or "hot water" running down the back. The patient may also have the ability to flex but not to extend the elbow.

There may be pain during palpation, local edema, or deformity. In addition, the patient may have "cough tenderness." (When the patient coughs, he or she has cervical pain.)

Look for ptosis, or mouth breathing (Gautman's position), or flaccid areflexia. The patient may be holding his or her head, may have a "cock-robin" appearance that may be indicative of a level C1-2 injury, or may have his or her arms folded across the chest, which may be indicative of a level C5-6 injury.

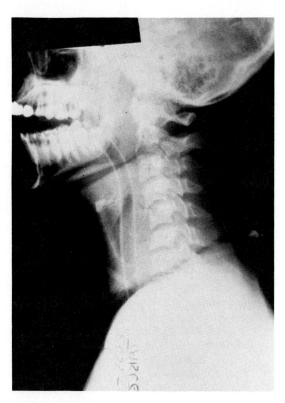

Fig. 22-6 Cross-table lateral cervical spine radiograph. All seven cervical vertebrae and the top of T1 must be visualized.

DIAGNOSIS

Diagnosis is based on clinical findings, the results of radiographs, computerized tomography, magnetic resonance imaging, and other diagnostic findings. Radiographs should include a cervical spine series, which includes a cross-table lateral film, an anteroposterior film, an oblique film, and an open-mouth odontoid film. On the cross-table lateral cervical spine film, all seven cervical vertebrae and the top of T1 must be visualized (Fig. 22-6). Radiographs may demonstrate subluxations, fractures, dislocations, and narrowing of paravertebral spaces.

To obtain an adequate cross-table cervical spine film, the nurse may find it necessary to drop the patient's shoulders by pulling downward on the patient's arms; this positioning allows for adequate visualization of the cervical vertebra and the top of T1. When positioning the patient, be sure that someone is maintaining alignment of the patient's head with manual traction.

The films must be assessed for evidence of the following: anteroposterior column alignment, the anteroposterior diameter of the spinal canal, the presence of bone fragments or bony displacement, the presence of linear fractures or comminuted fractures, soft tissue edema at or below the C3

cord level, the presence of a retropharyngeal hematoma, and vertebral inclination. If an adequate assessment of the films cannot be performed, the patient should be considered "uncleared" and should remain in a position of cervical protection and immobilization (maybe for days) until the cervical spine can be adequately assessed.

Other helpful diagnostic tests are the bulbocavernosus muscle reflex test and testing for an "anal wink," or contraction. The bulbocavernosus muscle reflex is tested by placing a finger in the patient's rectum and concurrently compressing the glans or the clitoris or tugging on a Foley catheter. If the anal sphincter contracts, this contraction is considered a normal finding. If the reflex is absent and then returns within 24 hours, the finding is considered a total lesion. The anal sphincter normally contracts ("winks") when there is a pin prick in the close vicinity of the anus. When a spinal cord injury is present, no response to the pin prick occurs.

PREVENTION OF FURTHER INJURY

A sufficient number of persons must be available when the patient is being moved, especially when the patient is being "log-rolled" or moved to another stretcher or table. Also the cervical, thoracic, and lumbar spine must be immobilized in accordance with local protocol.

THERAPEUTIC INTERVENTION

Therapeutic intervention is aimed at ensuring an adequate airway, ventilations, and prevention from further injury. In addition, considerable attention is being paid to minimizing postinjury edema: the airway may be at risk not only from a spinal cord injury that compromises the muscles of respiration but also from edema, which may cause obstruction. Endotracheal intubation should be considered. Ninety-six percent of persons with cervical spine injuries can be orally intubated safely.[5] Cricothyrotomy or tracheostomy should also be considered when the patient requires airway management and such management cannot be ensured by using conventional nonsurgical methods.

Problems with a patient's blood pressure may be directly related to the presence of spinal shock. First, before pharmacologic interventions such as the administration of atropine are instituted, consider elevating the patient's legs. Because of possible disruption of the sympathetic nervous system in cases of spinal shock, when blood pressure drops as a result of vasodilation the heart rate usually does not increase to compensate for the drop in blood pressure, whereas the heart rate does increase in cases of hypovolemic shock.

The procedure for immobilization of the cervical, thoracic, and lumbar spine is described in the box on p. 306. Placement of cervical tongs attached to cervical traction should also be considered; cervical tongs provide consistent traction (Fig. 22-7). If this intervention is used, apply no

CERVICAL SPINE IMMOBILIZATION PROCEDURE

1. Assess airway; ensure patency by using the jaw thrust or chin lift maneuver; do not hyperextend the neck; if endotracheal intubation is necessary and not possible without hyperextension, consider nasotracheal or digital intubation or cricothyrotomy to ensure the airway.

2. Evaluate the cervical spine by observation; palpate each spinous process, noticing deformity, crepitus, pain, and instability. Talk to the patient; inform the patient of each step of the process to alleviate anxiety and movement and to elicit his or her cooperation.

3. Gently apply in-line manual traction by placing the nurse's hands on either side of the head and stabilizing the neck in a neutral vertical position. In children, this is defined as the "sniffing" position. Once traction has been applied, it must be maintained until a comparable or better alternative has been implemented or until the possibility of cervical spine injury has been ruled out by radiographic findings or results of a computed tomography scan.

4. Have other members of the team assist by gently placing a spine board under the patient while one caregiver continues to maintain traction. Synchronize the log roll maneuver with absolute cervical spine protection.

5. Secure the patient to the long board. Undress the patient completely if possible, and pad bony prominences liberally. Remove any sharp or bulky objects. Place chest, hip, and leg straps across the patient, and snuggly attach the straps to handles or cutouts in the board. Secure the straps diagonally from the chest to the hips. Pad behind the head and neck to support the cervical spine, always maintaining a neutral position. Secure the patient's head to the spine board by using adhesive tape that is 2 inches wide. Tape across the eyebrows, and secure the ends of the tape to the spine board. Exercise extreme caution to ensure that the securing items do not interfere with respirations or emesis.

6. When you are satisfied with the absolute immobility of the patient's cervical spine, manual traction may be released.

7. Be prepared to perform logroll maneuver on the patient, using the back board, if emesis occurs. Be sure to have adequate suction equipment on hand.

8. If a short spine board or another short device is used, it should be used in conjunction with a long board or scoop stretcher. Short boards should be used only to facilitate extrication.

9. If the patient is wearing a helmet, leave it in place, as long as the airway is not compromised and immobilization can be accomplished. The procedure for helmet removal is described in the box above.

From Sheehy SB, Marvin JA, Jimmerson CL: *Manual of clinical trauma care: the first hour,* St Louis, 1989, Mosby–Year Book.

HELMET REMOVAL PROCEDURE

A variety of helmets is available for those who participate in sports for which head protection is recommended such as motorcycling, bicycling, kayaking, ice hockey, football, and automobile racing. The careful removal of this protective device is imperative for the protection of the cervical spine.

1. Never attempt to remove the helmet by yourself— it takes two persons to remove the helmet. Ensuring an adequate airway can usually be achieved with the helmet in place, and the potential exists for complicating an injury during a difficult removal.

2. One person applies in-line traction by placing hands on each side of the helmet with fingers on the patient's mandible, exerting careful pulling. Remember to cut or remove the chin strap.

3. A second person concurrently receives the weight of the patient's head by placing the fingers of both hands on the occipital region and the thumbs at the angles of the mandible. The second person is now in control of the head and neck.

4. The first person then removes the helmet by pulling laterally and carefully sliding it off. If the helmet has full face protection, special consideration must be given to the eye covering, which must be removed first. If it cannot be removed, tilt the helmet, *not the head,* back, to pass the face protector over the patient's nose. Then pull the helmet laterally.

From Sheehy SB, Marvin JA, Jimmerson CL: *Manual of clinical trauma care: the first hour,* St Louis, 1989, Mosby–Year Book.

more than 12 lbs of traction (the head weighs approximately 9 lbs), since too much traction may cause distraction (Fig. 22-8).[4]

Also consider the initiation of two large-bore (16-gauge or larger) intravenous (IV) catheters attached to warmed Ringer's lactate solution; administer the solution intravenously at a keep-open rate unless hemodynamic findings indicate otherwise. Place an indwelling urinary catheter to straight drainage, and carefully monitor hourly urine output. It is imperative that urinary retention and possible bladder rupture be prevented. Also, place a nasogastric or orogastric tube.

Although controversial, use of the pneumatic antishock garment should be considered for patients with hypotension, in accordance with local protocols.

In a randomized, controlled, double-blind study, high-dose methylprednisolone was used to treat acute spinal cord injuries.[1] If the methylprednisolone was started within 8 hours of the injury, patients demonstrated significant improvement in both touch and pin sensation and motor function at 6 weeks and 6 months after injury.

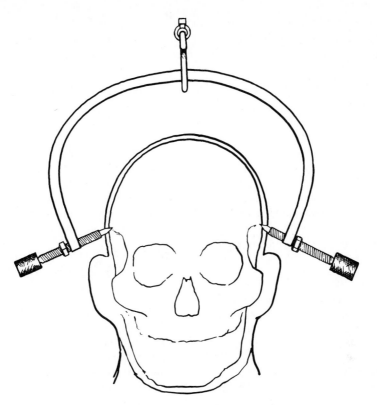

Fig. 22-7   Anatomic placement of cervical tongs.

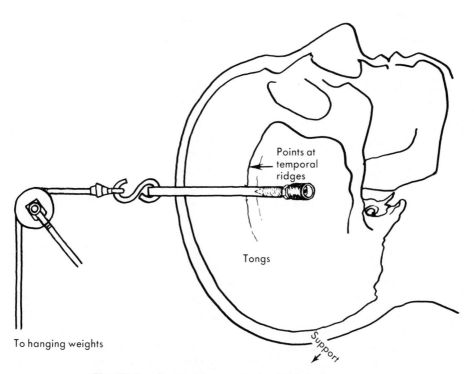

Points at
temporal
ridges

Tongs

To hanging weights

Support

Fig. 22-8   Cervical tongs attached to hanging weights.

The recommended dosage of methylprednisolone follows: 30 mg of methylprednisolone per kg of body weight, given over a period of 15 minutes, followed by a 45-minute pause, followed by a 23-hour continuous infusion of 5.4 mg per kg per hour via a large peripheral vein, a central line, or a Swan-Ganz catheter.

The formulas by which to calculate the dosage schedule include the following:

Bolus dose

$$\frac{(30 \text{ mg/kg}) \times (\text{patient's weight in kg})}{(50 \text{ mg/ml})} = \frac{\text{total bolus dosage}}{\text{(in milliliters)}}$$

- The infusion pump should be set to deliver a total bolus dose in 15 minutes.
- Keep the IV line open for an additional 45 minutes with normal saline solution.

Maintenance dose

$$\frac{(5.4 \text{ mg/kg}) \times (\text{patient's weight in kg})}{(50 \text{ mg/ml})} = \frac{\text{maintenance dose}}{\text{per hour}}$$
$$\text{(in milliliters)}$$

- The infusion pump should be set to deliver the hourly maintenance dose for 23 hours.

Because 1 hour spent on an unpadded board causes an 80% chance of significant skin problems later,[2] pressure points must be padded. Also ensure that tetanus prophylaxis and antibiotics are administered if appropriate.

Early neurosurgical consultation is important. Consider transferring the patient to a facility with neurosurgical rehabilitation capabilities or both capabilities. If the patient is transferred in tongs and traction, be sure that the hanging weights can hang freely: do not allow them to touch the floor or be taped.

For the patient's psychosocial welfare, provide positive support but do not offer false hope.

SOFT TISSUE INJURIES OF THE NECK
Fractured Larynx

The most common cause of a fractured larynx is blunt trauma such as impact from a steering wheel or dashboard, a rope, or a karate chop.

Signs and symptoms include a hoarse voice, cough with hemoptysis, progressive respiratory stridor, difficulty breathing, respiratory distress, and the presence of subcutaneous emphysema.

Diagnosis is made by clinical observation—palpating for subcutaneous emphysema and noting progressive respiratory stridor or respiratory distress. Therapeutic intervention includes emergency cricothyrotomy (performed in the ED) or tracheostomy (performed in the surgery department). (See Chapter 22.) Therapeutic intervention also includes the administration of high-flow oxygen both before and after the procedure and the administration of broad-spectrum antibiotics.

Penetrating Neck Wounds

Penetrating objects such as bullets, missile fragments, and knife blades can cause trauma to the structures of the neck. The extent of injury depends on the type of penetrating object, the force of the object, and the location and angle of the penetration.

Signs and symptoms include an obvious penetrating wound, airway obstruction, and signs of hypovolemia, hemothorax, or shock. Diagnosis is made by clinical observation, arteriography, or exploratory surgery.

Emergency therapeutic intervention includes airway management, ensuring adequate oxygenation, controlling bleeding, replacing blood loss with crystalloid solutions or blood products or both, and preparation for surgical intervention.

NURSING DIAGNOSES APPROPRIATE FOR PATIENTS WITH SPINAL CORD INJURY

High risk for injury, secondary to injury to the spinal cord with movement

Defining characteristics
- Fracture or dislocation of vertebrae
- Impalement of fragments into the spinal cord

Nursing interventions
- Place the patient with a suspected injury in a rigid cervical collar.
- Immobilize from head to hips.
- Turn patient using log roll technique.
- Apply in-line cervical traction as indicated.

Evaluation
- Patient will demonstrate no further progression of spinal cord injury.

Shock (neurogenic), potential for

Defining characteristics
- Injury to the spinal cord may result in decreased sympathetic tone and pooling of blood in the peripheral circulation, leading to shock.
- Warm, dry, flushed skin is the hallmark of neurogenic shock. (Refer to Chapter 19 for further information.)

Nursing interventions
- Monitor vital signs.
- Monitor urine output and fluid intake.
- Keep patient flat.
- Explain all procedures to patient and family.
- Administer fluids and pharmacologic agents as prescribed.

Evaluation
- The patient's vital signs will be within normal limits.

Urinary retention

Defining characteristics
- Absent sensory and motor impulses

Nursing interventions
- Monitor bladder for distention.
- Insert urinary catheter.
- Monitor urine output.

Evaluation
- The patient will be catheterized promptly.

High risk for impaired skin integrity

Defining characteristics
- Patient is unable to feel pressure and move to relieve that pressure.

Nursing interventions
- Bony prominences should be padded.
- Skin over bony prominences should be inspected frequently, and areas of pressure should be massaged to improve circulation.

Evaluation
- The skin will remain intact, without evidence of pressure.

Other nursing diagnoses that may be appropriate for the patient with a spinal cord injury are discussed in other chapters and include the following:

Ineffective airway clearance
Ineffective breathing pattern
Impaired verbal communication
Ineffective individual coping
Anticipatory grieving

SUMMARY

Trauma to the neck or cervical spine may result in life-threatening injuries or permanent paraplegias or quadriplegias. The goals in management of these types of injuries are to protect the airway, breathing, and circulation and to protect the patient from further harm. The nurse must be an astute observer and a meticulous giver of care. Injuries to the cervical spine are often extremely frightening to both the patient's family and his or her support group. Careful psychologic care must be given. If diagnostic and therapeutic interventions are not locally available, early transfer of the patient is essential to a favorable outcome.

REFERENCES

1. Bracken MB et al: A randomized controlled trial of methylprednisolone or naloxone in the treatment of acute spinal cord injury, *N Engl J Med* 322:1405, 1990.
2. Copass M: Lecture presentation, American College of Surgeons Advanced Trauma Life Support Course, University of Washington, Seattle, June, 1987.
3. Kraus JF et al: Incidence of traumatic spinal cord lesions, *J Chronic Dis* 28:471, 1975.
4. Shea J: Lecture presentation, Tacoma Fire Department Trauma Conference, Tacoma, Washington, Aug 2 and 3, 1987.
5. Shea J: Lecture presentation, Whatcom County EMS Conference, Bellingham, Washington, Oct 1988.

SUGGESTED READINGS

American College of Surgeons Committee on Trauma: *Advanced trauma life support provider manual,* Chicago, 1988, American College of Surgeons.

Ayuyao AM et al: Penetrating neck wounds, *Ann Surg* 202:563, 1985.

Balkany TJ et al: The management of neck injuries. In Zuidema GD et al, eds: *The management of trauma,* ed 4, Philadelphia, 1985, WB Saunders.

Campbell WH, Cantrill SV: Neck injuries. In Rosen P et al, eds: *Emergency medicine,* ed 2, St Louis, 1987, Mosby–Year Book.

Halpern JS: Administering methylprednisolone for acute spinal cord injuries, *JEN* 17(1):37, 1991.

Harris P: *Thoracic and lumbar spine and spinal cord injuries,* New York, 1987, Springer-Verlag.

Hockberger RS, Doris PE: Spinal injury. In Rosen P et al, eds: *Emergency medicine,* ed 2, St Louis, 1987, Mosby–Year Book.

Moulton RJ, Clifton GI: Injury to the vertebrae and spinal cord. In Mattox KL, Moore EE, Feliciano DV, eds: *Trauma,* East Norwalk, Conn, 1988, Appleton-Lange.

Susan Budassi Sheehy

$\mathbf{V}$ision is often considered the most important of the five senses. The ability to assess a patient who has an emergency eye problem and to plan and rapidly apply therapeutic interventions that reverse the problem or prevent further damage are important. A brief overview of the anatomy and physiology of the eye is presented in this chapter, along with a quick view of some of the more commonly seen eye emergencies encountered in the emergency care setting.

EYE

The eye is the organ of one of the most precious senses the human body possesses. Many times loss of vision can be prevented by rapid, careful treatment in the prehospital area and in the emergency department (ED).

To be able to deal with eye emergencies effectively and efficiently, the nurse must have a good understanding of the basic anatomy and physiology of the eye (Fig. 23-1).

Basic Anatomic Descriptions

Bony rim bony process that protects the eyeball
Eyelid closes to protect the eyeball, to distribute tears, and to regulate amount of light
Eyelashes minimize the amount of dirt particles that enter the eye area
Sclera tough, protective coating of the eyeball
Cornea front section of the eyeball that bulges; light passes through it to the lens
Retina inner lining of the posterior eyeball; collects light
Choroid middle layer of the eyeball; supplies the retina with blood, oxygen, and other nutrients
Macula area of the retina most sensitive to light and color
Lens disc through which light passes to the posterior chamber from the cornea and the anterior chamber; light passes through the cornea, the anterior chamber, the lens, and the vitreous humor to the retina
Iris controls the amount of light entering the posterior chamber by expanding and contracting the opening (the pupil)
Oculomotor muscles six muscles that control eyeball movement
Lacrimal glands (Fig. 23-2) secrete fluid (tears) to soothe the eyeball and decrease friction
Tears cover the eyeball; they are distributed by the eyelids (blinking) and exit through the lacrimal puncta into the lacrimal ducts and the nasolacrimal duct

Meibomian glands secrete oil that lines the eyelid margins and prevents tears from running out of the conjunctival sacs
Visual acuity central vision; stimuli on macula
Peripheral vision vision in which stimuli are on area of the retina other than macula

During triage for a patient with a complaint of trauma to the eye or a problem with the eye, the following conditions are given priority treatment:
1. Loss of sight without pain (may be caused by central artery or vein occlusion, intraocular hemorrhage, or retinal detachment)
2. Chemical burns
3. Foreign bodies
4. Painful eyes (may be conjunctivitis, iritis, or keratitis)
5. Penetrating objects

EYE EXAMINATION

Good lighting is essential during eye examinations, and the use of topical local anesthetics may be helpful. It is important to remember to be gentle and to explain to the patient what is happening and what you are about to do. It is essential to recognize an eye condition or trauma early so that further complications can be prevented whenever possible.

When examining a patient with an eye problem, perform a visual acuity examination before the actual eye examination, if possible.

Visual Acuity Examination

Perform the examination with the patient wearing glasses; then examine the patient again when the patient is not wearing glasses. If the patient's glasses are not available, have the patient read the visual acuity chart through a pinhole poked in a piece of cardboard.

Check each eye separately, then both eyes together.

Follow specific instructions for conducting the examination, choosing one of the following methods:
- The Snellen chart is read from a distance of 20 feet.
- The Rosenbaum Pocket Vision Screener (used for patients who cannot stand) is read at a distance of 14 inches from the nose.

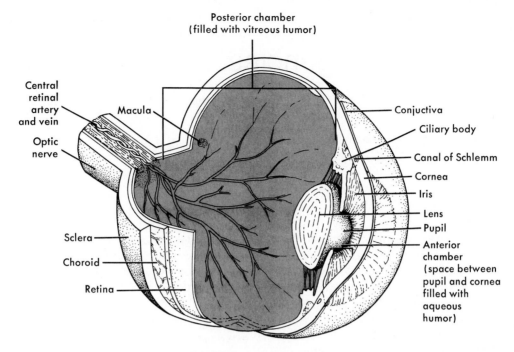

Fig. 23-1 Anatomy of eye.

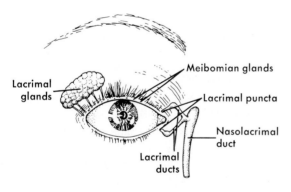

Fig. 23-2 Lacrimal glands.

- If a Snellen chart or other vision chart is not available, have the patient read newsprint and record the distance at which the paper must be held for the patient to be able to read it.
- If the patient cannot see newsprint, hold up a specific number of fingers and record the distance at which the patient can see your fingers and tell you how many you are holding up.
- If the patient cannot see fingers, record the distance at which he or she can perceive hand motion.
- If the patient cannot see hand motion, record the distance at which he or she is able to perceive light.
- If the patient is unable to perceive light, this finding must also be recorded on the chart.

Examples of Visual Acuity Examination

20/20	When the patient stands at 20 feet, he or she can read what the normal eye can read at 20 feet.
20/20 − 2	When the patient stands at 20 feet, he or she can read what the normal eye can read at 40 feet (but has missed two letters).
20/200	When the patient stands at 20 feet, he or she can read what the normal eye can read at 200 feet. The patient is considered legally blind if the reading is obtained while he or she is wearing glasses or contact lenses.
10/200	If the patient cannot read the letters on the Snellen chart, have him or her stand at half the distance to the chart and record the findings as the distance the patient is standing from the chart over the smallest line he or she can read.
CF/3 feet	The patient can count fingers at a maximum distance of 3 feet.
HM/4	The patient can see hand motion at a maximum distance of 4 feet.
LP/position	The patient can perceive light and determine the direction from which it is coming.
LP/no position	The patient can perceive light but is unable to tell the direction from which it is coming.
NLP	The patient is unable to perceive light.

Ophthalmoscope (Fig. 23-3). The ophthalmoscope is the basic tool used in examining the eye. It is used to observe the posterior chamber of the eye through the pupil with a beam of light. Ophthalmoscopes have differently shaped and differently colored light beams that are used to detect various conditions.

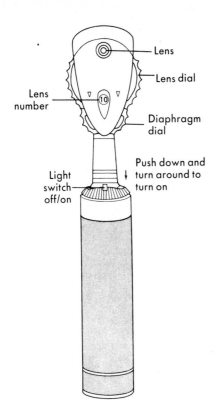

Fig. 23-3   Ophthalmoscope.

When recording information on a chart regarding the eye, simply use the words *right, left,* and *both* or use the following abbreviations:

OD	ocula dexter	right eye
OS	ocula sinister	left eye
OU	oculus uterque	both eyes
gtt	guttae	drops

TRAUMA TO THE EYE

When trauma to the eye is present, always assess the patient for associated trauma, which may be more life-threatening. When there is head or facial trauma, always search for associated eye injury.

Never put eye drops into the eye of a victim with eye trauma before examination and evaluation of the extent of injury. If the pain from trauma is severe, it can be minimized without medication by patching both eyes and decreasing the amount of movement of the globe. If a patient is unconscious, be sure to check for the presence of contact lenses and be sure to protect the cornea from drying by either instilling ophthalmic ointment and taping the eylids shut or instilling artificial tears frequently if the patient is unable to blink.

Industrial accidents account for more than half of all blindness to one eye and a fifth of all blindness to both eyes. Trauma to the eye occurs as the result of a large number of industrial accidents in which safety glasses are not worn

and is the number two cause of blindness in children, second only to amblyopia.

It is important to obtain a good history from a patient with eye trauma. Questions that assist in obtaining this history include the following:

What happened?

Were chemicals involved? Which ones?

Are there foreign bodies in the eye? What are they?

How did it happen?

Where did it happen?

Why did it happen?

Who witnessed it?

Was care given before arrival at the hospital? What? By whom?

Were safety glasses being worn at the time of the accident?

Is there any eye-related medical history, particularly of glaucoma, diabetes, or hormone therapy?

Eyelid injuries. The eyelid serves three purposes: to protect the eye, to distribute tears, and to regulate the amount of light entering the eyeball. The eyelashes offer extra protection to the eye by minimizing the amount of dirt particles that enter the eye area.

Because the eyelid has an excellent blood supply, trauma to the eyelid has a low incidence of infection and antibiotic treatment is rarely required.

Therapeutic intervention for eyelid injuries includes irrigation of the wound with normal saline solution and careful approximation of the wound edges in the early period after injury, before edema sets in. It is important to make efforts *not* to excise any tissue, since excision may cause a deformity in the eyelid and disrupt its function. If a large section of tissue is missing, request that a plastic surgeon perform plastic reconstruction to replace lid tissue so that the cornea is protected.

Be sure to check for a lacerated lacrimal duct when lid trauma is present. If there is such a laceration, the duct should be surgically repaired.

Orbital rim injuries. Orbital rim injury may occur as a result of a blunt or penetrating trauma to that area of the face. Periorbital ecchymosis ("black eye") may result, causing discoloration in and around the orbital rim area. Therapeutic intervention for periorbital ecchymosis includes application of an ice pack and examination of the orbital rim for fractures and eyeball damage and appropriate treatment for these. Assessment should include a visual acuity examination.

If there is a fracture of the prominent supraorbital rim and the frontal sinus, be sure to check for cerebrospinal fluid rhinorrhea. If the patient complains of a visual disturbance, there may be a fracture of the orbital roof, resulting in entrapment of the optic nerve.

Nonpenetrating blunt trauma to the eyeball. Blunt trauma to the eyeball may cause aqueous humor to depress the diaphragm of the iris or the ciliary bodies. When this occurs, the result is a hyphema or hemorrhage into the anterior chamber of the eye. Any patient who has a hyphema *must* be referred to an ophthalmologist immediately.

If the patient has a partial hyphema, therapeutic intervention includes strict bed rest, heavy sedation, and the use of bilateral eye patches for a minimum of 5 days. Some ophthalmologists choose to administer acetazolamide (Diamox), urea, or mannitol; osmotic diuretics decrease intraocular pressure. Ophthalmologists may also administer steroids and miotics or mydriatics or both.

Massive hyphema may occur at any time, from the time of injury up to 2 weeks afterward. This injury may cause corneal blood staining, secondary glaucoma, loss of vision, or even loss of the eye.

An "eight-ball" hemorrhage is a condition in which old clotted blood is found in the anterior chamber. Therapeutic intervention is to remove the clots surgically.

Retrobulbar hemorrhage may occur as a result of ruptured intraorbital vessels. It is evidenced by an eyeball that protrudes (exophthalmos) and diplopia (double vision).

A subconjunctival hemorrhage commonly occurs after trauma to the eye. It is usually left untreated and resolves itself within about 2 weeks.

Blow-out fracture. A blow-out fracture results from direct blunt trauma to the eyeball, causing an increased intraocular pressure that in turn causes a fracture of the orbit floor. It is diagnosed by obtaining a history of the incident and by observation of periorbital hematoma, subconjunctival hemorrhage, periorbital edema, enophthalmos, an upward gaze, and a complaint of diplopia; the latter three conditions are caused by trapping of the inferior rectus muscle and the inferior oblique muscle in the fracture. Radiologic diagnosis can be made based on the results of the standard facial radiographs.

When this fracture is present, apply a cold pack. If there is bony displacement, reduce the fracture and pack the maxillary sinus. Surgery may be required to free the trapped orbital muscle. Be sure to check for associated intraocular injuries, perform a visual acuity examination, and obtain an ophthalmology consultation.

Foreign bodies. Most commonly the foreign body in the eye is something small, causing the patient to complain that there is something in his or her eye. Foreign bodies and corneal abrasions feel almost alike to the patient. It is important to locate the foreign body, if there is one. Often local anesthesia is required to examine the eye adequately. General anesthesia is usually required to examine the eye of a child adequately *and to remove a foreign body*. Always ensure that there is good lighting and a magnification source when removing a foreign body from the eye. Avoid using sharp needles and eyespuds whenever possible.

Foreign body to the conjunctiva. The most common foreign body is the eyelash, and it usually can be found under the upper eyelid in the tarsal conjunctiva. Therapeutic intervention includes everting the upper eyelid and irrigating with normal saline solution, gently removing the foreign body with a moist cotton swab, or *very* carefully removing the foreign body with a 25-gauge needle at a tangential angle, and applying local antibiotics four times a day for 5 days. An eye patch may be applied, depending on the nature of the foreign body and on the amount of damage to the eyeball. It is also advisable to have the patient see an ophthalmologist within 1 day for a follow-up visit.

The main complication of a conjunctival foreign body is a scratched cornea. The cornea should be stained with fluorescein; if a scratch is present, treat the injury as you would a corneal abrasion.

Foreign body to the cornea. The presence of a body foreign to the cornea is painful to the patient. The patient usually complains that there is something under his or her eyelid because the moving lid rubs up and down on the foreign body. Therapeutic intervention includes irrigation of the eye with normal saline solution and removal of the foreign body with a moistened cotton swab or a 25-gauge needle (very carefully at a tangential angle to the eyeball). Always be sure to check for the presence of more than one foreign body. If the foreign body is metal, a rust ring forms within 12 hours. This rust ring must be removed by an ophthalmologist.

Everting the eyelid (Fig. 23-4)
- Have the patient look down.
- Grab the lashes of the upper eyelid and gently pull down.
- Apply gentle pressure on the upper lid with a cotton-tipped swab or other smooth instrument.
- Evert the eyelid over the swab or instrument.

Intraocular foreign bodies. Intraocular foreign bodies are easy to overlook, since they are usually small projectiles such as metal fragments that penetrate the eyeball at high speed and come to rest somewhere within the posterior chamber. Pain may be minimal. The actual opening to the chamber may be small and difficult to locate. One must suspect that a foreign body is there to be able to find it.

The presence of an intraocular foreign body is *an extreme emergency*, and therapeutic intervention must occur within early moments after the injury. If an external eye injury is present, the nurse must obtain a thorough history from the patient so that the presence of an intraocular foreign body may be ruled out.

The amount of damage to the eyeball depends on the size, shape, and composition of the foreign body. If surgery is required, fragments that can be magnetized are easier to remove. Surgical removal prevents further damage to the eyeball, such as hemorrhage, infection, detached retina, or loss of vision.

All foreign bodies should be considered contaminated, and patients should be treated with antibiotics and checked for current tetanus prophylaxis. Many intraocular foreign bodies may be seen only on a radiograph; it is therefore

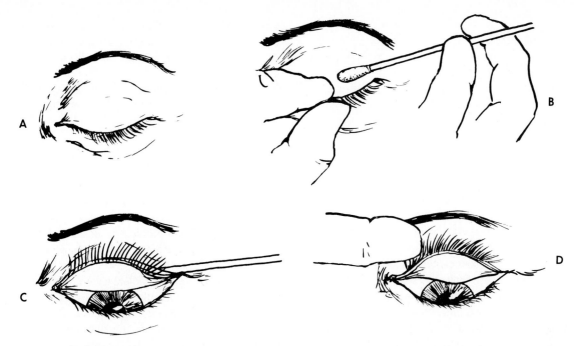

Fig. 23-4 Steps in everting eyelid. **A,** Eyelid. **B,** Placement of cotton swab (eyelashes are pulled down and back over swab). **C,** Eyelid everted over swab. **D,** Examination of inside of eyelid and eye.

mandatory that a radiograph be made of all suspected foreign bodies in the intraocular area.

Complications of intraocular foreign bodies may include infection, intraocular hemorrhage, detached retina, loss of vision, traumatic cataract, and loss of the eye.

Perforating and Penetrating Injuries to the Globe of the Eye

Penetrating injuries to the globe of the eye are usually a result of perforation by a sharp object such as a knife or dart. In this type of injury it is important to apply therapeutic intervention in the early stages of the injury to decrease the likelihood of further complications.

Emergency therapeutic intervention is to secure the impaled object if it is still penetrating the eyeball and to cover both eyes to decrease eye movement and reduce the possibility of further damage. Do not perform a detailed examination at this time; this examination should be reserved for an ophthalmologist. General anesthesia may be necessary to perform an adequate examination.

If eye tissue has not been eviscerated, an ophthalmologist usually removes the object during surgery and sutures the eye. If there is loss of vitreous humor and damage to the lens and ciliary body, enucleation may be required.

Other therapeutic intervention includes the administration of antibiotics, tetanus prophylaxis, and a regimen of corticosteroids.

Corneal lacerations. Small corneal lacerations are usually not sutured but rather left alone under a light pressure

dressing. If the laceration is large, an ophthalmologist should be consulted. The ophthalmologist usually places sutures of either 8-0 silk or 7-0 chromic, using a fine needle.

Corneal abrasions. Corneal abrasions are common injuries. They occur when a foreign body (such as a contact lens) denudes the epithelium. It is important to obtain a history of what caused the abrasion.

A patient with a corneal abrasion has a tearing eye and eyelid spasms and complains of pain on the surface of the eye. Corneal abrasion is diagnosed by staining the surface of the eye with fluorescein stain and observing the eyeball with a cobalt light and magnification. Use sterile, individually packaged fluorescein strips, because fluorescein solution is easily contaminated by pseudomonads.

Therapeutic interventions include the administration of local anesthesia while a visual acuity examination is being performed, the application of ophthalmic antibiotics, and patching of the injured eye for about 24 hours to prevent eyelid movement and to decrease the amount of light that enters the eye. These patients should receive follow-up care from an ophthalmologist within 1 day. Patients should be instructed *not* to use local anesthetic agents continuously.

Using fluorescein strips to stain the cornea
(Fig. 23-5)
• Explain the procedure to the patient.
• Moisten the end of a sterile fluorescein strip with normal saline solution.

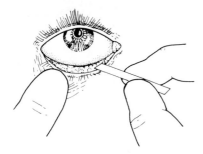

Fig. 23-5 Fluorescein staining. Touch moistened fluorescein strip to inner canthus of lower lid.

- Pull down on the lower eyelid.
- Touch the strip to the inner canthus of the lower eyelid.
- Ask the patient to distribute the staining solution by blinking (tears will spread the solution over the cornea).
- Using a cobalt lamp, examine the cornea.

Conjunctival lacerations. The most common cause of a conjunctival laceration is a fingernail. Signs and symptoms include swelling and bleeding from the conjunctiva. If the laceration is small (less than 5 cm), therapeutic interventions include applying ophthalmic antibiotics, patching, and observation of the eye. If the laceration is large (greater than 5 cm), an ophthalmologist should be called to suture the conjunctiva.

Corneal ulcers. Corneal ulcers commonly occur in the unconscious patient or in patients who have left their contact lenses in place for an inordinate period of time. The ulcer appears as a whitish spot on the cornea. The condition is painful, and the patient has photophobia, profuse tearing, and vascular congestion if he or she is conscious. With fluorescein staining the ulcer appears as a blue green cast. If *Pseudomonas aeruginosa* invades, the patient may lose the eye in a period of 48 hours. Therapeutic interventions include the administration of systemic antibiotics, the use of warm compresses, and the application of an eye patch.

Optic nerve avulsion. Optic nerve avulsion occurs infrequently. The injury usually results from a severe trauma in which the optic nerve enters the eyeball. A partial tear results in partial blindness, whereas a total tear results in total (permanent) blindness. Therapeutic intervention is surgical repair.

Iris injury. Traumatic iridocyclitis is an inflammation of the iris and ciliary body after contusion to the eye. It is evidenced by the presence of uveal pigment and lens tissue in the anterior chamber. Therapeutic intervention includes topical administration of cycloplegic agents and topical and systemic administration of corticosteroids. Complications include enophthalmos and loss of the eye.

Another type of iris injury is iris sphincter rupture. It is usually caused by trauma to the eyeball, which causes the pupil to dilate and the iris to notch at the edges.

Lens injury. Lens injuries can include partial dislocations (subluxations), total dislocations (luxations), and opacifications (cataracts). Therapeutic intervention for each is surgery.

Retina and choroid injury. Trauma to the retina and choroid may produce a white ellipse at which the sclera is visible through the rupture. If the macula is injured, decrease in visual acuity results.

Problems with Contact Lenses

All contact lenses float on tears and adhere to the cornea by means of capillary attraction. Lenses come in two forms: hard or soft (also known as hydrophilic lenses).

The most common problem associated with the wearing of contact lenses is the presence of chemicals or dirt particles under the lens, which causes irritation of the cornea. The second most common problem is wearing the lenses too long, which causes swollen, painful eyes. This condition usually occurs 6 to 8 hours after lens removal.

Therapeutic intervention for the presence of foreign bodies under the lens is lens removal and cleansing of the lens *and* eye before return of the lens to the eye.

If contact lenses have been worn too long, the lenses should not be worn for a period of 24 to 48 hours.

Sometimes a contact lens is lost in the cul-de-sac, most commonly the upper one. Therapeutic intervention is to evert the eyelid and remove the lens.

To determine whether the patient is wearing contact lenses, ask. If the patient cannot respond to your questions, check for an identifying (Medic-Alert) bracelet, or look at the eye tangentially, using a flashlight.

Removing a contact lens
Hard lenses
Use a suction cup designed especially for removing contact lenses; or use the two-handed method shown in Fig. 23-6.

Soft lenses
Locate the lens, grasp it between the thumb and index finger, and lift it off the cornea (Fig. 23-7).

Be sure to store lenses in separate, clearly marked ("right" and "left") containers filled with sterile saline solution.

Burns of the Eye

Chemical burns. Chemical burns commonly cause eye injuries in the home and in industrial settings. Chemical burns of the eye are (1) nonprogressive, superficial burns, usually caused by acids, (2) progressive burns caused by alkaline substances, and (3) irritants, caused by gases, such as tear gas and Mace.

In any type of chemical burn the immediate therapeutic intervention is copious irrigation with normal saline solution or tap water. Before examination of the eye is performed, local anesthesia may be required.

Acid burns are usually self-limiting, because when tissue is denatured as a result of the acid, the denatured tissue

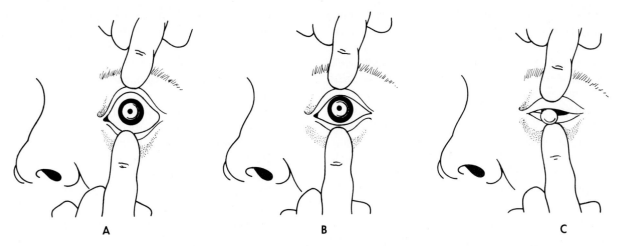

Fig. 23-6 Technique for removing hard corneal contact lens from eye. **A,** Spread eyelids apart. **B,** Push lids toward center of eye under contact lens. **C,** Remove lens.

neutralizes the acid. Therapeutic interventions include copious irrigation with normal saline solution, topical application of antibiotics, and administration of ophthalmic cycloplegic agents.

Alkali burns, such as those caused by lime or ammonia, present an *extreme emergency* because alkali causes much tissue destruction. Initially the burn may appear as white spots; severe damage is not evident until 3 to 4 days after the incident. Therapeutic interventions include copious irrigation with normal saline solution and the administration of antibiotics, cycloplegics, and corticosteroids.

When irrigating an eye, irrigate for 30 minutes and then check the pH of the conjunctiva, which is normally 7.0. If the pH is not normal after 30 minutes of irrigation, continue to irrigate the eye and periodically check the pH until it returns to normal.

Specific antidotes for chemical burns

Acid burns	Sodium bicarbonate 2%
Alkali burns	Citric or boric acid
Lime burns	Ammonium tartrate 5%

Complications of acid or alkali burns of the eye include adhesion of the globe to the eyelid, corneal ulcerations, entropion (eyelashes that turn in toward the eyeball), iridocyclitis, and glaucoma.

Delayed or latent action injury from direct contact with liquids and solids. The box below contains a list of substances that bind chemically with tissue and have delayed onsets of toxic action.

Thermal burns. When facial burns are present, it is quite common to find associated eyelid burns. It is not common, however, to see globe burns, unless the burn was produced by hot metal, steam, or gasoline. Burns to the eyelids may cause lid contractures. Therapeutic interventions should include analgesia, sedation, eye irrigation, antibiotics, cycloplegics, and bilateral eye patches.

Radiation burns. There are two types of radiation burns, ultraviolet and infrared. The severity of the burn depends on the wavelength and the degree of exposure.

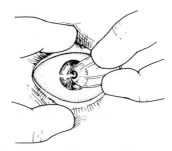

Fig. 23-7 Soft lens removal. Lift soft lens off cornea.

TOXIC SUBSTANCES WITH DELAYED ONSET OF ACTION

Cardiac glycosides	Methylchloracrylate
Colchicine	Methyldichloropropionate
Digitalis glycosides	Mustard gas
Dimethyl sulfate	Osmic acid
Dyes (cationic)	Podophyllum
Emetine	Poison ivy
Erythrophleine	Rare earth salts
Euphorbias	Squill
Formaldehyde	Sulfur dioxide
Ipecac	Surfactants
Manchanil	Triacetoxyanthracene
Methylbromide	

From Grant WM: Toxicology of the eye, ed 2, Springfield, Ill, 1974, Charles C Thomas.

Ultraviolet radiation burns. Ultraviolet radiation burns may be seen in welders (welder's arc flash), snow skiers, and ice climbers, people who read on the beach, and people who use a sunlamp. The burn is caused when ultraviolet radiation is absorbed by the cornea, producing keratitis, conjunctivitis, or both. It is usually 3 to 6 hours after the exposure before the patient demonstrates signs and symptoms of the burn, which include feeling as though there is a foreign body in the eye, tearing, and excessive blinking. This patient may also have associated facial and eyelid burns.

Therapeutic interventions include the administration of topical antibiotics, analgesics (systemic), and cycloplegics and the application of bilateral eye patches. All signs and symptoms of the injury should disappear, and the condition should improve within 24 hours.

Infrared radiation burn. Infrared radiation burn is a much more severe type of burn than ultraviolet radiation burn. Infrared radiation burns may cause permanent loss of vision, because the infrared rays are absorbed by the iris, which results in an increase of the temperature of the lens, causing cataracts.

Common types of infrared burns
- "Glass-blower's cataracts," resulting from prolonged exposure to intense heat
- Focal retinitis, caused by "eclipse blindness" or exposure to an atomic bomb, in which the lens condenses heat, causing a retinal scar and blindness
- X-ray burns, which are proportional to the penetration of the rays: grenz rays are soft rays that produce superficial keratoconjunctivitis and dermatitis; gamma rays are hard rays and overexposure produces retinal damage and cataracts

When the lens is damaged, the repair process is slow. The lens remains much more vulnerable to repeated injury during the healing process.

Irrigating the eye (Fig. 23-8, *A*)
- Cleanse the external area around the eye and eyelid.

- Prepare an irrigation basin or portable hairwashing tray, irrigation solution, and administration set.
- Have the patient lie down, or adjust the ear, nose, and throat (ENT) chair to a reclining position.
- Have the patient turn his or her head toward the affected side.
- Pull down the eyelid of the affected eye.
- Run irrigation fluid directly over the eyeball and lower-lid cul-de-sac from the inner to the outer canthus.
- Have the patient blink occasionally to distribute the irrigation solution over the eyeball.
- Irrigate for a minimim of 30 minutes (more if indicated by the levels of the pH).

Continuous eye irrigation with the Morgan therapeutic lens (Fig. 23-8, *B*). A Morgan therapeutic lens (Mortan, Inc., Missoula, Montana) is a specially designed lens that is placed on the eye and used to provide continuous ocular lavage or continuous ocular medication. The lens, which is a scleral lens, is made of a hard (polymethacrylate) plastic, and the tubing is made of a soft silicone plastic, with a female adapter at the distal end.

Placement (Fig. 23-8, *C*)
1. Explain the procedure to the patient.
2. Instill anesthetic ocular drops into the affected eye.
3. Ask the patient to look down.
4. Retract the upper lid.
5. Grasping the lens by the tubing and the small finlike projections, slip the superior border of the lens up under the upper eyelid.
6. Then have the patient look up.
7. Retract the lower eyelid, and place the lower border of the lens.
8. Have the patient turn his or her head toward the affected side, and place a folded towel under the patient's head to collect irrigation solution.
9. Attach the female adapter at the end of the lens tubing either to a syringe filled with the solution of choice, which is instilled at the desired rate, or to intravenous

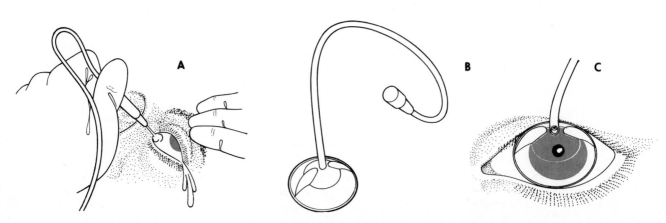

Fig. 23-8　**A,** Position for eye irrigation. **B,** Morgan therapeutic lens. **C,** Lens in place.

tubing that is connected to the solution of choice, which is instilled at a selected drip rate.

10. To remove the lens, follow steps 5 through 7 in reverse order.
11. Dry the patient's face and eye area with a towel.
12. Dispose of the lens.
13. Follow any additional orders for instillation of medication and dressing the eye.

MEDICAL PROBLEMS INVOLVING THE EYE

Some of the conditions discussed in this section, as well as ptosis, eyelid edema, entropion, ectropion, dacryocystitis, exophthalmos, pterygium, and convergent and divergent strabismus, are represented in Figs. 23-9 to 23-21.

Blepharitis

Blepharitis is an inflammation of the lid margin, usually caused by *Staphylococcus aureus*. Therapeutic interventions include application of cool, moist compresses and antibiotic ophthalmic ointment.

Hordeolum

Hordeolum, or stye, is an infection of the upper or lower eyelid at the accessory gland and is caused by *S. aureus*. The infection is evidenced by a small, external abscess, pain, redness, and swelling. Therapeutic intervention includes the application of warm compresses four times a day until the abscess "points." Antibiotic ophthalmic ointment should also be applied. The patient should be instructed *not* to squeeze the abscess, but rather to have it incised and drained by a physician when it comes to a point.

Chalazion

Chalazion is a sebaceous cyst that forms on the inside surface of the eyelid resulting from congestion of the meibomian gland. It is evidenced by a small mass beneath the conjunctiva of the lid that is red, swollen, and quite painful. Therapeutic interventions include the application of antibiotic ophthalmic ointment and incision and drainage by a physician.

Keratitis

Keratitis is an inflammation of the cornea that is light sensitive, red, and painful; it causes profuse tearing. A culture and sensitivity specimen is taken to determine the specific cause. Therapeutic interventions include application of warm compresses, antibiotic ophthalmic ointment, and topical corticosteroids, which should *not* be used for herpes simplex–type inflammations.

Keratoconjunctivitis

Keratoconjunctivitis is an inflammation of the outer layer of the eye. The inflammation can result from an allergic reaction, which appears as itching, redness, discharge, and tearing. Therapeutic intervention is usually administration

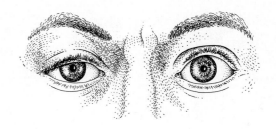

Fig. 23-9   Ptosis.

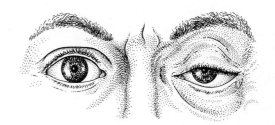

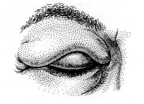

Fig. 23-10   Edema of eyelid.

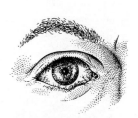

Fig. 23-11   Entropion.

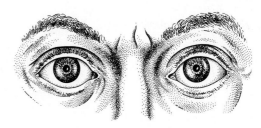

Fig. 23-12   Ectropion.

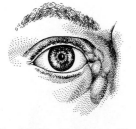

Fig. 23-13   Dacryocystitis.

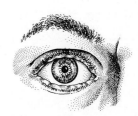

Fig. 23-14   Marginal blepharitis.

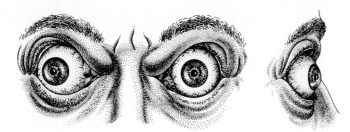

Fig. 23-15 Exophthalmos.

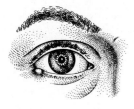

Fig. 23-16 Hordeolum.

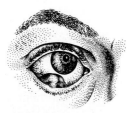

Fig. 23-17 Chalazion.

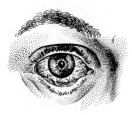

Fig. 23-18 Conjunctivitis.

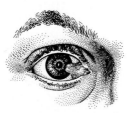

Fig. 23-19 Pterygium.

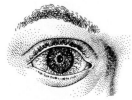

Fig. 23-20 Iritis.

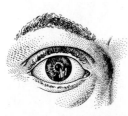

Fig. 23-21 Corneal abrasion.

of topical corticosteroids. Another cause of keratoconjunctivitis may be herpes simplex, in which case corticosteroids should *not* be used. Herpes keratoconjunctivitis is generally treated with idoxuridine (Stoxil) or vidarabine (Vira A).

Uveitis

Uveitis is an inflammation of the uveal tract that usually includes the iris, ciliary body, and choroid. Signs and symptoms of this condition are unilateral and include photophobia, tearing, pain, and blurred vision. Therapeutic interventions include application of warm compresses, analgesia (systemic), antibiotic ophthalmic ointment, corticosteroids (topical), and mydriatics (to dilate the pupil and prevent adhesions of the iris and the lens).

Acute Conjunctivitis

Acute conjunctivitis is a bacterial infection of the conjunctiva characterized by the eyelids sticking together when the patient wakes up in the mornings. It may be caused by staphylococcal, gonococcal, pneumococcal, *Haemophilus*, or *Pseudomonas* organisms. Therapeutic intervention is antibiotic ophthalmic ointment. Before antibiotic therapy is started, obtain a specimen for culture and sensivity testing.

Acute conjunctivitis is contagious. Thus detailed aftercare instructions must be given to the patient concerning how to prevent the disease from spreading.

One specific type of acute conjunctivitis is *Neisseria gonorrhoeae*; a copious amount of purulent discharge occurs, and the conjunctiva is extremely red and swollen. Therapeutic intervention for this type of conjunctivitis is application of penicillin ophthalmic ointment.

Acute Iritis

Acute iritis is an inflammatory condition of the iris characterized by photophobia and tenderness of the eyeball. Acute iritis is *not* an infectious process. Therapeutic interventions include application of cold compresses and topical corticosteroids, and the use of an eye patch and dark glasses.

Central Retinal Artery Occlusion

Central retinal artery occlusion produces sudden blindness, and prognosis is poor. Therapeutic interventions include amyl nitrate inhalation, sublingual nitroglycerin administration, inhalation of alternating carbon dioxide and oxygen to attempt to dilate the artery and return blood supply to the retina, or a combination of these.

Cavernous Sinus Thrombosis (Orbital Cellulitis)

Cavernous sinus thrombosis is an infection (pneumococcal, staphylococcal, or streptococcal) that has spread from an infected sinus to the orbit area. Signs and symptoms of this condition include facial and eyeball edema, vascular congestion in eyelids, aching pain, pain in eyeball, conjunctival chemosis, fever, decreased visual acuity, decreased pupillary reflexes, papilledema, and paralysis of the extraocular muscles. Therapeutic interventions are the application of antibiotic ophthalmic ointment and warm compresses and bed rest.

Retinal Detachment

The normal function of the retina is to perceive light and send an impulse to the optic nerve. When the retina is torn, vitreous humor seeps between the retina and the choroid, resulting in separation of the retina from the choroid, which decreases blood and oxygen supply to the retina. This loss of blood and oxygen supply renders the retina unable to perceive light.

Signs and symptoms of retinal detachment are flashes of light, a veil or curtain effect in the visual field, and a dark spot or particles in the vision. Therapeutic interventions include immediate strict bed rest, bilateral eye patches, administration of tranquilizers, and possibly surgery after ophthalmology consultation.

Glaucoma (Fig. 23-22)

It is estimated that approximately 1 million Americans have undiagnosed glaucoma. Glaucoma causes 1 out of every 10 cases of blindness in the United States. Acute glaucoma is a condition in which aqueous humor, secreted by the ciliary process epithelium in the posterior chamber of the eye and transported to the anterior chamber through the pupil, cannot escape from the anterior chamber, which causes a rise in the anterior chamber pressure.

Normally, aqueous humor leaves the anterior chamber and enters the vascular system via the Schlemm's canal at the junction of the iris and the cornea. This increase in anterior chamber pressure causes a decrease in circulation to the retina and an increased pressure on the optic nerve and may eventually cause blindness. *Acute glaucoma is an emergency situation* because it may cause blindness in just a few hours.

Acute glaucoma. Acute (closed-angle) glaucoma results when there is a blockage in the anterior chamber angle near the root of the iris. Signs and symptoms of this condition include severe eye pain, a fixed and slightly dilated pupil, a hard globe, a foggy-appearing cornea, severe headache, halos around lights, diminished peripheral vision, and occasionally nausea and vomiting. Therapeutic intervention is aimed at decreasing the pupil size to allow for aqueous humor drainage. This is accomplished by frequently (every 15 minutes) instilling miotic eyedrops— usually 1% or 4% pilocarpine (Table 23-1). The strength of the solution is not as important as the frequency of instillation is. Other therapeutic interventions include systemic administration of analgesia (usually morphine) and drugs such as acetazolamide (Diamox) to attempt to decrease intraocular pressure. Surgery may be indicated if pharmacologic intervention is unsuccessful.

Open-angle glaucoma. Open-angle (chronic or wide-angle) glaucoma is an obstruction of the Schlemm's canal that develops gradually. Because this condition is chronic and progresses slowly, the patient may be unaware of its presence. Therapeutic interventions for this type of glaucoma include instillation of miotic eyedrops and surgery.

Congenital glaucoma. Congenital (infantile or juvenile) glaucoma is a failure of the anterior chamber angle to develop normally. Early signs and symptoms are copious tearing and photophobia: a baby has a tendency to keep his or her eyelids shut more than usual. Therapeutic intervention is surgery.

Secondary glaucoma. Secondary glaucoma is an increase in intraocular pressure resulting from surgery, trauma, hemorrhage, inflammation, tumors, or various other conditions that may interfere with humor drainage. Therapeutic intervention varies, depending on the cause of the glaucoma.

Measuring ocular pressure with a tonometer. Tonometric examination is used to measure intraocular pressure. The Schiøtz tonometer, which is the most commonly used type, has a plunger that measures the amount of indentation pressure of the cornea when the tonometer is placed on it.

Before the tonometer is used, the eyeballs should be anesthetized with 1 to 2 drops of anesthetic ophthalmic drops, the patient should have the procedure thoroughly explained to him or her, and he or she should be placed in a lying position. A sterile tonometer, previously calibrated, is placed directly on the eyeball, and intraocular pressure is measured. With a Schiøtz indentation tonometer, if intraocular pressure is high, the tonometer scale reads low because the plunger cannot indent the eyeball very much. If

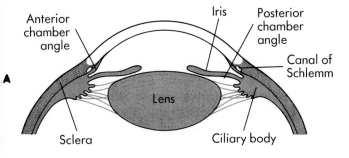

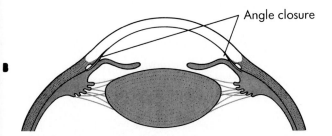

Fig. 23-22   Comparison of, **A,** normal angle of eye with, **B,** closed angle in closed-angle glaucoma.

Table 23-1 Ophthalmologic medications

Generic name	Common brand names	Action and use
MIOTICS		Constrict pupils; primarily used to treat glaucoma
Pilocarpine	Pilocar	Acts on myoneural junction
	Isopto Carpine	
	P.V. Carpine Liqui-film	
Carbachol	Carcholin	Acts on myoneural junction
	Carbamycholine	
	Isopto Carbachol	
	Doryl	
	P.V. Carbachol	
Echothiophate iodide	Phospholine	Cholinesterase inhibitor
Isoflurophate (diisopropyl flurophosphate)	DFP	Cholinesterase inhibitor
	Floropryl	
Acetazolamide	Diamox	Carbonic anhydrase inhibitor; decreases aqueous humor production
MYDRIATICS		Dilate pupils
Sympathomimetics		
Epinephrine	Adrenalin	Mydriasis and vasoconstriction
	Epitrate	
Phenylephrine	Neo-Synephrine	Mydriasis and vasoconstriction
Ephedrine	Epinedrine	Adrenergic vasoconstrictor and antiallergenic
Hydroxyamphetamine	Paredrine	Mydriasis
Parasympathomimetics		Paralyze ciliary muscles; accommodation; dilate pupils
Atropine sulfate	Isopto Atropine	Mydriasis and cycloplegia
Cyclopentolate	Cyclogyl	Mydriasis and cycloplegia
Homatropine	Homatrocel	Mydriasis and cycloplegia
	Isopto Homatropine	Anticholinergic and sedative
Scopolamine		Mydriasis and cycloplegia
Tropicamide	Mydriacyl	
	Mydriaticum	
Physostigmine	Physostol	Mydriasis and cycloplegia
Neostigmine		
CYCLOPLEGICS		Paralyze ciliary muscles; accommodation
Cyclopentolate	Cyclogyl	Mydriasis and cycloplegia
ANESTHETICS		Surface anesthesia
Proparacaine	Ophthaine	Local anesthesia
Tetracaine	Pontocaine	Local anesthesia
ANTIBIOTICS		
Tetracycline	Achromycin	Antimicrobial
Chloramphenicol	Chloromycetin	Broad-spectrum antibiotic
Plymyxin B with neomycin	Cortisporin	To treat nonpurulent, bacterial infections
	Neo-Polycin	
Gentamicin	Garamycin	To treat Gram-positive bacteria
Erythromycin	Ilotycin	For superficial topical infections
	Dista	
Sulfisoxazole	Gantrisin	Bacteriostatic
Sulfacetamide sodium	Sulamyd	Gram-negative and gram-positive bacteriostatic

Table 23-1 Ophthalmologic medications—cont'd

Generic name	Common brand names	Action and use
STEROIDS		Decrease inflammatory response
Dexamethasone	Decadron	Decreases inflammatory response
COMBINATION STEROID-ANTIBIOTICS		
Prednisolone acetate	Metimyd	Antiinflammatory, antibacterial
Prednisolone sodium phosphate with sodium sulfacetomide	Optimyd	Antiinflammatory, antibacterial
Neomycin sulfate and hydrocortisone acetate	Neo-Cortef	Antiinflammatory, antibacterial
Terramycin/oxytetracycline/hydrocortisone acetate	Terra-Cortril	Antiinflammatory, antibacterial
Neomycin sulfate with methylprednisolone	Neo-Delta-Cortef Neo-Medrol	Antiinflammatory, antibacterial
HERPES SIMPLEX VIRUS INHIBITORS		
Idoxuridine	Stoxil	Inhibits herpes simplex virus
Vidarabine	Vira-A	Inhibits herpes simplex virus when nonresponsive to Stoxil or if there is an allergic reaction to Stoxil
COMBINATION EYEDROPS		
Various combinations of phenylephrine hydrochloride, methylcellulose, boric acid, sodium borate, sodium chloride, ethylene diamine tetraacetate, and benzalkonium chloride	Ocusol Murine Visine Prefrin	Soothes tired eyes and decreases redness

intraocular pressure is low, the tonometer scale reads high because the plunger indents the eyeball more than normal.

A normal indentation tonometer reading is 11 to 22 mm Hg. A lower reading indicates increased intraocular pressure, and a higher reading indicates decreased intraocular pressure.

EYEDROPS AND OPHTHALMIC OINTMENTS

Eyedrops are instilled into the eye to decrease pain, for antibiotic therapy, to increase the size of the pupil, to decrease the size of the pupil, to reduce allergic reactions of the eye, or to cleanse the eye.

Procedure for Instilling Eyedrops

- Explain the procedure to the patient.
- Pull the lower eyelid downward.
- Instill 1 to 2 drops of the intended solution into the cul-de-sac (the center of the inner lower lid).
- Have the patient blink to distribute the solution.
- Instruct the patient *not* to squeeze his or her eyelids tightly shut because this causes the medication to leak out.

Procedure for Instilling Ophthalmic Ointment

- Explain the procedure to the patient.
- Pull the lower eyelid downward.

- Have the patient look up.
- Apply ointment in a thin line into the inner aspect of the lower lid from the inner to the outer canthus.
- Have the patient blink to distribute the ointment.
- Instruct the patient not to squeeze his or her eyelids tightly shut, since this repels the ointment.

SUMMARY

This chapter is not meant to be the definitive resource for care of all eye emergencies; rather, it provides a brief review of some of the more commonly seen eye emergencies. The care giver is advised to seek the advice of an ophthalmologist when he or she is uncertain of the immediate or follow-up care required for a given eye emergency.

SUGGESTED READINGS

Clark RB: Common ophthalmologic problems. In Rosen P et al: *Emergency medicine*, ed 2, St Louis, 1988, Mosby–Year Book.

Ellis PP: *Ocular therapeutics and pharmacology*, ed 7, St Louis, 1985, Mosby–Year Book.

Newell FM: *Ophthalmology principles and concepts*, ed 6, St Louis, 1986, Mosby–Year Book.

Perkins ES, Hansell P, Marsh RJ: *An atlas of diseases of the eye*, New York, 1986, Churchill-Livingstone.

Sheehy SB: *Mosby's manual of emergency care*, ed 3, St Louis, 1989, Mosby–Year Book.

CHAPTER 24

Ear, Nose, Throat, Facial, and Dental Emergencies

Susan Budassi Sheehy

Patients often come to the emergency department (ED) with an ear, nose, or throat emergency, especially during the evening, night, weekend, and holiday hours when it is difficult to get in touch with private practitioners. The nurse must be able to assess a patient and evaluate appropriate diagnostic tests and physical findings so that the severity of the problem can be determined.

EAR EMERGENCIES

The goal of treating a person with an ear injury is to prevent any further trauma to the ear, including the cartilage. During repair of the ear it is important to remember that circulation to this area is not great. When anesthetizing the area, therefore, be sure to use lidocaine *without* epinephrine. If there is a simple laceration that does not involve the cartilage, it should be irrigated and simple sutures placed. The wound may be left open to air if a light layer of antibiotic ointment is applied. If the wound involves cartilage, it should be minimally debrided, and the cartilage and perichondrial layer should be approximated; this is followed by closure and suture of the overlaying skin. Consider placing the patient on a regimen of oral antibiotic agents. The ear should be splinted with cotton balls behind it and a loose, bulky dressing over it.

If there is evidence of a subperichondrial hematoma, it should be aspirated to avoid formation of a cauliflower ear. Once it is drained, a pressure dressing should be applied and the wound checked frequently for recurrence of the hematoma, which, if it recurs, must be reevacuated.

Foreign Body

The patient with a foreign body in the ear usually has that as the chief complaint; but occasionally, especially in pediatric patients, a foreign body is discovered only after the detection of purulent drainage from the ear.

Before the ear is probed or irrigated, check to see if there is a history of a perforated tympanic membrane. When performing the examination, be sure that the light is good and that an appropriately sized speculum is available. Grasp the pinna and retract it to provide maximal visibility. Prepare the patient, since the ear is often sensitive to examination and manipulation. Nitrous oxide gas administration is often found to be useful in an examination or probe of the ear. If the patient is a child, be sure that the child is restrained. One may even have to administer a general anesthetic to examine the patient properly.

Once the foreign body is located, it may be removed by suction, irrigation, forceps, or a blunt 90-degree–angle hook, depending on the nature of the foreign body. Occasionally an insect flies into a patient's ear. If the insect is alive, it is best to attempt to remove it intact. The easiest way to do this is to drop mineral oil into the ear canal. Aim the canal upward and shine a light into it; the insect will crawl out toward the light. If one attempts to pull the insect out with forceps one might remove only a part of the insect, and removal of the remaining part(s) might cause much further irritation. If unable to remove the foreign body, refer the patient to an otolaryngologist.

Nontraumatic Emergencies

Otitis externa. Otitis externa (swimmer's ear) is a bacterial or fungal infection characterized by ear pain, an edematous canal, an exquisitely tender ear canal cartilage, purulent drainage, and hearing loss caused by accumulation of debris in the ear canal. It is differentiated from acute otitis media by the tenderness of the outer ear canal, which is absent in middle ear infection. This condition occurs most frequently during the outdoor-swimming season. Therapeutic intervention includes suctioning debris from the ear canal and placing a cotton wick saturated with a topical eardrop preparation (with or without corticosteroid ingredients). The wick should be left in place for 48 to 72 hours, with the solution instilled onto the indwelling wick three or four times a day. Once the wick is removed, the drops are continued for a total treatment time of 10 days. Narcotic analgesic agents may be necessary to relieve the pain for the first 24 to 48 hours.

Acute otitis media. Acute otitis media is generally preceded by an upper respiratory tract infection. Signs and symptoms are hearing loss, otalgia, "fullness" in the affected

325

ear, redness of the tympanic membrane, withdrawal or bulging of the tympanic membrane, white or yellow discoloration, and blebs on the tympanic membrane surface (bullous myringitis).

In the event of imminent perforation or bullae on the tympanic membrane producing severe pain, a myringotomy should be performed by an otolaryngologist. If the condition is not so severe, the patient may be treated with analgesic agents, antibiotics, and decongestants.

Vertigo. Most but not all cases of vertigo are otologic. Common causes of vertigo include a foreign body, head trauma with concussion, temporal bone fracture, acute labyrinthitis, infections of the middle ear, and mastoiditis. In addition to vertigo the patient may also complain of tinnitus, hearing loss, and nausea and vomiting. Spontaneous nystagmus associated with head movement can be detected during the physical examination. If the syndrome is disabling, hospitalization is recommended. Otherwise, the patient should be referred to an otolaryngologist for follow-up care after being treated symptomatically in the ED.

Motion sickness. Motion sickness is often accompanied by fatigue, dizziness, nausea and vomiting, blurred vision, nystagmus, diaphoresis, and cool clammy skin. It is usually caused by the motion of a plane, car, bus, or boat. It is thought to be caused by repeated stimulation of the semicircular canals of the ears.

Therapeutic intervention is primarily prevention by pretreatment. The patient may be placed on a regimen of transdermal scopolamine, oral meclizine, or dimenhydrinate. If the patient is already symptomatic, remove the patient from the cause of the motion sickness; this removal usually decreases signs and symptoms. The patient may also be treated with promethazine (Phenergan) and ephedrine in combination.

NOSE EMERGENCIES
Foreign Bodies

Foreign bodies in the nose are most commonly seen in children. They are usually discovered after a purulent discharge is noticed draining from one of the nostrils. Treatment consists of administering a decongestant nasal drop preparation, applying a topical anesthetic agent, placing the patient in Trendelenburg's position, and removing the object with alligator or ring forceps.

Epistaxis

An epistaxis, or nosebleed, is a frequently seen problem in the ED. Epistaxis can be minor or major, depending on the amount of bleeding and the response of the patient; it can be severe enough to become a life-threatening emergency. Epistaxis most commonly occurs in children, adults from 50 to 70 years of age, patients with blood dyscrasias, atherosclerotic heart disease, or hypertension, patients receiving anticoagulant therapy, patients with alcoholism, people with certain allergies, and patients with hereditary telangiectasia (Rendu-Osler-Weber disease).

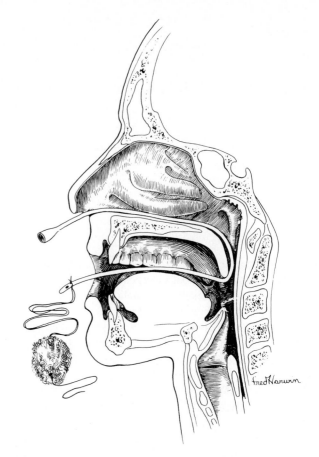

Fig. 24-1 Steps used in passing postnatal pack. (From DeWeese DD et al: *Textbook of otolaryngology,* ed 7, St Louis, 1987, Mosby—Year Book.)

Anterior epistaxis. Anterior epistaxis is common and is usually caused by bleeding from the anterior and inferior turbinates or at the area of Kisselbach. Therapeutic intervention is to place the patient's head in a slightly hyperextended position, suction clots, observe for the bleeding site, and apply a vasoconstrictor agent (via cotton balls) such as a 10% cocaine solution. After 5 to 10 minutes of pressure the bleeding sites should be cauterized with silver nitrate. During this entire period, reassure the patient; it may be a frightening time. If the patient has a blood dyscrasia or is receiving immunosuppressive agents, use a wedge of salt pork instead of the cocaine-soaked cotton balls; this method of treatment appears to be much more effective and much more comfortable.

Posterior epistaxis. Posterior epistaxis is a much more difficult problem to control. It is usually the result of a chronic condition, such as hypertension, atherosclerotic heart disease, blood dyscrasia, or a tumor. When bleeding occurs, it is usually from the sphenopalatine artery, the nasopalatine plexus (plexus of Woodruff), or the anterior ethmoid artery.

Therapeutic intervention includes ABCs, volume replacement if indicated, anesthetization of the nose with a 10%

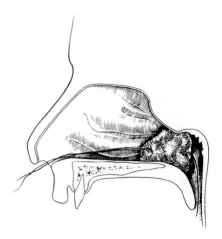

Fig. 24-2   Postnatal pack in place. (From DeWeese DD et al: *Textbook of otolaryngology,* ed 7, St Louis, 1987, Mosby–Year Book.)

cocaine solution, and packing of the bleeding site. The nurse should also check the patient's blood pressure and medical history. If the bleeding continues after packing, the internal maxillary artery or anterior ethmoid artery may have to be ligated.

When the posterior of the nose is packed, one must prepare the patient by anesthetizing the nose. One should also administer antibiotics and admit the patient for an observation period of 2 to 5 days once the packing is in place. The nose is packed by passing a rubber catheter (either a commercially available catheter used specifically for epistaxis or a Foley catheter with a balloon) through one nostril to the posterior palate. Tie a large pledget or a tampon to the catheter with two ties. Then pull the catheter out, pulling the tampon into place near the choana. Using your fingers, push the tampon firmly into place. If a commercial epistaxis catheter is used, it is not necessary to use a tampon, since the inflated balloon presses against the choana to tamponade the bleeding. If the tampon is being used, take one tie and pull it forward through the mouth. Tape the end of this tie to the outside of the patient's face. If the tampon should come loose and fall into the patient's throat, it can thus be easily removed by pulling on the string taped to the face. Once the balloon or tampon is in place, the nasal cavity should be placed bilaterally from the anterior openings using a nasal speculum, a bayonette forceps, and half-inch selvage-edged, petrolatum-impregnated gauze. It should be layered from front to back. Keep track of and record the number of packs used (Figs. 24-1 and 24-2). Both the commercial epistaxis catheter and the tampon should be secure through the nostril. The tampon should have a string tied to the petrolatum gauze; the catheter should be clamped with an umbilical clamp.

Be sure to tell the patient that if bleeding occurs again, he or she should keep his or her head up and tilted slightly forward. This helps to protect the airway. Instruct the patient not to blow his or her nose and to apply steady pressure to both nostrils with the fingers for at least 5 minutes. If the bleeding does not stop and the patient is not at the hospital or the private physician's office, the patient should immediately return to the office or ED.

THROAT EMERGENCIES

One of the most common throat emergencies is a foreign body to the throat. This foreign body may be penetrating or obstructing the airway, or it may be aspirated. The most common foreign bodies in an adult are chicken and fish bones. Often the point of lodgment is at the tonsils. Therapeutic intervention is aimed at clearing the airway. If the foreign body totally obstructs the airway, one must follow basic cardiac life support procedures for airway obstruction and administer 4 back blows, followed by 4 abdominal thrusts (Heimlich maneuver). Then one should attempt to breathe into the victim. If repeated attempts to clear the airway are unsuccessful, one should consider performing a cricothyrotomy.

Fractured Larynx

A fractured larynx is a life-threatening situation caused by a direct blow to the neck. Many times this type of patient is multiply injured, and this injury may be overlooked if not specifically checked. Upper airway obstruction from a fractured larynx is caused by the massive edema resulting from the fracture.

Signs and symptoms of a fractured larynx include severe shortness of breath, voice changes, respiratory stridor, and respiratory arrest with a history of trauma to the throat area. A fractured larynx is detected by feeling crepitus in the throat area; one cannot *see* it. Therapeutic intervention is to perform a cricothyrotomy, place the patient on antibiotics, and consider administering a regimen of corticosteroids. (See Chapter 13 for further discussion of the cricothyrotomy procedure.)

Upper Respiratory Tract Infection and Pharyngitis

An upper respiratory tract infection, also known as the common cold, appears with symptoms of fullness in the head, pain in the ears, a sore throat, elevated temperature, general malaise, possibly enlarged tonsils, enlarged cervical nodes, and a foul breath odor. Therapeutic intervention includes the administration of aspirin or acetaminophen and warm saline gargles; a regimen of antibiotics and forced fluids should also be considered.

Ingestion of Caustic Agents

Caustic agents that are most frequently ingested include household cleaning products such as lye, ammonia, sulfuric acid, and liquid drain cleaners. Initial examination usually reveals a reddened or bleeding surface with ulcerations or denuded tissue. It is difficult to determine the extent of the injury until endoscopic examination is performed. Therapeutic intervention goals are to reduce the amount of damage that will be done by any remaining caustic agent. This damage may be reduced by administering a specific antidote within 30 minutes of the ingestion. Avoid emesis and avoid passing a nasogastric or other indwelling tube whenever possible. Protect the ABCs and support respirations, if indicated. The patient should be admitted to the hospital for observation and further treatment, which may include dilatation, surgery, or both.

Neck Trauma

Auto accidents and assaults generate most of the neck injuries seen in the ED. The most serious sequelae to neck trauma are airway obstruction and cervical spine fractures and dislocations. A cervical spine trauma should be suspected in any patient with multiple injuries or severe injuries to the head or if the patient is complaining of tenderness and spasm, with or without neurologic tenderness. A cross-table lateral radiograph of the cervical spine should be obtained before ruling out this type of injury. The patient must have both the cervical and thoracic spines immobilized until this possibility is ruled out.

Penetrating neck wounds carry a 40% mortality if they are vascular. These injuries are recognizable by persistent bleeding from the wound, an expanding hematoma of the neck, a depressed airway, absence of extremity pulses, bruits, and central nervous system defects. If there is a severe laryngeal injury, the patient complains of hoarseness, dysphonia, aphonia, stridor, hemoptysis, neck tenderness, crepitus, and flattening of the laryngeal prominence. Indirect or direct laryngoscopy may reveal lacerations, hematomas, edema, or vocal cord immobility. In such cases the caregiver may consider endotracheal intubation or cricothyrotomy.

FACIAL TRAUMA

Patients with facial trauma are often seen in the ED. Although automobile and motorcycle accidents are the ma-

jor causes of facial trauma in the United States, sports injuries and domestic violence account for many others. It is far too easy to concentrate on the profuse bleeding of facial trauma (attributed to the vast amount of vascularity in this area) and overlook other not-so-obvious life-threatening problems, such as an obstructed airway or severe hypotension caused by trauma elsewhere. A patient with facial trauma may have other much more serious injuries such as hypovolemic shock, respiratory distress, a spinal cord injury, or an intracranial catastrophe. Facial injuries often involve four of the cranial nerves (Table 24-1). These should be carefully assessed. Assessment for facial trauma is shown in the box on the next page.

Facial Lacerations

Mostly for cosmetic reasons, immediate repair of facial lacerations is important. Facial lacerations, even the most severe, are *rarely* accompanied by facial fractures. Abrasions and contusions should be cleansed and debrided. If gravel or other small particles are present, carefully remove them, since they may cause "tattooing." If there is a powder ring from gunpowder, be sure to preserve it whenever possible. If preservation is not possible, take a picture of the ring before scrubbing it. If no camera is available, be sure to describe the mark in detail in your notes. Abrasions should be dressed with a topical antibiotic ointment.

Simple lacerations should be cleansed and debrided. The wound should then be sutured, with no tension, and dressed with a topical antibiotic ointment and a pressure dressing to reduce scar formation. To cleanse a facial wound properly, one may consider applying a local anesthetic to the wound, usually 1% lidocaine *with* epinephrine. Epinephrine produces vasoconstriction to reduce bleeding and also increases the absorption time of lidocaine. The full effects of the lidocaine and the epinephrine are achieved approximately 14 minutes after injection. If the wound is small, it can possibly be treated using local anesthetic. If it is large,

---

Table 24-1   Cranial nerves involved in facial trauma

Nerve	Name	Activity	Elicits	Test by
III	Oculomotor	Motor	Eyeball movement; supplies 5 of 7 ocular muscles	Pupil response; ocular movement to four quadrants
IV	Trochlear	Motor	Eyeball movement (superior oblique)	Same as above
V	Trigeminal	Motor and sensory	Facial sensation; jaw movement	Assessing pain, touch, hot and cold sensations, bite, opening mouth against resistance
VII	Facial	Motor and sensory	Facial expression; taste from anterior two thirds of tongue	Zygomatic branch: have patient close eyes tightly; temporal branch: have patient elevate brows, wrinkle forehead; buccal branch: have patient elevate upper lip, wrinkle nose, whistle

<table>
<tr><td>

SYSTEMATIC ASSESSMENT FOR FACIAL TRAUMA

Airway

Assess for an open airway. If there is an airway obstruction, it should be cleared. Avoid using the head-tilt method. Consider using airway adjuncts. The nasopharyngeal airway adjunct is particularly useful, especially when great amounts of edema are present.

Breathing

Ensure that adequate breathing is taking place. Consider administering supplemental oxygen. Remember that noisy breathing is obstructed breathing.

Circulation

Ensure that pulse rate and blood pressure are adequate.

Cervical spine

Protect the cervical spine and assume that there is an injury until proven otherwise (by cross-table lateral radiograph of the cervical spine). Of patients with severe head trauma, 10% have concurrent cervical spine trauma.

Control hemorrhage

Use direct pressure whenever possible. If the hemorrhage is into the airway, protect the airway.

Neurologic examination

Perform a brief neurologic examination, assessing for the level of consciousness, pupillary response and accommodation, the rate, rhythm, and depth of respiration, and motor movement.

Eyes

Carefully evaluate the eyes, checking for loss of vision, diplopia (double vision), foreign bodies, penetrating bodies, and hemorrhage.

Face

Check for malocclusion of teeth, tenderness to touch, asymmetry of the infraorbital rim; assess the zygomatic arch, anterior wall of the antrum, angles of the jaw, and lower borders of the mandible. Also check for a cerebrospinal fluid leak from the nose or face.

</td></tr>
</table>

one may elect to use a regional anesthetic such as a nerve block.

Facial lacerations may be sutured during the first 8 hours following the accident. If the injury is 8 to 24 hours old, the wound should be sutured and the patient placed on prophylactic antibiotics. If the wound is more than 24 hours old, saline soaks should be applied until the wound appears to be clear of infection, necrotic tissue, and debris. Once the soaking has been completed, the wound should be debrided and sutured, and the patient should continue to take systemic antibiotics. If facial wounds are punctures from glass fragments, the glass should be removed; usually no suturing is required.

Special Considerations

Certain areas of the face require special consideration. The eyelids should be sutured as soon as possible, since edema begins to develop soon after the injury: the eyelid may then be difficult to approximate. When the lips are sutured, one should pay particular attention that the vermilion borders are approximated. The eyebrows should be approximated and should never be shaved. If the cheeks are lacerated, one should pay particular attention to possible damage to the parotid gland and Stensen's duct before suturing takes place. Occasionally lacerations of the tongue can be left unattended. If, however, the laceration is deep and large, it should be sutured with absorbable suture material. One who is going to suture the tongue of a young child should consider sedating the child a half hour before suturing. In any patient with a soft tissue injury or an open fracture, a tetanus prophylaxis should be administered.

When discharging the patient from the ED, give the patient adequate aftercare instructions: to keep the wound clean and dry, to cleanse the wound around the area with warm, soapy water or a hydrogen peroxide solution, to apply a topical antibiotic ointment 2 or 3 times a day, to observe for signs of infection, and to return for suture removal in approximately 4 days. Once the sutures are removed, tape strips should be applied and kept in place for approximately 10 days.

Facial Fractures

When a patient is multiply injured, fractures are often given a low priority in terms of care. The repair of a facial fracture may be delayed for a week without severe consequences.

Nasal fractures. Fracture of the nose is the most commonly seen type of facial fracture. The mechanism of injury is usually a blunt trauma to the side or front of the nose. A radiograph is not usually required in making a diagnosis. By observing for swelling, deformity, and crepitus, one can make a clinical diagnosis. The fracture may be palpatable. Bleeding occurs both internally and externally. If there is a delay between the accident and the patient's arrival at the ED, fracture reduction has to be delayed until the swelling has subsided. Remember to treat a nasal fracture as if it were an open fracture: this means that the patient should be placed on antibiotics. If there is a septal hematoma, it should be excised. If it is not excised and packed, infection is likely.

There are three types of nasal fractures. The first is nasal bone fractures or depression with or without septal dislocation. This type of injury occurs as a result of a blow to the side of the nose. The second type of fracture is a fracture of both nasal bones with or without septal dislocation. This injury occurs as a result of a hard blow to the side or front of the nose. The third type of fracture is a comminuted fracture with flattening of the bridge and fracture of the septum. This injury occurs as a result of a severe blow with some type of a club or weapon.

Therapeutic intervention for a nasal fracture is to apply an ice pack to the bridge of the nose, splint the nose, and control bleeding. Once the patient is in a controlled environment, administer an anesthetic agent. Most commonly the infraorbital area, the nasal spine, and the dorsum of the nose are injected with 1% lidocaine *with* epinephrine. The mucosa should be packed in a 5% cocaine solution. Once the patient has been anesthetized, the impacted bone should be manipulated, freeing it from the cartilage with the fingertips and a pair of forceps. The fractured part should then be molded with the fingers. The inside of the nose should be packed to decrease the likelihood of bleeding. If there is a fractured septum, both sides of the nose should be packed. The nose should be splinted for 2 weeks.

Fracture of the zygomatic arch. A tripod (trimaleolar) fracture is a common type of zygoma fracture. In this type of injury the zygoma is fractured in three places: at the zygomatic arch, at the posterior half of the infraorbital rim, and at the frontal zygomatic suture. This injury occurs when there is blunt trauma to the front and side of the face. It is diagnosed by palpating the infraorbital rim fracture and by noticing swelling, limited eye movement in an upward gaze, and (using the mnemonic *TIDES*), *t*rismus (tonic contractions of the muscles of mastication), *i*nfraorbital hyperesthesia or anesthesia, *d*iplopia (double vision), *e*pistaxis, and *s*ymmetry absence (the appearance of a depressed cheek). Therapeutic intervention includes application of a cold pack, a check for a cerebrospinal leak, and surgical repair.

Maxillary fracture. Maxillary fractures are caused by severe forces. Many result from automobile accidents, domestic violence, or a direct blow to the face with a baseball bat or club. LeFort, a French pathologist, struck corpses with bats to see what types of fractures occurred. The three most common types of fracture patterns are the following:

LeFort I (Fig. 24-3). A LeFort I fracture is fracture of the transverse alveolar process involving the front teeth and a fracture that extends bilaterally up through the nose. Signs and symptoms include malocclusion of the teeth. Therapeutic intervention includes application of a cold pack and internal fixation.

LeFort II (Fig. 24-4). A LeFort II fracture is fracture of the pyramidal area, including the central part of the maxilla, into the nasal area. A sign and symptom is that the nose moves with the dental arch. Therapeutic intervention includes application of an ice pack, internal fixation, internal stabilization, and open reduction. These patients bleed profusely and require strict attention to their airways.

LeFort III (Fig. 24-5). A LeFort III fracture is a total craniofacial separation that includes a tripod fracture and craniofacial detachment. Signs and symptoms include the nose and the dental arch moving without frontal bone movement. Therapeutic intervention includes application of an ice pack, internal fixation, administration of antibiotics, and bed rest with the head

elevated. Fractures of the cribriform plate and the middle meningeal artery are common findings. Be sure to check for a cerebrospinal fluid leak from the nose or the ear.

Fractures of the mandible. A fracture of the mandible is the second most frequently seen type of facial fracture. Often a midline mandibular fracture is accompanied by other fractures, especially near the condyles. Many fractures of this type are open fractures. The mechanism of injury is usually a severe blow caused by a blunt force; this injury is commonly seen in contact sports. Signs and symptoms include malocclusion of the teeth, pain and trismus, displacement of the bony fragment, and palpatability. Therapeutic intervention includes application of an ice pack, immobilization, and surgical fixation (the unstable area being wired to a stable area).

Orbital blow-out fracture. An orbital blow-out fracture occurs when a blunt force hits the globe directly, causing an increase in intraocular pressure and a fracture of the orbit floor. Signs and symptoms include a history of head injury, periorbital hematoma and edema, subconjunctival hemorrhage, and enophthalmos. Therapeutic intervention includes application of an ice pack, and if the globe is displaced, packing of the maxillary sinus, reduction of the fracture, and a check for intraocular injury. A patient with this type of injury should also consult with an ophthalmologist.

Fractures that require no treatment. Certain fractures of the facial bones do not require any therapeutic intervention. These are nondisplaced facial fractures, fractures of the anterior maxillary antrum wall, fractures of the coronoid process of the mandible, and fractures of the condyles in children.

DENTAL EMERGENCIES

Patients with dental emergencies are not frequently seen in the ED; when they do come, they usually arrive in the evenings, at night, and on weekends and holidays—when the dentist's office is usually closed. These patients may have pain, trauma, or both. Ask questions about the pain to differentiate maxillofacial pain from dental pain. Pain of maxillofacial origin may be classified as a major or minor neuralgia.

Major Neuralgia

Trigeminal neuralgia. Trigeminal neuralgia (tic doloreux) is a degenerative process or pressure of the trigeminal nerve. It is most commonly seen in persons over 40 years of age. The patient describes the pain as excruciating, paroxysmal, and radiating in one of three patterns: along the eye and up into the forehead, from the upper lip through the nose and cheek into the eye, or into the lower lip along the outside of the tongue. The acute onset of this condition is known as Bell's palsy. Signs and symptoms of Bell's palsy include a droopy corner of the mouth, inability to close the mouth and the eyelid, and difficulty eating and

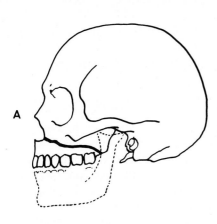

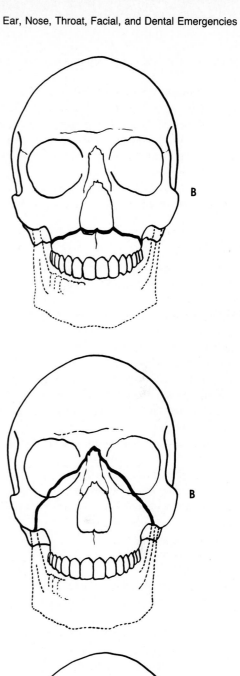

Fig. 24-3   LeFort I facial fracture. **A,** Lateral view. **B,** Frontal view.

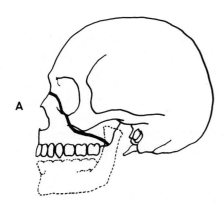

Fig. 24-4   LeFort II facial fracture. **A,** Lateral view. **B,** Frontal view.

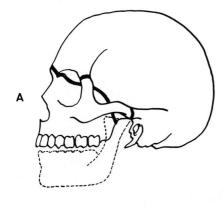

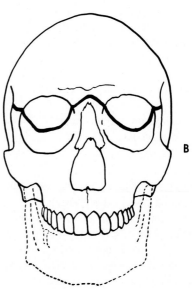

Fig. 24-5   LeFort III facial fracture. **A,** Lateral view. **B,** Frontal view.

swallowing. Therapeutic intervention is a trigeminal nerve block.

Glossopharyngeal neuralgia. Glossopharyngeal neuralgia resembles trigeminal neuralgia but is characterized by severe pain in the middle ear, the posterior throat, and the tonsils; it leads to a protrusion of the tongue. Therapeutic intervention includes administration of phenytoin (Dilantin) or carbamazepine (Tegretol).

Minor neuralgias. Minor neuralgias include sphenopalatine neuralgia, occipital neuralgia, and geniculate neuralgia.

Dental Pain

The most common cause of dental pain is decay of the teeth, also known as pulpal disease. Pulpal disease has the following phases:

1. Hyperemic. The vascular system responds to an external stimulus such as a cavity or dental trauma; at this point the condition is reversible.
2. Pulpitis. The pulp becomes infected.
3. Pulpal necrosis. The pulp dies, and fluid and pressure build up, causing severe pain.

Therapeutic intervention includes analgesia and referral to a dentist for repair.

Conditions that cause dental pain include the following:
Carcinoma
Causalgia (severe burning pain 2 to 3 weeks after tooth removal; usually related to stress)
Coronary artery disease (pain referred to the jaw)
Dry socket
Foreign body
Fractured styloid process
Fractured teeth
Glossodynia (a burning pain in the tongue usually caused by a fungal infection following antibiotic administration)
Hematomas (resulting from anesthetic injections)
Mandible fracture
Periocoronitis (erupting wisdom teeth)
Periodontal disease (gums)
Prosthetic device pressure
Sinusitis
Unerupted teeth (especially in children and especially wisdom teeth)
Vincent's angina, or "trench mouth" (ulceration of the pharynx and tonsils)

Toothaches

The most common cause of a toothache is pulpal disease (a dental caries or a cavity). The toothache occurs when the tooth becomes extremely sensitive to extremes of heat or cold. If the decay can be removed, the pain can be eliminated. This type of pain is paroxysmal and may be stimulated by an extreme temperature source. Irreversible pain indicates that a root canal (endodontics) or an extraction is necessary. The pain becomes worse at night as the patient is lying down and intracranial pressure increases. Therapeutic intervention consists of topical application of eugenol (oil of clove) or other analgesic agent and referral to a dentist for endodontics or extraction.

Chipped or Broken Teeth

The most frequently seen dental emergency in the ED is chipped teeth, an injury commonly seen in children and those involved in contact sports. The teeth most commonly injured are the four front upper center teeth. When a patient with this problem arrives at the ED, check for bleeding from the gums and the pulp. Bleeding from the pulp requires an emergency dental consultation. Often these injuries are accompanied by head injuries. If a patient has a head injury, look for associated dental trauma and pay particular attention to foreign bodies (such as broken teeth) that may obstruct the airway.

Avulsed Teeth

Avulsed teeth are teeth that have been removed from the mouth by trauma. If these teeth are found at the scene or are brought in by the patient, there is a chance that they may be reimplanted by a dentist. The likelihood of the teeth reanastomosing and not deteriorating depends on the age of the patient: children are more likely to have success with reimplanted teeth than are adults. The tooth (or teeth) should soak in saline solution until the dentist begins work.

SUMMARY

Although most ear, nose, and throat emergencies are not life threatening, they may cause pain. Sometimes facial trauma may be life-threatening because of subsequent airway problems, associated head trauma, or both. Rapid assessment, evaluation, and intervention is usually welcomed by the patient. Identification of life-threatening conditions and application of appropriate therapeutic interventions are essential.

SUGGESTED READINGS

American College of Surgeons: *Advanced trauma life support provider manual,* Chicago, 1985, The American College of Surgeons.

Amsterdam JT: Dental emergencies. In Rosen P et al, eds: *Emergency medicine: concepts and clinical practice,* ed 2, St Louis, 1987, Mosby–Year Book.

Amsterdam JT: General dental emergencies. In Tintinalli J et al, eds: *Emergency medicine: a comprehensive study guide,* New York, 1985, McGraw-Hill.

Buchanan RT, Haltman B: Severe epistaxis in facial fractures, *Plast Reconstr Surg* 71:768, 1983.

Cantrill S: Facial trauma. In Rosen P et al, eds: *Emergency medicine: concepts and clinical practice,* ed 2, St Louis, 1987, Mosby–Year Book.

DeWeese DD et al: *Textbook of otolaryngology,* ed 7, St Louis, 1987, Mosby–Year Book.

Emergency Nurses Association: *Trauma nurse care course provider manual,* ed 2, 1991, Chicago, The Association.

Kaban LB, Chung R: Maxillofacial skeletal fracture. In Callaham ML, ed: *Current therapy in emergency medicine,* Toronto, 1987, BC Decker.

Klein JO, Bluestone GD: Acute otitis media, *Pediatr Infect Dis J* 1:66, 1982.

Kruger GO: Fractures of the jaw. In Kruger GO, ed: *Textbook of oral and maxillofacial surgery,* ed 6, St Louis, 1984, Mosby–Year Book.

Okofor BC: Epistaxis: a clinical study of 540 cases, *Ear Nose Throat J* 63:153, 1984.

Sheehy SB: Mosby's manual of emergency care, ed 3, St Louis, 1989, Mosby–Year Book.

Stein HA, Slatt BJ, Stein RM: *The ophthalmic assistant: fundamentals and clinical practice,* ed 5, St Louis, 1988, Mosby–Year Book.

25 Chest Trauma

Susan Budassi Sheehy

One of the most life-threatening emergencies encountered in the ED involves a patient with chest trauma. Chest injuries resulting from traffic accidents and social violence have increased in recent years. Twenty-five percent of all trauma deaths in the United States are caused by chest trauma, and 25% to 50% of all major chest traumas result in death.[1] Trauma deaths account for the number one loss of lifetime working years—3.8 million working years annually. Heart disease accounts for a yearly loss of 2 million lifetime working years, and cancer for 1.8 million.[1] Head trauma is the number one cause of death, and chest trauma is number two.

The major causes of blunt trauma to the chest are automobile steering wheels and bicycle handlebars. Gunshot wounds and stabbings account for the majority of penetrating injuries.

Many of these are emergency injuries, and the nurse must assess the injury and apply therapeutic intervention concurrently.

ANATOMY AND PHYSIOLOGY

The thoracic cavity extends from the first rib and adjacent structures above, to the diaphragm, and includes 12 pairs of ribs. It contains intrathoracic structures such as the heart and pericardium, the lungs, the inferior and superior venae cavae, the aorta, and the esophagus.

The lungs are elastic structures and have a natural tendency to collapse. They are prevented from collapsing by negative pressure found between the lungs and the chest wall in the pleural space. When the chest wall expands, negative pressure increases, and at the same time the lungs fill with air from the upper airways and expand (Fig. 25-1). If negative pressure is lost, the lung(s) collapse (Fig. 25-2).

The chest wall expands with the assistance of the muscles of respiration. These are grouped into two categories: the main muscles and the accessory muscles. The main muscles of respiration are the diaphragm and the intercostal muscles. The diaphragm separates the thoracic cavity from the abdominal cavity and contains the phrenic nerve, which originates at the fourth cervical vertebra (C4). During expiration the diaphragm is located at about the sixth intercostal space. During deep inspiration it is located at about the fourth lumbar vertebra.

The accessory muscles used in respiration are the pectoralis major, which is a chest wall muscle that pulls on the anterior part of the chest, the sternocleidomastoid muscle, which has its main body in the neck and pulls on the upper chest, and the abdominal wall muscles.

When the intercostal muscles elevate the chest wall and the diaphragm drops down, negative pressure increases in the pleural space and the lungs expand with air entering the

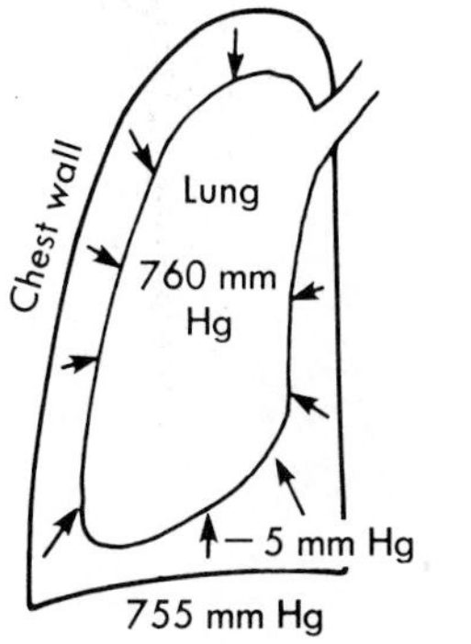

Fig. 25-1 Negative pressure in chest cavity.

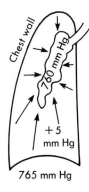

Fig. 25-2 Loss of negative pressure in chest cavity.

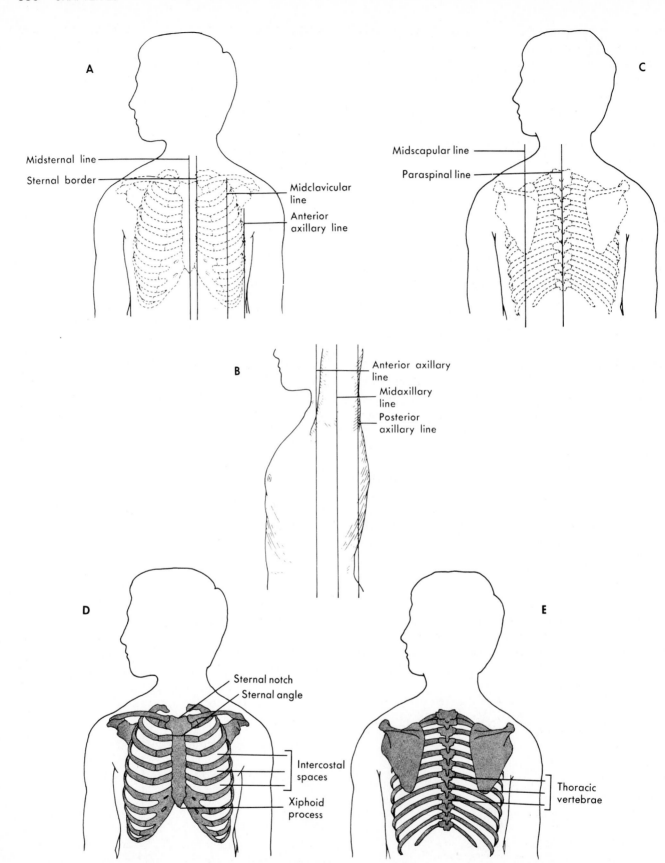

Fig. 25-3 Anatomic reference lines. **A,** Anterior. **B,** Lateral. **C,** Posterior. **D,** Anterior intercostal spaces. **E,** Posterior aspect.

airways—inspiration. When the intercostal muscles drop, the chest wall and the diaphragm rise, negative pressure decreases in the pleural space, and the lungs contract, with air exiting through the airways—expiration.

To describe an injury adequately and accurately, the nurse must be familiar with surface anatomy as described in Figure 25-3. Any wound between the nipples and the lower costal margin should be considered a chest injury, as well as an abdominal injury.

EVALUATION OF CHEST INJURIES

Any patient with chest trauma should be considered to have a serious injury until proved otherwise. Airway, breathing, circulation, and cervical spine should always be of primary concern. Chest injuries that may produce problems with any of these are flail chest, sucking chest wounds, pneumothorax, tension pneumothorax, hemothorax, and cardiac tamponade. Other injuries, such as esophageal rupture, tracheobronchial tree rupture, diaphragmatic rupture, aortic rupture, pulmonary contusion, and myocardial contusion, may not demonstrate immediate airway, breathing, or circulatory impairment but may eventually be fatal. Assessment of the chest trauma victim and therapeutic intervention are detailed in the box at right.

Nursing diagnoses appropriate to the patient with chest trauma are provided in the box on pp. 338 and 339.

Rib Fractures

Rib fractures are common chest injuries, particularly in the athlete involved in contact sports and in elderly individuals. These patients have a history of trauma to the chest, pain that increases with inspiration, and local pain and crepitus over the fracture site.

First rib fracture is often associated with clavicle fracture and sometimes with scapula fracture. One may see perforation of the subclavian artery or vein or tracheobronchial injury with first rib fracture. This rib is not well exposed, and trauma is not common. Great force is required for a fracture to occur. First rib fractures are associated with high mortality. With these fractures other injuries must also be considered.

When the lower ribs are fractured, the nurse should consider concurrent injury to the kidneys, the spleen on the left, and the liver on the right. If three or more ribs are fractured, the patient is treated as a multiple trauma victim and the nurse must search for other injuries.

Diagnosis can be made by palpation of the fractures or by radiograph. Therapeutic intervention is individual. If the fracture is simple and nondisplaced, rest, local heat, and simple analgesia are recommended. For elderly patients and those with jagged fractures, displaced fractures, known pulmonary disease, or multiple trauma, hospitalization is recommended. Rib fractures are particularly dangerous in elderly individuals, since their vital capacity is greatly decreased. Chest strapping for rib fractures is no longer

---

ASSESSMENT OF THE CHEST TRAUMA VICTIM AND THERAPEUTIC INTERVENTION

Maintain airway, breathing, and circulation
Perform quick (1-minute) evaluation
- Check for shortness of breath and cyanosis.
- Check vital signs.
- Check skin color and temperature.
- Check wound size and location.
- Check for paradoxic chest movement.
- Check for distended neck veins.
- Listen for respiratory stridor.
- Listen for bilateral breath sounds.
- Look for epigastric and supraclavicular indrawing.
- Give rough estimate of tidal volume.
- Check for tracheal deviation.
- Assess intercostal muscle use.
- Assess accessory muscle use.
- Check for subcutaneous emphysema.
- Look and listen for sucking chest sounds.
- Listen to heart sounds.

Obtain a quick history
- What happened?
- What was the mechanism of injury?
- How long ago did it happen?
- Where is the pain? Does it radiate?
- Is there anything that makes the pain better or worse?
- What does the pain feel like?
- How severe is the pain on a scale of 1 to 10?
- Is there any medical history?

Provide therapeutic intervention
- Maintain airway.
- Ensure adequate air movement.
- Administer oxygen.
- Cover any open chest wound.
- Insert needles or chest tube into anterior chest wall if tension pneumothorax is present.
- Initiate an IV line (two or more lines if possible, but do not delay transport to do this).
- Perform pericardiocentesis, if indicated.
- Obtain radiographic film of chest if more than three ribs are fractured, since victim is considered multitraumatized and other associated injuries must be sought. It is essential at this time to obtain cross-table lateral cervical spine film for detection of cervical spine injury before initiating any other diagnostic tests or moving the victim.
- Frequently recheck vital signs.
- Monitor heart rate for dysrhythmias.

---

recommended because it decreases ventilation and may cause atelectasis and pneumonia.

If chest pain is severe and ventilation is compromised, one may employ either local infiltration of an anesthetic solution directly into the fracture site or an intercostal nerve block above and below the fracture site. If an intercostal

NURSING DIAGNOSES APPROPRIATE TO PATIENT WITH CHEST TRAUMA

Ineffective airway clearance

CAUSES
- Airway obstruction
- Blood clot or foreign body
- Transection of trachea
- Distortion of trachea

DEFINING CHARACTERISTICS
- Decreased air movement
- Abnormal breath sounds (rales, crackles, rhonchi, or wheezes)
- Ineffective cough
- Change in rate or depth of respiration
- Dyspnea
- Cyanosis
- Alterations in blood gases
- Subcutaneous emphysema

NURSING INTERVENTIONS
- Remove obstruction if possible. Suction may be necessary.
- Administer oxygen.
- Control airway if necessary. Tracheostomy performed by physician may be necessary if trachea is transected.
- Continue to monitor vital signs and adequacy of air movement.

EVALUATION
- Patient is able to maintain adequate ventilation without assistance.
- Patient is maintaining adequate oxygenation by mechanical airway and ventilator.

Ineffective breathing pattern

CAUSES
- Flail chest
- Pneumothorax
- Hemothorax
- Tension pneumothorax
- Diaphragmatic rupture

DEFINING CHARACTERISTICS
- Dyspnea
- Paradoxic chest wall movement
- Use of accessory muscles, presence of stridor
- Epigastric or supraclavicular retractions
- Absence of bilateral breath sounds
- Presence of bowel sounds in chest
- Tachypnea
- Changes in depth of respiration
- Cyanosis
- Distended jugular veins
- Air fluid levels seen on radiograph of chest
- Alterations in arterial blood oxygenation

NURSING INTERVENTIONS
- Administer oxygen.
- If pneumothorax or hemothorax is suspected, prepare patient for insertion of flutter valve or chest tube. (If physician is not present and pneumothorax or tension pneumothorax is suspected, insert flutter valve or use 18-gauge needle and 50 ml syringe with three-way stopcock to remove air.)
- Set up Pleur-Evac system or other chest suction equipment.
- If flail chest is suspected, respiration should be stabilized by intubation and ventilation.
- Administer medication to relieve pain resulting from flail segment.
- Continue to monitor vital signs and assess for other problems.
- Draw or redraw blood gases to determine the adequacy of oxygenation.
- Insert nasogastric tube to decompress stomach and reduce pressure of thoracic cavity.
- Reassure patient and explain procedures.

EVALUATION
- Patient is able to maintain adequate oxygenation with or without intubation and mechanical ventilation.
- Vital signs return to normal.

nerve block is chosen, one must obtain a radiograph of the chest before and after the procedure to ensure that pneumothorax has not taken place.

Flail Chest

When two or more adjacent ribs are fractured in two or more places or when the sternum is detached, a flail chest occurs. Because significant force causes this injury, a resulting pulmonary contusion may also be present and may be life threatening. A myocardial contusion may also be present.

The diagnosis of flail chest is made by clinical observation of the paradoxic movement of a segment of the chest wall (Fig. 25-4), shortness of breath, and difficulty during breathing. Diagnosis is also based on a high clinical index of suspicion and a causative mechanism of injury.

The goals of therapeutic intervention are to provide oxygenation and to ensure good ventilation. This patient should be endotracheally intubated and ventilated with high-flow oxygen. The nurse should closely monitor fluid administration and lung sounds and be alert for the onset of pulmonary edema.

Sternal Fracture

A sternal fracture rarely causes problems unless it is totally detached from the ribs and becomes a flail segment.

NURSING DIAGNOSES APPROPRIATE TO PATIENT WITH CHEST TRAUMA—cont'd

Impaired gas exchange

CAUSES
- Impaired ventilation or perfusion resulting from injury to lung or hemodynamic instability (shock) or both
- Cardiac tamponade

DEFINING CHARACTERISTICS
- Dyspnea
- Agitation
- Confusion
- Somnolence
- Increased respiratory rate
- Cyanosis
- Increased pulse rate
- Decreased blood pressure
- Alterations in blood gases

NURSING INTERVENTIONS
- Administer oxygen.
- Suction airway.
- Intubate and ventilate as needed.
- Correct hypovolemia by IV therapy and replacement of fluid (balanced salt solutions and blood).
- If cardiac tamponade is suspected, prepare patient for pericardiocentesis.
- Insert nasogastric tube to relieve gastric distention and pressure on thoracic cavity.

EVALUATION
- Patient is able to maintain adequate oxygenation with or without mechanical intubation and ventilation.
- Vital signs return to normal.

Decreased cardiac output

CAUSES
- Tension pneumothorax
- Cardiac tamponade
- Hemorrhagic shock

DEFINING CHARACTERISTICS
- Increased pulse rate
- Decreased blood pressure
- Narrowed pulse pressure
- Flat or distended neck veins
- Agitation
- Confusion
- Cold, clammy skin
- Cyanosis
- Muffled heart sounds
- Tracheal deviation
- Decreased breath sounds unilaterally or bilaterally

NURSING INTERVENTIONS
- Restore effective breathing pattern.
- Continue to monitor vital signs.
- If cardiac tamponade is present, prepare patient for pericardiocentesis.
- Monitor for arrhythmias and possible component of cardiogenic shock from myocardial infarction.
- Patient is prepared immediately for necessary surgery.

EVALUATION
- Hemodynamic, cardiac, and respiratory values return to normal.

Nursing diagnoses that may be operant but are discussed in detail elsewhere include the following:
- Fluid volume deficit (1)
- Fluid volume deficit (2)
- Potential fluid volume deficit
- Pain
- Anxiety
- Fear

A sternal fracture, however, may be a clue to other underlying injuries, such as myocardial contusion. A detached sternum is commonly found after an automatic chest compressor has been used during cardiopulmonary resuscitation. Therapeutic intervention is identical to that for a flail chest.

Simple Pneumothorax

When air enters the pleural space, it causes a loss of negative pressure. This loss of negative pressure causes a partial or total collapse of the lung on the affected side (Fig. 25-5) and may result from a hole in the chest wall, the lungs, the bronchus, the trachea, or ruptured alveoli. This condition is known as a simple pneumothorax. Spontaneous pneumothorax usually occurs in men between the ages of 20 and 40 years and is probably caused by the rupture of subpleural blebs.

Diagnosis is made by obtaining a history of blunt trauma to the chest or sudden onset of sharp (pleuritic) chest pain, auscultating decreased breath sounds on the affected side, eliciting hyperresonance on percussion, finding shortness of breath and tachypnea, and discovering positive findings on radiographs of the chest. The patient may also demonstrate syncope and Hamman's sign, a "crunching" sound with each heartbeat that results from mediastinal air accumulation.

Therapeutic intervention may range from simply observing the patient, if the pneumothorax is small, to placing a

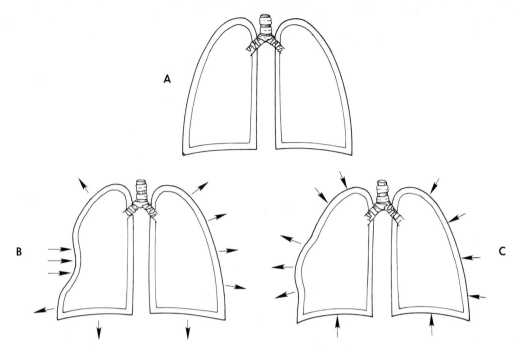

Fig. 25-4   Flail chest. **A,** Normal lungs. **B,** Flail chest during inspiration. **C,** Flail chest during expiration.

large-bore needle in the second intercostal space in the midclavicular line or the fifth intercostal space in the midaxillary line on the affected side or inserting a chest tube in the same location(s). These patients should be placed in a semi-Fowler's position, and high-flow oxygen should be administered.

Tension Pneumothorax

When air enters the pleural space during inspiration and cannot escape during expiration (similar to a one-way valve effect), a tension pneumothorax forms. As the positive pressure increases on the affected side, the lung on that same side collapses and a mediastinal shift occurs that compresses the heart and great vessels and the trachea. This shift in turn compresses the lung on the unaffected side and impedes venous return to the right atrium by putting pressure on the inferior and superior venae cavae (Fig. 25-6). Conse-

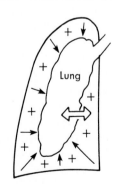

Fig. 25-5   Simple pneumothorax.

quently, neck vein enlargement is evident. The patient's ventilation decreases because of increased intrathoracic pressure, and the patient may become severely short of breath. Shock may ensue because of the lack of oxygenated blood flow to the heart. Other signs and symptoms of tension pneumothorax are a history of chest trauma, severe shortness of breath, paradoxic movement of the chest, a deviated trachea toward the unaffected side, cyanosis, distant heart sounds, and hyperresonance during percussion. Definitive diagnosis may be made by radiographic examination.

If the patient is severely symptomatic, do *not* delay therapeutic intervention until a radiograph is made—act immediately.

Therapeutic intervention includes maintenance of airway, breathing, and circulation; administration of oxygen at high flow under positive pressure; use of needle thoracotomy in the second intercostal space in the midclavicular line or the fifth intercostal space in the midaxillary line; placement of a chest tube; and initiation of intravenous (IV) therapy with Ringer's lactate or normal saline solution through a large-bore cannula.

If tension pneumothorax is not corrected, cardiac output continues to fall and the patient dies.

Open Pneumothorax (Sucking Chest Wound)

A sucking chest wound is an open pneumothorax with a chest wall defect. Air passes from the atmosphere through the chest wall into the pleural space and out again (Fig. 25-7). When an opening is made in the chest wall, loss of intrathoracic pressure results. If a flap forms and air can be

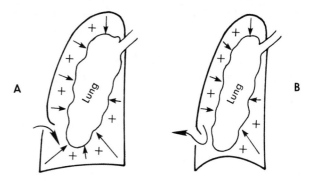

Fig. 25-7   Open pneumothorax. **A,** Air enters pleural cavity during inspiration. **B,** Air exits pleural cavity during expiration.

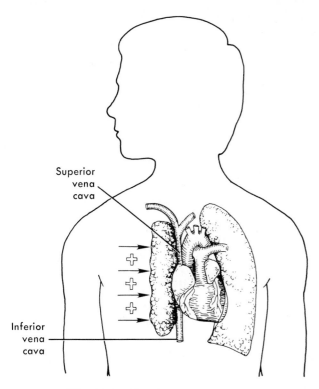

Fig. 25-6   Tension pneumothorax.

sucked into the pleural cavity but cannot be released, positive pressure begins to increase and a tension pneumothorax results.

If the diameter of the hole in the chest wall is greater than two thirds of the diameter of the trachea, there is preferential flow of air through the chest wall defect, which is the path of least resistance.[5]

The diagnosis of an open pneumothorax can be made by visualizing the defect or by hearing the sucking sound. The patient usually has dyspnea and chest pain and may demonstrate signs and symptoms of pneumothorax or tension pneumothorax.

Therapeutic intervention for an open pneumothorax is to administer oxygen. If the wound is large, greater than two thirds of the diameter of the trachea, seal the defect with a sterile occlusive dressing that has been taped on three sides to allow air to flow outward. If the wound is smaller than two thirds the diameter of the trachea and the patient is endotracheally intubated, it is better not to seal the wound, since a tension pneumothorax is likely to develop. When the wound is left open, the condition develops only into a pneumothorax. However, if the wound is sealed, an underlying lung injury is present, and air continues to leak into the thoracic cavity, a tension pneumothorax, which is life threatening, may develop. This patient should be observed closely for the development of a tension pneumothorax. If a tension pneumothorax develops and an occlusive dressing had been previously placed, the dressing should immediately

be removed. The patient may require chest tube placement: be prepared for this procedure. This patient may require blood. This is an ideal opportunity to consider autotransfusion. If the patient is bleeding intrathoracically, prepare the patient for surgery.

Pulmonary Contusion

A pulmonary contusion occurs commonly in cases of major trauma to the chest,[1] often in conjunction with flail chest. Pulmonary contusion is usually due to severe blunt trauma to the chest and is the most common life-threatening problem that results from trauma to the chest.[1] The pulmonary contusion may develop slowly, sometimes over a period of up to 4 hours.[4] Therefore patients with injuries that could potentially cause a pulmonary contusion must be closely observed for signs and symptoms of respiratory distress.

A contusion forms in the lung when blood extravasates into injured parenchyma, which causes hypoxia. A large contusion may cause tracheal obstruction. Depending on the amount of blunt force sustained, contusions may range from minor to massive.

This patient has an ineffective cough, increasing hyperpnea, and severe dyspnea and usually has other severe injuries. In addition, arterial blood gas levels demonstrate hypoxia.

The diagnosis of pulmonary contusion is based on a high index of suspicion, observation for obvious signs and symptoms, and radiographic visualization of the chest.

Therapeutic intervention is aimed at maintaining an adequate airway, administering humidified oxygen as prescribed, and limiting IV fluids during the resuscitative, early stages of care.[3] Whole blood and colloids should be used for volume replacement, to maintain oncotic pressure and to decrease pulmonary edema. Pulmonary contusion is a rare diagnosis in trauma care, when the use of diuretic agents and corticosteroids may also be considered.

Selective endotracheal intubation may be indicated based on arterial blood gas values and the facility of ventilation. Also, consider mechanical ventilation for this patient.

If the patient has pain, consider the administration of analgesics. Morphine sulfate can be given in increments of 1 to 2 mg intravenously (not intramuscularly). If respiratory rate and hypoxia result from the administration of morphine sulfate, consider administering naloxone (Narcan).

Hemothorax

A hemothorax is a collection of blood in the pleural cavity (Fig. 25-8). Blood accumulation may be mild (up to 300 ml), moderate (300 to 1400 ml), or severe (1400 to 2500 ml). Severe blood loss may be life threatening because of resultant hypovolemia and the tension that is forming.

Signs and symptoms of hemothorax are similar to those of pneumothorax and tension pneumothorax, with the addition of tachycardia, hypotension, dullness on chest percussion, and other associated signs of shock, such as cold, clammy skin, and tremors.

Therapeutic intervention is aimed at treating the shock condition with IV lines, oxygen, and Trendelenburg's position, and at relieving the pressure from the pleural cavity by inserting one or more chest tubes into the fifth intercostal space in the midaxillary line. Chest drainage should be measured and recorded. Surgery may be indicated if drainage is greater than 200 ml/hr during the course of 24 hours or if a massive amount of bleeding occurs initially.

If hemorrhage volume is high or if there is a shortage of whole blood, autotransfusion may be employed.

Chest Tubes and Chest Drainage

If air or blood is accumulating in the pleural cavity, a reduction of negative pressure occurs. Air and blood must be removed, and negative pressure must be restored. A method to remove both air and blood is insertion of a chest tube into the chest cavity. The chest tube is normally placed either through the second intercostal space in the midclavicular line (for air) or in the fifth intercostal space in the midaxillary line (for fluid). The tube is attached to a water-seal suction drainage system that acts as a one-way valve, allowing blood or air to escape but not allowing backflow.

Various types of chest drainage systems are available, either improvised or commercial. Regardless of the system chosen, the goal is the same: to remove blood or air from the pleural cavity and allow for lung reexpansion. The most

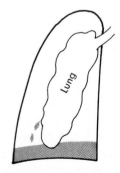

Fig. 25-8 Hemothorax.

commonly used types are plastic disposable systems equivalent to the three-chamber drainage system in which the first is the collection chamber for drainage from the patient's chest, the second chamber is the water seal, and the third is the pressure-regulating chamber (Fig. 25-9).

Ensure that the system is kept sterile and air-tight. Secure all connections with adhesive tape. The chest tube and connecting tubing should be "milked" periodically to evacuate any clots that may have formed. Be sure to measure the amount of drainage and record it both in nurses' notes and on the collection chamber itself.

LACERATION OF THE PARENCHYMA

Lacerations of the parenchyma are usually caused by penetrating trauma or fractured ribs. The lacerations are usually self-limiting and rarely require therapeutic intervention.

Tracheobronchial Injuries

Disruption of the tracheobronchial tree most commonly occurs near the bifurcation of the mainstem bronchus, approximately 1 inch from the carina. Disruption may be the result of blunt or penetrating trauma. Diagnosis is often delayed because onset may be delayed up to 5 days after trauma. If the disruption occurs below the carina, mediastinal air is evident on a radiograph of the chest. Bronchoscopy, however, is the definitive diagnostic tool.

The patient with a tracheobronchial injury may show signs and symptoms of an airway obstruction, hemoptysis, subcutaneous emphysema, or progressive mediastinal emphysema. An air leak may be present somewhere in the chest, and a tension pneumothorax may develop. Mortality is 50% in the first hour after injury for patients with these types of injuries.[1] Therapeutic intervention involves maintaining an open airway, administering high-flow oxygen, preparing for the placement of chest tubes, and preparing for surgery.

Diaphragmatic Rupture

A ruptured diaphragm may be life threatening.[4] The diaphragm is the main muscle of respiration; thus when it is ruptured, interference with the patient's ventilatory effort occurs. This injury may be present when a patient has had a traumatic injury at the levels of the fourth to the tenth ribs. Diaphragmatic rupture occurs as a result of the great force of a trauma to the abdominal cavity. When the trauma is blunt, the result is usually a large tear. When trauma is penetrating, the result is usually a small perforation such as that caused by a knife or a bullet. The patient with a ruptured diaphragm usually has other major injuries also.

The patient with a ruptured diaphragm may have chest pain that radiates to one shoulder and may have difficulty breathing. Breath sounds are decreased during auscultation, and rhonchi resulting from a hemothorax may be present.

Diagnosis is made when a bowel that has herniated can be visualized on a radiograph of the chest cavity. This film also demonstrates an elevated left hemidiaphragm, a nasogastric tube in the thoracic cavity, or loss of the costo-

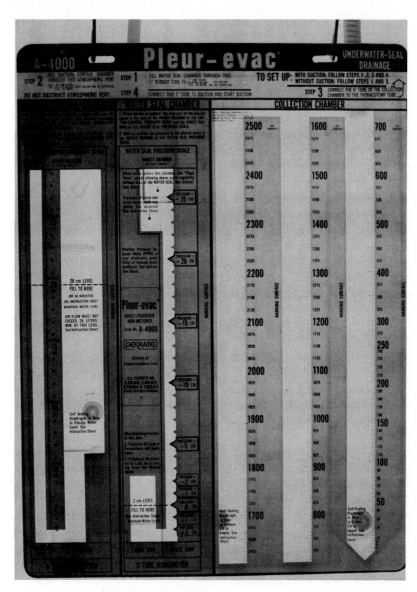

Fig. 25-9   Pleur-Evac system by Deknatel.

phrenic angle on the opposite side of the chest from the injury.[1] Diaphragmatic rupture can also be visualized on contrast radiography (a gastrointestinal series). Bowel sounds in the chest are audible.

Therapeutic intervention is aimed at decompressing the stomach with a nasogastric tube to prevent further herniation of abdominal contents into the thoracic cavity, administering high-flow oxygen, and preparing the patient for surgery.

Esophageal Rupture

A ruptured esophagus is a rare injury. If the diagnosis is missed, however, mortality is extremely high.[4] A ruptured esophagus usually results from a penetrating mechanism but may also result from severe epigastric blunt trauma. The injury is often seen in conjunction with a pneumothorax or a hemothorax and may be the result of an iatrogenic injury that occurs during esophagoscopy.

In a patient with a ruptured esophagus, mediastinal emphysema and a mediastinal crunching sound develop. The nurse may notice particulate matter, especially foodstuffs, in the chest tube drainage. The patient may be in shock but not complain of pain if he or she is conscious. The patient also usually has an elevated temperature.

Diagnosis of this condition is made by clinical observation, endoscopy, and contrast radiography (an upper gastrointestinal series). Therapeutic intervention is limited to emergency surgical repair.

CARDIAC INJURIES
Contusions

Cardiac contusions occur more frequently than they are diagnosed and are frequently associated with other injuries. The nurse should always suspect contusion in any patient with a history of blunt trauma to the chest, particularly an injury caused by a steering wheel or bicycle handlebars. Cardiac contusion should also be suspected in any patient after cardiopulmonary resuscitation.

The patient with a myocardial contusion usually has severe chest pain and chest wall contusions, and ecchymosis is evident. Dysrhythmias also develop within the first hour and up to 24 hours after trauma. The dysrhythmias are usually premature ventricular contractions, atrial fibrillation, right bundle branch block. ST segment elevation may appear on an electrocardiogram (ECG). If the contusion is significant, cardiac output may drop and cardiogenic shock may ensue.

Diagnosis is made based on a high index of suspicion and an identified mechanism of injury, such as a bent steering wheel, that suggests the possibility of this type of injury. Signs of injury may be seen on a 12-lead ECG. ST segment elevation, for example, may be seen in leads V_1, V_2, and V_3 if the injury is on the left side of the chest. Levels of cardiac isoenzymes are elevated, as they are in cases of myocardial infarction.

Therapeutic intervention is directed at preserving myocardial muscle. These patients should be given oxygen, narcotic analgesics for pain control, and appropriate therapy for dysrhythmias that occur. Patients should be admitted to a monitored bed for at least 48 hours of observation.

Penetrating Injuries

Most patients with penetrating injury to the heart die rapidly; few reach the hospital. If penetrating injury is identified, it is imperative to treat the shock aggressively and to transport the patient to a capable medical facility as soon as possible.

If the patient survives the trip to the ED, immediate thoracotomy is the appropriate treatment.

If myocardial rupture is present, the patient demonstrates severe hypotension, an elevated central venous pressure, distended neck veins, decreased ECG voltage, and decreased heart sounds. Mortality due to myocardial rupture is high. The right ventricle is more frequently ruptured than the left because of the superficial position of the right ventricle. Therapeutic intervention is aggressive pulmonary care, the administration of digoxin and diuretics, immediate thoracotomy, and repair of the rupture.

When the aortic valve ruptures, there is sudden onset of severe chest pain, severe shortness of breath, dyspnea, hemoptysis, a "roaring" loud murmur, and signs of congestive heart failure and pulmonary edema. Therapeutic intervention is immediate surgery for valve replacement.

Cardiac Tamponade

Many penetrating injuries of the heart may produce cardiac tamponade. The heart is surrounded by a fibrinous sac known as the pericardial sac. Tamponade occurs when a relatively minor wound of the heart bleeds into the pericardial space (Fig. 25-10). Blood begins to build up in the

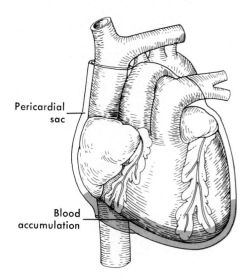

Fig. 25-10 Pericardial tamponade.

pericardial sac because either it cannot escape or it cannot escape as quickly as the bleeding occurs. Blood accumulation interferes with the filling of the ventricles and the pumping action of the heart, and cardiac output falls. The heart begins to compensate by becoming tachycardic; then the heart rate deteriorates.

As the heart rate increases, venous pressure increases, causing distended jugular veins; blood pressure falls; and heart sounds are muffled (Beck's triad). The patient becomes dyspneic and demonstrates Kussmaul's respirations. A paradoxic pulse and cyanosis are also evident.

Therapeutic intervention includes fluid administration to elevate central venous pressure, oxygen at high flow, placement in a high Fowler's position, pericardiocentesis, or pericardial window.

Pericardiocentesis. Pericardiocentesis is a procedure whereby a 16- to 18-gauge metal intracardiac needle is introduced into the pericardial sac to withdraw blood or fluid that is compressing the myocardium. The needle is attached to a large syringe, usually 30 to 50 ml. The hub of the needle is connected to the lead of an ECG machine by means of an alligator clip (Fig. 25-11). The needle is inserted about 3 cm to the left of the xiphoid process (the subxiphoid approach) and directed toward the left shoulder. The ECG machine should be running and recording continuously on the V-lead selector. The needle is advanced slowly until it penetrates the pericardial sac and reaches the myocardium. When the needle touches the myocardium, an electrical current of injury pattern appears on the V-rhythm strip; when this occurs, the needle is withdrawn a few centimeters, negative pressure is placed on the plunger, and the pericardial sac is aspirated. Withdrawal of as little as 15 ml of blood or fluid may be lifesaving.

After pericardiocentesis the patient should be observed closely for the possibility of further bleeding. If bleeding

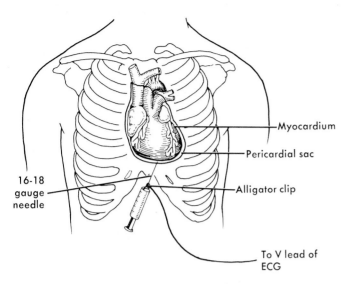

Fig. 25-11 Pericardiocentesis.

recurs, the pericardiocentesis may be repeated or thoracotomy for surgical repair may be recommended.

Complications of pericardiocentesis include laceration of a coronary artery, a lung, or a ventricle; dysrhythmias; and increase in the cardiac tamponade.

Pericardial window. A pericardial window is a procedure in which a small surgical incision is made below the zyphoid. The incision is spread to allow direct visualization of the pericardial apex. Aspiration of pericardial blood can then occur with direct visualization.

GREAT VESSEL INJURIES

The great vessels, the superior and inferior vena cavae and the aorta, are subject to both penetrating and blunt injuries. A penetrating injury to a great vessel is one of the most lethal injuries to the human body. If the victim reaches the hospital alive, immediate thoracotomy is indicated, as well as the administration of high-flow oxygen and the initiation of two or three large-bore IV lines.

Ten to twenty percent of victims of blunt trauma resulting in tears of the great vessels survive the initial accident and reach the hospital alive.[1] It is thought that this percentage survives because blood is contained by the adventitia, forming a false aneurysm. For those who survive the initial transport phase, mortality is 50% during each additional day that treatment is delayed.[2]

The most common cause of sudden death after an automobile accident is a ruptured aorta. The usual mechanism of injury is a rapid acceleration-deceleration force that causes a torsion and shearing force at the points of fixation of the aorta (ligamentum arteriosum or aortic root), resulting in a transverse tear and exsanguination or massive tamponade. This patient can rarely be saved.

Diagnosis can be made by observing signs and symptoms of cardiac tamponade or exsanguinating hemorrhage and mediastinal widening on an upright radiograph of the chest

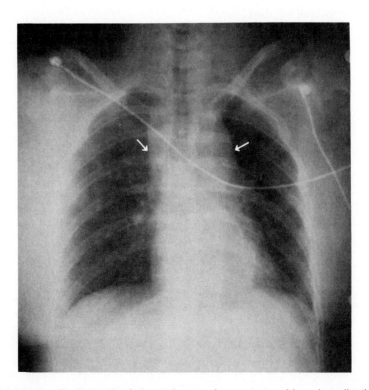

Fig. 25-12 Radiograph of chest. Arrows demonstrate widened mediastinum.

(Fig. 25-12). A left hemothorax, pseudocoarctation, a supraclavicular hematoma, or a combination of these may also be observed.[2] In addition, the aortic knob may be obliterated, and a pleural cap and nasogastric tube deviation may be observed on radiographs of the chest and abdomen.

Definitive diagnosis is made based on the results of thoracic aortogram or computerized tomography or at surgery. Therapeutic intervention includes the initiation of large-bore IV lines and the intravenous administration of crystalloid solution, which is run as rapidly as possible, early blood replacement, the administration of high-flow oxygen, and immediate surgery.

RUPTURED BRONCHUS

A ruptured bronchus, which occurs most commonly near the carina and the right mainstem, may be lethal if not diagnosed and treated immediately. Diagnosis is made by identifying the resultant tension pneumothorax and looking specifically for the rupture.

Therapeutic intervention is the administration of high-flow oxygen, chest tube placement, and immediate surgical repair of the rupture.

SUMMARY

The primary focus in any case of chest trauma should be the maintenance of airway, breathing, and circulation. Ensure an adequate airway, and administer oxygen at high flow. Initiate two large-bore IV lines with Ringer's lactate or normal saline solution if possible. Seal any open chest wounds and splint fractures. Rapid transport, diagnosis, and treatment are essential. The condition of these patients should be considered critical until proved otherwise.

REFERENCES

1. American College of Surgeons Committe on Trauma: *Advanced trauma life support instructor's manual,* Chicago, 1988, American College of Surgeons.
2. Clark D et al: Signs of high-risk blunt aortic trauma, *J Trauma* 30(6):701, 1989.
3. Davis JH: *Clinical surgery,* St Louis, 1987, Mosby–Year Book.
4. Lawrence P: *Essentials of general surgery,* Baltimore, 1988, Williams & Wilkins.
5. Sharar S: Lecture: chest trauma. Presented at the Advanced Trauma Life Support Course of the American College of Surgeons Committee on Trauma, Harborview Medical Center, University of Washington, Seattle, 1987.

SUGGESTED READINGS

Buckman RF Jr: Surgery of heart wounds: historical aspects, *Trauma Q* 4:2, 1988.

Budassi SA: *Mosby's manual of emergency care,* ed 3, St Louis, 1989, Mosby–Year Book.

Casale AS, Borkon AM: Penetrating cardiac trauma, *Trauma Q* 4(2), 1988.

Cohen S: How to work with chest tubes, Am J Nurs 80(4):685, 1980.

Failing T, Van Way CW: Ventilatory support in chest trauma, *Choices in Resp Management* 20(3):61, 1990.

Leonard DJ, Gens DR: Diagnosis of cardiac injury: pericardiocentesis vs. diagnostic pericardial window, *Trauma Q* 4(2), 1988.

Luchtefeld WB: Pulmonary contusion, *Focus Crit Care* 17(6):482, 1990.

Piano G, Turney SZ: Traumatic rupture of the thoracic aorta: surgical management, *Trauma Q* 4(2), 1988.

Rosen P et al: *Emergency medicine,* ed 3, St Louis, 1988, Mosby–Year Book.

Soutter DI, Rodriguez A: Cardiac contusion: diagnosis and management, *Trauma Q* 4(2), 1988.

Swanson J, Trunkey D: Failed diagnosis: pitfalls in chest trauma, *Topics Emerg Med* 10(2):81, 1988.

CHAPTER

26 Abdominal and Genitourinary Trauma

Susan Budassi Sheehy

The large abdominal cavity is frequently injured when a patient has been traumatized. Trauma to the abdomen and genitalia accounts for approximately 25% of all traumatic injuries.[1] There are two basic injury mechanism categories: blunt and penetrating. The abdomen or genitalia may be injured in a multiple trauma situation or with a mechanism of injury that may suggest the same. Be particularly alert for the presence of abdominal trauma in those patients who cannot identify pertinent signs and symptoms or in those who cannot communicate well, such as infants and children, elderly individuals, those who have used mind-altering substances, and those with an altered level of consciousness or a spinal cord injury.

Always consider the possibility of abdominal trauma when there has been a force to the area between the fourth rib and the hips. Remember that the diaphragm may rise as high as the fourth intercostal space during exhalation. The area between the fourth and tenth intercostal spaces should be considered both chest and abdominal trauma until either or both can be ruled out.

BLUNT TRAUMA

Blunt trauma usually results from a force to the abdominal wall, where energy is diffused into the abdominal cavity, either the intraperitoneal or retroperitoneal space, without causing an open or penetrating injury. Blunt trauma most frequently occurs as the result of a motor vehicle accident, a contact sport injury, a fall, or an intentional injury to a child (child abuse).

Diagnostic peritoneal lavage (DPL) can be performed to rule out intraabdominal injury, and abdominal computerized tomography (CT) is used to rule out both intraabdominal and retroperitoneal injury. If abdominal CT is performed, be sure to place a gastric tube before the study and instill a radiopaque dye in accordance with local protocol.

Other diagnostic examinations that can be performed to assess for abdominal and genitourinary trauma are arteriograms to rule out vascular injuries, cystograms to rule out urinary bladder injuries, IV pyelograms to rule out kidney and ureter injuries, and retrograde urethrograms to rule out penile shaft injuries. In addition, a rectal examination should be performed to determine the location of the prostate in men. When vascular supply to the stomach is diminished, acute gastric distention occurs, often causing the patient to have difficulty breathing and to vomit. Therefore a gastric tube should be placed to decompress the stomach, to check for the presence of blood, and to provide a route to place contrast dye if an abdominal CT scan will be performed.

Laboratory specimens routinely examined in cases of trauma should be collected. Particular attention should be paid to the complete blood count, serum amylase, and liver enzyme values, renal function studies, and other standard laboratory studies. A urinalysis should be included with laboratory studies, and a serum or urine pregnancy test should be considered for women of childbearing age. In addition to the routine pelvic radiograph usually obtained for all patients with multiple trauma injuries, radiographs that demonstrate specific types of abdominal trauma should also be made.

If the patient's hemodynamic condition remains unstable despite control of external bleeding and fluid replacement, the patient should be prepared for exploratory surgery. In fact, this decision is perhaps one of the most important aspects of care: to determine whether the patient requires emergency surgery, hospital admission for observation, or both before determining exactly which abdominal structures are injured. This decision can usually be accomplished by a team of astute clinicians from clinical observations and from the results of diagnostic studies. Close attention must be paid to stabilizing the patient's condition as much as possible while this decision is being made.

Some general signs and symptoms of possible abdominal trauma are observable bruises and abrasions, the presence of abdominal pain, rigidity, crepitus, palpable masses, or abdominal distention (not a reliable sign: 2 L of fluid in the stomach causes the abdomen to distend only three fourths of an inch), and signs and symptoms of shock: restlessness, anxiety, a decreased level of consciousness, cool clammy skin, cool distal extremities, delayed capillary refill, tachycardia, tachypnea, and hypotension. One should also con-

347

sider the strong possibility of abdominal trauma when other associated traumatic injuries are present.

When a patient has sustained blunt trauma to the abdomen, diagnosis may be difficult at best. It is essential to obtain a good history that includes details of the mechanism of injury. Close clinical observation is paramount. Pay particular attention to the patient's complaint of pain or response to abdominal palpation, including rigidity and guarding.

General therapeutic interventions for patients with abdominal trauma include airway management and administration of supplemental oxygen. Two large-bore IV lines should be initiated, and warmed crystalloids (Ringer's lactate solution) should be run at a rate that maintains blood pressure at an acceptable level. Be particularly careful to stabilize the cervical, thoracic, and lumbar portions of the spine until the possibility of injury to these areas can be ruled out.

At this point, if a gastric tube has not yet been placed, a gastric tube and an indwelling urinary catheter should be placed. One should also consider using the pneumatic antishock garment in accordance with local protocol.

DIAGNOSTIC PERITONEAL LAVAGE

Indications for diagnostic peritoneal lavage (DPL) include any patient who has sustained blunt trauma to the abdomen or the possibility of such trauma, or who is demonstrating signs and symptoms of shock or deteriorating vital signs but in whom surgery is not inevitable. DPL should also be considered for those patients who have an altered level of consciousness or sensation and cannot tell you about symptoms of abdominal pain or tenderness.

The bladder must be emptied before this diagnostic procedure. There are a few *relative* contraindications to this study: a gravid uterus, an abdominal wall hematoma, and the presence of abdominal scars from previous surgery. In each of these instances the location of the abdominal wall incision should be changed to avoid the area where complications could occur. The procedure, however, may still be performed. If a penetrating injury is evident, the abdomen should be explored during surgery.

Explain the procedure to the conscious patient, and instruct the patient concerning how he or she can cooperate during the procedure. Once again, ensure that the bladder is emptied via a Foley catheter. Decompress the stomach with a gastric tube. The anterior abdominal wall should be prepared by shaving and cleansing it with a surgical preparation solution such as 1% povidone iodine (Betadine) and should be draped with sterile towels. Lidocaine with epinephrine is used to anesthetize the incision area and minimize bleeding; it is usually injected 2 to 3 cm below the level of the umbilicus. A small laparotomy incision is made through the skin and subcutaneous adipose tissue to the linea alba. Absolute hemostasis must be maintained to avoid false-positive results. The

linea alba should be lifted with a forceps, and a small "nick" incision made with a scalpel. The incision should then be extended with a scissors.

The catheter should be introduced into the peritoneal cavity, with the tip directed toward the pelvis. Approximately 15 to 20 cm of the catheter should be placed into the peritoneal space. Attach a 20 cc syringe to the catheter, and aspirate for free blood. If the aspiration yields 20 ml of blood, the test is considered positive and the remainder of the procedure need not be performed. If little or no blood is obtained, attach the catheter to a container of 1000 ml warmed Ringer's lactate solution (10 ml/kg in a child) and infuse the solution rapidly.

Manually manipulate the abdomen to permit the solution to mix with peritoneal cavity contents. Place the solution container on the floor to siphon off the infused fluid. When the fluid no longer flows out, remove the catheter and repair the incision. Dress the wound with an antibiotic ointment and a small sterile dressing.

Specimens should be collected from the returned lavage fluid. They should be sent to the laboratory for determinations of hematocrit, red blood cell count, white blood cell count, serum amylase content, and the presence of bile, and for a culture and Gram stain. The result of lavage is considered positive if hematocrit is greater than 2 ml/dl, red blood cell count is 100,000 cells/mm^3 or more, white blood cell count is equal to or greater than 500 cells/mm^3, serum amylase content is 200 milliunits/ml or more, bile is noted, or any significant quantity of bacteria is present (which may indicate perforation of the intestines).

If the patient has unexplained hemorrhagic shock, peritoneal perforation, increasing abdominal tenderness or rigidity, evidence of peritonitis, visualized free air in the abdomen, positive results of DPL or abdominal CT scan, an enlarging abdominal mass in the absence of pelvic or vertebral fractures, or a progressive drop in hemoglobin concentration and hematocrit in the absence of hypotension, the patient should be prepared for an exploratory laparotomy.

PENETRATING TRAUMA

A large number of penetrating injuries in the United States can be attributed to the inner-city "knife and gun club"; they are the result of shootings and stabbings. Gunshot wounds account for about 15% of abdominal penetrating wounds, and stabbings account for about 2%.[2] Although two thirds of all stab wounds enter the anterior portion of the abdomen, only half of these cause serious injuries.[4] Seventy-six percent of patients with gunshot wounds to the abdomen require exploratory surgery, whereas only 33% of patients with stab wounds require surgery.[3]

When a patient has sustained a penetrating wound to the abdomen, the same basic principles of care as for all major trauma patients apply. Begin with management of the airway. Consider endotracheal intubation if the patient will require ventilatory assistance or if blood gas values indicate that the patient should be intubated. Be sure to provide supplemental oxygen via whatever method is appropriate. Control any external bleeding, and initiate two large-bore intravenous (IV) lines. Protect the cervical, thoracic, and lumbar portions of the spine. If an evisceration has occurred, cover the area with a wet-to-dry sterile dressing. Consider use of the pneumatic antishock garment in accordance with local protocol, and of course, consider the patient a candidate for surgery when the hemodynamic status deteriorates.

It is helpful, when obtaining a history of the event, to ascertain the type of weapon used, the caliber of the weapon, the time elapsed since the incident, and an estimate of external blood loss. Also, observe the patient closely for entrance and exit wounds.

ORGANS OF THE ABDOMEN AND THE GENITALIA
Stomach

The stomach is a huge, hollow organ. Because it is hollow, it can easily be displaced; therefore it is rarely injured in blunt trauma incidents. However, because the stomach is large and anterior, it is often injured as a result of penetrating mechanisms. Perhaps the easiest way to rule out the possibility of stomach injury is to insert a gastric tube, aspirate contents of the stomach, and examine the aspirate for the presence of blood. If free air is seen on an abdominal radiograph, one may also consider that either the stomach or the intestines have been perforated.

Liver

The liver is the largest solid organ in the body. Because of its size and anterior location, it is often injured as a result of both blunt and penetrating mechanisms. One should particularly suspect the presence of a liver injury when the eighth through twelfth ribs are injured on the right side of the body and when the upper or central part of the abdomen has been involved.

Patients with liver injuries may become hypotensive in a short time. An injury to the liver may be diagnosed on an abdominal CT scan and during exploratory laparotomy. Small lacerations may be left to heal by themselves. Large stellate lacerations must be surgically repaired.

Spleen

When major blunt trauma to the abdomen occurs, the spleen is injured approximately 41% of the time.[4] The spleen is dense and encapsulated. It is located just behind the eighth through tenth ribs in the upper left abdominal quadrant. The patient may have pain in the left shoulder, known as Kerr's sign, a type of referred pain. Definitive diagnosis of a ruptured spleen is usually made on an abdominal CT scan.

Patients who have had their spleens removed have a tendency for pneumococcal infections to develop. Because of this tendency, every effort is made to salvage the spleen whenever possible. If the spleen must be removed, the patient should receive pneumococcal polysaccharide vaccine (pneumovax). This procedure is especially important in children, who are particularly susceptible to the pneumococcal virus.

Pancreas

Pancreatic injury with blunt abdominal trauma is unusual, although it does occur. The pancreas is most likely to be injured with penetrating trauma. The pancreas is a semisolid organ, well protected by the stomach and liver, in the retroperitoneal space. Therefore splenic damage will not be evident as a result of PDL. However, an elevation of the level of serum amylase is seen during a 24-hour period. Because insulin is produced in the pancreas, removal of the pancreas causes insulin-dependent diabetes in the patient.

Kidneys

The kidneys are found in the flank area and are located retroperitoneally. They can be contused or lacerated (fractured) to varying degrees. A contusion may be self-limited, and a laceration may require surgical repair. A renal contusion may be treated with bed rest and forced fluids. Treatment of a lacerated kidney depends on the extent of the laceration. The kidney may be repaired, partially removed (a heminephrectomy), or totally removed (a nephrectomy). Diagnosis of the injury is made from results of IV pyelogram or CT scan. An indication of the injury is evident from urinalysis.

Ureters

Because the ureters are hollow and flexible, they are rarely injured in blunt trauma to the abdomen. However, they can be disrupted when penetrating trauma occurs. The diagnosis of a disrupted ureter is made from results of IV pyelogram. If disruption occurs, surgery to reanastomose the ureter should be performed.

Bladder

The bladder is a hollow organ. If it is empty, it is not usually injured in blunt trauma; however, if it is full of urine, it may rupture. The bladder also is often injured when pelvic fractures occur. A ruptured bladder is usually diagnosed from results of a cystogram; it is also evident from urinalysis, when gross blood is present without evidence of trauma at the urinary meatus or without difficult catheter placement. If the bladder is ruptured, the patient may be treated conservatively with a suprapubic catheter or may have surgical repair.

Urethra

Urethral disruption is more commonly seen in men because of the relatively unprotected anatomic location of the urethra in men. The mechanism of injury is usually a straddle-type injury caused by a crossbar on a bicycle or a motorcycle. The diagnosis of urethral injury is usually made by retrograde urethrogram. If a disruption is suspected, either by retrograde urethrogram or by the presence of blood at the meatus, a urologic consultation should be made. A Foley catheter should not be placed until the urologic consultation has been obtained and direction is given by the urologist.

Intestines

The intestines are hollow organs. Because of the extent of intestines (32 feet) and their anterior location and because they are relatively unprotected, fixed at certain points, and highly vascular, they are often injured in both blunt and penetrating trauma. When disruption of the intestines has occurred, surgical repair must be accomplished to control bleeding and to remove any intestinal contents that may have escaped into the abdominal cavity. This contamination of the abdominal cavity could cause peritonitis, severe infections, and sepsis.

Intestinal trauma may be diagnosed by a combination of radiographs, DPL, and abdominal CT scan. The definitive diagnosis, however, is made during exploratory laparotomy.

Diaphragm

When a diaphragmatic rupture occurs, complications may be severe and may include death. Problems ensue when the abdominal cavity contents herniate through the ruptured diaphragm into the chest cavity, causing severe compromise of breathing. In addition, negative pressure in the chest is lost and the diaphragm, which is the main muscle of breathing, is no longer functional. Diagnosis is made by observing some bowel or a gastric tube in the chest on a radiograph of the chest. Therapeutic intervention is immediate surgical repair. The insertion of a gastric tube to decompress the stomach may be somewhat therapeutic and may prevent the stomach from herniating into the chest cavity.

Abdominal Aorta, Inferior Vena Cava, and Hepatic Veins

The abdominal aorta, inferior vena cava, and hepatic veins are considered the major vessels of the abdomen. Disruption, which may occur from both blunt and penetrating trauma, causes severe hemorrhage. If the disruption is not corrected, death will quickly occur. Disruption of these vessels may be diagnosed by DPL and abdominal CT scan. The definitive therapeutic intervention is surgical repair.

ABDOMINAL TRAUMA AND THE PREGNANT PATIENT

When a pregnant woman is traumatized, abdominal trauma is often evident for obvious anatomic reasons. Certain things should be considered when caring for these women. If the woman is lying on her back, the fetus may be compressing the abdominal vasculature, which results in obstructive hypovolemia. Therapeutic intervention is to elevate the woman's right hip or to manually displace the uterus. These procedures allow for venous return to the right side of the heart and a return of blood pressure to normal. If the woman remains hypotensive and requires fluid volume replacement, blood products should be obtained as soon as possible because of the extreme need for both the mother and fetus to have fluids with oxygen-carrying capacity.

Whenever possible, when radiographs are being made, shield the uterus with a lead apron. Remember to continue monitoring the fetus throughout the resuscitation phase.

SUMMARY

The patient with abdominal trauma presents the caregiver with unique challenges. Among these is determining whether the patient should have surgery. If clinical observations are astute and history-taking is thorough, the nurse should be prepared to act rather than react. In other words, you should assume that an injury is present until you are able to rule it out as a possibility, instead of reacting to a situation in which the patient's hemodynamic condition suddenly becomes unstable and you are not prepared to deal with the situation. Always remember to consider the mechanism of injury to treat the patient's condition as a "worst case" scenario. In that way you will always be prepared to deal with clinical events as they happen.

REFERENCES

1. American College of Surgeons: *Advanced trauma life support provider manual,* Chicago, 1988, American College of Surgeons.
2. Cayten CG: Abdominal trauma, *Emerg Med Clin North Am* 2:799, 1984.
3. Papadopoulos R, Moore EE: Penetrating abdominal wounds. In Callaham ML, ed: *Current therapy in emergency medicine,* Toronto, 1987, BC Decker.
4. Marx JA: Abdominal trauma. In Rosen P et al: *Emergency medicine,* ed 2, St Louis, 1988, Mosby Year–Book.

SUGGESTED READINGS

Emergency Nurses Association: *Trauma nurse core course provider manual,* ed 2, Chicago, 1991, Emergency Nurses Association.
Gibson DE: Abdominal trauma, *Trauma Q* 4:1, 1987.
Sheehy SB, Marvin JA, Jimmerson CL: *Manual of clinical trauma care: the first hour,* St Louis, 1989, Mosby Year–Book.

Extremity Trauma

Susan Budassi Sheehy

Injuries to the limbs are some of the most commonly seen emergencies in the emergency department (ED). Commonly observed limb injuries are reviewed in this chapter, and the appropriate therapeutic interventions for each type of injury are discussed.

One of the greatest sources of disability in all age-groups in the United States is limb trauma. One must stress the importance of early management and correct therapeutic intervention to preserve life and limb, prevent disability, and promote good healing.

The skeleton is composed of 206 bones and provides the framework for the body. It also functions to provide support for the body, attachments for muscles, leverage, and protection to the vital organs (Fig. 27-1).

Two types of bones compose the skeleton. Cancellous (spongy) bone is found in the skull, the vertebrae, the pelvis, and the long bone ends; cortical (dense) bone is found in the long bones. Bones have blood, nerve, and lymphatic supply that allow the injured bone to repair itself. Bones are covered by a layer known as the *periosteum,* which provides an additional blood supply. Bones are labeled as long, short, flat, or irregular according to their shape.

Bone is connected to bone by bands of fibrous connective tissue known as *ligaments*. The fibrous cords that connect muscle to bone are known as *tendons*. The dense connective tissue found between the ribs, in the nasal septum, the ear, the larynx, the trachea, the bronchi, between the vertebrae, and on the articulating surface of the bone is known as *cartilage*. Cartilage has no neurovascular supply.

Joints are areas in which two bones are connected to provide mobility and stability, flexion and extension, medial and lateral rotation, and abduction and adduction. A joint consists of two articulating bone surfaces covered with cartilage, a two-layered sac containing synovial membranes for lubrication, and a capsule that becomes dense and forms a ligament. Movement is provided by muscles that overlie the joints and attach bone to bone with tendons.

When a victim with possible limb trauma is encountered, it is first essential to assess airway, breathing, and circulation (ABCs) before proceeding to treat the injured limb. One must also perform a rapid assessment to detect other major trauma, such as head, cervical spine, chest, or abdominal injury. If obvious head or cervical spine trauma is present or suspected, provide protection and preventive therapeutic intervention to these areas.

Once assured that no life-threatening injury has been left unattended, immobilize the traumatized extremity by splinting it both above and below the trauma site, as well as splinting the trauma site itself. Splinting is provided to prevent further damage and reduce the amount of pain in the injured limb. It is essential to evaluate the neurovascular status of the limb both before and after immobilization by assessing pulse rates distal to the trauma site, checking skin color, temperature, and capillary refill, and testing for sensation and movement distal to the trauma site. If neurologic or vascular status is compromised, attempt to apply traction to reduce the fracture and to allow for return of neurologic and vascular function.

Whenever possible, the injured limb should be elevated and a cold pack should be applied to the site of injury to keep the amount of swelling to a minimum. It may benefit the patient for the nurse to obtain a brief history of the circumstances surrounding the accident, the mechanism of injury, medical history, and any medications the patient is currently taking.

Careful observation must be made of any swelling, discoloration, contusions, abrasions, and obvious deformities. If an open fracture is evident or if a puncture site is present but no bone is protruding,* irrigate the wound with sterile normal saline solution and apply a dry sterile dressing over the wound; then apply a light compression dressing. The injury should then be splinted. *Never* attempt to reduce an open fracture in the prehospital care setting.

If bleeding is present, apply pressure either over the

Radiographs in this chapter are courtesy of Western Radiologic Medical Group, Inc., Los Angeles. Special thanks to Cindy Allen, RT, Administrative Secretary.

*If a puncture site is present but there is no bone end protruding, assume that the puncture site was made by a jagged bone end or a missile and treat it as an open fracture.

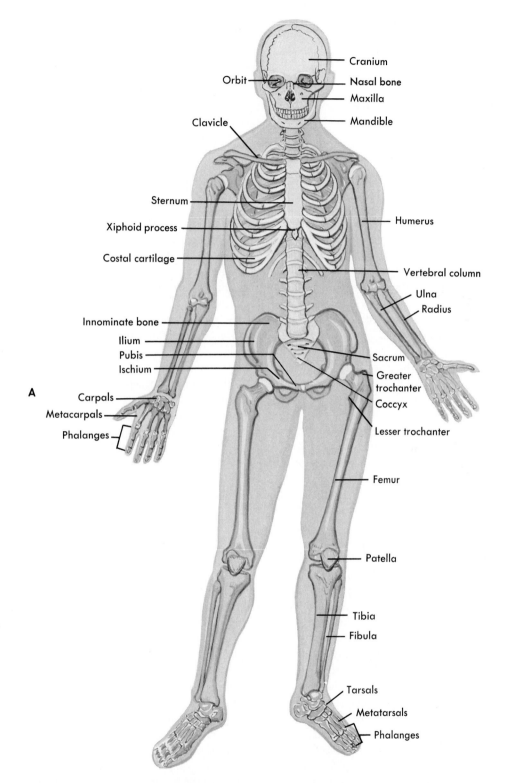

Fig. 27-1 Skeleton. **A,** Anterior view. (From Anthony C, Thibodeau G: *Textbook of anatomy and physiology,* ed 11, St Louis, 1983, Mosby–Year Book.)

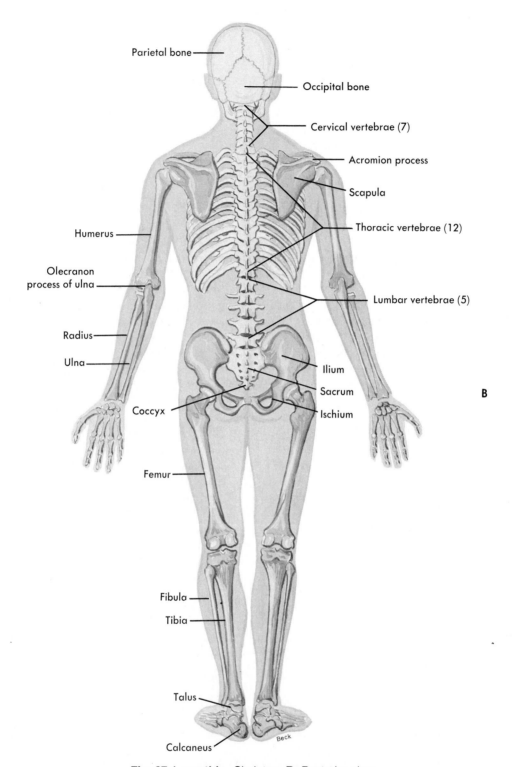

Parietal bone

Occipital bone

Cervical vertebrae (7)

Acromion process

Scapula

Humerus

Thoracic vertebrae (12)

Olecranon
process of ulna

Lumbar vertebrae (5)

Radius

Ulna

Ilium

Sacrum

Ischium

Coccyx

Femur

Fibula

Tibia

Talus

Calcaneus

Beck

B

Fig. 27-1, cont'd   Skeleton. **B,** Posterior view.

bleeding site or around the edges of the wound. A tourniquet should be used *only as a lifesaving measure* when bleeding cannot be controlled by other methods. If a tourniquet has been applied and all circulation to the limb has ceased for a prolonged period, the limb may have to be amputated.

At this point in therapeutic intervention, if the victim is still in the prehospital care setting, it is appropriate to transport him or her to a hospital facility.

Once the patient has reached the ED, provided that measures have been taken to ensure that the cervical spine has been protected, he or she should be totally undressed and examined both anteriorly and posteriorly for other associated injuries that may have been overlooked in the field.

SOFT TISSUE INJURIES

Soft tissue injuries frequently involve the limbs. They may consist of injuries to the skin and underlying tissues such as muscle, tendons, cartilage, ligaments, veins, arteries, and nerves.

The skin may be traumatized in several ways. If the epithelial layer is removed, exposing the dermal layer, an *abrasion* is created. A *contusion* is a bruise in which vessels are damaged but the skin is not disrupted; it is usually the result of a blunt force. A *hematoma* forms when blood escapes into the subcutaneous space. When skin is disrupted through the dermal layer, a wound known as a *laceration* is formed. Disruption of the skin by a sharp, pointed object is a *puncture* wound. If the puncturing object remains imbedded in the skin and tissues, it is an impaled object. It should not be removed until the wound and the object's location can be thoroughly evaluated.

When applying therapeutic interventions for soft tissue injuries, always first consider the ABCs. Once these three elements are ensured, control bleeding by applying direct or indirect pressure to the wound. If an impaled object is present, secure it so that it will not be removed accidentally. Place a dry sterile dressing over the wound, and evaluate the injured areas if possible. Apply a cold pack to the wound to minimize swelling. Be sure to check with the patient regarding the currency of his or her tetanus prophylaxis.

Abrasion

An abrasion is a soft tissue injury caused by the rubbing of skin against a firm surface. Scrape the epithelial layer away and leave the epidermal or dermal layer exposed; this technique is similar to intervention for a second-degree burn.

The type of wound should be scrubbed and irrigated. Remove any foreign bodies, apply topical antibiotic ointment, and affix a nonadherent dressing. Change the dressing daily until an eschar forms. The patient should avoid exposure of the area to sunlight for 6 months because of the possibility of hypopigmentation.

Avulsion

An avulsion is a full-thickness skin loss in which a section of skin is pulled away. Scrub, irrigate, and debride the wound. Deep structures such as muscle and tendons should be restored. If necessary, a split-thickness graft may be performed by a surgeon. Dress the wound with a bulky dressing.

Contusion

A contusion is extravasation of blood into tissues in which vessels are damaged but skin is not disrupted, usually as a result of blunt trauma. Apply a cold pack and provide analgesia. No dressing is required.

Laceration

A laceration is an open wound or cut through the dermal layers. It may be minor or major, extending to deep epithelium, and may vary in length and depth.

Control the bleeding (by means of pressure and elevation) and evaluate neurovascular status. Anesthetize and inspect the wound; then scrub and irrigate it and remove foreign bodies. Excise and approximate necrotic margins, using sterile adhesive bandages (tape strips) or sutures. Apply a dry dressing.

If the laceration is deep and there is uncertainty about the extent of underlying structural damage, the patient may require surgery.

Puncture

A puncture is a penetration of the skin by a pointed or sharp object. It may appear innocent, but it may have damaged underlying structures or be grossly contaminated. This type of wound rarely bleeds.

Treatment depends on depth of penetration and amount of contamination. Generally, soak the wound in surgical soap solution twice a day for 2 to 4 days; remove any foreign bodies and tape them to the chart. If the wound is contaminated, soak, anesthetize, and scrub and irrigate it. Then inspect the wound carefully, remove foreign bodies, excise necrotic tissue, and place a drain or packing.

If the foreign body is deep or if there is a question of vascular or neurologic compromise, the patient should have exploratory surgery and repair. If the object is impaling, leave it in place until it can be thoroughly evaluated.

Abscess

An abscess is a localized collection of pus. Anesthetize it, drain it with the affected limb in a dependent position, and remove any elliptic area. Apply loose packing to allow for drainage, and cover the area with a loose dressing. Administer antibiotics if the patient is febrile. Do not wait until an abscess "points." If an abscess is suspected, drain the site with a needle.

Hematoma

A hematoma is an escape of blood into subcutaneous space. It is usually the result of blunt trauma. Treatment varies, depending on location.

Crush Injuries

Although there are many types of soft tissue injuries, several are commonly seen in the ED. *Wringer injuries* were seen much more frequently in the days when wringer washing machines were commonly found in the home. A person with this type of injury may come to the ED after an industrial accident in which his or her arm was caught by the wringer of a commercial washing machine, causing a crush injury.

Treat this type of wound by cleansing it and dressing it with a sterile bulky dressing. Before dressing the wound, evaluate the limb for distal pulse rates and neurologic status. Elevate the limb above the level of the heart, order a radiograph, and determine current tetanus prophylaxis status. At this point, if the injury is isolated to a limb, consider analgesia. Depending on the extent of damage, consider consulting a specialist in orthopedics, neurosurgery, or vascular or hand surgery for further therapeutic intervention.

Other types of crush injuries occur when a heavy object falls on an extremity. Therapeutic intervention is the same as that for wringer injuries.

Impaling Injuries

Impaling injuries are seen often and usually result from an industrial accident in which the victim falls onto a sharp, immobile object. Assess the neurovascular status of the limb distal to the impaling object. Consider analgesia if the injury is isolated. Once again, check the current tetanus prophylaxis status. Order radiographs of the body parts involved, and call in appropriate surgical consultants if necessary.

Gunshot Wounds

Gunshot wounds usually result from acts of violence or hunting accidents. The amount of damage depends on the type of weapon used, the caliber of ammunition used, the distance from which the weapon was fired, and the part of the body that was hit. In general, a person who has been a victim of a gunshot wound, after assessment of the ABCs, should have the wound cleansed and dressed with a dry sterile dressing until it can be evaluated by a physician. Be sure to check for pulses and neurovascular status; assess the limb if possible. One item often overlooked in the excitement of the injury and other therapeutic intervention is the status of the patient's tetanus prophylaxis.

Knee Injuries

Knee injuries are a common form of soft tissue injury in which rotational or extraflexion trauma results in a medical meniscus, collateral ligament, or cruciate ligament strain or tear. Signs and symptoms of this type of injury include a history of trauma to the knee, swelling, ecchymosis, effusion, pain, and tenderness. Therapeutic interventions include use of a compression bandage, knee immobilizer, or cylinder cast, depending on the extent of the injury; elevation of the injured limb; application of a cold pack to the injured area for the first 24 hours (intermittently); and instructions to the patient concerning how to use crutches for the purpose of not bearing weight. If the injury is determined to be a ligament tear, it should be surgically repaired within 24 to 48 hours of the time of the injury.

Fingertip Injuries

Fingertip injuries are frequently seen in the emergency setting. The most common type of fingertip injury is a crush injury to the distal phalanx, resulting from a heavy object falling on the fingertip, or the fingertip being caught in a house or car door. Therapeutic intervention is to apply a soft, bulky, protective dressing. Radiographs should be obtained to rule out fractures. If a hematoma is forming under the fingernail, nail trephination should be carried out by penetrating the fingernail over the site of the hematoma with a nail drill, a scalpel, or a superheated paper clip to relieve the blood that is collecting under the nail.

Another type of fingertip injury that is seen with increasing frequency is one that is caused by a high-pressure paint or grease gun. This injury occurs when a person is cleaning the tip of a high-pressure gun and the gun releases a stream of paint or grease into the fingertip and up into the hand at high pressure. Particular attention must be paid to the history in this case, since the injury appears only as a small pinhole in the tip of the finger. Therapeutic intervention requires surgical debridement of the paint- or grease-injected limb after the patient receives general anesthesia.

Strains

A strain is a weakening or overstretching of a muscle at the point where it attaches to the tendon. Strains may occur as the result of almost any type of movement, from simply stepping off a step in the wrong way and twisting the ankle to a wrenching force as a result of an automobile accident. Most commonly, strains are seen as a result of athletic injuries.

A patient with a *mild* strain complains of local pain, point tenderness, and slight muscle spasms. Therapeutic interventions include use of a compression bandage, elevation of the limb above the level of the heart for 12 hours, application of a cold pack intermittently for the same period, and maintenance (by the patient) of light weight bearing on the injured part.

With a *moderate* strain the patient complains of local pain, point tenderness, swelling, discoloration, and inability to use the limb for prolonged periods. Therapeutic interventions include use of a compression bandage, elevation, and application of a cold pack for 24 hours; analgesia; and instructions for light weight bearing only.

When the strain is *severe,* the patient complains of local pain, point tenderness, swelling, and discoloration; he or she also offers a history of a "snapping noise" at the time of the injury. Therapeutic interventions include use of a compression bandage, elevation, and application of a cold pack for 24 to 48 hours; analgesia; and instructions for *no* weight bearing for 48 hours.

Sprains

A *sprain* is a ligament injury. The mechanism of inury may be the same as that of a strain, but in general a sprain is usually the result of a much more traumatic force. A sprain occurs when a joint exceeds its normal limit. The most common sprains are seen in the ankles, knees, and shoulders. A *mild* sprain produces slight pain and slight swelling. Therapeutic interventions include use of a compression bandage, elevation, application of a cold pack for 12 hours, and orders for light weight bearing. A *moderate* sprain causes pain, point tenderness, swelling, and inability to use the limb for more than a short time. Therapeutic interventions include use of a compression bandage, elevation, application of cold pack for 24 hours, and orders for light weight bearing with the use of crutches.

A *severe* sprain involves tearing of the ligaments, which causes pain, point tenderness, swelling, discoloration, and inability to use the limb. Therapeutic interventions include placement of a compression bandage or a cast, elevation, and application of a cold pack for 48 hours, and instructions for light to no weight bearing with the use of crutches.

Ruptured Achilles Tendon

With the advent of tennis and racquetball as major pastimes in the United States, one should expect to see an increasing incidence of ruptured Achilles tendon. This injury usually occurs in athletes over 30 years of age who actively participate in start-and-stop sports in which one steps off abruptly on the forefoot with the knee forced in extension. The patient complains of a sharp pain from the heel that extends into the back of the leg. There is a sudden inability to use the foot of the injured extremity; a deformity

develops, and the patient exhibits a positive Thompson's sign: when the calf muscle is squeezed, with the leg extended and the foot over the end of the table, the heel does not pull, and no upward motion is seen.

A patient with a ruptured Achilles tendon should have a compression bandage applied, along with elevation of the extremity and application of a cold pack until surgery can be performed to repair the tendon.

PERIPHERAL NERVE INJURIES

Throughout the text neurovascular function has been mentioned. Neurovascular function may be altered not only by mechanical, chemical, or thermal trauma to an extremity, but also by malignancies, toxins, metabolic factors, or collagen disease. The most common causes of peripheral nerve injuries are lacerations, penetrating wounds, fractures, and dislocations. The nurse should be familiar with the distribution of nerves, the origin of motor branches, and the muscles that they supply. When testing for motor loss, one should be able to visualize the tendon or muscle body that is being tested (Table 27-1).

Other, more sophisticated diagnostic tests such as electromyography, electrical stimulation, and nerve conduction tests are performed in the in-patient setting and are not appropriate for ED use. Likewise, peripheral nerve injury repair should take place in the operating room, not in the ED.

FRACTURES

A fracture is a disruption or break in the bone. In general, there are signs and symptoms that are common to most fractures. These include angulation, deformity, pain, point and region tenderness, swelling, lack of movement, and crepitus (grating of bone ends). Other findings are obvious bony fragment protrusion and decreased neurovascular status, including decreased distal pulse rates, decreased skin temperature distal to the fracture site, cyanosis, decreased sensation, and occasionally shock.

Fractures are divided into two general categories: closed or simple fractures, in which the bone is broken but the skin is not disrupted; and open or compound fractures, in which the bone is protruding, the bone has punctured the skin and returned into the limb, or a foreign object has penetrated the skin and bone, causing a fracture.

Table 27-1 Techniques for assessment of common peripheral nerve injuries

Nerve	Frequently associated injuries	Assessment technique
Radial	Fracture of humerus, especially middle and distal thirds	Inability to extend thumb in "hitchhiker's sign"
Ulnar	Fracture of medial humeral epicondyle	Loss of pain perception in tip of little finger
Median	Elbow dislocation or wrist or forearm injury	Loss of pain perception in tip of index finger
Peroneal	Tibia or fibula fracture; dislocation of knee	Inability to extend great toe or foot; may also be associated with sciatic nerve injury
Sciatic and tibial	Infrequent with fractures or dislocations	Loss of pain perception in sole of foot

Types of Fractures

- A transverse fracture results from an angulation force or a direct trauma (Fig. 27-2).
- An oblique fracture results from a twisting force (Fig. 27-3).
- A spiral fracture results from a twisting force while the foot is firmly planted (Fig. 27-4).
- A comminuted fracture results from a severe direct trauma. The fracture has more than two fragments (Fig. 27-5).
- An impacted fracture results from a severe trauma, causing the fractured bone ends to jam together (Fig. 27-6).
- A compression fracture results from a severe force to the top of the head or the os calcis, causing the vertebrae to be forced together (Fig. 27-7).
- A greenstick fracture is the result of a compression force. It usually occurs in children in the grammar school and junior high school age-groups (Fig. 27-8).
- An avulsion fracture is the result of a forceful contraction of a muscle mass, causing a bone fragment to break away at the insertion (Fig. 27-9).
- A depresson fracture is the result of a blunt trauma to a flat bone. This type of fracture is usually associated with a great deal of soft-tissue damage (Fig. 27-10).

Assessment

General assessment of a patient with a suspected limb fracture should include checking for pain or point tenderness, pulses distal to the fracture site, pallor (skin color) distal to the fracture site, paresthesia (tingling or numbness) of the extremity, and paralysis of the extremity. These indices are known as the five Ps. Other signs to check for are deformity, swelling, crepitus, discoloration, and associated wounds.

Therapeutic Intervention

Begin with the general assessment previously indicated. Determining the mechanisms of injury helps to determine the fracture diagnosis. Immobilize the fracture site by splinting the extremity, including the joints above and below the fracture site whenever possible. Once splinting has been accomplished, reassess the limb for neurovascular status. If compromise is present, apply traction in an attempt to restore integrity. Elevate the limb if possible, to decrease the amount of swelling and hemorrhage. Apply a cold pack to the injured area to cause vasoconstriction and decrease swelling, muscle spasms, and pain.

When a limb is traumatized, a fracture should be suspected until proved otherwise by radiographic studies, which are the definitive way to confirm a fracture. If possible, the radiograph should include visualization of joints above and below the trauma site, since these joints are often injured and frequently overlooked. The radiograph should also include both anterior and lateral views of the injured limb, since some fractures can only be visualized from one angle.

When limbs are fractured, they may cause damage to vessels that leads to hypovolemia and shock. A jagged bone may lacerate vital organs, arteries, veins, or nerves. Open fractures may lead to serious infections. Fractures may also cause fat emboli, which may occur from 24 to 48 hours

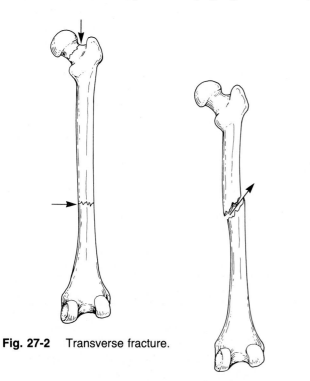

Fig. 27-2   Transverse fracture.

Fig. 27-3   Oblique fracture.

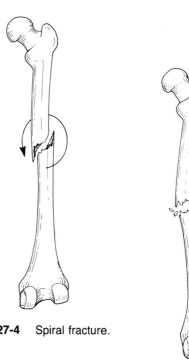

Fig. 27-4   Spiral fracture.

Fig. 27-5   Comminuted fracture.

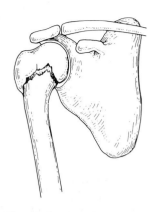

Fig. 27-6   Impacted fracture.

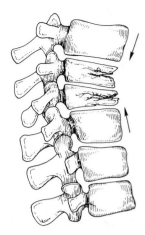

Fig. 27-7   Compression fracture.

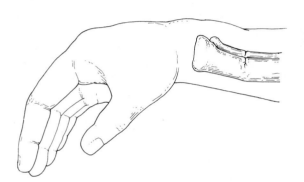

Fig. 27-8   Greenstick fracture.

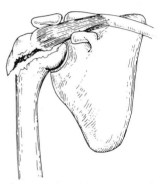

Fig. 27-9   Avulsion fracture.

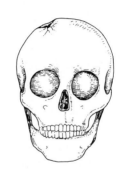

Fig. 27-10   Depression fracture.

after the fracture. They are most commonly seen in conjunction with pelvic, tibial, or femoral fractures but may also be associated with other types. Fat embolism is a life-threatening situation with a high mortality. The patient has a sudden onset of tachycardia accompanied by an elevated temperature, an altered level of consciousness, decreased respirations, cough, shortness of breath, cyanosis, petechiae, and pulmonary edema. Immediate therapeutic intervention includes oxygen delivery at a high flow rate, support of ABCs, and possible administration of corticosteroids and heparin according to physician or facility policy.

Victims with multiple fractures are frequently hospitalized. Many of these victims have had an accident resulting from alcohol abuse, in which they have fallen, been struck by an automobile, or been involved in a collision of two motor vehicles. If hospitalization is prolonged, these patients may begin to have delirium tremens. It is therefore essential to ask questions about alcohol use when obtaining the initial history. One must give appropriate attention to the patient with a history of chronic alcohol use. Therapeutic

intervention for a patient who has delirium tremens is based on local protocol and usually includes the administration of diazepam (Valium), chlorpromazine (Thorazine), paraldehyde, or IV alcohol.

Upper Torso Fractures

Bones in the upper torso that are common sites of fractures include the clavicle, shoulder, scapula, ribs, and sternum.

Clavicular fracture. Fracture of the clavicle is a common type of fracture that can be found in all age-groups (Fig. 27-11), particularly in children. It usually results from a fall on the arm or the shoulder or from direct lateral trauma to the shoulder such as contact injury in which athletes run into each other. The patient complains of pain in the clavicular area and point tenderness, and he or she will not raise the affected arm. Swelling, deformity, and crepitus are present. One also notices that the patient tilts his or her head toward the side of the injury, with the chin directed toward the opposite side. One should assess the neurovascular status of the arm, support the arm, and place the

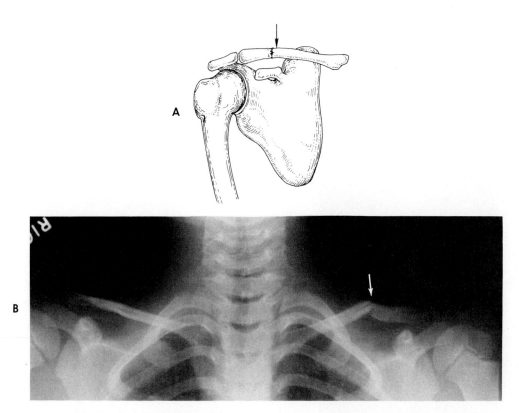

Fig. 27-11   A, Fracture of clavicle. **B,** Arrow on radiograph shows fracture.

shoulders in a figure-eight support (Fig. 27-12). The patient should be instructed to apply a cold pack to the injured area for 12 to 24 hours (intermittently) and to see an orthopedic specialist or be referred to the orthopedic clinic for follow-up care.

Shoulder fracture. A shoulder fracture is a fracture of the glenoid, humeral head, or humeral neck (Fig. 27-13). It is common to see shoulder fractures in elderly patients as a result of a fall on an outstretched arm or direct trauma to the shoulder. When this same mechanism of injury occurs in a younger person, it usually results in a shoulder dislocation. However, a fracture occurs in an elderly person because of a weaker bone structure.

When a patient has a shoulder fracture, he or she complains of pain in the shoulder area and point tenderness; he or she cannot move the affected arm; and gross swelling and discoloration occur. Therapeutic interventions include assessment of the neurovascular status, use of a sling and

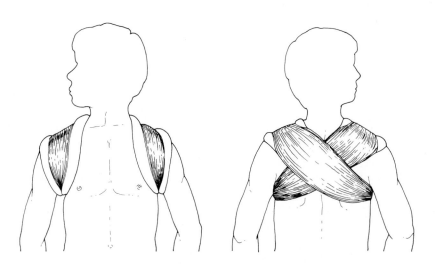

Fig. 27-12   Figure-eight support.

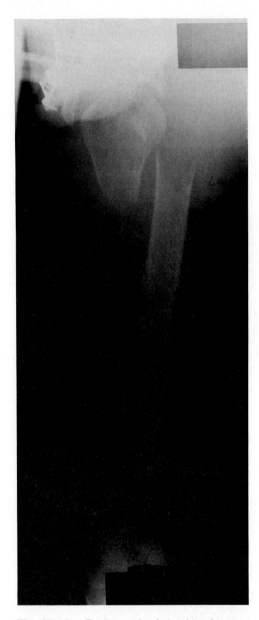

Fig. 27-13   Radiograph of shoulder fracture.

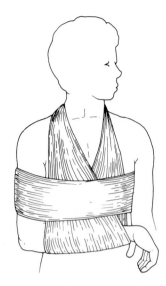

Fig. 27-14   Sling and swath.

There is usually bone displacement and swelling over the injured area. Therapeutic interventions include assessment of neurovascular status, placement of a compression bandage over the scapula if the bone is nondisplaced, use of a sling and swath bandage, and application of a cold pack for the first 24 hours. Complications include injuries to the underlying ribs or viscera.

Arm Fractures

Fractures of the upper arm. Fractures of the upper arm (humeral shaft) are commonly seen in children and in elderly persons (Fig. 27-16). This type of fracture results from a fall on the arm, a direct trauma, or in association with a dislocation of the shoulder. It is a painful fracture; the patient complains of point tenderness, and one notes swelling, the inability or hesitance of the patient to use the arm, a severe deformity or angulation, and crepitus. Therapeutic interventions include assessment of neurovascular status, use of a sling and swath bandage, application of a cold pack, and assessment for other injuries, since humeral shaft fractures are frequently associated with chest trauma. When the patient arrives in the ED, the fracture is usually reduced by closed reduction. If vascular or neurologic compromise is present, mild, steady, downward traction should be applied. The arm is casted: a long plaster splint is applied from the acromial process, down around the elbow, and back up to the acromial process. It is then wrapped with a compression elastic bandage to allow for swelling. The axilla should be padded with cotton, and the entire arm should be stabilized and supported with a sling. In addition to routine cast care instructions, the patient should be given instructions to exercise his or her wrists and fingers frequently. A danger of radial nerve damage accompanies a fracture of the middle or distal portion of the shaft. There is also a possibility of

swath (Fig. 27-14), and application of a cold pack over the area of injury. An orthopedic surgeon generally reduces the fracture and either immobilizes it with a sling and swath or admits the patient to the hospital, where skeletal traction is applied. If the fracture cannot be reduced by the manipulative method, an open reduction may be performed. One must pay particular attention to a humeral neck fracture, which may cause axillary nerve damage.

Scapular fracture. A scapular fracture (Fig. 27-15) may be seen in any age-group. This injury is usually the result of a violent, direct trauma; it may, however, be seen as the result of a severe muscle contraction. The patient complains of pain during shoulder movement and point tenderness.

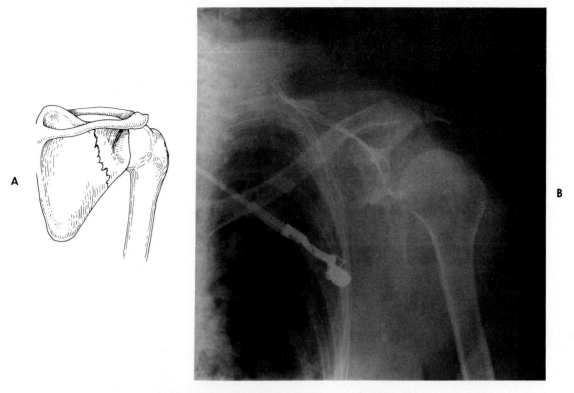

Fig. 27-15   **A,** Scapular fracture. **B,** Radiograph.

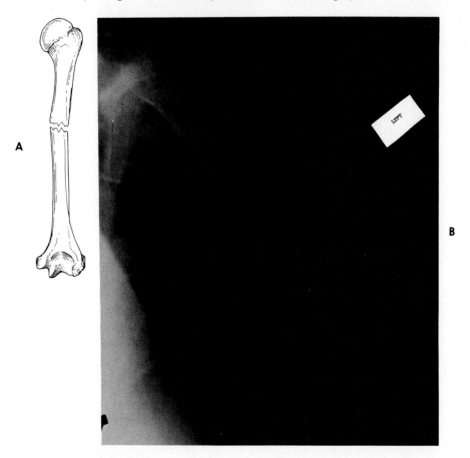

Fig. 27-16   **A,** Fracture of humerus. **B,** Radiograph.

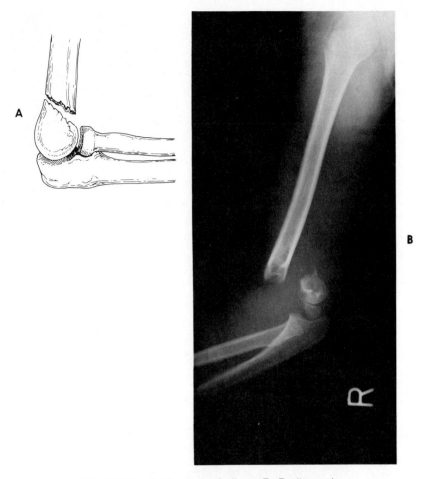

Fig. 27-17 **A,** Fracture of elbow. **B,** Radiograph.

hemorrhage if bleeding is not controlled within the early moments after injury.

Elbow fractures. Elbow fractures are seen most commonly in young children and young athletes. An elbow fracture results from a fall on an extended arm or on a flexed elbow (Fig. 27-17). This is a common result of a fall from a skateboard. The patient complains of pain and point tenderness. There is a great deal of swelling, since this injury is frequently associated with much soft tissue damage. The patient does not move his or her elbow, and a deformity is present. Because of the massive swelling, there may be vascular compromise, resulting in decreased circulation to the hand. Therapeutic intervention requires immediate assessment of vascular status. The arm should be splinted in the position in which it is found, which is not always an easy task. If possible, a sling and swath bandage should be applied, as well as a cold pack. If neurovascular compromise is evident, attempt to flex the arm at a greater angle. The fracture may be reduced manually, or it may have to be reduced by placement of a pin and traction. If the fracture is reduced in a closed manual fashion, it is usually casted

and placed in a sling. The complications associated with this type of fracture are brachial artery laceration, median or radial nerve damage, and Volkmann's contracture.

Volkmann's contracture results from ischemia to the muscles and nerves. Signs and symptoms of this condition are inability to move the fingers (manipulation of the fingers causes severe pain), severe pain in the forearm flexor muscles (even after reduction), inability to obtain a radial pulse rate, swelling, cold temperature of the extremity, cyanosis, and decreased sensation. Temporary therapeutic intervention includes removal of the cast and extension of the forearm with application of cold packs. It is essential to obtain immediate orthopedic consultation for further therapeutic intervention.

Forearm fractures. Forearm (radius and ulna) fractures are seen commonly in both adults and children. Forearm fractures usually result from a fall on an extended arm or as a result of a direct blow (Fig. 27-18). The patient exhibits signs and symptoms of pain, point tenderness, swelling, deformity and angulation, and occasional shortening of the extremity. Therapeutic interventions include assessment of

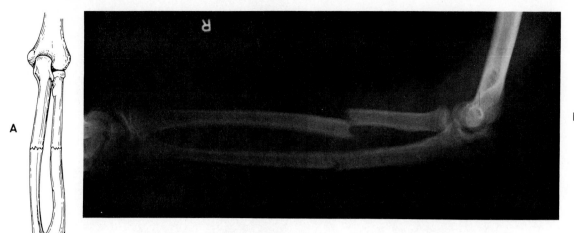

Fig. 27-18 **A,** Fractures of radius and ulna. **B,** Radiograph.

neurovascular status, placement of a splint to immobilize the fracture, use of a sling, and application of a cold pack. Many of these fractures can be manipulated with the closed reduction technique. They are then casted, with the elbow in 90 degrees of flexion. The shoulder and the fingers should be free of the cast and allowed to move freely. Complications include rare neurovascular compromise and Volkmann's contracture.

Wrist and Hand Fractures

Fractures of the wrist. Fractures of the wrist are common in elderly individuals but may occur in any age-group. The most common mechanism of injury is a fall onto an extended arm and an open hand. These patients complain of pain, swelling, and deformity. First assess the neurovascular status of the wrist and hand. The fractured limb should be splinted in the position in which it is found. The arm should be placed in a sling, and a cold pack should be applied. Because one can anticipate much swelling, one may place a compression bandage over the fracture site. Often these fractures can be manipulated in a closed reduction procedure and then casted and placed in a sling. Occasionally an open reduction is necessary to pin the fracture segments. Aseptic necrosis is a rare complication resulting from fractures of the wrist.

A fracture of the distal radius and ulna is known as a *silver fork deformity;* a silver fork deformity is the result of a fall onto an extended hand. This type of fracture is also known as a *Colles' fracture.* If a patient has a Colles' fracture, it is wise to check the mechanism of injury. Occasionally these victims fall from a height and fracture the os calcis (heel) and also sustain a compression fracture of the lumbodorsal vertebrae. The victim may then fall forward as a result of the pain from the lumbar fracture. As he or she falls forward, the hands are extended to break the fall, and the result is an associated Colles' fracture.

Carpal and metacarpal fractures. Fractures of the carpals (Fig. 27-19) and the metacarpals (Fig. 27-20) are common injuries in athletes, particularly in those involved in contact sports. Some of the more common types of fractures of the carpals and metacarpals result from such activities as fighting, which causes a fracture of the fifth metacarpal, known as a boxer's fracture. Another common type of fracture is an avulsion fracture, which results when someone throws a baseball and the distal attachment of the extensor tendon tears loose, bringing with it a segment of bone. Other common carpal and metacarpal fractures result from crush injuries in industrial settings.

Signs and symptoms of fractured carpals and metacarpals include pain, severe swelling, deformity, inability to use the hand, and frequently an open fracture. Therapeutic interventions include assessment of neurovascular status; control of bleeding; covering the open wounds with a dry, sterile, bulky dressing; splinting the fracture in a functional position; application of a cold pack; and application of pressure to the wound with a compression bandage. The fracture is usually casted in the ED.

Phalanx fractures. Fractured phalanges (fingers) are common in all age-groups (Fig. 27-21). Signs and symptoms are similar to those for carpal and metacarpal fractures, and therapeutic interventions are basically the same. Sometimes, a phalanx fracture has an associated hematoma beneath the fingernail (a subungual hematoma) and the patient complains of a severe, throbbing pain. Therapeutic intervention in this case is nail trephination. Therapeutic intervention for phalanx fractures is usually splinting the finger involved. Occasionally a surgical reduction is necessary to realign the fractured segments.

Pelvic Fractures (Fig. 27-22)

Pelvic fractures occur frequently in middle-aged and elderly adults. It is estimated that 65% of patients with pelvic fractures have other associated injuries. It is also estimated

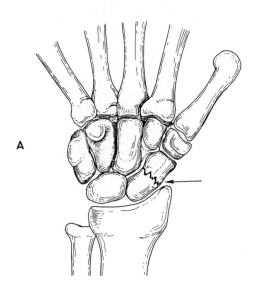

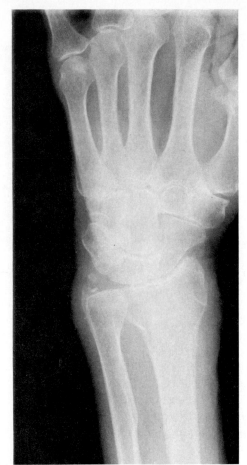

Fig. 27-19 **A,** Wrist fracture. **B,** Radiograph.

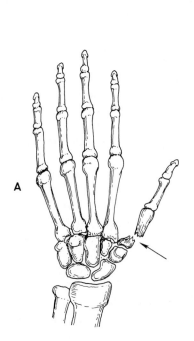

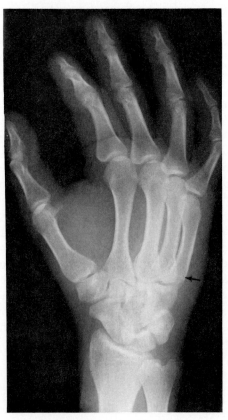

Fig. 27-20 **A,** Fractured metacarpals.
B, Radiograph.

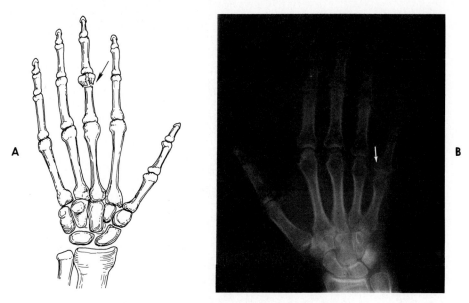

Fig. 27-21   **A,** Fractured phalanx. **B,** Radiograph.

that 8% to 10% of patients with pelvic fractures die. This injury commonly occurs as a crush injury from an automobile or motorcycle accident or as a result of direct trauma, a fall from a height, or sudden contraction of a muscle against resistance. The patient exhibits signs and symptoms of tenderness over the pubis when the iliac wings are compressed, paraspinous muscle spasm, sacroiliac joint tenderness, paresis or hemiparesis, pelvic ecchymosis, and hematuria. The patient may also demonstrate signs of blood loss, as evidenced by the presence of tachycardia, hypotension, and other signs of impending shock.

Therapeutic interventions include immobilizing the spine and legs with the use of a long board, flexing the knees to decrease pain, administering oxygen at high flow, monitoring vital signs every 5 minutes, initiating two large-bore intravenous lines for volume replacement (run at a rate in accordance with blood pressure and pulse rate measurements), placing the pneumatic antishock garment (PASG) under the patient, and inflating them as necessary. These patients should be transported to a hospital facility rapidly so that early radiographic studies, peritoneal lavage, and blood typing and crossmatching can be accomplished in minimal time. These patients have a tendency to bleed profusely, and blood should be typed and crossmatched to provide at least 5 units of whole blood. The average amount of blood lost is 2 units.

Complications of pelvic fractures include bladder trauma, genital trauma, lumbosacral trauma, ruptured internal organs, shock, and death.

In-hospital therapeutic intervention may include bed rest, with either pinning and traction or casting, after a closed or open reduction has been performed.

Hip Fractures (Fig. 27-23)

Hip fractures are common in elderly individuals; the fracture usually results from a fall or a minor trauma. When a hip fracture occurs in a younger person, it is usually the result of a major trauma. These patients complain of pain in the hip joint and the groin area, severe pain with movement of the leg, inability to bear weight, external rotation of the hip and leg, and minimal shortening of the limb. If the injury is extracapsular and associated with a trochanteric fracture, the patient complains of pain in the area of the lateral hip, one sees an increased shortening of the extremity, and the degree of external rotation is greater than with intracapsular injury.

Immediate therapeutic interventions include splinting the hip, either to a long board or to the opposite leg, checking pulse rates and neurologic status distal to the fracture site, and taking frequent vital signs, at least every 5 minutes. Once the patient reaches the hospital, early immobilization should be accomplished, and surgical intervention is often necessary.

Complications of hip fracture are the immediate complications of hypovolemia and shock and the later complications resulting from prolonged bed rest.

Leg Fractures

Femoral fracture (Fig. 27-24). Femoral fractures occur in all age-groups, usually as a result of major trauma. The patient complains of severe pain and an inability to bear weight on the injured leg. There is a noticeable deformity, swelling, and angulation. The limb shortens as a result of severe muscle spasms. Crepitus over the fracture site may also be evident.

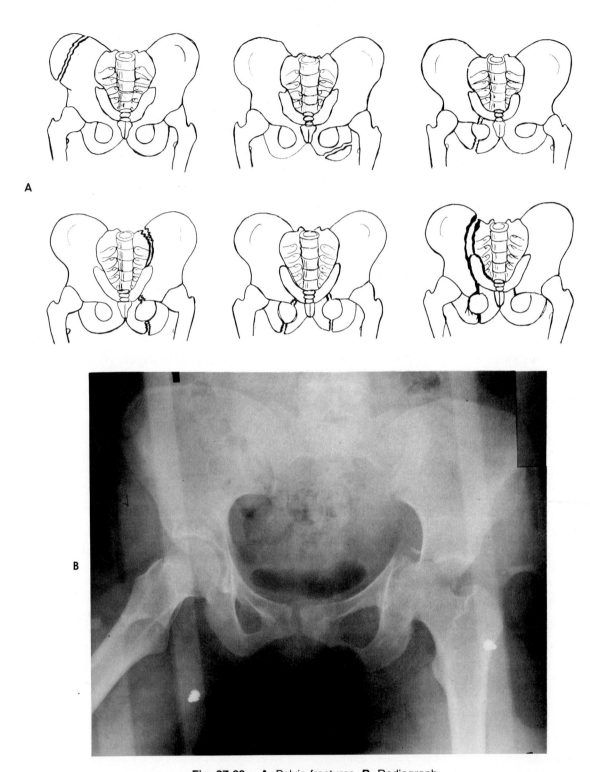

Fig. 27-22   **A,** Pelvic fractures. **B,** Radiograph.

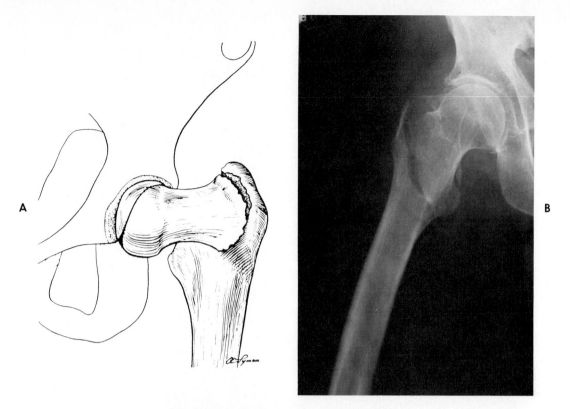

Fig. 27-23   A, Hip fracture. **B,** Radiograph.

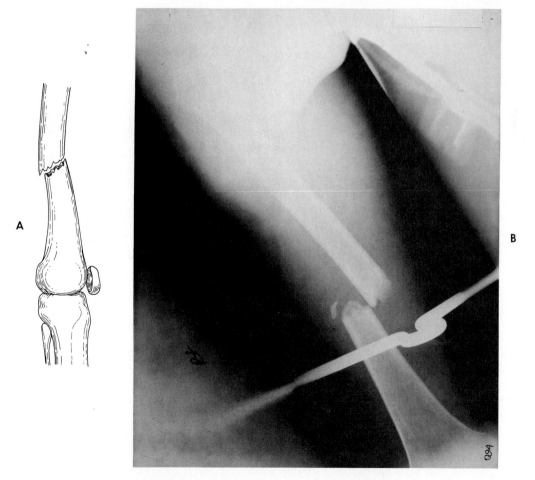

Fig. 27-24   A, Fracture of femur. **B,** Radiograph.

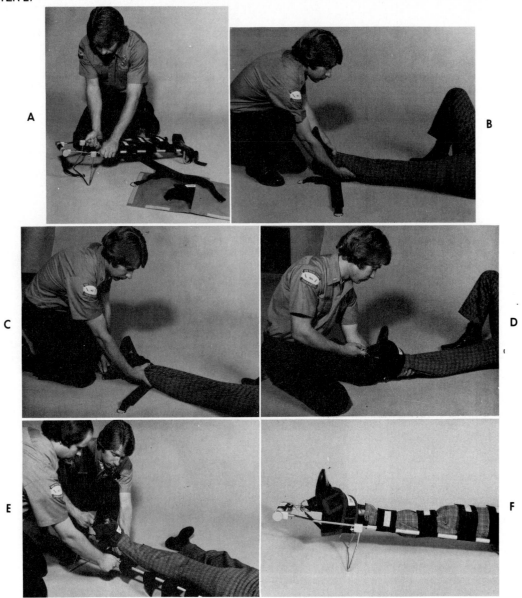

Fig. 27-25 Hare traction splint application. **A,** Remove cover. Twist collet sleeves to unlock. Place splint parallel to injured leg. Adjust splint to desired length, approximately 8 to 10 inches past foot. Twist collet sleeves to lock (excessive pressure not required). Fold down heel stand until it locks into place. Slide heel stand-up splint about 5 inches. Position Velcro support straps (two above knee and two below knee) and open. **B,** Remove tri-ring ankle strap from cover and place under patient's heel with padded side against foot. Place bottom edge of heel even with lower edge of sponge. **C,** Criss-cross top straps over instep, keeping straps high up on instep. **D,** Grasp all three rings, botton ring first, and exert manual traction to align leg using slow firm pull. Steady foot by placing one hand under heel. When establishing manual alignment, be sure to support lower portion of involved extremity just below point of fracture. **E,** While maintaining manual traction, have an assistant place splint under leg with half-ring placed just below the buttock. Secure half-ring strap. Once alignment is started, continue to maintain constant manual traction until alignment has been secured by splint. **F,** Insert S hook into three D rings, heel ring first. Twist knurled knob to apply traction. Tighten until strap is snug. Injured leg is then in traction. Fasten Velcro straps, which may also be used to apply pressure over any open wound. Position strap so it closes over bleeding area, apply gauze pad, and secure strap. Patient may then be moved. Adjust location of heel stand after patient has been placed on cot so that solid contact is established with cot. (Manufactured exclusively by Dyna Med, Inc., 6200 Yarrow Drive, Carlsbad, Calif. 92008.)

Therapeutic intervention includes use of the Hare traction splint (Fig. 27-25) or other type of long-leg splint, such as a Thomas splint, to apply traction to the limb. Do not use a long-leg air splint with a closed foot, since distal neurovascular status cannot be assessed. It is also not advisable to use the other leg as a splint. Whenever possible and as time permits, initiate two large-bore intravenous lines for volume replacement. Be sure to check for distal pulse rates and distal neurologic status. Check also for other associated injuries. Obtain frequent readings of vital signs, at least every 5 minutes. Apply a cold pack to the injured area. If the injury is isolated, consider analgesia. Once the victim arrives at the hospital, he or she should be prepared for traction, pin placement, or surgery.

Complications of femoral fracture include hypovolemia. It is not uncommon for a patient to lose 2 units of blood into the thigh of a fractured femur. As a result of severe muscle spasms that cause the bone ends to move, severe muscle damage may result. Also, knee trauma is often associated with femur fracture and could easily be overlooked. The greatest complication of femoral fracture is shock caused by hypovolemia. There is also a possibility of fat emboli.

Knee fractures. Knee fractures are either supracondylar fractures of the femur or intraarticular fractures of the femur or tibia (Fig. 27-26). This type of injury may occur in all age-groups and is usually the result of an automobile, motorcycle, or automobile-pedestrian accident that results in a direct trauma to the knee. The patient complains of knee pain, an inability to bend or straighten the knee (depending on the position of the knee after the accident), swelling, and tenderness. Therapeutic interventions should include providing a long-leg splint or securing one leg to the other, checking distal pulse rates, and assessing distal neurologic status. Depending on the extent of injury, the patient may have to be prepared for surgical repair, and the knee will most likely be casted. The most common complication of knee fracture is neurovascular compromise.

Patellar fractures. Patellar fractures are commonly seen in all age-groups (Fig. 27-27). These fractures usually occur as a result of a direct trauma from a fall or an impact with the dashboard of a car or from indirect trauma such as a severe muscle pull. The patient complains of pain in the knee. The fracture can often be palpated. Frequently there is an open fracture. Therapeutic interventions include covering the open wound and applying a cold pack and long-leg splint. When the patient arrives in the ED, radiographs of the affected limb should be made to determine the extent of the fracture. If the fracture is nondisplaced, the leg is usually placed in a long-leg cylinder cast. If the fracture is displaced, an attempt should be made to realign the parts. Sometimes it is necessary to

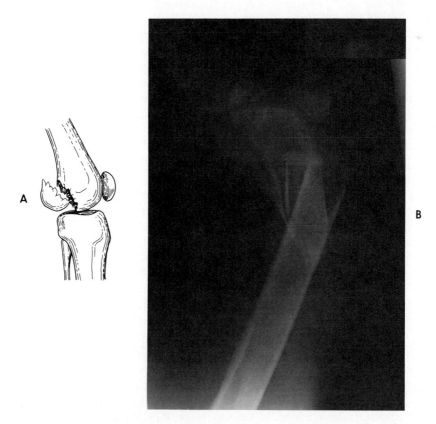

Fig. 27-26 A, Knee fracture. **B,** Radiograph.

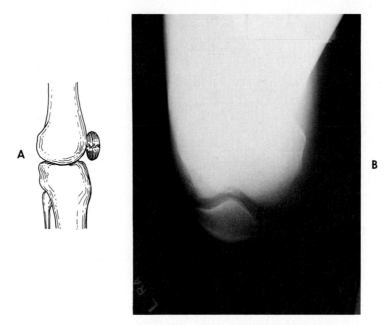

Fig. 27-27   A, Patellar fracture. **B,** Radiograph.

send the patient to surgery for an open reduction and perhaps even a pinning. Remember that the patella is an important part of the knee in that it aids in leverage of the knee and protects the knee joint.

Tibial and fibular fractures. Tibial and fibular fractures are seen commonly in all age-groups (Fig. 27-28). These fractures result from direct or indirect trauma or a rotational force. The patient complains of pain in his or her leg, point tenderness, swelling, deformity, and crepitus. Many tibial and fibular fractures are open fractures. These injuries should be splinted as they are found, and no attempt to realign them should be made unless there is neurovascular compromise. Be sure to check for neurovascular status before and after splinting. Most of the time the leg can be splinted with a long-leg splint. If there is an open fracture, it should be irrigated with sterile normal saline solution and covered with a dry sterile dressing. Apply a cold pack to the area of the wound. When the patient arrives in the ED, radiographs should be obtained and the extent of the injury should be determined. Open or closed reduction may be necessary. The patient's leg is almost always casted. If the fibula alone is fractured, which is unusual, a walking cast is usually applied, since the fibula is not a weight-bearing bone.

Complications of tibial and fibular fractures can include soft tissue damage, infection, neurovascular compromise, and Volkmann's contracture.

Ankle fractures. Fractures of the ankle are commonly seen in all age-groups (Fig. 27-29). These types of injuries occur as a result of direct trauma, indirect trauma, or torsion. The patient complains of pain in the area of the injury, inability to bear weight on the extremity, point tenderness, swelling, and deformity. Therapeutic interventions include use of a soft splint, assessment of neurovascular status, application of a cold pack, and elevation. Radiographs are obtained when the patient arrives in the ED. Depending on the extent of damage, the patient may need a closed or open reduction and pinning and most likely a cast. Depending on the extent and location of the injury, the patient may be placed in a walking cast. The most common complication that results from this type of injury is neurovascular compromise.

Foot Fractures

Tarsal and metatarsal fractures. Fractures of the tarsals and metatarsals are common in all age-groups (Fig. 27-30). These fractures occur as a result of automobile accidents, athletic injuries, crush injuries, or direct trauma. The patient complains of pain in his or her foot and hesitates to bear weight on it. Point tenderness, deformity, and swelling are present. Therapeutic intervention includes placement of a compression dressing and a soft splint. When the patient arrives in the ED, a radiograph is obtained to determine the extent of the injury. The fracture(s) should be reduced if necessary, and the patient should have his or her foot placed in a cast. He or she may be allowed to walk on crutches without weight bearing. Complications from this type of injury are rare.

Heel (os calcis) fracture. Fractures of the heel are usually seen in young adults and usually result from a fall from a height in which the victim lands on his or her feet (Fig. 27-31). The patient complains of pain in the heel area and point

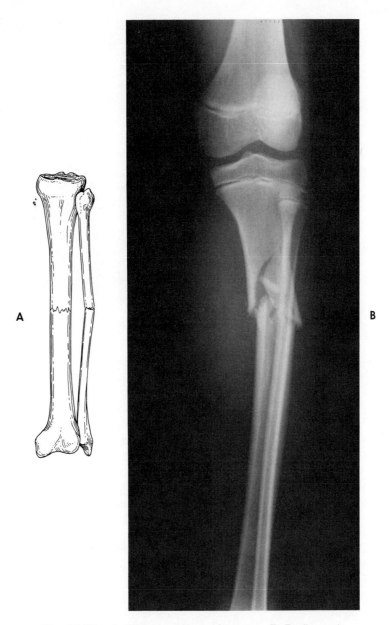

Fig. 27-28   A, Tibial and fibular fractures. **B,** Radiograph.

tenderness and demonstrates swelling and perhaps dislocation. Therapeutic interventions include placement of a compression dressing, elevation of the injured extremity, and application of a cold pack. When the patient arrives in the ED, radiographic studies should be performed. Management usually includes reduction of the fracture if necessary and application of a below-the-knee, weight-bearing cast. Occasionally open reduction is necessary. Complications of this type of injury are, frequently, an associated lumbosacral compression fracture and, rarely, a Colles' fracture.

Toe (phalangeal) fractures. Fractures of the toes (phalanges) are commonly seen in all age-groups (Fig. 27-32).

They are usually caused by kicking a hard object or running into an immovable object (stubbing the toe). The patient complains of pain in the toe area, and swelling and discoloration can be observed. Therapeutic interventions include placement of a compression dressing, use of a rigid splint, elevation, and application of a cold pack. After radiographic studies have been performed in the ED, felt or cotton is placed between the fractured toe and the toe next to it. The two toes are then taped together so that the uninjured toe acts as a splint. The patient may bear weight as tolerated and is instructed to wear shoes that do not put weight on the toes from the anterior aspect. Complications from this type of injury are rare.

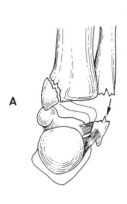

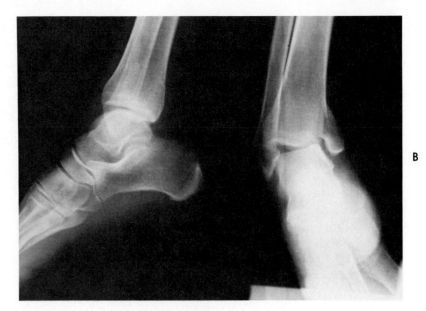

Fig. 27-29 **A,** Ankle fracture. **B,** Radiograph.

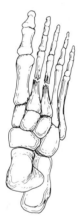

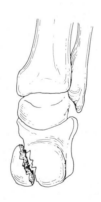

Fig. 27-30 Foot fracture.   **Fig. 27-31** Heel fracture.

Fracture Healing

Fractures may heal poorly as a result of improper immobilization, poor reduction, insufficient immobility, too much traction on the injured extremity, a decreased neurologic or vascular supply, and infection.

DISLOCATIONS

Dislocations occur when a joint exceeds its range of motion and the joint surfaces are no longer intact. Soft tissue injury within the joint capsule and surrounding ligaments, severe swelling, and possible vein and artery damage are commonly observed with this type of injury. One can frequently project a diagnosis before confirming radiographs are obtained by soliciting information about the mechanism of injury.

In general, dislocations produce severe pain, deformity at the joint, an inability to move the joint, swelling, and point tenderness. Therapeutic interventions include careful palpation of the joint and splinting the injury as it is found. Do *not* attempt to relocate the joint in the prehospital setting unless there is severe neurovascular compromise. It is important to transport the patient as soon as possible so that the ED physician or orthopedic surgeon can administer adequate anesthesia and reduce the dislocation immediately. Be careful to check for associated fractures.

Acromioclavicular Dislocation

Acromioclavicular separations are commonly seen in athletes (Fig. 27-33). They are caused by a fall or a force on the point of the shoulder. The patient complains of great pain in the joint area. He or she cannot raise the affected arm or bring it across his or her chest. One notes a deformity and point or area tenderness, swelling, and possibly a hematoma over the injury site. Therapeutic interventions include neurovascular assessment, application of a cold pack, and use of a sling and swath. The separation is usually reduced, and the arm and shoulder are then immobilized. Occasionally the patient requires surgery for an open reduction and wiring. Complications from this type of injury are rare.

Shoulder Dislocation

Dislocations of the shoulder usually occur in the young and in athletes. There are two general categories: anterior and posterior dislocations. Each type has several variations, but these are not discussed in this text. For more information, the reader is referred to the readings at the end of the chapter.

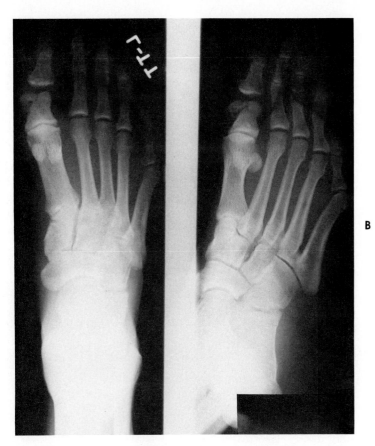

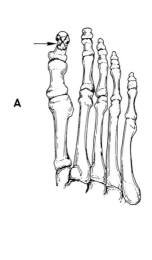

Fig. 27-32   A, Toe fracture. **B,** Radiographs.

Anterior shoulder dislocations usually occur as the result of an athletic injury in which the athlete falls on an extended arm that is abducted and externally rotated. The result is a force that pushes the head of the humerus in front of the shoulder joint (Fig. 27-34).

Posterior dislocations are rare. They are usually found in patients who have had seizures in which the arm was abducted and internally rotated.

In all shoulder dislocations, the patient complains of se-

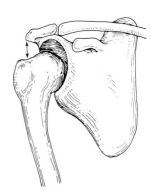

Fig. 27-33   Acromioclavicular separation.

vere pain in the shoulder area, an inability to move his or her arm, and a deformity, which is sometimes difficult to see in a posterior dislocation. It is estimated that 55% to 60% of shoulder dislocations seen in the ED are recurrent. Therapeutic intervention includes support of the extremity in the position in which it is found or in the position of greatest comfort. A cold pack should be applied. If the dislocation is recurrent and relocation is easy to do, it may be performed in the field; however, this is not advisable. Check for distal pulse rates, skin temperature and moisture, and distal neurologic status. When the patient arrives in the ED, radiographs should be made before the joint is relocated, unless there is neurovascular compromise. Once the joint is relocated, immobilize it by placing a sling and swath bandage or other commercially available device on the injured side. The patient should be referred to an orthopedic surgeon. Complications from this type of injury are neurovascular compromise and associated fractures.

Elbow Dislocation

Dislocations of the elbow joint are seen most commonly in children, teenagers, and young adults. Elbow dislocation is a common athletic injury (Fig. 27-35). It may result from a fall on an externally rotated arm or as a result of a young

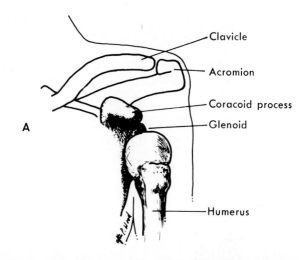

Clavicle

Acromion

Coracoid process

Glenoid

Humerus

A

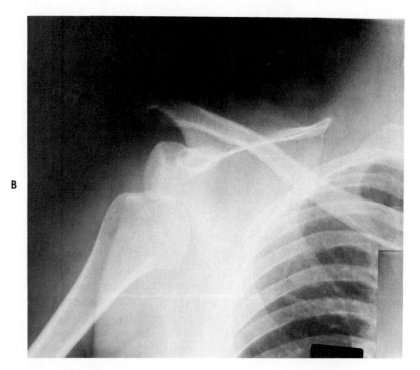

B

Fig. 27-34 **A,** Anterior shoulder dislocation. **B,** Radiograph.

child being jerked or lifted by a single arm (known also as nursemaid's elbow). The patient complains of pain in the joint area. The area may feel "locked," and any movement may produce severe pain. Swelling, deformity, and displacement are noted. Therapeutic interventions include immobilization in the position of greatest comfort for the patient, assessment of neurovascular status, and application of a cold pack. When the patient arrives in the ED, after studies of the injured extremity have been performed, the joint should be relocated. Once the joint is relocated, it is immobilized. The position of immobilization depends on the type of dislocation. The most common complication of this type of injury is neurovascular compromise.

Wrist Dislocation

Dislocation of the wrist is an injury seen most frequently in athletes; it may be seen in all age-groups. It usually results from a fall on an outstretched hand (Fig. 27-36). The patient complains of severe pain in the wrist area. Swelling, deformity, and point tenderness are evident. Therapeutic interventions include placement of a splint, use of a sling and swath bandage, and application of a cold pack. On arrival in the ED, the patient should have radiographic studies of the injured extremity performed, followed by relocation of the joint. Casting to immobilize the joint is then performed. Complications of this type of injury are neurovascular compromise, especially median nerve damage.

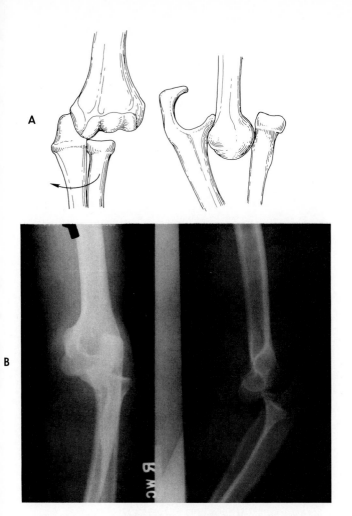

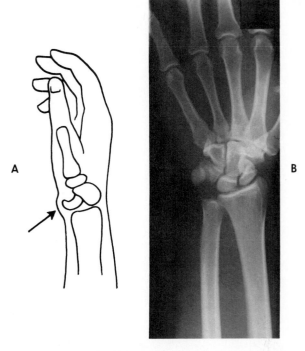

Fig. 27-36   A, Dislocation of wrist. **B,** Radiograph.

Fig. 27-35   A, Dislocation of elbow. **B,** Radiograph.

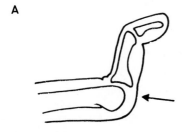

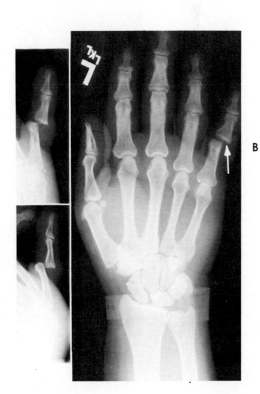

Fig. 27-37   A, Finger dislocation.
B, Radiographs.

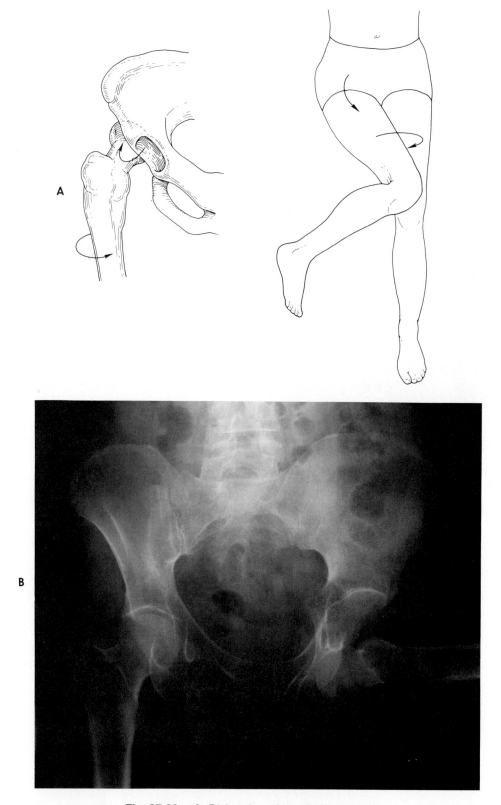

Fig. 27-38 **A,** Dislocation of hip. **B,** Radiograph.

Hand or Finger Dislocation

Hand or finger dislocations are most commonly seen in athletes. This injury usually results from a fall on an outstretched hand or finger. It may also result from direct trauma to the tip of the finger (Fig. 27-37). The patient complains of pain in the area of the injury and inability to move the joint. Deformity and swelling are noted. Splint the injury in the position of comfort and apply a cold pack until radiographs are obtained and interpreted and until relocation of the joint is attempted. The injured area is then usually splinted to immobilize the joint.

Hip Dislocation

Hip dislocations are common to all age-groups. This injury usually results from a major trauma in which the leg is extended before impact (Fig. 27-38). This injury is commonly seen in head-on collisions in which the leg is extended and the foot is on the brake pedal just before impact or in which the knee jams into the dashboard (Fig. 27-39). This type of injury also occurs as a result of falls and crush injuries. The dislocation may result in either anterior or posterior displacement. The patient complains of pain in the hip area and in the knee area. The hip is flexed, adducted, and internally rotated in cases of posterior dislocation and flexed, abducted and externally rotated in cases of anterior dislocation. The joint feels locked, and the patient is not able to move his or her leg.

Splint the extremity in the position in which it is found or in the position of greatest comfort. Be sure to check for neurovascular status and other associated injuries. Apply a cold pack and transport the patient to an ED, where the hip joint can be relocated. Necrosis of the femoral head may occur if the joint is not relocated within 24 hours.

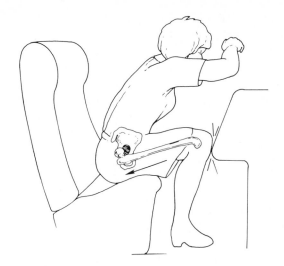

Fig. 27-39   Knee impact with dashboard.

Once the hip joint is relocated, the patient is usually placed on a regimen of bed rest in traction. Children may be placed in a spica cast. Complications from this type of injury are femoral artery and nerve damage.

Leg Dislocation

Knee dislocation. Knee dislocations are common in all age-groups (Fig. 27-40). The mechanism of injury is usually a major trauma. The patient complains of severe pain in the knee area, inability to move the leg, much swelling, and deformity. Immediate therapeutic intervention consists of splinting the limb in the position of comfort or in the position in which it is found. Check for distal neurovascular compromise, and apply a cold pack. When the patient arrives

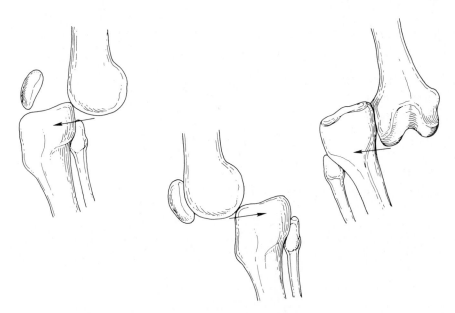

Fig. 27-40   Knee dislocation.

in the ED, after radiographs are obtained to determine the extent of damage, the joint must be relocated. Early reduction is essential to avoid damage to the arteries and nerves. Complications include peroneal, popliteal, and tibial nerve damage. A fractured tibia is also frequently associated with knee dislocation. Almost all persons who have a dislocation of the knee joint have associated and usually severe damage to the capsule (muscles, ligaments, or tendons).

After reduction, the patient is admitted to the hospital, where he or she is placed on a regimen of bed rest; the knee is kept elevated, and cold packs are applied intermittently for 7 to 10 days. After this period, the patient is usually provided with a cast.

Patellar dislocation. Dislocations of the patella are commonly found in all age-groups (Fig. 27-41). Patellar dislocation is a common injury in athletes and in those individuals who have had a direct trauma to the lateral aspect of the knee or a rapid rotation on a planted foot. These patients usually demonstrate signs of pain, keep the affected knee in a flexed position, and are unable to use that knee. There is a great deal of tenderness and swelling in the patellar area. Therapeutic interventions include splinting the leg in the position in which it is found and applying a cold pack. After radiographs have been obtained, the patient should have the patella reduced. This reduction is usually accomplished spontaneously when the leg is placed in extension. After relocation, the knee is placed in a compression bandage and a cylinder cast is applied.

The patella may relocate itself before its dislocation has been discovered. If a mechanism of injury and signs and symptoms of this injury are present, therapeutic intervention should be the same whether or not the patella is currently dislocated.

Ankle dislocation. An ankle dislocation is usually the result of an athletic injury and is commonly associated with a fracture (Fig. 27-42). Such a dislocation results from lateral stress motion in which the normal range of motion of the ankle is exceeded. The patient complains of severe pain in the ankle area and inability to move the joint. There is much swelling and deformity. Therapeutic intervention includes splinting the ankle and foot in a position of comfort. Neurovascular status should be checked and a cold pack should be applied. Further management includes obtaining radiographs to determine the extent of injury. The ankle may be relocated by either the closed or the open method, depending on the degree of injury and associated fractures. The primary complication of this type of injury is neurovascular compromise.

Foot dislocation. Dislocations of the foot occur in all age-groups. This is a rare injury and is usually the result of an automobile or motorcycle accident in which a combination of forces has acted at the same time. This type of dislocation is almost always associated with an open wound. The patient complains of severe pain in the foot region. Point tenderness is present, and the patient cannot use his or her foot. Much swelling and deformity are evident. If there is an open wound, it should be covered with a sterile dressing. Apply a soft splint, check neurovascular status, and apply a cold pack. Radiographs should be obtained to determine the extent of injury. Once the foot is relocated, a cylinder cast is usually applied, and the patient is instructed to elevate the limb and apply cold packs for 24 hours. There should be no weight bearing on the foot.

Toe (metatarsophalangeal) dislocation. Dislocations of the metatarsophalangeal joints (toes) are rare. When they do occur, they are commonly associated with open fractures.

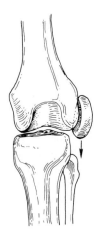

Fig. 27-41   Dislocation of patella.

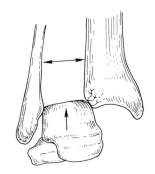

Fig. 27-42   Dislocation of ankle.

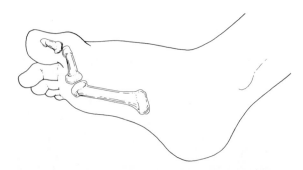

Fig. 27-43   Dislocation of metatarsophalangeal joint.

It is important to reduce these dislocations immediately, since delay may result in inability to perform a closed reduction of the dislocation (Fig. 27-43). The patient complains of pain and point tenderness in the area of the joint. There is a great deal of swelling and noticeable deformity. Therapeutic interventions consist of covering the area with a bulky dressing to prevent further damage, elevating the extremity, and applying a cold pack. After radiographs have been obtained, the dislocation should be reduced; the foot and toes should then be immobilized.

PEDIATRIC LIMB TRAUMA

If a fracture occurs at the epiphysis (growth center), early closure of the epiphyseal plate may occur. As the child continues to grow, there will be no growth of this particular bone in which a fracture at the epiphyseal plate has occurred. As a result, the child has one extremity that is shorter than the other. If the fracture of the plate is only partial, there may be an angular deformity because the bone beneath the nonfractured section continues to grow, whereas the section under the fracture segment does not. Epiphyseal fracture should be closely followed up by an orthopedic surgeon for several months, since the outcome is difficult to predict at the time of the injury.

TRAUMATIC AMPUTATIONS

Traumatic amputations are common in farm workers as a result of accidents that occur with the use of heavy farm machinery, in factory workers, as a result of a limb being caught by a heavy machine, and in motorcyclists, as a result of a limb being amputated when the motorcycle and driver are involved in a collision with another vehicle. Body parts that are frequently amputated are the digits (fingers, toes), the distal half of the foot (transmetatarsal), the lower leg below the knee, the lower leg at the knee, the lower leg above the knee, the hand, the forearm, the arm, the ears, the nose, and the penis.

Therapeutic interventions for any type of amputation include control of the ABCs; control of bleeding; support of the limb in a functional anatomic position if the part is only partially amputated; initiation of two large-bore intravenous lines; administration of oxygen at high flow, usually by nasal cannula; and rapid transport to a facility at which the patient can be further evaluated.

Preservation of the Amputated Part

Whenever possible, the amputated part should be preserved as though it were being prepared for reimplantation. The part should be kept at a hypothermic temperature of about 40° F (4.4° C). *Do not freeze the part.* Hypothermia can be accomplished by immersing the part in a container of normal saline solution and placing the entire container in a bag filled with ice. *Do not place the part directly on ice.* If this type of equipment is not available, dress the part in a wrap saturated with normal saline solution or Ringer's lactate solution. Attempt to keep the limb in correct anatomic position.

Reimplantation

Occasionally reimplantation is possible. Limiting factors are the availability of a reimplantation team, the amount of damage to the attached part and to the amputated part, the time elapsed since the accident, the overall predicted outcome of the reimplantation, and the general physical condition of the victim. Historically upper-extremity reimplantations have been more successful than lower-extremity reimplantations. One physician treated fingertip amputations conservatively, without reimplantation, and found that the fingertips regenerated within 1 year.

SPLINTING

Splinting is performed to prevent further damage to soft tissues, prevent damage to nerves, arteries, and veins, and to decrease pain. Always splint above and below the injury site. For example, when the elbow is injured, a splint should be applied not only to the elbow but also to the forearm and the upper arm.

Application

When applying a splint, be sure to immobilize the injured part. If there is severe angulation, correct it only if splinting is impossible or if neurovascular compromise is present. Whenever possible, do not try to apply a splint to an extremity alone; have the second rescuer place the padding and the splint while you support the extremity. Secure the injured part inside the splint, but do not use an elastic bandage.

When applying an air splint, provided that the splint is open at both ends, slip the splint over your own arm backwards. Grasp the distal portion of the injured limb with the hand of the arm that has the air splint on it. Then, slide the splint from your arm onto the injured extremity. Once the splint is in the proper position, inflate it.

Always remember to recheck neurovascular status after splint placement.

Types of Splints

Four basic types of splints are available. Those include soft splints such as a pillow; hard splints such as a board or other object that has a firm surface; air splints, which are inflatable and provide support without being hard; and traction splints, which decrease angulation and provide support and traction.

Many varieties of splints are available to rescue personnel. These include the Thomas splint and the Hare traction splint (Fig. 27-44), which are used for fractures of the midshaft of the femur or upper third of the tibia. These types of splints should *not* be used on hip, lower tibial or fibular, or ankle fractures or in fractures of the femur in which there are associated tibial or fibular fractures.

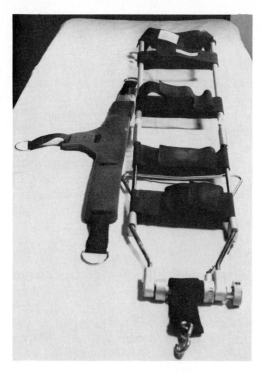

Fig. 27-44   Hare traction splint. (Photo by Richard Lazar.)

Other types of splints are short boards and long boards, which are used for extrication or immobilization, particularly for those patients suspected of having a cervical spine or thoracic spine fracture. Several commercial variations are available; these perform the same functions as the short boards and long boards.

Also available are aluminum long-leg splints, cardboard splints, ladder splints, padded boards, air splints, vacuum splints, and a host of commercially available products. In addition, the creative rescuer can improvise to provide a splint.

PLASTER CASTS

A brief overview of plaster casting and care of casts is presented here. The reader should refer to a text for orthopedic assistants for a complete description of techniques and types of casts.

Applying the Cast

Before applying the plaster to the injured extremity, gather all needed equipment. The limb should be covered with stockinette, and bony prominences should be padded with cotton. Soak the plaster in cool to warm water, and apply it rapidly before it has a chance to harden.

Aftercare Instructions for Patients with Casts

- Return to the ED, the orthopedic clinic, or your private physician within 24 hours for follow-up care.
- Keep the cast dry.

- Keep the limb elevated above the level of the heart for 24 hours after the injury.
- If any of the following abnormalities are present, return to the follow-up clinic immediately: (1) change in temperature of the digits; it is abnormal if they are very cold or very hot, (2) change in color of the digits; it is abnormal if they are blue, or (3) absence of feeling in the digits.
- Wiggle the digits at least once each hour.
- If a foreign object is dropped into the cast, return to the follow-up care facility immediately.
- If swelling recurs or if a foul odor is present, return to the follow-up clinic.

Pressure Ulcers

If a pressure ulcer is developing, the patient has an elevated temperature, he or she continues to have pain after the first days after the injury, and he or she complains of being unable to get sleep at night. If this occurs, the cast should be removed and the situation should be evaluated immediately.

CRUTCH AND CANE FITTING

First of all, when fitting a patient for crutches or a cane, measure with the shoe he or she will be wearing when ambulating with the crutches or the cane. The shoe should fit well, have a 1-inch heel, and tie or buckle. Instruct the patient that he or she not wear a slip-on shoe while ambulating.

Axillary Crutches

Axillary crutches should be fitted so that each armpiece is 2 inches from the axilla with no weight on the axilla. The tips of the crutches should be placed 6 to 8 inches to the side, and the front of the foot should be positioned at a 25-degree angle. Each handpiece should be fitted so that the elbow is at a 30-degree angle of flexion.

Loftstrand Crutches

Loftstrand crutches should be fitted so that the tips of the crutches are placed 6 inches to the side and the front of the foot is positioned at a 25-degree angle. Each handpiece should be fitted so that the elbow is at a 30-degree angle of flexion.

Cane

A cane should be fitted so that when it is held next to the heel, the elbow is at a 30-degree angle of flexion. A cane should be used for minimal support, particularly in patients with hip injuries, and should be used to assist balance only.

GAIT TRAINING

1. Have the patient stand and balance (Fig. 27-45, *A*).
2. Have the patient hold the crutches 4 inches to the side of and 4 inches in front of the feet (Fig. 27-45, *B*).

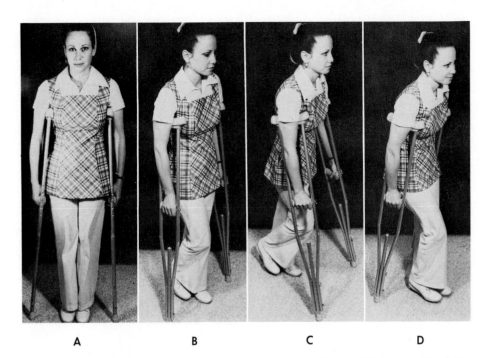

A   B   C   D

Fig. 27-45 Gait training series. Three-point gait. **A,** Standing and balancing. **B,** Holding crutches. **C,** Straightening elbows to carry weight on hands. **D,** Three-point gait. (Photos by Richard Lazar.)

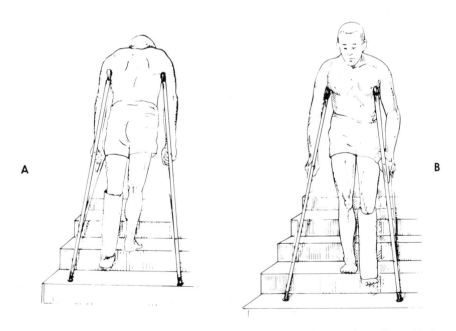

Fig. 27-46 **A,** Going upstairs and, **B,** going downstairs with crutches. (From Barber J, Stokes L, Billings D: *Adult and child care,* ed 2, St Louis, 1977, Mosby—Year Book.)

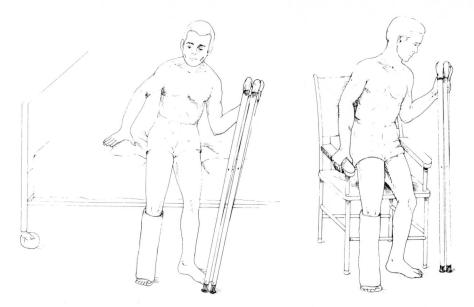

Fig. 27-47 Transferring from sitting to standing with crutches. (From Barber J, Stokes L, Billings D: *Adult and child care,* ed 2, St Louis, Mosby—Year Book.)

3. All weight is carried on the hands by straightening the elbows. Instruct the patient *not to place any weight on the axillae,* not even while resting (Fig. 27-45, *C*).
4. In the ED a three-point gait is usually taught, since this type of gait is used when little or no weight bearing is desired (Figs. 27-45, *D*, 27-46, and 27-47).

SUMMARY

The key to care of the patient with a limb injury is to preserve or restore normal neurovascular status and motor function. Although attention to limb injuries is a secondary priority when caring for the victim of multiple trauma, it is important to protect the limb from further harm and to assess the situation and apply appropriate therapeutic interventions as soon as it is feasible to do so.

SUGGESTED READINGS

American College of Surgeons Committee on Trauma: *Advanced trauma life support,* Chicago, 1988, The American College of Surgeons.

Connolly, JF, ed: *DePalma's the management of fractures and dislocations,* ed 4, Philadelphia, 1985, WB Saunders.

Dobyns JH, Linocheid RL: Athletic injuries of the wrist, *Clin Orthop* 198:141, 1985.

Emergency Nurses Association: *Trauma nurse care course,* Chicago, 1991, The Association.

Ferhel RD, Hedley AK, Eckhart JJ: Anterior fracture dislocation of the shoulder: pitfalls in treatment, *J Trauma* 24:363, 1984.

Fisk G: The wrist, *J Bone Joint Surg* 66:396, 1984.

O'Brien ET: Acute fractures and dislocations of the wrist, *Orthop Clin North Am* 15:237, 1984.

Parisien JD: Fractures and dislocations of the elbow. In Edlich RF, Spyker DA, eds: *Current emergency therapy '85,* Rockwell, Md, 1985, Aspen Publishers.

Schneider FR: *Orthopedics in emergency care,* St Louis, 1984, Mosby—Year Book.

Sheehy SB: *Mosby's manual of emergency care,* ed 3, St Louis, 1989, Mosby—Year Book.

Cindy LeDuc Jimmerson

As people become more active outdoors, the incidence of environmental trauma will increase. Along with the benefits of increased activity come the problems of increased exposure to environmental hazards. Some of the more commonly seen environmental emergencies are discussed in this chapter.

DROWNING AND COLD WATER NEAR-DROWNING

Drowning is a significant contributor to accidental deaths in the United States, claiming approximately 8000 lives per year. Typically the victims are young, with 40% of them under the age of 5.[1] In cases of near-drowning, when the victim survives a drowning event, rapid identification and initiation of resuscitative measures are vital. It has been documented in recent years that many drowning victims have a good chance of survival without neurologic sequelae if the conditions surrounding the incident are specific and the emergency care team is prepared for this kind of event.

Physiology of Drowning

Although the course of drowning can stimulate many physiologic responses, death by drowning is simply caused by asphyxiation. The victim who goes through the stages of struggling, relaxation, and loss of consciousness usually aspirates large amounts of water into the lungs. In about 15% of drownings, the victim has an intense laryngospasm and does not aspirate water but dies instead of airway obstruction. This is known as *dry drowning*.

One might assume that victims of dry drowning have a better chance of survival than do *wet drowning* victims because their lungs are spared the injury of aspiration. In persons who do aspirate water, the lethal factor is pulmonary edema. Depending on whether the aspirated water was fresh or saline, changes in circulating blood volume can be expected. With freshwater near-drownings, the water is absorbed into the bloodstream because of its relative hypotonicity compared with plasma, and *hyper*volemia occurs. Red cells may also absorb this excess water, and lysis may occur; this can account for the hemoglobinuria found in some freshwater near-drowning victims. Dilutional electrolyte problems accompany even mild hypervolemia, but all these problems are reversible when blood volume normalizes. Of greater significance is damage to the delicate membranes of the alveoli themselves. Surfactant activity is decreased with freshwater aspiration and lung compliance is impaired, often causing rupture or engorging of the alveoli and subsequent pulmonary edema. Reduced gas exchange, hypoxemia, and acidosis ultimately cause death.

Seawater aspiration causes *hypo*volemia as a result of the hypertonic nature of seawater relative to plasma. Plasma is drawn through the alveoli into the lungs, and pulmonary edema, impaired gas exchange, and hypoxemia result. In contrast to aspiration of fresh water, in seawater aspiration hemoconcentration increases the concentration of electrolytes. During resuscitation of a seawater drowning victim, these electrolyte problems can be reversed with restoration of adequate circulating volume.

Although many near-drowning victims may recover after rescue and respiratory resuscitation at the scene, all drowning incidents should be reported and all patients taken to a hospital for observation. Although the patient may look fully recovered immediately, *postimmersion syndrome,* or pulmonary edema resulting from an inflammatory reaction to lung injury and disturbances to surfactant function, can cause adult respiratory distress syndrome from 1 to 72 hours after the event. Therefore *every* drowning victim should be observed in the hospital for at least 24 hours after the event.

Sudden death from contact with cold water is known as *immersion syndrome* and is usually attributed to vagally induced bradycardia or cardiac arrest. Alcohol use has been shown to contribute significantly to this reaction.

Identification of Cold-Water Near-Drowning Victim

History
Length of immersion
Temperature and quality of the water
Associated injuries
When cardiopulmonary resuscitation (CPR) was initiated
Patient's response to CPR

383

Physical examination

Deathlike appearance

Blue or gray color

No respirations

No blood pressure

Pulseless (or a rate as slow as 4 or 5 beats/min; must monitor the pulse rate for a full minute to detect pulse rate or observe the pulse rate on a cardiac monitor)

Cold skin

Dilated pupils ("fish eyes")

Temperature (Taking a deep rectal temperature reading with a low-reading thermometer is important.)

Field Resuscitation

Field resuscitation of the near-drowning victim is crucial to survival; immediate initiation of CPR after removal from the water has been cited as one of the most significant lifesaving factors. Whether or not advanced life support is available, good results have been realized with excellent, prompt, field-initiated CPR. In light of the surprisingly good results of resuscitation attempts for victims submerged up to 1 hour, the following steps should be followed at the scene and en route to the hospital:

1. Ascertain duration of submersion; if unknown, assume duration of less than 1 hour.
2. Clear the airway and perform a 5-second pulse check; if negative, start CPR immediately and do not interrupt if possible.
3. Assess the patient carefully for associated injuries; immobilize the patient on a backboard and protect the cervical spine, especially if the history and mechanisms of injury suggest that other injuries may be present.
4. Determine the rectal temperature with a low-reading thermometer if possible (15 cm inside rectum).
5. Remove wet clothing and *gently* wrap the victim in dry blankets.
6. If the medical facility is less than 15 minutes away, do not add heat.
7. If the hospital is more than 15 minutes away, add heat (warm oxygen, warm intravenous [IV] fluids, or *well-padded* heat packs).
8. *Always* transport the patient to a medical facility, even if the patient recovers at the scene.

Hospital Resuscitation

Resuscitation of a near-drowning victim in the clinical setting should be a smooth continuation of the efforts in the field. Quality CPR must be continued with as few interruptions as possible. Rewarming efforts should be aggressive if the victim's core body temperature is below 32° C (90° F). The heart is resistant to drug therapy and electroconversion when the core body temperature is lower than 32° C (86° F), and early rewarming may prevent ventricular fibrillation. Hospital resuscitation includes the following steps:

1. Obtain a good prehospital history of the event, treatment, and progress.
2. If CPR is in progress, continue CPR and begin active rewarming (warm IVs, lavage, oxygen, enemas, or cardiopulmonary bypass). Do not submerse the victim in a warm bath. *Rewarm the patient only until circulation has been established; then perform only passive rewarming.*
3. Handle the victim *gently:* a cold heart is an irritable heart, and rough handling may induce ventricular fibrillation when body temperatures are below 32° C (90° F).
4. Continuously monitor the core temperature with a rectal probe.
5. Be prepared for the patient to become *hyper*thermic.
6. Anticipate pneumonitis and pulmonary edema and treat with corticosteroids, penicillin, or furosemide (Lasix).
7. Anticipate profound neurologic depression; cerebral resuscitation with intraventricular monitoring, diuretics, and possibly barbiturates is recommended.
8. Anticipate possible hemolysis, disseminated intravascular coagulation, and renal insufficiency; treat the patient as you would any other patient with those complications.

Guidelines for transfer to a higher-level medical facility. Generally, patients should be transferred to a higher-level facility if there is a lack of nursing and support staff or a lack of the equipment necessary to properly provide care for this type of critically ill patient. More specifically, the near-drowning patient should be transferred to a higher-level facility if any of the following is present:

- No capability for rapid arterial blood gas analysis
- Deterioration of pulmonary status
- Renal insufficiency
- Hemolysis
- Profound neurologic depression
- Significant associated trauma
- Accident has involved diving, and the patient requires hyperbaric treatment. (The aircraft should be pressurized to match sea level pressure; it may be necessary to increase oxygen supplementation, depending on the level of pressurization in the aircraft cabin.)

Factors that increase the victim's chances of survival

- Immediate and quality CPR
- Younger age
- Colder water (Cold water is water of less than 70° F.)
- Cleaner water
- Shorter immersion time
- Less struggle

Associated injuries vastly decrease survival rate.

Factors that do not affect the victim's chances of survival

- Sex
- Race
- Swimming ability

- Eating a meal before the event
- Nature of the water, that is, salt water or fresh water
- Use of the Heimlich maneuver during resuscitation attempts
- Concurrent illnesses (such as heart disease or pulmonary disease)

DIVING EMERGENCIES

In the past few decades, self-contained underwater breathing apparatus (scuba) diving has increased in popularity as improvements in the comfort and safety of equipment have been made and the recreational market has expanded. Although there are thousands of commercial and military divers, most of the approximately 4 million scuba divers in the United States are recreational divers. Along with the increase in the number of divers has come an increase in dive-related accidents. Most of those accidents occur as a result of the marine environment, for which humans are not ideally designed. Cold water, lack of available oxygen, and the alternative mode of escape from hazard (swimming as opposed to running) are intrinsic problems for which the diver must compensate. Diving accidents are occurring more frequently in all areas of the country, not just in warm coastal resort areas.

As emergency care givers it is our responsibility to be able to recognize the special problems that complicate dive-related injuries and to be familiar with those resources we may need to use that are beyond the scope of the community hospital emergency department (ED). Treatment of injuries that occur at uncommon levels of atmospheric pressure may require the special facilities of hyperbaric pressurization. If the patient is very cold, rewarming devices and low-reading thermometers are essential during the initial resuscitation. Taking a history and obtaining details about the dive (for example, length and depth) and information concerning the accident (Have other physical injuries occurred?) are essential to planning the resuscitation and treatment of the diving accident victim. Good witness information obtained by prehospital personnel should be included with the patient's record and sent with the patient if interhospital transfer is required.

Because water is so much denser than air, pressure changes are greater under water, even at reasonably shallow depths (Table 28-1).

Boyle's law states that the volume of a gas is inversely related to its pressure at a constant temperature. Table 28-1 demonstrates this law. The principle of this law is the basic mechanism of all types of barotrauma. For example, if a normal pair of lungs contains 2000 cc of air at sea level, the volume of air decreases as the diver descends. Decreases are the following:

Depth (feet)	Air in each lung (cc)
Sea level	1000
33	500
100	250
233	123

When a diver uses a scuba tank of pressurized air, the volume of air in the lungs remains constant at various depths.

If the diver ascends but does not exhale on the way up, the water pressure decreases and the gas in his lungs expands, greatly increasing the pressure in the lungs.

Depth (feet)	Air in each lung (cc)
233	1000
100	2000
33	4000
Sea level	8000

As the gas expands, the lungs expand to the limit; then the lungs rupture, and pneumothorax results. The high-pressure air is also forced into the circulatory system, producing air embolism. Air embolism is normally prevented by exhaling on controlled, slow ascents. Divers risk injury when they ascend from depths too rapidly or when they hold breath during ascent.

Air Embolism

Signs and symptoms
Tightness of chest
Shortness of breath
Pink, frothy sputum
Vertigo
Limb paresthesias or one-sided paralysis
Seizures

Table 28-1 Pressure-volume relationships according to Boyle's law

	Depth (feet)	Gauge pressure (atmospheres)	Absolute pressure (atmospheres)	Gas volume (%)*	Bubble diameter (%)*
Air	0	0	1	100	100
Sea water	33	1	2	50	79
	66	2	3	33	69
	99	3	4	25	63
	132	4	5	20	58
	165	5	6	17	54

*Bubble diameter is probably a more important consideration than gas volume when considering the ability of recompression to restore circulation to a gas-embolized blood vessel.[1]

Table 28-2 Gas toxicities in diving

Gas	Signs and symptoms	Therapeutic interventions
Oxygen (from breathing 100% oxygen)	Twitching, nausea, dizziness, tunnel vision, restlessness, paresthesias, seizures, confusion, pulmonary edema, atelectasis, shock lung	Maintain airway, breathing, and circulation; intubation, controlled ventilation to reduce FIO_2, decompression, positive end expiratory pressure
Carbon dioxide (from inhaling expired air; 8%-10% causes toxicity)	Dizziness, lethargy, heavy labored breathing, unconsciousness	Ascent to surface, ABCs, 100% oxygen
Carbon monoxide (from contaminated tank—filled too close to internal combustion engine)	Dizziness, pink or red lips and mouth, euphoria	Ascent to surface, ABCs (CPR if necessary), 100% oxygen in hyperbaric chamber at 3 atmospheres for 1 hour

Loss of consciousness

Other signs and symptoms of simple pneumothorax and tension pneumothorax are discussed in Chapter 25.

Therapeutic interventions

Death is an immediate threat to the diver with air embolism; this patient must be considered at grave risk and must receive immediate therapy. Interventions include the following:

Administration of positive-pressure oxygen

Needle thoracentesis for tension pneumothorax (see Chapter 25)

Placement of patient in left lateral Trendelenburg's position to avoid cerebral embolism

Prompt recompression and controlled decompression in a hyperbaric chamber

To prevent air embolism, divers should exhale during ascent.

Nitrogen Narcosis

Henry's law states that at a constant temperature the solubility of any gas in a liquid is almost directly proportional to the pressure of the liquid. Nitrogen narcosis is a condition in which nitrogen, which is 79% of the composition of room air, becomes dissolved in solution because pressures are greater than normal. Dissolved nitrogen produces neurodepressant effects similar to those of alcohol. Symptoms of nitrogen narcosis usually begin to appear at depths between 75 and 100 feet. Experienced divers seem to have less problem with this syndrome than novices, although nitrogen narcosis is an inescapable problem for all divers. At depths below 200 feet the effects of nitrogen narcosis are significant enough to render the diver unable to work; loss of consciousness occurs at a depth of approximately 300 feet. Individual divers seem to have various levels of tolerance for nitrogen narcosis. Nitrogen narcosis has no real metabolic significance; the risk lies in the impairment of the diver's judgment and the incidence of accidents that occur when divers are "narked." Jacques Cousteau quite aptly describes this condition as "rapture of the deep" (Table 28-2). The diver becomes euphoric, silly, and unaware of the dangerous situation and the need to surface.

Signs and symptoms
Impaired judgment

Feeling of alcohol intoxication

Slowed motor response

Loss of proprioception

Euphoria and sillyness

Therapeutic intervention. Ascent to the surface causes symptoms to disappear; no land therapy is required. Nitrogen narcosis can be avoided by limiting depths of dives.

Decompression Sickness

Decompression sickness ("the bends," dysbarism, caisson disease, diver's paralysis) occurs when the partial pressure of respirable nitrogen changes as a diver ascends from depth too rapidly and the nitrogen converts back from solution to gas, forming bubbles in the tissue and blood. "Too rapidly" is defined at each dive, depending on the depth-time relationships of the dive, which are calculated in the standard U.S. Navy air decompression tables (Table 28-3). Normally, during a gradual ascent, the nitrogen is allowed to reach an equilibrium that permits the escape of nitrogen through respired air; decompression sickness happens only during ascent and only when that equilibrium cannot be established and bubbles are squeezed into the blood and tissue. The mechanical and biophysical effects that result from those bubbles are complex and best treated when identified early and treated with correct recompression.

The most significant mechanical effect of bubbles is vascular occlusion. Because nitrogen bubbles can develop in any tissue such as lymphatic tissue and cells, mechanical results of supersaturation of nitrogen also include lymphedema, cellular distension, and cell rupture. Biophysical effects of bubbles are multiple, although the end result is poor tissue perfusion and ultimately ischemia. A good history of the length and depth of the dive helps the emergency team use the dive tables and properly calculate the patient's treatment needs.

Signs and symptoms
Shortness of breath

Itch

Rash

Table 28-3   U.S. Navy standard air decompression table*

Depth (feet)	Bottom time (min)	Time to first stop (min:sec)	Decompression stops (feet) 50	40	30	20	10	Total ascent (min:sec)	Repetitive group
40	200	....	......	......	......	......	0	0:40	(†)
	210	0:30	......	......	......	......	2	2:40	N
	230	0:30	......	......	......	......	7	7:40	N
	250	0:30	......	......	......	......	11	11:40	O
	270	0:30	......	......	......	......	15	15:40	O
	300	0:30	......	......	......	......	19	19:40	Z
50	100	....	......	......	......	......	0	0:50	(†)
	110	0:40	......	......	......	......	3	3:50	L
	120	0:40	......	......	......	......	5	5:50	M
	140	0:40	......	......	......	......	10	10:50	M
	160	0:40	......	......	......	......	21	21:50	N
	180	0:40	......	......	......	......	29	29:50	O
	200	0:40	......	......	......	......	35	35:50	O
	220	0:40	......	......	......	......	40	40:50	Z
	240	0:40	......	......	......	......	47	47:50	Z
60	60	....	......	......	......	......	0	1:00	(†)
	70	0:50	......	......	......	......	2	3:00	K
	80	0:50	......	......	......	......	7	8:00	L
	100	0:50	......	......	......	......	14	15:00	M
	120	0:50	......	......	......	......	26	27:00	N
	140	0:50	......	......	......	......	39	40:00	O
	160	0:50	......	......	......	......	48	49:00	Z
	180	0:50	......	......	......	......	56	57:00	Z
	200	0:50	......	......	......	1	69	71:00	Z
70	50	....	......	......	......	......	0	1:10	(†)
	60	1:00	......	......	......	......	8	9:10	K
	70	1:00	......	......	......	......	14	15:10	L
	80	1:00	......	......	......	......	18	19:10	M
	90	1:00	......	......	......	......	23	24:10	N
	100	1:00	......	......	......	......	33	34:10	N
	110	0:50	......	......	......	2	41	44:10	O
	120	0:50	......	......	......	4	47	52:10	O
	130	0:50	......	......	......	6	52	59:10	O
	140	0:50	......	......	......	8	56	65:10	Z
	150	0:50	......	......	......	9	61	71:10	Z
	160	0:50	......	......	......	13	72	86:10	Z
	170	0:50	......	......	......	19	79	99:10	Z
80	40	....	......	......	......	......	0	1:20	(†)
	50	1:10	......	......	......	......	10	11:20	K
	60	1:10	......	......	......	......	17	18:20	L
	70	1:10	......	......	......	......	23	24:20	M
	80	1:00	......	......	......	2	31	34:20	N
	90	1:00	......	......	......	7	39	47:20	N
	100	1:00	......	......	......	11	46	58:20	O
	110	1:00	......	......	......	13	53	67:20	O
	120	1:00	......	......	......	17	56	74:20	Z
	130	1:00	......	......	......	19	63	83:20	Z
	140	1:00	......	......	......	26	69	96:20	Z
	150	1:00	......	......	......	32	77	110:20	Z

*Courtesy United States Navy.

†See Table 21-4 for repetitive groups in no-decompression dives.

Continued.

Joint pain
Crepitus
Fatigue
Dizziness
Unconsciousness
Paresthesias
Paralysis
Seizures
Localized signs of thrombosis
Factors that increase severity of symptoms
Extremes of water temperature
Increasing age
Obesity
Fatigue
Poor physical condition
Alcohol consumption
Peripheral vascular disease
Heavy work during diving
Therapeutic intervention
Immediate transfer to recompression facility (If the location of the nearest recompression chamber or the procedure for transfer is unknown, a 24-hour assistance number can be called to reach the National Divers Alert Network at Duke University. Sources of advice and information concerning dive-related emergencies are provided in the box below.)
Administration of high-flow oxygen
Intravenous (IV) fluid replacement
Regimen of corticosteroids

Any complaint of joint pain within 24 to 48 hours after a dive should be treated by decompression. A simple test for "joint bends" is to inflate a blood pressure cuff to high pressure (250 to 300 mm Hg) around the affected joint; pain from the bends in that joint should subside for as long as the cuff remains inflated.

REFERENCES FOR DIVE ACCIDENT ADVICE AND LOCATION OF DIVE CHAMBERS

U.S. Navy Experimental Diving Unit, Washington, D.C., (202) 433-2790
This telephone number is operational 24 hours a day, 7 days a week. Ask to speak to the duty officer, who will give you the name, location, and telephone number of the nearest decompression chamber.

National Divers Alert Network, Duke University, (919) 684-8111
When calling this number, alert the person answering the phone that a dive-related emergency has occurred and request to speak to the dive physician on duty. A physician familiar with dive-related emergencies will advise you of emergency care techniques and the location of the nearest decompression chamber.

Bends can occur at depths of less than 33 feet (1 atmosphere) if ascent is too rapid. Errors that commonly occur during treatment of decompression sickness include the victim's failure to report symptoms, failure to treat the patient when the cause is unclear, and failure to identify severe symptoms that result from a dive-related accident.

Prevention
Follow the recommendations given in the U.S. Navy's repetitive dive tables (Figs. 28-1 and 28-2) for staying within a safe range of depth and time during repeated dives.
Limit depth of dives.
Limit length of dives.
Carry a scuba identification card for at least 48 hours after a dive.

Use of decompression tables. Gradual ascent with delays at certain depths to allow nitrogen to be desaturated can be safely achieved with the use for decompression tables. These tables calculate the rate of nitrogen absorption by the body. Any dive performed within 12 hours of a previous dive is considered a repetitive dive, and the repetitive dive table should be used.

Other Medical Problems Encountered in Diving

The squeeze. The squeeze results from a compression of air trapped in hollow chambers, which produces severe, sharp pain, when external pressure is greater than internal pressure. The squeeze may occur in the following cavities:
Ears
Sinuses
Lungs and airways
Gastrointestinal tract
Thoracic cavity
Teeth
Added air spaces (face mask or diving suit)
Signs and symptoms
Pain
Edema
Capillary dilation
Rupture of space
Bleeding.
The squeeze occurs when the diver descends to depth without exhalation, or as a result of other trapping of air in body spaces without release.

The treatment for all squeeze-related problems is gradual ascent to shallower depths, which decreases pressure, and maintenance of airway, breathing, and circulation (ABCs).

Ear squeeze or sinus squeeze. The cause of the middle-ear squeeze is a blocked eustachian tube or paranasal sinus and an inability to equalize pressure in those spaces. This condition can be avoided by not diving when these chambers are congested from colds or allergies and by making descents gradually to allow pressures in air-filled chambers to equalize.

A more serious but less common type of aural squeeze

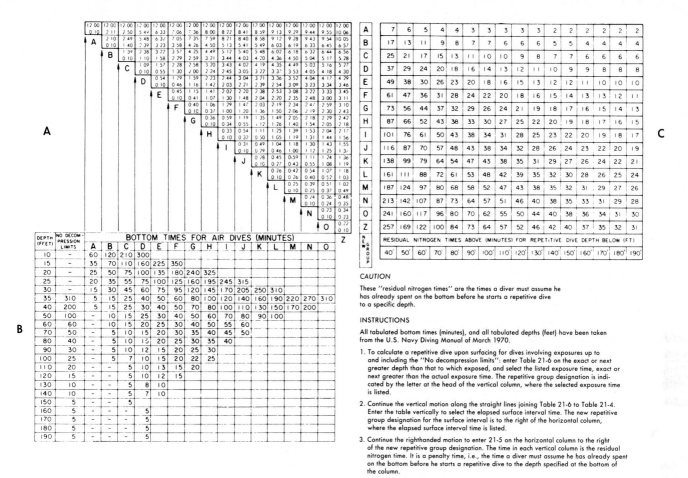

Fig. 28-1 *The Nu-way* repetitive dive tables. **A,** Surface interval credit table (times in hr:min). **B,** "No decompression" limits and repetitive group designation table for "no decompression" air dives. **C,** Repetitive dive timetable for air dives. (Copyright 1970 by Ralph Maruscak. Reprinted courtesy of Ralph Maruscak.)

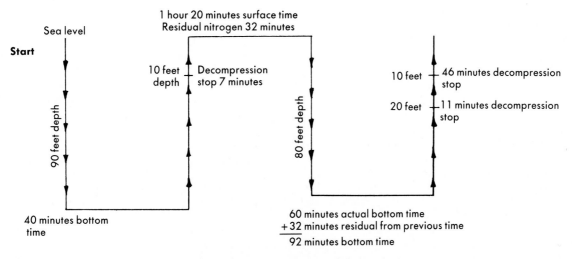

Fig. 28-2 Sample dive plan.

is inner-ear barotrauma, in which the structures of the inner ear may rupture because of sudden pressure changes between the middle and inner ear. This condition may lead to permanent nerve damage and deafness. Consultation with an otolaryngologist should be sought for the dive patient who complains of tinnitus, vertigo, and deafness.

Barotrauma of ascent. Barotrauma of ascent occurs in reverse of the squeeze. Assuming that the air-filled chambers of the body have equalized pressure during the diver's descent, air trapped in those spaces will expand as atmospheric pressure decreases during ascent, if the air is not allowed to escape because of obstruction. Although this condition is uncomfortable, usually no treatment is required, since the condition subsides with time and eventual equalization.

Hyperpnea exhaustion syndrome. Diver fatigue is usually responsible for hyperpnea exhaustion syndrome. Symptoms include the following:

Tachypnea
Anxiety
Feeling of impending doom
Difficulty during floating
Exhaustion
Treatment consists of resurfacing and rest.

CARBON MONOXIDE POISONING

Carbon monoxide (CO) is the most frequent source of poisoning in the United States. Carbon monoxide poisonings include accidental and intentional poisonings and account for approximately 3500 deaths annually in this country. While most of the severe cases of CO intoxications are associated with inhalation of smoke from house fires, engine exhaust and improperly vented and faulty home heating systems are significant contributors to accidental poisoning.

Hypoxia resulting from three mechanisms of CO poisoning creates the risk of death and CNS depression in the patient who has been exposed to CO. Because CO has 200 times more affinity for hemoglobin than oxygen has, CO binds the hemoglobin and makes oxygen-carrying deficient, even in an environment where oxygen is available. Carbon monoxide works in three ways to contribute to hypoxic results.

By competing with oxygen for hemoglobin binding, CO reduces the ability of the blood to carry oxygen to the tissues. Carboxyhemoglobin (HbCO) is formed by this binding and can be measured to determine the severity of oxygen-carrying interference. Carboxyhemoglobin is measured in parts per million, and concentrations are indicated by percentages (Table 28-4). Carbon monoxide also binds with myoglobin at a rate 40 times greater than oxygen's. Thus hypoxia occurs at the tissue level, as well as in the oxygen transport system.

The second mechanism by which CO causes hypoxia occurs in the oxygen delivery system. Generally, oxygen is diffused from the blood to the tissues. Carboxyhemoglobin

Table 28-4   Signs and symptoms of carbon monoxide exposure levels

Exposure level	Signs and symptoms	Treatment
MILD 10% to 25% HbCO when no cardiac or neurologic involvement is present	Throbbing headache, nausea, impaired function of complex tasks	Maintain airway; administer IV fluids; cardiac monitor oxygen administration by tight-fitting mask for 4 hours or until HbCO < 5%
MODERATE 20% to 30% HbCO; *less* if cardiac or neurologic involvement is present	Severe headache, irritability, weakness, visual problems, palpitations, loss of dexterity, nausea and vomiting, decreased mentation	Hyperbaric oxygen administration at 3 atmospheres for 46 minutes; repeat in 6 hours if full CNS recovery does not occur; maintain airway; administer IV fluids; cardiac monitor
SEVERE 40% to 50% HbCO	Tachycardia, tachypnea, collapse, syncope	As above
LIFE THREATENING 50% to 60% HbCO	Coma, Cheyne-Stokes respirations, intermittent convulsions, cherry red mucous membranes	As above
LETHAL Greater than 60% HbCO	Cardiac and respiratory depression, likely cardiac arrest	CPR and as above

shifts the oxyhemoglobin curve, and the partial pressure of oxygen necessary to unload oxygen from the blood to the tissue will be lower than in normal tissue. Thus hypoxia that results from this second complication is more significant than hypoxia that results from a simple reduction of the amount of functional hemoglobin. Even though oxygen is available in the blood, the pressure necessary to push it off the hemoglobin and into the tissue is impaired.

The third effect of CO that results in hypoxic states occurs during the utilization of oxygen by the tissues. Carbon monoxide interferes with the cytochrome oxidase systems. This interference impairs cellular respiration by displacing oxygen, particularly in high-rate metabolic organs such as the brain and heart. Oxygen displacement is responsible for the development of dysrhythmias and many central nervous system (CNS) symptoms.

All patients with HbCO levels greater than 25% should be admitted to the hospital for observation. They should be discharged with instructions that include reexamination in 7 to 10 days. Signs of neurologic sequelae should be explained to the patient before discharge, since headaches, loss of memory and concentration, irritability, personality changes, and excessive fatigue may require hyperbaric treatment if they recur.

SNAKEBITES

There are more than 3000 species of snakes in the world. Of these, 375 species, from five different families, are venomous. The five families are crotalidae (copperheads, rattlesnakes, cottonmouths), elapidae (coral snakes, cobras, mambas), viperidae (puff adders), hydrophidae (sea snakes), and colubridae (boomslangs). More than 45,000 snakebites occur in the United States each year. Of these, 8000 are inflicted by poisonous snakes. However, fewer than 15 deaths result from these snakebites each year.

Venom is a complex substance containing enzymes, gly-coproteins, peptides, and other substances that are capable of causing tissue destruction. Some venoms contain substances that are cardiotoxic, neurotoxic, hemotoxic, or a combination of any two. The venom is injected into a victim by the snake's fangs. Venom is stored in the ducts of the fangs but is manufactured in the salivary glands. In the United States, crotalidae cause most of the serious injuries and deaths. Crotalidae have two long fangs that originate in the anterior maxilla. They also have teeth and may bite (Fig. 28-3). Other kinds of snakes have small, fixed fangs that do not retract into the mouth. Nonpoisonous snakes have fangs that retract into the mouth and rows of several small teeth (Fig. 28-4). Snakes usually bite in self-defense. The area snakes most commonly bite is an extremity.

Signs and symptoms of snakebite depend on the size and kind of the snake, the size and age of the patient, the location and depth of the bite, the number of bites, and the amount of venom injected. The patient may have a sensitivity to the venom that makes the reaction worse. A secondary infection may also occur as a result of a bite from the snake's teeth, which may contain many microorganisms. Many signs and symptoms can be divided into local and systemic reactions. Local reactions include fang marks, teeth marks, edema around the bite site occurring from 1 to 36 hours after the bite, pain at the site of the bite, petechiae, ecchymosis, loss of function of the limb, and necrosis 16 to 36 hours after the bite. Systemic reactions include nausea and vomiting, diaphoresis, syncope, and a metallic or rubber taste in the patient's mouth. The patient may also have paralysis, excessive salivation, difficulty in speaking, visual disturbances, muscle twitching, paresthesias, epistaxis, blood in the urine, stool, vomitus or sputum, and ptosis. Neurologic symptoms may include constricted pupils and seizures. Life-threatening systemic reactions include severe hemorrhage, renal failure, and hypovolemic shock.

Therapeutic interventions include ensuring the ABCs, keeping the patient calm, and keeping the limb dependent and immobilizing it. One should place a moderately constricting band *only* to impede lymphatic flow, not to interfere

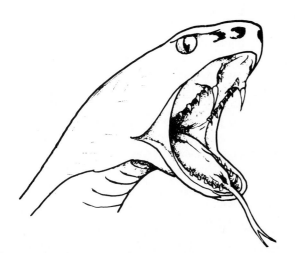

Fig. 28-3   Pit viper. Fangs originate in anterior maxilla.

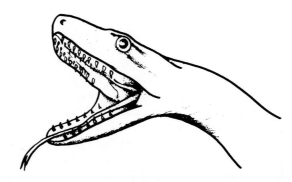

Fig. 28-4   Nonpoisonous snake. Rows of short, small teeth are evident.

with arterial or venous flow.[4] Place the band 4 inches proximal to the bites, and remove any potentially constricting jewelry. The bite wound should be cleansed, but incision for venom suction is rarely indicated. If incision and suction are performed immediately, 25% to 30% of the venom may be removed; the effectiveness of incision drops dramatically 30 minutes after the bite. An intravenous infusion of Ringer's lactate should be initiated to prepare for the emergency administration of medications and for fluid administration in case of hypovolemia. An analgesic may be administered. If the patient's condition warrants concern regarding impending shock, a central line should be employed for monitoring central venous pressure. Tetanus prophylaxis should be administered if the patient's immunization history is incomplete or outdated. It is important to accurately document the time of the bite injury and all interventions that were employed in the prehospital and emergency department phases of the patient's care. The use of ice has not been proven beneficial and may in fact impair the absorption of antivenin and increase the area of necrosis because of decreased circulation. The patient should not drink coffee or alcohol and should not be allowed to smoke.

Antivenin Therapy

Antivenin therapy should be reserved for life-threatening snakebites only, since the antivenin carries a high incidence of sensitivity reactions and the possibility of anaphylaxis. If antivenin is administered, it should be given in the hospital setting with a physician at hand; antivenin therapy is *not* a prehospital procedure. The patient must be closely monitored, and resuscitation equipment and medications must be readily available.

Obtain a careful allergy history. Antivenin is prepared in horse serum, and the patients who are allergic to this medium usually carry some identification or are able to tell you about this sensitivity. Perform skin testing for antivenin *only* if it is determined that the patient will receive the medication and only if the patient has had no previous antivenin treatments and has a negative history of allergy to horse serum. Inject 0.02 ml of a 1:100 dilution of antivenin intradermally. Observe the patient for 15 to 20 minutes; then check the site for the development of wheals. Record the skin response on the patient's chart. If the patient has a positive skin reaction and the physician elects to administer the antivenin, be alert to possible systemic reactions such as urticaria, wheezing, or any symptom of progressing anaphylaxis. Meticulous observation of the patient and slow administration of the medication are paramount. The patient should be advised by the physician of the risks of the treatment, and a consent should be signed for its administration. Again, resuscitation equipment and medications, including epinephrine 1:1000 for subcutaneous use, and epinephrine 1:10,000 for intravenous use should be ready for administration. Even if the results of the skin test are negative, both the patient and the family should be informed of signs and symptoms of delayed reaction when the patient is discharged. Because the administration of antivenin is not a common ED procedure in most areas of the country, consultation with a professional poison center is advised for detailed handling of this unique population.

DOG BITES

Dog bites account for 84% of all bites occurring to humans in the United States and occur at a rate of 500 bites per 100,000 population. There are more than 1.2 million dog bites in the United States each year. Children comprise the population most at risk. Most bites occur on the extremities. Many dog bites are provoked incidents. There is a higher incidence of dog bites in urban areas than in rural areas.

Wounds can range from simple punctures to major deforming lacerations and tears and soft tissue crush injuries. The type of injury usually depends on the size of the dog and the body area in which the wound is afflicted. If a bite is not treated, complications such as infection, cellulitis, osteomyelitis, and residual neurovascular damage may occur.

Therapeutic intervention is aimed at reducing the possibility of infection by soaking and irrigating puncture wounds and irrigating lacerations and other open wounds. Potentially disfiguring wounds of the delicate tissue on the face, particularly eyelids, lips, and ears, should be cleansed gently before evaluation for repair by a reconstructive surgeon. A good tetanus immunization history is important to ensure protection, and local animal control and public health authorities should be involved with quarantine of the dog to monitor the risk of rabies. Good aftercare instructions for wound care should be given to the patient and family, and a careful explanation of how to recognize signs and symptoms of infection should be included.

CAT BITES AND SCRATCHES

Cat bites account for 3% of the total number of bites inflicted on humans in the United States each year. Wounds may involve tendons and joint capsules because cat teeth are sharp, narrow, and long. There is a greater incidence of wound infections from cat bites than from dog bites, since cats are hunters and often come into contact with bacteria-infested rodents. Cats also use their paws to groom themselves and may have a considerable amount of bacteria on their claws.

Therapeutic intervention includes soaking and irrigating puncture wounds and scrubbing and irrigating lacerations and scratches. One should be sure that the patient has current tetanus prophylaxis. Both surgical debridement and antibiotic therapy may be required for patients with cat bite injuries.

HUMAN BITES

Of all the bite injuries, human bites carry the highest rate of infection. The most common sites for bites are the fingers, hands, ears, and tips of noses. If a patient arrives at the ED with a boxer's fracture, look for an open wound over the knuckles that may have occurred when the fist impacted with another person's teeth. The result of a human bite may be a laceration, a puncture, a crush injury, soft tissue tearing, or possibly amputation.

Therapeutic intervention includes scrubbing and irrigating the wound, exploring the wound, and considering debridement of devitalized tissue and the possibility of antibiotic therapy. If the appearance of the wound suggests bony injury, radiographic examinations are indicated. Keep the injured part elevated, and be sure that the patient's tetanus immunization is current. If the wound is over a joint, the joint should be splinted until the wound is well healed. As with all bite injuries, the patient and family should receive concise verbal and written discharge instructions concerning observation of the wound for signs of developing infection.

SPIDER (ARACHNID) BITES

All spiders inject a venom when they bite. Most venom induces itching, stinging, swelling, or a combination of these in the local area. Black widow spider venom and brown recluse spider venom may cause systemic reactions. In a 10-year period, only 65 deaths were reportedly caused by spiders in the United States; of these, 63 were from the black widow spider.

Black Widow Spiders (Latrodectus mactans)

Black widow spiders are usually found in damp, cool places such as under rocks or in woodpiles. They are recognizable by their black bodies and the bright red hourglass marking on their abdomens. Their venom is neurotoxic. Signs and symptoms of black widow bites include painful sting, tiny red marks at the point of entry of the venom, nausea and vomiting, hypertension, and elevated temperature. The patient may also have respiratory difficulty, headache, syncope, weakness, and chest and abdominal pain, and seizures and shock may develop.

Therapeutic intervention includes treating the patient symptomatically, cooling the area of the bite with ice packs to slow the action of the neurotoxin, administration of muscle relaxants such as methocarbamol (Robaxin) or diazepam (Valium), administering calcium gluconate for muscle spasms (administer 10 ml of a 10% solution mixed in a 100 ml solution of normal saline intravenously over a period of 15 minutes). Consider the administration of narcotic analgesics and antivenin therapy. If antivenin therapy is chosen, follow the precautions outlined earlier in this chapter in the discussion of snakebite and contact a poison center for personal coaching if still uncertain. If aggressive supportive therapy is given, the signs and symptoms of black widow spider bites usually subside within 48 hours.

Brown Recluse Spiders (Loxosceles reclusa)

Brown recluse spiders are found in the southeastern, south central, and southwestern United States. They prefer inhabiting dark areas such as basements, garages, closets, and boxes. For this reason it is not uncommon to see these bite injuries in any part of the country, when one of these spiders accompanies a traveller home in the luggage. This type of spider can be identified by the light brown color and the dark brown fiddle-shaped mark on the back.

Signs and symptoms of brown recluse spider bites include mild stinging at the time of the bite, local edema, a bluish ring around the area of the bite, and a bleb formation. Erythema, local ischemia, and tissue necrosis appear on the third or fourth day. An eschar forms on the fourteenth day, and there is a possibility of an open sore. The wound should be healed within 21 days. Systemic reactions include fever and chills, nausea and vomiting, weakness, general malaise, arthralgias and joint pain, and petechiae. Severe systemic reactions include seizures, disseminated intravascular coagulation, renal failure, hemolysis, and cardiopulmonary arrest.

Therapeutic intervention includes consideration of administration of antihistamines, antibiotics, and systemic or local corticosteroids. Local debridement, skin grafting, rehydration, and possibly blood transfusion should also be considered.

SCORPION STINGS

Scorpions are found primarily in the warm southwestern states and in exotic pet shops in every state. There are more stings in the early evening and night hours. Scorpions appear to sting in self-defense, when they are provoked; they are not aggressive creatures. There are several kinds of scorpions, but only one is considered lethal, the *Centruroides sculpturatus*. The tail of a scorpion contains a telson, where the venom is produced and stored, and a stinger, which injects the venom.

Signs and symptoms of scorpion stings include local pain at the sting site, edema, discoloration, hyperesthesia, numbness, and agitation; then drowsiness, itching, speech disturbances, tachycardia, hypertension, and tachypnea may occur. The patient also has wheezing, respiratory stridor, profuse salivation, visual disturbances, an ataxic gait, incontinence, muscle spasms of the jaw muscles, nausea and vomiting, dysphagia, seizures, and anaphylaxis.

Therapeutic intervention includes treating the patient's symptoms, supporting the ABCs, ensuring tetanus prophylaxis, and the remote possibility of administering antivenin therapy. A scorpion sting antivenin is being tested at the Poisonous Animal Research Laboratory, Arizona State University, Tempe, Arizona.

BEE, WASP, HORNET, AND FIRE ANT (HYMENOPTERA) STINGS

Hymenoptera stings can cause a variety of reactions ranging from mild local reactions to anaphylactic shock. These reactions can occur from the time of the sting up to 48 hours later. The stings are cumulative: the greater the number of stings, the more severe the reaction.

Signs and symptoms vary from mild stinging or burning

Table 28-5 Bites and stings

Type of arthropod	Signs and symptoms	Management
STINGING		
Honeybee *(Apis mellificus)* Bumblebee *(Bombus)*	Painful injection wound with stinger often visibly protruding; edema and itching may be apparent.	Remove stinger by scraping with dull object. Do not grasp and pull, since this contracts the venom sac, releasing more toxin. Cleanse site and apply antiseptic. Apply ice and elevate part. Oral antihistamines and steroids may be indicated.
Yellow jacket *(Vespula maculifrons)*	Painful injection wound. Does not leave stinger behind: stings repeatedly.	See bee sting, *above*. Watch for anaphylaxis.
Wasp *(Chlorion ichneumonica)*	Wheal formation, edema, and itching may be present.	
Hornet *(Vespula maculata)* Velvet ant *(Mutilla sacken)* Fire ant *(Solenopsis geminata)*	Painful injection wound with wheal, which expands into large vesicle; as purulence develops, reddening of area occurs; scarring and crusting follow reabsorption of pustule.	See bee sting, *above*. Watch for anaphylaxis.
Scorpions *(Centruroides sculpturatus, Centruroides vittatus,* and *Centruroides gertschi)*	Lethal: No visible local effect. Sharp pain, hyperesthesia followed by hypoesthesia, itching, and speech disturbances are common. Jaw muscle spasms, nausea, vomiting, incontinence, and seizures follow. Death may occur from cardiovascular or respiratory failure.	Apply tourniquet as near to sting site as possible, and pack area in ice well beyond the tourniquet. After 5 minutes loosen tourniquet and reapply.
	Nonlethal: Sharp burning pain at sting site with edema and discoloration; anaphylaxis is rare.	Caution: Morphine and opiates are contraindicated, since they enhance toxic effects.
BITING AND PIERCING		
Tick *(Dermacentor variabilis)*	Victim unaware of presence; local irritation and possible infection when body is pulled off and head remains in tissue; some species (which transmit Rocky Mountain spotted fever) cause flaccid paralysis from neurotoxin. Initial symptoms are paresthesias and pain in lower extremity. Respiratory failure results from bulbar paralysis.	Remove offending ticks. Apply gasoline, ether, or hot (not burning) match to the body. Wait 10 minutes for disengagement. Do not manually remove, since squeezing the body may inject more virus into the victim. Paralysis will dramatically subside.
Centipedes Eastern house centipede *(Scutigera cleoptratu)* Western house centipede *(Scolopendra heros)*	Wound site is red, edematous, and painful; sometimes tissue necrosis occurs.	Cleanse wound. Employ analgesics and antibiotics if indicated.
Spiders Black widow *(Latrodectus mactans)* (Hourglass spider, female)	Pricking sensation is followed by dull, numbing pain. Edema and tiny red fang marks may become visible. Chest and abdomen pain may be evident adjacent to the site of the bite. Pain and rigidity of muscles subside after 48 hours. Blood pressure, temperature, and white blood count may be elevated. Hematuria rarely develops. Spinal fluid has been known to be under increased pressure.	Use ice locally to slow absorption of toxins. Employ muscle relaxants and 10% calcium gluconate IV to reduce spasms. Use antivenin *(Latrodectus mactans)*. Do skin test before administration of the horse serum. Symptoms subside 1-3 hours after antivenin administration.

Table 28-5   Bites and stings—cont'd

Type of arthropod	Signs and symptoms	Management
BITING AND PIERCING—cont'd		
Brown recluse *(Loxosceles reclusa)* (Fiddleback)	Local reactions begin 2-8 hours after bite with pain, edema, bleb formation, and ischema. On third or fourth day after bite, central area turns dark and is firm to touch. In the second week the central area becomes depressed and demarcated with open ulceration formation. Healing may take place in about 3 weeks. Fever, chills, malaise, weakness, nausea, vomiting, joint pain, and petechiae may also be noted. Blood dyscrasias such as hemolytic anemia and thrombocytopenia rarely occur.	Immediate excision of wound with toxins may be useful. Steroids, antihistamines, and antibiotics are to be employed as indicated. Skin grafting may be necessary if healing does not take place.
True bugs		
Kissing bug *(Conenose triatoma)*	Mild or no pain at wound site. Redness, edema, itching, or nodular hemorrhagic lesions, depending on sensitivity.	Cleanse wound with soap and water. Oral antihistamines may be indicated. Anaphylaxis has been reported.
Assassin bug *(Arilus christatus)* (Wheel bug)	Intense pain at wound site. Usually lasts 2-5 hours. Localized edema, itching, and redness.	Cleanse wound with antiseptic solution. Anaphylaxis rare.
VESICATING OR URTICATING		
Blister beetles	Clear amber fluid (cantharidin) is released from the insects' knee joints, prothorax, and genitalia. Mild burning sensation may become apparent due to fluid released at site.	Cleanse area with soap and water as soon as possible.
Lepidoptera (larva) Lo caterpillar *(Automeris lo)* Puss caterpillar *(Megalopyge opercularis)* Saddle back caterpillar *(Sibine stimulea)* Range caterpillar *(Hemileuca oliviae)*	Distinct row of released spines may be seen at site of intense pain. Nausea, vomiting, headache, and fever may be present.	Remove spines with adhesive tape if possible. Apply ice to the wound; analgesics may be indicated. Unremoved spines could cause infection.
Aquatic organisms*		
Stingray	Wound contains venom sacs from furrowed spine of stingray tail. Fainting, nausea, vomiting, and diarrhea occur with occasional progression to muscle paralysis, respiratory distress, seizures, and even death.	Immediately irrigate wound to remove venom sacs (that is, flush with normal saline). Follow initial irrigation with immersion in hot water for 30 minutes (43.3°-45.5° C) to inactivate venom. Antibiotics are recommended; antihistamines and steroids may also be indicated. For severe cases have ventilatory support and resuscitation equipment at hand. Surgical closure of wounds may be necessary in some instances.
Catfish	Wound from dorsal spine causes pain and infection.	Use deep irrigations of hydrogen peroxide. Employ antibiotics as indicated.

*Antivenins for most aquatic bites and stings (stonefish, jellyfish, sea snake, and so on) are available from Commonwealth Serum Laboratories, Melbourne, Australia.

Continued.

Table 28-5   Bites and stings—cont'd

Type of arthropod	Signs and symptoms	Management
VESICATING OR URTICATING—cont'd		
Portuguese man-of-war (*Physalia physalis*)	Tentacles become embedded in skin. There may be welts, burned areas, or streaks. Pain may be intense enough to produce shock and collapse. Headache, cramps, and paralysis are also noted.	Tourniquet may be tried. Remove tentacles with alcohol and sodium bicarbonate scrub (prevents further stinging and neutralizes acid). Leave alcohol on for 6-8 min. Follow with sodium bicarbonate, allowing it to dry. Employ antihistamines and steroids locally and systemically. General anesthesia may be necessary to control pain.
Stings (cone shell snails, sea anemones, corals, and jellyfish)	Acid wound produced.	Cleanse wound with alkali (ammonia, sodium bicarbonate).
Bites (sea snake and octopus)	Wounds contain neurotoxin. Muscle stiffness, paralysis, myoglobinuria, and death from respiratory arrest can occur.	Apply tourniquet. Control shock. Use indicated resuscitation measures.
Scorpion fish	Intense pain, edema, shock, and ECG changes.	See stingray injuries, *above,* for wound cleansing and heat application. Give antivenin.
Sea urchins	Painful injection site with erythema, edema, numbness, and paralysis. Respiratory distress and death may occur.	Use heat as described under stingray. Do not attempt to remove spines initially but do attempt to locate them using x-ray films. Granulomatous lesions often develop from embedded spines.

sensations, swelling, and itching to severe local reactions such as edema of the entire extremity. The patient may also have severe systemic reactions demonstrated by urticaria, pruritus, edema, bronchospasm, laryngeal edema, and hypotension.

Therapeutic intervention varies depending on the severity of the reaction. If there is a mild reaction, first remove the stinger by scraping it away with a dull object; a credit card or piece of thin, stiff cardboard works well. Do *not* grasp the stinger with a forceps; this squeezes the venom sac and injects more venom. Cleanse the site of the sting, and apply an antiseptic cream. Apply ice and elevate the limb. Consider the administration of oral antihistamines and corticosteroids. If the reaction is severe, support the ABCs, and administer epinephrine 1:1000 subcutaneously or 1:10,000 intravenously. If the patient becomes hypotensive, initiate intravenous administration of Ringer's lactate to maintain adequate blood pressure, and apply the pneumatic antishock garment (PASG). Consider the use of vasopressors, antihistamines, corticosteroids, and theophylline. The doses of these vary, depending on the size and age of the patient and the severity of the sting reaction.

Fire ants have a painful sting that causes a wheal to form. This wheal expands into a large vesicle. The area then begins to redden, and a pustule forms. When the pustule is reabsorbed, crusting and scar formation occur.

There is always a possibility of anaphylaxis in any patient with a history of allergy to bee stings. Therapeutic intervention is the same for all hymenoptera stings.

TICK BITES

A tick may cause flaccid paralysis as a result of neurotoxins contained in their venom. This condition is commonly called "tick toxicosis" and may present a confusing picture if the tick is undiscovered. Symptoms range from pain and paresthesias in the lower extremities to ataxia and rarely respiratory failure from bulbar paralysis.

Patients usually seek medical advice with the tick still embedded in the skin, and removal of the insect is required to stop the envenomation. Many colloquial "tricks" for tick removal are popular, such as smothering the tick with petroleum jelly (encouraging him to retreat on his own) and killing the tick with ether or a hot (not flaming) match. The important issue in tick removal is to remove the entire tick. *Gently* grasping the tick with forceps (gentle enough to not squeeze the tick in half) at the point of entry into the skin is usually the best method. Sometimes the patient arrives at the ED and has the symptoms listed previously but is unaware that a tick is embedded in the skin. Close examination may be required to discover the insect, usually found in the hair, on the neck or back, or in any warm area inside the clothing. The neurologic symptoms reverse and disappear rapidly after the tick is removed.

The bites and stings of arthropods are described in Table 28-5.

Cooling Power of Wind on Exposed Flesh Expressed as an Equivalent Temperature (under calm conditions)

Estimated wind speed (in mph)	Actual Thermometer Reading (°F)											
	50	40	30	20	10	0	-10	-20	-30	-40	-50	-60
	EQUIVALENT CHILL TEMPERATURE (°F)											
calm	50	40	30	20	10	0	-10	-20	-30	-40	-50	60
5	48	37	27	16	6	-5	-15	-26	-36	-47	-57	-68
10	40	28	16	4	-9	-24	-33	-46	-58	-70	-83	-95
15	36	22	9	-5	-18	-32	-45	-58	-72	-85	-99	-112
20	32	18	4	-10	-25	-39	-53	-67	-82	-96	-110	-124
25	30	16	0	-15	-29	-44	-59	-74	-88	-104	-118	-133
30	28	13	-2	-18	-33	-48	-63	-79	-94	-109	-125	-140
35	27	11	-4	-21	-35	-51	-67	-82	-98	-113	-129	-145
40	26	10	-6	-21	-37	-53	-69	-85	-100	116	-132	-148
(wind speeds greater than 40 mph have little additional effect)	LITTLE DANGER In < 5 hr with dry skin Maximum danger of false sense of security			Increasing Danger Danger from freezing of exposed flesh within one minute			GREAT DANGER Flesh may freeze within 30 seconds					
	Trenchfoot and immersion foot may occur at any point on this chart.											

INSTRUCTIONS

MEASURE local temperature and wind speed if possible, if not, ESTIMATE. Enter table at closest 5° interval along the top and with appropriate wind speed along left side. Intersection gives approximate equivalent chill temperature. That is, the temperature that would cause the same rate of cooling under calm conditions. Note that regardless of cooling rate, you do not cool below the actual air temperature unless wet.

Fig. 28-5   Wind chill chart.

INJURIES CAUSED BY COLD

When determining ambient temperature, refer to the "wind chill" calculation chart (Fig. 28-5). The chart allows you to calculate the ambient temperature based on the thermometer readings and the wind speed.

Chilblains

Chilblains are localized areas of itching and painful redness accompanied by recurrent edema that usually occur on the ears, fingers, and toes. Chilblains are usually seen in climates that are cool and damp. A chilblain is thought to be a mild form of frostbite. Prevention of exposure to this type of climate is the best recommendation: the symptoms are treated by removal from the climate.

Immersion Foot

Immersion foot usually occurs when there is constant contact between foot moisture and cold temperatures, usually when the patient is wearing a watertight boot that does not allow normal evaporative "breathing." This condition is seen commonly in hunters and soldiers on maneuvers. At first the skin appears only cold, damp, and wrinkled, but gangrene can develop if the conditions are prolonged and repeated. Therapeutic intervention includes drying the feet, changing into dry socks frequently, and when in a controlled environment, soaking the feet in warm water.

Frostbite

Frostbite occurs when ice crystals form in the body's intracellular spaces. These crystals enlarge and compress the cells, resulting in cell membrane rupture and interruption of enzymatic activity and metabolic processes. Histamine is released, causing an increase in capillary permeability, red cell aggregation, and microvascular occlusion. After frostbite has occurred, the condition is irreversible. One should, however, protect the areas around the frostbitten area so that the area of injury does not extend. It is often impossible to estimate the extent of the injury until several days after exposure. Remember that this patient may also have hypothermia. While we must be aware of the presence of frostbite and handle frostbitten limbs gently, hypothermia takes treatment priority over frostbite because hypothermia is a life-threatening condition.

Superficial frostbite. Superficial frostbite usually involves the fingertips, ears, nose, toes, and cheeks of the face. Signs and symptoms include tingling, numbness, burning sensation, and a whitish color. The skin feels cold to touch. Treatment includes *very gentle handling* (Do not rub the injured part.) and application of *warm* (not hot) soaks (104° to 110° F; 40° to 43° C). The extremities should be elevated on pillows and the patient should have bed rest for several days, until the full extent of the injury has been evaluated and normal circulation has returned. The patient's room should be kept warm, and the use of heavy blankets should be avoided. Friction and weight on the injured parts should be strongly avoided. Remember that the injured tissue is friable and that the success of recovery significantly depends on careful handling.

Deep frostbite. When the actual temperature of a limb is lowered, there is a possibility of sustaining deep frostbite. When ice crystals form, local vascular and tissue changes can lead to the death of cells. The degree of frostbite depends on several factors. Among these are the ambient temperature, the wind chill factor (Fig. 28-5), the amount of time exposed, whether or not the patient was wet while exposed or was in direct contact with metal objects, and the type and layers of clothing worn. Other factors that may contribute to the severity of frostbite are the color of the skin (darker people are more prone to have frostbite), a lack of acclimatization, history of previous frostbite injury, poor peripheral vascular status, anxiety, exhaustion, and a frail body type.

Signs and symptoms of frostbite are a white discoloration of the skin that is followed by a waxy appearance and slight, burning pain that is followed by a feeling of warmth, then numbness. Blisters appear 1 to 7 days after injury; edema of the entire extremity occurs, and grey black mottling discoloration eventually results in gangrene.

Treatment of the affected part before arrival at a medical facility includes transport with gentle handling and moderate elevation of the part, *without* rewarming, unless one can ensure that the temperature of the water that is thawing the part can be kept constant. Keep in mind that thawing frozen tissue is extremely painful and that analgesia must be available for the patient. *Do not* rub the part with snow or ice; if the extremity has been thawed, do not allow the patient to exercise the part. Prevent further heat loss by removing wet clothing, covering the patient with dry blankets, and removing him or her from the cold environment. Mylar or wool head covers should be placed on every cold patient to prevent heat loss from the vascular scalp. If the patient is being transported in a ground or air ambulance, administration of *warmed* oxygen is recommended. Rewarming of a patient with hypothermia and severe frostbite should occur under controlled conditions and strict medical control. Recording core temperatures (deep rectal or esophageal) as soon as practical can be helpful in developing a plan for definitive care of the cold patient. Once the patient reaches the ED, the frostbitten part should be immersed in warm water at a temperature of 104° to 110° F (41° to 43° C). If the patient's only problem with cold is frostbite and system hypothermia is not a medical problem, administer warm liquids by mouth. Cover the patient with warm blankets, but be aware of friction and pressure on the affected parts. Protect the thawed part with a large, soft, bulky dressing, and keep the part elevated. *A frostbitten limb should never be in a dependent position.* Narcotic analgesics should be given by IV route, and all IV fluids should be prewarmed. Be sure that the patient has current tetanus prophylaxis, and consider antibiotic therapy. If severe vascular constriction is present, an escharotomy may be required. Amputation is not an emergency procedure but may have to be performed several weeks after injury.

Hypothermia

Hypothermia is defined as a condition in which the core temperature of the body drops below 95° F (35° C). Severe hypothermia is defined as a core temperature of less than 90° F (32.2° C). In severe hypothermic conditions many physiologic changes occur, some of which may cause irreversible problems. Death usually occurs when the core temperature falls below 78° F (25.6° C). Early signs and symptoms of hypothermia are fatigue, a slow gait, apathy, and muscle incoordination.

Many metabolic responses in the body depend on temperature. When hypothermia occurs, cellular activity decreases. When temperature drops by 18° F (10° C), the body's metabolic rate drops by two to three times. Renal blood flow decreases and there is a decrease in the glomerular filtration rate, which causes water to not be reabsorbed, and dehydration results. Respirations decrease, carbon dioxide retention occurs, and hypoxia and acidosis result. Also, because of the lack of glucose, hypoglycemia occurs. Heart muscle cells become more sensitive when cold and are prone to developing dysrhythmias. The characteristic Osborne or "J" wave may be seen on the electrocardiogram of cold patients. The most common dysrhythmias are atrial and ventricular fibrillation. The cold patient is in great danger of ventricular fibrillation when the core temperature falls below 82° F (28° C). It is generally understood that the heart that fibrillates at these very cold temperatures does not respond to conventional treatment without rewarming. One attempt at defibrillating may be considered but should be performed simultaneously with aggressive rewarming and should not be repeated until the patient is warmer than 85° F (30° C). Careful handling of very cold patients, especially when temperatures reach this vulnerable mid-80s range, is imperative because even turning the patient may induce ventricular fibrillation. Careful handling includes cautious driving over rough roads and obstacles during transport. If the patient has mild hypothermia (that is, is still shivering, alert, and oriented) he or she should be moved to a warm environment, treated with warmed oxygen, and given (orally) warmed fluids that contain glucose or other sugars to provide more heat through calories.

Core rewarming is essential to prevent rewarming shock. Rewarming shock occurs when the peripheral areas are rewarmed faster than the core. This condition causes a large amount of lactic acid, which was located in the extremities, to be rapidly shunted back to the heart and may induce fibrillation. There is also the possibility of peripheral vasodilation and hypotension occurring as a result of relative hypovolemia.

Above all else, the simple measure of gentle handling must be exercised. Protection of the airway should be cautiously performed; endotracheal intubation should be performed only if necessary. It is important to protect the patient from unnecessary physical stimulation until rewarming is successful. Intubation is usually considered unnecessary if adequate ventilation can be achieved with an oral airway adjunct and a bag-valve-mask device and attentive care by a respiratory therapist. It is essential that we consider all of the aspects of resuscitation and ventilate the patient's lungs with warmed, humidified oxygen. Blowing cold oxygen into the lungs and into the close proximity of the heart can drop the core temperature even lower in the already hypothermic patient.

Many methods are used for core rewarming of the hypothermic patient. Success with rewarming depends on the age and general condition of the patient before the hypothermic event, the length of exposure, and the careful handling that the patient has received since rescue. As mentioned previously, warm oxygen that is blown into the lungs through the vascular airways and in the vicinity of the heart should be the first effort to rewarm the patient and prevent further heat loss. It makes good sense to warm the blood that is most accessible and that will travel first to the core areas of the body and eventually to the muscle, skin, and gut as the patient rewarms. As previously discussed, rewarming the heart early in the resuscitation dramatically reduces the risk of ventricular fibrillation.

It has been found that in the cold patient, shivering can increase oxygen consumption by as much as 50%; controlling shivering, especially in the cold patient with other high oxygen demand problems (such as trauma), can be accomplished by intravenous administration of 25 mg meperidine.

INJURIES CAUSED BY HEAT
Heat Cramps

Heat cramps occur in hot weather when a person performs strenuous tasks and drinks large volumes of water, causing a dilutional electrolyte imbalance. He or she is probably also losing electrolytes from excessive perspiration. Signs and symptoms are cramps (especially in the shoulders, thighs, and abdominal wall muscles), weakness, nausea, tachycardia, pallor, profuse diaphoresis, cool moist skin, and a history of ingestion of large amounts of water or other hypotonic fluids. Therapeutic intervention is to provide sodium chloride by mouth or intravenously. The patient must be removed from the hot environment and should rest during adequate electrolyte replacement. The consumption of Gatorade, a readily available oral electrolyte supplement, should be encouraged for individuals who either work in hot weather or undertake strenuous recreational activities in hot weather.

Heat Exhaustion

Heat exhaustion occurs when a prolonged fluid loss is caused by perspiration, diarrhea, or diuretics and by a warm to hot ambient temperature and inadequate fluid and electrolyte replacement. This condition is seen most commonly in the very young and the very old. Patients with heat exhaustion have thirst, general malaise, muscle cramping, headache, and nausea and vomiting. The patient may be anxious, tachycardic, and dehydrated. The dehydration may cause orthostatic hypotension and temperature elevation (98.6° to 105° F; 37° to 40° C). The patient with heat exhaustion usually has diaphoresis. The patient should be moved to a cool, quiet environment, all constricting or tight clothing should be removed, and he or she should be watched closely for further complications of dehydration. The patient's temperature should be monitored, and fluid and electrolyte replacement should be initiated with either an oral balanced salt solution (such as Gatorade) or an intravenous infusion of 0.9% saline solution. The use of salt tablets is not recommended because of the possibility of gastric irritation and the potential for hypernatremia. Hypotension may be corrected initially by administering boluses of 300 to 500 ml of normal saline. Subsequent infusion solutions should be chosen based on the patient's serum electrolyte levels, since it may be necessary to decrease the salinity or add electrolytes such as potassium. Patients with hypotension or a history of cardiac disease should be placed on a cardiac monitor. Older patients or those with known cardiac disease require careful observation and fluid administration, and a patient who does not improve significantly in 3 to 4 hours of emergency treatment should be considered for admission to the hospital.

Heat Stroke

Heat stroke is a life-threatening condition in which the patient's body temperature exceeds 105° F (40.6° C). Many conditions affect the outcome of hyperthermia of this magnitude; some of those are environmental, but most significant is the patient's ability to dissipate heat. The most common predisposing factors are old age, alcoholism, and preexisting illness, particularly cardiovascular disease. The environmental conditions that complicate the outcome are high environmental temperature, high relative humidity, and low wind. Individuals who have one or more of the physical conditions are at a much greater risk if the exacerbating environmental conditions are also present. Use of recreational drugs and some medications may also predispose an individual to heat stroke. The most common street drugs with which we associate this problem are lysergic acid diethylamide (LSD), amphetamines, phencyclidine (PCP), and alcohol. Prescription medications that can also precipitate the problem are anticholinergics (phenothiazines, butyrophenones, tricyclic antidepressants, antihistamines, antispasmodics, Jimson weed, and antiparkinsonian drugs). Diuretics and beta-blockers such as propranolol can also precipitate the problem. Patients with large-area burn scars, as well as those with any skin disorder that impairs conduction heat loss, are at a greater risk. Usually the onset of heat stroke is sudden, although elderly individuals and patients who are in predisposing environments may have the symptoms of heat exhaustion for several hours before heat stroke.

The patient with heat stroke may be awake or unconscious but most certainly has some CNS symptoms, including anxiety, confusion, hallucinations, loss of muscle coordination, and combativeness. Because of the direct thermal damage to the cells of the brain and the low-flow state of cerebral circulation, cerebral edema and hemorrhage may develop. Because the brain, particularly the cerebellum, is so sensitive to thermal injury, the range of neurologic symptoms is broad. In addition to those described, the emergency nurse should be prepared to deal with seizures, psychosis, and decerebrate posturing and be aware that if the brain stem is involved, the patient may have fixed and dilated pupils. Rapid cooling and restoration of adequate circulation must be a priority to prevent neurologic damage or death.

In addition to the symptoms previously described, the patient may have dry skin, although more than 50% of patients with heat stroke do perspire.[1] This fact is not in keeping with theories that heat stroke victims are always "dry." Respirations almost always are increased, as is the pulse rate. All hyperthermic patients should receive supplemental oxygen by the method most appropriate for the level of consciousness. Blood pressure is usually low as a result of dehydration and peripheral vasodilation. High-output cardiac failure may develop, and all critically "hot" patients should be placed on the cardiac monitor in the ED. Monitoring of central venous pressure and pulmonary capillary wedge pressure should be considered in the critical care phase to monitor fluid status. Protection of the kidneys and liver from thermal and low-flow damage is critical. It is important to monitor and encourage urinary output if appropriate. Myoglobinuria and poor perfusion of the kidneys may put the kidneys at risk for failure, and close monitoring of urinary output for color, amount, and pH is important. Administration of mannitol 0.25 g/kg is recommended in patients whose urine output is less than 50 ml per hour.

The treatment for heat stroke is immediate and rapid cooling, which should be initiated by the prehospital care providers. Cooling can be accomplished by cool bathing, especially with a fan overhead, using well-padded ice packs in vascular areas such as the groin, axillae, and neck. Cooling blankets may be used, but it should be remembered that cooling from wet skin is 25 times more effective than cooling from dry skin: bathing is the method of choice. More aggressive measures should be considered when lowering the temperature is difficult or if the temperature is extremely high initially. These measures include ice water lavage of the rectum and stomach. The core temperature must be monitored and recorded carefully during the cooling phase to prevent inadvertent hypothermia. Intravenous administration of 10 to 25 mg chlorpromazine (Thorazine) helps prevent shivering, which is uncomfortable and increases oxygen consumption dramatically. Aspirin and acetaminophen are *not* effective in reducing temperatures in heat stroke. The fluid volume in most victims of hyperthermia is not greatly depleted, and administration of 1 to 2 L of isotonic saline solution or Ringer's lactate during the first 4 hours is usually adequate. Again, close hemodynamic monitoring is indicated until normal vital signs have been recovered. Corticosteroid therapy (usually with methylprednisolone) may be used to treat cerebral edema, and intracranial pressure monitoring is helpful.

SUMMARY

Environmental emergencies will continue to occur for as long as people expose themselves to environmental hazards. A knowledge of some of the more commonly seen environmental emergencies allows the emergency nurse to practice effectively and confidently.

REFERENCES

1. Nelson RK: *Environmental emergencies,* Philadelphia, 1985, WB Saunders.
2. Nemirof M: Cold water near-drowning. Lecture, Trauma and Emergency Nursing Conference, Anaheim, California, Aug 1989.

SUGGESTED READINGS

Auerbach PA, Geehr EC, eds: *Environmental emergencies,* St Louis, 1988, Mosby–Year Book.

Budassi SA: *Mosby's manual of emergency care,* ed 3, St Louis, 1989, Mosby–Year-Book.

Cardona V et al: *Trauma nursing: from resuscitation through rehabilitation,* Philadelphia, 1989, WB Saunders.

Rosen P et al: *Emergency medicine: concepts and clinical practice,* St Louis, 1987, Mosby–Year Book.

Schwartz G et al: *Principles and practice of emergency medicine,* ed 2, Philadelphia, 1986, WB Saunders.

State of Alaska hypothermia and cold water near-drowning guidelines, Emergency Medical Services Division of Public Health, Juneau, Alaska, 1989, Alaska Department of Health and Social Services.

CHAPTER

29 Disaster Preparedness

Jean R. Callum and Norman M. Dinerman

The emergency department (ED) is only one area of the hospital that is affected by a sudden influx of patients from a disaster. However, the ED provides a critical interface with the disaster scene and it is the first "clinical domino" of the institution to sustain the burden of patient care. The consequences of staff performance in the ED are felt throughout the organization during the acute phases of a disaster response. It is of pivotal importance, therefore, that emergency nurses and their physician colleagues participate in the design, development, testing, evaluation, and modification of the hospital and community disaster plans.[1]

This chapter provides a framework for disaster preparedness by showing how individual participation and the ED's disaster planning efforts fit into the broader scheme of hospital, community, state, and national planning efforts. Functional definitions for disaster planning and preparedness are also presented. With this framework in mind, four aspects of the dynamic process of disaster preparedness are discussed in detail (Fig. 29-1). The primary focus of this chapter is hospital and ED preparedness. For those interested in community and regional planning, a list of additional readings at the end of the chapter provides opportunity for further study.

A FRAME OF REFERENCE
The Big Picture

One might think of disaster preparedness in terms of a series of concentric circles. All the circles have a common center—the individual—and each depends on those contained within to provide a successful disaster response (Fig. 29-2).

On the national and state levels, the Federal Emergency Management Agency (FEMA) is the central point of contact within the federal government for a wide range of emergency management activities. Among FEMA's activities are the following[4]:

- Ensuring continuity of government and coordinating mobilization of resources during national security emergencies
- Supporting state and local governments in disaster plan-

ning, preparedness, mitigation, response, and recovery efforts
- Coordinating federal aid for events declared disasters and emergencies by the President
- Providing training and education to enhance the professional development of federal, state, and local emergency managers
- Developing community awareness programs for weather emergencies and home safety

Hospitals and their disaster preparedness managers are well advised to become familiar with local and state FEMA representatives and the services they provide. Their consultative advice can be helpful, and they are sure to become involved in most actual disaster situations.

Also at the federal level is the National Disaster Medical System (NDMS). Formed in 1981 to respond to major catastrophic disasters, the NDMS has the following primary objectives[7]:

1. To provide medical assistance to a disaster area in the form of medical assistance teams and medical supplies and equipment
2. To evacuate patients that cannot be cared for in the affected area to designated locations elsewhere in the nation
3. To provide hospitalization in a national network of hospitals that have agreed to accept patients in the event of a national emergency

The NDMS currently consists of 75 disaster medical assistance teams (DMATs) from throughout the United States. A DMAT is made up of about 30 volunteer physicians, nurses, and other personnel who are trained in disaster response. A DMAT might be used by local authorities, for mass casualty search-and-rescue operations; by state authorities, for medical response in their home state; or by national authorities, to provide interstate aid.[7] For example, in 1989 the NDMS responded to Hurricane Hugo by sending a DMAT from Albuquerque, New Mexico, to the U.S. Virgin Islands. The effectiveness of this disaster response system relies heavily on the enthusiasm and participation of individual emergency nurses and physicians.

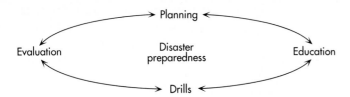

Fig. 29-1 Four aspects of dynamic process of disaster preparedness.

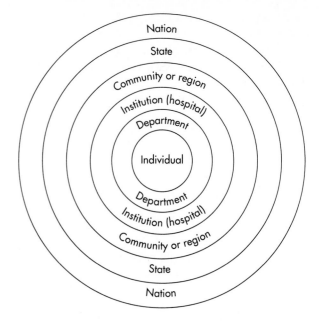

Fig. 29-2 Disaster preparedness.

At the regional and community level, effective disaster planning and response requires participation by hospital, emergency medical service (EMS), and police and fire department personnel. In addition, local media, airports, and industries (often the site of disaster incidents), mental health workers, clergy, public utilities, the Red Cross, and governmental agencies (for example, the National Guard and FEMA) should be involved. In southern Penobscot County, Maine, such a group recently planned and executed a disaster drill that required participation from many public and private agencies—a true test of our community preparedness. Although the rest of this chapter focuses primarily on hospital planning, the concentric circles of disaster preparedness and the larger context to which we are all accountable must be kept in mind.

Functional Definitions

What is a disaster? FEMA[3] defines disaster as

. . . an occurrence of a severity and magnitude that normally results in deaths, injuries and property damage and that cannot be managed through the routine procedures and resources of government. It usually develops suddenly and unexpectedly and requires immediate, coordinated, and effective responses by multiple government and private sector organizations to meet human needs and speed recovery.

A more memorable definition of disaster might be the following: "Many people trying to do quickly what they do not ordinarily do, in an environment with which they are not familiar."[11] Both definitions address the disparity between casualties created and the coordinated application of resources to manage them. A successful disaster response is one that resolves this disparity.[1]

Disasters may be broadly and beneficially classified based on their functional impact on the system. Those disasters which create a situation of *multiple casualty overload* situation or those which involve *paralysis* of hospital function are the two fundamental categories. The latter may be further subdivided to include disasters that involve partial or complete destruction of the six critical substrates of the institution and nondestructive disasters. Clearly, combinations of these types of disaster may occur.

The multiple casualty overload type of disaster imposes a volume of patients on the system in such a way that modifications of routine diagnostic and therapeutic inter-

ventions must be undertaken. It is assumed that the integrity of the physical plant, the organizational structure for administration, and the employees themselves have not been affected by the disaster. All the personnel, supplies and equipment, communications, and structural attributes of the physical plant may thus be augmented to bring about a successful resolution to the crisis.

In contrast, the paralytic type of disaster precludes the augmentation of the routine staff and structure of the institution. Even in nondestructive forms of paralytic disasters such as snowstorms or employee strikes the normal load of patients imposes severe burdens on the institution and creates a situation of relative patient overload. In destructive paralytic disasters such as earthquakes, tornadoes, floods, internal explosions, or riots the paralysis of the institution may be virtually complete. Even the normal flow of patients to a hospital that is paralyzed in either a destructive or nondestructive type of disaster creates severe burdens on the system and threatens to compromise patient care.

In paralytic disasters of both types, reconstitution of the following critical substrates is mandatory to restore institutional function: (1) personnel, (2) the physical plant, (3) supplies and equipment, (4) communications, (5) supervision, and (6) transportation.

Because the variety of paralytic disasters is so diverse, disaster preparedness for this eventuality entails a knowledge of the means by which each of the six critical substrates of institutional function may be acquired in modified form. For example, professional personnel may have to be acquired from other agencies that are as yet untouched by the disaster. A knowledge of sources of acquisition of the six substrates of institutional function is imperative if adaptation to the disaster is to be successful.

Disasters may also be described as static or dynamic. These terms are so-called dimensional modifiers. *Static* disasters are those which are within a self-contained geographic area and generally produce a fixed number and type of casualties in a relatively brief period, for example, an aircraft accident. In contrast, a *dynamic* disaster is geographically widespread and produces an increasing number of diverse casualties over a prolonged period. Examples include floods, earthquakes, and tornadoes. The dynamic type of disaster involves modification of institutional function to allow an extension of the initial disaster efforts. The static disaster by definition requires an intensive response for a well-defined period.

Most hospital disaster plans describe institutional response to an incident of multiple casualty overload. Adaptation of hospital function during a paralytic type of disaster may require deliberation of various leaders within and outside the organization to identify suitable alternatives for institutional function. Thus the disaster response in the paralytic form of disaster is difficult to articulate in advance. Redundancy of resources is fundamental in meeting the challenge of the paralytic disaster. In contrast, the multiple casualty overload disaster may be successfully managed by augmenting existing resources and making extensive changes in procedures.

PLANNING
Hospital Disaster Committee

The hospital disaster committee provides the focus for institutional disaster planning. Broadly speaking, this committee has the following purposes: (1) to ensure institutional preparedness for disaster situations through planning, education, drills, and evaluation, and (2) to ensure compliance with disaster preparedness regulatory standards. The many responsibilities of this committee include the following:

- Reviewing and updating the hospital disaster plan
- Assisting departments and services in developing individual plans
- Integrating hospital planning with community planning
- Ensuring that the hospital plan and preparedness systems are in accord with Joint Commission on Accreditation of Healthcare Organizations (JCAHO), federal, state, and local regulations
- Integrating disaster policies and procedures with hospital policies and procedures
- Educating and orienting hospital personnel and medical staff
- Planning, executing, and evaluating exercises and drills
- After a drill, completing plan changes and follow-up evaluation
- Maintaining an awareness of recent developments and research in disaster preparedness
- Serving as an internal and external resource to others

A number of factors should be considered when choosing members of the disaster committee. All key departments,

both clinical and nonclinical, must be represented. Medical staff and management representation is always essential. Hospital staff with specialized knowledge in disaster preparedness should also be appointed. In addition, members must have enough authority within the hospital organization to make needed policy changes and a commitment to meeting the objectives of the committee.

The chairperson of this committee may come from any discipline, so long as he or she has an ability to understand the big picture, the power (or knowledge) to turn ideas into policy, and the stamina to keep this dynamic and sometimes tedious process going.

More About Regulatory Compliance

The JCAHO has explicit requirements for hospital disaster preparedness. During the accreditation process, the JCAHO will look for the following[8]:

- Evidence of a plan to manage the consequences of a disaster
- A description of the hospital's role in community-wide emergency preparedness plans
- Evidence of staff training
- Evidence of semiannual plan implementation resulting from drills or actual disaster situations

Those responsible for ensuring regulatory compliance must review not only the JCAHO standards but also the *scoring guidelines* that the Commission uses to determine compliance. The scoring guidelines are far more concrete than the standards and reveal requirements in much greater specificity. The scoring guidelines suggest the need to perform a variety of procedures, including the following[8]:

- Identify and test alternate sources of essential utilities.
- Identify and test an emergency communication system.
- Develop and test a procedure for identifying an alternate care site.
- Develop and test a plan for total facility evacuation.
- Complete two drills per year, at least 4 months apart, with one of the drills involving an actual influx of "patients."
- Complete and document emergency preparedness training programs so that at least 91% of a random sample of hospital staff can adequately describe such training.
- Complete and document critiques of each drill, giving evidence of problem identification and subsequent corrective action.

A good hospital disaster preparedness program generally meets and exceeds regulatory standards. Although we must be aware of these standards, focusing our energies toward "doing the right thing" almost always results in regulatory compliance.

The Hospital Disaster Plan

Entire books have been written about developing hospital disaster plans. The box on p. 406 provides a checklist of key disaster plan elements that many authors have used and recommended. However, a variety of different approaches to disaster planning have been taken. Those charged with developing a plan might consider some additional reading to ensure that the unique needs of their hospital and community are adequately addressed.

More About Department Plans

All hospital departments and medical staff services that would be involved in responding to a disaster situation must develop individual disaster plans. The department or service plan defines the specific responsibilities of hospital staff and physicians. All departments and services should use that same format or template for writing their plans. The box on p. 407 provides an example of a template successfully used in two large hospitals.

It is important to ensure that medical staff plans are integrated with plans of related hospital departments. For example, the operating room disaster plan must mesh with those of the surgery and anesthesiology services. In some instances, particularly with the laboratory, radiology, and ED departments, hospital and physician services are so interdependent that a single plan suffices for both. In addition, many members of a hospital's medical staff may have staff privileges at other local institutions. In this instance, interhospital cooperation during planning is vital.

If you have responsibility for developing or contributing to your hospital's ED plan, consider the following questions:

- How is the plan activated?
- Does the community-wide plan call for personnel from the ED to be sent to the scene? Who will go? How will they get there? What will they do?
- Who is in charge? What if the persons in charge are unavailable?
- What patient classification system will be used for triage at the hospital?
- Where will the ED command post be?
- How will additional personnel be notified?
- How will you augment your space?
- What are the responsibilities of staff (by job classification)?
- What will you need from ancillary and support departments?
- How will you keep the area clear of all but essential personnel?
- How will you keep patient care records?
- How will you deal with visitors, family members of victims, and the media?
- How will you communicate pertinent patient information to other hospital departments (registration, nursing units, operating room, laboratory, community relations, administration, and so on)?
- What additional supplies and equipment are needed? How will you get them?

Just as each hospital, each ED is unique, so are the answers to these questions.

KEY ELEMENTS OF THE HOSPITAL DISASTER PLAN

1. Table of contents—critical for quick referencing
2. Letter of authorization—generally signed and dated by the hospital CEO; gives the authority to implement the plan
3. Purpose and scope—described in the box on p. 407
4. Definition of terms—such as those defined in the first section of this chapter
5. Chain of command—clearly identifies disaster response leadership by title
6. Activation process—procedures for putting the plan into action
    Mobilization and staging—described in the box on p. 407
        Normal readiness
        Increased readiness
        Warning
        Response
        Recovery
    Notification—describes steps taken to notify key personnel
7. Patient management plan—overview (see no. 8)
8. Area use modification plan—a one-page reference guide identifying locations of key functions
    Patient care
        Triage (for example, at ED entrance)
        Critical, salvageable patients (ED)
        Dead patients (morgue)
        Uninjured patients (auditorium)
        Minor injuries (outpatient clinic)
        Medical emergencies (intensive care unit)
        Fractures (orthopedics)
        Surgical emergencies (operating room)
        Unsalvageable patients (outpatient surgery)
        Hysteria; behavioral emergencies (psychiatry)
        Pregnant women with injuries (labor and delivery)
        Patients being discharged to accommodate victims (discharge unit)
    Command posts—provide points of coordination and communication
    Labor pool—to augment personnel where needed
    Families of victims
    News media
9. Communication plan—must ensure smooth flow of information and options for system failures
10. Individual department plans—organized in alphabetical order
11. Paralytic disasters
    Procedures for special incidents (such as bomb threats, fires, or chemical spills)
    Evacuation plan
12. Interagency agreements (for example, water suppliers, or Red Cross assistance)

From Seliger JS, Simoneau JK: *Emergency preparedness disaster planning for health facilities,* Rockville, Md, 1986, Aspen Publishers.

SAMPLE TEMPLATE

Author (Name)
Associate Editor (Name)
Revision (Date)
Department/Service (Name)

Purpose

To outline in a sequential fashion the procedures, duties, and responsibilities of the (department name) in the event of a mass casualty incident. This plan outlines those operations to be performed during all phases of such an incident.

Scope

All mass casualty incidents within (hospital name) service area. At the request of the (state) Emergency Management Agency, those mass casualty incidents outside (hospital name) service area.

Chain of command

(Listing of supervisory chain of command by title)

Personnel notification mechanism

(Steps taken to notify personnel within department)

Specific plan

Normal readiness

A written disaster plan will be maintained and used as follows:

Reviewed yearly

Presented at new-employee orientation seminar

Presented yearly on each unit

Located in an accessible place on each unit, in the nursing office, and with the on-call administrator

A current telephone call list will be kept in the (name location).

The call list will be reviewed and redistributed quarterly by the (name responsible person by title).

All (department name) staff will keep their phone numbers current with the (name responsible person).

(List any other relevant information.)

(List any other steps taken to ensure that department is prepared for a disaster response.)

Increased readiness

(List steps taken when notified that a *possible* disaster situation exists, for example, an airliner with engine trouble will be landing at a local airport.)

Warning

(List steps taken when notified that a *probable or likely* disaster situation exists, for example, a disabled airliner has landed at a local airport but it is not known whether there are any injured.)

Response

(List steps taken to responses to *actual* incoming disaster victims, for example, more than 80 injured people from an airline crash will be transported to local hospitals.)

Recovery

(List steps taken to return to normal operations.)

Evaluation

(List steps taken to evaluate the disaster response.)

"Getting it Done"

The task of developing a hospital disaster plan is far less overwhelming if many authors are involved. Department directors and medical service chiefs can be given a template, previously described, for plan development. Each plan is assigned to an associate editor who is a member of the hospital disaster committee. The associate editor ensures that department plans follow the approved format and meet the objectives of the hospital plan. The editor (usually the same person who chairs the committee) must see that the plan is coordinated both internally and externally with the community-wide plan. The editor and associate editors usually write the parts of the plan that are not department specific. Members of the disaster committee should remember three things: organization is critical to success, deadlines must be set and met, and the process is dynamic and ongoing, that is, you never really "get it done."

Special Considerations

Among the many issues that emerge during disaster plan development, a few need special attention.

The media. Every disaster plan should contain a detailed plan for management of the news media. In the hospital setting we look to the public relations department to provide leadership in this area. The role of the public information officer of the hospital is critical at all stages of a disaster situation. In general, the clinician should follow usual policies regarding patient confidentiality as closely as possible and refer press inquiries to the hospital's public information officer.[5] In turn the public information officer must be prepared to provide a response to such inquiries. If the hospital does not assist the media by providing timely and accurate information, good reporters (who are inquisitive and aggressive) will certainly get the story by other means. It is suggested that the hospital plan to set up a media center nearby but outside the patient care areas, where telephones, rest rooms, and food can be provided. Erik Auf der Heide's excellent book, *Disaster Response: Principles of Preparation and Coordination,* provides a particularly enlightening chapter on media management and is highly recommended reading.

Families. Families and loved ones of victims deserve special care and handling. One or more hospital departments (patient relations, chaplaincy services, and so on) should assume responsibility for family care. A written plan should address, at a minimum, the chain of command, personnel, special supplies and equipment (tissues, diapers, phone books, telephone access, and so on), the location of the waiting area, the way in which patient information will be provided, and how families will be reunited with discharged patients. Remember that the media will want to interview family members.

Mental health services. Disasters produce psychologic casualties. At the time of the incident, hysteria or other behavioral emergencies may require immediate assistance of mental health workers. The hospital plan should provide for this eventuality. In addition, it is important to recognize that both victims and emergency response team members may have a delayed reaction to the stress of the incident. Many communities have developed "critical incident stress debriefing teams" to assist emergency service personnel in overcoming emotional reactions that have the potential to interfere with their ability to function at the scene or later on the job. If your community has such a team, they should be integrated with the community and hospital disaster plans.

Patient information and record keeping. The possibility that large numbers of victims will arrive in rapid succession (and perhaps without identification) necessitates special provisions for record keeping. Specially prepared and numbered "disaster packets" containing clinical forms and registration forms expedite patient care and admission. Our own hospital plan calls for an admissions supervisor (stationed at the triage area) to develop a master patient identification list. This list, referred to as the mass casualty incident (MCI) key, includes the patient's MCI number (which may be the patient's only identifier until a name can be determined), name, medical record number, age, sex, and the disposition of the patient's case. Each patient is assigned to an admissions employee, who is to seek out the previously listed information and report it to the admissions supervisor coordinating the master list. This system was developed after various ancillary and patient care departments reported having problems with patient identification during drills. The master list is distributed at least every hour to those who need it until more routine identification procedures can be employed. Alternative solutions may be more workable in other institutions.

Communications. Any veteran of disaster planning knows that communication and information flow during drills and actual incidents are at the root of most of the problems that will be identified in a subsequent critique. Redundancy of technology is very important: the probability is high that normal systems of communication will break down during a disaster situation. A good hospital disaster plan recognizes this probability and identifies as many options as possible. Our own disaster plan assigns from the management staff no less than six "communication officers," whose sole responsibility is to make rounds between the administrative command post and a specific group of departments, providing two-way information updates.

Supplies and equipment. A mass casualty incident of any consequential size places stress on the operation of the hospital materials management department; good planning can help reduce the degree of stress. First-response departments (ED, operating room, intensive care unit, and so on) should work with the materials management department to develop a specific plan for augmenting their supplies. The hospital should also recognize that it will be seen as a supply resource for the disaster site itself. The community-wide plan should specifically identify the hospital's role in providing supplies and equipment to the scene. Hospital personnel should participate in the development of this community-wide plan.

EDUCATION

A paper plan is only that if staff and physicians do not understand their responsibilities during a disaster. Disaster education can take a variety of forms. In planning educational opportunities, remember that enthusiasm for disaster planning is directly related to the intensity of the most recent disaster and inversely related to the distance from it.[1a]

Lectures. The most informative and interesting educational sessions tend to be those presented by someone who was intimately involved in an actual disaster incident. Pictures, anecdotes, and personal experiences emphasize the importance of disaster planning in a way that nothing else can. Scheduling such lectures periodically and before drills or plan updates is a good way to generate more enthusiasm for the process.

New-employee orientation. New employees usually go through a general hospital orientation and a department-specific program. Disaster preparedness should be discussed broadly during general orientation, when the chairperson of the disaster committee can briefly describe the hospital's program. Department directors can use the orientation period to have the new employee read and ask questions about the department disaster plan. There are many things for employees to learn during the first 2 weeks on the job: their role in a disaster response is one of those things.

Disaster games. Disaster education can be fun. In our own hospital, members of the disaster committee have taken turns being the "Disaster Master." Each had to develop a disaster scenario, write down the actions they would expect the administrator-on-call or the nursing supervisor to take, and then spring a 15-minute pop quiz (including critique) on an unsuspecting colleague. What about a disaster game show with teams of competing departments? A tabletop game of "place the patient" for nursing and registration? We need be limited only by our good sense and creativity.

Drills. Next to an actual incident, disaster drills are perhaps the best tool available for education. They are discussed in detail in the next section.

Critiques. The evaluation process, discussed in greater detail later in the chapter, provides an opportunity for feedback, interaction, and plan changes. The educational significance of critiques should not be overlooked.

DRILLS
Why Drills?

Disaster drills provide an opportunity to educate hospital employees about emergency preparedness; they allow us to take a practical look at our paper plans. They help us create options and alternatives for disaster response. They allow us to develop interagency relationships so that working together during a crisis will be easier. All these elements enable us to be better prepared for an actual disaster. If these reasons are not compelling enough, remember that your hospital's accreditation will be at risk if regular drills are not completed.

Types of Drills

Orientation seminar. An orientation seminar is an orientation to the hospital disaster plan, to a new procedure within the plan, or perhaps even to the concept of disaster preparedness. The orientation seminar generally focuses on something new, bringing together individuals who have a role or interest in the topic. Methods such as lecture, film, slides, or panel discussion might be used. An orientation seminar is a good place to start if drills have not been a regular event or if you have just made a major update to your disaster plan. Such a seminar would not be considered a drill by JCAHO.

Tabletop exercise. A tabletop exercise is an activity that presents key disaster response personnel with a simulated disaster without time constraint. This type of drill is usually held in an informal conference room setting. It is intended to allow participants an opportunity to evaluate their plans and resolve issues of coordination in a nonthreatening environment and under minimal stress. A tabletop exercise is a good next step after the orientation seminar is completed. You might also choose to conduct one or more tabletop exercises each year to fulfill educational and regulatory requirements.

Functional exercise. The functional exercise is designed to evaluate one or more plan functions or complex activities. These exercises are fully simulated disaster situations: stress is introduced by intense activity, complex decisions, and significant requirements for coordination. This type of exercise may be held in a conference room setting but will require increased preparation time and resources.

Full-scale exercise. The full-scale exercise is intended to evaluate all major aspects of the disaster preparedness program. This type of exercise requires actual mobilization of personnel, supplies, and equipment to determine coordination and response capability. The process is an interactive one that occurs over a substantial period. This type of drill should be attempted only after other, less intense exercises have been successfully completed.[2]

Planning a Drill

The degree and type of planning required for a drill depend on the scope and type of exercise. An orientation seminar at a single hospital can be adequately planned by a single individual; a full-scale exercise involving the entire community requires months of interagency planning. Therefore for a larger drill, your first step is to form or become involved in a drill planning committee. After you set the date and time for the exercise, the group must consider the following issues.

Goals. It is important to specifically identify the goals of the exercise. What do you want to test, and what criteria will you use to assess the outcome? For example, if you choose to test only the notification portion of your plan, you must develop a way to determine how many individuals or departments in the target group were contacted and if contact occurred promptly.

The scenario. A reasonably detailed disaster scenario must be developed that identifies the type of incident and the circumstances that lead to it, the number of victims, type and severity of injuries, and any other relevant information.

The scene. The site of the incident must be determined, and preparations must be made for scene organization and coordination.

Victims. Solicit volunteers to act as victims, and organize an adequate number of moulage artists. Be sure to instruct your volunteers regarding their role.

Transportation. If prehospital care providers are involved in the drill (they might not be involved in a single-hospital exercise), transportation of victims from scene to hospital will be no problem. However, do not forget that "victims" must be transported back to the scene after the exercise is completed.

The hospital. The scope and type of drill assist hospital managers in identifying which departments will be involved. If the drill is announced, department directors may ask for advice about which personnel should be called in. Steps must also be taken to ensure that routine care proceeds as smoothly as possible during the drill. It can be difficult for staff to separate real victims from moulaged victims. Think about how you can do this effectively, but do not forget that you will have an audience. In a recent drill at our hospital, shouting "this is a real one" seemed to work for caregivers, but it probably did not give the patients' family members a feeling of confidence.

Tips and pointers

- Organize volunteers to be mock family members. Tell them who they are trying to locate and set them loose. This exercise really helps test your family management plan.
- The media will be happy to participate. Organize a mock press conference. Remember that a drill is a media event; a "real" press team is likely to cover it.
- Do not always conduct your drills on a Saturday morning in the summer. Test all shifts. Remember that disasters occur in the winter, too.
- An announced drill is good for those who are just getting started learning disaster preparedness. Once staff members have more experience, make the drill a surprise.
- Keep meticulous records. If something is not documented, you did not do it.
- Take care of your volunteers. Remind them to wear old clothes, have a clinician brief victims on their injuries ("behavioral moulage"), give them written and verbal

instructions, provide food and rest rooms, tell them what to do if they have a real illness or injury (you might use a special code word known to all), tell them where to go on completion, be polite, and say thank you.

EVALUATION
Critiques

Planning, education, and drills have little meaning if an evaluation process is not completed. Just before or immediately after a disaster drill, leadership from key departments should be provided with a critique form. This form should be easy to fill out; questions should be aimed at those components of the plan that are tested in the drill. In addition, drill planners might consider assigning observers. These individuals can provide an objective written evaluation of actions taken during the exercise. It is also advisable to schedule a verbal critique after the drill so that participants are able to interact and discover thematic problems and concerns.

Follow-Up Actions

After written and verbal critiques have been summarized, the hospital disaster committee should be convened. Each problem or concern that was raised in the critique process should result in corrective action. This action may be simple (for example, updating a call-in list) or quite complex (for example, completely revising the area use modification plan). In either case, follow-up actions should be timely and well documented. Revising the hospital disaster plan is the last step in the process, bringing us full circle. Education, another drill, evaluation, and more planning follow. Disaster preparedness is a dynamic and continuous process.

CASE STUDY

If there is any doubt about the importance of disaster planning and regular disaster drills, the response to the crash of Flight 1713 should dispel it (see Case Study 29-1, above).[9] A disaster plan for the city and county of Denver has been in place for many years. Twice-yearly disaster drills contribute to its success. In fact, one of the two annual drills always take place at Stapleton International Airport. On September 23, 1987—only weeks before the crash—a drill at Stapleton was completed. The similarities between the drill and the actual crash were amazing. Twenty-seven passengers "died" during the drill, whereas 26 were killed in the crash. The exercise called for 77 victims to be transported to hospitals; 56 victims were transported on the day of the crash. The same physician coordinator who participated in the drill was, by chance, the medical coordinator at the crash scene. Ironically, Continental Airlines had also been the subject of the September drill.

Although this story may make some drill planners feel a bit uneasy about their predictive power, the important point is that a well-developed and tested disaster plan was con-

---

CASE STUDY 29-1

Continental Airlines Flight*

On November 15, 1987, Continental Airlines Flight 1713 crashed at Stapleton International Airport, Denver, Colorado (Fig. 29-3). The DC-9, carrying 82 passengers and crew, had taken off in a blinding snowstorm. Seconds after takeoff, one of the wings touched the ground, flipping the plane over. The wreckage was devastating—the plane broke apart and collapsed; more than 7 hours of intensive efforts were required to remove entrapped victims. Injuries to passengers were primarily caused by the impact, deceleration, and the effects of entrapment. Of 28 victims, 9 succumbed exclusively to mechanical asphyxiation. Fortunately, the fire that erupted at impact was relatively minor and burn injuries were insignificant. In all, 26 people died at the scene and 56 were transported to local hospitals. Two more people subsequently died.

*From McCann B: Denver airplane crash highlights effectiveness of medical disaster planning and drilling, *Emerg Med Ambul Care News,* Jan 1988.

---

ducted in Denver and these efforts paid off when the stakes were the highest. For example, it was pointed out earlier that one purpose for drills is to develop interagency relationships so that improvisation and creation of options may occur. At the Denver crash, medical personnel knew that because of an 8° F (-22.2° C) wind chill factor, hypothermia posed a major threat to entrapped victims and rescue personnel. Medical coordination asked for heat, and the airlines, fire department, and maintenance personnel were able to locate and set up auxiliary power units that blew warm air through the airplane. Because of the auxiliary power units, hypothermia was not a serious problem.

Certainly, some problems did occur, not the least of which was the weather. All the major concerns were identified in one of the eight separate critiques that took place after the crash. That intensive scrutiny allowed disaster planning officials to make needed changes to their plan. Be assured that annual drills are still going on in Denver.

A PERSONAL MISSION

What can one person do to make a difference? You can start by knowing your role in your ED's plan. Read your hospital's entire plan; see how it relates to community disaster preparedness efforts. Participate in drills and the critiques that follow them. Volunteer to assist your nurse manager in updating the department's plan and ensuring that supplies and equipment are available. Share your knowledge with others in the department, especially new employees. Work with your nurse manager to organize a disaster exercise or game for ED staff that will test their knowledge of the plan. Find out about the NDMS and local FEMA activities.[6] Get involved. Disaster preparedness begins with you.

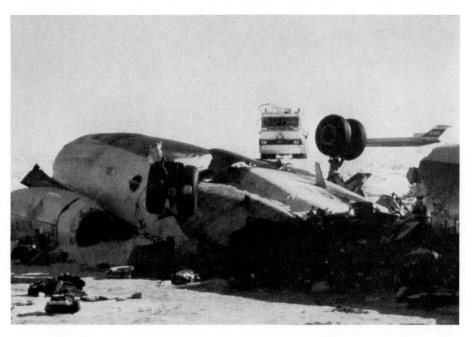

Fig. 29-3 Crash of Continental Airlines Flight 1713, Denver, Colorado.

REFERENCES

1. Dinerman N: Disaster preparedness: observations and perspectives, *JEN* 16(4):252, 1990.
1a. Dinerman N: Personal communication, Aug 1990.
2. Federal Emergency Management Agency: *Exercise design course: guide to emergency management exercises,* SM 170.2, Washington, DC, 1984.
3. Federal Emergency Management Agency: *Objectives for local emergency management,* CPG 1-5, Washington, DC, 1984.
4. Federal Emergency Management Agency: *This is the Federal Emergency Management Agency,* L-135, Washington, DC, 1983.
5. Gough R, Gulliver LS: Anchors, bites, and choppers: media relations and legal issues in disasters, *JEN* 16(4):259, 1990.
6. Hanson C: Disaster preparedness: becoming involved, *JEN* 16(4): 74A, 1990.
7. Hogan J, Rega P, Forkapa B: A civilian-sponsored DMAT: a community's collaboration among three hospitals, *JEN* 16(4):245, 1990.
8. Joint Commission on Accreditation of Healthcare Organizations: *Accreditation manual for hospitals,* 1989, The Commission.
9. McCann B: Denver airplane crash highlights effectiveness of medical disaster planning and drilling, *Emerg Med Ambul Care News,* Jan 1988.
10. Seliger JS, Simoneau JK: *Emergency preparedness: disaster planning for health facilities,* Rockville, Md, 1986, Aspen Publishers.
11. Tierney KJ: Emergency medical preparedness and response in disasters: the need for interorganizational coordination. In Petak WJ: Emergency management: a challenge for public administration, special issue, *Public Admin Rev* 45:77, 1985.

SUGGESTED READINGS

Auf der Heide E: *Disaster response: principles of preparation and coordination,* St Louis, 1989, Mosby–Year Book.
Numerous articles on disaster preparedness, *JEN* 16(4), 1990.

CHAPTER 30

Burns and Thermal Injuries

Janet A. Marvin

The evaluation of the patient with a major burn injury is the same as for any other trauma victim. Initially the patient should be evaluated for problems with airway, breathing, and circulation (ABCs). A careful assessment using the ABC4 Primary Survey should also aid in the identification of other life-threatening injuries. A secondary head-to-toe assessment is necessary to diagnose other injuries such as fractures, abdominal injuries from blunt trauma, or closed head injuries. The *burn wound itself should receive low priority during the initial survey* except that all clothing should be removed, and if the wound is the result of a chemical, the would should be thoroughly rinsed with water to stop the burning process. This should be done with caution so that staff members do not get the chemical on themselves and thus sustain an injury.

CAUSES AND INCIDENCE

Burn injuries occur as a result of exposure to flame, flash, hot liquids, hot objects, chemicals, electrical current, or radiation (Fig. 30-1). Since there is no national reporting system for burn injuries, many injuries go unreported. The best estimates suggest that there are approximately 60,000 hospitalizations and 10,000 deaths annually. Most of the available data come from the National Fire Data Center, under the auspices of the National Fire Prevention and Control Administration. Most of their data are related to fires and the injuries they cause and do not take into account burn injuries related to scalds, chemicals, or electrical current. Thus although fires, especially residential fires, result in the majority of burn-related deaths, scald injuries are by far the single most common burn injury, accounting for 40% to 50% of injuries seen in most burn centers. The most common cause of death in the first 48 hours after injury is respiratory complications related to smoke inhalation. After 48 hours, sepsis is the most common cause of death.

ASSESSMENT OF DEPTH AND EXTENT OF BURN

Depth of Burn

The depth of the injury may be referred to as first, second, or third degree or partial thickness or full thickness injury (Table 30-1). Identification of the depth of injury is often

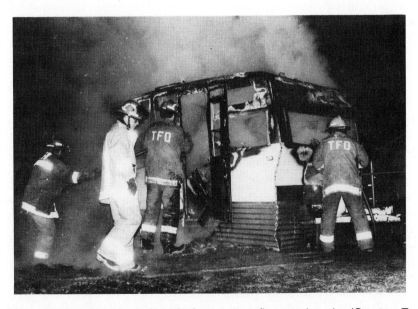

Fig. 30-1 Burn injuries occur as result of exposure to flame and smoke. (Courtesy Tacoma Fire Department, Tacoma, Wash.)

Table 30-1 Classification of burn injury

Depth of burn	Sensitivity	Appearance	Healing time and results	Treatment
PARTIAL THICKNESS				
FIRST DEGREE				
Epidermal	Hyperalgesia	Erythema	3 to 5 days; no scarring	Moisturizers
Superficial dermal	Hyperalgesia to pink	Blisters, red, moist	6 to 10 days; minimal scarring	Topical antibacterial agents or biologic dressings required
SECOND DEGREE				
Moderate dermal	Normal algesia	Blisters, pink, moist	10 to 18 days; some scarring	Topical antibacterial agents or biologic dressings required
Deep dermal	Hypoalgesia or analgesia	Blisters, opaque, with less moisture	>21 days; maximal scarring if not excised and grafted	Topical antibacterial agents and early excision and grafting
FULL THICKNESS				
THIRD DEGREE				
Loss of all dermal elements with extension into fat, muscle, and bone	Analgesia	White, opaque, brown, or black, occasionally deep red; very dry, leathery; may or may not have blisters or thrombosed veins	Never heals if area is larger than 3 cm^2; the longer the wound is open, the more hypertrophic the scar	Topical antibacterial agents and early excision and grafting

difficult initially, and unless it is superficial, as with a first-degree burn, or deep, as with a third-degree burn, there is little need to identify the depth of injury during the initial survey and treatment. The depth of the injury may actually increase over time as edema forms and circulation to the area of tissue injury is compromised. This process usually peaks at about 48 hours, and at 48 to 72 hours a more accurate determination of depth can be made.

Extent of Burn

The extent of injury for thermal and chemical injuries is assessed by using formulas such as the Rule of Nines (Fig. 30-2), the Berkow, or the Lund and Browder formula (Figs. 30-3 and 30-4).[2] For the Rule of Nines it is important to remember that the formula must be modified for children. As noted in Fig. 30-2, *B*, the head and neck of an infant represent 19% of the body surface area (BSA), whereas the legs represent a correspondingly smaller percentage, that is, 13% for each lower extremity. To correct for age, one should subtract 1% from the head for each year of age, up through 10 years, and add 0.5% to each lower extremity. To obtain a more accurate estimate of the extent of burn, it is helpful to calculate both the area of burn and the unburned areas. The two estimates should then be compared and if the total is more or less than 100%, the areas should be reestimated.

When estimating burn size, one should remember to assess the posterior aspects of the body as well. In electrical injuries it is more difficult to assess the extent of injury because the surface damage may be minimal when compared with the underlying damage. Thus when describing an electrical injury, it is more important to describe the injury anatomically than to try to calculate a percentage of burn.

Severity of Burn

The severity of burn injury is based on an assessment of the extent and depth of injury, as well as the age of the patient, the presence of concomitant injuries, smoke inhalation, or preexisting diseases. The American Burn Association's categories for burn injuries are listed in Table 30-2.

Care of patients with burns of different severity is determined by the availability of specialized care facilities. The initial stabilization of any burn patient should be available in any community hospital with 24-hour emergency capabilities. Patients with minor burns may be treated as outpatients or be admitted to the community hospital. Patients with moderate burns may be treated either in a community hospital with appropriate staff and facilities to deliver burn care or in a hospital with a specialized burn care facility. Patients with major burns should be cared for in a hospital

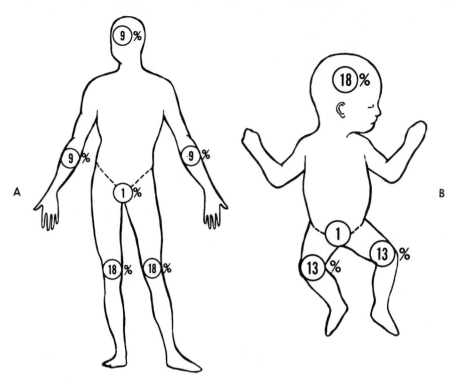

Fig. 30-2   Rule of Nines. **A,** Adult. **B,** Child.

with specialized burn care facilities. Transfer agreements with special care units should be developed in advance to facilitate timely and uneventful transfer.

PHYSIOLOGIC RESPONSE TO BURN INJURY
Initial Circulatory Changes

With major electrical burn injuries and thermal or chemical injuries greater than 15% to 20% BSA, fluid shifts may result in hypovolemia. Problems with circulatory deficits

Table 30-2   Categories of burn injuries

	Major burn* (%BSA)	Moderate burn† (%BSA)	Minor burn† (%BSA)
ADULTS			
Second degree	>25%	15% to 25%	<15%
Third degree	>10%	3% to 10%	<3%
CHILDREN			
Second degree	>20%	10% to 20%	<10%
Third degree	>10%	3% to 10%	<3%

Data from the American Burn Association, eighth annual meeting: Specific optimum criteria for hospital resources for care of patients with burn injuries, San Antonio, Tex, April, 1976.
*In both adults and children, burns involving hands, face, feet, or perineum, or burn injuries complicated by smoke inhalation, major associated trauma, or preexisting illnesses.
†Not involving face, hands, feet, or perineum.

are directly proportional to the extent of injury. Thus the more extensive the injury, the greater the amount of fluid that will shift and the more severe the physiologic derangements. A simplistic view of the physiologic response is presented in Fig. 30-5. With injury to the skin, the normal host defense response is set in motion. This response involves the release of histamines and other vasoactive substances that cause an increase in capillary permeability and localization of white blood cells and plasma proteins in the area to fight infection. If the wound is greater than about 15% BSA, the capillary leak may involve other areas of the body besides the injured area. In this way, generalized edema develops and results in a loss of intravascular volume. With the translocation of the fluid portion of the blood (plasma) from the intravascular to the interstitial space, the patient's hematocrit increases and the blood becomes more viscous. The body's compensatory mechanism to this functional fluid loss is to increase peripheral resistance so that blood is shunted from the peripheral to the central circulation. This process gives rise to the cool, pale, clammy extremities seen in the burn patient. This response acts to maintain central circulation for a short period, but eventually the patient has a decrease in cardiac output and shows signs of hypovolemia.

Response of the Lung to Smoke Inhalation

Inhalation injury or smoke inhalation is a syndrome composed of three distinct problems: carbon monoxide intoxi-

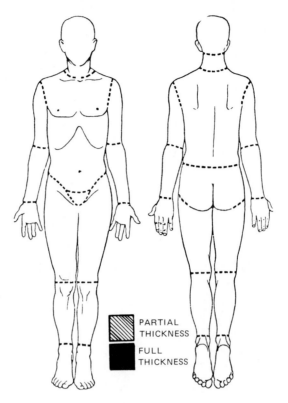

Percent Surface Area Burned

AREA	1 YEAR	1-4 YEARS	5-9 YEARS	10-14 YEARS	Y 15 YEARS	ADULT	2°	3°
Head	19	17	13	11	9	7		
Neck	2	2	2	2	2	2		
Ant. Trunk	13	13	13	13	13	13		
Post Trunk	13	13	13	13	13	13		
R. Buttock	2½	2½	2½	2½	2½	2½		
L. Buttock	2½	2½	2½	2½	2½	2½		
Genitalia	1	1	1	1	1	1		
R. U. Arm	4	4	4	4	4	4		
L. U. Arm	4	4	4	4	4	4		
R. L. Arm	3	3	3	3	3	3		
L. L. Arm	3	3	3	3	3	3		
R. Hand	2½	2½	2½	2½	2½	2½		
L. Hand	2½	2½	2½	2½	2½	2½		
R. Thigh	5½	6½	8	8½	9	9½		
L. Thigh	5½	6½	8	8½	9	9½		
R. Leg	5	5	5½	6	6½	7		
L. Leg	5	5	5½	6	6½	7		
R. Foot	3½	3½	3½	3½	3½	3½		
L. Foot	3½	3½	3½	3½	3½	3½		
TOTAL								

Fig. 30-3 Lund and Browder formula. (From Artz CP, Moncrief JA: *The treatment of burns,* ed 2, Philadelphia, 1979, WB Saunders.)

cation, upper airway obstruction, and a chemical injury to the lower airways and lung parenchyma.

Carbon monoxide intoxication is the most common killer of victims of fires. Most people who die in a fire will have been overcome by carbon monoxide before they sustain their burn injury. In the body, carbon monoxide has a 200 times greater affinity for hemoglobin than oxygen, thus causing inadequate tissue oxygen delivery. Carbon monoxide also combines with myoglobin in muscle cells, which results in muscle weakness. These two factors, tissue hypoxia resulting in mental confusion and muscle weakness, are said to be the major reasons most fire fatalities occur. In addition,

carbon monoxide combines with the cytochrome oxidase system of the brain and may result in prolonged coma in some fire victims.

Upper airway obstruction is the result of intrinsic or extrinsic edema that may lead to airway occlusion at or above the vocal cords (Fig. 30-6). This injury is primarily a thermal injury, resulting in tissue damage in the posterior pharynx. Actual thermal injury below the vocal cord is rare because the posterior pharynx is an efficient heat exchange system. True thermal injury below the vocal cords is usually the result of a live steam injury, in which water vapor carries the heat into the lungs, or injuries that occur in either an

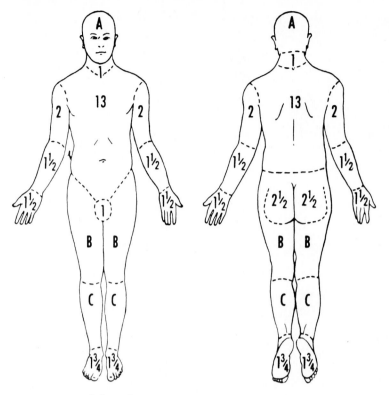

Relative Percentage of Areas Affected by Growth

	Age in Years					
	0	1	5	10	15	Adult
A—½ of head	9½	8½	6½	5½	4½	3½
B—½ of one thigh	2¾	3¼	4	4¼	4½	4¾
C—½ of one leg	2½	2½	2¾	3	3¼	3½

Fig. 30-4 Lund and Browder formula. (From Artz CP, Moncrief JA: *The treatment of burns,* ed 2, Philadelphia, 1979, WB Saunders.)

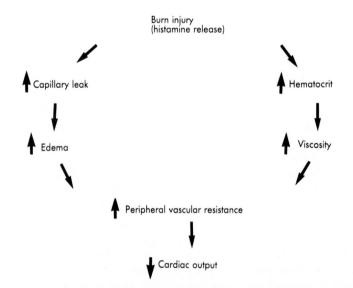

Fig. 30-5 Physiologic response to burn injury.

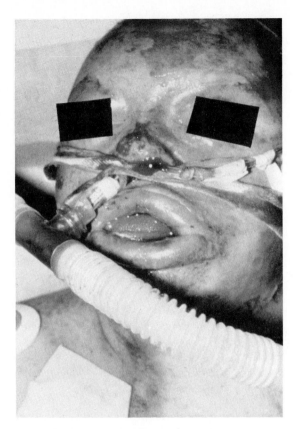

Fig. 30-6   Patient with face burns and inhalation injury.

oxygen-enriched atmosphere or one in which the person was inhaling explosive gases, such as during inhalation anesthesia. True thermal injury to the lungs is almost always fatal. Thermal injury to the upper airway is usually associated with facial burns. The edema progresses rapidly, totally occluding the airway in minutes to hours. The management for airway edema is early intubation.

Chemical injury to the lower airways is a common problem with the inhalation of smoke. Chemical injury from acids and aldehydes in the smoke may damage the lung parenchyma. These chemicals are attached to carbon particles in the smoke, and because they are heavier than air, they are readily inhaled and find their way down the bronchi into the alveoli. This chemical injury results in hemorrhagic tracheobronchitis, increased edema formation, decreased surfactant levels, and decreased pulmonary macrophage function. This condition leads to the rapid development of adult respiratory distress syndrome (ARDS) over a period of 24 to 48 hours. Severe inhalation injury may increase the patient's fluid needs in the first 24 hours by as much as 50% of calculated values.[2]

GENERAL MANAGEMENT CONSIDERATIONS

The patient should initially be assessed using the ABC4 survey for trauma. Then assessment for specific burn injuries should be performed.

Airway

Assessment
- High index of suspicion or history of smoke inhalation
- Visual inspection of the oropharynx and vocal cords for redness, blisters, and carbonaceous particles
- Increasing restlessness
- Complaints of difficulty in breathing and swallowing
- Increasing difficulty in handling secretions
- Increasing hoarseness
- Rapid shallow respiration

Measurement of blood gas levels, although appropriate to assess oxygenation problems related to chemical injury to the lower airway, reveals little about impending airway obstruction.

Therapeutic intervention
- Early intubation (before complete occlusion)

Tracheostomies can and should be avoided initially in these patients. The edema formation of the neck makes these procedures especially difficult.

Breathing

Circumferential chest wall burns
Assessment
Initially the major, specific, burn-related problem that may impair breathing is a circumferential full thickness burn of the thorax. This problem may limit chest wall excursion and prevent adequate gas exchange. Visually inspect the chest for the following:
- Tight leathery eschar circumferentially around the chest
- Inadequate expansion of chest
- Rapid shallow respirations
- Restlessness or confusion
- Decreased oxygenation
- Decreased tidal volume

Therapeutic intervention
Escharotomies of the chest are surgical incisions made along the lateral borders of the chest halfway between the midaxillary line and the midnipple line. If the abdomen is also involved, an incision can be made over the diaphragm to connect the two lateral incisions.

These incisions are made only deep enough to release the eschar and expose the underlying subcutaneous tissue. This depth should allow for immediate improvement in the excursion of the chest wall.

These incisions cause bleeding. One should have an electrocautery unit or 10 to 20 small hemostats available to control the bleeding.

General anesthesia is not necessary, since the incisions are made only in the area of the full thickness burn. Narcotic analgesia given intravenously is sufficient to relieve any pain.

Carbon monoxide (CO) intoxication
Assessment
- Decreased respirations or apnea at the scene
- Cherry red normal skin

- Confusion or coma
- Increased CO level in measurement of carboxyhemoglobin (HgbCO) level
- Carbonaceous sputum

Therapeutic intervention

- Administer oxygen at 100% or at as high a percentage as possible
- If not breathing, intubate and ventilate
- If unconsciousness continues after 1 to 1½ hours with adequate resuscitation and no evidence of head injury, the use of hyperbaric oxygen therapy may be considered
- Radiograph of chest

Chemical injury or ARDS

Assessment

This condition is usually not a problem for at least 8 hours after injury. Clinical findings include the following:

- Decreased oxygenation
- Increased secretions
- Rapid respirations
- Increased patchy infiltrates on radiograph
- Confusion

Therapeutic intervention

- Intubation and ventilation
- Positive end-expiratory pressure
- Bronchodilators as indicated
- No corticosteroids (Corticosteroids given to patients with burns and smoke inhalation increase the morbidity and mortality at least threefold.)[3]

One should assess for other trauma-related causes of problems in breathing, especially pneumothorax or hemothorax, tension pneumothorax, and flail chest. These problems should be expected when burn victims have been in car accidents or explosions or have jumped or fallen. History of chronic pulmonary problems that may complicate therapy should also be noted.

Circulation

Assessment

The following assessment guidelines should be followed closely; if present, they indicate a low-flow state:

- Increased pulse
- Decreased blood pressure
- Increased respirations
- Central venous pressure (CVP) below 3 cm H_2O
- Decreased urine output
- Hematocrit above 50 mg/dl
- Diminished capillary refill
- Restlessness or confusion
- Nausea or vomiting
- Ileus

Therapeutic intervention

- Start one or two large-bore intravenous (IV) lines (one if less than 40% BSA; two if greater than 40% BSA or if the patient is to be transferred).

- Avoid using leg veins for IV sites when possible in adults because of the increased risk of thrombophlebitis.
- Administer fluid replacement by one of the many accepted formulas; two of the more popular are the Baxter formula and the modified Brooke formula.

Baxter formula

First 24 hours: 4 ml of Ringer's lactate/kg body weight per percentage of BSA

- ½ of calculated amount during first 8 hours
- ¼ of calculated amount during second 8 hours
- ¼ of calculated amount during third 8 hours

Time is calculated from the time of injury, not the time IV therapy was initiated.

Second 24 hours:

- D_5W in sufficient quantities to keep serum Na^{++} level below 140 mEq/L
- Potassium to maintain normal serum K^+ level
- Plasma or plasma expander to maintain adequate volume with normal pulse rate, blood pressure, and urine output

Modified Brooke formula

First 24 hours: 2 ml of Ringer's lactate/kg body weight per percentage of BSA

- ½ of calculated amount during first 8 hours
- ¼ of calculated amount during second 8 hours
- ¼ of calculated amount during second 8 hours

Time is calculated from time of injury, not the time IV therapy was initiated.

Second 24 hours: Same as Baxter formula

NOTE: These and other formulas are intended only as a guideline for fluid replacement and may need to be adjusted up or down as one monitors the signs of adequate resuscitation. These signs are the following:

- Pulse rate in upper limits of normal range for age
- Blood pressure normal for age
- Urine output
    - 30 to 50 ml/hour for adults
    - 20 to 30 ml/hour for children
    - 1 to 1.5 ml/kg body weight per hour in infants
- Urine glucose level less that 2+
- Mental alertness
- Absence of ileus or nausea

For electrical injuries there is no formula for fluid resuscitation. Ringer's lactate is administered rapidly, 1 to 2 L per hour in the average adult, until the patient shows signs of adequate resuscitation.

- Urine output is usually maintained at 2 to 3 times the normal volume to facilitate the excretion of myoglobin.
- Once urine output is established, mannitol may be given to increase urine flow and aid the excretion of myoglobin.
- Acidosis (pH 6.8 to 7.0) is a common early complication, and repeated administration of sodium bicarbonate may be required ($NaHCO_3$) to prevent dysrhythmias until fluid therapy can correct the acidosis.

- Draw blood for complete blood count and measurement of electrolyte levels, and type and crossmatch blood.
- Place Foley catheter; send urine for urinalysis and measurement of myoglobin level.
- Monitor hourly urine output.
- Monitor urine glucose level and acetone level every 2 to 4 hours.
- Monitor cardiac rhythm.
- Obtain a 12-lead electrocardiogram.

Prevention of Infection

Aseptic technique
- Gloves, mask, cap, and gown are required for all personnel.
- *All* invasive procedures should be treated as sterile procedures.
- Wounds should be kept covered with clean sheets while other care is being provided.

Antibiotics
- Topical antibiotics should be applied as soon as possible after the wound is debrided.
- Systemic antibiotics are rarely indicated even in severe burns until the patient has a culture-proven infection. Exceptions to this guideline may be young children, elderly patients, diabetic persons, or patients with immunodeficiency diseases.

Tetanus prophylaxis
- For minor or moderate burns, give tetanus immunization if previous immunization had been given more than 10 years ago.
- For major burns or grossly contaminated burns, give tetanus immunization if previous immunization had been given more than 10 years ago.
- In patients who have never been immunized or in whom there is no clear history of immunization, give tetanus hyperimmune globulin (Hypertet) in addition to tetanus immunization.

Management of Pain

Assessment
- Patient complains of pain specific to burn injury or other injuries.
- Patient is restless and has tachycardia with rapid respirations. (Rule out other potential causes.)
- Ask patient to rate pain on a scale of 1 to 5 or another frequently used scale.

Therapeutic intervention
- Administer morphine in small doses (3 to 5 mg in adults) frequently (every 20 to 40 minutes).
- Always administer IV analgesia in burns greater than 15% BSA.
- Explain procedures to the patient.
- Administer antianxiety drug such as diazepam (Valium) if patient is severely agitated for no apparent reason.

NOTE: Burn wounds are exquisitely painful, especially partial thickness injuries. Careful titration of morphine, either as needed or as a morphine drip, can be used effectively to control pain initially.

Obtain a History
- How did injury occur (flame, scald, or the like)?
- Was smoke involved? Was it in a closed space?
- Who was involved? What happened to others?
- What was the patient doing before the accident? (This question may lead to early diagnosis of stroke or myocardial infarction.)
- What previous medical problems or allergies did the patient have?

Burn Wound Care

Burn wound care can wait until patient's condition is stabilized.

Circumferential full thickness injuries
Assessment
- Assess all patients with full thickness circumferential burns for circulatory problems.
- Check distal pulse rates with Doppler device.
- Assess capillary refill.
- Note paresthesia.

Therapeutic intervention
- If patient has signs of circulatory compromise, an escharotomy is performed (Fig. 30-7 illustrates placement of surgical incisions).

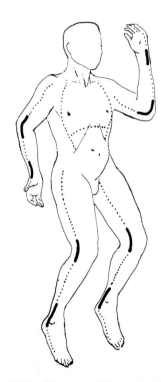

Fig. 30-7   Placement of escharotomies.

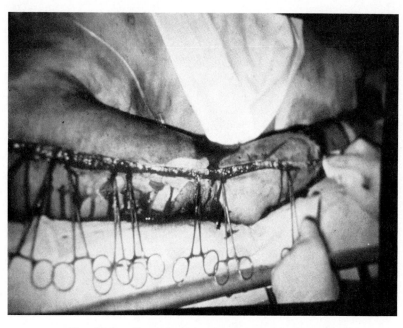

Fig. 30-8 Control of bleeding from escharotomy.

- Be prepared to respond to significant bleeding with either an electrocautery unit or 10 to 20 small hemostats to control bleeding (Fig. 30-8).
- Once procedure is completed, apply a topical antibacterial agent to open wound, dress with a light pressure dressing, and keep the patient's arms and legs slightly elevated.

Thermal burns resulting from flames, flash, scalds, and hot objects (Fig. 30-9)

- Cleanse wounds with sterile or clean water, 0.25 strength povidone iodine (Betadine), and clean cloths or coarse mesh gauze dressings.

- Break and remove outer covering of blisters larger than half-dollar size, except on palms of hands and soles of feet.
- Shave all hairy areas of burns and adjacent areas.
- Cover wound immediately with prescribed topical antibacterial agent with or without a dressing.
- Elevate extremities slightly to reduce swelling.

Chemical burns

- Thoroughly rinse these wounds immediately with tap water or saline solution to remove the chemical. Remember to remove clothing and jewelry and rinse the nonburned areas as well, since some areas of chemical

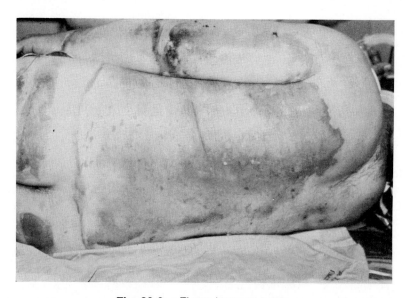

Fig. 30-9 Flame burns to back.

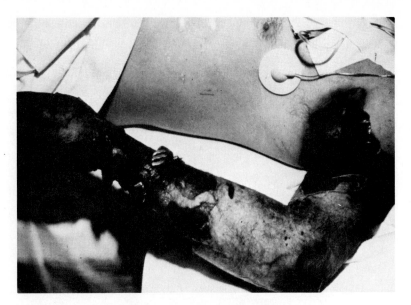

Fig. 30-10 Electrical injury.

exposure may not begin to hurt, blister, or even become red immediately.

- Then treat the wound as if it were a thermal burn.
- Chemical burns of the eyes are ophthalmologic emergencies. As with other chemical wounds, thoroughly rinse the eye with copious amounts of water or saline solution. If the patient is wearing contact lenses, wash the eye before trying to remove lenses. If the lens does not come out during irrigation, carefully remove the lens with a lens removal suction cup. If lens is adherent, leave it in place for an ophthalmologist to remove and continue irrigation of the eye. When the lens is removed, the eye should be thoroughly irrigated again.

Electrical injuries

- Electrical injuries are different from thermal or chemical wounds; in electrical injuries there may be little superficial tissue loss with massive muscle injury underlying normal-looking skin (Fig. 30-10).
- These wounds should be gently cleansed with water or saline solution and 0.25 strength povidone iodine (Betadine).
- There is rarely any need to debride the wound immediately.
- These wounds should be handled minimally. Cadaver-like limbs should not be moved about or manipulated because large patent vessels may be torn and massive hemorrhage may occur.
- Topical agents that penetrate deeply, such as mafenide acetate (Sulfamylon), should be used to cover the wound.
- Light dressings may be applied to cover these often grotesque wounds; however, do not apply dressings if

they impair observation of extremities for the development of compartment syndrome.

- Because of possible muscle damage, injured extremities should be observed for compartment syndrome. Symptoms may include the following:

  Pain

  Pallor

  Paresthesia

  Decreased motor function

  Decreased pulse

- Fasciotomies are performed to relieve compartment syndrome. These procedures are usually performed when the patient has received general anesthesia so that all compartments can be completely explored. This procedure can be painful, since the incisions are often made through normal skin.
- Fasciotomies are left open, covered with a topical antibacterial agent, and dressed with a light dressing after surgery.

Tar or asphalt burns

- Tar or asphalt burns may be deep or superficial, depending on the temperature of the tar, which may range from 150° to 600° F or more (Figs. 30-11 and 30-12).
- Cool the tar with cool liquids.
- Do not try to peel off the tar.
- Remove the tar by loosening with mineral oil, petroleum jelly (Vaseline), or a solvent such as Medi-Sol. Removal can be accomplished in areas of noncircumferential burns by applying the oil or ointment and a light dressing, removing the dressing after 4 to 12 hours, and reapplying the oil or ointment and a dressing.
- For circumferential areas, the oil or ointment can be

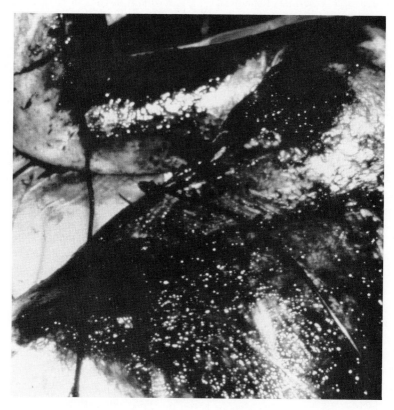

Fig. 30-11   Tar burns of chest before removal of tar.

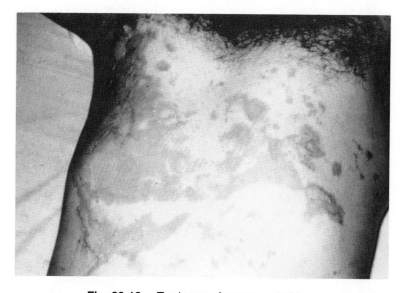

Fig. 30-12   Tar burns after removal of tar.

applied with light dressings and changed every 20 to 30 minutes until the tar is removed.
- Then the wound can be treated as a thermal or chemical wound.

NURSING DIAGNOSES FOR THE PATIENT WITH THERMAL INJURY
Fluid Volume Deficit

Defining characteristics

The following parameters should be assessed closely; if present, they indicate a low-flow state:
- Increased pulse
- Decreased blood pressure
- Increased respirations
- Central venous pressure below 3 cm H_2O
- Decreased urine output
- Hematocrit above 50 mg/dl
- Diminished capillary refill
- Restlessness or confusion
- Nausea or vomiting
- Ileus

Nursing interventions
- Monitor assessment guidelines.
- Initiate IV therapy.
- Adjust intravenous flow rates or administer fluids.
- Maintain accurate fluid intake and output record.
- Ensure safe and accurate function of all monitoring equipment.
- Notify physician if assessment guidelines cannot be maintained without an increase of more than 20% of ordered flow rates or quantities of fluid.
- Secure all IV lines to prevent dislodgement. (IV lines that must penetrate a burn wound should be sutured in place.)
- Apply aseptic technique when handling and maintaining invasive lines to reduce chance of infection.

Evaluation
- Assessment guidelines are maintained within normal limits.
- Patient receives prescribed or needed volume of fluid during an appropriate time period.

Fluid Volume Excess

Fluid volume excess may be a significant complication in children or patients with preexisting cardiac disease.

Defining characteristics
- Increased central venous pressure
- Increased pulmonary capillary wedge pressure
- Decreased pulse
- Dyspnea

Nursing interventions
- Monitor assessment guidelines, especially central venous pressure, pulmonary capillary wedge pressure, confusion, dyspnea, and inadequate oxygenation.
- Report significant changes in assessment guidelines.
- Adjust intravenous fluid flow rates.
- Administer oxygen as necessary.

Evaluation
- Volume excess is recognized promptly and treated.

Impaired Gas Exchange

Impaired gas exchange could result from carbon monoxide intoxication, upper airway obstruction, inhalation of chemical irritants, or circumferential chest wall burns.

Defining characteristics
- Dyspnea
- Agitation
- Confusion
- Somnolence
- Increased respiratory rate
- Cyanosis
- Increased pulse rate
- Decreased blood pressure
- Alterations in blood gas levels
- Increased carbon monoxide level on carboxyhemoglobin measurement
- Hoarseness
- Edema and redness of posterior pharynx
- Carbonaceous sputum
- Full thickness circumferential burns of the chest wall

Nursing interventions
- Recognize risk factors (possible smoke inhalation or chest wall burns).
- Monitor the following respiratory guidelines:
  Rate and character of breathing
  Increasing hoarseness
  Difficulty in handling secretion
  Difficulty with chest wall expansion
- Monitor patient for signs of airway obstruction.
- Observe for carbonaceous sputum.
- If appropriate, measure blood gas levels and evaluate partial pressure of oxygen, partial pressure of carbon dioxide, and pH concentration.
- If patient is intubated, secure tube to prevent extubation. (Prevent excessive pressure on lateral wall of nares to prevent necrosis. Also, pad injured areas on face and ears to eliminate pressure necrosis.)
- Maintain ventilator settings for appropriate function.
- Explain procedure to allay patient's fears of procedures or equipment.
- Provide patient with a method to communicate his or her needs.
- Suction as necessary to assist with elimination of secretions.
- Perform aseptic maintenance of all suction and ventilation equipment.
- Administer sedatives or pain medication as appropriate to allay anxiety and assist patient to cooperate with ventilator.

Evaluation
- Impending respiratory problems are recognized promptly and corrected.
- Assessment guidelines are returned to normal limits.
- Patients requiring intubation are managed safely, and fear and anxiety are diminished.

Potential for Infection

Defining characteristics
- Presence of burn wound
- Need for invasive procedures

Nursing interventions
- Provide an aseptic environment.
- Cleanse and debride wound.
- Apply topical antibacterial therapy.
- Cleanse nonburned areas.
- Administer tetanus prophylaxis and systemic antibiotics as prescribed.
- Provide aseptic management of all invasive lines and procedures.
- Avoid IV lines in leg veins to avoid risk of thrombophlebitis.

Evaluation
- Patient's wounds and environment are managed aseptically.
- Topical and systemic antibiotics are administered in a timely, safe manner to prevent infection.

Altered Tissue Perfusion

Altered tissue perfusion could result from circumferential full thickness burns, compartment syndrome, or general low-flow state.

Defining characteristics
- Edema of extremities
- Full thickness circumferential burns of the extremities
- Electrical injuries

Nursing interventions
- Recognize potential risk factors in patients (full thickness circumferential burns, electrical injury, other muscle trauma, or low-flow states) and the frequent combination of several risk factors.
- Restore adequate fluid volume state as prescribed
- Monitor extremities for the following:
  Capillary refill
  Pulses distal to area of injury
  Pain or paresthesias
  Decreased nerve and muscle function
  Cyanosis of unburned distal areas
- Elevate extremities slightly to reduce edema unless compartment syndrome is suspected. Elevating arms and legs more than 30 to 40 degrees may lead to increased edema formation.
- If compartment syndrome is suspected, keep extremities level but not dependent.
- If escharotomies or fasciotomies are needed, prepare

patient by explaining the procedure and perform the following procedures:
  Administer pain medication or sedatives as prescribed.
  Prepare sterile equipment and assist with the procedure.
  If patient is to go to the operating room for a fasciotomy, prepare the patient for surgery.
- Protect extremities with decreased circulation and neurologic functions from additional injury. (Avoid pressure from constricting bed clothing or restraints.)

Evaluation
- Signs of decreased tissue perfusion are prevented or diagnosed quickly and treated quickly.
- Additional tissue loss is prevented.
- If escharotomies or fasciotomies are required, these are accomplished under aseptic conditions with the least discomfort possible to the patient.

Pain

Defining characteristics
- Complaint of pain
- Nonverbal expression of pain
- Agitation

Nursing interventions
- Observe for and record objective and subjective data consistently.
- Administer medications as prescribed and as requested.
- Assist patient and family to understand various pharmacologic and nonpharmacologic therapies that may help to relieve pain.

Evaluation
- Objective signs and subjective complaints of pain diminish.
- Patient feels that he or she has control over pain management.

Fear, Anxiety, and Spiritual Distress: Secondary to Potential Loss of Life, Body Image Change, or Ability to Work

Defining characteristics
- Verbalization of fear of loss of life, disfigurement, or other losses
- Restlessness
- Increased muscle tension
- Increased verbalizations
- Increased information-seeking
- Narrow focus of attention
- Expressions of anger
- Expressions of anger with God

Nursing interventions
- Encourage the patient to discuss fears or anxiety.
- Explain why painful procedures must be performed, and give patient a time frame for when the pain will lessen.

- Maintain an accepting but hopeful outlook when the patient discusses problems or lashes out at staff.
- Encourage family, friends, and business associates to maintain close contact with the patient.

Evaluation

- Patient is able to talk freely about fears and anxiety.
- Patient and family feel supported by the staff.

REFERENCES

1. Artz CP, Moncrief JA: *Burns: a team approach,* Philadelphia, 1979, WB Saunders.
2. Dimling RH: Early pulmonary abnormalities from smoke inhalation, *JAMA* 251:771, 1984.
3. Moylan JA, Chan CK: Inhalation injury: an increasing problem, *Ann Surg* 188:34, 1978.

Interfacility Transport

Sidney Salvatore

STABILIZATION AND TRANSPORT

Interfacility transport becomes necessary when a seriously ill or injured patient requires advanced skills or equipment not available at an institution. The emergency department (ED) must be prepared to make rapid assessments to identify those who need definitive care at another facility. To make appropriate decisions about transport, one must have current knowledge of resources, including tertiary facilities and emergency medical service (EMS) systems. Advance organization ensures that the patient is transported according to established standards that provide an optimal outcome.

ORGANIZATION BEFORE TRANSPORT
Knowledge of Resources

Every ED is occasionally involved with organizing and carrying out an interfacility transfer. Effective organization should include assessment of the facility's capabilities, understanding of other facilities' capabilities, and in-depth knowledge of available EMS systems. Integrating these factors into the transfer system requires work well in advance of the actual transport.

Assessing your own institution. To recognize patients who would benefit from transfer, an objective assessment of the referring institution's personnel and facilities must be made. The qualifications and availability of physicians and nurses needed to care for all patients who come to the ED must be examined. Facilities to be assessed include the intensive care unit, the operating room, and pediatric, obstetric, neonatal, and psychiatric units. The ability to perform advanced diagnostic testing and to provide adequate blood and blood products must be analyzed. All these factors influence the level of care available to sick or injured patients. Changes in any of these factors must be communicated to the ED staff to ensure prompt recognition of patients requiring transfer for proper management of their care.

Assessing receiving institutions. Understanding the capabilities of the receiving institution's personnel and facilities is part of the responsibility of the referring institution. Determining which facility best meets the patient's needs can be expedited by creating guidelines for transfer in advance. The care of trauma patients at centers designated for that purpose improves patient outcome. Trauma center designation by the American College of Surgeons Committee on Trauma predetermines the response capabilities of receiving centers. An adequate system for trauma care should include access to the proper trauma center.

Neonates at high risk are best cared for in the neonatal intensive care unit (NICU) designated for that purpose. Hospitals not having a neonatal intensive care unit may need to transfer neonates to obtain optimal care.

A coordinated plan between the transferring and receiving institutions should include criteria for transfer, contact phone numbers, and requirements for stabilization and effective transfer. Having a plan avoids unnecessary delays. Other special areas to assess in advance are limb reimplantation centers, burn care, and eye care.

In addition to careful assessment of the medical assessments of the medical resources available to patients at the referring and receiving institutions, there must be a clear plan for emergency transportation for patients in need of interfacility transfer. It is the responsibility of the referring institution to be thoroughly familiar with the modes of transport and their capabilities, available equipment, and length of time for transfer.

Transfer time may make the difference in the outcome for a critically ill or injured patient. The decision whether to use air or ground transport for interfacility transport must be made on the basis of many factors. An informed decision can be made if the advantages and disadvantages are examined carefully. Factors such as out-of-hospital time, weather, terrain, work space, equipment, personnel, and proximity of landing site to the facility influence such decisions. Many institutions have hospital-based flight programs with a staff ready to respond when needed. Other communities have aircraft that can be used with advance notice. A close examination of the resources available allows for a more organized approach when an emergency arises. (See Chapter 32 for information about aeromedical transport.)

To provide advanced care for the patient with a critical

illness or injury, the transport team may need to have personnel prepared to provide a higher level of care than is available through their community's EMS. Personnel might include nurses, physicians, or a respiratory therapist. Each situation may require particular expertise. Advance training for these transports is advantageous. Hospital personnel accompanying patients should have forms for documenting the care delivered en route.

Legal Responsibilities

The act of transferring a patient from one facility to another should be well documented and should be within the legal guidelines established by each institution. Transfer protocols that satisfy the requirements of federal legislation (COBRA) should be established by each hospital. These requirements state that there must be physician-to-physician contact before the transfer and that the receiving institution agrees to accept the patient. The risks and benefits of a transfer must be explained to the patient (or his or her legal representative), and a consent form must be signed to indicate that the patient has been informed. A copy of the consent form and records of care must accompany the patient to the receiving hospital.

Financial Considerations

The financial considerations that affect the transfer of patients often influence where and how patients are transferred. Third-party reimbursement usually provides coverage for a medically needed transfer to another institution. Knowledge of potential financial problems helps avoid unnecessary delays at the time of the transfer decision. The patient's chart should reflect the need for services that are not available at the referring institution to justify the transfer for reimbursement.

STEPS IN ARRANGING TRANSFERS

The patient who must be transferred needs stabilization and a plan for effective transfer. While the patient is being medically stabilized, the transfer system should be initiated. The following is a list of the components that make up an interfacility transfer:

1. Physician-to-physician communication
2. Selection of proper transport mode
3. Appropriate personnel to accompany patient
4. Plan of care during transfer, including physician's orders
5. Specific drugs and equipment needed for patient care
6. Explanation of transfer given to patient or relative
7. Consent for transfer signed by the patient or relative
8. Patient care data, including record of care, medical findings, interventions, radiographs, consent forms, and specimens
9. Travel directions and maps to the receiving facility, given to relatives
10. Communication with the receiving nursing unit

STABILIZING THE PATIENT IN PREPARATION FOR TRANSFER

The preparation necessary for the interfacility transfer of ill or injured patients depends on the specific illness, injury, age, and circumstance. Potential problems during transport must be anticipated before departure and proper interventions made at the referring institution so that patients are sent in stable condition. The special needs of trauma patients, as well as the needs of cardiac, elderly, neonatal, and obstetric patients, must be recognized. Most of the following interventions can be applied to any situation.

Airway

Airway patency during transport is of primary importance. Potential airway compromise must be anticipated before transport so that the proper interventions can be accomplished under controlled circumstances rather than in the transport vehicle.

Endotracheal intubation should be considered in patients who have the potential to aspirate, have difficulty with chest expansion, or are in need of hyperventilation. Examples of patients with the potential for airway compromise as a result of secretions include those with an altered level of consciousness, facial fractures, epiglottitis, or inhalation burns. Difficulty with chest expansion is another indication for intubation before transfer. Patients with a chest wall injury, spinal cord injury, or neurologic dysfunction may require ventilatory assistance.

Chest Tubes

Chest tube placement may be accomplished before transport if there is potential for a pneumothorax or hemothorax. A closed drainage system or flutter valve should be in place and secured to avoid retrograde recurrence of a pneumothorax.

Gastric Tubes

The need for gastric tube placement must be considered to protect the airway from stomach contents being aspirated, as well as to prevent ineffective ventilation resulting from an elevated diaphragm when the stomach fills with air (gastric dilation). The nasogastric tube is contraindicated in cases such as nasal trauma or suspected cribriform plate fracture. (An orogastric tube should be considered in such cases.) Gastric contents can be suctioned en route by using ambulance suction equipment. A second suction device must be available for airway suction. The gastric tube should be well secured before departure.

HEMODYNAMIC STABILIZATION

To stabilize patients adequately before interfacility transport, one must intervene as necessary to maintain an adequate pulse rate and blood pressure. Patients in shock or at risk for developing shock require the following interventions.

Control of Bleeding

Control of external bleeding sites with pressure or wound closure may be necessary. The use of splints for long bone fractures and the pneumatic antishock garment (PASG), if not contraindicated, for pelvic injuries provide stability and pressure to control bleeding. Applying the PASG before loading the patient and inflating the garment as needed are preferable to attempting to apply the garment in a moving vehicle.

Correction of Hypovolemia Resulting from Fluid Loss

Proper intravenous (IV) access is needed to replace fluid loss as part of the stabilization process. Large-bore IV cannulas (14-gauge or 16-gauge peripherally or 8.5-gauge subclavian) with blood or trauma tubing provide rapid fluid resuscitation routes as needed. Having more than one IV route during transport avoids the need for a restart while in a moving vehicle. The use of plastic IV bags for fluid enables one to use pressure bags when they are required. Blood that has been prepared for transport and placed in a cooler accompanies the patient.

Insertion of a Bladder Catheter

Patients requiring fluid management should have a bladder catheter placed and attached to a urimeter to properly measure urinary output. Catheterization is contraindicated when there is blood at the meatus, indicating possible urethral damage. In this case a urethrogram should be performed before catheter insertion. In addition to permitting measurement of output, bladder drainage decreases patient discomfort during a long transport.

Cardiac Monitoring

The cardiac status of the patient who is about to be transferred must be determined before transport. An electrocardiogram and rhythm strip should be obtained before departure to determine whether the patient needs any intervention before transport. Continuous monitoring should take place en route.

CENTRAL NERVOUS SYSTEM STABILIZATION

All attempts should be made to stabilize the patient's neurologic condition by attempting to maintain normal intracranial pressure, controlling seizure activity, and preserving the integrity of the spinal cord. Precautions may include consultation with the receiving neurologist to determine proper interventions such as medications, patient position, and ventilation regimen.

Hyperventilation

Control of intracranial pressure in the head-injured patient should include hyperventilation. Ventilation is adequate when the carbon dioxide level is maintained at 28 torr for adults and 20 to 22 torr for children.

Medication

The use of diuretics to control intracranial pressure is determined by the neurosurgeon at the receiving center. Patients with spinal cord involvement may receive methylprednisolone to prevent spinal cord edema as soon after their injury as possible. Patients requiring seizure control should initially be managed with medications in the ED, and appropriate safety precautions should be taken before transport.

Immobilization

Trauma patients who have received injuries that may involve the spinal column should be immobilized on a backboard with a rigid cervical collar, 2-inch tape, and other immobilization devices. The patient should be strapped to the board in such a way that he or she could be turned if vomiting occurs. Spinal precautions should be taken whenever there is the slightest possibility of spinal injury.

SKELETAL SYSTEM STABILIZATION

Care of patients with skeletal injuries should include pain management and immobilization of fractures to prevent blood loss, neurovascular damage, and microembolization.

Immobilization

Appropriate splints permit assessment of distal pulse rates during transport. Air splints have pressure changes during air transport and should not be used. Pelvic fractures may be immobilized with the use of the PASG. Traction splints for femur fractures provide comfort and prevent microembolization. Be aware that traction splints, because of their length, can sometimes be difficult to fit into the transport vehicle. This possibility should be determined in advance.

Preservation of Amputated Parts

Patients being transferred for limb reimplantation need special care. The amputated part should be wrapped in gauze moistened with normal saline solution and placed in a container that can be kept on ice in a cooler. It is important that the amputated part not be placed directly on the ice or in solutions, to avoid tissue destruction.

Wound Care

Depending on the severity of the patient's other injuries, wound care should be limited to the control of bleeding, initial cleansing, and application of sterile dressings. Wounds that will be sutured at the receiving institution may require sterile saline dressings to keep the tissues moist.

Burn Care

Estimation of the percentage of body surface burned should be completed and recorded. Burns should be dressed with dry sterile dressings in accordance with local burn protocols. Moist dressings promote heat loss, and sterility is difficult to maintain. Remove rings or constricting clothing. Constriction and impairment of circulation of burned extremities and chest can occur in severe burns. The need for a fasciotomy before transfer should be considered.

Medications

Tetanus prophylaxis, including tetanus immune globulin, should be administered before transport as necessary. The use of antibiotics is indicated in some cases and should begin as soon as possible after the injury. A culture of the wound before administration of antibiotics is appropriate in some cases.

EMOTIONAL STABILIZATION AND PSYCHOSOCIAL SUPPORT

The patient who is about to be transferred and has been physically stabilized has many needs. Nurses can address these needs by recognizing that the patient may have many fears and questions. Providing information about what is happening and explaining what will take place during transport may decrease the level of fear. Speaking in a calm manner reassures the patient that the situation is under control. Maps and written directions to the receiving facility should be given to the family. Advise them concerning speed and distance from the transport vehicle to avoid an accident. If the patient is unstable, advise the family to stay at the original hospital until the patient is actually transported, in case the patient worsens and cannot survive the transport.

To reduce the patient's stress, the family should be allowed to visit before the patient is transferred. Parents should be allowed to hold or touch their children before the transport. If possible, a picture should be taken of a newborn so that the mother who cannot accompany her child has something to keep and the bonding process can continue while the two are separated.

BASELINE DIAGNOSTIC STUDIES

The studies necessary for stabilization depend on the severity and type of the illness or injury. Each situation has different priorities. Baseline studies that are needed to make proper decisions regarding transfer should be performed while the system of transfer is being put into effect. In severely injured patients, only those tests which affect the airway, breathing, and circulation should be performed.

The American College of Surgeons Committee on Trauma recommends performing the following studies, as time permits:

1. Radiographs of the cervical spine, chest, pelvis, and extremities that may be injured.
2. Laboratory tests, including measurements of hemoglobin content, hematocrit, and arterial blood levels, urinalysis, toxic screens and measurement of blood alcohol content, and blood typing and crossmatching
3. Electrocardiogram

Copies of all the data and radiographs should be properly labeled and sent with the patient. Samples of peritoneal fluid, blood, and spinal fluid, when indicated, should accompany the patient. Laboratory data not completed at the time of transfer should be called or sent by "fax" machine to the receiving center.

DOCUMENTATION THAT ACCOMPANIES THE PATIENT

Records that should accompany the patient include the following:

1. Prehospital care record
2. ED record of care
3. Medical history if available
4. Results of laboratory studies
5. Copies of radiographs
6. Transfer record
7. Protocol or orders used during transfer
8. Transfer consent form

EQUIPMENT

The following equipment is needed for maintaining stability in ill or injured patients during transport. The nurse should be familiar with the operation of the equipment in the vehicle and extra equipment that is brought to provide care for particular patients.

Equipment Needed for Transport

Airways
  Nasal airway adjuncts
  Oropharyngeal airway adjuncts
  Endotracheal or nasotracheal tubes
Oxygen delivery system
  Oxygen
  Oxygen tubing
  Oxygen cannulas
  Oxygen masks
  Bag-valve-mask device
  Demand valve
  Ventilator
  Pulse oximeter
Suction equipment
  Suction catheters
  Catheter-tip syringe for gastric tube
IV equipment
  IV fluids and pump
  IV restart equipment
  Pressure infusion bag
PASG
Doppler device or sensitive stethoscope
Cardiac monitoring and resuscitation equipment
  Cardiac monitor and defibrillator
  Defibrillator pads
  Recording paper

Table 31-1   Duration of cylinder flow

Cylinder	2 L/min	4 L/min	6 L/min	8 L/min	10 L/min	12 L/min	15 L/min
E	5.1 hr	2.5 hr	1.7 hr	1.2 hr	1.0 hr	0.8 hr	0.6 hr
H	56 hr	28 hr	18.5 hr	14 hr	11 hr	9.2 hr	7.2 hr

Emergency medications
Restraints

Oxygen supply must be available for the duration of the transfer in sufficient amounts to care for the patient (Table 31-1).

MANAGEMENT OF CARE DURING INTERFACILITY TRANSFER

The emergency nurse accompanying the ill or injured patient must coordinate the care of the patient during the transfer. The care taken to properly stabilize the patient in the ED prepares for a smoother transfer for the patient. Continual assessment and intervention must take place to keep the patient as stable as possible. Proper communication and documentation while en route provides continuity of care.

Assessment

Continual assessment of the patient during transport may be limited as a result of noise and vibration. The use of oximeters to determine oxygenation and cardiac monitors to determine pulse rate and rhythm is of great benefit. Observation of color, temperature, and distal pulse rates of injured extremities is necessary. An ultrasound stethoscope is helpful when auscultation is difficult. One may have to rely on palpation for blood pressure measurement. Observing the patient's urinary output during transfer is another assessment tool. The patient's level of consciousness should be evaluated and recorded frequently. Lung sounds, temperature of the neonate and Isolette, fetal heart tones, and motor function should also be monitored.

Interventions

To maintain patient stability, the nurse must be prepared to undertake proper interventions as needed during transport. Protocols and physician's orders regarding these interventions clarify for the transporting team what is expected of them. Examples of interventions that may be needed include the following: securing the airway, suctioning, turning the patient to avoid aspiration, emptying gastric contents, administering fluid, changing the fluid administration rate, restarting a malfunctioning IV line, performing an emergency needle thoracotomy, applying the PASG, administering medications, performing advanced life support measures, and restraining the patient for safety. It is also necessary to plan the course of action if the patient's condition deteriorates while en route. Facilities that are located between the referring and receiving facilities could be used in case of unforeseen circumstances.

Evaluation

The patient must be assessed after each intervention. Response to interventions should be documented. Patient comfort needs should be assessed often, and measures should be taken to alleviate the patient's discomforts and fears.

Communication

Ideally the transport team is able to communicate adequately during the transport to keep the receiving facility aware of the patient's condition. Any interventions needed at the referral center can then be planned.

Documentation

Having a form that is used specifically for transfer (Fig. 31-1) enables proper documentation of the care rendered during transport and the patient's response to interventions. Keep a copy of this document, and return it to the patient's record at the referring facility. This procedure ensures that the record of care is complete.

TRANSFER OF CARE ON ARRIVAL AT THE RECEIVING FACILITY

To ensure that transfer of care of the patient is complete, the nurse should accompany the patient to the receiving unit. A report concerning the patient's condition, recent assessment, and interventions should be given to the nursing staff. Copies of the transfer data, history, laboratory values, radiographs, electrocardiograms, consent forms, and specimens should be included. Information about which relatives have been informed and which ones are expected to arrive would be helpful information to the nurse receiving the patient. Delivering care in the receiving hospital is the responsibility of the employees at the receiving facility and should not be delegated to the transferring nurse after arrival. Be sure to have a closing interaction with the patient, and provide an update concerning the patient's condition to the family before departing. If the nurse wishes to receive a follow-up report on the patient, it should be requested, and the nurse's name and phone number should be left with the nurse who receives the patient.

Name _____

Address _____

Transferring hospital _____

Referring physician _____

Contact person for follow-up care _____

_____

Receiving hospital _____

_____

Notified by _____

Receiving physician _____

Patient report called to _____

By _____

Date of transfer _____   Time _____

Date of birth _____

Telephone _____

Telephone _____

Telephone _____

Accepted ☐ Yes ☐ No

Time _____

Family notified
ID band placed
Valuables sent
Transfer consent
IV sites labelled

Emergency medical condition   Mechanism of injury   **History and allergies**

Management

C-spine control _____ Backboard _____

NG _____ Chest Tube (R) _____ (L) _____

Airway _____

Oxygen _____ % _____

Procedures _____

_____

Other _____

_____

Intake Total _____ Foley _____

Output Total _____ Other _____

Crystalloid _____ Colloid _____

Medication summary
List meds, total dose, time of last dose

D.T. _____

Sent with patient

CAT Scan   ED Record
X-ray Films   EKG
Med. Record   DPL Results
Nsg. Flow Sheet   Ex. Spec.
Lab Results

Enroute vital signs

Temperature _____

Date Time	B/P	P	Resp	Mntr Ptrn	Pupils	Enroute therapy and response

Transfer team members and titles _____

Form completed by _____

Patient has been informed and agrees to transfer. _____

(Patient signature)

Fig. 31-1   Interhospital transfer form. (From Maine Emergency Nurses Association.)

SUMMARY

Transferring patients routinely or urgently requires a great deal of organization and communication between facilities. Having in place a working system that is evaluated frequently ensures a safe and beneficial transfer of the patient.

SUGGESTED READINGS

American College of Surgeons: *Advanced trauma life support student manual,* Chicago, 1988, The College.

American College of Surgeons Committee on Trauma: *Resources for optimal care for the injured patient,* Chicago, 1990, The College.

American Heart Association: *Advanced cardiac life support manual,* Dallas, 1981, The Association.

American Heart Association: *Pediatric advanced life support student manual,* 1988, The Association.

Boyd CR, Corse KM, Campbell RC: Emergency interhospital transport of the major trauma patient: air versus ground, *J Trauma* 29:789, 1989.

Chatburn RL, Lough MD, Schrock WA: *Handbook of respiratory care,* Chicago, 1983, Mosby–Year Book.

Cogbill TH, et al: Acute gastric dilatation after trauma, *J Trauma* 27:1113, 1987.

Emergency Nurses Association: *Emergency nursing core curriculum,* ed 3, 1987, WB Saunders.

Emergency Nurses Association: *Standards of emergency nursing practice,* St Louis, 1990, Mosby–Year Book.

Harrahil M, Bartkus E: Preparing the trauma patient for transport, *JEN* 16:25, 1990.

Martin GD, et al: Prospective analysis of rural interhospital transfer of injured patients to a referral trauma center, *J Trauma* 30:1014, 1990.

Omnibus Budget Reconciliation Act of 1989, Pub. L. No. 101-239, Washington, DC, Government Printing Office.

Sheehy SB, Marvin JA, Jimmerson CL: *Manual of clinical trauma care: the first hour,* St Louis, 1989, Mosby–Year Book.

Wayne R: Rural trauma management, *Am J Surg* 157:463, 1989.

CHAPTER 32

Aeromedical Transport

Susan Engman Lazear

Aeromedical transport of patients has developed into a subspecialty of emergency care. Caring for the sick and injured during transport should be performed by skilled individuals who have a knowledge of flight physiology and the nursing interventions instituted to reduce the impact of complications that may develop.

Air transport is regulated, in part, by the Federal Aviation Administration (FAA) and is accomplished by using either fixed-wing (airplane) or rotary-wing (helicopter) vehicles. The advantage of fixed-wing transport is the ability to travel long distances at speeds of more than 250 miles per hour. Care is provided in a pressurized cabin with sophisticated on-board medical equipment. Many aircraft have the capability of transporting multiple patients, and in some instances family members are allowed to accompany the patient. All-weather navigational equipment allows for the transfer of patients during inclement weather.

Fixed-wing transport requires suitable airfields to ensure the safety of the crew and patient. Accessibility to such fields may be a problem in isolated areas. Rarely are patients injured at an airfield; thus their transfer by ground ambulance to the aircraft is necessary. However, the benefits of air transport greatly outweigh the delays these transfers may cause.

Rotary-wing vehicles provide rapid point-to-point transport. Helicopters can reach most areas and can bypass difficult terrain. Landing zones can be made at or near the site of the patient to prevent lengthy ground transport times. Most helicopters operate within 150 miles of their base station to allow for routine trips without refueling.

One of the disadvantages of helicopters is the dependence on certain minimum conditions of weather; if these conditions are not met, the weather can cause delay or cancellation of the flight. Helicopter cabin size often restricts access to the patient, limiting in-flight interventions. Weight limitations restrict the number of passengers and amount of equipment that can be put on board. In transfers by rotary-wing vehicles, comprehensive stabilization of the patient is required before departure.

Patients who benefit from air transport are those whose medical needs exceed the capabilities of the local hospital, including patients requiring specialized medical or surgical interventions, equipment, or personnel. Rotary-wing vehicles are also used to expedite transfer of a patient from a remote area to the nearest health care facility. All patients can be cared for during air transport, and no patient should be excluded from consideration based on illness or injury.

FLIGHT PHYSIOLOGY

Exposure to environmental factors occurs during the air transport of patients. The problems encountered depend on changes in atmospheric conditions, vehicle design and configurations, motion of the aircraft, and the patient's condition. Some of these can be detrimental to the patient, but with proper nursing care before and during transport, these harmful effects can be minimized or eliminated.

Atmospheric changes occur when the aircraft's altitude changes. Ascending into the atmosphere from sea level causes a decrease in the atmospheric pressure, which in turn causes a decrease in the partial pressure of gases, a decrease in temperature, and an expansion of gases. The opposite occurs during descent. Many of these effects are minimal unless the change in altitude is greater than 5000 feet.

Fixed-wing and rotary-wing vehicles are designed according to different principles. Most fixed-wing aircraft used in patient transport are pressurized, which allows for a comfortable cabin atmosphere when flying at high altitudes. Pressurization differentials allow for different cabin pressures at different atmospheres. Generally the lower the altitude at which a plane is flying, the lower the cabin pressure that can be achieved. This ability to maintain a physiologically comfortable environment within the aircraft is a benefit when transporting patients who may have been affected by atmospheric changes. Although pressurization allows for flights at high altitudes, even subtle changes in the environment may be harmful to a person whose condition is severely compromised.

If the pressurization system were to fail, the pressurization within the cabin might be lost, causing a sudden change in atmospheric pressure. This rapid decompression causes the interior of the cabin to equalize with the pressures outside the cabin, resulting in sudden and often detrimental effects on the human body. There would be a rapid loss of oxygen, a sudden drop in temperature, and an expansion of gas. A healthy individual may be able to withstand these changes, but the condition of an individual who is compromised may deteriorate quickly. It is in the best interest of those transporting patients to be aware of these effects and do all that can be done before departure to minimize complications.

Rotary-wing vehicles are not pressurized; therefore these atmospheric changes are felt whenever the helicopter ascends and descends. Thus patients who are transported by helicopter may be at greater risk than those transported by fixed-wing aircraft.

There are four problems that develop in transport as a result of changes in atmospheric pressure: hypoxia, gas expansion, dehydration, and decreased temperature. Other problems that affect patient outcomes are influenced by the motion of the vehicle and the constraints resulting from vehicle design.

Hypoxia

Many of the patients transported by air are hypoxic as a result of their disease state. This hypoxic state is potentiated when changes in atmospheric pressure are encountered. As an aircraft ascends in altitude, the partial pressure of oxygen (PO_2) decreases, thereby causing a decreased diffusion gradient for the oxygen molecule to cross the alveolar membrane. Table 32-1 shows the effects of altitude on the PO_2.

Simple calculation of the diffusion gradient is accomplished by using the following formulas:

(Atmospheric pressure − Water pressure) ×

(percentage of oxygen) = PO_2

and

Alveolar PO_2 − Venous PO_2 = Diffusion gradient

Assuming that the water pressure is equal to 47 mm Hg, the PO_2 at sea level would be 150 mm Hg: $(760 − 74) \times (0.21) = 150$. At an altitude of 6000 feet the calculated PO_2 would be 118 mm Hg: $(609 − 47) \times (.21) = 118$ mm Hg.

The decrease in PO_2 that occurs in the respiratory tree is approximately 45 mm Hg. Therefore, at the alveolar level, the PaO_2 at sea level would be approximately 105 mm Hg and the PaO_2 at 6000 feet would be about 73. The PO_2 of venous blood is approximately 40 mm Hg. Therefore the diffusion gradient at sea level is equal to 65 mm Hg (105 − 40) and at 6000 feet is equal to 33 mm Hg. Patients with congestive heart failure and adult respiratory distress syndrome (ARDS), among others, would be severely compromised when this drop in the diffusion gradient occurs.

Transporting patients by pressurized fixed-wing aircraft can limit the complications that develop as a result of this drop in the PO_2. Most aircraft used for air transport are able to maintain a sea level cabin pressure when flying below 7000 to 10,000 feet. At higher altitudes the cabin can be pressurized; the maximum cabin pressure altitude is generally maintained below 9000 feet. Therefore, when cabin pressures are controlled the atmospheric changes that occur are limited, controlled, and within a tolerable range.

Patients with disease-induced hypoxia are at increased risk of compromise during aeromedical transport. These patients include those with congestive heart failure, ARDS, and carbon monoxide poisoning; those in hypovolemic shock with an adequate amount of circulating hemoglobin; and those with stagnant hypoxia induced by low-flow states such as hypothermia. Altitude-induced reduction in the PO_2 causes further deterioration in these patients if interventions are not performed to correct the problems related to hypoxia.

Signs and symptoms of hypoxia include changes in vital signs, tachycardia, pupillary constriction, confusion, disorientation, and lethargy. All these signs may be caused by a number of other illnesses and injuries, making the diagnosis of hypoxia more difficult. Astute observation of the patient is necessary to detect and correct the problems of hypoxia.

Before transporting the patient, stabilization measures can be taken to help reduce the effects of atmospheric changes in oxygenation. Supplemental oxygen can be provided, and if the patient has previously been requiring oxygen, the percentage of oxygen can be increased. This increase in oxygen delivery is performed as a prophylactic, temporary measure during the transport; when the patient arrives at the

Table 32-1 Effects of altitude on partial pressure of ambient oxygen

Altitude (feet)	Atmospheric pressure (mm Hg)	Partial pressure of ambient oxygen (PO_2)
0	760	150
500	746	146
1000	733	144
1500	720	141
2000	707	138
2500	694	135
3000	681	133
3500	669	130
4000	656	128
4500	644	125
5000	632	123
5500	621	120
6000	609	118
6500	598	115
7000	586	113
8000	564	108
9000	543	104
10,000	523	100

receiving institution, the oxygen can be decreased or terminated pending the outcome of the arterial blood gas test.

Proper positioning of the patient combats the effects of hypoxia. Ensuring proper chest excursion by loosening the chest restraints on the stretcher allows the patient to breathe easier. In certain aircraft the head of the stretcher can be elevated to an angle of at least 30 degrees; however, in many rotary-wing transports this elevation is not possible because of limited head room.

The hypovolemic patient can receive transfusions to increase the hematocrit and oxygen-carrying capacity of the blood. Patients who are alert are generally anxious regarding their outcome, and this anxiety causes an increased respiratory rate and a decrease in their oxygenation. Providing a calm environment and thoroughly explaining all procedures, noises, and so on can help reduce the patient's feeling of helplessness. Case Study 32-1 demonstrates the effects of altitude changes on a patient.

Calculating the PO_2 of patients in various environments and situations will tell only part of the story: the patient described in the case study, whose cardiac history is extensive, may also be anxious about leaving his loved ones behind and about the prognosis. In addition, although he may feel most comfortable in the sitting position, he must lie flat during the transport. Assessing the patient's vital

---

CASE STUDY 32-1

Effects of Altitude Changes on a Patient

A 58-year-old man requires transport from a small rural hospital to a university medical center for evaluation. He has a long history of cardiac disease and is currently receiving vasopressors for blood pressure support. The referring hospital is located at an altitude of 500 feet, whereas the medical center is at a 4000-foot elevation. During transport the helicopter must fly over a mountain range with peaks at altitudes of more than 6000 feet.

At the referring hospital the patient had a PO_2 of 150 mm Hg when breathing room air. When nasal prongs were used, the PO_2 rose to 178 mm Hg, and the patient's pretransport blood gas levels during use of the nasal prongs were adequate. During transport the helicopter must fly at an altitude of 6500 feet to ensure clearance of the mountains. During the time the patient is at this altitude his PO_2 will drop to 138 mm Hg if use of the nasal prongs is continued. However, to ensure that altitude-induced hypoxia does not develop, a nonrebreather mask can be applied; use of this mask would raise the patient's PO_2 to approximately 400 mm Hg. At the medical center, at an altitude of 4000 feet, the patient's PO_2 when nasal prongs are used would be calculated to be 152 mm Hg; this PO_2 may be inadequate for his current condition, necessitating the use of other oxygen delivery systems.

Table 32-2   Effects of gas expansion on patient condition and medical equipment

	Complications	Therapeutic interventions
PATIENT CONDITION		
Pneumothorax	Air expansion within pleural cavity, causing dyspnea	Insert flutter valve chest tube with water seal drainage
Bowel obstruction	Air expands, causing rupture	Insert nasogastric tube to suction; elevate head of bed
Plugged middle ear	Unable to equalize pressure	Valsalva maneuver in awake patient; ascend and descend slowly
Congested sinuses	Trapped air expands, causing pain	Vasoconstrictor sprays
Open skull fracture	Air in cranial cavity expands, causing herniation	Implement hyperventilation measures to reduce intracranial pressure
Colostomies, ileostomies	Air in bowel expands, causing increased motility	Insert rectal tube for decompression; change bag frequently
Gas gangrene	Air expands within tissues, leading to necrosis	Incision and drainage
Dental caries	Pain caused by air expansion	Administer local anesthetic
EQUIPMENT		
PASG, air splints	Air expands: pressure within garment or splints increases	Decrease volume at altitude
IV bottles	Air within bottle expands: fluid does not flow	Use plastic IV bags
Endotracheal tube cuffs	Air expands, causing tracheal necrosis	Decrease volume at altitude
Foley catheters	Air within drainage system expands: urine does not flow	Use a vent system Irrigate catheter
Oxygen flowmeters	Flow is increased under pressure	Monitor oxygen supply frequently
Volume ventilators	Volume of gas delivered increases	Measure tidal volume

signs and level of consciousness provides the best indicator of how he or she is tolerating the transport. All interventions that can be performed to improve the patient's oxygenation status must be undertaken.

Gas Expansion

According to Boyle's law, a volume of gas is inversely proportional to its pressure. As the transport vehicle ascends, the atmospheric pressure decreases and gas expands. One hundred cubic centimeters of gas at sea level expands to 130 cc at an altitude of 6000 feet, to 200 cc at 18,000 feet, and to 400 cc at 34,000 feet. Gas expansion is a potential problem in all transports in which the aircraft ascends but is especially significant in an unpressurized fixed-wing aircraft flying above 12,000 feet.

Air, which can expand, is found in many places, including the pleural space when a pneumothorax is present, air splints, endotracheal tube cuffs, intravenous fluid bottles, and the pneumatic antishock garment (PASG). Table 32-2 lists various conditions and situations in which gas can expand and the nursing measures that can be taken to reduce the risk of complications.

If measures are taken during ascent to prevent gas expansion, such as removal of air from the PASG, an *opposite* measure must be taken during the aircraft's descent. For example, a patient with multiple traumas requires long-distance transport from a village in Alaska to a trauma center in Washington. The condition of the patient has been stabilized with the use of the PASG before transport. As the aircraft departs from Alaska and ascends to a cruising altitude of 28,000 feet, the cabin pressure rises to approximately 8000 feet. The air that was in the PASG is now increased in volume by at least one third, and most likely the PASG pants are now too tight and are compromising the circulation to the patient's lower extremities. By monitoring the patient's blood pressure, transport personnel can adjust the volume of air in the garment to ensure maximal benefit. During transport the PASG should be monitored continually for changes in pressure to detect both underinflation and overinflation. As the aircraft descends for landing at the receiving airfield, the PASG must be evaluated once again for effectiveness; usually air must be added.

Rotary-wing vehicles that are flying low, over flat terrain, encounter few problems with gas expansion during transport. However, if the transport requires traversing high-altitude areas, the interventions described are essential.

Dehydration

Another problem encountered during an increase in altitude is the drop in ambient humidity. This loss of humidification is enhanced in a pressurized fixed-wing aircraft, since system pressurization is achieved by recycling the air and removing the moisture from it.

Patients who are dehydrated or diaphoretic are at increased risk for dehydration, which can affect fluid volume.

Supplemental intravenous fluids are administered to prevent dehydration.

Other groups of patients affected by dehydration are mouth-breathers and those who are intubated. These patients have lost the natural respiratory humidification mechanisms, and secretions become quite tenacious and difficult to mobilize. Ensuring that humidified oxygen is provided not only prevents this drying of the respiratory tree but also counters the effects of hypoxia.

Decreased Temperature

The standard lapse rate for temperature is that for each 1000-foot gain in altitude, there is a drop of 2 centigrade degrees in temperature until the temperature reaches $-55°$ C. During the aircraft's ascent into the atmosphere, this temperature drop causes a cooling of the aircraft. Although the transport vehicles are heated, the fuselage becomes quite cold and radiates the cold into the interior of the cabin. The coldest area of the aircraft is against the outside walls. This cooling, although most significant during the cold-weather months, is noticeable at all times of the year.

In addition to altitude-induced temperature changes, a number of different environmental conditions affect air transport of patients. Interhospital transports require that the patient be removed from the hospital, transported outside to the helipad or into an ambulance for transfer to the airfield, and subsequently transferred into the transport vehicle. The opposite occurs at the receiving end of the transfer. These multiple transfers expose the patient to constantly changing environmental conditions, including cold weather. The patient whose condition is compromised is less able to tolerate these stresses and exhibits signs and symptoms of cold stress, including a decrease in level of consciousness, increase in heart rate, and shivering. These symptoms increase the patient's oxygen demands, and the previously hypoxic patient becomes increasingly hypoxic.

Awareness of an environmental drop in temperature allows for adequate stabilization before the transport. Minimizing the exposure to environmental conditions by means of efficient transfers is of utmost importance. The interior temperature of the transport vehicle can be controlled and should be set in accordance with the patient's needs, not the needs of the transport crew. Maintaining an adequate supply of linen and wrapping the patient in a rescue (Mylar) blanket is useful in cold environments. Caution should be used with Mylar blankets because their function is to reflect the patient's radiated heat back to him or her; if wrapped too tightly, the patient can become overheated. A cap can be put on the patient to reduce radiated heat losses from the head.

Another effect that occurs with changes in temperature is that gas molecules contract while ambient air cools. This change in gas molecules is similar to that which occurs with a decrease in altitude. The changes in environmental temperature that occur during transport affect the gas expansion within body cavities and equipment, according to Boyle's law. This effect is most notable in the PASG and air splints. When the patient is transferred from a warm hospital interior to the cold air outside, the volume of gas within the garment decreases and the peripheral vasoconstriction effect on the venous system is decreased. As the ambient temperature warms, the garment expands, causing an increase in the patient's blood pressure. This change in gas volume must be compensated for during each change in the environmental conditions.

Other problems that develop with cold environments include the cooling of IV solutions and the crystallization of medications, most notably mannitol. A patient who has cold stress resulting from changes in the environment requires warm IV fluids. Solutions stored in the aircraft or solutions that have been exposed to the environment are quite cold and must be warmed before administration. If possible these solutions should be stored in the warmest spot in the cabin. However, if the solutions remain cold, heat packs can be wrapped around the IV bag to warm the fluid. Some transport programs employ heating pads to keep the fluids warm; the only drawbacks with such a system are the need for electricity to operate the pad and the risk of overheating the fluid, which may render the fluids useless. Mannitol should not be stored in an aircraft that is quite cold; instead, it must be placed in the aircraft before departure.

Acceleration and Deceleration Forces

Acceleration forces occur during takeoff and "climb-out." Blood pools in dependent areas, most commonly the lower extremities, causing fluid shifts that may not be tolerated by the severely compromised patient. Restoration of hemovolemia and proper positioning of the patient can help minimize the effects of these forces.

Deceleration forces occur during slowing, stopping, or rapid descent. For the patient who is lying with head forward in an aircraft, deceleration forces cause blood to pool in the head and upper body. This pooling of blood produces what is known as "redout" as blood rushes to the head, causing an increase in blood within the ocular cavity. Deceleration forces are most harmful to the patient with increased intracranial pressure; the phenomenon may also be severely compromising to the patient with congestive heart failure.

The effects of acceleration and deceleration forces vary with the speed, angle, and duration of the forces. These forces are much more pronounced in a fixed-wing aircraft, although in certain instances the pilots can control these effects, as long as safety measures and regulations are met. If a patient is known to be severely compromised, the transport personnel should discuss this problem with their flight crew. A slow descent is often an option, and if the airfield is long enough, a longer landing roll can be performed to decrease some of the deceleration forces occurring when the aircraft is slowed to a stop.

Positioning of the patient is crucial to counter these forces.

In many aircraft the stretcher restraints are not interchangeable; therefore the patient must be loaded head-first into the cabin. However, if the patient can tolerate a head-elevated position, the effects of these forces can be minimized, since fluid shifts are centered at the core of the body rather than in the periphery.

Rotary-wing vehicles are also subject to acceleration and deceleration forces but these are of much less magnitude than in fixed-wing aircraft. In addition to forward and rearward movement, helicopters are capable of lateral movement; however, forces resulting from these movements are of little consequence. Because of the confined space of the helicopter, positioning of the patient to counteract these forces is usually more difficult, if not impossible; however, pilot control is much greater.

Motion Sickness

Changes in inner ear equilibrium caused by excessive motion can cause motion sickness. Nausea and vomiting may develop in the patient. In addition, the flight crew and transport personnel are also subject to the effects of motion sickness. Prophylactic premedication is the best intervention available to limit these unwanted complications.

Other causes of motion sickness include hypoxia, excessive visual stimuli (such as the blinking lights on the aircraft control panel), stress, fear, unpleasant odors, heat, and poor diet. Gastric gas expansion occurring during ascent can worsen the problem. To prevent or limit these symptoms, transport personnel should provide adequate oxygenation, stare at a fixed visual reference, cool the cabin interior, attempt to limit stressors and fear, and have the patient lie in the supine position.

For crew members who have motion sickness, premedication with transdermal scopolamine is the best treatment. However these patches must be applied within a few hours of departure, and since aeromedical transports are not usually scheduled, this preventive measure may not be possible. Often the crew members "recover" from their motion sickness when they have a patient to care for; it seems to be a question of "mind over matter."

Noise

Transport vehicles are inherently noisy. Engine noises create a constant loud hum that not only is distracting but also can cause an increased level of stress. Reducing extraneous noise is often impossible, but limiting the sound input can be accomplished by the application of earplugs, cotton balls, or headphones. However, when noise reduction devices are used for the patient, all noise is reduced, including communication. The patient who is not able to hear all the conversation may become increasingly agitated, believing that the crew is talking about him or her. It is important to remember to include the conscious patient in as much conversation as is appropriate. In a helicopter, which is extremely noisy, the earpieces of the stethoscope can be inserted into the patient's ears and the crew can speak at the diaphragm to allow for communication with the patient.

Noise also interferes with the ability to hear breath sounds, heart sounds, and blood pressure. Doppler devices are available to assist with detecting blood pressure but are of little use for hearing breath or heart sounds. Other assessment techniques are important in ascertaining adequate ventilation, such as observing for bilateral chest wall movement, using pulse oximetry, and placing the stethoscope over the trachea to listen for air movement.

Although the flight crew may be familiar with noises of the aircraft, it is important to explain all sounds to the patient. Many aircraft have audible warning signals to prevent accidents, but to the patient these alarms may signal that the aircraft is in danger of crashing. A preflight briefing should include the patient, and continual reminders help to alleviate these fears.

Vibration

As a result of vehicle design, aircraft vibrate. The effects of vibration are much more noticeable in a helicopter, especially during takeoff and landing. This constant motion can cause equipment to loosen and become a danger during flight. FAA regulations require that all equipment must be secured during takeoff and landing, but it is wise to keep equipment secured at all times in the event of any unexpected turbulence.

The patient should also be secured to the stretcher at all times. Before loading and unloading the patient from the aircraft, the stretcher restraints should be checked for proper fit. During transport the straps may be loosened to allow the patient to move; however, the restraints should never be fully released.

Continual vibration can also cause changes in equipment settings. Constant jostling can cause knobs to slip, changing the functioning of the machinery. Ventilators are especially prone to this complication, and settings should be checked frequently during flight.

Immobilization

As a result of long transport times, prolonged immobilization of the patient can lead to the development of pressure sores and venous stasis. Space limitations and the inability to change the patient's position exacerbate these problems. The patient at greatest risk is the patient with a suspected spinal injury who is secured to a backboard.

Before departure, all splints, casts, and pressure areas should be padded. The patient secured to a backboard for a suspected cervical spinal injury can have a small towel or pad placed under the coccyx area to prevent pressure sores. In transport, proper positioning and assessment of range of motion should be performed within the space constraints. Assessing for areas of compromised perfusion should be included as part of the assessment of vital signs.

The length of the transport includes not only the time it takes to fly from the referring location to the receiving hospital; ground transport times, unexpected delays, and transfer times must all be considered. For example, a patient is injured in a motor vehicle accident at a remote site and is secured to a backboard to protect the cervical spine. This patient is then transported by ground ambulance to the nearest hospital. After evaluation of the injuries, it is decided that the patient requires the facilities of a major trauma center. The radiographs of the cervical spine are inconclusive, so the patient must remain on the backboard during transport. Subsequently the patient is taken by ground ambulance to the nearest airport, flown to the receiving airfield, and again transferred by ground ambulance to the trauma center. The total length of time that the patient is secured to the backboard exceeds 5 to 6 hours. Although the flight took only 1½ hours, the patient was immobilized for five times that long.

Consideration of injuries must take precedence during stabilization of the patient, but using padding splints, traction devices, and so on and protecting bony prominences help limit the preventable problems associated with immobilization.

Psychosocial Effects

Transport of patients affects the patient, his or her family, and the transport personnel. Removing the patient from home, family, and a familiar environment increases the stressors placed on him or her. The patient can exhibit fears of flying, fears of dying, and anger, which is often directed at the referring hospital for being, in the patient's mind, unable to care for him or her. The need for the transport is often translated in the patient's mind to mean that he or she is dying, since only "sick" people need to be transported. All these stressors increase the patient's anxiety level, causing an increase in heart rate and respiratory rate, diaphoresis, nausea, and vomiting, and a general worsening of the patient's condition.

The referring hospital personnel and transport crew should work together to alleviate the patient's fears, by thoroughly explaining all procedures, noises, and reasons for the transport. A team member should interact with family members and include the family in all explanations. The transport personnel should work to instill confidence in the patient concerning the referring hospital. This confidence is important; if the patient survives, he or she will be returning to the home community and will be cared for at the referring hospital in the future.

The patient's family also have tremendous fears. If the patient is acutely ill or injured, this interaction may be the last that they have with their loved one. The family may not understand the need for the transport, and time must be spent with them to explain all requirements and the necessity of immediate transfer. The family may also have what is called the "Mecca syndrome," an inflated idea of what can be done for the patient at the receiving facility. The family may believe that the receiving hospital will save the life of a patient, when in fact that may not be possible.

A family member may also want to accompany the patient. In helicopter transports this possibility is usually out of the question because of space and weight limitations. However, depending on the type of fixed-wing aircraft, there may be an extra seat for a family member. The transport personnel should make the decision to allow the family member to come with the patient, although final decision is the responsibility of the pilot-in-command. It is important to remember that if the patient's condition deteriorates during flight, there is no place for the family member to go and he or she must watch all interventions. On the other hand, the family member's presence may help alleviate some of the patient's anxiety, especially when the patient is a child. The decision should not be made until the time of the transport, since the patient's condition changes and promises may not always be able to be kept.

To alleviate the anxiety of the family, they should be provided with as much information as possible about the receiving hospital. Maps, plans for patient admission, and a telephone contact will give them some direction after the patient departs. They should be informed of the estimated length of transport and the expected time of arrival at the receiving hospital. This time should be calculated taking into consideration the weather, unexpected delays, changes in time zone, and other factors. Overestimation of the time is always best—if the transport is completed sooner than anticipated, the family will feel relief. On the other hand, if the transport takes longer than expected, the family will begin to feel fear about the outcome of the transport itself.

One of the last things that should be done before departure with the patient is to allow the family time together with the patient. The last remarks and the last kiss goodbye may be the most important few minutes of the transport.

The transport personnel are also affected by their jobs. The interactions with the patient are short term and often rushed. The patients who are transported have an increased mortality, and the transport crew may begin to question the effectiveness of their work. The flight crew (pilot and copilot) may have little experience with sick or injured people; the flight crew, as well as the patient's family, may need to receive an explanation of the transport.

Following the patient's progress in the receiving hospital helps the crew alleviate the anxieties related to dealing with patients for the short term. Transport personnel must remember that they are often the only personal contact that the family has with the receiving hospital; the crew can remain in contact with the family, explaining interventions and other procedures. Maintaining contact and follow-up with the referring personnel also provides the transport crew with opportunities to communicate about the patients and helps instill a sense of commitment and pride in their job.

REQUIREMENTS FOR TRANSPORT
Equipment

Equipment used in air transport of patients must be based on the level and type of medical care the patient requires during transport. Because of space and weight limitations, not all equipment can be carried in the transport vehicle. Before departure a decision must be made concerning what equipment and how much equipment should be taken. However, a limited amount of backup supplies must be on hand in the event of unexpected delays.

All medical equipment must be easily secured. Equipment requiring an alternating current (AC) power source should have a backup battery source, or an alternative, hand-operated device should be available. All equipment should be protected from electromechanical interference. Equipment with diaphragms (such as oxygen analyzers) may not function in the pressurized cabin of a fixed-wing aircraft. All equipment should be tested in-flight before it is used on a patient.

Required vehicle equipment and medical equipment usually include the equipment listed in the box below. Specialized equipment is now available for transport vehicles,

---

EQUIPMENT REQUIRED FOR AEROMEDICAL TRANSPORT

Vehicle equipment
Communication system
Adequate lighting with ability to isolate pilots from lights
Electrical outlets (110 v AC)
Locking hooks for IV bags and bottles
Fire extinguisher
Survival gear appropriate to environment over which transport will occur
Sharps disposal container
Trash receptacle

Medical equipment
Oxygen tanks with flowmeters
Air cylinders (if ventilator is to be used)
Portable and permanent suction devices with regulators
Cardiac monitor with defibrillator
Radio-shielded Doppler device
Stretcher with approved securing mechanisms
Blood pressure cuffs
Emesis basin
Urinal and bedpan
Additional items
    Infusion pumps
    Backboards
    PASG
    Cervical collars
    Heimlich valves
    Water seal drainage sets
    Cervical spine immobilizer

Universal precautions equipment
    Goggles
    Gloves
    Gowns
    Masks

Patient-specific equipment

but before such equipment is purchased, a trial should be performed. The disadvantages of some types of equipment are specialized accessories, which make the equipment difficult and costly to use. For example, some IV infusion pumps require specialized infusion tubing that must be changed before the transport; the time spent repriming tubing can delay the transfer.

Expendable items should be placed in soft packs whenever possible. Product packing materials may be removed to eliminate extraneous bulky material. Various types of efficient equipment packs include burn, neonatal, IV, trauma, and medication packs. Pediatric equipment may be kept in a separate pack to reduce the quantity of equipment taken on all transports.

When arranging equipment it is best to have the equipment prepared for use. Intravenous solutions should be in plastic bags, tubing should be secured to the bag with a rubber band. Nasogastric tubes should be banded together with gloves, lubricant, benzoin, tape, and the appropriate connectors. This organization, which is completed before the transport, can expedite interventions and limit the need to open many compartments to find one or two items.

Equipment of any type should be lightweight and compact. Aluminum cylinders of oxygen, which weigh one third of the weight of steel tanks, are available. Pocket-type Doppler devices can be removed from the aircraft and taken with the transport personnel.

Adequate equipment should be available to care for the patient during the entire transport and during any unexpected delays. To calculate the amount of equipment necessary, estimate the length of the transport, including the transfer times, then multiply that figure by one half. To estimate the amount of oxygen remaining in a standard "E" cylinder, the following formula is used:

$$\frac{\text{PSI} \times 0.3 \text{ L/min}}{60 \text{ minutes}} = \text{Hours in cylinder}$$

However, altitude and pressure changes cause changes in flow rates. Table 32-3 shows the effects of altitude on flow rates.

Medications are commonly carried in hard plastic cases to prevent breakage of vials and bottles. The types and amount of medications carried depend on the types of patients transported and the medical protocols of the transport program. Narcotics should be in locked carrying cases that can be secured and should be counted at each shift change.

Personnel

Flight team configurations are many and varied. Emergency department (ED) and critical care nurses are generally chosen to become flight nurses. They can work alone, as a member of a two-nurse team, or with a paramedic, an emergency medical technician, or an emergency physician. Respiratory therapists are also used, either as a second member of the team or as a third member when the patient is intubated and requires ventilatory support.

Flight nursing has developed into a subspecialty of emergency nursing. Flight nurses now go through rigorous training before joining a flight team. The National Flight Nurses Association (NFNA) is developing a flight nurse core course to provide standardized training in such areas as flight physiology, stabilization, communications, and medicolegal issues. Initial training includes both classroom and clinical experience. Preceptor programs are used frequently to allow the new flight nurse exposure to the transport environment. Recurrent training is also needed to maintain skills, update information concerning current therapies, and review current policies and procedures. Monthly "run" reviews provide for quality assurance as well as the sharing of learning experiences among other staff members.

Training requirements include review of patient assessment techniques, especially techniques that are most beneficial in a noisy environment; patient handling considerations; field stabilization; oxygen therapy and ventilatory support; safety, crash, and survival procedures; communications; equipment use and maintenance; documentation; and flight physiology. Specialized advanced life support measures are reviewed, including care of burns, neonatal care, high-risk obstetrics, and pediatrics. Length of training depends on the types of patients transported and the level of care provided during flight.

In addition, many flight nurses are trained to perform advanced invasive procedures such as intubation, chest tube placement, and so on; frequent proficiency checks are required in these cases to maintain a high standard of care. These nurses are under the direction of a medical director but usually function without direct medical control during the transport itself. This expanded role increases the liability of the flight nurse and requires extra attentiveness to standards of care.

PREFLIGHT RESPONSIBILITIES

Before the transport of patients, arrangements and stabilization measures must be undertaken. Permission from the family must be obtained, although permission is usually obtained by the referring personnel. A physician must accept the patient at the receiving facility, and if possible, per-

Table 32-3 Effects of altitude on flow rates

Flowmeter (L/min)	Flow rate at altitude (calculated)		
	2000 ft	5000 ft	8000 ft
2	2.1	2.4	2.6
4	4.2	4.7	5.3
6	6.3	7.1	7.9
8	8.4	9.4	10.6
10	10.5	11.8	13.2
12	12.6	14.1	15.8

INFORMATION TO ACCOMPANY PATIENT

Name, age, sex, height, and weight
Family information—name, address, telephone number
    for contact person
Patient chart, to include:
    History and physical findings
    Radiographs and laboratory reports
    Vital signs record
    Medication record
    Prehospital care record (history of illness, injury)
    Discharge note with synopsis of care
Signed permission to receive care at receiving facility
Name and telephone number of contact individual at
    referring facility

---

mission to receive care should be signed by the next of kin.

Information to accompany the patient should include those items listed in the box above. To ensure safe and efficient transfer of care, all items must be included. Pertinent laboratory specimens should also be transferred with the patient, including a tube of mother's blood for neonates, peridialysis fluid, blood, urine, and gastric samples for the overdose patient, and other body secretions as pertinent. Radiographs and the results of special studies should also be sent with the patient to save the time and money involved in unnecessarily repeated studies.

Stabilization of patients is discussed in depth in Chapter 31. Oxygen, intravenous fluids in plastic IV bags, cardiac monitoring, nasogastric suctioning, and Foley catheter drainage are standard interventions for the majority of patients transferred by air. To stabilize the patient for air transport, the 10 problems discussed in this chapter concerning flight physiology should be reviewed and interventions should be undertaken to prevent or counteract the problems that may occur.

IN-FLIGHT RESPONSIBILITIES

During transport of patients, vital signs should be obtained at least every 15 minutes. Depending on the patient's condition, vital signs may be taken as frequently as necessary. Changes in patient condition usually occur during ascent and descent, when pressure changes are occurring within the aircraft. It is important to monitor the patient's response to transport during these times.

The advantage of air transport is that the transport personnel are never farther than a few feet away from their patient. This closeness allows for astute observations of the patient and the ability to pick up on subtle changes in condition. However, because of the noise, distractions, and space limitations within the transport vehicle, certain cues are distorted and the crew must pay particular attention to monitoring the patient closely for any of the problems that

may develop as a result of changes in atmosphere or the transport itself.

Patients with Respiratory Distress

Warm, humidified oxygen should be administered to all patients, and the percentage of oxygen should be increased for those who were receiving oxygen therapy before the transport. Gas expansion within the pleural cavity can cause the size of a previously undetected pneumothorax to increase, which may result in respiratory embarrassment. A flutter valve should be placed to reduce the pressure within the chest cavity (Table 32-2). If the patient had a chest tube placed before transport, the tube should never be clamped during flight. A one-way (Heimlich) valve can be placed between the chest tube and the drainage set to prevent air from reaccumulating in the chest cavity in the event of an accidental disruption of the system.

Pulmonary secretions become more tenacious with dehydration and a decrease in ambient humidity. Instillation of sterile saline before suctioning will enhance removal of secretions. Hyperventilation can accompany cold stress or be caused by excessive noise and vibration. Measures should be taken to warm the patient and allay the patient's fears and anxieties.

Immobilizing the patient on the stretcher prevents adequate chest expansion and can lead to underventilation and subsequently atelectasis. Elevating the head of the patient improves oxygenation and gas exchange and helps limit the pulmonary congestion that occurs as a result of acceleration and deceleration forces.

Mechanical volume ventilators used in the transport environment must be constantly monitored for delivery of adequate tidal volumes, since gas expansion can affect the volume of gas delivered. Oxygen flow rates of at least 15 L/min are required to operate ventilators and can rapidly increase oxygen supply. Should the ventilator fail, the patient must be ventilated with a resuscitation bag.

Patients with Cardiovascular Conditions

Hypoxia presents the greatest risk to the cardiac patient during transport. Hypoxia leads to increased myocardial irritability and ventricular ectopy. Providing supplemental oxygen and positioning the patient for optimal gas exchanges is imperative. Interventions to decrease oxygen demands include keeping the patient warm, allaying fears, and preventing motion sickness.

Placement of a nasogastric tube can help prevent a decrease in venous return, which occurs with gastric distention. However, placement must be performed with caution because vagal stimulation and bradycardia can develop. The decision to employ a nasogastric tube should be made on a patient-by-patient basis.

Acceleration forces cause a pooling of blood in the lower extremities and subsequent poor cardiac return. The opposite effect develops as a result of deceleration forces, when cardiac congestion and transient fluid overload develop. The patient having congestive heart failure is severely compromised by these factors, and pretransport diuresis can help prevent these problems.

Specialized equipment associated with cardiac patients needs special attention. Patients with pacemakers need to be monitored for pacer malfunctions that may occur as a result of radio and navigational equipment signals. Intraaortic balloon pumps are now available for use during transport. Only trained personnel should use these devices, since the risk of balloon dislodgment and equipment malfunction is increased in the transport environment. During the transport, close monitoring of the pressures within the balloon is imperative to detect changes that may result from gas expansion.

Patients with Multiple Traumatic Injuries

Examples of in-flight care of the patient who has sustained multiple traumatic injuries have been presented. Hypoxia and gas expansion can rapidly cause deterioration of the pulmonary and cardiovascular systems. Pulmonary embolus must be considered a possibility when increasing dyspnea develops. Thoracic injuries must be identified and stabilized before transporting the patient.

The effect of gas expansion on the PASG, air splints, and endotracheal tube cuffs has been discussed previously. Free air in the peritoneal cavity resulting from either bowel injury or peritoneal lavage should be aspirated if possible.

Adequate resuscitation of the trauma patient usually includes fluid and blood support. Measures must be taken to ensure that blood products are properly stored. In the event that their use is unwarranted, they can be returned to the blood bank for future use.

Patients with Head Injuries

Patients who have sustained head injuries, either isolated or in conjunction with other injuries, are especially at risk for compromise resulting from air transport. Increased intracranial pressure causes a decrease in the level of arterial oxygen saturation, which may result in hypoxia caused by changes in the partial pressure of oxygen. Subsequently, hypoxia can result in seizure activity, and seizure precautions should be instituted at all times.

Noise, vibration, vomiting, and an increase in metabolic rate associated with cold stress all cause an increase in intracranial pressure. In-flight measures, including hyperventilation, should be taken to reduce these untoward effects and prevent unnecessary rises in intracranial pressure. Induction of paralysis can also help control intracranial pressure; however, posturing and other clinical indicators of patient status are forfeited. Positioning of the patient has been discussed previously. Efforts to minimize the effects of gravitational forces should be undertaken.

Burn Victims

Burns of the face, head, and neck may cause massive swelling and may compromise the airway. Prophylactic intubation before transport prevents having to perform an intubation in the poorly lit, cramped interior of the aircraft. Supplemental oxygen should be administered to all patients with suspected smoke inhalation; supplemental oxygen combats the effects of hypoxia in all patients. Providing cool humidified oxygen to the patient with suspected oropharyngeal burns helps reduce swelling.

Loss of the skin causes massive fluid shifts and loss of the temperature-regulating mechanism. Evaporative heat loss increases in the burned area, and the burn victim becomes increasingly dehydrated and cold. All wounds should be covered with absorbent dressings to help control heat loss and to limit contamination of the wounds. Dressings should not be moistened with saline solution or other fluids, because this procedure enhances hypothermia. Using a Mylar blanket to cover the patient also helps limit heat loss.

Patients with burns require a large amount of fluids and dressings; therefore adequate supplies must be available throughout the transport. A burn pack that contains extra IV fluids, dressings, and an escharotomy pack should be taken on each transport of a burn victim. Escharotomies may become necessary when fluid shifts occur during take-off and descent.

Maintaining sterility of the transport environment is impossible. Meticulous care to prevent contamination should be performed at all times. Wearing masks and gowns over the transport clothing helps limit the transfer of bacteria. Topical antibiotics may be applied before the transport; however, this procedure will delay evaluation of the burn wound when the patient arrives at the receiving hospital, since the antibiotic must be removed.

Patients with High-Risk Obstetric Conditions

Hypoxia and fluid shifts increase the irritability of the uterus and can lead to premature labor. Hypoxia of short duration has little effect on the fetus, but prolonged maternal hypoxia can lead to fetal distress and subsequent fetal demise. Supplemental oxygen should be provided to the patient throughout the transport.

Pressure from a distended stomach increases irritability of the uterus and increases pressure on the diaphragm, causing dyspnea. Nasogastric tube placement is uncomfortable for the pregnant woman; however, the tube assists with decompression of the stomach and decreases the risk of aspiration resulting from delayed gastric emptying.

Pregnancy increases the blood volume by approximately 45% to 50%. This increased volume must be replaced if the woman is hypovolemic. In addition, fluid shifts accompanying acceleration and deceleration forces can cause decreased uterine blood flow and should be prevented by means of proper positioning.

The pregnant patient should be placed in the left lateral decubitus position during transport. It is often difficult to safely secure the patient to the stretcher in this position, and it may be necessary to secure the patient in the supine position during loading and unloading. The woman should be returned to the left lateral decubitus position as soon as the aircraft has reached its cruising altitude or whenever there are signs of fetal distress.

Preeclampsia and eclampsia can cause an increase in nausea and vomiting associated with motion. These patients are also sensitive to extraneous stimulation, and the noise and vibration may cause increases in blood pressure. Dim lighting and earplugs for the patient help prevent overstimulation of the patient.

All personnel who transport high-risk obstetric patients must be familiar with the techniques of childbirth and neonatal resuscitation. Equipment for delivery and resuscitation must be readily available. Imminent delivery requires reaching the nearest hospital to avoid in-flight delivery, although this facility may not be the final destination. Keeping a newly delivered infant warm, dry, and oxygenated is the priority of newborn care.

Pediatric Patients

The problems associated with transport of children are the same as those for adults. However, interventions must take into account the unique anatomic and physiologic features of children. Since equipment of the appropriate size for the age and weight of the child must be available, a large assortment of choices must be available.

Pediatric patients have smaller vital capacities than do adults and are more prone to the effects of hypoxia. Children may not be able to tolerate or cooperate with the application of an oxygen mask; however, the oxygen mask can be placed in front of the child's face and oxygen can be blown at the child. If a family member has accompanied the child, he or she can assist with administration of oxygen by holding the mask and encouraging the child to cooperate.

The gastric cavity of the child is small; therefore the child has a greater tendency to develop complications from gastric gas expansion. Many nasogastric tubes for children do not have a sump port. These tubes should not be used if possible, since the absence of the sump port makes emptying the stomach more difficult.

The greater ratio of surface area to body mass in children makes them more susceptible to evaporative heat losses. The proportionally larger surface areas of the head and neck also enhance radiated heat loss, putting the child at great risk for hypothermia. A stocking cap and extra linen help keep the child warm.

To secure children to the standard stretcher is difficult; the stretcher restraints are not easily moved, and extra straps may be necessary to keep the child secured. One method of transporting a child less than 4 or 5 years of age is to place the child in his or her car seat and secure the car seat to the stretcher restraints. Using and providing familiar items such as car seats, toys, and security blankets also helps to alleviate the child's fear of the unknown.

If the child's condition is stable, it may be advantageous to include a family member in the transport. The family member can comfort the child and help explain the procedures. In addition, the family member can provide diversionary activities, as warranted, to keep the child occupied.

Other in-flight responsibilities include documentation of all interventions, vital signs, and changes in the patient's condition. Changes in environmental conditions such as takeoff, landing, and so on should also be documented, since changes in the patient's condition may be secondary to the effects of transport rather than changes in the disease process itself. Throughout the transport, safety must be the number one consideration.

POSTFLIGHT RESPONSIBILITIES

On arrival at the receiving hospital, the flight crew must brief the personnel who will be caring for the patient. The flight team is the vital link between the referring and receiving facilities and can provide information about mechanisms of injury, previous interventions, and changes in patient status. The nurses and physicians who will take over care of the patient may not be able to immediately review the complete hospital record of the patient because other interventions take priority; therefore the shared information is of upmost importance.

After the transfer of patient care is completed, the flight crew should notify the referring personnel of the safe arrival of the patient. Liability is shared among these two parties and is terminated when the patient is accepted at the receiving facility. Information about patient status should be given, and plans for care should be outlined. Follow-up information concerning patient outcomes should be provided by the receiving staff or the flight crew on a weekly basis.

The family should also be notified of the safe arrival of the patient at this time. They are often waiting by the telephone for word on the patient and appreciate prompt notification.

Cleaning, restocking, and charting must all be performed before the transport is considered complete. The timing of the next transport is often unknown, and the aircraft and crew must be ready to respond immediately.

SAFETY

Safety in air transport should be the primary concern of all individuals. Most accidents occur in conjunction with helicopter transports; however, risk is also associated with fixed-wing transports.

The safety of the patient depends on the flight crew. The patient must be restrained at all times by means of at least two restraints. If the patient is uncomfortable during the flight, his or her position can be changed and the straps can be loosened but they should never be removed.

All equipment must be secured in accordance with FAA regulations. Meeting these stringent requirements ensures that passengers and crew are not injured by flying objects during any turbulence that is encountered or when a crash occurs. Equipment that is not secured to the airframe itself should be kept in soft packs and placed on the floor during takeoff and landing. Emergency exits should never be blocked by equipment or extraneous items.

The crew should also be strapped in at all times. Seat belts may have to be removed for a short time during certain interventions (such as when starting an IV line) but should be refastened when the intervention is completed. Knowledge of the location of emergency exits and how they function is imperative. Location of fire extinguishers should be clearly marked, and all personnel should be trained to use them. Emergency procedures for rapid egress should be practiced regularly.

Everyone involved in the transport should be briefed before departure, including not only the medical personnel and the pilots but also the patient and family members. Flight conditions, expected flight times, possible anticipated problems or delays, and emergency procedures should be discussed.

Medical personnel are responsible for the safe transport of the patient. These team members are responsible for the safe use of medical equipment and decision making concerning patient needs. The pilot-in-command of the aircraft has ultimate responsibility for the transport. The pilot has "the final say" concerning who should be transported and when the transport will occur. Weather and mechanical delays take precedence over the transport of the patient. During an emergency, the pilot will dictate procedures to be followed, even if they are at odds with the goals of the medical personnel.

Ground personnel must also be trained and briefed regarding the safety of the aircraft. This briefing is especially important when a helicopter is approaching an accident scene and untrained individuals and bystanders are in the vicinity. Before approaching a scene landing, radio communications should be initiated with ground personnel. The pilot or flight crew member should relay all safety information to the site coordinator. If the pilot has any concerns about the safety of ground personnel, the helicopter will not be set down until these problems are rectified.

A safe landing zone should be in a clearing that measures 100 feet by 100 feet. All wires, trees, and possible hazards should be *both* marked and verbally described to the pilot. Smoke flares can be ignited to assist the pilot to identify the location of the landing zone, as well as wind direction and velocity. All bystanders and the patient should be at least 500 feet from the landing site, because the rotor blades create a large amount of swirling dust, dirt, and gravel, which can cause injury to those on the ground.

The ground personnel should be instructed to wait to approach the helicopter until the pilot has given the sign that is safe to do so. Many accidents occur because individuals approach the helicopter while the blades are still rotating; when the blade rotation begins to slow, the blades drop and may cause unexpected injury. A "hot" loading or unloading (one that is performed with the rotor blades turning at idle power) should be made only in extreme circumstances and only by experienced personnel.

The pilot or medical personnel should direct the loading and unloading of the patient. Weight distribution is critical in aircraft, and ground personnel may not be aware of these requirements.

Ensuring the safe transport of the patient is the responsibility of all individuals involved in the transport. All personnel should remain conscious of safety at all times: safety should be the number one priority.

SUMMARY

Air transport of the sick and injured has improved outcomes of many patients. Proper stabilization procedures should incorporate anticipation of the problems encountered during air transport. Employing specialized equipment and personnel trained in transporting patients by air ensures that the patient is transported in a highly sophisticated environment. In-flight responsibilities include monitoring the patient for changes in condition that develop as a result of changes in the transport environment. Although patient care is of utmost importance, safety of all personnel is the number one priority.

SUGGESTED READINGS

Lee G: *Flight nursing: principles and practice,* St Louis, 1991, Mosby–Year Book.

Tissue and Organ Donation

Mary Ellen McNally Pederson

A critical issue faced by emergency nurses is that of tissue and organ donation. In the past the emergency nurse was peripherally involved with the donation of organs and tissues, but as technology and availability of professionals to recover tissue and organs increase, donation is an everyday happening in the emergency department (ED). Emergency nurses and other health care professionals must be prepared and are responsible for offering the family or next of kin of a patient who dies the opportunity to consider donation.

Each time a patient dies in the ED, the patient can be considered a potential tissue donor. Almost any person who dies can become a tissue donor, excluding persons with a systemic infectious disease. The most common donor is a tissue donor, yet this potential is frequently overlooked by health care professionals. Many needed tissues are lost because no one remembered to offer the family the option of donation. More important, the family of the person who has just died are not provided with the opportunity to carry out the wishes of their family member. This individual may have expressed the wish to donate tissues and organs by signing a donor card or may have previously discussed these wishes with his or her next of kin. At a time when family stress is greatest, the wish to donate is not considered a first priority and is frequently forgotten. It is up to the health care professional to provide the opportunity for donation.

Countless individuals are waiting for a new cornea, bone, or other tissue. The lives of these individuals may not hang in the balance, as when one is waiting for a heart, liver, lung, or heart and lung transplantation, but their quality of life can be greatly enhanced as a result of transplantation. Transplantation has been found to surpass the efficacy of conventional means of treatment and is clearly superior to no treatment at all.

As common as tissue donation is or can be, the special situation of organ donation may be available to some families. This option is possible when an individual suffers a severe brain injury or a prolonged anoxic event. Such situations result in the eventual death of brain tissue, rendering the patient dead and supported only by mechanical means.

These patients are typically the victims of traumatic injuries that commonly occur as the result of a motor vehicle accident, gunshot wound to the head, a ruptured cerebral aneurysm, arteriovenous malformation, a severe stroke, or a severe anoxic event resulting from prolonged cardiac arrest.

An individual who is declared dead by brain-death criteria and who is a potential organ donor can also be considered a tissue donor, unlike the patient in a state of asystole, which allows for tissue donation only. Visceral organ donation requires an intact circulatory system; the donor is placed on a ventilator and may require other physiologic supports such as vasopressors or other medications to maintain blood pressure, fluid balance, and adequate arterial blood gas levels. Before a patient can be considered for potential organ donation, he or she must meet the criteria for brain death or be in the process of evaluation for these criteria. Ultimately he or she must be declared dead as determined by brain-death criteria for actual donation to take place.

All too often the family of the patient who is declared dead according to brain-death criteria are not offered the option of organ and tissue donation. For example, a 1985 Gallup poll described a situation in which 20,000 potential donors were identified and only 3000 became actual organ donors.[10] The most commonly cited reason for this situation is that the health care professional is uncomfortable dealing with death and broaching the subject of donation[4] and does not wish the family to suffer a greater loss as a result of a request of such a sensitive nature: He or she may feel that the family and the patient have suffered enough. The result of this hesitation, however, is that the supply of organs and tissues does not meet the demand. Because of the widening gap between donors and recipients, legislation in the form of "required request law" has been enacted. Many states mandate that the health care professional or hospital designee offer to each family, at the time of the patient's death, the option of tissue and organ donation as deemed appropriate. Sensitivity to the family's cultural, religious, and emotional situation must be considered. More often than not the family appreciate that the option is offered because something positive can result from the death of a loved one.[3]

The family may not wish to hear more about the option of donation and may decline to donate, but as a family they are given the choice to make that decision and should be supported in their decision, whatever it might be.

HISTORICAL PERSPECTIVE

Throughout time humanity has been intrigued with the idea of finding a way to maintain and extend life to its fullest. Today's technologies permit replacement of a diseased organ with one that is healthy, using transplantation techniques to restore life and health.

Tissue transplantation is described in the historical literature as early as 1682, when Meekren made an attempt to replace a portion of a soldier's cranium with the skull bone of a dog.[8] Corneal graft surgery was undertaken by Wolf in 1800,[15] and in 1881 skin grafting was tried as a temporary means of treating a severe burn.[14] Further work in skin grafting was carried out by Sir Peter Medawar, who used skin grafts treated with cold refrigeration in the 1940s.[11] Medawar was also awarded the Nobel Prize for his work in immune response and the rejection phenomenon,[7] which to a great extent has been the basis on which further study in transplantation has been realized. Advances in the last 15 years in immunosuppressive therapies have greatly enhanced the potential for many transplantation procedures that were previously hampered by tissue rejection complications.

Work in whole organ transplantation began somewhat later than in tissue transplantation. However, in 1902 Ullman[8] attempted the transplantation of kidneys in a goat model, spurred on by the degree of kidney failure.

Many attempts at dialyzing patients whose kidneys had failed were made as early as the 1860s by Grahm who used his wooden hoop dialyzer.[5] However, in the 1940s Kolft designed the dialysis machine on which current dialysis is based.[13] Merrill and his colleagues at the Peter Bent Brigham Hospital in Boston implemented dialysis therapy in 1954.[6] This work was based on Kolft's work as the method of choice for treating patients in end-stage renal failure.

Simultaneously research in renal transplantation was being carried out because great numbers of persons were requiring dialysis. Dialysis remains a lengthy, expensive, and limited modality for patients with kidney failure. The first kidney transplantations were carried out at the Peter Bent Brigham Hospital in 1954 between living, identical twins by Murray (Nobel Prize winner, 1990) and Harrison.[1] These autografts were successful. Further work with living, related (sibling, parent) donors and cadaveric donors continued with moderate success.

As kidney and tissue transplantation became a more effective treatment modality, the possibilities of other whole organ transplantation became a reality. The first liver transplantation was performed in 1963 in Denver, Colorado, by Thomas Starzl.[12] The first lung transplantation was performed by Hardy at the University of Mississippi in 1963,[9] and the first kidney and pancreas transplantation was by Lillehei at the University of Minnesota in 1967. The historical literature describes pancreatic transplantation and details the transplantation of a sheep's pancreas into a human, a xenograft, by Williams in 1893. This took place before a description and isolation of islet cells in the pancreas had been made.

Most sensational of all in the arena of transplantation was the transplantation of the first heart in 1967 by Christiaan Barnard in Cape Town, South Africa. The first heart and lung transplantation was performed by Shumway in 1981 at Stanford University. Each of these extrarenal transplantations was somewhat limited in restoring life for the individual receiving the new organ. However, each transplantation was the beginning of a new technologic era. This activity and further innovative research resulted in several new areas of concern. Of greatest consequence was the prevention of rejection, infection, and other issues related to allograft survival. These issues and others such as the determination of death by brain-death criteria, inclusive of the professional's comfort level with the concept and the lack of available organs and tissues for transplantation, are diligently being addressed by the medical and transplantation community.

LEGISLATIVE OVERVIEW

Transplantation is a thriving technology. Survival rates have improved, and legislators began taking notice of this unique medical practice in the late 1960s. Two key documents were developed in 1968, one legislative and the other relating to effective medical practice. These were known as the Uniform Anatomical Gift Act and the Harvard Criteria for Determination of Brain Death.[5]

The Uniform Anatomical Gift Act of 1968 was adopted as law in all 50 states. Organ and tissue donation became an accepted legal and medical practice. This law allowed an individual to decide whether he or she wished to become an organ or tissue donor. Each person may carry a donor card; a sticker is affixed to the driver's license signifying the individual's intent to donate in the event of death. Next of kin are notified of the person's intent to donate. The donor card has become a tool of communication to ED professionals to let them know of an individual's wish to donate. A person filling out the donor card must be 18 years of age or older and must have two witnesses (preferably known to the card carrier) who sign the card on behalf of the donor.

The most important aspect of this process is that the next of kin must be aware of the donor's wishes. In the donation process the next of kin have the integral role of giving final permission for the donation. The order of priority of the next of kin is (1) spouse, (2) adult child, (3) parent, (4) sibling, and (5) guardian. The next of kin acting for the deceased must be 18 years of age or older. In most situations of a traumatic death, many family members are involved in the care and decision making for the patient. Decision making on behalf of the patient is difficult at best. When the issue of donation is addressed, many families become confused about the wishes of their loved ones, particularly if discussion has not taken place regarding donation. Often dissension exists among family members, which can be painful and distressing. However, the best decision is one with which all family members are comfortable. The next of kin with highest priority has the final decision-making power. Finally, if the patient had ever expressed the desire either to donate or not to donate, the family should be encouraged to honor the deceased's wishes.

The Uniform Anatomical Gift Act not only provides the individual with the opportunity to donate organs and tissues if he or she so desires but also protects the individual if he or she had chosen not to donate. The act established guidelines for prevention of the donation process as desired.

Throughout the years the Uniform Anatomical Gift Act has been amended to assist in meeting the growing need for transplantation organs and tissues. The amendment of greatest note was the development of the required request or required referral clause. The concept of required request was the direct result of a congressional investigation in the early 1980s surrounding the difficulties that a private citizen might have in obtaining an organ for transplant because of a shortage of organs and lack of third-party funding for an organ transplant. Senator Albert Gore of Tennessee spearheaded an inquiry by a committee of experts to determine the shortcomings and inequities of the organ transplant process, and the Organ Transplantation Act (P.L. 98-507) was enacted. The law mandated the formation of the Organ Transplantation Task Force, which was directed to critically review the medical, ethical, economic, and legal issues surrounding donation and transplantation. The report of the Organ Transplantation Task Force, published in 1986,[8] outlines a number of recommendations for the donation and transplantation community. Key conclusions that affect the emergency nurse and other health care professionals were (1) that families were not being approached consistently concerning their option to donate tissues and organs for transplantation and (2) that health care providers were hesitant to approach families with the option of donation. Recommendations were (1) to encourage states to enact some form of required request legislation, mandating that hospitals implement and develop organ and tissue donation policies, (2) to encourage states to enact the Uniform Determination of Death Act, and (3) to encourage and support the need for increased professional and public education.

Aside from the development of the task force, the Organ Transplantation Act required the Department of Health and Human Services (DHHS) to establish a single national network for the distribution and management of organs and tissues for transplantation. The Organ Procurement and Transplantation Network, to be administered by the secretary of the DHHS, was created. A private, nonprofit agency would be employed to serve as the network and accomplish the objectives of the secretary. The United Network of Organ Sharing (UNOS) was engaged to fulfill this obligation.

UNOS is located in Richmond, Virginia, and serves as a clearinghouse for organs and tissues recovered for transplantation.

As a consequence of the task force recommendations, required request legislation evolved in 44 states in the form of amendments to the respective state Anatomical Gift Acts. The rationale behind the legislation is summed up nicely by ethicist Arthur Caplin, PhD[2]:

In enacting required request legislation, our society has indicated its collective desire that people routinely be given the option of organ and tissue donation as a last act of respect for the dead and their families and as an expression of concern for those who will die unless more organs and tissues are made available.

The goal of the required request law is to ultimately increase the number of organs and tissues available for transplantation and at the same time, and more important, to provide the grieving family with the option of considering tissue and organ donation for a family member. Each state law has its own idiosyncrasy and each state's requirements are a bit different, but essentially all ascribe to these purposes and goals. In response to state legislation throughout the United States, Congress incorporated into the federal Consolidated Omnibus Budget Reconciliation Act (COBRA) of 1986 (P.L. 99-506) a requirement that hospitals receiving Medicare funding develop policy to achieve the following[10]: (1) Ensure that families of potential donors are made aware of the option of organ or tissue donation and their option to decline to donate, (2) encourage discretion and sensitivity with respect to the circumstances, views, and beliefs of such families, and (3) require that an organ procurement agency designated by the secretary of DHHS be notified of potential donors.

Ten UNOS regions have been designated in the United States by DHHS. Within each region, a single designated Organ Procurement Organization theoretically serves to advise hospital administration, nurses, and medical professionals concerning new issues related to tissue and organ donation and to provide the respective hospital with the services necessary for recovery and placement of organs and tissues. In many regions, however, a number of isolated Organ Procurement Organizations (OPOs) joined together as a consequence of the legislation to share the responsibility of the organ and tissue donation process and to eliminate competition for organs. (Fig. 33-1). When an emergency nurse is attempting to make a referral for donation regardless of the type of donation, and is unsure of which region or organ procurement agency to contact, the nurse can dial the 24-hour telephone number of UNOS: 1-800-666-1884.

THE DONATION PROCESS

When a patient dies in the ED, he or she should be considered for donation of some tissue or organ.

Three key pieces of information that must be documented in the medical record for the donation to take place are the

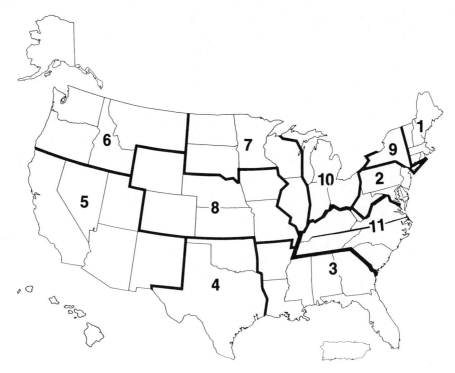

Fig. 33-1 UNOS regional map.

following:
1. Determination and declaration of death
2. Consent from the next of kin
3. Medical examiner's approval (as appropriate according to individual state law)

Determination of Death

A patient must be declared dead for the process of donation to begin. The Uniform Determination of Death Act plays an integral role in the process of identifying which criteria must be met for determining death. Death in an individual is defined when either of the following criteria are met[10]:

I. An individual with irreversible cessation of circulatory and respiratory function is dead.
   A. Cessation is recognized by an appropriate clinical examination.
   B. Irreversibility is recognized by persistent cessation of functions during an appropriate period of observation or trial of therapy or both.
II. An individual with irreversible cessation of all functions of the entire brain, including the brainstem, is dead.
   A. Cessation is recognized when evaluation discloses two findings.
      1. Cerebral functions are absent.
      2. Brainstem functions are absent.
   B. Irreversibility is recognized when evaluation discloses three findings.

1. Cause of coma is established and is sufficient to account for the loss of brain functions.
2. Possibility of recovery of brain functions is excluded.
3. Cessation of all brain functions persists for an appropriate period of observation or trial of therapy or both.

These commonly accepted criteria have been adopted as the standard. Traditionally, death has been determined when an individual's heart stopped beating. As technology evolved, a patient could be maintained on mechanical support devices, and determination of death by brain-death criteria became a recognized practice. Determination of death by brain-death criteria has been described by many neuroscience professional groups, most notably the Harvard Group, in the *Harvard Criteria for Determination of Brain Death*.[5] The process of determining death by brain-death criteria when appropriate has become more specific as a result of (1) a restating and updating of the criteria by the President's Commission for the Study of Ethical Problems in Medicine and Biomedical and Behavioral Research, (2) the evolution of the definition of brain death, and (3) increased levels of comfort and experience with application of the criteria on the part of neuroscience physicians and hospital personnel.

After death has been determined, it must be documented in the patient's medical record, including the time of death. Then the patient must be evaluated as a potential tissue and organ donor. The criteria used to determine whether a patient is a suitable candidate for donation are changing constantly, and it is recommended that emergency nurses and other health care professionals always contact their respective organ procurement agency to determine from a medical perspective whether donation is possible.

Medical criteria that may eliminate a patient from candidacy for donation of organs and some tissue include the presence of a documented septicemia or communicable disease or the possibility that the patient is at high risk for human immunodeficiency virus. Many eye recovery programs recover corneas from patients with septicemia solely for the purpose of research. All other persons can be considered potential candidates for donation of tissues or organs. An error commonly made occurs when a patient who is diagnosed with metastatic cancer is determined to be ineligible for donation: any person with a metastatic disease can be a donor of corneas for research and transplantation, depending on the clinical history and findings during the physical examination of the corneas.

Emergency nurses referring potential donors to the re-

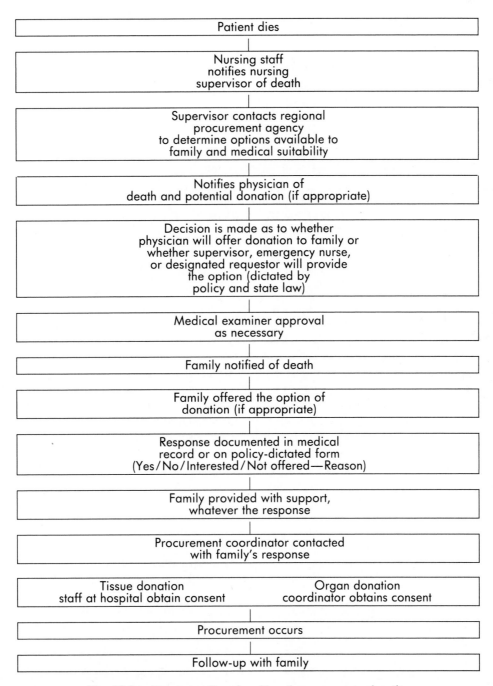

Fig. 33-2   Referral pattern for either tissue or organ donation.

Name of procurement agency
24-hour hot line phone (phone number of local organ procurement organization)
WORKSHEET

Name of patient: _____

Age: _____

Cause of death: _____

Time of death: _____

Family status: _____

(Next of kin, location of family; have family been offered donation?)

Medical Examiner's Case: YES [ ]   NO [ ]

(Phone number
for Medical Examiner)   Has the medical examiner been called? YES [ ]   NO [ ]

Approval for donation given?   YES [ ]   NO [ ]

Attending physician _____ Phone number _____

Physician status: Notified of death   YES [ ]   NO [ ]

Will offer donation option to family   YES [ ]   NO [ ]
Determined donation not an option YES   [ ]   NO [ ]
Reasons documented in record   YES [ ]   NO [ ]

CONTACT LOCAL PROCUREMENT AGENCY FOR ALL PATIENTS WHO DIE

Fig. 33-3   Organ and tissue donor referral guideline.

gional procurement agency must be prepared to employ the referral policies that have been approved within their respective institutions. If no policy exists, contacting the local procurement agency can be of benefit; the agency will help the hospital design a program to suit its needs and comply with state law.

A typical referral pattern for tissue or organ donation is outlined in Fig. 33-2.

Why is the regional procurement agency called so early in the process? The answer to this often-asked question is that (1) the possibility of a medical ruleout can be addressed before discussion with the family ensues and (2) discussion with the physician regarding this issue may be essential to clarify whether the patient is a potential donor.

When the nurse calls the local procurement agency, the guideline shown in Fig. 33-3 for required information is recommended.

Medical Examiner's Approval

The medical examiner must be notified when donation is to take place under certain circumstances, including the following:
1. Homicide
2. Suicide
3. Accidental death
4. Death within 24 hours of admission

5. Patient is admitted in comalike state and dies
6. Death of an individual 3 years of age or less

Each state has its own specific criteria, and before these criteria are included in a donation policy, the hospital should contact the state medical examiner for more information. For example, the medical examiner's office in Rhode Island requires notification of death and request for approval of donation *without* exception, for all persons who are potential tissue or organ donors. Documentation of this notification is essential for the donation to take place. Notation of the communication with the medical examiner should be included in the patient's medical record.

Documentation of the next of kin's consent must be included in the medical record. Usually permission for donation of tissues and organs is written on a specific consent form provided by the local organ procurement organization or a state-mandated form with hospital-specific amendments. The consent process is a delicate one and requires an individual with the sensitivity and knowledge to handle the grieving family's questions and concerns. The process of consent is discussed in more detail later in this chapter.

THE DOCUMENTATION PROCESS

General practice in health care dictates the presence of excellent documentation. There are three essential elements to the documentation process when a donation of tissues or

1. Name of donor _____ Date of death __ / __ / __

2. Medical record number _____

3. Next of kin not offered donation   YES [ ]

         Reason donation not offered _____
         If not offered, stop here

4. Name of person making the request for anatomic gift

         Name _____ Professional role _____

5. Name of next of kin granting or refusing consent for donation

         Name _____ Relationship Spouse   [ ]
                                                Adult child [ ]
                                                Parent   [ ]
                                                Sibling   [ ]
                                                Guardian   [ ]
                                                Other   [ ]

6. Next of kin consent: consented to donation   YES [ ]   NO [ ]
         IF NO, STOP HERE; IF YES, GO ON TO No. 7.

7. Directions for documentation
     a. For each tissue or organ offered document (check) if consent granted or denied.
     b. If specific tissue or organ not offered for donation, make no entry on that line.
     c. If consent given but tissue or organ not procured, enter reason not procured.

               a   b   c

Reason not procured (reasons 1 to 3)
(1) Clinically unsuitable
(2) Technician unavailable
(3) Other

Tissue/organ	Consent outcome		Tissue/organ procured		Reason not procured
	Granted	Denied	Yes	No	
Eye/cornea	1 [ ]	2 [ ]	1 [ ]	2 [ ]	[ ] _____
Heart for valves	1 [ ]	2 [ ]	1 [ ]	2 [ ]	[ ] _____
Bone	1 [ ]	2 [ ]	1 [ ]	2 [ ]	[ ] _____
Kidneys	1 [ ]	2 [ ]	1 [ ]	2 [ ]	[ ] _____
Liver	1 [ ]	2 [ ]	1 [ ]	2 [ ]	[ ] _____
Pancreas	1 [ ]	2 [ ]	1 [ ]	2 [ ]	[ ] _____
Heart	1 [ ]	2 [ ]	1 [ ]	2 [ ]	[ ] _____
Lungs	1 [ ]	2 [ ]	1 [ ]	2 [ ]	[ ] _____
Heart/lungs	1 [ ]	2 [ ]	1 [ ]	2 [ ]	[ ] _____
Other	1 [ ]	2 [ ]	1 [ ]	2 [ ]	[ ] _____

ONE COPY TO MEDICAL RECORDS AND ONE COPY TO BE PLACED IN THE MEDICAL RECORD

Fig. 33-4   Record of request for anatomic gift. (Adapted from Maine state law, recommended documentation form.)

organs takes place. Once family members have been apprised of their option to donate, an anatomic gift form must be completed (Fig. 33-4) stating that the next of kin have been provided with the option of donating organs and tissues. Such document should be filed for every person who dies in the hospital. A copy of this document should be placed in the patient's medical record and in a central hospital location or log book. Examples of this central location might be the medical records department and the admitting and discharge office, or this information can be placed on a computer for future statistical evaluation and analysis. The design of this form depends on hospital policy and require-

---

Patient Identification   Donation by Next-of-Kin

_____

I, _____ of _____
              (next-of-kin)   (address of next-of-kin)

_____, hereby give my permission to
       (relationship to deceased)

The New England Organ Bank, and _____
                                                     (hospital/other tissue bank)

the medical staffs thereof to remove and I authorize the subsequent donation of the following organ(s) and/or tissue(s):

[ ] eye/cornea   [ ] heart for valves   [ ] bones   [ ] kidneys   [ ] liver   [ ] other
[ ] pancreas   [ ] heart   [ ] lungs   [ ] heart/lungs   [ ] blood for testing
For organ donation only: [ ] spleen   [ ] lymph nodes   [ ] pre-typing lymph node dissection

of _____ to be used for such purposes, including organ
       (patient/deceased)

transplant, medical institutions located outside the state of Maine. Permission is further granted for the transfer of the patient to the hospital where removal of the above-mentioned organ(s) will occur. Tissue recovery will take place in the hospital where death occurs. Permission is also granted for the performance of any procedures that are deemed necessary in association with the removal of these organs and/or tissues.

I further understand that an evaluation, including blood testing, will be performed under the direction of the institution that receives the tissue, organs, and blood sample in order to assess the suitability of the tissue for transplantation. I further understand that all information regarding any test results will be kept confidential, even from me, to the extent provided by law, unless disclosure is deemed necessary to protect the health and welfare of others. Organs and/or tissues deemed not to be medically acceptable will not be used for transplantation, may be destroyed through normal procedures or referred to an established research center for the sole purpose of research.

I have been given the opportunity to ask questions and have had my questions answered to my satisfaction.

I further understand that if permission is being given prior to the actual death of _____,
I understand that death will occur shortly.   (patient/deceased)

Accordingly, it is understood that if this permission is given before death it will become effective only upon the death and then automatically, and such permission may be relied upon by the Medical Center, the Community Hospital, the New England Organ Bank, and members of their medical staffs, and any medical institution which may ultimately receive these organs unless permission is revoked by me by communicating with a representative of the New England Organ Bank, or medical center or with the attending physician prior to the removal of the organs donated.

_____   _____
Signature of Next-of-kin   Witness

_____   _____
Street   Witness

_____   Witnessed to obtaining signature
City   State   Zip   this _____ day of _____, 19___.

Permission obtained by:

_____
Name   Title   Phone #

Fig. 33-5 Permission for organ or tissue removal and donation. (Adapted from Maine state law, recommended consent form.)

ments of state law. After this form has been completed, noting in particular that the option to donate has been offered, a consent form must then be completed if the family wishes to donate tissues and organs (Fig. 33-5).

Each state and hospital have the option of creating consent forms. However, most procurement agencies provide forms and prefer that the consent form they have developed be used. This document is modified periodically to comply with changing laws. If consent forms are not available in the ED, the local procurement agency or UNOS will provide them promptly.

The last form of documentation required is dictated by state law. Many states have enacted an annual reporting mechanism for donation data. These data must be tabulated and submitted to the state department of health or other state regulatory body for review, licensure, and certification of the institution. Keeping records of data also provides the hospital with much-needed feedback concerning how best to provide donation education within the hospital community. These data can also be coordinated with data that must be reported annually for verification of Medicare and Medicaid funding, which may be required by federal regulations pertaining to COBRA of 1986 and 1990. (This verification has not yet been mandated.)

A policy or program to manage the process of tissue and organ donation must be developed in each institution. The program can only be as strong as those who manage and are committed to it. Whether this program is managed by a donation liaison staff member who works with the procurement agency's donation coordinator, a donation committee, or a dedicated emergency nurse, it must be recognized that the process does not begin and end with the development of a policy. With a significant commitment, the program will evolve successfully. Documentation of what occurs during the year after the program's inception is the best measure of the program's strengths and permits ongoing assessment and correction of shortcomings. The successes can and should be shared with other institutions as a contribution to the overall tissue and organ donation process; the failures should also be shared, when successful solutions have been developed.

OBTAINING CONSENT: WHO SHALL ASK?

Offering the family or the next of kin the option of donation is one of the more difficult yet potentially rewarding responsibilities that emergency nurses assume in their professional careers. Providing a family with this option may give them a measure of comfort and consolation. The comfort is not necessarily experienced at the time of the death. When the shock of the death has been realized, the family's knowledge that their loved one has been able to help another often encourages the family to cope and continue with their lives. The following statement expresses the positive effect of donation during one family's grief[11]:

At the time of our daughter's death it was difficult to think and make choices. Now, it has helped our grieving to know that in spite of our tragedy and loss several other people are blessed with health, hope and the promise of life.

Rob and Jan Rivera
Denver, Colorado

The best person to approach the family about donation is a professional who has developed a rapport with the family, for example, the primary nurse, the primary care physician, or a member of the clergy who has spent time with the family. The person who has been designated to carry out this responsibility should be familiar with the donation process and comfortable with his or her feelings about death and the donation of tissues and organs; to assume this responsibility, much thought and knowledge are required.

Emergency nurses are in the ideal position to offer the family the option of donating tissues and organs. They have been working with the family and patient throughout the admission and have in most situations developed the greatest rapport with the family. It is quite important, however, to discuss with the attending physician the potential for donation and the probability that the emergency nurse will offer the option of donation if appropriate unless the physician wishes to do so. If the physician does not wish that the family be offered the option of donation, he or she must document the reason in the medical record. If the physician is not comfortable with the process of offering the option of donation to the family, the emergency nurse may be obliged to offer donation to the family. Be aware that your institution may have an established protocol for offering donation to a family and that this protocol should be given consideration before proceeding.

Many institutions have developed a program in which staff are educated in the art of obtaining consent and are available to offer donation to the family. These staff members are referred to as *requestors* or *initiators* of consent for donation. The emergency nurse caring for the patient who has just died may not be familiar with the process of obtaining consent. The requestor can be a great resource and can assist with the process. If no one is available, the nurse can contact the local organ procurement organization for support. An ED educational program can be requested concerning the methods of obtaining consent and initiating the donation process.

Before the family is made aware of their option to donate a family member's tissues or organs, the family must be told that the patient has died. The family must be comfortable with the knowledge that everything possible was done to prevent death and that all available treatments were given to maintain life and health.

When family members have been informed that a member has died, their sense of devastation is extreme. They are in grief and disbelief. Discussion of anything immediately after the discussion of the death may be impossible. Family members need time to absorb and react to the news and should be given all the time they need.

Waiting until the family gives a verbal or nonverbal cue that they are ready to discuss what is to happen next is essential to provide them with an opportunity to grieve. In the case of potential brain death, when tissues and organs may be donated, the situation usually involves a sudden, unexpected event, and the person who dies may be young and previously healthy. This patient is usually transferred to an intensive care setting, where a series of tests is administered to establish that criteria for determining brain death have been met. Death is declared, and the family has more time to adjust to the idea that death has taken place. Understanding that death has occurred in the patient who has met the brain-death criteria is most difficult for families; their loved one is breathing and warm and looks alive. The family must come to accept that mechanical ventilatory support of the patient with brain death is strictly that, mechanical, and has nothing to do with life and survival. If the support systems were removed, the patient's heart would stop beating and all signs of life would be absent. Helping the family to understand that death has occurred is difficult. This information must be provided for the family by the primary physician in terms that they can understand and educationally reinforced by the primary nurse and other available health care professionals.

When the patient in the ED is declared dead by the more conventional criterion of cardiac asystole, it is less difficult for the family to grasp the reality of the event. Death as a result of cardiac arrest is more commonly recognized than brain death, and the heart's arrested activity is a tangible end point. However, in these cases, the family members have less time to consider possible options or treatments and less time to adjust to their loss.

Emotions can be labile: adjusting to the idea of the death is always difficult. Many emotions may be engulfing the family at this time. They may have had little to do with this particular family member recently, or they may be feeling responsible for the one who has just died. Families often ask themselves what could have been done to prevent death or how this death might have been made easier. Before the option of donation is broached, the family members need time to gain control of their thoughts and adjust if possible to the reality that a family member has died and is not going to return home. Their lives will never be the same, and as difficult as it may seem, they must continue to live without this loved one.

The first step in the initiation process of donation, identifying the next of kin, can be straightforward or complex, depending on the family situation. It would be prudent to review the order of priority of the next of kin outlined earlier in the chapter. One must also differentiate between the next of kin and the family spokesperson. For example, the wife of a 70-year-old man in cardiac arrest may not come to the hospital when her husband is admitted and dies. However, in the absence of a son or daughter, a close family friend accompanies the patient and is relaying all information to the next of kin by telephone. It is not appropriate in this case to offer the family friend the option of donation. One must initiate the process of donation by talking with the wife on the telephone and if appropriate, obtain consent over the telephone. The nurse must keep in mind that when obtaining consent over the telephone, two witnesses are required to assist in the process and must sign the consent form indicating that the next of kin has given permission to donate tissues and organs.

If family members choose to come to the ED to see the patient who has just died, they will need time to say goodbye to the patient and to begin to make plans and arrangements.

It is critical that the family be provided with a private room or location that is comfortable, quiet, and gives them an opportunity to share their feelings of loss and grief with each other or experience that grief alone. Realizing that the family member is dead is the greatest hurdle that the family must overcome. (Viewing the body of the person who has just died is a critical step in this process.)

An assessment of what the family knows or what they have been told is of great importance in offering them the option of donation. If they are not yet able to accept that death has occurred, then it is not time to talk about donation. The family must hear the words *death* and *dead* when references are made to the status of their family member. A common error in health care is to refer to the death euphemistically. For example, the nurse may say that the patient "has just expired" or "passed on" or "will no longer be with us," or that "there is no hope" or "it is over." Saying the word *dead* when talking to the family is straightforward and prevents misinterpretation. Because they are shocked and may be in a state of denial, the family may not comprehend the impact of the message that there is "no hope for their loved one." This understanding is critical in the case of the family of a patient who is considered dead by brain-death criteria. If they do not yet comprehend the death, the subject of donation should not be broached.

The family essentially "becomes the patient" after death of their loved one. It is important to determine how the family members are working together as a unit. Who is the "strong right arm" of the family? Who is asking the questions? Who is the spokesperson or next of kin? What was the family's relationship to the deceased? How does the family make decisions? These and other general observations of the family's behavior are essential in initiating the process of donation in a way that is comfortable both for the family and for the nurse.

Other goals in assessment of the family should include assessment of the family's cultural and religious background and its impact on how they will handle the concept of donation. A decision not to offer donation because of religious and cultural biases based on assumptions about the family's last name and background has no place in the process. The choice belongs with the family.

When is it appropriate not to ask the family about donation? What if the family says no to donation? These difficult questions should be dealt with on an individual basis.

The appropriate time to ask a family about donation depends on circumstance. There is no perfect time to ask. The nurse's clinical judgment may be the best resource. The family's emotional stability and ability to comprehend the death and its meaning to them may direct the entire process. The ability to recognize the verbal or nonverbal cues concerning when the family is ready to be asked about donation is developed after time and experience in dealing with families who face death.

The family should not be offered the option of donation only when, in the clinical judgment of the emergency nurse, the family is unable to cope with hearing one more piece of information. Offering the option of donation may increase the family's pain and heighten the crisis; donation should not be offered in this case.

When a family says no to donation, that response is perfectly reasonable. Donation is not an option for every family or every individual. Whatever the decision about donation, it is the right one for that family or individual and should be accepted. The nurse's role is to give the family the choice and support the family's decision.

EDUCATION OF THE FAMILY

The family needs to be given information about donation so that they can decide what is right for them and what the family member would have wished. Detailed, understandable information is essential. The family must never be coerced about donation and its benefits.

The family needs to know that if they grant permission for donation, it will be carried out promptly. The family should also be told that although there is always the chance of slight deformities, in general, donations will cause no body deformity. Even after donation of bone, for instance, the body can be prepared for an open-casket funeral.

In the case of multitissue donors such as the donor described in the case study below, donation of all tissues is not always possible in all areas of the country because of a lack of resources. However, donation should be offered to the family if the option is available. This donation will take place shortly after the family has returned home from the hospital and teams can be arranged to recover the tissue. The tissue recovery teams may be in the same facility, or they may be 500 miles away and transportation arrangements may be complex. When eyes and corneas, heart for valves, and skin are the only tissues to be recovered because of specific medical concerns about bone donation, the entire donation could take place in the morgue, since an operating room would not be needed. However, if bone were included in the donation, an operating suite and sterile aseptic technique are the protocols for most bone procurement teams across the country.

Procurement of internal organs takes place in an operating suite. The multitissue, multiorgan procurement procedure is usually completed in about 4 to 5 hours. Delays in the procurement process should be reported to the family promptly. Recovery of eyes or corneas, heart for valves, and skin can be carried out in the morgue or other private room away from other hospital activity and patients. The regional procurement agency will provide the technical staff to recover the eyes, valves, and skin. If the family has made special plans regarding funeral arrangements, they should inform the emergency nurse or coordinator of those plans.

A donation coordinator from the local organ procurement organization is available for support in the case of any donation. In most donations of internal organs the coordinator attends to the patient and family at the hospital, obtains consent from the family, explains the process of donation to the family, and coordinates the entire donation from start to finish. In the case of tissue donation only, the coordinator is less likely to be at the hospital but is available for consultation and ensures that necessary support is available. The coordinator works with the emergency nurse, other contact staff at the hospital, and the respective procurement teams.

THE PROCUREMENT PROCESS
Tissue Procurement: Eyes, Corneas, Bone, Heart for Valves, and Skin

Tissue procurement is less complex than internal organ procurement.

The coordinator from the procurement agency arranges for the arrival of the recovery teams and works with the nursing staff in the operating suite of the hospital to set up surgery time and conditions convenient for all parties involved.

The maximum time allowed for recovery of tissue after asystole is approximately 10 hours for bones, 6 to 10 hours for valves, and 24 hours for corneas and skin. These time limits vary, depending on the procurement agency. The preferred time of recovery is that time closest to asystole.

The process of recovering bones is usually carried out

CASE STUDY

Multitissue Donor

A 54-year-old man is admitted to the ED in cardiac arrest at 2:30 A.M. He is in asystole and is declared dead at 3:15 A.M. His wife gives permission to donate organs and tissues. "Anything he can donate is fine. . . . He always wanted to be an organ donor." The medical examiner approves the donation for eyes, corneas, bone, skin, and heart for valves.

using sterile technique. Usually all four limbs, including both femurs, proximal tibia, fibula, and proximal humerus, are prepared for recovery. Occasionally a mandible, hemipelvis, every other rib, tissues from the limbs such as tensor fasciae latae, Achilles tendon with a block of calcaneus, and others are recovered.[25] The surgical procedure lasts approximately 1½ to 4 hours, depending on the experience of the team and the number of tissues to be recovered. A single incision is made along each limb so that the respective bones can be extracted. A prosthetic device made of polyvinyl chloride telescopic tubing or in some cases wooden dowels is used to replace the bones as a means of reconstruction. Aside from the single incision made along the inner aspect of the limb, there should be no deformity associated with the procurement process. After procurement of the bone, it is stored in a freezer at −70° F or is freeze-dried or processed into chips for later use. The uses of bone are extensive, ranging from replacement of bone that has been invaded by a tumor to replacing bone in neurosurgical cases in which bone has been removed.

The bone recovery process is difficult to observe and participate in, particularly if the staff in the operating room are not accustomed to this type of procedure. If this is the case, before the procurement procedure is performed, an educational in-service program should be provided for the staff by the regional procurement agency. The donation coordinator who oversees the development of the hospital's program in conjunction with the hospital's liaison should organize an educational program of this type to facilitate the education and comfort level of operating room staff who will eventually be involved in this process.

After death the eye donor should be maintained in a refrigerated room if available, the head should be elevated at an angle of 20 degrees, and the eyes should be taped shut with paper tape. Cool compresses can be placed over the eyes to prevent swelling and to ease the procurement process. The recovery of eyes is a clean procedure using sterile technique; it requires 20 to 30 minutes. Two methods of recovery are commonly used: recovery of the entire globe of the eye and a corneal punch procedure. The eye tissue is packed in preservative solution. The container is placed on ice and dispatched to the respective eye recovery center for processing. The corneas are generally transplanted within 24 to 48 hours. They are used in the treatment of keratoconus and other diseases of the cornea. If the globe of the eye has been recovered, the orbit is filled with ample cotton and a cap similar in contour to the eye, eliminating any deformity resulting from the absence of the globe. The technical staff recovering the eyes must be skilled in these procedures and in many states must be certified in the techniques of recovery.

For recovery of the heart for valves, the entire heart is removed from the donor. The aortic and pulmonary valves are dissected from the heart and are eventually used as replacement valves. Aortic root replacement, repair of tetralogy of Fallot, and pulmonary atresia can also be performed using valve parts. The chest is opened from the xyphoid process to the sternal notch. The ribs and sternum are retracted and the heart is mobilized. The cardiectomy of the heart includes dissection along the great vessels extending distally from the heart as far as possible. The heart is then removed from the chest, placed in sterile Ringer's lactate solution, packed in a sterile container, double-bagged sterilely, and packed on ice for shipping to the processing center. The valves are dissected from the heart, their integrity is examined, and the entire heart is examined for pathologic conditions. Serologic examinations are performed, and after a brief period of quarantine the valves are released for homograft transplant according to size and need. The donor will have a single incision on the chest; this incision will not prevent the possibility of an open casket if the family so wishes.

If the process of skin recovery is available in the region, this procedure can also take place in the morgue. A clean room and sterile technique are required. Using a dermatome, skin is recovered from the buttocks, thighs, back, and abdomen. A split-thickness graft is removed from the top surface of the body; it is barely visible unless the donor has a dark tan or is of high pigment. Once the skin is recovered, it is treated with antibiotics, prepared surgically for grafting, and stored in freezers at −70° F. The recovered skin is used for temporary grafts in the care of severely burned patients to provide protection from infection, fluid shifts, and other complications of burns.

Solid-Organ Procurement: Heart, Lungs, Liver, Pancreas, and Kidney

The recovery of solid organs for transplant may be complex and requires the cooperation of team members representing many different disciplines. Before the process can begin, the family or next of kin must give their consent for the specific organs and tissues to be donated. The time of death, as determined by brain-death criteria, must be documented in the record, and the medical examiner's approval must be in place before proceeding.

Many hours of hemodynamic maintenance of the donor may be necessary before the actual procedure takes place. The donation coordinator works with the family to address their concerns and with the intensive care unit staff to manage the donor until the time of the procurement. The hemodynamic parameters of donor management have been worked out over time and if met, facilitate the procurement of the healthy organs for transplant. The hemodynamic parameters of donor management include the following:

1. Maintain a systolic blood pressure of 100 mm Hg
2. Manipulate the ventilatory setting to maintain a PO_2 of 100 or better
3. Maintain a urine output of 100 to 500 ml/hour
4. Maintain hematocrit of 30 or more

These parameters are for the adult donor. The goals are

the same in the pediatric patient but are specifically based on weight and size of the potential donor. The potential donor may not necessarily exhibit these parameters, but the patient must be considered for donation.

Once the patient is declared dead by brain-death criteria, management for preservation of organs for transplantation can begin. The donor's blood pressure is extremely labile, and diabetes insipidus develops as a result of herniation of the brain. This results in an imbalance of fluids and electrolytes. Management of the donor includes the balancing of fluid and electrolytes and the use of pressors such as dopamine and dobutamine, along with treatment of the developing diabetes insipidus. Antidiuretic hormone replacement using a pitressin supplement via an intravenous drip, intranasally, or by injection is frequently instituted. Management of the pulmonary status of the donor should also occur so that blood gas levels reflect extremely well oxygenated organs. Hematocrit is monitored closely to prevent lowered oxygen transport, which may have resulted from excessive bleeding caused by a related trauma. It is essential to review all laboratory values, including fluid status, and to evaluate these for overhydration or underhydration. Numerous laboratory studies, including electrolyte measurements, hematologic studies, liver function tests, cardiac enzyme assessment, electrocardiogram, echocardiogram, cardiology consultation, arterial blood gas tests, and evaluation of radiographs of the chest, are carried out to determine the health of the organs that are to be recovered.

After the patient has been accepted as a donor and all organs to be recovered have been assigned to a receiving patient, all recovery teams convene at a stated time convenient to all parties. The host hospital has final determination of operating time. Most donations of organs occur during the late hours of the night and the hospital will be asked to provide operating room staff and anesthesia support.

The donor is transported to the operating room fully supported by mechanical means and is hemodynamically maintained in the operating room according to the goals outlined previously.

The donor is maintained throughout the organ dissection and mobilization of the respective tissue until organs and tissues are freed for immediate removal and preservation. After the last aspects of the dissection have been completed, the aorta is clamped and cardioplegia takes place. Quick cooling and in situ flushing of the organs is then accomplished. After flushing of the organs has been completed, they will be removed from the donor, examined individually in a sterile back basin, flushed again if required, and packed in a sterile container for transport and immediate transplant (in the case of heart, heart and lung, and single lung). For kidneys, approximately 24 hours may elapse before transplantation takes place. For the pancreas and liver, the number of hours that may elapse before transplantation ranges

from 6 to 20 hours. This flexibility of preservation time in the case of the kidneys, liver, and pancreas is largely the result of the development of the preservation fluid "U.W." by Dr. Folkert O. Belzer of the University of Wisconsin during the late 1980s. This preservation fluid has greatly enhanced the procurement process, allowing time for transportation of organs and prospective tissue typing of the donor with the recipient. Prospective tissue typing is primarily carried out between kidney donor and recipient and in some cases between heart, heart and lung, and single-lung donor and recipient.

WHO WILL PAY?

The process of donation of tissues and organs is an expensive one. The family of the donor should never be issued the hospital bill that has accrued during the hospital stay until the organ procurement agency has had an opportunity to review the charges and take care of all charges related to the donation process. Families must be made aware of this, if at all possible, when they speak with the coordinator. If the family members receive a bill, they are encouraged to contact the organ procurement agency, which will ensure proper payment of the bill.

In the United States, payment for the organ transplant is usually made by third-party payors. In 1972 the End-Stage Renal Disease Act was enacted, allowing patients with end-stage renal disease to be covered by Medicare for treatment of dialysis and kidney transplantation. All persons were given the opportunity for treatment essential to life. For liver and heart transplantation most third-party payors cover the cost of the transplantation surgery and postoperative care, although in many states, third-party reimbursement is not available in the case of heart and lung, pancreas, and lung transplantation, since these transplants are still considered experimental. There has been a great deal of controversy regarding the expense of transplantation, with emphasis on the number of individuals helped, cost, and life expectancy after the graft and the transplantation. Table 33-1 presents the cost range for solid-organ transplantations.

These costs vary from center to center but serve as a guideline for actual costs. It has been difficult for many states to justify the cost of transplantation in the time of

Table 33-1   Solid-organ transplantation costs

Organ	Approximate cost ($)
Heart	57,000 to 110,000
Heart and lung	130,000 to 200,000
Kidney	25,000 to 30,000
Liver	135,000 to 238,000
Pancreas	30,000 to 40,000

From American Council on Transplantation: From here to transplant, Alexandria, Va, 1987, The Council.

cost containment when so few individuals are benefited. Oregon, for example, has reallocated Medicaid monies previously designated for transplantation, except in the case of kidneys and corneas, to other areas of the governmental budget that were felt to better serve a greater number of individuals such as pregnant mothers and infants and mothers at high risk.[14] How the money is spent and who pays for these highly specialized, technologically advanced procedures are questions considered daily, and the ethics of choosing between one cause to benefit another is grappled with continuously.

ETHICAL ISSUES

There are numerous ethical issues related to donation and transplantation of organs and tissues. Those that affect the daily practice of the emergency nurse include the nurse's role in offering the family the option of donation, the comfort level of the emergency nurse in this area of nursing care, and how best to deal with examination of one's feelings regarding this option. Occasionally the emergency nurse is also faced with a death determined by brain-death criteria, maintaining the patient who has been declared dead so that others may benefit, and dealing with a family's grief and confusion. These and other questions, including determining who shall receive the organ and who shall pay for the transplant, and including issues related to the sale of organs and tissues, required request and presumed consent, and how far the art of transplantation should be extended to extend life, are routinely reviewed on a global level and addressed in numerous forums. The answers are always complex and are of ongoing concern.

The key to effective nursing care is to individually access one's personal and professional feelings, examine the literature on the respective issues, and make a decision that is consistent with personal beliefs. If the nurse is uncomfortable with donation and with offering the family the option of donation, it is best for the nurse to separate himself or herself from that aspect of practice and pass the responsibility on to a peer who is more comfortable with the process. Thus families, potential donors, and potential recipients will be better served.

SUMMARY

There are many issues surrounding the role and responsibility of the emergency nurse related to tissue and organ donors. It is the emergency nurse's responsibility to provide the family with the option of tissue and organ donation when a patient dies in the ED. The *Emergency Nurses Association Position Statement of 1987* clearly indicates this responsibility[15]:

The Emergency Nurses Association believes emergency nurses should be knowledgeable in identification of potential donors and life support of donor patients, and in accessing resource personnel from state and/or local transplant teams. It is within the role of

the emergency nurse, and is now mandated by federal law, to initiate discussions regarding organ donation and to facilitate, coordinate, and intervene with families as appropriate.

Most potential donors are patients who are admitted to the hospital by ED staff and eventually die in the ED. For too long the concept of donation has been associated solely with the trauma victim, the patient who is maintained and declared dead by brain-death criteria in the intensive care setting. Almost any person who dies can be a donor of some tissue or organ for transplantation. This is a new concept and a new responsibility that is an integral part of the practice of the emergency nursing care for patients and families in crisis.

REFERENCES

1. American Council on Transplantation: *From here to transplant*, Alexandria, Va, 1987, The Council.
2. American Hospital Association, American Medical Association, and United Network for Organ Sharing: *Required request legislation: a guide for hospitals on organ and tissue donation*, Chicago, 1988, American Hospital Association, American Medical Association, and United Network For Organ Sharing.
3. Batten HL, Prottas JM: Kind strangers: the families of organ donors, *Health Affairs* Summer 1987, p 38.
4. Caplin AL: *Professional arrogance and public misunderstanding*, Hastings Center Report, April 1988, p 37.
5. *Defining death: medical, legal, and ethical issues in the determination of death*, President's Commission for the Study of Ethical Problems in Medicine and Biomedical Research, Washington, DC, 1981.
6. Dekker ML: Bone and soft tissue procurement, *Orthop Nurs* 8(2):33, 1989.
7. Department of Health and Human Services: *Organ transplantation: issues and recommendations*, Report of the Task Force on Organ Transplantation, Washington, DC, 1986, US Department of Health and Human Services.
8. DeBoer H: The history of bone grafts, *Clin Orthop* 226:292, 1988.
9. Emergency Nurses Association: *Role of the emergency nurse in organ procurement: ENA position statement*, Chicago, 1987, The Association.
10. Gallup Poll 1985: *The US public's attitudes toward organ transplant/organ donation*, 1985, The Gallup Organization.
11. Grenvik A: Ethical dilemmas in organ donation and transplantation, *Crit Care Med* p 1012, 1988.
12. Laudicina SS: *Medicaid coverage and payment policies for organ transplants: findings of a national survey*, George Washington University, 1988, US Department of Health and Human Services.
13. National Kidney Foundation: *For those who give and grieve: a booklet for donor families*, Washington, DC, 1990, The Foundation.
14. Newberry MA: *Textbook of hemodialysis for patient care personnel*, Springfield, Ill, 1989, Charles C Thomas.
15. Tilney NL: Renal transplantation between identical twins: a review, *World J Surg* 10(3):381, 1986.

Barbara Bennett Jacobs

Injury or trauma continues to be one of the major public health problems in the United States. In the broadest sense, injuries to human beings are influenced by and ultimately have an impact on society. In particular, however, the injury process as described by Haddon[11] is a combination of influences and factors before the injury event, during the event, and after the injury has been sustained. These factors are associated with the human *host,* for example, the amount of ingested alcohol; the *vehicle* or vector of energy transfer, for example, the type of motor vehicle; and the *environment,* such as obstacles near the roadway.

An injury is the damage to tissues and structures of the human body that has resulted from an exchange with environmental energy and that is beyond the body's resistance or resilience.[12] This definition is universal enough to include all the injuries resulting from mechanical energy, electrical energy, heat and fire, chemicals and poisons, radiation, radiant energy, and drowning or asphyxiation. The epidemiology of injuries, the determinants and distribution of this event in populations, is a method of identifying the specific characteristics of those persons who sustain specific types of injuries. Frequent variables associated with epidemiologic study are age, race, gender, socioeconomic status, geographic location, and specific exposure circumstances, such as smoking and alcohol use.

Humanity's encounter with environmental energy and the resulting injury that may occur has been recorded since ancient times. The ubiquitous presence of injuries, however, may dilute their importance and fosters an attitudinal acceptance of their occurrence. Since the decline of the use of the word *accident,* more focus is now placed on prevention and less focus is placed on chance, fate, and blame as contributors to the injury process. Efforts are emerging to focus on the injury problem and to direct research activities toward developing countermeasures that reduce injuries by targeting specific types of hazards within specific populations.

The publication of *Injury in America* in 1985 provided the template for future federal funding for research into the prevention of trauma.[5] Since this landmark publication, the Division of Injury Control of the Centers for Disease Con-

trol, funded by appropriations through the Department of Transportation's National Highway Traffic Safety Administration (NHTSA), has funded injury research centers and extramural grant programs across the country. With the annual budget increasing during the last 5 years, more funds are now available to continue the much needed research in the five areas of injury: epidemiology, acute care, prevention, rehabilitation, and biomechanics. In 1986 and 1987 the Division of Injury Epidemiology and Control received an annual average of $11.3 million.[4] The 1990 budget was $22.7 million. Following are the currently operational injury research centers:

1. University of Alabama, Birmingham
2. Harvard School of Public Health
3. University of California, Los Angeles
4. University of California, San Francisco
5. University of Iowa
6. University of Washington, Harborview Medical Center
7. University of North Carolina School of Public Health
8. The Johns Hopkins University School of Hygiene and Public Health

FEDERAL DATA SOURCE

This discussion of the epidemiology of injuries or trauma will derive data mostly from national sources such as the National Center for Health Statistics to provide an overall view of the extent of the injury dilemma. Published data in journals tend to focus on small patient populations such as those patients treated with a specific injury at a specific hospital. The purpose and goal of this chapter, however, are to provide population-based figures that present the epidemiologic foundation of trauma.

The National Center for Health Statistics publishes a yearly mortality report that summarizes data related to all deaths in the United States.[22-27] For the 8 years of data that are reviewed in this chapter, accidents and their adverse effects have ranked as the *fourth* leading cause of death, preceded by diseases of the heart, malignant neoplasms (cancer), and cerebrovascular diseases (stroke). Table 34-1 shows the death rates for the four leading causes of death

Table 34-1 Death rates and percentages of total deaths for four leading causes of death in the United States, 1981-1988

	Rate per 100,000 population (% of total deaths)				
Year	All causes	Heart disease	Malignant neoplasms	Cerebrovascular disease	Accidents and effects
1981	862.4 (100)	328.7 (38.1)	184.0 (21.3)	71.3 (8.3)	43.9 (5.1)
1982	852.0 (100)	326.0 (38.3)	187.2 (22.0)	68.0 (8.0)	40.6 (4.8)
1983	863.8 (100)	329.2 (38.2)	189.3 (21.9)	66.5 (7.7)	39.5 (4.6)
1984	862.3 (100)	323.5 (37.8)	191.8 (21.8)	65.3 (7.6)	39.3 (4.4)
1985	873.9 (100)	323.0 (37)	193.3 (22.1)	64.1 (7.3)	39.1 (4.5)
1986	873.2 (100)	317.5 (36.4)	194.7 (22.3)	62.1 (7.1)	39.5 (4.5)
1987	872.4 (100)	312.4 (35.8)	195.9 (22.4)	61.6 (7.0)	39.0 (4.5)
1988	882.0 (100)	311.3 (35.3)	197.3 (22.4)	61.2 (6.9)	39.5 (4.5)

Table 34-2 Rankings of six leading causes of death by age-groups in the United States, 1988

	Age-groups (yr)					
Cause of death	1-4	5-14	15-24	25-44	45-64	>65
Accidents and effects	1	1	1	1	4	
Heart diseases	5	5	5	3	2	1
Cerebrovascular diseases	—	—	—	—	3	3
Congenital diseases	2	3	—	—	—	—
Malignant neoplasms	3	2	4	2	1	2
Homicide	4	4	2	6	—	—
Suicide	—	6	3	5	—	—
Chronic pulmonary diseases	—	—	—	—	5	4
Pneumonia and influenza	6	—	—	—	—	5
Human immunodeficiency virus	—	—	6	4	—	—
Diabetes	—	—	—	—	—	6
Chronic liver diseases	—	—	—	—	6	—

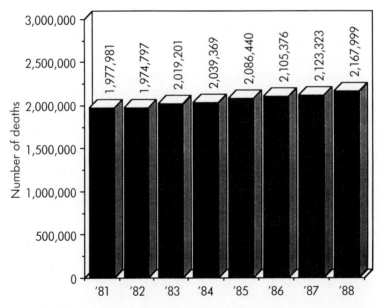

Fig. 34-1   Total number of deaths in United States, 1981-1988.

and the percentage of deaths for each cause. A rate rather than a raw number is more useful because the rate adjusts for the population and is more useful in making comparisons. The death rate is the number of deaths per 100,000 population.

To adjust the death rate by age lends even more clarity to the analysis. Fig. 34-1 does, however, show the actual number of deaths for the years 1981 to 1988, with deaths increasing each year with the population. Accidents and their adverse effects are the leading cause of death for the persons between the ages of 1 and 44 years. The phrase *accidents and their adverse effects* includes International Classification of Diseases codes E800 to E949. Additional injuries are separated and classified as suicides (E950 to 959), homicide and legal intervention (E960 to 978), and other external causes (E980 to 999). Table 34-2 demonstrates the rankings of the six leading causes of death for individual age-groups in 1988, the most current year of final statistics available. In the 15- to 24-year age-group, the three leading causes of death are all injury related, that is, accidents and their adverse effects followed by homicide and suicide. For persons older than 65 years, accidents are the seventh leading cause of death. Figs. 34-2 to 34-4 show the increasing numbers of deaths from categories of death associated with injury. The deaths caused by trauma are recorded on death certificates, which are later tabulated into the annual U.S. report on mortality by E-code. All other deaths are recorded by N-code. The difference is that N-codes depict the actual *nature* of the death by clinical category, such as diabetes and heart diseases. In contrast, the E-code does not explain the anatomic fatal injury, that is, head or chest injury, but depicts the *external cause* of the death, such as motor vehicle, homicide, or suicide. In a large population, such as the entire United States, the percentage of deaths from actual body systems injured is unknown and can be estimated only on the basis of smaller patient populations reported in the literature.

Gender and Age

Because the previously described differences in death are unevenly spread across age-groups, age becomes an important epidemiologic determinant of death caused by trauma. Gender is also significant in explaining differences in trauma mortality. In 1988, of the 38,167 deaths of persons between the ages of 15 to 24 years, 18,507 (48.5%) were caused by accidents and their adverse effects. This is a slight decrease from 1986, when the percentage was 50%. In 1988, 78% of all deaths of persons 15 to 24 years old were due to all injuries (accidents and adverse effects, homicide, suicide, and other external causes). A similar situation exists for people between the ages of 25 and 34 years, with all injuries ($n = 31,328$) causing 53% of the deaths. As age increases from this point, the percentage of deaths caused by trauma begins to decline. Table 34-3 shows the death rates for all trauma deaths according to age-groups, and Table 34-4 shows rates according to gender. Death caused by trauma is more prevalent among males. In 1988, 71.3% of the 152,572 deaths resulting from all injuries occurred in males and 28.7% in females. Other differences between rates in males and females are discussed in the following sections related to specific mechanisms of injury.

Geographic United States

The region of the United States with the highest death rate caused by accidents and their adverse effects is the East South Central region (Kentucky, Tennessee, Alabama, Mis-

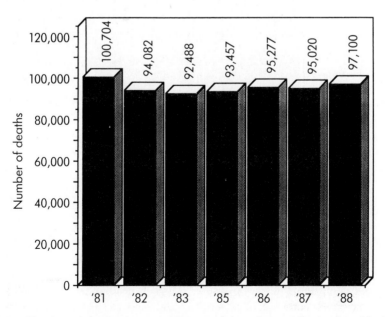

Fig. 34-2   Number of deaths from accidents and the adverse effects of accidents (E800 to 949).

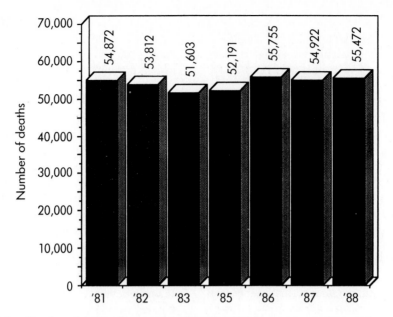

Fig. 34-3 Number of deaths from suicide (E950 to 959), homicides and legal interventions (E960 to 978), and other causes (E980 to 999).

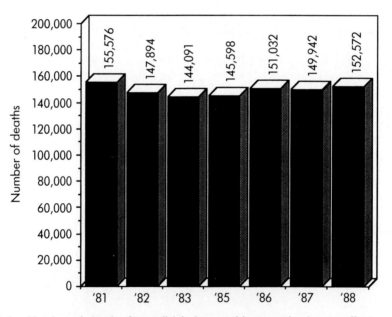

Fig. 34-4 Number of deaths from all injuries: accidents and adverse effects, suicide, homicide and legal intervention, and others.

sissippi). The rate is 50.9 per 100,000 population compared with 31.2, the lowest death regional rate, seen in New England (Maine, New Hampshire, Vermont, Massachusetts, Rhode Island, Connecticut). The East South Central region also has the highest death rate for motor vehicle crashes, 26.7 per 100,000 population, compared with the lowest, 14.8, in the Middle Atlantic region (New York, New Jersey, Pennsylvania). The Mountain region, comprising Montana,

Idaho, Wyoming, Colorado, New Mexico, Arizona, Utah, and Nevada, has the highest death rate resulting from suicide, 19.0 per 100,000 population, compared with the lowest rate, 8.6, in the Middle Atlantic region.

In descending order, the individual states with the five highest death rates (per 100,000 population) from accidents and their adverse effects are Alaska (74.4), New Mexico (56.7), South Carolina (55.9), Mississippi (54.8), and Idaho

Table 34-3 Number and age-specific death rates for all accidents (E800-999) in the United States, 1988

| Age-group (yr) | No. of deaths (rate per 100,000 population) | | | | |
	Total deaths	Accidents and effects	Suicides	Homicide and legal intervention	All other external causes
All	2,167,999 (882.0)	97,100 (39.5)	30,407 (12.4)	22,032 (9.0)	3033 (1.2)
<1	38,910 (1008.3)	936 (24.3)	—	315 (8.2)	42 (1.1)
1-4	7429 (50.9)	2858 (19.6)	—	381 (2.6)	55 (0.4)
5-14	8925 (25.8)	4215 (12.2)	243 (0.7)	459 (1.3)	73 (0.2)
15-24	38,167 (102.1)	18,507 (49.5)	4,929 (13.2)	5771 (15.4)	449 (1.2)
25-34	59,137 (135.4)	16,728 (38.3)	6710 (15.4)	6992 (16.0)	898 (2.1)
35-44	77,454 (219.6)	11,551 (32.8)	5205 (14.8)	3834 (10.9)	636 (1.8)
45-54	117,472 (486.2)	7514 (31.1)	3532 (14.6)	1727 (7.1)	288 (1.2)
55-64	269,749 (1235.6)	7663 (35.1)	3406 (15.6)	1130 (5.2)	206 (0.9)
65-74	488,545 (2729.8)	8971 (50.1)	3296 (18.4)	760 (4.2)	197 (1.1)
75-84	601,914 (6321.3)	10,145 (106.5)	2,462 (25.9)	433 (4.5)	104 (1.1)
>85	459,170 (15,594.0)	7880 (267.3)	605 (20.5)	139 (4.7)	61 (2.1)
Unknown	587	132	19	91	24

Table 34-4 Number of accidental deaths and death rates by gender in the United States, 1988

| Cause of death | No. of deaths (rate per 100,000 population) | | |
	Both genders	Male	Female
Accidents and effects	97,100 (39.5)	65,821 (55.0)	31,279 (24.8)
Suicide	30,407 (12.4)	24,078 (20.1)	6329 (5.0)
Homicide and legal intervention	22,032 (9.0)	16,712 (14.0)	5320 (4.2)
Other external causes	3033 (1.2)	2208 (1.8)	850 (0.7)
Total (%)	152,572	108,819 (71.3%)	43,753 (28.4%)

(54.6). Those with the five lowest rates are New Hampshire (27.6), Hawaii (28.7), Massachusetts (29.7), Rhode Island (29.7), and Connecticut (30.7).

MOTOR VEHICLE CRASHES

Although the word *accident* appears in the government-generated mortality documents, few epidemiologists, preventionists, or persons concerned with the devastation caused by trauma use it. The once-phrased "motor vehicle accidents" are referred to as motor vehicle crashes (MVCs). Of all the deaths caused by accidents and their adverse effects in 1988, 51% were due to MVCs. The age-adjusted death rate for MVCs was 19.7 per 100,000 population in 1988, a 1% increase from 1987 but a 15.1% decrease from 1979. The age-group with the highest death rate (38.5) caused by MVCs in 1988 was between 15 and 24 years of age; 14,406 persons in this age-group were killed.[10] Fig. 34-5 shows the distribution of fatalities from MVCs according to specific age-groups. The age-group of 25 to 34 years had an increase in the MVC death rate from 16.6 per 100,000 persons in 1986 to 23.9 per 100,000 persons in 1988, the largest increase of any other age-group.

Fatal Accident Reporting System

Another source of information regarding fatalities associated with motor vehicle crashes is the Fatal Accident Reporting System (FARS). The National Center for Statistics and Analysis of the NHTSA garners data on all MVCs in which there was a fatality that occurred on a publicly accessed roadway, when the death occurred within 30 days of the event. All states including Puerto Rico and the District of Columbia contribute to this useful data base. The report is generated annually. The following facts concern fatal accidents in 1988 that were related to motor vehicles[39]:

1. There were 42,119 fatal MVCs.
2. Of these, 47,093 people were fatally injured.
3. Although fatalities increased by 1.5% in 1988, the number of vehicle miles traveled also increased. In 1988 the traffic fatality rate was the lowest recorded since 1960. The rate was 5.1 in 1960, reached its highest rate, 5.5, in 1966, and dropped to 2.3 in 1988. This means that 2.3 fatalities occurred per 100 million vehicle miles traveled.
4. Fatality rates per 100,000 population were as high as 26.08 in 1972, with a steady decline occurring

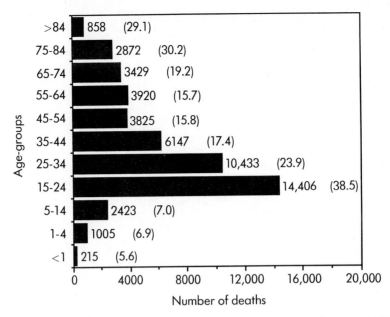

Fig. 34-5 Motor vehicle–related deaths, by age-groups: United States—1988 (death rates per 100,000 population).

from 1979 (22.75) through 1983 (18.18). In 1986 the fatality rate began to increase again (19.12), dropped in 1987 (19.06), and increased again to 19.16 in 1988.

5. Table 34-5 shows the number of fatalities according to the type of vehicle involved, with passenger cars being the vehicle of death for 25,802 persons; of these, 17,216 (67%) were drivers.

6. The number of fatally injured drivers increased by 1.6% from 1987 to 1988. The age-groups with in-

creases (percent increase over 1987 shown in parentheses) in the number of fatalities were as follows: under 15 (3.3%), 18 to 20 (4.9%), 35 to 44 (3.6%), 45 to 54 (8.9%), and over 65 (6.6%).

7. There were 32,945 males (70%) fatally injured compared with 14,124 females (30%) and 24 fatalities of unspecified gender.

8. Of all single-vehicle crashes, 48.1% were a result of some sort of collision with a fixed object, such as a pole, tree, or sign.

9. Of those fatalities involved in multivehicle crashes, 78.9% were either head-on (34.7%) or angled collisions (43.25%).

10. The frequency of fatalities is greatest on Saturdays, followed by Fridays, Sundays, Mondays, Thursdays, Wednesdays, and Tuesdays.

11. During weekends more fatalities are at night, whereas during the weekdays more fatalities occur during the day.

12. Of the 42,119 fatal crashes, 57% of the fatalities were in rural areas, with 42% in urban areas.

13. The types of roadway where fatal crashes occurred were as follows: major collector, 26.3%; minor arterial, 20%; other principal arterial, 18.3%; local, 17%; interstate, 10%; minor collector, 7.1%; and unknown, 1.4%.

14. Of the 62,686 vehicles involved in the 1988 fatal crashes, 69% were "going straight," 15% were negotiating a curve, 6% were involved in a turn, 2.5% were stopped or parked, 2.3% were passing, and 1.7% were avoiding a pedestrian or animal; the few

Table 34-5 Type and number of vehicles involved in 47,093 fatal motor vehicle crashes in the United States, 1988

Type of vehicle	No. involved
OCCUPANT CRASHES	
Passenger cars	25,802
Light trucks	7265
Multipurpose vehicles	1041
Motorcycles and other motorized vehicles	3661
Heavy trucks	785
Buses	53
Other	435
Unknown	136
NONOCCUPANT CRASHES	
Pedestrians	6869
Pedal cyclists	910
Other	136

remaining crashes involved starting or stopping, changing lanes, and unknown maneuvers.

15. Seat position in the vehicle involved in a fatal crash is an important characteristic of all fatal crashes. The following lists the occupant position and the percentage of persons sitting in those positions who perished during a fatal crash: front left (driver, usually), 47%; front right, 38%; rear left, 23%; rear right, 23%; front middle, 21%; rear middle, 18%; and other and unknown, 27%.

16. In 1988, 3661 motorcyclists (including those driving other motorized vehicles such as mopeds) were killed; 67% were as a result of frontal collisions.

17. In those states with helmet laws for motorcyclists, 64% of those *involved* in a fatal crash were wearing helmets. In those states without helmet laws, 28% of those *involved* in such a crash were wearing helmets. Of the 3486 drivers or passengers killed on motorcycles, 43% wore helmets, 56% did not. (Because these data report only fatalities, no conclusions can be made regarding the effectiveness of helmets without data regarding nonfatalities.)

MVCs claim the lives of more than 49,000 persons each year, with young men being the prime victims. The highest fatality rate is for those between the ages of 15 and 24 years. Preventive strategies targeting this specific age-group are obviously desperately needed.

FALLS

Although considerable data are available regarding fatal injuries, less is recorded regarding nonfatal injuries. However, in a 1989 report to Congress highlighting the cost of injury, it was reported that falls account for the largest number of hospitalizations resulting from injury.[29] The elderly population is at highest risk for death from falls; those more than 75 years of age have a death rate 12 times greater than the death rate for persons of all ages.[29]

HOMICIDE

Because homicide is listed by E-code as a specific cause of death, the numbers associated are readily available. Homicides, however, evoke concern about the issues related to firearms, even though not all homicides result from firearm use. In 1988, there were 22,032 homicides and legal intervention deaths compared with 21,103 in 1987. The homicide-only rate per 100,000 persons from 1970 to 1983 peaked in 1974 (9.9), declined in 1975 and 1976, and increased steadily with another peak in 1980 (10.5). The 1983 death rate per 100,000 persons was 8.5.

In 1986 homicide was the leading cause of death for blacks between the ages of 15 and 34 years, the third leading cause of death of white persons between the ages of 15 and 24 years, and the fourth for white persons between the ages of 25 and 34 years (Table 34-6 and Fig. 34-6). Homicide is the fifth leading cause of death for black persons overall and the fourteenth for white persons. The National Center for Health Statistics reports a 55% increase in the rate for firearm homicides in black male teenagers between the ages of 15 and 19 years (31.7 to 49.2 per 100,000) from 1983 to 1987.[21] The 1988 homicide and legal intervention death rate for black males is reported as 58.0 and 47.5 per 100,000 persons for all other nonwhite males. In 1987, 11% of all deaths of children between the ages of 1 and 19 years were firearm related, leading to 3392 deaths.

The weapons used to commit a homicide are overwhelmingly handguns (Fig. 34-7). The percentage of homicide victims who know their assailant is higher among blacks (59.8%) than whites (48.4%). Black female victims know their assailant in 65.8% of the incidents compared with 55.8% for white females. Fewer males know their assailant: 58.3% for blacks and 45.7% for whites.[6]

Gun control issues are paramount in the political agenda. During the 1990 session, Congress discussed a bill related to curbing semiautomatic assault weapons with more than 300 pending amendments and provisions spanning such is-

Table 34-6 Ranking by race and age of injury-related causes of death (if among the 10 leading causes) in the United States, 1986

Age (yr)	Accidents and effects			Suicide			Homicide and legal intervention		
	Black	White	Other	Black	White	Other	Black	White	Other
<1	5	3	5	—	—	—	8	10	7
1-14	1	1	1	—	8	9	3	5	5
15-24	2	1	1	3	2	2	1	3	3
25-34	2	1	1	5	2	4	1	4	2
35-44	3	3	2	8	4	5	4	6	6
45-54	4	3	3	—	6	7	6	9	6
55-64	5	6	4	—	8	9	10	—	—
>65	7	8	7	—	—	—	—	—	—
OVERALL RANKING FOR TOTAL POPULATION	4	4	3	—	8	6	5	14	9

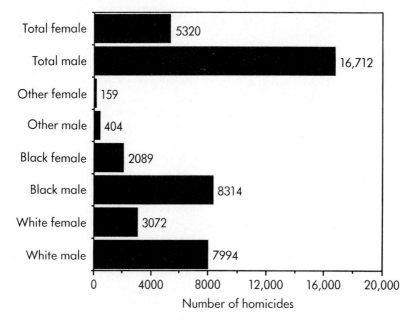

Fig. 34-6 Number of homicides, by race and gender: United States—1988.

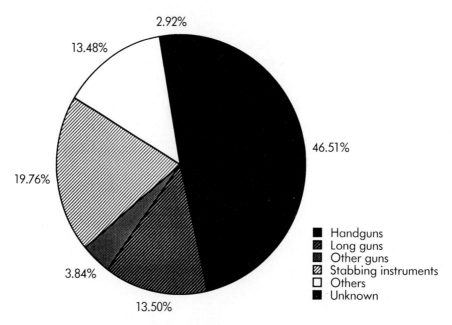

Fig. 34-7 Weapons used in homicide.

sues as death penalty requirements for 30 federal crimes. The debate continues, with numerous organizations dividing the issues. Countermeasures that would address the need for prevention of firearm- and handgun-related deaths, such as longer waiting periods for gaining a permit to own a gun, are being introduced.

BURNS

Approximately 5600 persons died from all types of burns in 1985, and an additional 54,400 persons were hospital-

ized.[29] The National Fire Protection Association claims that residential fires in 1988 claimed 6277 lives, an increase of 7% from 1987.[17] The largest number of burn-related deaths are due to residential fires. The Centers for Disease Control reported on fatalities in residential fires between 1978 and 1984 and demonstrated that the southern United States has the highest incidence of deaths and the highest death rate per 100,000 population. In all four regions those less than the age of 5 years and more than the age of 65 years were at highest risk. Seasonally, more fatal residential fires occur during the winter months, followed by spring, fall, and summer.[3]

Einhorn and Grunnet[7] reported that 200,000 serious injuries are a result of fire, and of those injured, 50,000 are hospitalized from 6 weeks to more than 2 years. Death and injury from fire can be a result of contact with the actual flame, yet most damage to the body is a result of exposure to carbon monoxide and to the decomposition and combustion of synthetic and natural materials that yield hydrogen cyanide, nitrogen oxides, acid gases, aldehydes, and alcohols.[7]

The National Burn Information Exchange (NBIE), a data base originally started at the University of Michigan in 1964, now has 130 burn care facilities contributing data. The data base includes information on burn victims treated at approximately 35% of the 1740 designated burn beds in hospitals across the United States. This data base and others like it are designed to monitor the variables associated with a particular injury to identify factors that contribute to survival, to develop national norms, and to be a means for data exchange to promote the optimum care for patients and to identify methods of prevention. For example, the NBIE has documented that size and depth of burn, and patient age, are significant in determining the severity of the burn.[8] Medical history is also related to mortality. Patients who sustained a 40% to 49% total body surface area (TBSA) burn, who had no significant medical history, have an 88% survival rate, whereas those with one past disease process have a 76% survival rate; for those with three or more diseases the survival rate drops to 40%.[8]

This large data base also documents the relationship of the percentage of TBSA burned to length of stay with dramatic decreases in length of stay for the same percentage of burn from 1964 to 1984. For example, between 1964 and 1972 a patient with a 30% TBSA burn had a mean length of stay of 60 days. The mean dropped to 41 days between 1973 and 1978 and down to 35 days between 1979 and 1984. Of concern for patients and clinicians is the difference between survival rates for patients with the same injury at different facilities. The NBIE documented that patients whose wounds were closed earlier have better survival rates and that survival rates are also better in facilities where burn care was more organized (burn team time with patients and active medical directors).[8]

SUICIDE

Death as a result of suicide presents significant consequences to society as a whole and to individual families in particular. In 1988, 30,407 suicides occurred, according to government statistics.[27] Figs. 34-8 and 34-9 demonstrate that white males have a suicide death rate almost twice that of black males (21.7 vs 11.5) and that the suicide death rates since 1979 have dropped for almost every age-group except for those older than 65 years. Since the late 1950s, however, the death rate from suicide of those between 15 and 24 years has tripled.

Depression is the leading psychiatric illness to be associated with suicide, followed by alcoholism.[2] Hopelessness has also been associated with suicide.[19] Risk factors for suicide are marital status (more suicides in unmarried persons), age, gender, unemployment, history of previous suicide attempts, family history of suicide attempts, and other

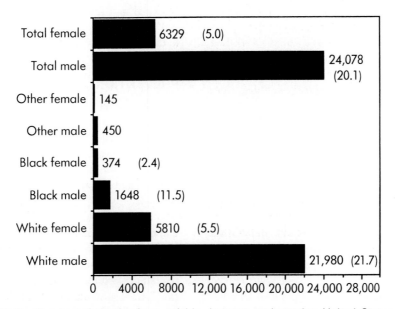

Fig. 34-8 Number of deaths from suicide, by race and gender: United States—1988 (rates per 100,000 population).

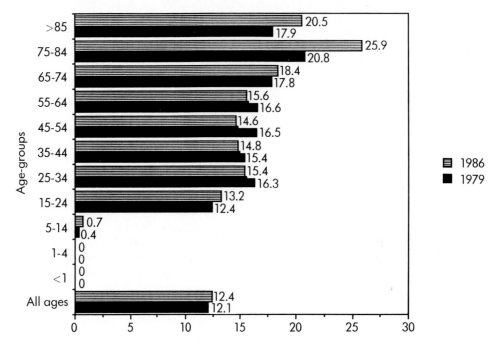

Fig. 34-9 Death rates from suicide, by age-groups: United States—1979 and 1988.

medical illnesses. Depression and antisocial behavior are two of the psychiatric illnesses associated with 90% of youth suicides.

THE RELATIONSHIP OF ALCOHOL TO INJURY

The 1990 report to Congress concerning alcohol states that nearly 18 million adults in the United States have alcohol-related problems and that 150,000 deaths per year are in some way related to alcohol use. Additionally, the report states that the cost of alcohol abuse per year is $128.3 billion.[36] The most studied relationship of alcohol to injury is in the area of MVCs. The FARS uses a statistical method to *estimate* the involvement of alcohol in crashes, because not all states provide information regarding blood alcohol content (BAC). The estimates are computed with data from cases in which the BAC is known. The use of alcohol in BAC concentrations of 0.10% for drivers, whether or not killed in a collision where a fatality occurred, has been steadily declining. In 1982, 30% of the drivers involved in a fatal crash had a BAC of 0.10% or greater, compared with 24.6% in 1988. In 1982, 43.8% of drivers fatally injured in a MVC had BACs of 0.10% or greater compared with 37.4% in 1988. From 1982 to 1988 the percentage of drivers under the age of 18 years who were involved in fatal crashes decreased by 35%, the largest decrease for any age-group during the same time period.[39] The number of fatalities in those crashes where at least one driver or nonoccupant was intoxicated decreased by 12% from 1982 through 1989.[20]

If a fatal crash occurred between midnight and 6 AM,

49.5% of the drivers were estimated to be intoxicated, whereas only 6.6% were intoxicated if the crash occurred between 6 AM and noon. There are varying estimates of alcohol involvement in drivers involved in fatal crashes. Motorcycle drivers involved in fatal crashes have the highest estimated alcohol use, with 36.3% of 3703 drivers estimated to have BACs of 0.10%. This is in contrast to drivers of passenger cars involved in fatal crashes, of whom 24.7% have BACs of the same level. The drivers of heavy trucks involved in a fatal crash have the lowest BAC estimate, at 2.6%. These estimates reflect drivers of vehicles involved in fatal crashes, whether they were killed or survived (Table 34-7).

PREVENTION

A discussion of the epidemiology of trauma must include a discussion of prevention. The advances in scientifically documenting the failure and success of various injury countermeasures are rapidly growing. The injury process, control strategies, and the influences on those strategies as a result of social and behavioral attitudes and practices are a complex network.

A leader in injury prevention, William Haddon, was the first director of the (now) NHTSA and also president of the Insurance Institute for Highway Safety.[1] His research scientifically documented the influence of alcohol on fatally injured drivers and pedestrians.[9,16] He defined the following strategies for reducing injuries, which form the basis of developing many injury prevention programs:

1. Preventing the creation of hazards

Table 34-7 Percentage of drivers involved in fatal* motor vehicle crashes by blood alcohol concentrations: United States—1988

Vehicle	No alcohol	0.01%-0.09%	≥0.10%	Total No. of drivers
Passenger cars	67%	8.3%	24.7%	36,736
Vans	77.1%	5.2%	17.7%	2407
Motorcycles	50.2%	13.5%	36.3%	3703
Light trucks	61.1%	7.9%	31%	11,066
Heavy trucks	95.7%	1.7%	2.6%	4477

*Driver may or may not have been the fatality.

2. Reducing the number of hazards
3. Preventing the release of existing hazards
4. Modifying the rate or spatial distribution of release of hazards
5. Separating the hazard from potential hosts in terms of time or space
6. Separating hosts from hazards with the use of material barriers
7. Modifying the basic qualities of hazards
8. Making hosts more resistant to damage
9. Countering the damage that has already occurred
10. Stabilizing, repairing, and rehabilitating the injured person

The primary role of emergency nursing in caring for trauma victims has been within the last strategy, which is the actual, direct patient care provided to trauma victims by both prehospital- and hospital-based emergency nurses. As evidenced by position statements from the Emergency Nursing Association, these nurses and other nursing epidemiologists and researchers are beginning to focus attention on the prevention of trauma by being involved in legislative issues and injury prevention programs, and by being proponents and participants in injury control strategizing at the local, state, and national levels.

Haddon also suggests avoiding emphasis on the single cause of an injury so as not to exclude others.[10] As mentioned earlier, the use of the word *accident* is declining. Haddon is also a proponent of not using the word *accident* to describe injuries. Haight[13] suggests *not* discussing cause and subsequent blame in the safety research vocabulary. Strategies for injury control used to classify most injury countermeasures are the following[28,31]: (1) education and persuasion, (2) laws and administrative rules, and (3) altering environment by technology and engineering.

Education and persuasion strategies are designed to alter the behavior of those who may be exposed to certain hazards. An example is teaching high school students the perils of driving while intoxicated. The second countermeasure, laws and administrative rules, is also designed to alter behavior but not through an educational forum. The change in behavior is primarily generated by requirements and penalties imposed by laws or rules, such as mandatory seat belt use and speed limit laws. The third strategy deals with protecting the potential host by adjusting the agents, vehicles, or the environment through laws, administrative rules, or persuasion addressed to manufacturers. The law regulating the installation of automatic restraining devices in automobiles is an example. In terms of effectiveness, research indicates that education is the least effective and automatic protection is the most effective.[5]

Education and Persuasion

To educate potential hosts of injury is to attempt to alter their risk-taking behavior in such a way that will prevent subsequent trauma. Police and fire educational programs to teach young children safe play and what to do in the case of a potential injury threat are examples of educational countermeasures. There are some barriers to this strategy, including available research to document its efficacy. People must first perceive that they are at risk before they will use risk-prevention behaviors. It has been suggested that there is an optimism bias whereby people perceive themselves to be less vulnerable than others.[33] However, the landmark publication, *Injury Prevention: Meeting the Challenge,*[28] concludes, "Education/behavior change approaches to prevent childhood injuries have been tested, but evidence of their effectiveness is weak." The authors also suggest that to "combine a simple, targeted message in conjunction with legislation/enforcement and engineering/technology interventions" increases the effectiveness of injury prevention programs. For example, teaching young children how to behave in a fire ("stop, drop, roll"), together with regulating the installation of smoke detectors in homes, is more effective than the educational component in isolation.

Another barrier to behavior change by education is the number of times a person has to perform a countermeasure for protection. Few would deny that the use of a seat belt can reduce the risk of injury. Yet seat belts that must be buckled each time one rides in a car may not be used as often as those that are automatically placed as the driver or front-seat passenger gets in the car and closes the door. In comparison, the installed air bag requires no action on the part of the passenger or driver to engage its usefulness and protection.

Legal Regulations of Behavior

The regulation of a speed limit is an example of attempting to alter a driver's behavior by making it illegal to behave in a certain manner. The behavior also benefits others as well as the person exhibiting the behavior.

One example of the history of legal regulation is the enactment and eventual repeal of laws related to the use of motorcycle helmets. Between 1967 and 1969, 37 states enacted laws that required motorcyclists to wear protective helmets. These laws were necessary if states wanted to qualify for state highway funds. By 1975, only three states did not have such a helmet law (California, Utah, and Illinois). Because Congress removed the law as a fiscal qualifier for highway funds in 1976, 26 states repealed or weakened their helmet laws. In 1960 the deaths per 10,000 motorcycles was 13.8. By 1975, at the peak of helmet laws, the rate had dropped dramatically to 6.5. By 1979, after many states had repealed or weakened laws, the rate once again increased to 9.2.[37] Full helmet laws are now in effect in 23 states and the District of Columbia. This means that drivers and passengers are required to wear protective headgear. Twenty-three other states have some form of helmet law but these laws are not all-inclusive. For example, some states have age requirements. Usually those under the age of 18 years must wear helmets.

The rate of head injuries in riders without helmets was two to three times greater than that of those with helmets.[37] Of fatally injured motorcyclists the head injury rate for those not wearing helmets was three to nine times greater than for those wearing them.[38] Hurt and others[14] demonstrated that the motorcyclist who is the least likely to wear a helmet is the motorcyclist who has consumed alcohol and is most likely to be involved in a fatal crash. NHSTA, in its report after the repeal of the Kansas motorcycle helmet law, found a statistically significant increase in the severity of head injuries after the repeal.[38] However, there is still opposition to these laws, mostly from motorcyclists themselves. Some of the arguments against helmet use are obstruction of vision, cause of neck injuries, discomfort inside the helmet, and a sense of safety when wearing a helmet such that the driver may take other risk-taking behaviors.

The use of laws to protect persons from harm is fraught with concerns for freedom, individual rights, and consumer naivete. Robertson[31] described some of the factors that influence compliance with laws and rules. Compliance is greater if the required behavior would be performed whether or not the law was in effect; if detection and conviction are highly probable; if the behavior does not interfere with pleasure, convenience, or comfort; if there are few exemptions in the law; if the time between detection and conviction are close; if compliance is easily observed by enforcers; and if the punishment is severe.

Some laws are considered deterrence laws, such as the speed limit of 55 miles per hour. Not exceeding the speed limit is related to how one perceives the appropriateness of the law and to whether one will risk violation. Such laws may deter unwanted behavior for two basic reasons. One is that the driver does not exceed the speed limit because doing so would be illegal; a second is that the driver complies with the law because it is believed that it is safer to drive at slower speeds.

The attempts to regulate the consumption of alcohol before a vehicle is driven are currently a pressing national and state issue. The drunk driving problem is ubiquitous in its penetration into social, judicial, medical, moral, legal, political, business, economic, and recreational arenas. Consumption of alcohol is legal. However, limits are placed to determine intoxication levels that, if reached, are illegal if one then drives a vehicle while intoxicated. In 1988, Surgeon General C. Everett Koop conducted the Surgeon General's Workshop on Drunk Driving.[35] To demonstrate the magnitude of coping with this behavior, the workshop participants developed recommendations in 11 different areas: pricing and availability; advertising and marketing; epidemiology and data management; education; judicial and administrative processes; law enforcement; transportation and alcohol service policies; injury control; youth and other special populations; treatment; and citizen advocacy. It is clear from the delineation of these areas that the prevention of this one behavior to control the devastation it causes spans a number of disciplines and requires coalitions of concerned researchers, scientists, legislative officials, law enforcement agencies, advocacy groups, and others, to derive a reasonable and useful injury prevention network.

Technology and Engineering Changes in Environment

The first effort to make the environment safer for roadway travel was the National Traffic Vehicle Safety Act and the Highway Act enacted in 1966. NHTSA was founded in the Department of Transportation and set safety standards for the manufacture of new cars, particularly in three areas: crash avoidance such as glare reduction and braking systems, injury severity reduction (such as seat belts, head restraints, and energy-absorbing steering columns), and postcrash features (such as fire retardants). One injury severity reduction standard, seat belts, was studied, and it was found that the death rate of those who wore seat belts was reduced by 40% to 50% over those who did not.[30]

As states embark on legislation for overall mandatory use of seat belts, all states have passed mandatory laws for infants and children. Child restraint laws vary from state to state in a number of factors, such as age of the child, exemptions, and registration of the vehicle.[36] Enforcement of these laws is variable. Fortunately, automatic protection is becoming more prevalent. All new cars manufactured after 1990 must have some form of *passive* restraint system. This means that the consumer does not have to engage a restraining system *actively*. The passive restraint system may be an automatic belt system (motorized shoulder belt, nonmotorized shoulder belt, or nonmotorized three-point lap and shoulder belt) or an inflatable air bag in the steering wheel or dashboard. The research related to positive prevention effects of air bags has been available for many years, yet only recently have manufacturers been installing them.

Protecting people from hazards is exemplified by the restriction of sale of motorized all-terrain vehicles (ATVs) in the United States. After the Consumer Product Safety Commission estimated that there were 340,000 ATV-related injuries and 1000 ATV-associated deaths, they authorized the U.S. Justice Department to file an action. A complaint and preliminary consent agreement were filed in U.S. District Court to end sale of the new three-wheel ATVs and to announce the risk of injury to known ATV owners. The final consent decree was approved in 1988.[15,40]

The degree of responsibility for safety and protection of the users of products is balanced by the manufacturers with the cost of implementation or installation. Robertson has written that manufacturers oppose new safety regulations because of cost or unproved effectiveness.[32]

The three injury prevention strategies form the basis of developing injury prevention programs. The elements for developing an injury prevention program are as follows[28]:

Injury problem identification	Description of problem
Program identification	Coordinated effort
Establishment of goal	Changes needed
Establishment of objectives	Measured changes
Establishment of outcome objectives	Impact on mortality and morbidity

COSTS

Together with discussions of epidemiology and prevention of injuries is the concern of economic impact on the injured person and of the costs associated with prevention, acute care, and rehabilitation. The cost of trauma was given in a recent report to Congress.[29] This report uses a lifetime cost of injury that is estimated by incidence of injuries and per-person costs. The per-person cost is a calculation of direct costs (sum of the discounted cost in each year, multiplied by the survival probability) and two indirect costs: morbidity costs (average earnings by gender and age and cost of lost housekeeping services because of the injury) and mortality costs (number of deaths and future expected earnings considering gender and age). Tables 34-8 and 34-9 summarize the incidence of injuries, fatalities, number of hospitalizations, the average lifetime costs per person, average cost per fatal injury, average cost per hospitalization, average

Table 34-8   Types of injuries, fatalities and hospitalizations: United States

Type of injury	No. of total injuries	No. fatalities	No. of hospitalizations
Motor vehicle	5,372,000	45,923	523,028
Falls	12,289,000	12,866	783,357
Firearms	268,000	31,556	65,129
Poisonings	1,702,000	11,894	218,554
Fires and burns	1,463,000	5,671	54,397
Drowning and near-drowning	38,000	6,171	5,564
All other	35,726,000	28,487	699,707
Total	56,859,000	142,568	23,499,736

From Rice DP et al: *Cost of injury in the United States: a report to Congress, 1989,* Institute for Health and Aging, University of California, San Fancisco; Injury Prevention Center, Johns Hopkins University, Baltimore,1989.

Table 34-9   Direct and indirect cost per injury: United States

Type of injury	Lifetime cost per person injured (mean $)	Cost per fatal injury (mean $)	Cost per hospitalization (mean $)	Cost per nonhospitalization (mean $)	Lifetime cost (billion $)
Motor vehicle	9,062	352,042	43,409	1,570	48.7
Falls	3,033	99,669	38,174	499	37.3
Firearms	58,831	373,520	33,159	458	14.4
Poisoning	5,015	372,691	17,631	171	8.5
Fire and burns	2,619	249,367	35,303	347	3.8
Drowning	64,993	362,292	31,408	—	2.5
All others	1,187				42.4
Total lifetime cost, all injuries					157.2

From Rice DP et al: *Cost of injury in the United States: a report to Congress, 1989,* Institute for Health and Aging, University of California, San Fancisco; Injury Prevention Center, Johns Hopkins University, Baltimore,1989.

Table 34-10 Costs per fatal motor vehicle crash and costs for all motor vehicle injuries (abbreviated injury scores 1 to 6)

Cost category	Cost, per fatal injury ($)	Cost, all injuries (million $)
Property damage	7,708	5,423
Medical costs	1,471	4,873
Productivity	383,284	20,941
Services		
Emergency	334	
Legal	11,825	
Administrative	21,580	
Total		7,193
Total	425,406	38,430

Miller TR, Luchter S, Brinkman CP: Crash costs and safety investment, *Accident Ann Prev* 21(4):303, 1989.

Table 34-11 Costs per injury and "estimated rational investment" to prevent injuries by abbreviated injury score

Abbreviated injury score	Cost per injury ($)	Investment for prevention of injury ($)
AIS 1	2,860	4,000
AIS 2	8,058	31,000
AIS 3	19,489	115,000
AIS 4	155,832	375,000
AIS 5	391,314	1,525,000
Fatal	425,406	2,000,000

Miller TR, Luchter S, Brinkman CP: Crash costs and safety investment, *Accident Ann Prev* 21(4):303, 1989.

cost per nonhospitalization, and the lifetime cost for specific injuries. The total cost calculated, by 1985 data, was $157.2 billion.

Miller and others[18] reported costs related to MVCs and safety investment, a project done for the Federal Highway Traffic Safety Administration. An "estimated rational investment" to prevent crashes (according to the Abbreviated Injury Scale) in comparison with the calculation of the cost of the crash was calculated. Using property damage, medical costs, loss of productivity in household and workplace, emergency service costs (police, fire, ambulance), and legal and administrative costs as the measures of an individual injury, they concluded that the cost for one fatal injury is $425,406 (Table 34-10). Of this figure, 90% is related to lost productivity. When all severities are considered crashes cost $38 billion per year, of which 50% is lost productivity at home and/or at work. Table 34-11 shows the rational investment levels to prevent injuries. The rational investment computed by this research is a figure derived from the following: multiplying the value of life-years and function-years lost by the value of a life-year ($120,000), plus the addition of societal versus individual costs (such as federal and state taxes, medical costs as borne by insurance, and legal and court costs). The National Safety Council has suggested the use of that $225,000 as the cost per life in strategizing resource allocations for prevention, whereas NHSTA has suggested a figure of $358,000. Miller's research suggests that the cost is considerably more, that is, $2 million for each fatality (Table 34-11). The purpose of such research is to demonstrate that, although it is difficult to determine the monetary value of a person's life, it is important to perform such analyses as a foundation for deriving prevention strategies that will come under the scrutiny of cost-benefit analyses. If the initial cost-per-life estimate is too low, there may be a tendency to keep prevention costs correspondingly low.

The cost of trauma is also related to the problems associated with American society. The urban issues of drug use, escalated violence, and uninsured and underinsured persons have all affected the stability of designated trauma systems across the country.

SUMMARY

Because trauma is a preventable occurrence in a number of circumstances, the number of young lives lost is truly a national tragedy. The epidemiology or study of the determinants and distribution of disease in populations enables us to define the injury problem and to identify those target populations where special attention and implementation of injury prevention programs may be useful.

REFERENCES

1. Baker S: Injury science comes of age, *JAMA* 262(16):2284, 1989.
2. Barklage NE: Evaluation and management of the suicidal patient, *Emerg Care Q* 7(1):32, 1991.
3. Centers for Disease Control: Regional distribution of deaths from residential fires—United States; 1978-1984, *MMWR* 36:38, 1988.
4. Committee to Review the Status and Progress of the Injury Control Program, National Academy of Sciences, National Research Council: *Injury control: a review of the status and progress of the injury control program of the Centers for Disease Control,* Washington, DC, 1988, National Academy Press.
5. Committee on Trauma Research, Commission on Life Sciences, National Academy of Sciences, National Research Council and the Institute of Medicine: *Injury in America: a continuing public health problem,* Washington DC, 1985, National Academy Press.
6. Division of Injury Epidemiology and Control, Center for Environmental Health: *US Department of Health and Human Services, Public Health Service, Centers for Disease Control Homicide Surveillance,* Atlanta, 1986, Centers for Disease Control.
7. Einhorn IN, Grunnet ML: The toxicology of combustion products, *Emerg Care Q* 1(3):60, 1985.
8. Feller I, Jones C: The national burn information exchange: the use of a national burn registry to evaluate and address the burn problem, *Surg Clin North Am* 67(1):167, 1987.
9. Haddon W et al: A controlled investigation of the characteristics of adult pedestrians fatally injured by motor vehicles in Manhattan, *J Chron Dis* 14:655, 1961.

10. Haddon W Jr: The changing approach to the epidemiology, prevention and amelioration of trauma: the transition to approaches etiologically rather than descriptively based, *Am J Public Health* 58:1431, 1968.

11. Haddon W Jr: A logical framework for categorizing highway safety phenomena and activity, *J Trauma* 12:197, 1972.

12. Haddon W Jr: Advances in epidemiology of injuries as a basis for public policy, *Public Health Rep* 95:411, 1980.

13. Haight FA: Road safety: a perspective and a new strategy, *J Safety Res* 16(3):91, 1985.

14. Hurt H, Ouellet J, Thom D: Motorcycle accident cause factors and identification of countermeasures. In *Technical report,* Vol 1, Washington, DC, 1981, US Department of Transportation, National Highway Traffic Safety Administration.

15. Kutzes WF: ATVs: the hidden danger, *Law Med Health Care* 17(1):86, 1989.

16. McCarroll JR, Haddon W Jr: A controlled study of fatal automobile accidents in New York City, *J Chron Dis* 15:811, 1961.

17. Medical news and perspectives, *JAMA* 262(16):2195, 1989.

18. Miller TR, Luchter S, Brinkman CP: Crash costs and safety investment, *Accident Ann Prev* 21(4):303, 1989.

19. Minkoff K, Bergman E, Beck A: Hopelessness, depression and attempted suicide, *Am J Psychiatry* 130:455, 1973.

20. Morbidity and Mortality Report: Alcohol-related traffic fatalities—United States: 1982-1989, *MMWR* 39(49):889, 1990.

21. National Center for Health Statistics: *Advance data from vital and health statistics: firearm mortality among children and young adults,* No. 178, Hyattsville, Md, 1989, National Center for Health Statistics.

22. National Center for Health Statistics, US Department of Health and Human Services, Public Health Service: *Monthly vital statistics report: advance report of final mortality statistics, 1981,* 33:3, 1984.

23. National Center for Health Statistics, US Department of Health and Human Services, Public Health Service: *Monthly vital statistics report: advance report of final mortality statistics, 1982,* 33:9, 1984.

24. National Center for Health Statistics, US Department of Health and Human Services, Public Health Service: *Monthly vital statistics report, advance report of final mortality statistics, 1983,* 34:6, 1985.

25. National Center for Health Statistics, US Department of Health and Human Services, Public Service: *Monthly vital statistics report: advance report of final mortality, 1986,* 39:6, 1988.

26. National Center for Health Statistics, US Department of Health and Human Services, Public Health Service: *Monthly vital statistics report: advance report of final mortality statistics, 1987,* 38:5, 1989.

27. National Center for Health Statistics, US Department of Health and Human Services, Public Health Service: *Monthly vital statistics report: advance report of final mortality statistics, 1988,* 39:7, 1990.

28. National Committee for Injury Prevention and Control: Injury prevention: meeting the challenge, *Am J Prev Med* 5(3) (suppl), 1989.

29. Rice DP et al: *Cost of injury in the United States: a report to Congress, 1989,* Institute for Health and Aging, University of California, San Francisco; Injury Prevention Center, Johns Hopkins University, Baltimore, 1989.

30. Robertson LS: Estimates of motor vehicle seatbelt effectiveness and use: implications for occupant crash protection, *Am J Public Health* 66:85, 1976.

31. Robertson LS: *Injuries: causes, control strategies, and public policy,* Lexington, Mass, 1983, Lexington Books.

32. Robertson LS: Motor vehicle injuries: the law and the profits, *Law Med Health Care* 17(1):73, 1989.

33. Svenson O, Fischoll B, MacGregor D: Perceived driving safety and seat belt usage. *Accident Anal Prev* 17(2):119, 1985.

34. Teret SP et al: Child restraint laws: an analysis of gaps in coverage, *Am J Public Health* 76(1):31, 1986.

35. US Department of Health and Human Services, Public Health Service, Office of the Surgeon General: *Surgeon general's workshop on drunk driving proceedings,* Washington, DC, 1989.

36. US Department of Health and Human Services: *Seventh special report to the US Congress on alcohol and health,* Washington, DC, 1990, US Government Printing Office.

37. US Department of Transportation, National Highway Traffic Safety Administration: *A report to Congress on the effect of motorcycle helmet use law repeal—a case for helmet use,* Department of Transportation HS 805-312, April 1980.

38. US Department of Transportation, National Highway Traffic Safety Administration: *The effect of motorcycle helmet usage on head injuries and the effect of usage laws on helmet wearing rates: a preliminary report,* Washington, DC, 1989.

39. US Department of Transportation, National Highway Traffic Safety Administration, National Center for Statistics and Analysis: *Fatal accident reporting system, 1988: a review of information of fatal traffic accidents in the United States in 1988,* Washington, DC, 1987.

40. *USA vs American Honda Motor Co, Inc., Honda Motor Co, Ltd, Honda Research & Development Co, Ltd, Yamaha Motor Co, Ltd, Yamaha Motor Corp, USA Suzuki Motor Corp, Kawasaki Heavy Industries, Ltd, Kawasaki Motor Corp, USA Polaris Industries LP,* CA 87-3535, District Court, Washington, DC, 1987.

Susan Budassi Sheehy and Deborah M. Amos

Several types of neurologic emergencies are encountered in the ED. In this chapter a neurologic emergency is defined as a state of neurologic injury or disease that poses an immediate threat to life or that can result in a permanent neurologic deficit if untreated.

HEADACHE

Headache is one of the most common chief complaints of patients in the ED. Headache is a symptom of some underlying disorder, not a diagnosis. Carefully examine these patients because their problem may range from minor to the most serious, such as subarachnoid bleeding. Headache may indicate intracranial involvement, especially if the onset is sudden and the patient has no history of headaches. Be careful to question the patient with chronic headaches; find out whether the present headache is different from the others and how it is different. Obtain answers to the questions listed in the box at right.

Causes of Headaches

Headaches may be extracranial or intracranial. Many causes of headache are not emergency conditions. Extracranial causes of headache include acidosis, dehydration, hypoglycemia, and uremic and hepatic disorders. Ophthalmic causes of headache include glaucoma (see Chapter 23), refractory errors, and inflammatory or allergic problems. Toxicologic emergencies and poisonings (see Chapter 40) may cause headaches. Additional causes of headaches include ear infections (see Chapter 24), upper respiratory infections, sinus congestion, facial trauma (see Chapter 24), temporomandibular joint syndrome, toothaches (see Chapter 24), anemias, polycythemias, electrolyte disturbances, and viral or bacterial systemic infections. Each of these is treated according to the cause.

Migraine

The diagnosis of migraine is made on the basis of the patient's history. Headache is *never* the only symptom of a migraine, nor is it a required feature of a migraine attack. It is better to think of migraine as a complex that includes an assortment of symptoms, which may or may not be

followed by long-lasting neurologic deficits. About 10% to 20% of the U.S. population have fairly common and readily recognized migraine headaches. Before migraine is diagnosed, other causes of headaches must be ruled out.

Headaches may be classified as vascular or nonvascular. Vascular headaches are thought to have three separate

---

QUESTIONS TO ASK ABOUT HEADACHES

Is this the first headache?
When did this headache start?
Did the patient sustain any trauma?
Does the patient have any personality changes?
Has the patient exhibited any memory loss?
Has the patient had a recent infection?
Has the patient had any eye problems?
Has the patient had any recent neurologic problems?
Does the patient have hypertension? How long has the patient had it?
Has the patient had any emotional problems?
Is the patient currently taking any medications?
Has the patient ever had a seizure or a seizure disorder?
Using the PQRST mnemonic, assess the chief complaint of pain.

P (*Provoking factor*)
What provokes the pain? What makes it better? What makes it worse?

Q (*Quality*)
What does the pain feel like? Have the patient describe it.

R (*Radiates*)
Where is the pain? Where does it go?

S (*Severity*)
How bad is the pain? Give it a number from 1 to 10 with 1 being the mildest and 10 being the most severe.

T (*Time*)
How long has the patient had the pain? When did it start? When did it end? How long did it last?

phases. In the initial phase, the prodromal phase, any one of a number of stimuli can act as a trigger, resulting in biochemical changes within the blood vessel. Platelets clump and substances such as serotonin are released, resulting in severe vasoconstriction. During this phase patients may have an aura. Auras or prodromes may take the form of scotomata (blind spots), teichopsia (zigzag patterns resembling forts), photopsia (flashing, colored lights), paresthesias, or visual or auditory hallucinations. The writer Lewis Carroll, who had migraines, saw the distorted figures in his book *Alice in Wonderland* as part of his migraine attack. Prolongation of this prodromal or vasoconstrictive phase can result in ischemic changes to neurologic tissue located beyond the area of vasoconstriction.

In the second phase of vascular migraine, platelet clumping and levels of neurotransmitters such as serotonin are decreased. Inflammation and dilation of cerebral blood vessel walls result. The headache component of a migraine is seen in this phase.

The third phase of a vascular migraine is the recovery phase. Blood vessels return to normal size. Levels of circulating neurotransmitters return to normal. Inflammation and edema persist around the blood vessels, and nerve endings are sensitized, which can result in extreme tenderness to touch.

Vascular migraines include classic migraine, common migraine, cluster headache, hemiplegic migraine, ophthalmoplegic migraine, facial migraine, and migraine equivalents. Nonvascular migraines include the muscle contraction of tension headache. In nonvascular migraine the force of skeletal muscle contractions in the head or neck produces a characteristic steady, nonpulsatile pain.

Some of the more commonly recognized triggers for migraines include changes in sleep patterns, physical exertion, sudden weather changes resulting in rise or fall in barometric pressure, increased stresses of daily life, dieting (especially fasting modes), heat, lights, cyclic estrogen levels, and certain foods. Food products linked to migraine attacks include alcoholic beverages, excessive caffeine, meats containing nitrates, monosodium glutamate, yeast products, ripened cheeses, and chocolate. Fermented fruits or juices may also contribute to migraine attacks.

Pharmacologic therapy used during a migraine attack can include analgesics, antiinflammatory medications, beta adrenergic blockers, serotonin antagonists, vasoconstrictors (ergotamine derivatives), and antidepressants. For ergotamine derivatives to be effective, they must be taken fairly early in the migraine attack. One danger in the use of ergotamines is the possibility of onset of action before the patient enters the vasodilator phase, thereby *worsening* the vasoconstriction that already exists. Drug therapy may also include diuretics, antihistamines (such as Benadryl), anticonvulsants (such as Dilantin), and short courses of corticosteroids. Oral contraceptives should be avoided in patients with classic, hemiplegic, or ophthalmoplegic migraines.

Oral contraceptives should not be used concurrently with ergotamines.

In addition to drug therapy, medical and nursing interventions may include biofeedback therapy, relaxation training, assertiveness training, family counseling, dietary counseling, allergy testing, and patient, family, and community education.

Heredity plays a strong role in the migraine phenomenon, with more than 90% of patients reporting a family history of migraine. More women than men tend to have migraine attacks. First attacks usually seem to occur when the patient is less than 40 years old. With increasing age, frequency of attacks decreases. It is not uncommon for persons who have migraine to have more than one type of migraine phenomenon.

Most vascular headaches seem to occur suddenly. The pain may be described as either intense, sharp, and piercing, or pounding and throbbing. Nausea, vomiting, generalized weakness or fatigue, and eye pain may also be described.

Classic migraine. Patients with classic migraine have some form of aura. The aura may last for 15 to 20 minutes. It clears more rapidly than it develops and may disappear shortly after the headache component begins. The headache component is generally severe and unilateral, although it may become bilateral. This headache may last from 30 minutes to several days. Patients are also prone to photophobia, or sensitivity to light, and to a sensitivity to sound. A sound as minor as the buzzing of a fly in the room may become intolerable to the client. Ninety percent of patients have nausea, vomiting, and anorexia during the attack. Pain can be worsened by walking, straining, or any sudden change in body position. Classic migraine is seen during periods of increased stress, during the school years, and during pregnancy.

Common migraine. Eighty-five percent of persons who have migraine have common migraine. Prodromal symptoms tend to be not focal in origin but generalized. Symptoms may include euphoria, hunger, depression, irritability, or periods of intensive yawning. Generalized edema and recent weight gain may also be present. Photophobia is also present. In contrast to classic migraine, pregnancy provides some relief from common migraine. Ergotamines are effective for treatment of this type of migraine pain.

Cluster headache. Patients with cluster headache have closely grouped attacks that last for several weeks and are followed by remission that may last several months or even years. Sometimes the person may have as many as a dozen attacks a day. Patients who have annual bouts of cluster headaches tend to have them in the spring and in the fall. The pain is excruciating and unilateral, and may be felt in the temple region or behind the eye. Occasionally pain also travels to the ear, nose, and cheek areas. Additional localized signs and symptoms include facial flushing, nasal congestion, lacrimation, rhinorrhea, salivation, and generalized autonomic symptoms. Partial or complete Horner's syndrome may be seen on the affected side. Usually the attacks wake the client from a deep sleep or tend to occur during periods of rest from exhaustion. Sometimes an alcohol sensitivity develops immediately before a cluster attack. Ergotamine-induced relief is only temporary and does not break the cluster cycle. This form of migraine is 10 times more common in men. Another hallmark of a cluster migraine may be noted in the patient's behavior during the attack. In most migraines, clients tend to remain as still as possible. It is not unusual in cluster migraines to witness a patient pacing up and down, holding the affected side of the face. Clients have been seen to beat their heads against the wall during their attack in an effort to break the cycle and interrupt the pain. The pain may also cause the patients to attempt or succeed in attempting to commit suicide. Treatment for cluster headaches may include administration of oxygen or intramuscular injection of dihydroergotamine mesylate. The prophylactic treatment of choice may be methysergide maleate (Sansert) or combination trials of prednisone and ergotamine tartrate. Some physicians consider a trial of lithium during this period to be appropriate.

Ophthalmoplegic migraine. Ophthalmoplegic migraines usually begin during infancy or early childhood. They contain a headache component, as well as evidence of a third-nerve paralysis. If untreated, prominent visual field defects or blindness may occur. Therapy during the attack includes ergotamines and corticosteroids, and prophylactic treatment consists of administration of methysergide.

Hemiplegic migraine. Sensory changes during hemiplegic migraine include visual field defects, arm, mouth, or leg numbness, and miscellaneous paresthesias. Motor changes can include onset of aphagia, upper and lower extremity unilateral weakness, or paralysis. Family history is often positive for migraine phenomena, and the patient history may include presence of classic or common migraine. Treatment of choice is rest, sedation, analgesia, and an increase in carbon dioxide levels. Ergotamines are contraindicated in this form of migraine. Prophylactic therapy may include the use of aspirin and papaverine.

Facial migraine. Facial migraine is usually a unilateral episodic facial pain associated with symptoms of cluster headache or common migraine. This form of migraine is also called "the lower-half" headache.

Migraine equivalents. Migraine equivalent describes complexes that have features of migraines but that lack a specific headache component. They may include cyclic vomiting and bilious attacks, abdominal migraines, periodic diarrhea, periodic fever, periodic sleep and trancelike states, periodic mood changes, menstrual syndromes, and precordial migraines.

Muscle contraction headaches. Muscle contraction or tension headache is usually associated with some period of emotional or physical stress. The patient is unable to relax muscle contractions of the scalp and neck. Some researchers have indicated that low blood levels of serotonin may play a role in the onset of the muscle contraction headache. The headache is described as a steady tightness around both temporal areas or in the occipital area. The patient may have limited motion of the head, neck, and jaws because of the discomfort. Pressure over contracted muscles may worsen the pain. The occurrence of a depressive state may be linked to variations in serotonin blood levels. In other forms of migraines vasodilation of cerebral blood vessels is treated with vasoconstrictive drugs. In muscle contraction headache, no vasodilation phase occurs. Pain only worsens with the use of vasoconstrictive drugs and is relieved by the use of vasodilators. Other treatment includes administration of mild analgesics and identification and treatment of the cause of the pain.

Traumatic headaches. Headaches that result from craniocerebral trauma can be either emergency or nonemergency conditions. Postconcussion or contusion headaches, as well as headaches that are part of the posttraumatic syndrome, are nonemergency conditions. Potentially life-threatening situations that can result in the symptom of headache include conditions of cerebral edema, increased intracranial pressure, epidural hematomas, subdural bleeding, intercerebral bleeding, leaking aneurysms, and leaking atrioventricular malformations (see Chapter 21).

Temporal arteritis. When the patient has severe stabbing pains in one or both temporal regions, it is possible that the problem is caused by temporal arteritis. This is an inflammatory condition that affects the branches of the carotid artery, usually in patients older than 50 years of age. The condition is more common in women. Headache is its most prominent and severe symptom. Because of the pain, the patient may have difficulty sleeping and opening and closing the mouth. A history of rheumatoid arthritis or frequent complaints of muscle pains may be present. Additional complaints may include weight loss, night sweating, aching of the joints, fever, and red nodules over the temporal region. Early diagnosis of this condition and treatment with corticosteroids is necessary, to prevent the development of visual symptoms caused by a decrease in blood supply in the optic nerve. Left untreated, this condition can result in blindness. In most patients with temporal arteritis the sedimentation rate is above normal. A biopsy of a specimen from the superficial temporal artery can confirm this diagnosis.

HYPERTENSION

When cardiac output or peripheral vascular resistance is greatly increased, hypertension results. A systolic blood pressure between 140 and 160 mm Hg is considered potentially dangerous. This patient should be referred for follow-up to recheck his or her blood pressure. A patient with a blood pressure of 160/90 mm Hg or more should be considered to have hypertension. If the patient also has one of the following, the condition should be considered an absolute emergency:

1. Cerebrovascular accident

2. Myocardial infarction
3. Angina pectoris
4. Congestive heart failure
5. Aortic dissection
6. Renal insufficiency
7. Grade 3 or 4 retinopathy

Pay attention to the systolic, as well as the diastolic, blood pressure reading; this reading is just as important and diagnostic. If hypertension is present, make a differential diagnosis to determine the causative agent or problem. If the patient is less than 25 years of age, he or she probably has renal vascular disease. Obtain results of urinalysis, and determine blood urea nitrogen, creatinine, serum electrolyte, uric acid, serum calcium, lipid, and glucose levels to assist in diagnosis. Also obtain an electrocardiogram and a radiograph of the chest. If the problem is thought to be renal vascular disease, obtain an intravenous (IV) pyelogram.

Occasionally a patient has elevated blood pressure without evidence of end-organ damage. This blood pressure increase may be caused by another problem, such as drug withdrawal, especially from clonidine or propranolol; a drug interaction, such as monoamine oxidase (MAO) inhibitors and Chianti wine; a direct effect of drugs, such as amphetamines, tricyclics, or phencyclidine; pheochromocytoma; head trauma with increasing intracranial pressure; or Guillain-Barré syndrome. Therapeutic intervention is to treat the underlying cause.

Essential Hypertension

Essential hypertension originates from the kidneys and adrenal glands or results from neurogenic causes, coarctation of the aorta, or toxemia of pregnancy. Signs and symptoms include headache, epistaxis, syncope, tinnitus, and unconsciousness.

Table 35-1 presents a comparison of benign and malignant hypertension.

Minor Complications

Complications from essential hypertension vary. Minor ones include left ventricular hypertrophy, dysrhythmias, bundle branch blocks of varying degrees, and grade 3 retinopathies.

Major Complications

1. Congestive heart failure
2. Pulmonary edema, which may result from many causes, including severe hypertension. Signs and symptoms include dyspnea, production of pink frothy sputum, rales, and bronchospasm. Pulmonary edema is treated with morphine sulfate, high-flow oxygen, diuretics (usually furosemide), aminophylline, and positive pressure. Sitting upright may produce some relief.
3. Renal insufficiency
4. Myocardial infarction
5. Peripheral vascular insufficiency

Table 35-1 Comparison of benign and malignant hypertension

Characteristic	Benign (gradual phase)	Malignant (accelerated phase)
Duration	>10 yr	<2 yr
Onset	Gradual; frequently asymptomatic	Sudden; symptomatic
Encephalopathy	Rarely	Often

6. Grade 4 retinopathy
7. Aortic dissection (see Chapter 25). Patients with a dissecting aneurysm in the thorax demonstrate chest pain that radiates to the back, hypertension, pulse rate discrepancies between the femoral areas, and blood pressure discrepancy between each arm. Therapeutic intervention is the administration of sodium nitroprusside and a beta-blocking agent and consideration for surgical intervention.
8. Hypertensive encephalopathy, in which the patient demonstrates fluctuating levels of consciousness and while conscious, may have a headache, have seizures, and/or demonstrate a grade 4 retinopathy. Therapeutic intervention consists of administering diazoxide and sodium nitroprusside and treating the underlying condition.
9. Cardiovascular accident (See following section.)
10. Sudden death

Table 35-2 lists the stages of complications in hypertension.

Hypertensive Crisis

When a patient has a diastolic blood pressure greater than 130 mm Hg, he or she is considered to be in hypertensive crisis. Several of the more common causes of this condition are discussed here.

Drug overdose. Many drugs can cause a hypertensive crisis when taken in overdose. Therapeutic intervention is the administration of sodium nitroprusside.

Drug withdrawal. The sudden withdrawal of certain drugs causes hypertensive crisis. Therapeutic intervention is the administration of agents for specific medications. Alpha-blocking and beta-blocking agents should be given for clonidine (Catapres) withdrawal; bed rest, nitroglycerin, and propanolol are recommended for propranolol (Inderal) withdrawal.

MAO inhibitors. If MAO inhibitors and Chianti wine are taken together, a severe hypertensive crisis results. Therapeutic intervention includes the administration of phentolamine (Regitine) and phenoxybenzamine (Dibenzyline).

Glomerulonephritis. Glomerulonephritis often causes a severe hypertensive crisis. Therapeutic intervention includes administration of hydralazine, diazoxide, and furosemide.

Table 35-2   Stages of complications of hypertension

Area involved	1	2	3	4
Fundi	Vascular spasms	Vascular sclerosis	Hemorrhage and/or exudates	Papilledema
Heart	Left ventricular hypertrophy	Congestive heart failure	Myocardial ischemia	Myocardial infarction
Aorta and branches	Atherosclerosis	Aneurysm with or without rupture	Dissection of aneurysm	Rupture of aneurysm
Brain	Cerebrovascular insufficiency	Encephalopathy	Cerebral thrombosis	Intracranial or subarachnoid hemorrhage
Renal	Benign nephrosclerosis	Malignant nephrosclerosis	Impaired renal function; low specific gravity; proteinuria; hematuria	Elevated creatinine and blood urea nitrogen levels

Hyperthyroidism. Hyperthyroidism causes a severe hypertensive crisis when in the acute stages. Therapeutic intervention includes administration of alpha-blocking and beta-blocking agents, iodine, and prophylthiouracil.

Antihypertensive Medications

Commonly used antihypertensive medications are listed in Table 35-3.

SEIZURES

Seizure is one of the most common disorders seen in the ED. Approximately 1% to 2% of the U.S. population have seizure disorders. Remember that seizures are symptoms, not a diagnosis. A seizure is defined as an abnormal period of electrical activity in the brain. The international classification of epileptic seizures places seizures into three major categories: partial, generalized, and unclassified seizures.

Partial Seizures

In partial seizures the seizure activity is usually limited to one specific body part. It may consist only of focal motor activity in that area, or the activity may spread in an orderly fashion to surrounding areas (Jacksonian seizure). Partial seizures may also be limited to somatic sensory symptoms such as tingling or numbness of a body part. They may also consist of visual, auditory, olfactory, or taste symptoms only. With this type of seizure the patient's mental status is relatively normal. These are all described as simple partial seizures. In complex partial seizures the symptoms usually include a loss of consciousness. Temporal lobe seizures (psychomotor seizures) are often preceded by an aura. The aura can take the form of a foul smell, a metallic or bitter taste, sensations of buzzing, ringing, or hissing, or vague visceral feelings in the thorax and abdomen. Commonly the patient describes feelings of being in a twilight state, having a sensation of time standing still, or having to force himself or herself to think. Individuals may say that they feel fa-

miliar in what they know is an unfamiliar environment (déjà vu) or the reverse, a feeling of unfamiliarity with a known environment (jamais vu). Affect of symptoms such as inappropriate fear or laughter may also occur. The most characteristic symptom of a temporal lobe seizure is the occurrence of automatisms. Automatisms are semipurposeful patterned repetitive movements such as lip-smacking, chewing, patting of hands, facial grimacing, rubbing one's clothes, or plucking at bed sheets. The last subcategory of partial seizures includes partial seizures with secondary generalized seizures. These seizures originate locally and progress until the seizure involves the entire body. The client loses consciousness during this type of seizure activity. This progression to generalized seizures is possible with any of the partial seizures previously discussed.

Generalized seizures

Generalized seizures include the following types.

Absence (petit mal) seizures. Absence seizures usually occur in children between the ages of 4 and 12 years. These seizures involve an abrupt cessation of activity with a momentary arrest of consciousness. These spells usually last less then 15 seconds, during which the patient is unaware of his or her surroundings. Sometimes the spell may be accompanied by automatisms.

Tonic-clonic (grand mal) seizures. Tonic-clonic seizure begins with a sudden loss of consciousness and major tonic contractions of the muscle groups, causing the arms and legs to extend stiffly as the client falls to the ground. Sometimes a shrill cry may precede the event. During this tonic phase of a grand mal seizure the patient is apneic, has dilated and unresponsive pupils, may bite the tongue, and has bowel or bladder incontinence. During the clonic phase strenuous and rhythmic muscle contractions are seen. The patient may undergo hyperventilation, profuse sweating, rapid pulse, and excessive salivation with frothing from the mouth. A postictal state then occurs with muscle relaxation, deep

Table 35-3 Rapid-acting antihypertensive agents

Drug	Route	Dose	Onset	Notes	Given for
Sodium nitroprusside (Nipride)	IV	Titrate 50 mg in 500 ml D₅W (100 μg/ml); run at 3 μg/kg/min	1-2 min	Requires constant monitoring; most effective; most controllable; relaxes smooth muscle and increases venous capacity; decomposes in light; no direct heart action; requires concomitant diuretic	Aneurysm; drug-induced pheochromocythemia; acute encephalopathy; hypertension with acute or chronic glomerulonephritis; malignant hypertension; eclampsia; hypertension with left ventricular failure; intracranial hemorrhage
Trimethaphan camsylate (Arfonad)	IV	Titrate 1 g in 1,000 ml D₅W (1 mg/ml) run at 1-2 mg/min, titrated	3-4 min	An automatic ganglionic blocking agent; decreases cardiac output; requires constant monitoring; requires CircOlectric bed; may cause tachyphylaxis; no direct heart action; requires concomitant diuretic	Aneurysm; acute encephalopathy; malignant hypertension; intracranial hemorrhage; hypertension with left ventricular failure; do not use in acute or chronic hypertension with glomerulonephritis or eclampsia
Diazoxide (Hyperstat, Proglem, Proglycem)	IV	300 mg (5 mg/kg) rapidly (<30 sec); repeat at 4-24-hr intervals as needed	1-2 min	May cause hypercalcemia and sodium retention; give concurrently with diuretic; may cause nausea and vomiting; blood pressure will fall initially, then rise slightly	Acute encephalopathy; hypertension with acute or chronic glomerulonephritis; intracranial hemorrhage; malignant hypertension; do not use in eclampsia, left ventricular failure, or aneurysm
Hydralazine (Apresoline, Dralzine, Hydralyn, Norpres 25, Rolazine)	IV, IM	10-20 mg slowly; repeated every 4-6 hr	15-20 min	Relaxes smooth muscle, causing peripheral vascular dilatation and reflux tachycardia; causes headache and flushing; less rapid than other drugs; consider propranolol; requires concomitant diuretic	Eclampsia; malignant hypertension; hypertension; with acute or chronic glomerulonephritis; do not use in left ventricular failure or aneurysm
Reserpine (Serpasil)	IM	2.5 mg	1½-2 hr	Depletes catecholamines; may cause drowsiness; lack of precise control	Malignant hypertension; do not use in hypertensive encephalopathy or intracranial bleeding
Methyldopa (Aldomet, Dopamet, Medimet 250, Novomedopa)	IV	500 mg in 50 ml D₅W over 30-60 min	30-60 min (maximum 3-6 hr)	Decreases cardiac output and peripheral vascular resistance; response is variable; may cause drowsiness	Hypertension with acute or chronic glomerulonephritis; malignant hypertension; do not use in hypertensive encephalopathy or intracranial bleeding

breathing, and a depressed level of consciousness. The patient awakens confused and disoriented, with complaints of headache, muscle aching, and fatigue. There is general amnesia for the attack. Affected individuals may sleep for several hours afterward. Therapeutic intervention is to protect the patient's airway and head, protect the patient from further injury, and administer 50% dextrose and 0.8 mg of naloxone if the cause is unknown.

Myoclonic seizure. Myoclonic seizure consists of a single jerk of one or more muscle groups and usually lasts for a few seconds.

Atonic seizure. Atonic seizures, also known as drop attacks, are sometimes associated with myoclonic jerks. They involve a sudden loss of muscle tone.

Akinetic seizures. Akinetic seizures involve a loss of movement without atonia.

Unclassified Epileptic Seizures

Unclassified epileptic seizures are those that cannot be placed in either of the previously mentioned general categories.

Therapeutic interventions. Treatment for seizures depends on the underlying cause of the event. Treatment is also directed toward management of the seizure activity. Treatment can involve pharmacologic intervention, surgical intervention, dietary therapy, cerebellar stimulation, and biofeedback therapy. Drug therapy varies according to the particular type of seizure activity. Use of IV dilantin, phenobarbital, and diazepam (Valium) is commonly seen in the ED. All seizure patients should receive a brief neurologic examination. Also determine whether the patient has a history of seizures or any other suspect medical history. Check for the presence of an identifying (Medic-Alert) tag or other type of medical information identification, and check the patient carefully for signs of trauma.

Status Epilepticus

Status epilepticus is defined as a series of consecutive seizures or a continuous seizure that has not responded to traditional therapy. Therapeutic intervention is to determine the cause of the seizure and to treat this cause, if possible. Maintain an open airway and administer 100% oxygen through an endotracheal tube. Administer naloxone, 0.8 mg IV; 50% dextrose, 50 ml IV; thiamine, 100 mg IV (if the patient may be an alcohol abuser); diazepam (Valium) in 5 mg IV increments; phenytoin (Dilantin), 25 to 50 mg/min IV in normal saline solution; phenobarbital, 140 mg every 10 to 15 minutes IV; or paraldehyde, 1 to 4 ml IV or intramuscularly. If all else fails, consider general anesthesia.

UNCONSCIOUSNESS (COMA)

Unconsciousness is the depression of consciousness and the total lack of awareness of self and surroundings. There is little or no response to a stimulus. The major causes are (1) structural and (2) metabolic and toxic. Determine whether the unconsciousness is focal or diffuse and whether it is organic (95% of cases) or functional. Determine whether the patient's condition is improving or deteriorating as time passes. Perform a brief neurologic examination (see Chapter 20).

Therapeutic intervention is to ensure airway, breathing, and circulation (ABCs), draw blood samples for glucose determination, and administer naloxone (Narcan), 0.8 mg IV, 50% dextrose, 50 ml, and thiamine, 100 mg IV. Place the patient in a left lateral swimmer's position with the head dependent to prevent emesis and aspiration. Be sure to protect the cervical spine until the possibility of injury can be ruled out. Hyperventilate the patient with 100% oxygen if head trauma or intracranial hemorrhage is suspected.

When assessing the patient, check temperature, respiration rate, blood pressure, pulse rate, skin vital signs (color, temperature, moisture), pupils, lung sounds, and deep tendon reflexes. Check for breath odor, needle tracks, petechiae, and posturing. Find out whether the patient has had any recent trauma. Examine the abdomen, chest, and extremities. Check for Babinski's sign, Battle's sign, hematotympanum, raccoon eyes, Kernig's sign, Brudzinski's sign, lacerations of the tongue, and incontinence.

Assistance with diagnosis may be made by obtaining a complete blood cell count, platelet count, serum electrolyte and serum glucose levels; blood urea nitrogen and creatinine levels; serum toxicologic values; and serum cholesterol, magnesium, calcium, phosphorus, and bilirubin levels. Also obtain a urinalysis; monitor electrocardiogram readings and cerebrospinal fluid (pressure); obtain skull, face, chest, or abdominal radiographs; and consider a computed tomographic scan of the head. Not all these diagnostic tools should be used, but all may be considered, depending on the findings in the patient.

GUILLAIN-BARRÉ SYNDROME

Guillain-Barré syndrome is an acute disease that causes paralysis because of a decrease of myelin at the nerve roots and in the peripheral nerves. Signs and symptoms are a tingling sensation in the extremities lasting for hours to weeks, severely decreased deep tendon reflexes, and a symmetric paralysis that begins in the lower extremities and ascends, affecting the muscles of respiration and causing respiratory paralysis. Therapeutic intervention is to support the ABCs, consider endotracheal intubation and ventilator support, and provide general supportive care until the disease has worked its course. Patients who survive this disease usually require a long program of rehabilitation.

MYASTHENIA GRAVIS

Myasthenia gravis is a defect in neuromuscular transmission. It occurs at any age but is predominant in adults between the ages of 20 and 30 years. It occurs more frequently in women. In a crisis state onset may be sudden and it may cause respiratory paralysis and arrest. Signs and symptoms include increasing fatigue; delayed muscle strength recovery; weak eye, facial, and jaw muscles; weak pharyngeal muscles; diplopia; dysphagia; and inability to swallow. Therapeutic intervention is to support the ABCs, consider endotracheal intubation and ventilator support, and administer neostigmine (Prostigmin), 1 mg IV, for crisis states and barbiturates, opiates, quinidine, quinine, corticotropin, corticosteroids, aminoglycosides, antibiotics, and muscle relaxants.

BOTULISM

Botulism is caused by eating improperly canned foods. These foods usually have a high bacterial content before canning and have not been sterilized properly. Botulism can also occur in infants who have been given raw, unprocessed honey. Signs and symptoms are dry mouth, diplopia, urinary retention, distended abdomen, difficulty chewing, difficulty swallowing, a nasal tone to the voice, and respiratory paralysis; the patient remains awake throughout all this. He or she may have postural hypotension and then may have dilated and fixed pupils. Therapeutic intervention is to support ABCs, lavage the stomach if there has been recent food ingestion, and administer antitoxin.

PARALYTIC SHELLFISH POISONING

Saxitoxin is produced by marine protozoans and interferes with neuron membrane permeability to sodium ions. This toxin is consumed by shellfish such as clams, oysters, and sea snails and produces the condition known as "red tide." If shellfish containing saxitoxin are consumed by human beings, paralytic shellfish poisoning results. Signs and symptoms are progressive paresthesias of the mouth and head, dysphagia, tremors, vertigo, flaccid quadriplegia, dysarthria, and respiratory paralysis. Therapeutic intervention is to support the ABCs, consider endotracheal intubation and ventilatory support, and provide good supportive care. The prognosis is usually good after 24 hours.

CEREBROVASCULAR ACCIDENT

Oxygen and glucose deprivation can result in cell death. This can occur through a decrease in cerebral blood flow or cerebral perfusion pressure. The area of cerebral infarction is called a stroke or cerebrovascular accident (CVA). Clients at risk for cerebrovascular occlusive diseases include those with the following risk factors:

1. Hypertension
2. Diabetes mellitus
3. Atherosclerosis
4. Hyperlipidemia
5. Polycythemia
6. Cardiac diseases, including myocardial infarction, congestive heart failure, left ventricular hypertrophy, dysrhythmias, and cardiac valve disease, congenital abnormalities of the circle of Willis, sedentary work

habits, family history, cigarette smoking, the use of oral contraceptives, and increased life stress.

Approximately half of all cases of stroke are caused by the occurrence of cerebral thrombosis. Occlusion of cerebral vessels can occur through the deposit of atherosclerotic plaque. In this case signs of neurologic deficit may appear slowly. Neurologic deficits are limited to the same area but become progressively worse over time. The client should be assessed for loss or decrease of carotid pulse rates and for the presence of a bruit over the carotids. The patient may have had a headache before the onset of neurologic symptoms. Neurologic deficits depend on which area of the brain is deprived of blood flow.

Another major cause of stroke is the cerebral embolus. An embolus is a free-floating substance in the bloodstream that travels to the brain, where it becomes lodged in the cerebral blood vessel. Embolic substances include blood clots, calcified plaque from blood vessels outside the brain, air, tumor particles, fat, vegetation from diseased heart valves, or air. Such substances tend to fragment as they float, resulting in multiple areas of occlusion. The patient shows signs of multifocal neurologic deficits.

Intracranial bleeding can also cause interruptions to cerebral blood flow. The onset of symptoms may be much more rapid than those caused by cerebral thrombus. Possible causes include ruptured arterial aneurysms, leaking arterial venous malformations, hemorrhage related to tumors, or hemorrhages related to hypertensive vascular disease.

Classification

Cerebrovascular accidents may be classified as transient ischemic attacks, reversible ischemic neurologic deficits, strokes in evolution, or completed strokes.

Transient ischemic attacks. A temporary disturbance of blood supply may cause a transient neurologic deficit. Symptoms may be present for only several minutes or may last up to 24 hours. The patient has no permanent neurologic deficit.

Reversible ischemic neurologic deficit. In reversible ischemic neurologic deficit the neurologic deficits last longer than 24 hours. Symptoms may continue for several days or weeks. There may be minimal, partial, or no residual neurologic deficit beyond this time.

Stroke in evolution. In stroke in evolution, once again, symptoms persist after the first 24 hours; however, a progressive neurologic deterioration may be seen. Residual neurologic deficits are present.

Completed stroke. In completed stroke the patient appears stable and the neurologic deficit is permanent and unchanging.

Signs and Symptoms

Presenting signs and symptoms and appropriate treatments vary according to the cause of interruption of cerebral blood flow. In all cases therapeutic interventions include maintenance of an adequate airway, optimum ABCs, and close monitoring of blood pressure, pulse rate, respiration rate, and neurologic vital signs. Anticoagulant therapy such as the use of heparin or coumadin is indicated in the patient having a series of transient ischemic attacks and in the person showing evidence of cardiac embolization (mitral stenosis, atrial fibrillation). Anticoagulant therapy is contraindicated in the person having a hemorrhagic stroke or in the person with extreme hypertension. After a stroke has completely evolved, anticoagulant therapy should be avoided, regardless of the cause, because of increased risk of future hemorrhage into the now necrotic area of brain tissue. Platelet antiaggregation medication such as aspirin or dipyridamole (Persantine) may be used to prevent or minimize thrombus formation.

The patient with severe hypertension may require IV hydralazine, nitroprusside, or nitroglycerin. Care should be taken that blood pressure is not reduced too rapidly or to too low a level. With decreases in pressure of more than 30 mm Hg risk of an adequate perfusion to the brain is increased. In the patient with subarachnoid hemorrhage, prolonged vasospasm could result in cerebral infarction. Treatment methods therefore include the use of calcium channel blockers such as nifedipine. Such therapy allows for relaxation of cerebral vasculature, thereby preventing an extension of an infarcted area.

Other causes of cerebral ischemia can include conditions resulting in systemic hypotension, cardiac arrest, severe ce-rebral edema, and hemorrhagic shock. Therapeutic intervention should include treatment modalities that restore a normal systemic blood pressure, decrease cerebral edema, restore a normal circulating blood volume, and ensure adequate oxygenation in as short a time as possible.

SUGGESTED READINGS

American Association of Neuroscience Nurses: *Core curriculum for neuroscience nursing,* vols 1 and 2, Chicago, 1991, The Association.

Bannister SR: *Brain's clinical neurology,* London, 1985, Oxford University Press.

Barnett HJM et al: *Stroke: pathophysiology, diagnosis and management,* New York, 1986, Churchill Livingstone.

Biller J et al: Spontaneous subarachnoid hemorrhage in young adults, *Neurosurgery* 21:664, 1987.

Carpenter MB: *Core text of neuroanatomy,* Baltimore, 1985, Williams & Wilkins.

Hennings R, Jackson DL: *Handbook of critical care neurology and neurosurgery,* New York, 1985, Praeger.

Millikon CH, McDowell F, Easton JD: *Stroke,* Philadelphia, 1987, Lea & Febiger.

Plum F, Posner JB: *Diagnosis of stupor and coma,* ed 3, Philadelphia, 1983, FA Davis.

Purchase G, Allen D: *Neuromedical and neurosurgical nursing,* London, 1984, Bailliere-Tindall.

Ropper AH, Kennedy SK: *Neurological and neurosurgical intensive care,* ed 2, Rockville, Md, 1988, Aspen.

Taylor JW, Ballenger S: *Neurological disfunctions and nursing interventions,* New York, 1980, McGraw-Hill.

Teasdale G, Jennett B: Assessment of coma and impaired consciousness, *Lancet* 2:81, 1974.

Wirth EP, Racheson RA, eds: *Neurosurgical critical care,* Baltimore, 1987, Williams & Wilkins.

Susan Budassi Sheehy

Cardiac emergencies are some of the most commonly seen emergencies in the emergency department (ED). Of primary concern is to identify those conditions which are potentially life threatening and to apply appropriate therapeutic interventions. In addition, the patient should be made comfortable and anxiety should be reduced.

CHEST PAIN OF CARDIAC ORIGIN

Of the 600,000 people who die from myocardial infarction (MI) each year, 200,000 to 300,000 die within the first 2 hours after the initial onset of the infarction, before reaching the hospital. MI may be medically treatable. Mortality from infarction can be reduced significantly if the patient receives proper medical care in the early phases of the infarction. Thus major campaigns to introduce the public to the signs and symptoms of MI and the advent of the mobile intensive care unit were initiated. Early care can be brought to the victim at home or at the scene of the infarct.

Certain factors can increase the incidence of MI. As these risk factors are compounded, the risk of MI is also compounded. Known risk factors are cigarette smoking, hypertension, obesity, diabetes mellitus, type A personality, lack of exercise, aging, poor diet, a family history of coronary artery disease, and a high serum cholesterol level. For example, a person who smokes two packs of cigarettes a day increases the risk of MI by a multiple of 4. It has been demonstrated that the greater the number of risk factors a person has, the greater are the person's chances of having an MI.

It has been conservatively estimated that more than 5.5 million people over 18 years of age have coronary artery disease. *Atherosclerosis* is a combination of two words: *atheroma,* which means lipid deposits, and *sclerosis,* which means smooth cell fibrosis.

Angina Pectoris

When the myocardium becomes hypoxic, a retrosternal discomfort occurs, which is known as angina pectoris. This is thought to occur as the result of an increased oxygen demand, an increased cardiac output, and the inability of that oxygen to reach the myocardium because of blockage in the coronary artery. The prevalent cause of coronary artery occlusion is atherosclerosis. Other causes of this condition are emboli, coronary artery spasm, and dissecting aortic aneurysm.

Differential diagnosis of angina (Table 36-1) can be made by the history obtained from the patient. It is important to obtain answers to the following questions, with use of the PQRST mnemonic:

P (*provoking*)

What provokes the pain? What makes it better? Worse?

Q (*quality*)

What is the quality of the pain? It is sharp? Dull? Pressure?

R (*radiating*)

Where is the pain? Does it radiate to any other area?

S (*severity*)

How severe is the pain, on a scale of 1 to 10?

T (*time*)

What time did the pain start? When did it end? Has it ever occurred before? How long did it last then?

Types. There are two types of angina: stable and unstable. Stable angina, also known as typical angina, occurs as a predictable event after such activities as exercise or body strain. There are two subcategories of unstable angina: typical unstable angina and Prinzmetal's angina. The attacks of typical unstable angina, or preinfarction angina, are prolonged and occur more frequently, and the episodes become more severe. Prinzmetal's angina, or variant angina, occurs when the patient is at rest. This pain usually occurs at the same time each day. During the attack the patient may have an elevated ST segment during electrocardiography. The prognosis in Prinzmetal's angina is poor, with a 50% mortality during the first year. In the early stages of the disease, if coronary catheterization results are diagnostic of blockage, coronary artery bypass surgery is usually recommended.

Treatment. The purpose of treating angina is to increase coronary artery blood flow and to reduce myocardial oxygen demand. Nitroglycerin is the drug of choice in the treatment of angina pectoris. It is administered sublingually in $\frac{1}{100}$-, $\frac{1}{150}$-, and $\frac{1}{200}$-grain tablets. Nitroglycerin acts by dilating coronary arteries, reducing afterload (thereby decreasing

Table 36-1 Differential diagnosis of angina

Characteristic	Stable angina	Unstable (preinfarction) angina
Location of pain	Substernal; may radiate to jaws and neck and down arms and back	Substernal; may radiate to jaws and neck and down arms and back
Duration of pain	1-5 min	5 min; occurring more frequently
Characteristic of pain	Aching, squeezing, choking, heavy burning	Same as stable angina, but more intense
Other symptoms	Usually none	Diaphoresis; weakness
Pain worsened by	Exercise; activity; eating; cold weather; reclining	Exercise; activity; eating; cold weather; reclining
Pain relieved by	Rest; nitroglycerin; isosorbide	Nitroglycerin, isosorbide may give only partial relief
ECG findings	Transient ST depression; disappears with pain relief	ST segment depression; often T wave inversion; but ECG may be normal

Table 36-2 Coronary arteries in MI

Right coronary artery	Left coronary artery

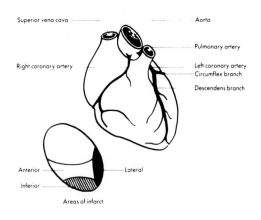

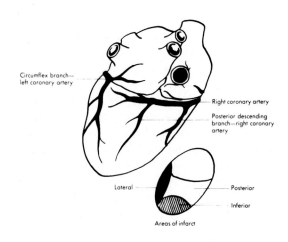

Supplies
  Right atrium
  Right ventricle
  Posterior surface of left ventricle
  50%-60% of sinoatrial node
  Bundle of His
Block causes
  Infarction of posterior wall of left ventricle
  Infarction of posterior wall of interventricular septum
In inferior MI (leads II, III, aVF) anticipate second-degree heart block, Mobitz type 1 block, Wenckebach block

Left circumflex branch
Supplies
  Left atrium
  Free wall of left ventricle
  40%-50% of sinoatrial node
  8%-10% of arteriovenous node
  Bundle of His
  Right bundle
Block causes
  Lateral wall infarction
  Posterior wall infarction (near base)
Left anterior descending branch
Supplies: interventricular septum
Block causes
  Infarction of anterior wall of left ventricle
  Effect on papillary muscle (which attaches to mitral valve)
  Infarction of anterior wall of septum
  In anterior MI (leads V₂, V₂, V₃) anticipate second-degree heart block, Mobitz type 2 block

blood pressure), reducing preload (venous return to the heart), and reducing left ventricular–end diastolic pressure.

Myocardial Infarction

Myocardial infarction (MI) a localized ischemic necrosis of an area of the myocardium, is caused by a narrowing of one or more of the coronary arteries, possibly resulting from a spasm, hemorrhage, thrombus, or other known cause. The primary causes of coronary artery narrowing are thought to be atherosclerotic plaques or thrombi, myocardial contusion, hypovolemic shock, coronary artery spasms, and dehydration. The location and size of the infarct depend on which coronary artery is affected and the level at which it is blocked (Table 36-2).

Most commonly MI is a result of blockage of the anterior descending coronary artery, causing involvement of the anterior wall of the myocardium. If the circumflex branch of the left coronary artery is involved, an anterolateral infarction occurs. Posterior infarction is caused by a block in the right coronary artery. Inferior wall MI can be caused by a block in either the left anterior descending artery or right circumflex artery.

Pain characterized as crushing, burning, sharp, heavy, or by a variety of other descriptions is described by one third of the victims of MI. The pain has been said to last anywhere from several minutes to several weeks. It is theorized that local hypoxia, lactate buildup, and sensory response of the hypoxic myocardium contribute to pain. The location of pain varies. It may localize in the substernal area, or it may radiate into the jaw and down the left arm. The patient may have nausea, vomiting, and hiccups caused by phrenic nerve stimulation.

Blood pressure decreases because poor pump action of the heart causes a decreased cardiac output. Sodium and water retention may occur as the result of decreased cardiac output and increased venous pressure. When MI occurs, a proportional amount of ventricular failure occurs. When ventricular failure is severe, the stroke volume decreases, resulting in an increased ventricular diastolic pressure. The body's sympathetic response decreases blood flow to the periphery. A decrease in blood flow and pressure to the kidneys leads to a slow glomerula filtration rate. Because of this rate, the renal cells are stimulated and renin production begins. With the increase in renin production, angiotensin levels increase. Angiotensin causes secretion of aldosterone. The combination of increased aldosterone and decreased glomerular filtration rate causes sodium and water retention and produces edema.

When auscultating the heart, one may hear a decreased first heart sound because of decreased myocardial contractility. One may also hear an increased second sound because of an increase in pulmonary artery pressure. An S_3 sound may be heard as the result of ventricular dilation and increased ventricular fluid pressure. A pericardial friction rub may be heard as the result of transient pericarditis.

Table 36-3   Serum enzymes in MI

Enzyme (normal values)	Elevation (hr after infarction)	Peak (hr)	Return to normal (days)
CPK (60-30)	2-5	24-48	2-3
SGOT (12-40)	6	24-48	3-4
LDH (150-300)	6-12	48-72	5-6
	6-12	48-72	10+
SGPT (6-53)	6-10	24-48	5

CPK, Creatinine phosphokinase; *LDH,* lactic dehydrogenase; *SGOT,* serum glutamic-oxaloacetic transaminase; *SGPT,* serum glutamic-pyruvic transaminase.

One may elicit an alternating pulse rate as a result of left-sided heart failure. Increased pressure because of congestion causes a backflow of blood into the jugular veins, which causes them to remain distended when the patient is sitting at a 45-degree angle. One also notes a prominent V wave with a rapid, deep Y-wave descent. The patient may also have an elevated temperature caused by inflammation and necrosis of myocardial tissue. As myocardial cells die and become necrotic, enzymes leak into the serum (Table 36-3).

Diaphoresis results from an autonomic nervous system response. The patient may show signs of anxiety as a result of pain and fever. The pulse rate increases because of low cardiac output causing a compensatory sympathetic nervous system response. The patient may also have cyanosis caused by a decreased oxyhemoglobin concentration and a decreased blood supply to the peripheral vascular system.

Traditional treatment of MI includes administration of oxygen, nitroglycerin, sublingually or by IV drip, morphine sulfate for pain control, and prophylactic lidocaine, and dysrhythmia therapy. Recent advances in thrombolytic therapy for the treatment of MI have proven most advantageous (see Chapter 13).

New Antidysrhythmic Agents

Several relatively new antidysrhythmic agents are now available. They can be characterized into two groups: those which are used to treat supraventricular dysrhythmias and those which are used to treat ventricular dysrhythmias.

Supraventricular agents

Adenosine (Adenocard). Adenosine acts to slow the conduction of the atriovenous (AV) node. Its primary use is in paroxysmal supraventricular tachycardia. It is given via rapid bolus. Advantages are its safe use in patients who have received digitalis and in patients with Wolff-Parkinson-White syndrome. It has been found to be ineffective in atrial fibrillation, atrial flutter, and ventricular tachycardia. It is contraindicated for use with sick sinus syndrome and second- or third-degree heart blocks. Some patients have facial flushing, dyspnea, or chest pressure when the medication is given. Rarely, heart blocks and asystole have occurred.

Esmolol (Brevibloc). Brevibloc is a beta-blocking agent that is cardioselective. It is given via IV bolus, 500 mg/kg for 1 minute, followed by an IV drip of 50 µg/kg/min for 4 minutes, up to 300 µg/kg/min. If there is no effect, repeat 50 µg/kg/min loading dose and follow it with 100 µg/kg/min. It may be repeated to a 200 µg/kg rate and occasionally to 300 µg/kg. A dose of 200 µg/kg/min is equivalent to 4 mg of IV propranolol (Inderal). At this same dosage level, hypotension is commonly seen.

The primary uses of esmolol are in cases of atrial fibrillation, atrial flutter, and noncompensatory sinus tachycardia. It should not be used in patients with bradycardia, heart blocks, diabetes, bronchospasm, or congestive heart failure. It may cause dizziness, nausea, phlebitis, and tissue necrosis.

Ventricular agents

Amiodarone (Cordarone). Amiodarone widens the transmembrane action potential without affecting phase zero. It is used for recurrent, refractory ventricular fibrillation and refractory unstable recurrent ventricular tachycardia. A loading dosage of 800 to 1600 mg/per day should be given. The patient should be monitored for 1 to 3 weeks because it may take this long for the drug to take effect. Once an effect is seen, the dosage should be decreased to 600 to 800 mg per day for a month, then to 400 to 600 mg per day. There are many toxic or adverse reactions to amiodarone including alveolitis, ventricular tachycardia, bradycardia, ventricular fibrillation, torsades de pointes, sinus arrest, visual disturbances, photosensitivity, hypothyroidism, thyrotoxicosis, fatigue, loss of coordination, peripheral neuropathy, nausea and vomiting, anorexia, and constipation.

Encainide (Enkaid). Encainide is given in cases of sustained ventricular tachycardia to slow conduction rate through the His bundle, the Purkinje system, and the AV node. Encainide causes an increase in the refractory factors of the atria, the AV node, and the ventricles. There appears to be an increase in mortality when this drug has been used for treatment of non–life-threatening dysrhythmias. It is contraindicated for use when bifascicular block or second- or third-degree blocks are present or when the patient is in cardiogenic shock. Dosage is 25 mg 3 times a day, increased in 3- to 5-day increments to a maximum of 75 mg 3 times a day. The dosage should be reduced when renal or hepatic disease is present.

Mexiletine (Mexitil). Mexitil is an analog of lidocaine that is given to treat ventricular dysrhythmias, such as frequent premature ventricular contractions, couplets and triplets, and ventricular tachycardia. Mexiletine is frequently known to cause gastrointestinal upset, syncope, tremors, and loss of coordination. Careful administration is recommended in the presence of hepatic disease. The usual dosage is 200 mg every 8 hours initially to a maximum of 1200 mg/day.

Propafenone (Rhythmol). Propafenone prolongs conduction through the AV node but does not affect the sinoatrial node. It should be given only when life-threatening ventricular dysrhythmias are present. The dosage is usually 150 mg every 8 hours. Adverse effects include bronchospasm and heart blocks. Less commonly, congestive heart failure, increased dysrhythmias, and pacemaker threshold increases have been reported.

Flecainide (Tambocor). Flecainide decreases intracardiac conduction, especially in the AV node, the atria, and the His-Purkinje system. It is used to treat life-threatening dysrhythmias, ventricular tachycardia, and ventricular fibrillation. Contraindications for use of this drug are the same as those for encainide. Flecainide can occasionally cause first-degree block or bundle branch block. The initial dosage is 100 mg every 12 hours, gradually increased over 3 to 5 days. Serum drug levels should be less than 1 µg/ml.

Tocainide (Tonocard). Tocainide is an analog of lidocaine that is used to decrease myocardial cell irritability in the presence of life-threatening dysrhythmias. Adverse reactions are rare, but when they do occur, they are severe and may include blood dyscrasias, interstitial pneumonitis, fibrosis, AV blocks, nausea, syncope, tremors, and paresthesias. The initial dosage is usually 400 mg every 8 hours (1200 to 1800 mg/per day). Caution should be used when administering this drug to a patient with renal disease.

Congestive Heart Failure

Congestive heart failure occurs when the heart fails to function adequately as a pump. This inadequacy results in venous congestion, decreased stroke volume and cardiac output, and an increase in peripheral systemic pressure. Onset may be gradual or sudden. Congestive heart failure may be seen alone or in conjunction with pulmonary edema. The onset of congestive heart failure is a *symptom* of an underlying problem, which may include hypertension, fluid overload, intracranial injury, MI, or valvular heart disease. Congestive heart failure may also be seen as a result of coronary artery disease, cardiomyopathy, and dysrhythmias, especially tachycardias at a rate greater than 180 beats/min and bradycardias of less than 30 beats/min. Sometimes fever, hyperthyroidism, and adult respiratory distress syndrome may result in congestive heart failure. It may also be seen in oxygen toxicity syndromes and after pneumothorax, uremic pneumonia, intracranial tumors, and the administration of drugs such as methotrexate, busulfan, hexamethonium, and nitrofurantoin.

Congestive heart failure is identified by severe shortness of breath, dyspnea, weakness, dependent edema, distended neck veins, bilateral rales, an increased circulation time, and hepatomegaly.

While obtaining a brief history from the patient or the family or friends, be sure to assess the patient for the adequacy of the airway, breathing, and circulation (ABCs). Once these priorities are established, check vital signs, monitor the heart rate for dysrhythmias, auscultate the lungs and the heart, and observe the patient for the presence of distended neck veins and peripheral edema.

Therapeutic intervention includes keeping the patient in bed and in a high Fowler's position; administering oxygen therapy, digitalis, and diuretics; maintaining an IV line at a keep-open rate or by placing a heparin lock; monitoring intake and output; and weighing the patient.

Acute Pericarditis

Acute pericarditis is an inflammation of the pericardial sac. It may occur as a result of trauma, infection, coronary artery disease, or neoplasms. Coxsackievirus, streptococci, staphylococci, tuberculosis, and *Haemophilus influenzae* are generally the causes in younger people. There are other causes in the middle-aged and elderly population.

These patients have severe chest pain, which increases during inspiration and increased activity, fever, chills, and dyspnea. Patients appear diaphoretic, and they may be hypotensive. Tachycardia or other dysrhythmias may be present, as well as pericardial friction rubs that increase in intensity when the patient leans forward. The patient has general malaise and demonstrates ST segment elevations of 1 to 3 mm in all electrocardiogram (ECG) leads except aVR and V_1.

Therapeutic intervention should include the administration of oxygen by nasal cannula at 4 to 6 L/min, sedation and analgesia, bed rest, and much reassurance. This patient may also be given antibiotics. Be aware that if pericardial effusion results, there is great danger of pericardial tamponade.

Pericardial Tamponade

Pericardial tamponade is a condition in which blood leaks into the pericardial sac from a disruption in the heart and causes a compression of the heart when the sac fills with blood. The condition may result from trauma, infection, or other rarer causes such as neoplasms. The pericardial sac is nondistensible and, when filled with blood, compresses the heart until cardiac output is greatly compromised.

A positive effect of tamponade is that it may slow the rate of bleeding or may actually stop the bleeding. However, when the tamponade is rapid or large, cardiac output is greatly diminished and the patient goes into shock and dies if this condition is not corrected.

Tamponade causes a decreased venous return to the heart, which causes an elevated central venous pressure, distended jugular veins, and a decreased cardiac output. This decreased cardiac output causes compensatory vasoconstriction together with increased peripheral vascular resistance, which initially appears as a slightly elevated blood pressure.

As little as 150 to 200 ml of blood in the pericardial sac may cause profound shock to develop. Removing as little as 10 to 20 ml of blood from the pericardial sac may be enough to reverse the shock condition.

Common signs and symptoms of pericardial tamponade

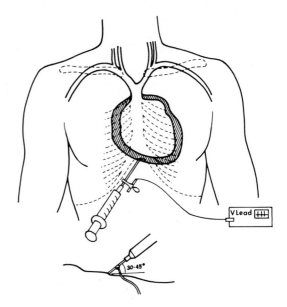

Fig. 36-1 Pericardiocentesis.

are Beck's triad: a decreased blood pressure, distended jugular veins, and distant heart sounds. Other findings are tachycardia and a central venous pressure greater than 15 mm Hg. If these signs are identified, suspect tamponade. Other signs and symptoms include a decreased arterial pressure, a weak, thready pulse rate, cyanosis, increased respiratory rate, dyspnea, paradoxic pulse rate, restlessness, a widened cardiac silhouette, and finally, shock.

Therapeutic intervention includes initiation of an IV line of Ringer's lactate or normal saline solution, administration of oxygen at 6 L/min by nasal cannula, and pericardiocentesis (Fig. 36-1), or a peri-cardial window.

Paradoxic pulse rate. Paradoxic pulse rate is a finding in one third of patients with pericardial tamponade. Its cardinal sign is an abnormal fall in systolic blood pressure during inspiration. To check for the presence of a paradoxic pulse rate, apply a blood pressure cuff to the patient's arm and inflate the cuff until systolic sounds disappear. Slowly deflate the cuff until the first systolic sounds can be heard. During normal inspiration the systolic sound disappears. Deflate the cuff until all systolic sounds can be heard during both inspiration and expiration. The difference in millimeters of mercury between the pressure at which the systolic sound disappears during inspiration and the pressure at which *all* systolic sounds can be heard is called the *paradox*. A difference of more than 10 mm Hg indicates the presence of a paradoxic pulse rate.

CHEST PAIN OF AORTIC ORIGIN
Aortic Dissection

One of the most commonly seen life-threatening disorders of the aorta is a dissecting aneurysm. It occurs primarily in men and is frequently seen in conjunction with hypertension

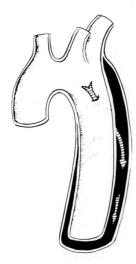

Fig. 36-2   Dissecting aortic aneurysm.

and atherosclerotic heart disease. It may also be seen after chest trauma and with Marfan's syndrome.

An aortic dissection is a tear in the intimal layer of the aorta (Fig. 36-2). As a result of this tear, blood leaks between the intimal layer and the medial layer. A type 1 dissection occurs in the ascending aorta and extends beyond the aortic arch. A type 2 dissection is a dissection of the ascending aorta alone. A type 3 dissection begins beyond the left subclavian artery.

As the aorta dissects, it may occlude the major vessels that branch off of the aorta. These include the myocardial, cerebral, mesenteric, and renal vessels. Rupture of a dissection may cause either pericardial tamponade or a rupture into the thoracic cavity, resulting in exsanguination, shock, and eventually, death.

Signs and symptoms of aortic dissection include excruciating or tearing chest pain that is substernal and is felt through to the posterior thoracic cavity, dyspnea, orthopnea, diaphoresis, pallor, apprehension, syncope, tachycardia, unilateral absence of major arterial pulses or bilateral blood pressure differences, hypertension, pulsation at the sternoclavicular joint, a murmur of aortic insufficiency (in ascending aortic dissection), hemiplegia or paraplegia, and

Table 36-4   Differential diagnosis of chest pain

Cause	P (*provokes*): Pain worsened by	Pain relieved by	Q (*quality*): Characteristic of pain
Acute MI	Movement, anxiety	Nothing; no movement, stillness, position, or breath holding; only relieved by medication (morphine sulfate)	Pressure, burning, aching, tightness, choking
Angina	Lying down, eating, effort, cold weather, smoking, stress, anger, worry, hunger	Rest, nitroglycerin	Aching, squeezing, choking, heaviness, burning
Dissecting aortic aneurysm			Excruciating, tearing
Pericarditis	Deep breathing, trunk movement, maybe swallowing	Sitting up, leaning forward	Sharp, knifelike
Pneumothorax	Breathing		Tearing, pleuritic
Pulmonary embolus	Breathing		Crushing (but not always)
Hiatus hernia	Heavy meal, bending, lying down	Bland diet, walking, antacids, semi-Fowler's position	Sharp, severe
Gastrointestinal disturbance of cholecystitis	Eating, lying down	Antacids	Gripping, burning
Degenerative disk (cervical or thoracic spine) disease	Movement of neck or spine, lifting, straining	Rest, decreased movement	Sharp, severe
Degenerative or inflammatory lesions of shoulder, ribs, anterior scalenus	Movement of arm or shoulder	Elevation and arm support to shoulder, postural exercises	Sharp, severe
Hyperventilation	Increased respiratory rate	Slowing of respiratory rate	Vague

shock. The chest pain may be confused with that of MI, severe back strain, pericarditis, or peptic ulcer. A widened mediastinum is evident on radiographs. When a chest radiograph is taken, it should be made with the patient in an upright position to validate the widened mediastinum, which may appear widened in the presence of no aortic dissection if the radiograph is made with the patient in a supine position.

Therapeutic intervention includes placing the patient in a high Fowler's position, administering high-flow oxygen, initiating two large-bore IV lines with Ringer's lactate, nitroprusside (Nipride), and propranolol (Inderal), and much support and reassurance of the patient. Most likely the dissection will be ruled out after angiography, and if dissection is present, the patient may be taken to surgery immediately, depending on the location and extent of the dissection.

CHEST PAIN OF OTHER ORIGINS
Hyperventilation Syndrome

Hyperventilation is one of the most commonly seen conditions in the ED. It may occur as the result of an anxiety disorder, or it may be the response to a disease process such as MI, salicylate overdose, or intracerebral hemorrhage. It

is of utmost importance to treat this patient with extreme caution and to pay close attention to other evident signs and symptoms of an underlying disorder.

A patient who comes to the ED with a chief complaint of hyperventilation presents a difficult diagnostic problem. It is important to avoid labeling the patient as simply a "hyperventilation" and to consider the possibility that the hyperventilation may be caused by something other than anxiety. Remember that hyperventilation may be a response to an organic process—one in which the treatment of having the patient breathe into a paper bag may be extremely detrimental to the patient. Medical and surgical illness must be ruled out before the assumption is made that the patient is hyperventilating in response to a psychologic problem.

Hyperventilation can be a sign of many illnesses and conditions, including anxiety, pregnancy, fever, liver disease, trauma, hypovolemia, pulmonary embolus, stress, ketoacidosis, high altitude, thyrotoxicosis, pulmonary hypertension, pulmonary edema, anemia, stroke, central nervous system lesion, and fibrotic lung disease. Hyperventilation causes partial arterial carbon dioxide pressure to drop (hypocapnia) and cerebral vasculature to constrict, resulting in respiratory alkalosis, which is evident because of symptoms

R (radiates): Location of pain	T (time): Onset of pain	History	Other
Across chest; may radiate to jaws and neck and down arms and back	Sudden onset; lasts 30 min to 1 hr	Age 40 to 70 yr; may or may not have history of angina	Shortness of breath, diaphoresis, weakness, anxiety
Substernal; may radiate to jaws and neck and down arms and back	Sudden onset; lasts only few min	May have history of angina; circumstances precipitating; pain characteristic; response to nitroglycerin	Unstable angina appears even at rest
Center of chest; radiates into back; may radiate to abdomen	Sudden onset	Nothing specific except that pain is usually worse at onset	Blood pressure difference between right and left arms, murmur of aortic regurgitation
Restrosternal; may radiate up neck and down left arm	Sudden onset or may be variable	Short history of upper respiratory infection or fever	Friction rub, paradoxic pulse rate >10 mm Hg
Lateral side of chest	Sudden onset	None	Dyspnea, increased pulse, decreased breath sounds, deviated trachea
Lateral side of chest	Sudden onset	Sometimes phlebitis	Cyanosis, dyspnea, cough with hemoptysis
Lower chest; upper abdomen	Sudden onset	May have none	
Lower substernal area, upper abdomen	Sudden onset	May have none	
Substernal; may radiate to neck, jaw, arms, or shoulders	Sudden onset	May have none	Pain usually on outer aspect of arm, thumb, or index finger
Substernal; radiates to shoulder	Sudden onset	May have none	
Vague	Sudden onset	Hyperventilation, anxiety, stress, emotional upset	Be sure hyperventilation from nonmedical cause

of tetany. Signs and symptoms of hyperventilation include anxiety and panic, shortness of breath, paresthesias of the fingers and toes and periorbital area, carpopedal spasms, confusion, syncope, and occasionally, chest pain.

Therapeutic intervention includes calmly and reassuringly explaining to the patient what is happening and why it is happening. Have the patient talk to you: it is difficult to hyperventilate while talking. As a last therapeutic intervention, have the patient breathe into a paper bag (carbon dioxide rebreathing). Remember to look for underlying causes of the hyperventilation before treating it as a reaction to an emotional state.

OTHER CAUSES OF CHEST PAIN

Other causes of chest pain may be abdominal in origin. With such illnesses as hiatal hernia, gastric or peptic ulcer, pancreatitis, esophageal spasms or other entities such as Mallory-Weiss syndrome or Boerhaave's syndrome, the patient may have chest pain. Additional problems that can cause chest pain are musculoskeletal disorders involving trauma, degenerative disk disease, xiphoidalgia, costrochondritis, Mondor's disease, and postherpetic syndrome (Table 36-4).

ELECTROCARDIOGRAM MONITORING AND PLOTTING AN AXIS
Monitoring

Monitoring on a four-lead monitoring system with an automatic lead switch button is shown in Fig. 36-3, *A*.

Monitoring on a three-lead electrocardiogram (ECG) monitor without an automatic lead switch button is shown in Fig. 36-3, *B* and *C*. Leads II and MCL$_1$ are the best leads to monitor for dysrhythmias.

Standard 12-lead ECG. The standard 12-lead ECG "records" 12 views of the heart's electric activity and records it on a wax-coated, standardized ECG paper (Figs. 36-4 and 36-5).

Before you begin
1. Check to be sure that all leads are placed correctly.
   a. "Green and white on the right," "Christmas trees (red and green) below the knees."
   b. Ensure that there is a conduction medium between the electrodes and the patient.
   c. Avoid placing the electrodes over large muscle masses.
2. Ensure that lead wires are not touching anything metal. This placement will cause 60-cycle interference.
3. Explain what you are doing to the patient.

When you begin
1. Standardize the machine at the beginning of each lead.
2. Record at least four complexes in each lead.
3. If 60-cycle interference occurs, check for the following:
   a. Loose leads
   b. Leads and wires against metal
   c. Other electric machines that could be unplugged
4. If the patient will be transferred to a coronary care or intensive care unit where a daily ECG will be done,

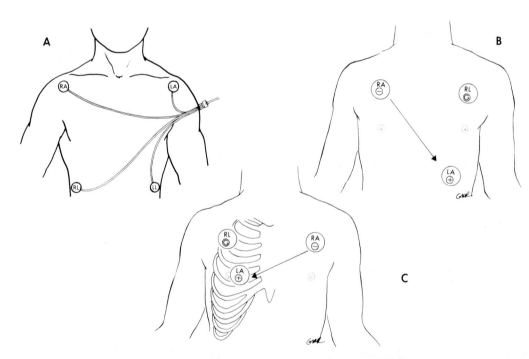

Fig. 36-3 **A,** Lead placement for four-lead monitoring system, with automatic lead switch button. Monitoring on three-lead system without automatic lead switch button. **B,** Lead II. **C,** Lead MCL$_1$.

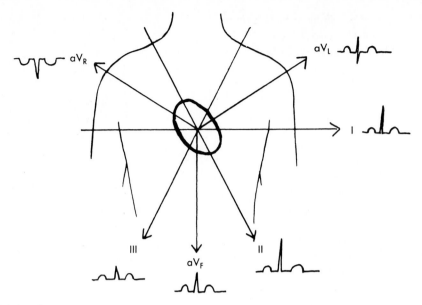

Fig. 36-4   Six-limb lead (leads I, II, III, aVR, aVL, and sVF) would normally appear as shown.

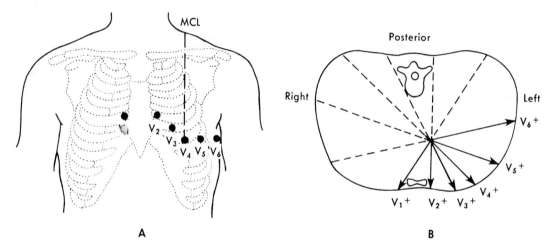

A   B

Fig. 36-5   Graphic representation of precordial or chest (V) leads, the last six leads of 12-lead ECG.

mark the chest site where the chest leads are placed (with methylene blue or another dye) to ensure that the leads will have the same placement each time an ECG is recorded.

5. Attempt to maintain the patient's modesty.

Conclusion

1. End the ECG with at least 15 seconds of lead II recording (used for dysrhythmia detection).
2. Record the patient's name, the date, and the time the ECG was taken directly on the ECG strip.

3. Interpret the strip, or relay it to the appropriate person for interpretation.

Interpretation. When current flows toward a lead (arrowheads, positive electrode), an upward ECG deflection occurs. When current flows away from a lead (arrowhead, positive electrode), a downward deflection of the ECG occurs. When current flows perpendicular to a lead (arrowhead, positive electrode), biphasic deflection of the ECG occurs.

When examining a 12-lead ECG, examine each of the 12 leads individually and note any of the following:

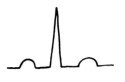
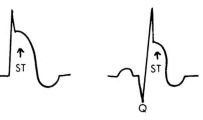

Normal	Ischemia	Injury	Infarct
	Decreased blood supply T wave inversion May indicate ischemia without myocardial infarction	Acute or recent; the more elevated the ST segment, the more recent the injury	Significant Q wave greater than 1 mm wide and half the height + depth of the entire complex Indicates myocardial necrosis

The leads directly recording the area of infarct demonstrate changes. An anterior wall myocardial infarction appears in leads V_1, V_2, and V_3:

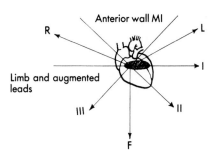
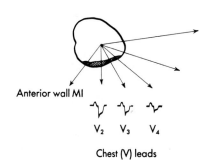

An inferior wall myocardial infarction appears in leads II, III, and aV_F:

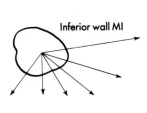
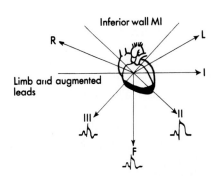

A lateral wall myocardial infarction appears in leads, I, $aV_L, V_5,$ and V_6:

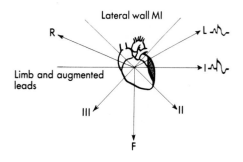

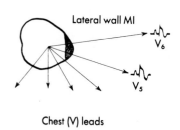

A posterior wall myocardial infarction appears in leads V_1 and V_2. The first R wave is tall, there is a depressed ST segment, and there is an elevated T wave:

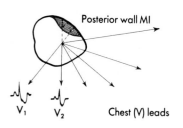

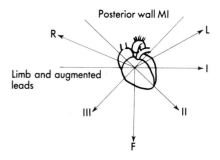

Plotting a Sample Axis

An axis is a graphic representation of the main vector in the heart.

Equipment

12-lead ECG
Graph paper
Ruler
Writing instrument

Procedure

1. Draw leads I and aV_F lines on graph paper.

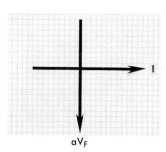

2. Examine lead I of the ECG.
   a. Determine if it is positive or negative.
   b. Determine by how much.

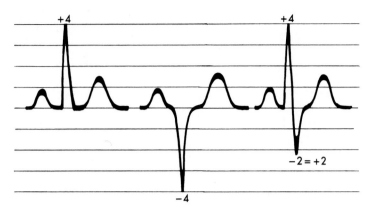

---

3. Plot the positive infection or negative deflection on the
   graph paper by drawing a perpendicular line.
   a. Positive goes *toward* the lead.
   b. Negative goes *away from* the lead.

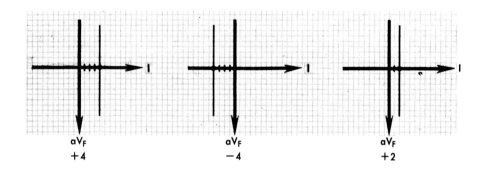

---

4. Examine lead aV$_F$ of the ECG.
   a. Determine if it is positive or negative.
   b. Determine by how much.

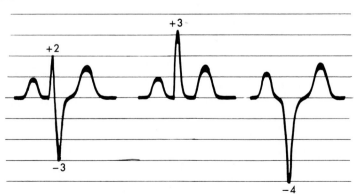

5. Plot the positive inflection or negative deflection on the
   graph paper by drawing a perpendicular line.
   a. Positive goes *toward* the lead.
   b. Negative goes *away from* the lead.

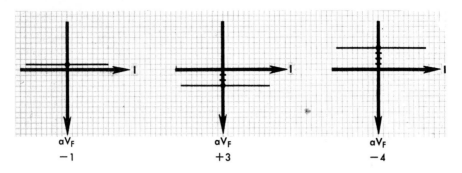

6. The intersection of the plots of lead I and aV$_F$ is the axis.

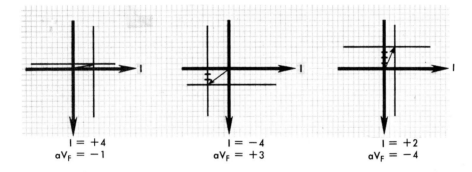

7. Superimpose a protractor compass over the graph paper
   to determine the exact degree of axis or estimate the
   degree of axis by quadrants.

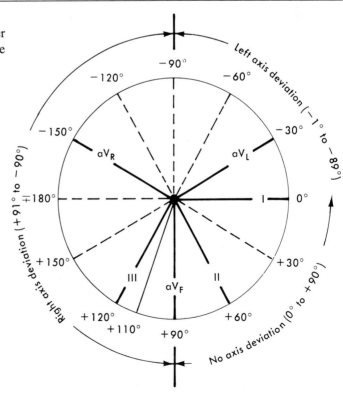

SUGGESTED READINGS

AIMS Trial Study Group: Long-term effects of intravenous anistreplase in acute myocardial infarction: final report of the AIMS study, *Lancet* 335:427, 1990.

Andreoli K et al: *Comprehensive cardiovascular nursing,* ed 7, St Louis, 1991, Mosby–Year Book.

DeBakey ME et al: Dissection and dissecting aneurysms of the aorta: twenty-year follow-up of 526 patients treated surgically, *Surgery* 92:1118, 1982.

Fowler NO, ed: *The pericardium in health and disease,* Mt Kisko, NY, 1985, Futura Publishing.

Goldberger AL: *MI: ECG differential diagnosis,* ed 3, St Louis, 1984, Mosby–Year Book.

Lee G: *Flight nursing,* St Louis, 1991, Mosby–Year Book.

ISIS-2 (Second International Study of Infarct Survival), Collaborative Group: Randomized trial of intravenous streptokinase, oral aspirin, both or neither among 17,187 cases of suspected acute myocardial infarction: ISIS-2, *Lancet* 2:349, 1988.

Italian Group for the Study of Streptokinase in Myocardial Infarction (GISSI): Effectiveness of intravenous thrombolytic treatment in acute M.I., *Lancet* 1:397, 1986.

TIMI Study Group: Thrombosis in Myocardial Infarction (TIMI) Trial: phase I findings, *N Engl J Med* 312:932, 1985.

TIMI Study Group: Comparison of invasive and conservative strategies after treatment with intravenous tissue plasminogen activator in acute myocardial infarction: results of the Thrombolysis in Myocardial Infarction (TIMI) phase II trial, *N Engl J Med* 320:618, 1989.

Roberts R: Patient selection for thrombolytic therapy: reexamining the criteria. *Clin Challenges Acute Myocardial Infarct* 1(4):4, 1990.

Wilkerson JT: Acute M.I. In Wyngaarten JB, Smith LH Jr, eds: *Cecil textbook of medicine,* ed 7, Philadelphia, 1985, WB Saunders.

PULMONARY EMERGENCIES

Susan Budassi Sheehy

Patients who arrive at the ED with pulmonary emergencies are considered to be, in most cases, triaged as emergent or urgent patients, since compromise of the airway or breathing may be life-threatening. Most of these patients, if conscious, are extremely anxious and gasping for breath. This adds stress to the emergency care provider's already stressful environment.

Many emergency pulmonary conditions are readily reversible if assessment and interventions are careful and prompt. Many of the common pulmonary emergency conditions are reviewed in this chapter.

RESPIRATORY PROBLEMS

It is important to be familiar with the meaning of terms that are used frequently in respiratory disorders:

ventilation—the amount of air passing into and out of the lungs

hypoventilation—too little air going in and out of the lungs

hyperventilation—respirations that are too deep and too rapid

tidal volume—amount of air breathed in with each normal breath

tachypnea—a respiratory rate greater than 20 breaths/min

dyspnea—shortness of breath (objective)

orthopnea—difficult breathing except in an upright position

stridor—crowing sound heard with upper respiratory obstruction

To assess the tidal volume without the assistance of a sophisticated piece of equipment, place the back of your hand near the patient's mouth and nose to feel for air movement, and then place your hands on the patient's lower rib margin and feel for chest movement. With a little practice, you can become very accurate at assessing tidal volume this way.

Begin assessment of any patient complaining of respiratory distress by first ensuring the ABCs. Then listen for noises. If there is noise, obstruction is present. Check the patient's level of consciousness. Check skin vital signs (color, moisture, and temperature). What do the respirations sound like? What do they look like? Are they shallow? Deep? Is the patient using accessory muscles of respiration such as the sternocleidomastoid or abdominal muscles, or is there supraclavicular indrawing? Finally check for paradoxic movement of the chest wall.

Dyspnea

Dyspnea is the objective finding that the victim is short of breath. It is one of the most frequently seen complaints in both the prehospital and emergency care settings and is one of the findings in many diseases and cases of trauma. It is essential to make a rapid and accurate assessment of the problem and intervene therapeutically as fast as possible before disaster sets in.

To be able to accurately assess the problem, one must determine when the shortness of breath began, and what, if known, caused it to happen. It is important to know whether the episode came on gradually or suddenly. Ask the patient if the problem is in getting air *into* the lungs or in getting air *out* of the lungs. This may be a repeated episode, and he or she may be able to tell you what happened the last time this occurred and how it was treated. The patient may also be able to tell you if this episode is worse or less severe than previous episodes.

Ask the patient about a history of lung disease or heart disease. Ask if he or she has a history of asthma or hypertension. Be sure to use terms with which he or she is familiar. Ask the patient if he or she smokes, is taking any medications, or has difficulty walking short distances or up stairs.

Look for the objective signs of obvious respiratory distress—flaring of the nostrils, cyanosis, pallor, and decreasing level of consciousness.

If a patient is indeed short of breath, be sure that the ABCs are present or have been established. If the patient is still conscious, place him or her in a high Fowler's position and administer oxygen. If the patient has a history of chronic obstructive lung disease, run the oxygen at 2 L/min. If there is no history of lung disease, administer oxygen at 6 to 8

L/min via nasal cannula or mask, if the victim will tolerate it. Initiate an intravenous (IV) line of D_5W to keep the vein open.

Asthma

Asthma is an obstruction of airflow to or from the lungs that may be caused by secretions, swelling, or spasms that may be caused by antigens, infections, environmental pollutants, exercise, medications, or stress. This produces bronchospasm, hypoxia, and anxiety. Between attacks the lungs and the bronchial tree are normal.

It is estimated that more than 8 million persons in the United States have asthma. It may occur at any age and is believed to be caused by a bronchial tree that is sensitive to inhaled substances such as pollen, molds, feather dust, animal dander, dust, gases, insecticides, and foods such as chocolate, milk, or seafood.

In addition, asthma attacks may be caused by excessive stress, depression, cigarette smoke, a pulmonary embolus, nasal polyps, other allergies, or cardiovascular problems.

Signs and symptoms include cough, dyspnea, and wheezing. The patient may also be diaphoretic and experience tachycardia.

Therapeutic intervention is aimed at reducing bronchospasm and improving oxygenation. The traditional drug of choice in acute episodes of asthma is epinephrine. It is given in a 1:1000 solution subcutaneously in a dose of 0.1 to 0.3 ml. This dosage may be repeated at 40-minute intervals up to a total of three doses.[4]

Terbutaline sulfate is an alternative medication that can be given in acute or stable asthma. It is a longer acting drug than epinephrine and has equivalent bronchodilatory action.

After the administration of epinephrine or terbutaline, consider administering aerosolized adrenergic agonists. This method of administration allows for rapid effects without undesirable systemic side effects. Medications available for this use are isoetharine hydrochloride, isoetharine mesylate, isoproterenol hydrochloride, metaproterenol sulfate, and albuterol.

If epinephrine, terbutaline, or aerosolized agents have not been effective, consider administering aminophylline or theophylline. Determine whether the patient has been taking these medications and follow hospital protocols for dosage calculations.

Other medications that have been used to treat asthma are corticosteroids and parasympathetic antagonists. Corticosteroids are given to cause an antiinflammatory effect. Stimulation of cholinergic lung receptors causes mast cell degranulation and the contraction of smooth muscle. Parasympathetic antagonists block these events and relieve bronchospasm.

In the patient with asthma, sedation should not be used as a treatment for the acute attack. Patients should, however, be hydrated. Most patients with acute asthma attacks have lost fluid from such conditions as hyperventilation or from inadequate fluid intake. If the patient is unable to take fluids by mouth, consider IV fluid replacement.

If arterial pH demonstrates severe acidosis, administer sodium bicarbonate until pH is above 7.3.[6] Remember that oxygen should be administered to maintain an arterial oxygen saturation of at least 90%.[2]

If a patient has been resistant to pharmacological therapy, consider the use of endotracheal intubation and assisted ventilation. Although there are no strict guidelines as to when this would be appropriate, consider the clinical picture of the patient. If PA_{CO_2} continues to rise, and the patient is becoming exhausted, then consider intubation and assisted ventilation.

Bronchitis

Bronchitis is a chronic irritation of the bronchial mucosa, causing a frequent and productive cough. It is caused by recurrent exposure to cigarette and cigar smoke, air pollution, or chronic inhalation of irritating substances. It is commonly seen in middle-aged persons, more frequently in men than in women, and it may be a precursor to chronic obstructive lung disease.

The patient has dyspnea and a productive cough that increases in the evenings and in damp, rainy weather.

Therapeutic intervention includes removing the cause of the irritation and having the patient rest and drink plenty of fluids. You may also employ bronchodilators, expectorants, and antibiotics if necessary. If the problem is a chronic one, the patient may choose to move to a dry, warm, dust-free climate.

Chronic Obstructive Lung Disease

Chronic obstructive lung disease, also known as chronic obstructive pulmonary disease (COPD) and emphysema, is a process in which the alveoli of the lungs enlarge and lose their elastic property and the alveolar wall begins to destruct. Because of the inelasticity of the alveoli, the patient is unable to exhale adequately, and there is much difficulty with adequate gas exchange at the alveolar level.

The exact cause of COPD is not known, but it is believed to have a positive connection to cigarette smoking, since 90% of patients who have this disease are smokers with a history of smoking more than one pack of cigarettes per day for many years. Other causative factors are thought to be pulmonary irritants such as air pollution, industrial inhalants (especially silicone), and tuberculosis.

When a patient with COPD comes to the ED, he or she usually relates a history of emphysema and dyspnea that has increased in severity over the past several days. He or she appears cyanotic, especially in the lips, fingernails, and earlobes. The patient's fingers are probably clubbed, since this process has gone on for a prolonged period. Assessment shows that the patient has a prolonged expiratory phase of respiration, and breath sounds are faint, with wheezes and rales present. He or she demonstrates a prolonged expiratory phase of respiration and uses accessory muscles of respiration. You will notice subclavicular and tracheal indrawing on inspiration. The patient's cough is productive, and he or she offers a history of many years of smoking. He or she may have a barrel chest.

Therapeutic intervention in the acute phase of this disease includes placing the patient in a high Fowler's position, administering oxygen at low liter flow (2 L/min by nasal cannula), initiating an IV line of D_5W, and administering aminophylline, 250 mg in 25 ml D_5W to run over 5 to 10 minutes. When administering oxygen, be very careful to observe the patient for a positive response. Remember that the most serious, life-threatening event to the patient is hypoxemia. So if the patient is not responding favorably to the initial therapy, do not hesitate to administer oxygen at a higher flow rate.

Smoke Inhalation

When a person is exposed to a fire, besides being burned, he or she may also suffer from smoke inhalation or inhalation of a noxious gas that was created as a product of combustion. Although the burns may be minor, the inhalation of smoke may be life-threatening, because severe pulmonary damage may result in chemical pneumonitis, asphyxiation resulting from increased carboxyhemoglobin levels, or pulmonary edema.

When synthetic materials burn, the products of combustion usually include noxious gases (Table 37-1). Exposure to these gases may cause additional pulmonary problems.

It is important to obtain a good history if a patient has been exposed to smoke or noxious gases. Find out how long the victim was exposed, if he or she was in a confined space, the type of material that was burning, and how much of the material was burning.

The primary manifestation of smoke inhalation is pulmonary edema, which may not manifest for 24 to 48 hours. Signs and symptoms of smoke inhalation include a mild irritation of the upper airway and a burning pain in the throat or chest. The patient may have singed nasal hairs, carbonaceous sputum, facial burns, and hypoxia. Pulmonary auscultation may reveal rales, rhonchi, or wheezes. He or she may be dyspneic and restless. The patient may cough, have a hoarse voice, and show other signs of pulmonary edema. If a patient has a history of exposure to smoke or other noxious gases without other signs of pulmonary irritation, he or she should be observed for several hours before being allowed to leave the hospital.

Therapeutic intervention for victims of smoke inhalation includes maintenance of the ABCs, administration of high-flow humidified oxygen, and placement of an IV line of D_5W to be kept open. Arterial blood gases should be drawn, and appropriate therapy should be administered in accordance with results. Encourage the patient to cough and breathe deeply and provide for chest physical therapy and tracheal toilet. Victims of smoke inhalation should be admitted to the hospital and observed for 24 to 48 hours. They may require endotracheal intubation, cricothyroidotomy, or tracheostomy. Also consider the use of bronchodilators, steroids, and a nasogastric tube.

Table 37-1   Data on toxic products of combustion

Material	Use	Major toxic chemical products of combustion
Polyvinyl chloride	Wall and floor covering, telephone cable insulation	Hydrogen chloride (P) Phosgene (P) Carbon monoxide
Polyurethane foam	Upholstery	Isocyanates (P) (toluene, 2,4-diisocyanate) Hydrogen cyanide
Lacquered wood, veneer, wallpaper	Wall covering	Acetaldehyde (P) Formaldehyde (P) Oxides of nitrogen (P) Acetic acid
Acrylic	Light diffusers	Acrolein (P)
Nylon	Carpet	Hydrogen cyanide Ammonia (P)
Acrilan	Carpet	Hydrogen cyanide Acrolein (P)
Polystyrene	Miscellaneous	Styrene Carbon monoxide

From Genovese M et al: *Chest* 71:441, 1977.
P, Pulmonary irritant.

Pulmonary Edema

Pulmonary edema, also known as "backward failure" or circulatory overload, is a result of back pressure into the lungs and left atria, which causes an increased pressure in the pulmonary capillaries. This increase in pressure causes fluid to leak out of the capillaries and into the alveoli, producing what is known as pulmonary edema. Pulmonary edema is a commonly seen acute medical emergency that requires prompt recognition and rapid management. When it is recognized and treated early, results of the treatment are usually dramatic and favorable. Normally, fluid content in relation to the lung mass is 20%. In acute pulmonary edema, fluid content sometimes reaches greater than 1000%.

It is important to remember that pulmonary edema is a *symptom* of some other underlying disorder and should not be considered a diagnosis. Pulmonary edema is most commonly of cardiac origin, although there are several other conditions that may also cause it. Some of the more frequent causes of pulmonary edema are myocardial infarction with left ventricular failure (the box below displays the mechanism of pulmonary edema of cardiac origin), aortic insufficiency, aortic stenosis, mitral stenosis, amyloidosis, myocarditis, hypertension, coronary artery disease, dysrhythmias (particularly tachycardia of greater than 180 beats/min and bradycardia of less than 30 beats/min, hyperthermia, near drowning, hyperthyroidism, exercise, and severe congestive heart failure. Other causes are adult respiratory distress syndrome, heroin overdose, methadone overdose, inhalation of toxic substances, pulmonary embolism, high altitude, neurogenic problems, volume overload, anemia, uremia, disseminated intravascular coagulation, renal impairment, lymphatic obstruction, bacteremic sepsis, beriberi, and general anesthesia.

MECHANISM OF PULMONARY EDEMA OF CARDIAC ORIGIN

Myocardial infarction
↓
Left ventricular failure
↓
Increased pressure in left ventricle
↓
Increased pressure in pulmonary venous system
↓
Loss of plasma oncotic pressure
↓
Leak of fluid into interstitial tissue
↓
Reflex spasm of airways (cardiac asthma) and pulmonary alveoli
↓
Pulmonary edema and interference with gas exchange
↓
Decreased P_{O_2} and acidosis

The onset of pulmonary edema is usually sudden, even though the underlying process may have been going on for a prolonged time. The initial complaint is usually shortness of breath. The patient may also complain of tightness across the chest, anxiety, inability to lie down, a decreased exercise tolerance, paroxysmal nocturnal dyspnea and orthopnea, cough, Cheyne-Stokes respirations, central and peripheral cyanosis, rales, rhonchi, wheezes, distended neck veins, and S_3 gallop and decreased heart sounds, peripheral edema, tachycardia, and pink, frothy sputum.

The goals of therapy in pulmonary edema are to decrease hypoxia, improve ventilation, decrease pulmonary capillary wedge pressure, and improve myocardial contractility.

While obtaining a brief history from the patient or the family, ensure that ABCs are adequate. Check the patient's vital signs. The patient will usually be tachypneic, tachycardic, and hypertensive. It is estimated that 75% of patients who have pulmonary edema with congestive heart failure are hypertensive. Monitor the patient carefully for dysrhythmias. Pulmonary edema may be the result of a dysrhythmia, or the dysrhythmia may be present because of hypoxia.

Lung auscultation may reveal rales and rhonchi; wheezes suggest cardiac asthma, which is caused by a reflex spasm of the airways.

When auscultating the heart, you often hear an S_3 gallop rhythm of ventricular distension and/or muffled heart sounds.

Because there are no valves in the internal jugular veins, they act as "manometers" for the right atrium. To observe the jugular vein, the head should be turned to the patient's left or right and the vein should be observed at the posterior border of the sternocleidomastoid muscle. Place the patient in a semi-Fowler's position. If the vein is distended more that 2 inches above the sternal notch when the patient is sitting up at an angle of at least 30°, this suggests right atrial congestion. Examine the patient for peripheral edema, especially in dependent parts of the body such as the arms, legs, feet, and sacral area.

Therapeutic intervention. It should be remembered that the following therapeutic interventions are meant to improve circulatory and ventilatory dynamics and will not alter the underlying disease process. After initial life-threatening therapeutic interventions, it is necessary to study the cause of the pulmonary edema further and treat the cause.

High Fowler's position. The initial step in treatment of pulmonary edema is to place the patient in a high Fowler's position. The patient should have his or her legs over the edge of the bed in a dependent position whenever possible. You will find that it is not necessary to convince the patient to do this: he or she will insist on sitting up because lying down cannot be tolerated. This position, with legs dependent, decreases venous return to the heart, decreases the work of breathing, and increases tidal volume.

Oxygen therapy. Administer oxygen to treat the hypoxic

state. When the patient is in a controlled environment, administer 100% oxygen by mask with intermittent positive pressure breathing. This type of oxygen administration requires much reassurance and direction, since the patient has the sensation that he or she is suffocating.

IV line. Initiate IV therapy with D_5W at a keep-open rate. This line is for the administration of medications. Attach a controlled volume measuring device to the IV bag.

Morphine sulfate. The patient should be medicated with morphine sulfate, 8 to 15 mg in 2 mg to 3 mg increments, slow IV push every 3 minutes. Morphine is given to cause venous dilatation and venous pooling, thereby causing a decreased venous return to the heart. It also has the effect of sedation, which causes the patient to be less anxious and slows his or her rate of breathing. Morphine should be given with much caution, since it may cause respiratory depression. Attention must be paid to the rate and depth of respirations after administration, especially in patients with a history of chronic obstructive respiratory disease. Naloxone (Narcan) is a narcotic antagonist that may be administered (titrated to effect by IV push) if the patient has respiratory distress as a result of morphine administration.

Nitroglycerin. Nitroglycerin, $\frac{1}{150}$ grain, may be given sublingually if the patient has a systolic blood pressure of above 100 mm Hg. By dilating peripheral vasculature, nitroglycerin acts as a "chemical tourniquet" to pool blood. Administration of nitroglycerin may be repeated as long as systolic blood pressure remains above 100 mm Hg. Do not use vasodilators if the patient is hypotensive.

Diuretics. Diuretics are given to decrease intravascular volume and produce a fluid loss in the form of urinary output. The diuretic of choice is furosemide (Lasix). Furosemide usually elicits a response within 5 to 15 minutes after administration.

Digitalis. To increase myocardial contractility and improve cardiovascular function, administration of digitalis may be considered.

Aminophylline. Aminophylline may be used for its effect on the lungs, where it produces bronchodilation and decreases bronchospasm. It also increases heart rate and myocardial contractility. The hazard of aminophylline administration is that it may produce life-threatening ventricular dysrhythmias.

Arterial blood gas analysis. Arterial blood gas values should be measured; the following blood gas values are desirable: PO_2, 80 mm Hg; PCO_2, 30 to 40 mm Hg; and pH, 7.4.

Reassurance. In addition, offer patients as much reassurance as possible. Patients with pulmonary edema are very frightened and often have the feeling that they are suffocating and dying. Verbal and touch reassurance are very important. Your words and touch can help patients to relax and improve the effects of therapeutic interventions.

Foley catheter. Placement of a Foley catheter should be done only if the patient cannot urinate by himself or herself or if he or she is unable to control urination.

If the patient's systolic pressure is less than 90 mm Hg, consider initiating a dopamine drip at a rate of 10 μg/kg/min. The dose should then be titrated at up to 40 μg/kg/min until the systolic pressure is greater than 90 mm Hg.

If inotropic agents are to be used, prepare the patient for the placement of an invasive monitoring line as soon as possible. If dysrhythmias are a concern, consider administering prophylactic antidysrhythmic agents, such as lidocaine.

If the patient must be endotracheally intubated to gain control of his or her airway, this is usually best accomplished via the nasal route with the patient sitting in a high Fowler's position.

Mnemonic for Treatment of Pulmonary Edema: MOST DAMP

M	= *m*orphine	D	= *d*iuretics
O	= *o*xygen	A	= *a*minophylline
S	= *s*it up	M	= *m*onitor
T	= *t*ourniquets*	P	= *p*ositive pressure

High-altitude pulmonary edema. Besides being the result of a medical illness, pulmonary edema can result from exposure to a high altitude without the benefit of acclimatization. High-altitude pulmonary edema occurs when there is a rapid ascent to altitudes above 10,000 feet and the person is performing heavy physical activity for the first 3 days while at this altitude, or if there is underlying disease. Signs and symptoms of this disorder occur 6 to 36 hours after the initial exposure. It may also be seen in those who normally dwell at high altitudes, go to sea level for 2 or more weeks, and then return to the high altitude. This condition may occur in the absence of underlying cardiovascular disease or pulmonary disorders. It demonstrates itself as marked pulmonary hypertension and is treated with a return to sea level, bed rest, and oxygen therapy.

Pulmonary Embolus

The signs and symptoms of pulmonary embolus are frequently confused with those of myocardial infarction, pneumothorax, rib fractures, or other phenomena in which the chief complaint is chest pain. Because of this, pulmonary embolus is one of the most difficult conditions to diagnose in the emergency care setting. Pulmonary embolus is the third leading cause of death in the United States and the most common form of respiratory death among patients who are hospitalized.

Pulmonary embolus is the complication of a disease or condition in which a venous thrombus forms, usually in the deep veins of the legs, and becomes detached to form an embolus. The embolus lodges in a branch of the pulmonary artery, usually in the lower lobes of the lungs, causing a partial or total occlusion, and therefore, a pulmonary infarct.

---

*Rotating tourniquets are no longer used. The term "tourniquets," as used in this mnemonic, refers to nitroglycerin, a "chemical tourniquet."

The degree of hemodynamic compromise depends primarily on the extent of blood flow that has been obstructed. The embolus may consist of blood, fat, air, bone, amniotic fluid, or a foreign body. Sixty-six percent of deaths from pulmonary embolism usually occur within less than 30 minutes from the time the thrombus becomes an embolus.

Pulmonary embolus is most commonly seen as a result of trauma, surgery, or long-bone fractures. It is also seen occasionally with obesity, a decreased peripheral circulation, congestive heart failure, or thrombophlebitis. Cardiac diseases such as congestive heart failure or prolonged bed rest may cause pulmonary emboli to form. Pulmonary emboli may also appear in conjunction with acute infections, blood dyscrasias, childbirth (amniotic fluid emboli), scuba diving (air emboli), poor IV initiation techniques (air emboli), and with oral contraception use, the presence of neoplasms, and central venous pressure lines.

Pulmonary embolus is usually underdiagnosed. Common signs and symptoms of pulmonary embolus may be nonspecific and cause the emergency nurse to think of other reasons for the signs and symptoms. More common signs and symptoms include shortness of breath, tachypnea, tachycardia, and angina-like chest pain. Patients with pulmonary emboli may also have pallor or cyanosis or both, anxiety, occasionally decreased blood pressure, and wheezes. An embolus may be demonstrated by electrocardiography as right bundle branch block and a right axis deviation with peaked P waves in the limb leads and a depressed T wave in the right precordial leads (V_1, V_2, V_3). Occasionally, however, there may be no signs or symptoms that precede the terminal event, or symptoms may be vague and unrecognized.

Diagnosis is usually made by history of the event and by arterial blood gas values, chest radiograph results, electrocardiographic findings, the presence of an elevated temperature, results of a ventilation-perfusion scan or pulmonary angiography, the presence of an S_3-S_4 gallop murmur, and the presence of crackles and rales on auscultation.

Arterial blood gas values may be variable, and therefore, not very useful. An abnormal electrocardiogram will only be seen if there is a massive pulmonary embolus. Good diagnostic blood tests are not available. Chest radiographs may demonstrate a widened right pulmonary artery and lack of perfusion, the presence of atelectasis or infiltrates, or a pleural effusion or an elevated hemidiaphragm.

A ventilation-perfusion scan is used to determine the absence of a pulmonary embolus. A pulmonary angiogram is the best diagnostic test and may actually visualize the embolus. Other diagnostic procedures include digital subtraction pulmonary angiography, computerized tomography, magnetic resonance imagery, and fiberoptic angioscopy.

Therapeutic intervention is generally supportive and includes maintenance of the ABCs, the administration of oxygen at high flow rates, insertion of an IV line with D_5W, and the administration of an analgesic agent such as me-peridine. Morphine should *not* be given because it causes respiratory depression. You should also consider administering bronchodilators and managing dysrhythmias. Clotting times should be monitored and anticoagulant therapy should be started to prevent recurrent emboli and to lyse current clots. Heparin is usually the anticoagulant of choice. The dosage depends on the extent of the embolus. For massive pulmonary emboli, give 10,000 U in an IV bolus, followed by 1500 U per hour IV until the patient's partial thromboplastin time is 1.5 to 2.5 times the control value. Partial thromboplastin time should be measured every 4 hours. If the embolus is not massive, give 5000 U of heparin IV bolus, followed by 1000 U every hour (IV) until partial thromboplastin time is 1.5 to 2.5 times control.

In addition, low-molecular-weight dextran should be given to prevent continuing thrombosis. Long-term anticoagulation should be achieved with warfarin (Coumadin).

Some institutions are considering thrombolytic therapy for pulmonary embolus. Tissue plasminogen activator (t-PA) (Activase/t-PA) has recently been approved by the Food and Drug Administration for the thrombolysis of emboli in cases of pulmonary embolus. One institution's protocol for t-PA administration for a pulmonary embolus is outlined in the box on p. 507.

Studies have shown that embolus lysis has occurred in 82% of those patients treated with t-PA (by pulmonary angiography 2 hours after infusion).[3] Streptokinase-urokinase has not proven as effective as t-PA because of its antigenic properties and because of excessive bleeding after infusion. Currently, t-PA appears to be more effective and safer than other thrombolytic agents.

Other possibilities for therapeutic intervention for pulmonary embolus are the surgical interventions of pulmonary embolectomy or inferior vena cava interruption. In order to perform pulmonary embolectomy, the cardiovascular bypass pump team must be available. This procedure is usually reserved for the patient who is in profound shock or cardiovascular collapse. Inferior vena cava interruption is used when the patient has an absolute contraindication to anticoagulation therapy. It is done to prevent recurrent pulmonary emboli. In this procedure, an inferior vena cava filter (a Kimray-Greenfield filter) is placed. This filter prevents lower-extremity emboli from reaching the lungs.

In terms of prevention, when discussing the possibility of pulmonary embolus formation with a patient or family, instruct the patient to ambulate frequently, especially when taking long trips where he or she may be sitting for a long period of time. He or she should also avoid long periods of standing to avoid venous pooling. Patients should be encouraged to ambulate early during the postoperative phase of care. If a patient must be on a regimen of bed rest, devices should be used to intermittently compress the lower extremities or a bed should be used that can change the patient's position frequently. In addition, range of motion exercises should be performed several times each day.

TISSUE PLASMINOGEN ACTIVATOR PROTOCOL FOR PULMONARY EMBOLISM

Thrombolytic therapy promotes clot dissolution, which leads to reversal of right ventricular dysfunction, dilation, and elevated pulmonary artery pressures. The simultaneous lysis of thrombi in leg veins may also occur. Thrombolytic therapy is recommended for the hemodynamically compromised patient with massive pulmonary embolus (PE) and for patients with significant cardiopulmonary disease with predisposed risk.

Patient selection

INDICATIONS AND INCLUSION CRITERIA

Yes No

— — Symptoms compatible with PE (* most common)

Dyspnea* (acute/unexplained onset)	Tachypnea*
Crackles, rales, friction rub	Cyanosis
Pleuritic pain,* chest discomfort, splinting	Cough
Anxiety, restlessness, apprehension*	Hemoptysis*
Fever	Syncope*
Gallop heart rhythm	Diaphoresis
Increased pulmonic component to S_2	Tachycardia
Clinical findings DVT/thrombophlebitis	

— — Onset of symptoms ≤ 14 days

— — History of PE does not preclude treatment

— — ≥ 18 years of age

— — Results of arterial blood gases indicate: hypoxemia, hypercapnia, hypocapnia, respiratory alkalosis

— — Electrocardiographic changes (only massive PE may show right axis deviation and/or $S_1 Q_3 T_3$ pattern, right bundle branch block, tall peaked P waves in leads II, III)

— — Chest radiograph (usually nonspecific, but findings suggestive of PE: elevated hemidiaphragm, atelectasis, localized infiltrate, plural effusions)

The above compatible clinical picture in conjunction with the following invasive and noninvasive tests:

— — Pulmonary angiography positive for: intravascular filling defect or vessel cutoff

— — Noted elevation in hemodynamic pressures (right atrium, right ventricle, PAP)

  or

— — V/Q lung scanning abnormality

— — Impedance plethysmography (IPG) deep vein obstruction (optional)

  or

— — Other imaging modalities (e.g., Doppler ultrasonography, magnetic resonance imaging)

CONTRAINDICATIONS AND EXCLUSION CRITERIA

Because thrombolytic therapy increases the risk of bleeding, Activase is contraindicated in the following situations:

  Active internal bleeding

  History of cerebrovascular accident

  Recent (within 2 months) intracranial or intraspinal surgery or trauma

  Intracranial neoplasm, arteriovenous malformation, or aneurysm

  Known bleeding diathesis

  Severe uncontrolled hypertension

* Also see *Warnings*

Preprocedure protocol and tests

1. Establish two peripheral IVs in separate arms
     Document where IVs were started
     Document any other sites where IVs were attempted or puncture sites
     Pressure dressings/Amicar to all sites
2. Lab studies
     Label all tubes
     Complete blood count with differential
     Prothrombin time, partial thromboplastin time, fibrinogen, FDP, thromboplastin time—baseline and posttreatment
     Serum electrolytes, blood urea nitrogen, creatine clearance, blood sugar
     Type and screen 2 units—red blood cells
3. Perform either a diagnostic invasive (e.g., pulmonary angiogram) or noninvasive (e.g., V/Q lung scan, IPG) procedure to confirm PE, unless not required for positive diagnosis

From Samuel Goldhaber, MD, Brigham and Women's Hospital, Boston.   *Continued.*

4. Establish baseline hemodynamic pressures: right atrial, right ventricular, PAP (if pulmonary angiogram performed) or right atrial, PAP, PCWP if preexisting central line in place
5. Establish baseline VS, H & H, PaO_2 saturation

Treatment

STANDARD SUPPORT THERAPY (ORDERS PER PHYSICIAN)

Supplemental oxygen ⎯⎯⎯⎯⎯⎯⎯⎯⎯⎯⎯⎯⎯⎯⎯⎯⎯

Hemodynamic support ⎯⎯⎯⎯⎯⎯⎯⎯⎯⎯⎯⎯⎯⎯⎯⎯

⎯⎯⎯⎯⎯⎯⎯⎯⎯⎯⎯⎯⎯⎯

Pain medication ⎯⎯⎯⎯⎯⎯⎯⎯⎯⎯⎯⎯⎯⎯⎯⎯⎯⎯

Other medication ⎯⎯⎯⎯⎯⎯⎯⎯⎯⎯⎯⎯⎯⎯⎯⎯⎯

ACTIVASE DOSAGE AND ADMINISTRATION FOR PE

Reconstitution: Tissue plasminogen activator (t-PA) is available in both 20 mg and 50 mg vials. Each vial is packaged with 20 ml or 50 ml sterile water for injection to be used as diluent for reconstitution. (Only use nonbacteriostatic sterile water for injection, United States Pharmacopeia, without preservatives. Bacteriostatic water should not be used.) Activase may be administered as reconstituted at 1.0 mg/ml, or as an alternative, the reconstituted solution may be diluted further in 5% dextrose or 0.9 NS solution (up to a 1:2 dilution). After reconstitution, reconstituted tissue plasminogen activator (rt-PA) is stable for 8 hours.

DOSAGE REGIMEN

100 mg IV/2-hour controlled infusion

50 mg IV/hr over 1st hour ⎯⎯⎯⎯⎯⎯⎯

50 mg IV/hr over 2nd hour ⎯⎯⎯⎯⎯⎯⎯

ADMINISTRATION

1. Purge IV line with mixed drug.
2. Administer as controlled infusion.
3. To ensure completion of second hour dose, add 20 to 30 ml flush to empty IV bag when pump alarms.
4. Do not admix any other medications to t-PA line.

ANTICOAGULATION

Heparin therapy is not instituted until after the completion of t-PA therapy (or if infusing, discontinue before therapy)

DOSE

1. Based on maintaining partial thromboplastin time or thromboplastin time 1½-2½ times control
2. Given without a bolus dose
3. Continuous infusion of 1000 U/hr or 15 U/kg/hr or as prescribed by physician

Monitor and follow up

Repeat baseline lab tests per institution protocol (aprotinin should be used to prevent in vitro degradation of fibrinogen in blood samples drawn during or immediately after therapy)

Repeat hemodynamic parameters to assess for change/improvement

Monitor/assess for changes in baseline signs and symptoms

Monitor for signs of bleeding complications

Repeat pulmonary angiogram or V/Q lung scan on completion of therapy and/or before patient discharge for final clinical evaluation (If no improvement, consider surgical options available, i.e., embolectomy, inferior vena cava interruption or filter)

WARNINGS

The presence of any of the following conditions does not rule out use of Activase, but the risks of therapy may be increased and should be weighed against the anticipated benefits.

Recent (within 10 days) major surgery (e.g., thoracic, coronary artery bypass graft, obstetrical delivery, organ biopsy, previous puncture of noncompressible vessels)

Cerebrovascular disease

Recent gastrointestinal or genitourinary bleeding (within 10 days)

Recent trauma (within 10 days)/nontraumatic CPR

Hypertension: systolic blood pressure $\geq$ 180 mm Hg and/or diastolic blood pressure $\geq$ 110 mm Hg

High likelihood of left heart thrombus (e.g., mitral stenosis with atrial fibrillation)

Acute pericarditis

Subacute bacterial endocarditis

Hemostatic defects including those secondary to severe hepatic or renal disease

Significant liver dysfunction

Pregnancy

Diabetic hemorrhagic retinophathy or other hemorrhagic ophthalmic conditions

Septic thrombophlebitis or occluded arteriovenous cannula at seriously infected site

Advanced age (i.e., over 75 years old)

Patients currently receiving oral anticoagulants (e.g., warfarin sodium)

Any other condition in which bleeding constitutes a significant hazard or would be particularly difficult to manage

Pneumothorax (Spontaneous)

A spontaneous pneumothorax is usually caused by the rupture of a pulmonary bleb. These blebs are found in the younger population, from ages 16 to 26 years, as congenital anomalies. They are seen in the older population as the result of COPD. Some other causes of spontaneous pneumothorax may be the use of mechanical ventilation, the rupture of a cyst or abscess, fungal disease, cancer, or tuberculosis. Spontaneous pneumothorax can also result from trauma, chest compressions (in CPR), tracheostomy, or subclavian line placement.

Signs and symptoms may be minimal if the pneumothorax is small. If it is greater than 40%, the patient is dyspneic, tachypneic, and cyanotic and has sudden onset of pleuritic chest pain. Breath sounds are decreased, and the patient usually appears agitated.

If the simple pneumothorax develops into a tension pneumothorax, a decreased motion of the chest wall, a deviated trachea, distended jugular veins, a mediastinal shift, tympany on percussion, and eventually, shock are evident.

The goal of therapeutic intervention for spontaneous pneumothorax is to reexpand the collapsed portion of the lung. To do this, you must administer oxygen at high-liter flow, initiate an IV line of D_5W, place the patient in a high Fowler's position, and either insert a needle through the anterior chest wall or place a chest tube in the second intercostal space in the anterior plane, midclavicular line, or the fifth intercostal space in the midaxillary line. (For more information on pneumothorax, see Chapter 25.)

Pleurisy

Pleurisy is an inflammation of the lining of the chest cavity. It results from tuberculosis, pneumonia, trauma, or tumors. Dry pleurisy (fibrinous) manifests as sharp chest pain that increases with inspiration; the patient takes short, quick breaths and sometimes lies on his or her affected side. Therapeutic intervention includes bed rest, analgesia, sedation, and oxygen administration.

Exudative pleurisy with effusion usually results from an infectious process. The patient has dyspnea, an elevated temperature, and a history of dry pleurisy. Therapeutic intervention includes bed rest, analgesia, a thoracentesis to remove fluid, antipyretics, and oxygen at moderate flow rates.

Pneumonia

Pneumonia results from an acute bacterial, viral, or fungal infection. It may be preceded by an upper respiratory tract infection, an ear infection, or an eye infection, or it may occur as the primary illness, without other medical precipitating causes. Pneumonia occurs primarily in younger children, elderly persons, and those who are debilitated.

Pneumonia may be classified according to the causative organism (pneumoccocal or streptococcal) or according to location (bronchial or lobar). Persons who have pneumonia often have been bedridden or have rib fractures, or an underlying cardiac or pulmonary disorder. Other causes include smoking, diabetes mellitus, exposure to extreme changes in environmental temperatures, steroids, or immunosuppressive therapy. Pneumonia is often seen in persons who abuse alcohol or drugs, and thus have a tendency to aspirate. It is also seen in other cases in which the victim has aspirated, such as postarrest/CPR situations.

A patient with pneumonia has an elevated temperature of 39.4° C to 40° C. He or she is diaphoretic and may complain of chest pain that may be referred diaphragmatically and mistaken for a gastrointestinal disorder. He or she may have a productive cough and may be tachypneic, tachycardic, cyanotic, and apprehensive. He or she may also complain of abdominal distension, vomiting, and headache.

The aim of therapeutic intervention is to relieve respiratory distress and control infection. This can be accomplished by administering humidified oxygen and antibiotics, controlling fluid and electrolyte balance, and encouraging the patient to cough, turn, and breathe deeply frequently.

Occasionally pneumonia is complicated by rupture of a pneumatocele, which produces a pneumothorax or an empyema. Therapeutic intervention for both is placement of a chest tube.

Adult Respiratory Distress Syndrome

Adult respiratory distress syndrome, also known as ARDS, shock lung, pulmonary contusion, Da Nang lung, congestive atelectasis, wet lung, and posttraumatic lung, is pulmonary congestion that occurs suddenly and causes atelectasis and hyaline membrane formation because of a decrease in surfactant and the build-up of mucus along the alveoli. It is acute and progressive respiratory failure that may be caused by a variety of conditions such as a cardiopulmonary bypass, infection, pulmonary edema, and inhaled toxins. ARDS may also be caused by hemorrhagic shock and multiple transfusions, contusions of the lung itself, fat emboli, aspiration, overdose, or eclampsia. It is also seen frequently in conjunction with disseminated intravascular coagulation.

The lungs initially appear normal, and then there is progressive atelectasis, increased interstitial and alveolar edema, and a marked ventilation-perfusion abnormality that results in progressive hypoxemia and difficulty breathing as lung compliance decreases.

Signs and symptoms of ARDS include dyspnea and tachypnea, cyanosis, hypoxemia, hypocapnia, pulmonary hemorrhage, and hypotension.

Therapeutic intervention includes maintenance of the ABCs, endotracheal intubation or tracheostomy, ventilation with a volume-cycled ventilator with positive end-expiratory pressure (PEEP) at 5 to 15 cm water pressure, administration of diuretics and salt-poor albumin, fluid restriction, and possibly administration of steroids and/or anticoagulants.

You must also pay strict attention to providing meticulous pulmonary toilet.

PEEP prevents alveoli collapse, increases functional residual capacity, improves the ventilation-quotient relationship, combats pulmonary edema, and enhances forced inspiratory oxygen (FIO_2). PEEP is dangerous to use, however, because it increases the chance of oxygen toxicity and fluid overload, and it decreases cardiac output. It may cause a pneumothorax and infection. If you have chosen to use PEEP and it has not proved effective, you may use hyperbaric oxygen. Some practitioners choose to employ the bypass oxygenator.

Near-Drowning

Each year in the United States more than 6500 deaths result from drowning.[1] Over half of these occur in home swimming pools. Worldwide statistics indicate that over 140,000 drowning deaths occur each year. Drowning is the second leading cause of accidental death in the United States and the second leading cause of death in children and adolescents. It accounts for 10% of all accidental deaths, and 47% of these are children under the age of 4. The highest incidence of drowning occurs in adolescents who are 15 to 19 years old, an age at which alcohol use and risk-taking are prevalent behaviors. It is interesting to note that the incidence of drowning deaths is 5 times higher in males than in females.

Near-drowning or drowning may result when a person cannot stay afloat because of fatigue, panic, or an acute medical emergency such as myocardial infarction, seizures, or trauma. It may also result from hyperventilation before a long underwater swim, or it may be an attempted or successful suicide.

When near-drowning occurs, voluntary breathholding occurs for a short time, followed by an involuntary gasp, when water is aspirated into the hypopharynx. Signs and symptoms include progressive dyspnea, auscultatory wheezes, rales and rhonchi, tachycardia, cyanosis, and a cough that produces a pink, frothy sputum. The victim may eventually have a fever but may initially be hypothermic because of cold water temperatures. The patient who comes into the ED may complain of chest pain and demonstrate mental confusion. He or she may have seizures and increased muscle tone. The patient may lapse into a coma or have cardiopulmonary arrest.

Therapeutic intervention for the near-drowning victim includes maintenance of the ABCs. If indicated, use advanced cardiac life support measures. Be sure to protect the cervical spine, since cervical-spine trauma may be the cause of the near-drowning incident. Initiate an IV line and carefully administer fluids on the basis of hemodynamic status at usually one third of the normal maintenance rate. Oxygen should be administered under positive pressure. The patient should be endotracheally intubated if PAO_2 is below 60 mm Hg with an FIO_2 greater than 0.50, if he or she has acute pulmonary edema or acute respiratory distress, or if his or her level of consciousness decreases. If the patient is intubated and mechanically ventilated, be sure to add PEEP to the ventilatory cycle. Suction the airway frequently. Correct any acid-base imbalance in accordance with arterial blood gas values. Administer antibiotics, steroids, and isoproterenol (Isuprel) for bronchospasm. It would be wise at this point in therapeutic intervention to place a gastric tube and a central venous pressure line or a balloon-tipped thermodilution catheter. This patient should be admitted to the intensive care unit for close observation and monitoring for at least 24 hours. Refer to Fig. 37-1, *A* to *D* for an algorithm on therapy for patients without respiratory distress, with respiratory distress, with an altered level of consciousness, and with hypoxemia. Hyperventilate the patient to a PCO_2 of 30 mm Hg. Consider barbiturate coma, muscle paralysis, and intracranial pressure monitoring.

Near-drowning and drowning may be categorized into three types: *dry, wet,* and *secondary. Dry drowning* occurs in 10% to 20% of cases. The victim asphyxiates because he or she cannot inspire oxygen as a result of laryngotracheal spasm, which prevents the entrance of water as well as oxygen into the lungs. This results in cerebral anoxia, edema, and unconsciousness. The victim of dry drowning has the best chance of surviving.

The second type, *wet drowning,* occurs in 80% to 90% of cases. This victim usually makes a violent respiratory effort and consequently fills his or her lungs with water.

The third type of drowning is *secondary drowning,* which occurs with the recurrence of respiratory distress after a successful resuscitation and recovery from the initial incident. This may occur when pulmonary edema or aspiration pneumonia happens. It may happen at any time from minutes to days after the initial incident. Pulmonary edema that occurs as a result of a near-drowning incident may be caused by either fresh or salt-water aspiration. Salt water is a hypertonic solution that causes fluid to traverse the alveolar-capillary cellular membrane, which results in pulmonary edema. This type of near-drowning also causes hemoconcentration and hypovolemia.

Fresh water is a hypotonic solution. Fluid rapidly traverses out of the alveoli by diffusion. Fresh water contains contaminants such as chlorine, algae, and mud, which cause surfactant breakdown and fluid seepage into the alveoli, also resulting in pulmonary edema. This type of near-drowning causes hemodilution and hypervolemia and its consequences. Pulmonary edema in both salt-water and fresh water near-drownings is complicated by the inflammatory response of the body.

In all types of near-drowning incidents, pay close attention to electrolyte abnormalities and correct them as they occur (Table 37-2). Also, be sure to serially record a Glasgow coma score. Modell[5] states that, if a patient is awake, there will be a 100% neurological recovery. If consciousness is blunted there is a 90% to 100% chance of recovery. If

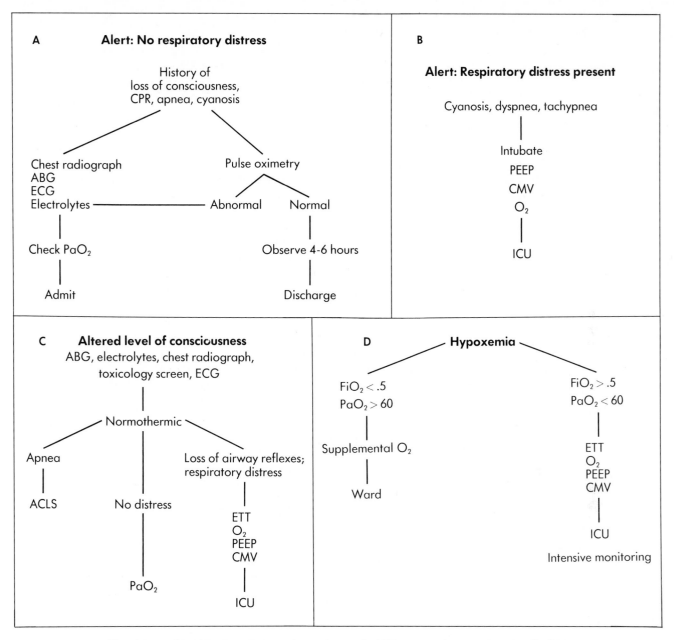

Fig. 37-1 Algorithm on therapy for patients. **A,** Without respiratory distress. **B,** With respiratory distress. **C,** With an altered level of consciousness. **D,** With hypoxemia. (From Stephen Ludwig, MD, Medical College of Pennsylvania. Modified.)

the patient is comatose, a 19% to 55% chance of recovery can be expected on the basis of the level of coma, with nonpurposeful movement having 55%, abnormal flexion having 50%, abnormal extension 57%, and flaccidity 19%.

MEASUREMENT AND MONITORING
Drawing Blood for Blood Gas Measurement

Selection of site
Choose the radial, brachial, or femoral artery (Figs. 37-2 to 37-4).

Avoid limbs that demonstrate poor circulation.

Avoid limbs in which hematomas are present.

If the radial artery is selected, check for the presence of a positive Allen test.

Allen test. To assess for Allen's sign, palpate both the radial and ulnar pulses. Occlude both arteries with firm pressure and raise the arm to balance the hand. Release the ulnar artery and assess for return of color to the hand. If the hand *does not perfuse* (negative Allen's sign), this in-

Table 37-2 Significant differences between salt and fresh water aspiration

Salt water	Fresh water
HYPOXIA	
Greater degree of hypoxia; fluid in alveoli interferes with ventilation	Alteration of normal surface tension properties of surfactant with subsequent collapse of the alveoli; atelectasis; uneven ventilation and recurrent collapse continue until surface active material regenerates
BLOOD VOLUME	
Hypertonic fluid draws water into the alveolar spaces, causing a persistent hypovolemia; increase in blood osmolarity and viscosity	Hypotonic water rapidly absorbed into the circulation; transient hypervolemia; decrease in blood osmolarity and viscosity; elevated CVP
SERUM ELECTROLYTES	
Changes usually insignificant; hyperkalemia may result from severe hypoxia and acidosis; picture may be complicated by ingestion of large amounts of salt water	
HEMOGLOBIN	
Hemolysis occurs after aspiration of at least 11 ml of fluid/kg body weight, with a possible decrease in hemoglobin	
HEMATOCRIT	
Technical problems make correct measurements almost impossible and interpretation difficult	
CARDIAC CHANGES	
Sufficient water to cause ventricular fibrillation is seldom aspirated	
CENTRAL VENOUS PRESSURE	
An increase in CVP coincides with hyperventilation; falls rapidly to normal when only small amounts of liquid have been aspirated	
Aspiration of large amounts of fluid results in initial rise in CVP, followed by a rapid drop to zero	Aspiration of large quantities of fluid results in a persistent rise in CVP
NEUROLOGIC EFFECTS	
When salt water is ingested in large quantities, the magnesium ion may cause lethargy, drowsiness, and coma	
URINARY SYSTEM	
Acute renal failure caused by tubular necrosis, resulting from hypoxia and hypotension	Acute renal failure caused by hemolysis and hypotension

From Warner CG ed: *Emergency care: assessment and intervention*, ed 3, St Louis, 1983, Mosby–Year Book.

dicates that the ulnar artery is not capable of maintaining circulation to the hand. Therefore do not attempt a radial artery puncture in the extremity (see Fig. 14-15).

Suggested equipment

Container of crushed ice (plastic bag or emesis basin is inadequate)
Rubber or cork stopper or commercial blood gas cap
5 ml *glass* syringe or specially treated plastic syringe
Two 22-gauge 1.5-inch needles
Two alcohol swabs
Sodium heparin, 0.5 ml (1000 U/ml)
One small, dry, gauze pad
Gummed label for syringe

Laboratory requisition slip with the following information: concentration of oxygen patient is receiving and by what route (FIO_2) and patient's rectal temperature at the time the specimen is collected (both parameters affect calculation of values)

Drawing the specimen

1. Explain the procedure to the patient.
2. Draw up 0.5 ml heparin into the syringe; flush the syringe with heparin (expel all air bubbles).
3. Use a commercially prepared blood gas syringe.
4. Wear gloves.
5. Replace the needle.

Fig. 37-2 Brachial artery and continuation of axillary artery. Advantages: radial and medial nerves in proximity and venous system in proximity, making venous sampling possible.

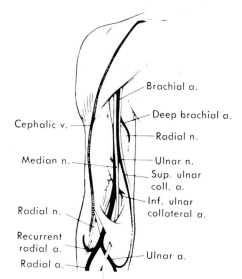

Fig. 37-3 **A,** Radial artery extends from neck of radius to median side of styloid process. Advantage: not close to nerves or veins; thus venous sampling is unlikely. Disadvantage: puncture may produce spasm; artery is small. **B,** Anatomic location of radial artery.

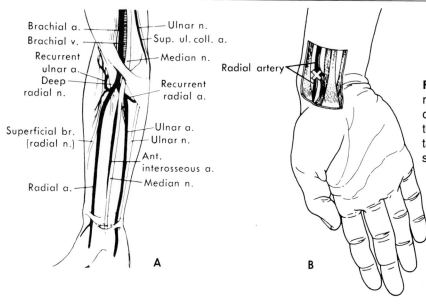

Fig. 37-4 Femoral artery branches from abdominal aorta and branches to superficial epigastric, superficial circumflex iliac, external pudendal, deep femoral, and descending genicular arteries. Advantage: easily accessible. Disadvantage: may have large amount of interstitial bleeding before it is noticed. Proximity to vein makes venous sampling possible.

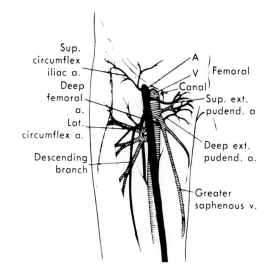

6. Select the puncture site.
7. Straighten the limb of the selected puncture site; position on a firm surface.
8. Palpate the artery: assess the pulse and position of the artery.
9. Cleanse area over the puncture site with an alcohol swab. (Be sure to use plenty of friction and allow alcohol to dry before actual puncture.)
10. Immobilize the artery between two fingers. (Be careful not to contaminate the puncture site.)
11. Penetrate both the skin and the artery at a 45- to 90-degree angle, holding the syringe like a pencil (Fig. 37-6).
12. If the syringe begins to fill and the plunger begins to move spontaneously, this usually indicates that the needle is in the artery.
13. If the syringe does not begin to fill spontaneously, withdraw the needle slightly—you may have gone all the way through the artery.
14. If systolic blood pressure is less than 100 mm Hg, the syringe may not fill spontaneously and it may be necessary to manually withdraw the plunger (e.g., during CPR).
15. If the blood sample is not bright red or bluish, it may indicate that the specimen is venous, and another attempt at an arterial specimen should be made.
16. Obtain 3 to 5 ml of arterial blood sample. (Some laboratories will accept less for analysis.)
17. Withdraw the needle quickly.
18. Apply direct pressure with dry gauze.
19. Maintain pressure for 5 minutes. (Make certain to time it on your watch or the wall clock: it is difficult to estimate 5 minutes.)

Care of specimen
1. Expel all air bubbles from the sample.
2. Stick the needle into a cork or rubber stopper, using one hand, without holding the stopper, or remove the needle and cap the syringe, taking precautions to prevent contaminating yourself with blood.
3. Place the gummed label containing patient's name and hospital number on the syringe.
4. Place the syringe in the container of ice.
5. Send to laboratory immediately along with completed laboratory request form. (If you have a small laboratory, it frequently will help if you call the laboratory before obtaining the arterial specimen so that the blood gas analyzer can be calibrated before the arrival of the specimen.)

Aftercare
Ensure that pressure is maintained over the puncture site for at least 5 minutes. (Sandbags will not do—use fingers.)

Do not use dressings or Band-Aids that interfere with visualization of the puncture site. Patients with blood dyscrasias or those who are anticoagulated may require a longer period of pressure to ensure that bleeding has ceased.

Observe the puncture site for at least 1 minute after manual pressure has ceased for formation of a hematoma.

Reassess pulse.

Interpretation of arterial blood gas values (Fig. 37-7)

Notice the pH value: 7.35 to 7.45 = normal; above 7.45 = alkalosis; below 7.35 = acidosis.

Note the bicarbonate level: 22 to 26 mEq = normal; above 26 mEq = metabolic alkalosis; below 22 mEq = metabolic acidosis.

Notice the Pco_2 value: 35 to 40 mm Hg = normal; above 45 mm Hg = respiratory acidosis; below 35 mm Hg = respiratory alkalosis.

Make an acid/base "diagnosis" on the basis of these criteria. Consider the effect on blood gas values of compensatory mechanisms. Although the values are abnormal, they may not all fit the criteria. The variance is caused by the compensatory action; see the following examples:
1. Acid. Hydrogen ion donor; carbonic acid (H_2CO_3) is an acid.
2. Base. Hydrogen ion acceptor; bicarbonate (HCO_3) is a base.
3. Acidosis. Increased acid concentration and/or decreased base concentration; a pH of less than 7.4 is considered acidosis; a pH less than 7.3 is considered within the danger range; severe acidosis is a central nervous system depressant; *signs and symptoms:* judgment errors, lethargy, disorientation.
4. Alkalosis. Increased base concentration and/or decreased acid concentration; a pH greater than 7.4 is considered alkalosis; a pH greater than 7.6 is considered within the danger range; severe alkalosis is a

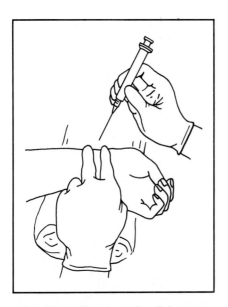

Fig. 37-5 Puncture of radial artery.

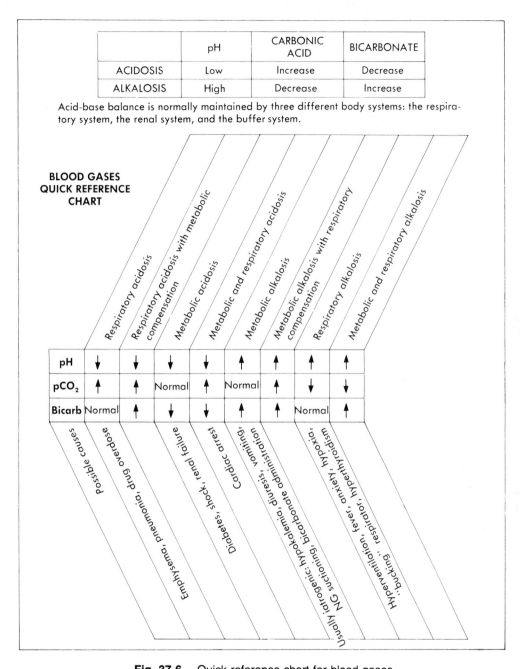

	pH	CARBONIC ACID	BICARBONATE
ACIDOSIS	Low	Increase	Decrease
ALKALOSIS	High	Decrease	Increase

Acid-base balance is normally maintained by three different body systems: the respiratory system, the renal system, and the buffer system.

Fig. 37-6   Quick reference chart for blood gases.

central nervous system excitant; *signs and symptoms:* tingling of fingers, muscle spasms, seizures.

5. pH. Hydrogen ion concentration of a solution; the relationship of carbonic acid (H_2CO_3) and bicarbonate (HCO_3) determines the pH of human serum; acid/base balance is a function of the ration of carbonic acid (H_2CO_3) to bicarbonate (HCO_3).

SUMMARY

Patients with pulmonary emergencies may arrive at the ED with conditions that are life threatening. Accurate as-

sessment and prompt interventions may reverse an otherwise disastrous situation.

REFERENCES

1. Centers for Disease Control: Drowning in the United States: 1978-1984, *MMWR* 37:27, 1988.
2. Cherniak RM: Comprehensive approach to asthma, *Chest* 87:54, 1985.
3. Goldhaber SZ et al: *t-PA protocol for pulmonary embolism,* Boston, 1987, Brigham and Women's Hospital.
4. Gotz VP, Brandsetter RD, Marr DD: Bronchodilatory effect of subcutaneous epinephrine in acute asthma, *Ann Emerg Med* 10:518, 1981.

5. Modell JH, Graves SA, Kuck EJ: Near-drowning: correlation of level of consciousness and survival, *Can Anesth Soc J* 27:211, 1980.
6. Summer WR: Status asthmaticus, *Chest* 87:87, 1985.

SUGGESTED READINGS

Allman FD et al: Outcome following cardiopulmonary resuscitation in severe pediatric near-drowning, *Am J Dis Child* 140:571, 1986.

Arabian AA: Embolic pulmonary disease. In Spagnolo SV, Medinger A, eds: *Handbook of pulmonary emergencies,* New York, London, 1986, Plenum.

Bell TS, Ellenberg L, McComb JG: Neuropsychological outcome after severe pediatric near-drowning. *Neurosurgery* 17:604, 1985.

Bohn DJ et al: Influence of hypothermia, barbiturate therapy and intracranial pressure monitoring on morbidity and mortality after near-drowning, *Crit Care Med* 14:529, 1986.

Bordow RA, Moser KM, eds: *Manual of clinical problems in pulmonary medicine*, Philadelphia, 1985, Little, Brown.

Conn AW, Barker GA: Fresh water drowning and near-drowning — an update. *Can Anesth Soc J* 31:538, 1984.

Gonzales-Rothi RJ: Near-drowning: consensus and controversies in pulmonary and cerebral resuscitation, *Heart Lung* 16:474, 1987.

Orlowski JP: Drowning, near-drowning and ice water submersions, *Pediatr Clin North Am* 34:75, 1987.

Pearn J: The management of near-drowning, *Br Med J* 291:1447, 1985.

Thompson BT et al: Pulmonary emergencies. In Wilkins EW Jr, ed: *Emergency medicine: scientific foundations and current practice*, Baltimore, 1989, Williams & Wilkins.

Williams SM: The pulmonary system. In Alspach JG et al, eds: *Core curriculum for critical care nursing*, Philadelphia, 1985, WB Saunders.

CHAPTER 38

Abdominal and Genitourinary Emergencies

Susan Budassi Sheehy

Abdominal pain is one of the most commonly heard chief complaints in the emergency care setting. The pain may be caused by an acute event or from a chronic process. There are three types of abdominal pain: visceral, somatic, and referred.

Visceral pain may be caused by the stretching of hollow viscus. The patient describes the pain as cramping or "like gas." This type of pain intensifies, then decreases, and is usually centered on the umbilicus or lower in the midline. The pain is difficult to localize during examination because the pain is diffuse. The patient probably is also diaphoretic and has nausea and vomiting. He or she may also have hypotension, tachycardia, and abdominal wall spasms. Many conditions have as a symptom a visceral type of pain. Among them are acute appendicitis, pancreatitis, cholecystitis, and intestinal obstruction.

A bacterial or chemical irritation of the nerve fibers produces somatic pain. The pain is sharp and can usually be localized to a specific area. A patient with this type of pain usually lies with the legs flexed and the knees pulled into the chest to prevent any stimulation to the peritoneal area, which may cause an increase of the pain. This patient also demonstrates involuntary guarding and rebound tenderness.

Referred pain occurs at a distance from the original source of the pain. This type of pain is thought to be caused by the development of nerve tracts during fetal growth and development. Biliary pain is referred to the subscapular area. For example, renal colic is usually referred to the genitalia and flank area; problems involving the uterus and rectum often refer pain to the low back; a peptic ulcer may cause back pain.

When assessing the patient with a chief complaint of pain, it is important to remember that each person reacts differently to pain. Elderly individuals do not seem to react as much to pain as do younger people. Also, men have a tendency to hide their pain because the expression of pain is not considered masculine in many cultures. The patient's ethnic background may also play a large part in how the patient reacts to pain. However pain is described, remember that it is a symptom and not a diagnosis. The object of care

is to identify the cause, treat the cause, and eliminate the pain.

When assessing a patient whose chief complaint is pain, one should consider whether the patient requires hospitalization, what the cause is, and whether the patient requires surgery.

Of key importance to understanding issues related to the chief complaint of abdominal pain is a thorough understanding of the peritoneal cavity. The peritoneum is a serosal membrane that covers the liver, spleen, stomach, and intestines. It provides a semipermeable membrane, perceives acute pain, and provides proliferative cellular protection. Technically, all abdominal organs are behind the peritoneum and thus are retroperitoneal, but the liver, spleen, stomach, and intestines are suspended into the peritoneum and are functionally considered intraperitoneal organs.

The peritoneum is permeable to fluid, electrolytes, urea, and toxins. It contains somatic afferent nerves, which make it extremely sensitive to all types of stimuli. In acute abdominal conditions the peritoneum helps us to localize an irritable focus by producing sharp pain and tenderness; it also produces voluntary and involuntary abdominal muscle rigidity and rebound tenderness.

ASSESSMENT OF THE PATIENT WITH ABDOMINAL PAIN

When assessing someone with a chief complaint of abdominal pain, one should be systematic about the approach. A good history and information about the pain are important. The use of the following mnemonic, *PQRST*, is helpful:

P (*provocation*)
What makes the pain better? Worse? Position? Vomiting?
Q (*quality or character*)
What does the pain feel like? Is it burning? Tight? Crushing? Tearing? Pressure? Crampy?
R (*radiation, location, referral*)
Where does the pain radiate? Where is it most intense? Where does it start? The appendix, gallbladder, stomach, and duodenum usually are point specific for pain. When localized pain becomes generalized, rupture may have occurred.

517

DIFFERENTIAL DIAGNOSIS BASED ON LOCATION OF PAIN IN THE QUADRANTS OF THE ABDOMEN

Right upper quadrant
Cholecystitis
Hepatic abcess
Hepatitis
Hepatomegaly
Pancreatic
Duodenal ulcer perforation

Left upper quadrant
Pancreatitis
Splenic rupture
Myocardial infarction
Gastritis
Left renal pain
Left lung pneumonia
Right renal pain
Myocardial infarction
Pericarditis
Right lung pneumonia

Right lower quadrant
Appendicitis
Cholecystitis
Perforated ulcer
Intestinal obstruction
Meckel's diverticulum
Abdominal aortic dissection or rupture
Ruptured ectopic pregnancy
Twisted right ovary
Ovarian cyst
Pelvic inflammatory disease
Endometriosis
Right ureteral calculi
Incarcerated hernia
Gastric ulcer perforation
Aortic aneurysm dissection or rupture
Colon perforation

Left lower quadrant
Appendicitis
Intestinal obstruction
Diverticulum of the sigmoid colon
Ruptured ectopic pregnancy
Twisted left ovary
Ovarian cyst
Pelvic inflammatory disease
Endometriosis
Left ureteral calculi
Left renal pain
Incarcerated hernia
Perforated descending colon
Regional enteritis

S (*severity*)
How severe is the pain, on a scale of 1 to 10?
T (*time*)
When did the pain start? When did it end? How long did it last? Severe abdominal pain that lasts more than 6 hours *usually* requires surgical intervention.

Ask about any associated symptoms, such as nausea, vomiting, diarrhea, fever, or chills.

Carefully inspect the abdomen, then *gently* palpate the abdomen for the presence of pain, tenderness, spasm, or masses. Ask the patient to cough (to rule out rebound tenderness). Auscultate bowel sounds. To determine that bowel sounds are absent, one must auscultate for a full 5 minutes. Ask the patient whether he or she has any signs or symptoms other than pain. Does the patient appear sick? Note the facial expressions and the body position.

Pain that begins suddenly and is associated with colic usually indicates a visceral obstruction (partial or complete) or a vascular obstruction. If perforation occurs, pain is usually acute and severe, and does not vary in intensity; this type of pain occurs in conditions such as a rupture, torsion, strangulation, or vascular occlusion.

Pain that is gradual in onset is usually caused by an inflammatory process. As a general rule, the more acute the pain, the more acute the problem. Remember that if a large amount of blood volume has been lost, the patient will most likely have an altered level of consciousness and may not be able to express that pain is present.

When assessing a patient with pain, pay particular attention to a description of the location of pain, because this may offer some useful information for diagnosis. Differential diagnosis based on the location of pain in the four quadrants of the abdomen is listed in the box at left. Ask the patient where the original pain occurred because the pain may now be diffuse. Sometimes the location of the pain can be directly correlated with its cause. For example, stomach problems are almost always associated with epigastric pain. Gallbladder pain is almost always in the right upper quadrant of the abdomen, and pain from the appendix is almost always in the right lower quadrant.

In certain conditions, including the following, referred pain may be the clue to diagnosis:

Problem area	Location of referred pain
Fluid collection under diaphragm	Top of shoulder
Ruptured peptic ulcer	Back
Pancreas	Midline back or directly through to back
Biliary tract	Around right side to scapula
Dissecting ruptured aortic aneurysm	Chest through to back (thoracic) or low back and thighs (abdominal)
Renal colic	Groin and external genitalia
Appendix	May be epigastric region
Uterine disease	Low back
Rectal disease	Low back

The following description of pain may also offer a clue to the diagnosis:

Severe sharp pain	Infarction or rupture
Severe pain controlled by medication	Pancreatitis, peritonitis, small-bowel obstruction, renal colic, biliary colic
Dull pain	Inflammation, low-grade infection
Intermittent pain	Gastroenteritis, small-bowel obstruction

Signs and Symptoms Associated with Abdominal Pain

Nausea, vomiting, or anorexia. Sometimes the chief complaint of nausea, vomiting, or anorexia may offer clues to the cause of the abdominal pain. If the most prominent signs and symptoms are nausea and vomiting, the most likely causes are acute gastritis, gastroenteritis, pancreatitis, or a high intestinal obstruction. Intractable vomiting or feces in emesis usually indicates an intestinal obstruction. Blood in emesis suggests gastritis or upper gastrointestinal (GI) bleeding. In appendicitis pain usually precedes vomiting.

Diarrhea, constipation, and stool color. Diarrhea and constipation also offer clues to the cause of abdominal pain. Diarrhea usually indicates an inflammatory process. Constipation or a lack of flatus expulsion indicates dehydration, a paralyzed ileus, or an intestinal obstruction. Stools that are clay colored indicate a biliary tract obstruction. Black tarry stools indicate lower intestinal bleeding. Bloody diarrhea suggests amebic dysentery, Crohn's disease, or ulcerative colitis.

Chills and fever. Chills and fever indicate that bacterial infection, pyelonephritis, or appendicitis may be present, especially if the fever and chills are repeated. Intermittent fever and chills may indicate acute cholecystitis.

Urinary tract symptoms. A burning sensation during urination may indicate a urinary tract infection. If there is pain during urination, an obstruction may be somewhere along the urinary tract. Hematuria or dysuria may be indicative of a urinary tract infection or renal colic.

Gynecologic symptoms. If signs and symptoms are gynecologic, the origin of the problem is usually gynecologic. The pain may indicate a ruptured corpus luteum or ovarian cyst, a ruptured ectopic pregnancy, or pelvic inflammatory disease, among other conditions. Vaginal bleeding may suggest any of a number of gynecologic disorders (see Chapter 45).

Gastrointestinal upset. Gastroenteritis, or gastrointestinal (GI) upset, is suggested when a person has abdominal pain after eating a meal, especially if several other people have eaten the same meal and the patient is the only one who has the discomfort. Pain followed by the ingestion of fatty foods indicates cholecystitis. Pancreatitis is common in persons with a history of alcohol abuse. If the pain begins just before mealtime and is relieved by eating, it is probably caused by a gastric ulcer or other gastric disorder.

Age. Sometimes the age of the patient offers a clue to the cause of the pain. For example, intussusception is rarely seen in patients older than 2 years of age and intestinal obstruction is usually seen in patients more than 40 years of age.

Physical Examination and Laboratory Tests

Often a patient's physical appearance offers a clue to the diagnosis. Note the position in which the patient is lying and the expression on his or her face. Note skin color, temperature, and moisture. If the condition is acute, the temperature may be normal for a while and then elevate as a response to the process. If an accurate temperature is desirable, take the temperature rectally. Temperature may be elevated if there has been rupture or peritonitis. Usually when patients are in pain, they have tachycardia; occasionally, however, one sees a reflux bradycardia.

Rapid and shallow respirations indicate shock, pancreatitis, or peritonitis. Inflammations cause the patient to allow minimal movement of the abdominal wall consciously.

Hypotensive blood pressure may indicate shock, rupture, or another acute condition that requires surgery.

Inspection. Pay close attention to the patient's abdominal wall. Note whether there is much movement. The finding of very little movement suggests peritonitis. If the patient is in a position with the hips flexed and knees drawn up, acute appendicitis, pelvic abscess, or a psoas abscess are likely diagnoses. If there is peristaltic movement, one should suspect intestinal obstruction. If ascites is present, be suspicious of hepatic involvement. If there is a palpable and visible abdominal mass, suspect an abdominal aneurysm.

Palpation. When palpating the abdomen, be as gentle as possible. Be alert to spasms, tenderness, and masses. While palpating, pay attention to the patient's facial expressions, because they may give clues to the severity and increasing intensity of the pain.

Percussion. Percussion is a difficult art to learn. Even the most astute diagnostician often has difficulty interpreting percussive findings. One useful percussive finding, however, is tympany. Tympany is a sign that some sort of gas is present; some conditions with this sign are appendicitis and sigmoid obstruction. Ascites sounds like shifting dullness where it normally should not be. Ascites can be suggestive of a tumor, congestive heart failure, or free blood in the peritoneal cavity. Dullness over the suprapubic area indicates urinary retention.

Auscultation. Bowel sounds are often a problem in the emergency setting because it takes a full 5 minutes of auscultation without hearing sounds before one can state that bowel sounds are absent—and often in the ED one is not afforded this amount of time. In the normal bowel 10 to 20 peristaltic sounds occur per minute.

Laboratory Tests and Radiographic Examinations

The following laboratory tests should be performed on the patient with abdominal pain:
1. Electrolyte level
2. Serum amylase level

3. Urinalysis
4. Urine amylase level
5. Complete blood cell count (include hematocrit and hemoglobin level)
6. Blood urea nitrogen (BUN) level

The following radiographic studies should be taken:

1. Upright chest film
2. Upright abdominal film
3. Left lateral decubitus film
4. Plain abdominal film
5. IV pyelogram if indicated
6. IV cholangiogram if indicated
7. Upper GI series if indicated
8. Lower GI series if indicated

Consider the following:

1. Abdominal ultrasound
2. Abdominal CT scan

Conditions requiring that surgery be considered include the following:

Appendicitis	Cholecystitis
Bowel obstruction or infarction	Pancreatitis
	Salpingitis
Ruptured ectopic pregnancy	Perforation of viscus
	Ruptured intraabdominal aneurysm
Ureteral stone	Massive GI bleeding
Peritonitis	
Diverticulitis	

Chronic conditions that may have abdominal pain as a symptom include the following:

Ulcerative colitis	Irritable bowel syndrome
Crohn's disease	Regional enteritis
Reflux esophagitis	

Conditions outside the abdomen that may have abdominal pain as a symptom include the following:

Hepatitis	Pleurisy
Rheumatic fever	Hip joint disease
Myocardial infarction	Spinal tumors
Pneumothorax	Empyema
Pneumonia	

Conditions That Cause Abdominal Pain

Inflammatory conditions that cause abdominal pain

Peritonitis. Peritonitis is an inflammation of the peritoneal membrane. It is actually a symptom of an acute situation or a chronic condition. The most common cause of peritonitis is an inflammatory process caused by a contaminant, such as an acute bacterial process (usually pneumococci or hemolytic streptococci). When bacteria invade, peritoneal cells begin to secrete fluid. Common causes of peritonitis are acute appendicitis, necrotizing enterocolitis, GI tract disruption, or intravascular visceral obstruction or devascularization or both.

In addition to symptoms of rebound tenderness and pain, a patient with peritonitis usually has tachycardia, an elevated temperature, and vomiting. If there is irritation of the posterior diaphragmatic area, pain is referred to the lateral shoulder area. If there is anterior diaphragmatic irritation, pain is referred to the subclavicular area. Usually the patient lies with the knees flexed and drawn up toward the chest in an attempt to relax the abdominal musculature. During abdominal auscultation bowel sounds are found to be diminished in adults. This is not a reliable sign in infants and children. A rectal examination should be performed on all patients, and a pelvic examination should be performed on most women.

Primary peritonitis indicates that the cause of the condition is intraperitoneal. Secondary peritonitis indicates that the condition originates in an organ or area outside the peritoneal cavity. Aseptic peritonitis refers to a foreign agent that enters the peritoneal cavity, such as a wood sliver, a surgical sponge, or blood.

Pneumoperitoneum indicates that gas is in the peritoneal cavity. Pneumoperitoneum may have occurred as the result of a perforation of the GI tract, from *Clostridium* (a gas-forming organism), or by iatrogenic means.

Appropriate diagnostic studies are a complete blood cell count (CBC), urinalysis, chest and abdominal radiographs, peritoneal lavage, or a combination of these. Therapeutic intervention is cause specific and ranges from the administration of antibiotics to abdominal surgery.

Acute appendicitis. Acute appendicitis occurs when the appendix becomes obstructed, blood supply is impaired, and bacteria invade. If allowed to persist, the appendix becomes nonviable and gangrenous, and ruptures intraperitoneally.

The patient has abdominal pain or cramping or both, nausea and vomiting, tachycardia, and anorexia. Usually the abdominal pain is initially diffuse and periumbilical and later becomes intense and localized to the right lower quadrant, just inside the iliac crest, at a point known as McBurney's point. There can, however, be aberrancies in the location of the pain. Chills and fever also usually develop. The patient usually prefers to lie with the hips and knees flexed.

If the appendix ruptures, peritoneal signs increase, and involuntary guarding develops. At this point the appendix either abscesses or ruptures. Increased fever and rebound tenderness are present.

Diagnosis is made by clinical signs and symptoms and by an elevation of white blood cells to greater than 10,000 cells/mm^3 with a neutrophil fraction of greater than 75%.[2] Laboratory studies, such as BUN and serum electrolyte levels, and an abdominal radiograph can be useful for the differential diagnosis of abdominal pain. Occasionally ultrasound demonstrates an enlarged appendix.

Therapeutic intervention for appendicitis is appendectomy. If the diagnosis is uncertain, hospital admission, close observation, and repeated assessments are usually appropriate. Morphine sulfate given in small increments is also recommended to relieve pain and reduce anxiety.[1]

Acute pancreatitis. Pancreatitis causes a severe epigastric pain after the ingestion of alcohol or a large amount of food, nausea and vomiting, abdominal distension, abdominal tenderness, and abdominal rigidity.

Therapeutic intervention includes an IV line of Ringer's lactate, administration of an analgesic for pain management, insertion of a nasogastric tube, administration of an antibiotic, and a chest radiograph to check for pulmonary involvement. Of patients with pancreatitis, 20% to 50% have pulmonary complications.

Diagnostic tools to assist in the diagnosis of pancreatitis are a CBC, measurements of serum electrolytes, alkaline phosphatase, serum glucose, serum amylase, and serum bilirubin, a monitoring of cardiac activity and central venous pressure, and insertion of a Foley catheter for the measurement of hourly urine output.

If there is perforation, fever, tachycardia, and signs of generalized sepsis will occur.

To diagnose ulcerative colitis, obtain a CBC and measurements of serum electrolytes, serum amylase, BUN and creatinine, serum glucose, and bilirubin; place the patient on a cardiac monitor, measure central venous pressure, obtain an abdominal radiographic series, place a Foley catheter, and measure hourly urine output.

Therapeutic intervention includes initiation of an IV line with Ringer's lactate, antibiotics, and hospital admission.

Toxic megacolon. Toxic megacolon is associated with colitis and is highlighted by a severe dilation of the colon. Signs and symptoms are fever, explosive bloody diarrhea, a very quiet abdomen on auscultation, prostration, and possibly the appearance of shock.

Therapeutic intervention includes initiation of an IV line of Ringer's lactate and hospital admission.

Esophagitis. Esophagitis is an inflammation of the hiatal esophagus usually caused by regurgitation of gastric acids. It is often seen in conjunction with a gastric ulcer or a hiatal hernia. It may be caused by the ingestion of a caustic substance such as lye or another alkaline or acid agent. Signs and symptoms are a steady, substernal pain that is increased when swallowing, occasional vomiting, weight loss, esophageal obstruction, esophageal bleeding, and a foul breath odor. It is diagnosed by an upper GI series or by observation of the effect of the administration of 15 ml of viscous lidocaine and 20 ml of antacid (if the patient has esophagitis, the lidocaine and antacid give instant relief from pain).

Therapeutic intervention includes a bland diet, antacids, and surgery to correct an existing anatomic defect. If the problem has been caused by the ingestion of a caustic material, one must pay attention to the airway, breathing, and circulation (ABCs) and consider dilation of the esophagus and the administration of antibiotics.

Gastritis. Gastritis is an inflammation of the gastric mucosa. It can result from hyperacidity, bile reflux, shock, or the ingestion of a gastric irritant. Signs and symptoms are epigastric pain, nausea and vomiting, mucosal bleeding, and epigastric tenderness on palpation of the abdomen at the epigastric area. It is diagnosed by relief of pain after the administration of an antacid, by gastroscopy, or by an upper GI series.

Therapeutic intervention includes antacids, a bland diet, a sedative for severe nausea, fluid replacement if vomiting has been severe, placement of a nasogastric tube, and administration of anticholinergic medications.

Peptic ulcer. A peptic ulcer can occur anywhere in the stomach or duodenum. The primary cause of the condition is usually hyperacidity. Signs and symptoms include a burning pain in the epigastric region that usually occurs early in the morning or just before meals. The pain is relieved by antacids, bland foods, or vomiting. Symptoms may occur during stressful periods and especially when production of gastric acids is increased. Diagnosis is confirmed by the relief of pain upon administration of antacids, by gastroscopy, or by an upper GI series.

Therapeutic intervention includes antacids, a bland diet in several small feedings, sedation, placement of a nasogastric tube (if the patient is vomiting severely), and replacement of fluids through an IV line or by mouth, if the patient can tolerate it. Check the serum electrolyte level, because the patient may need electrolyte replacement.

Obstructive conditions causing abdominal pain

Intestinal obstruction. Intestinal obstruction has a large variety of causes, such as hernia, fecal impaction, adhesions, tumors, paralyzed ileus, gallstones, regional enteritis, intussusception, volvulus, abscesses, or hematomas. The obstruction may be primary or secondary, as a result of an inflammation or central nervous system problem. The most significant danger of an obstructive condition is dehydration. Other significant dangers are infarction or perforation of the bowel. Signs and symptoms include nausea and vomiting, abdominal pain, constipation or obstipation, and abdominal distention. Diagnosis is made by observing filled bowel loops proximal to the block (filled with fluid), obtaining serum electrolyte levels, serum amylase levels, CBC, serum glucose, and a urinalysis. Therapeutic intervention includes an IV of Ringer's lactate, antibiotics, a nasogastric tube, hospital admission, and consideration of surgery (Table 38-1).

Cholecystitis. Cholecystitis is an inflammation of the gallbladder that may be exacerbated by gallstones. Signs and symptoms include abdominal pain of sudden onset (especially after the ingestion of fried or fatty foods), pain that radiates from the epigastrium to the right upper quadrant, a low-grade fever (38° C or 100.4° F), nausea and vomiting, local and rebound tenderness, pain referred to the right supraclavicular area, and possibly slight jaundice. Findings show that the patient is often a light-complexioned, fortyish, overweight woman. Diagnosis is made by urinalysis, CBC, serum electrolytes, BUN and creatinine, serum glucose, and serum bilirubin levels. Therapeutic intervention is placement of a nasogastric tube, initiation of an IV line with

Table 38-1 Radiographic and clinical evidence of specific bowel obstructions

Type	Radiographic findings	Clinical signs and symptoms
Bowel obstructions (general)	Air-fluid levels may appear as "string of beads" and thus serve as important diagnostic clue to mechanical obstructions. More than two fluid-air levels reflect mechanical obstruction, adynamic ileus, or both. Fluid-filled loops form proximal to impediment and are indicative of bowel obstruction. Routine films or contrast studies show air-fluid levels, distortion, abscess formation, narrow lumens, mucosal destruction, distension, and deformities at site of torsion.	Pain, distension, vomiting, obstipation, and constipation
Strangulation obstruction	"Coffee bean" sign appears on radiograph (dilated bowel loop bent on itself, assuming shape of coffee bean). Gas- and fluid-filled loops may have unchanging locations on multiple projection films. Pseudotumor (closed-loop obstruction filled with water that looks like tumor) may be present.	Abdominal tenderness, hyperactive bowel sounds, leukocytosis, rebound tenderness, fever
Gallstones	Air in gallbladder tree, distension of small bowel, and visualization of stone.	
Hernia		Extraabdominal or intraabdominal hernia may be present: in men, most commonly inguinal; in women, right-sided femoral hernias
Volvulus		Torsion of mesenteric axis creating digestive disturbances
Intussusception	"Coiled spring" appearance seen on contrast radiograph	

Ringer's lactate or normal saline solution, hospital admission, and possible surgery that is either traditional through laparotomy or through laparoscope. Lithotripsy may also be a consideration.

Esophageal obstruction. The most common cause of an esophageal obstruction is a foreign body. Signs and symptoms are a history of foreign body ingestion, subcutaneous emphysema in the cervical area (if perforation has occurred), and the complaint that something is stuck in the esophagus. Occasionally the foreign body can be visualized on a chest radiograph or by esophagoscopy. Therapeutic intervention includes observation (if the object has no sharp edges and can easily pass through both the upper and lower GI systems) or retrieval of the foreign body through use of esophagoscopy.

Incarcerated hernia. One of the most common causes of a chief complaint of abdominal pain is an extremely incarcerated hernia, which is a protrusion of bowel or other abdominal viscera through the abdominal musculature but not through the skin. Unless the hernia is strangulated, blood supply is usually good. They are most commonly found in the inguinal, femoral, and umbilical areas. Pain usually occurs after exertion. Therapeutic intervention is a manual attempt at replacement of the hernia. If it is strangulated, surgical intervention is recommended.

Hemorrhagic conditions that cause abdominal pain

Upper GI bleeding. Several conditions cause upper GI bleeding. Upper GI bleeding is defined as bleeding proximal to the Treitz's ligament. Signs and symptoms are hematemesis, melena, possibly a history of chronic alcohol abuse, epigastric tenderness, possible jaundice, possible hepatomegaly and splenomegaly, and possible shock.

Types of upper GI bleeding

Bleeding peptic ulcer. Two thirds of all upper GI bleedings are caused by peptic ulcers. They are generally thought to be caused by the granulation of an ulcer and the erosion of the ulcer through a vessel.

Therapeutic intervention is first to provide for the ABCs. An IV of Ringer's lactate should be initiated, and the patient placed on bed rest, receiving supplemental oxygen. The patient should also be placed on a cardiac monitor. If the bleeding is active, an iced saline solution gastric lavage should be performed with a large-bore tube. If the patient is in shock, type and crossmatch the patient for blood replacement and prepare the patient for surgery.

Bleeding esophageal varices. Esophageal varices are

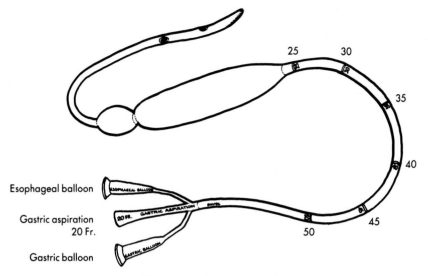

Esophageal balloon

Gastric aspiration
20 Fr.

Gastric balloon

Fig. 38-1   Blakemore tube.

common in patients with chronic hepatic disease. Portal hypertension causes the collateral channels of blood to develop between the stomach and the systemic veins of the lower esophagus. When these channels rupture, the patient is in a critical situation. More than one third of patients with cirrhosis of the liver die from bleeding esophageal varices. Signs and symptoms are massive, bright red bleeding of the GI tract and a history of chronic alcohol abuse with portal hypertension.

Therapeutic intervention is to ensure ABCs, balloon tamponade the bleeding areas in the esophagus with a Sengstaken-Blakemore tube (Fig. 38-1), and possibly perform surgical intervention.

Mallory-Weiss syndrome. Mallory-Weiss syndrome was first described in 1929 by Mallory and Weiss. It is a tear at the cardioesophageal junction that has been caused by retching and vomiting unsynchronized with regurgitation. Signs and symptoms are a history of retching and vomiting with emesis followed by hematemesis on subsequent vomiting episodes. It is diagnosed by visualization on celiac arteriography or endoscopy.

Therapeutic intervention includes balloon tamponade with a Sengstaken-Blakemore tube, intraarterial vasopressin, and whole blood transfusions.

Boerhaave's syndrome. Boerhaave's syndrome is small tears of the esophagus caused by vomiting after a large meal; it is thought to be caused by dilation of the esophagus. Signs and symptoms include bloody expectoration, possible massive bleeding if the tears are severe, and pain in the esophageal area. Therapeutic intervention includes the ABCs, close observation, and possible surgery.

Lower GI bleeding. Bleeding from the large bowel and the rectum is usually caused by diverticulitis, carcinoma, cecal ulcers, hemorrhoids, polyps, or ulcerative colitis. The cardinal sign of lower GI bleeding is bright red blood from the rectum. Therapeutic intervention depends on the cause of the bleeding. Surgical intervention may be required if the bleeding is severe. Most of the time the bleeding stops spontaneously.

How to insert a nasogastric tube

1. Measure the length of the tube required by measuring from the tip of the patient's earlobe to the tip of the nose and from the tip of his nose to the umbilicus; mark the tube at this point.
2. Explain the procedure to the patient.
3. Lubricate the tube at the tip and a few inches up from the distal end with a water-soluble lubricant.
4. Place the patient in high Fowler's position.
5. Have the patient place his or her head in a sniffing position.
6. Check the patient for a deviated septum.
7. Insert the tube through the nares; instruct the patient to swallow as the tube is being passed; using a small amount of water and having the patient sip and swallow during this process usually helps (unless water is contraindicated).
8. Continue to pass the tube until it is at the level previously marked; if the patient begins to choke or cough during the procedure, stop and allow him or her to rest; if coughing and choking continue, remove the tube and begin again. The tube may have inadvertently passed into the trachea.
9. Check to be sure the tube is in the stomach; while air is being injected into the tube, auscultate the epigastric region for the sound of air movement or aspirate the tube for the presence of stomach contents.
10. Secure the tube by taping it to the nose and the forehead.
11. Connect the distal end of the tube to intermittent suction

if the tube is single lumen and to continuous suction if the tube is double lumen. (Single-lumen tubes are rarely used anymore.)

How to insert a Sengstaken-Blakemore tube

1. Explain the procedure to the patient.
2. Check the tube balloons for patency.
3. The pharynx may be anesthetized.
4. Lubricate the tube with a water-soluble lubricant at the tip and several inches up from the distal end.
5. Insert the tube through the nares for approximately 50 cm.
6. Check to be sure the tube is in the stomach; while air is being injected into the tube, auscultate the epigastric region for the sound of air movement or aspirate the tube for the presence of stomach contents.
7. Fill the gastric balloon with 200 to 250 ml of radiopaque (Hypaque) dye and double-clamp it.
8. Apply gentle traction to check for placement and to wedge the balloon into the cardioesophageal junction.
9. Aspirate the stomach contents to check for continued bleeding; if bleeding is present, inflate the esophageal balloon to a pressure between 25 and 45 mm Hg by attaching the distal end of the balloon to a sphygmomanometer.
10. Double-clamp the tube.
11. Obtain an abdominal radiograph to verify the tube's position.
12. A small nasogastric tube may be passed to the upper end of the gastric balloon to allow upper esophageal aspiration if required.
13. The esophageal balloon should be deflated every 8 hours to prevent necrosis.
14. Be sure to monitor the patient closely for airway obstruction and keep equipment near in case the balloons must be deflated rapidly.

Intraarterial vasopressin. Vasopressin given intraarterially is used to control bleeding from lesions that are caused by erosive processes, from tears, from peptic ulcers, and from esophageal varices. Vasopressin is usually chosen after identification of the lesion on an angiogram. It is infused at a rate of 0.1 to 0.4 U/min for a 15-minute period. Once the infusion is completed, the angiogram is repeated. The dose of vasopressin is then repeated in accordance with arteriogram findings. While the infusion is running, closely monitor the patient's heart rate and rhythms and arterial pressure. The infusion will continue for 24 hours and then will be reduced for the second 24 hours. After 48 hours of vasopressin the patient should be given normal saline solution IV for the next 24 hours to check for bleeding.

GENITOURINARY EMERGENCIES
Medical Genitourinary Emergencies

There are many types of medical genitourinary emergencies. Many of the most common are reviewed here.

Pyelonephritis. Pyelonephritis is an inflammation of the kidneys that involves the tubules, glomeruli, and pelvis. The most common cause is a bacterial infection. Signs and symptoms are severe flank or back pain, urinary urgency, nocturia, dysuria, tenderness over the flank area, fever, chills, and urinary frequency. It is diagnosed by the finding of leukocytosis, pyuria, bacteriuria, and hematuria. Therapeutic intervention includes forcing fluids, bed rest, broad-spectrum antibiotics, and possible hospital admission in cases of abscess or gram-negative septicemia or if signs and symptoms are severe.

Perinephric abscess. When perinephric abscess appears, the patient usually offers a history of a recent skin infection (within 1 month) or a urinary tract infection that has lasted a long time. Signs and symptoms include a fever, extreme tenderness in the flank area, palpation of a mass in the flank area, and spinal scoliosis that is concave on the affected side. It is diagnosed by visualizing an elevated diaphragm on the affected side and a decreased psoas shadow on radiographic examination. Therapeutic intervention includes incision and drainage of the abscess and administration of antibiotics.

Renal carbuncle. A renal carbuncle is an abscess in the periphery of the kidney. Signs and symptoms are severe flank tenderness or pain, fever, and chills. Often these signs and symptoms are present, but urinalysis is normal; this is how the diagnosis of renal carbuncle is made. Therapeutic intervention includes incision, drainage, and administration of antibiotics.

Renal colic and renal calculi (Fig. 38-2). Pain caused by renal colic radiates from the flank into the right or left lower quadrant and also radiates occasionally to the leg. This pain occurs as a result of ureteral distention caused by the movement of a renal stone (calculus) or blood clots. The location of the stone may vary (Fig. 38-2). The size of the stone or clot does not relate to the severity of the pain. Signs and symptoms include restlessness and severe flank pain that radiates to the right or left lower abdominal quadrant, which is sudden in onset. The patient also has urinary urgency and frequency, diaphoresis, low-grade fever, hematuria, dysuria, and decreased blood pressure.

Diagnosis is made by IV pyelogram, straining urine, and urinalysis and by observing the calculi on an x-ray film of the kidneys, ureter, and bladder. Therapeutic intervention includes analgesic agents, IV fluids, antiemetics, urology consultation, possible hospital admission, lithotripsy, or possible surgical intervention.

Urinary retention. An inability to void is known as urinary retention. It may be caused by urethral strictures, an enlarged prostate, blood clots, renal stones, a reflex neurogenic bladder (usually associated with a cerebrovascular accident), multiple sclerosis, congenital stenosis, foreign bodies, bladder stones, hysteria, or as a side effect of a parasympatholytic agent and certain other medications. Signs and symptoms are lower abdominal pain and a mass that can be palpated just above the symphysis pubis. Ther-

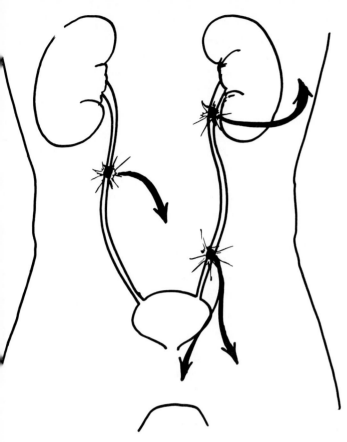

Fig. 38-2   Areas of renal stone lodging and patterns of pain radiation.

apeutic intervention is the insertion of an indwelling catheter and possibly a urology consultation.

Hematuria. There are many causes of blood appearing in the urine. Some of these are trauma, renal calculi, anticoagulant therapy, blood dyscrasias, prostatectomy, ruptured scrotal varices, and renal or bladder tumors. Check with the patient to see when bleeding is occurring. Bleeding that occurs at the beginning of the urination period suggests bleeding from the anterior portion of the urethra. Bleeding that occurs at the end of the urination stream indicates bleeding from either the posterior urethra or the point where the bladder connects to the urethra. Bleeding that occurs throughout urination is probably from the upper urinary tract or the bladder.

Be cautioned that not all reddish urine contains blood. It may be caused by food coloring, certain medications, and possibly the ingestion of beets. If bleeding occurs in a woman, one should be sure to check the source of the bleeding, since it may be from the vagina.

Diagnosis in hematuria is made on the basis of the patient's history, a urinalysis, and a CBC. Therapeutic intervention for hematuria depends on the cause of the bleeding.

Be sure to check vital signs carefully and to pay attention to other clues.

Oliguria and anuria. Oliguria is the excretion of less than 500 ml of urine per day. Anuria is the absence of urine excretion. The chief complaint of these patients is the inability to void. If one catheterizes these patients for diagnostic reasons, one will find that little or no urine is present. Either of these conditions may be caused by fluid and electrolyte imbalances, urinary tract obstructions, acute tubular necrosis, tumors, or accidental occlusion during surgery, especially sterilization surgery. Signs and symptoms are possibly marked dehydration, weakness, and uremic frost. Therapeutic intervention includes an IV pyelogram and urologic consultation. If the cause is severe dehydration, therapeutic intervention is the administration of fluids and electrolytes in accordance with serum electrolyte values. If the case is caused by hypotension from any cause, therapeutic intervention should be aimed toward elevating blood pressure to an acceptable value. One must isolate the cause and administer therapeutic interventions accordingly. Peritoneal or renal dialysis may be necessary.

Acute cystitis. Cystitis is more common in women than in men. It is an infection of the bladder that occurs as a result of migration of bacteria from the urethra to the bladder. It is commonly known as "honeymoon cystitis." It may also occur as a result of acute prostatitis. Signs and symptoms include urinary urgency, nocturia, mild hematuria, and fever (usually in men).

In women it is diagnosed by a urinalysis demonstrating white blood cells and bacteria. In men it is diagnosed by the finding of a tender prostate, urinary retention, and fever. Therapeutic intervention differs for men and women. For men, administer a sulfa combination drug (Septra) or tetracycline. In addition, the abscess should be drained, if present. Bed rest and increased fluid intake are necessary. Women should be treated with nitrofurantoin or sulfonamides, increased fluids, and warm baths.

Genitourinary Problems Unique to Males

There are several genitourinary problems that are unique to males. Some of the more common ones are presented here.

Cryptorchidism. Cryptorchidism is the condition of an undescended testicle. It is diagnosed by history, a mass in the inguinal region, and the absence of a testicle in the scrotum. Therapeutic intervention is to administer gonadotropins and/or perform surgery.

Penile scrotal edema. Penile scrotal edema is a common finding in men with congestive heart failure. It is identified by a pitting edema of the scrotum. Therapeutic intervention is aimed at treating the congestive heart failure.

Acute epididymitis. Acute epididymitis is an infection of the epididymis, a section of the male reproductive system. Sometimes it occurs as a result of physical exertion, after a cystoscopic examination or prostate surgery, or in patients with a history of urethral discharge or urinary bladder catheterization. Signs and symptoms include swelling and enlargement of the epididymis, sudden tenderness radiating up the spermatic cord, an elevated temperature, and possibly sepsis. Therapeutic intervention includes antibiotics, bed rest, elevation of the scrotum, and forced fluids.

Hematospermia. Hematospermia is a condition in which blood is present in semen. This is a condition common in middle-aged men. The most common cause is the rupture of a varicose vein. Therapeutic intervention is to offer much reassurance and possibly a urology consultation if the condition is recurrent.

Hydrocele. A hydrocele is the condition in which fluid collects in the tunica vaginalis. Generally there is no pain or tenderness, and the only sign is the presence of a large scrotal mass. Surgery is performed only if the hydrocele is large and uncomfortable.

Acute orchitis. An inflammation of the testicle is known as orchitis. It may result from parotiditis (mumps) or other viral infections. Signs and symptoms are unilateral testicular swelling, unilateral testicular tenderness, and an elevated temperature. Therapeutic intervention is antibiotics, bed rest, and a scrotal support.

Peyronie's disease. Peyronie's disease is a syndrome in which a fibrous plaque forms on the corpora cavernosa. When an erection occurs, the penis is curved, and there is considerable pain. Signs and symptoms include a curved penis on erection and painful intercourse. Therapeutic intervention is relatively nonexistent. One should provide much psychologic support.

Priapism. Priapism is a prolonged erection that is not relieved by ejaculation. Common causes of this condition are spinal cord injury, sickle cell crisis, tumor, hematologic disorders, and unknown causes. Signs and symptoms are a prolonged erection and occasionally pain. Therapeutic intervention is analgesia or sedation and possible surgical intervention if the condition persists.

Prostatitis. Prostatitis is an inflammation of the prostate gland. It is often accompanied by cystitis. Signs and symptoms are extreme tenderness on examination, an elevated temperature, and possibly urinary retention. Therapeutic intervention includes antibiotics, bed rest, forced fluids, and surgical intervention.

Testicular torsion. Testicular torsion is the twisting of the testicle in the tunica vaginalis; it usually twists at the spermatic cord. It is most commonly seen in children and adolescents. When the testicle is elevated, there is increased pain. Signs and symptoms include severe scrotal pain, swelling, and nausea and vomiting that increases during physical activity. The patient also has an elevated temperature, a high-riding testicle, and a tense scrotal mass. Therapeutic intervention is ice packs, manual manipulation to try to reduce the torsion, and possible surgical intervention if the manual manipulation is unsuccessful.

Testicular tumor. The most common age group for a testicular tumor is between 20 and 30 years. This patient's chief complaint is a scrotal mass without pain. Other signs and symptoms include swelling and a hard testicular mass with a normal epididymis. Therapeutic intervention is surgery.

Nonspecific urethritis. Patients with nonspecific urethritis are commonly seen in the emergency department with a chief complaint of urethral discharge. Signs and symptoms are burning on urination, urinary frequency, dysuria, and urethral discharge. A Gram stain does not demonstrate gram-negative intracellular diplococci. Therapeutic intervention includes trimethoprin-sulfonamide combination or tetracycline.

Varicocele. A varicocele is a dilation of the spermatic cord caused by vascular congestion. Signs and symptoms are a scrotal mass just above the testicle and disappearance of the mass when the patient is supine. Therapeutic intervention may be surgery.

Sexually Transmitted Diseases

Chancroid. A chancroid demonstrates as inguinal adenopathy 3 to 4 days after sexual intercourse, a discharge, and a positive skin test. Therapeutic intervention is treatment with tetracycline.

Gonorrhea. Gonorrhea is actually a form of urethritis that is infectious and contagious. Signs and symptoms are burning on urination, a white, creamy discharge 3 to 7 days after sexual intercourse, gram-negative diplococci on Gram stain, and a positive gonococcus culture. Therapeutic intervention is to treat the patient with antibiotics (penicillin or tetracycline) and to arrange for follow-up care.

Granuloma inguinale. Granuloma inguinale is a chronic venereal disease in which the skin and subcutaneous tissue of the genitalia, perineum, and inguinal region are affected. Signs and symptoms are swelling, ulceration, and pain. Therapeutic intervention is administration of tetracycline.

Lymphogranuloma venereum. Lymphogranuloma venereum is a venereal disease caused by a virus. Signs and symptoms are a transient genital lesion and, in women, lymphadenopathy and rectal strictures 1 to 3 weeks after exposure through sexual intercourse. Painful nodes also appear. Therapeutic intervention is administration of tetracycline.

Syphilis. The most common chief complaint in the ED of a patient with syphilis is painless ulcerations. They appear several weeks after exposure through sexual intercourse. Therapeutic intervention is penicillin.

Dialysis Emergencies

Dialysis patients often arrive at the ED with a variety of complaints. A few complaints, however, are more common than others and are presented here.

Clotted shunts. There are two common types of shunts

used for hemodialysis: the external Scribner shunt and the internal Brescia-Cimino fistula. The latter is an arteriovenous fistula. If a shunt is clotted, therapeutic intervention depends on which type of shunt is in place. A Scribner shunt can be declotted in the emergency department; a Brescia-Cimino fistula must be evaluated at surgery.

Shunt infections. The most common infecting agent in a Scribner shunt is staphylococci. A sample taken from the site of the shunt should be cultured. Therapeutic intervention is to administer antibiotics. If a Brescia-Cimino fistula is infected, there are usually also signs of systemic infection. Therapeutic intervention is the administration of antibiotics and evaluation of the infection by obtaining blood cultures.

In many dialysis patients dysrhythmias, hypotension or hypertension, pericardial disease, and cardiac arrest develop. Most of these emergencies are treated as they are for a nondialysis patient. Dysrhythmias usually occur as a result of hyperkalemia. If dysrhythmias begin to develop shortly before a scheduled dialysis session, one could probably assume that the problem is hyperkalemia. Often this condition is caused by the patient deviating from strict dietary regulations. Cardiac arrest may even develop. If the arrest does occur, chances are that it has been caused by either hypovolemia or hyperkalemia. For the latter, large doses of calcium chloride are required before the arrest situation can be changed. One is also advised to provide all the other basic and advanced life support measures indicated for any patient.

REFERENCES

1. Doherty GM, Lewis FR Jr: Appendicitis: diagnostic challenge, *Emerg Med Clin North Am* 7:3, 1989.
2. Young GP: CBC or not CBC? That is the question, *Ann Emerg Med* 15(3):367, 1986.

SUGGESTED READINGS

Berry J, Malt RA: Appendicitis near its century, *Ann Surg* 200:567, 1988.

Bongard F et al: Differential diagnosis of appendicitis and PID, *Am J Surg* 150:90, 1985.

Buchman TG, Zuidema GD: Reasons for delay of the diagnosis of acute appendicitis, *Surg Gynecol Obstet* 158:260, 1984.

Hatch E: The acute abdomen in children. *Pediatr Clin North Am* 32(5):1151, 1985.

Neblett WW et al: Acute abdominal conditions in children and adolescents, *Surg Clin North Am* 68(2):415, 1988.

Robinson JA, Burch BH: An assessment of the value of the menstrual history in differentiating acute appendicitis from pelvic inflammatory disease, *Surg Gynecol Obstet* 159:149, 1984.

Silen W: *Cope's early diagnosis of the acute abdomen*, New York, 1983, Oxford University Press.

Stevenson RJ: Abdominal pain unrelated to trauma, *Surg Clin North Am* 65(5):1181, 1985.

Way LW: *Current surgical diagnosis and treatment*, ed 8, Los Altos, Calif, 1988, Lange Medical Publications.

CHAPTER 39

Metabolic and Endocrine Emergencies

Dianne Danis

Endocrine, metabolic, and fluid and electrolyte disturbances are commonly seen in emergency care, yet they are often not the first diagnoses to come to the emergency nurse's mind. Patients with depressed consciousness, coma, or bizarre behavioral disturbances may be having a metabolic crisis and are in jeopardy unless the conditions are managed correctly. It is therefore important that a metabolic or endocrine problem be systematically considered an etiologic factor in any patient whose symptoms are not easily explained.

These disorders are complex and sometimes subtle: they often coexist. The most common metabolic problems are alcohol- and diabetes-related emergencies. However, acute adrenal and thyroid crises should not be overlooked, since they can be life threatening if not managed aggressively. Finally, the emergency nurse should also consider fluid and electrolyte imbalances a metabolic problem, since they create a wide range of signs and symptoms and potentially endanger life. An awareness of classic manifestations and associated causes can alert emergency personnel to these emergencies and ensure prompt, definitive therapy.

ALCOHOL-RELATED EMERGENCIES

The emergency nurse is likely to encounter alcohol-related emergencies daily. Nurses should clearly understand that these problems can be *true* medical emergencies: do not permit the behavioral manifestations to distract you from an underlying metabolic threat to life. The following general guidelines should be carefully considered by all emergency personnel:

1. Realize that alcohol intoxication and alcohol withdrawal can be fatal.
2. Differentiate alcohol-related problems from head injury, drug overdose, and hypoglycemia.
3. Do not be misled by the appearance of the patient: a well-dressed, refined, elderly woman can also be intoxicated; a white, middle-class teenager can be an alcoholic.
4. Obtain a careful history. Be aware of denial about alcohol consumption.

5. It is the amount of alcohol consumed, not the type of beverage, that determines the level of intoxication.
6. Consider social services or alcohol counseling referral for patients with alcohol-related problems who are seen in the emergency department (ED).
7. Always take the opportunity to confront a patient with the effects of his or her drinking; health crises may render patients and families less likely to engage in denial and more receptive to the need for treatment.

The Disease of Alcoholism

Alcoholism affects the lives of Americans and the practice of emergency nurses to an almost unimaginable extent, as the following facts demonstrate:

1. There are an estimated 10 million individuals with alcoholism in the United States.
2. More than 200,000 Americans die of alcoholism every year.
3. Alcohol abuse costs Americans $60 billion annually.
4. A strong relationship exists between alcohol use and child abuse, domestic violence, rape, traffic fatalities, fire-related deaths, drownings, homicide, and suicide.
5. In one ED, one third of all patients seen between 9 PM and midnight and two thirds of those arriving between midnight and 3 AM had positive results of breath tests for the presence of alcohol.[16]

Assessment for Alcohol-Related Conditions

Identifying the patient with alcoholism. One would think that an emergency care provider would be able to identify an individual with alcoholism every time, but studies have shown that many signs and symptoms of alcoholism are overlooked in practice.

Tweed[14] has summarized the conclusive, probable, and possible signs and symptoms of alcoholism. The *conclusive* indicators are occurrence of alcohol withdrawal syndrome, alcoholic cirrhosis, job loss or promotion loss as a result of drinking, marital or family disruption because of drinking, three or more arrests for intoxication or driving while intoxicated, and admission of inability to control drinking.

The *probable* indicators are alcoholic hepatitis, pancreatitis, and gastritis, tolerance to alcohol intake, blackouts, frequent references to drinking, sustained "therapeutic" use of alcohol, significant others' complaints about a person's drinking, frequent job changes, unexplained changes in business relationships, job loss as a result of increased interpersonal difficulties, frequent fights and assaultiveness while drinking, frequent automobile accidents while intoxicated, and loss of interest in activities not directly associated with drinking. One last indicator: according to West,[17] "The patient who is brought to the hospital drunk is probably a chronic alcoholic."

The emergency nurse may find it difficult to elicit an honest drinking history from the alcoholic patient because denial and concealment are inherent aspects of the disease. A patient who has more than four drinks per day is likely to have a drinking problem, but few patients admit to having this problem. Mayfield, McLeod, and Hall[10] have developed the CAGE questionnaire, which consists of questions that have been identified as helpful and relatively unthreatening, including the following:

1. Have you ever had a problem with alcohol?
2. When was your last drink? ("Yes" to the former and "within 24 hours" to the latter are 90% sensitive and specific responses.[5])
3. Have you ever tried to *Cut* down on your drinking?
4. Are you *Annoyed* by criticism of your drinking?
5. Do you feel *Guilt* about your drinking?
6. Have you ever felt the need to take an *Eye opener?*

A positive response to two questions on the CAGE test is virtually diagnostic of alcoholism.[10]

Complications of Acute and Chronic Alcohol Ingestion

No part of the human system is untouched by chronic alcohol misuse. The following sections discuss alcohol intoxication, alcohol-related seizures, alcohol withdrawal syndromes, Wernicke-Korsakoff syndrome, and Antabuse reactions. The box below provides a comprehensive listing of the complications of alcoholism. A thorough head-to-toe examination of alcoholic patients is essential to avoid overlooking potentially serious complications and associated illnesses or injuries.

Ethanol intoxication. Ethanol (ethyl or grain alcohol) is the intoxicating agent in fermented and distilled liquors. Intoxication after ethanol ingestion is a common phenomenon among ED patients. Intoxication may constitute a patient's initial problem, may have aggravated or caused the problem, or may coexist with an unrelated problem. In addition to being a clinical entity, intoxication is also a legal

---

CLINICAL CONDITIONS ASSOCIATED WITH ACUTE AND CHRONIC ALCOHOL USE

Injury
Abuse and assault
Homicide
Suicide
Unintentional injury
Burns
Hypothermia

Neurologic
Seizures
Cerebellar atrophy
Cortical atrophy
Wernicke's encephalopathy
Hepatic encephalopathy
Korsakoff's psychosis
Peripheral neuropathy

Eye, ear, nose, and throat
Poor dental health
Cancer of oral cavity and larynx

Cardiovascular
Dysrhythmias
ECG abnormalities
Alcoholic cardiomyopathy
Ischemic heart disease
Hypertension

Pulmonary
Lung cancer
Chronic obstructive pulmonary disease

Gastrointestinal
Gastritis
Gastrointestinal hemorrhage
Peptic ulcer disease
Esophageal varices
Mallory-Weiss syndrome
Fatty liver
Zieve's syndrome
Alcoholic hepatitis
Cirrhosis
Hepatoma
Cancer of esophagus, stomach, and bowel
Pancreatitis
Malnutrition

Genitourinary and obstetric
Testicular atrophy
Fetal alcohol syndrome

Hematologic
Anemia
Leukopenia

Splenic sequestration
Hemorrhage

Metabolic
Hypoglycemia
Alcoholic ketoacidosis
Lactic acidosis
Hypokalemia
Hypomagnesemia
Hypocalcemia
Hemachromatosis
Hypertriglyceridemia
Hyperuricemia
Delirium tremens

Infectious
Pneumonia
Tuberculosis
Cellulitis
Cutaneous ulcers
Meningitis
Bacteremia

entity defined by measurement of a certain level of alcohol content in blood (blood alcohol level), most commonly 100 mg/dl, equivalent to 0.10%.

The primary short-term effects of alcohol are those exerted on the central nervous system. Alcohol acts as a depressant and, in large doses, as an anesthetic. Both motor performance and mental functioning are adversely affected, and emotional responses are altered. The manifestations of intoxication may be correlated with the blood alcohol level (Table 39-1). The correlation is not precise, however, since systemic concentration depends of many variables such as weight, sex, age, rate of absorption from stomach and small intestine, and ingestion of food, carbonated beverages, and other substances. Also, a certain tolerance to alcohol develops in persons with chronic alcoholism; this tolerance results in symptoms becoming evident at proportionately higher blood levels. Maximum blood alcohol levels occur between 30 minutes and 3 hours after drinking has stopped, so it is possible for the condition of a patient with alcoholism to continue to deteriorate after arrival in the ED. Another rule of thumb is that the rate of absorption, distribution, metabolism, and excretion of alcohol is approximately 1 oz per hour. The blood alcohol level of a person who drinks at or below this rate will be measured as low to nonexistent. Heavier drinking results in rising blood alcohol levels and prolonged recovery time. Ethanol has been shown to be metabolized at a constant rate of 12 mg/dl/hr in persons who do not have alcoholism; in persons with alcoholism the rate is 17 mg/dl/hr. Undeniably, it would be a boon to EDs everywhere if an antagonist to alcohol were discovered.

Assessment. Assessment of the person with presumed alcohol intoxication must be thorough. It is tempting to assume that these patients are just drunk, give them the "once-over," then consign them to a back room while they "sleep it off." However, failure to take these patients seriously may have disastrous results for three reasons: patients do die of simple alcohol intoxication; intoxication may mask other more serious problems; and patients who appear to be intoxicated may actually have a medical condition that mimics intoxication.

When a patient has acute alcohol intoxication, a history may be difficult or impossible to obtain. Valuable collateral sources of information include family, first responders, and medical records. When possible, relevant history should be obtained and focused particularly on the chief complaint, drinking history, and health history.

A brief but comprehensive head-to-toe assessment must be performed. Since the intoxicated patient literally does not "feel any pain" and is a particularly unreliable historian, there is no substitute for inspection, including particular attention to the respiratory, cardiovascular, and neurologic status.

Specific laboratory assessment consists of measurement of blood alcohol level, with a variety of other tests obtained as indicated. Rapid and reliable alcohol level assessment is now possible with the use of a hand-held breath analyzer[86] (Fig. 39-1). When a test of blood alcohol content is being requested for legal rather than medical purposes, the nurse must be careful to adhere to state law and hospital policy. Although using an alcohol wipe to prepare the skin before phlebotomy is unlikely to influence the reported alcohol level, using an alcohol wipe is best avoided when any potential legal issues are present.

In more advanced stages when alterations in mental status are dominant, alcohol intoxication is a diagnosis of exclusion: all other possible diagnoses must be considered and excluded before the diagnosis can be made. Accurate diagnosis is more than an academic exercise, since many of the alternative diagnoses require rapid treatment. A suggested approach to evaluating and treating the comatose patient is shown in Fig. 39-2.

Management. Intervention for alcohol intoxication is generally supportive and usually limited to the period of acute intoxication. With comatose patients a standard treatment approach, sometimes called "the cocktail," often yields both diagnostic and therapeutic results: 1 ampule of 50% dextrose solution, 100 mg of thiamine, and 1 or 2 ampules of naloxone are administered intravenously.

Frequent reassessment is necessary. The patient's condition should gradually improve if the only problem is intoxication. If the patient's condition does not gradually improve, emergency personnel should be alerted to consider the other causes of altered mental status.

In pure intoxication the biggest problem is respiratory depression, which occurs when blood alcohol levels are 400 mg/dl or greater; respiratory depression may necessitate intubation and ventilation. These patients should be placed

Table 39-1 Approximate correlation of blood alcohol levels and symptoms*

Blood alcohol level	Signs and symptoms
50 mg/dl	Rarely produces symptoms
100-200 mg/dl	Emotional and affective changes, such as exhilaration, talkativeness, boastfulness, belligerence, remorse, sentimentality; slurred speech; ataxia; decreased inhibitions; slowed reaction time; confusion
250 mg/dl	Sedation; decreased response to stimuli; nausea and vomiting; muscular incoordination; appears "acutely intoxicated"
300-400 mg/dl	Stupor or even coma; impaired deep tendon reflexes; peripheral vascular collapse; seizures; nystagmus; hypoventilation
Above 500 mg/dl	Usually fatal as a result of cardiac or respiratory arrest

*Chronic users of alcohol require higher blood alcohol levels before associated symptoms are noted; the lethal dose, however, is approximately the same.

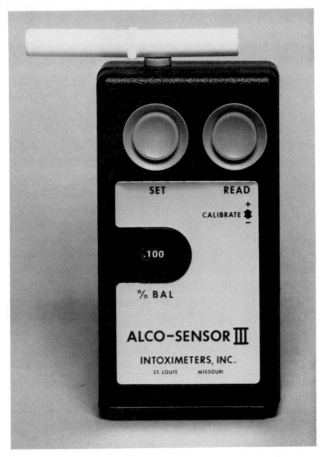

Fig. 39-1   Alco-Sensor III. (From MiniMed Technologies, Inc., Sylmar, Calif.)

in the acute care area of the ED, where they can be closely monitored.

When acutely intoxicated patients are agitated and combative, restraint or sedation may be necessary. The use of haloperidol (Haldol) has been shown to be effective and usually does not lower blood pressure.[9]

Rarely, blood alcohol levels must be lowered rapidly. The only methods of lowering blood alcohol level rapidly are hemodialysis and peritoneal dialysis. Indications for dialysis include blood alcohol levels greater than 600 mg/dl, blood alcohol levels greater than 400 mg/dl in conjunction with severe acidosis, ingestion of methanol or ethylene glycol, and severe intoxication in children.

Addressing a patient's substance abuse and social and emotional problems is often frustrating and difficult. Fig. 39-3 offers a possible triage plan for dealing with intoxicated patients.

Nursing diagnoses. Nursing diagnoses and interventions are often more important than the patient's underlying medical problems. In addition to an ineffective breathing pattern, the risk for ineffective airway clearance exists: a patient's tongue may obstruct the airway, or the patient may vomit and aspirate. A side-lying position is recommended. Suction and an oral airway adjunct should be available at the bedside. A nasogastric tube and gastric evacuation should be considered, especially in those patients who must be kept supine. (The need for cervical spine immobilization is common with these patients.) Oximetry is a quick way to determine oxygen saturation levels.

Another major nursing diagnosis is *high risk for injury*. The patient who is too intoxicated to walk (or drive) is a great danger to self and others. Compromised driving ability may occur in patients with blood alcohol levels of anywhere from 50 to 400 mg/dl. The danger is that this individual is incapable of recognizing the risk and often insists on being allowed to leave the ED. Staff are justified in restraining the intoxicated patient. Ideally, patients should not be released until the risk for injury has subsided and they are reasonably sober. Some authors advocate the use of written "driving prescriptions" that tell patients when they will be able to safely drive.[12]

When patients have a knowledge deficit, teaching before discharge is difficult. All important aftercare instructions should be in writing, and the family should be included in teaching whenever possible. With some patients a follow-up telephone call the next day may serve to reinforce the discharge teaching and also allow an opportunity for discussion of the patient's drinking pattern and substance abuse problem.

Alcohol-associated seizures. Seizures often occur in patients with alcoholism, for many reasons. Seizures within a 12- to 48-hour period after cessation of drinking are not unusual. The seizures are usually limited to this period and cease spontaneously. They do not indicate a seizure disorder per se; they may be related to withdrawal, although the relationship is not entirely clear. A person with alcoholism who does have a seizure disorder as a result of idiopathic epilepsy is likely to have an increased number of seizures because alcohol lowers the seizure threshold. If anticonvulsants have been prescribed, individuals with alcoholism are prone to noncompliance. Also, individuals with alcoholism are at a high risk for posttraumatic epilepsy because of their increased incidence of head trauma. Status epilepticus may occur as a result of alcohol withdrawal, and this possibility should always be considered in the differential diagnosis of seizures. Pharmacologic management is usually not required for isolated alcohol-related seizures, and phenytoin (Dilantin) does not seem to prevent recurrent alcohol-associated seizures.

Alcohol withdrawal syndrome. Alcohol withdrawal syndrome results from a decrease or cessation in alcohol intake. It has been theorized that physiologic mechanisms develop in patients with alcoholism to compensate for the depressant effect of alcohol. When the blood level drops, the protective mechanisms appear unmasked as autonomic hyperactivity.

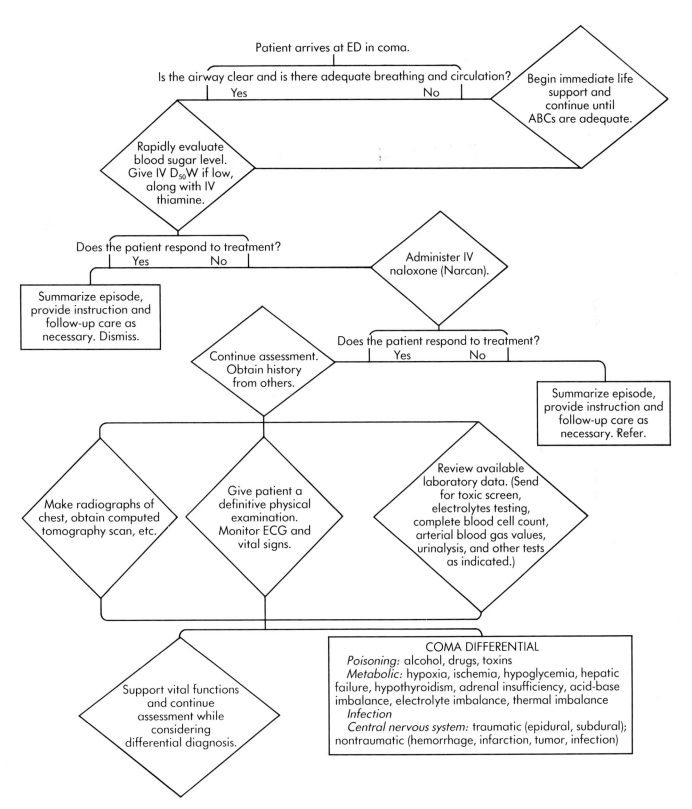

Patient arrives at ED in coma.

Is the airway clear and is there adequate breathing and circulation?

Yes / No

Begin immediate life support and continue until ABCs are adequate.

Rapidly evaluate blood sugar level. Give IV D$_{50}$W if low, along with IV thiamine.

Does the patient respond to treatment?

Yes / No

Summarize episode, provide instruction and follow-up care as necessary. Dismiss.

Administer IV naloxone (Narcan).

Does the patient respond to treatment?

Yes / No

Continue assessment. Obtain history from others.

Summarize episode, provide instruction and follow-up care as necessary. Refer.

Make radiographs of chest, obtain computed tomography scan, etc.

Give patient a definitive physical examination. Monitor ECG and vital signs.

Review available laboratory data. (Send for toxic screen, electrolytes testing, complete blood cell count, arterial blood gas values, urinalysis, and other tests as indicated.)

Support vital functions and continue assessment while considering differential diagnosis.

COMA DIFFERENTIAL
Poisoning: alcohol, drugs, toxins
Metabolic: hypoxia, ischemia, hypoglycemia, hepatic failure, hypothyroidism, adrenal insufficiency, acid-base imbalance, electrolyte imbalance, thermal imbalance
Infection
Central nervous system: traumatic (epidural, subdural); nontraumatic (hemorrhage, infarction, tumor, infection)

Fig. 39-2 Management of comatose patient.

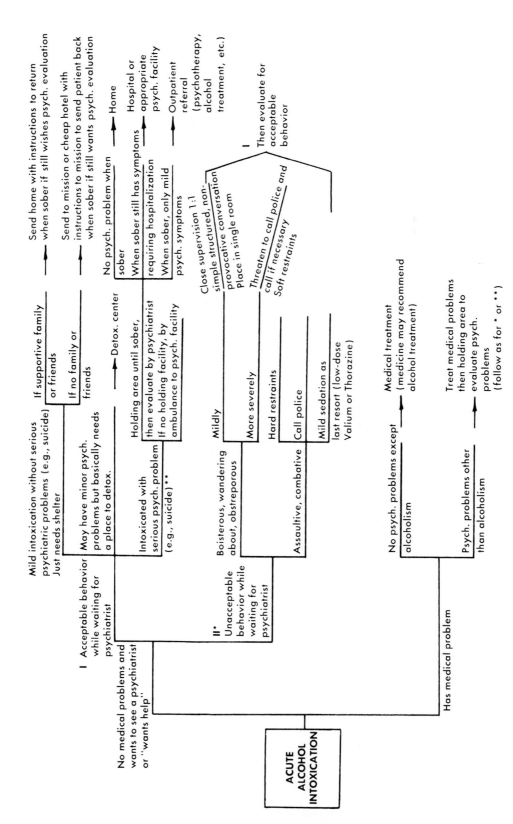

Fig. 39-3 Plan for triage of patient with acute alcohol intoxication. (Courtesy Dr. Regina Pally, Los Angeles, Calif.)

Minor withdrawal. Minor withdrawal develops within the first 24 hours after a change in drinking pattern. Manifestations include low-grade fever, hypertension, tachycardia, anxiety, irritability, agitation, tremor, insomnia, anorexia, nausea, and vomiting. As withdrawal advances, hallucinations (usually visual) or seizures may occur.

Withdrawal can easily be treated pharmacologically (Table 39-2). Of course, many persons with alcoholism "self-treat" by resuming the consumption of alcohol. For those who wish detoxification, withdrawal may be treated on an outpatient basis or admission to a detoxification facility or hospital may be needed.

Outpatient treatment is feasible for mild cases, when the person is able to care for himself or herself and social supports are available. All patients should receive thiamine. One suggested protocol uses chlordiazepoxide (Librium) therapy. Beta blockers and clonidine may also be helpful. Referral to an alcohol treatment program is mandatory.

Patients who require inpatient treatment are those with severe autonomic symptoms (temperature of more than 100.6° F; heart rate of 120 beats/min; or blood pressure of 150/100); serious concomitant medical, traumatic, or surgical condition; Wernicke's encephalopathy; seizures; hallucinations; or history of previous episodes of delirium tremens. Benzodiazepines seem to be the most effective agents in managing more severe withdrawal, probably because of the cross tolerance of these drugs and alcohol.

Delirium tremens. Delirium tremens is the end point of the continuum of alcohol withdrawal and occurs 2 to 5 days after the last drink. About 5% of those with untreated alcohol withdrawal progress to full-blown "DTs." Even when this dangerous illness is treated appropriately, mortality is approximately 2%.

Delirium tremens is characterized by delirium or disorientation in conjunction with agitation and autonomic arousal. Patients are acutely disturbed, usually actively hallucinating, and exhibiting gross tremors. They are diaphoretic, tachycardic, and febrile.

Diazepam (Valium) is most often recommended for managing delirium tremens. Lorazepam (Ativan) has been recommended for elderly patients or those with liver disease. The drug is given intravenously (IV) in sufficient amounts to suppress agitation. Table 39-2 details the drugs used to manage alcohol withdrawal.

Other interventions include protective restraints, initiation of IV lines, fluid replacement for dehydration, correction of electrolyte, metabolic, or nutritional abnormalities, and provision of a quiet, low-stimulus environment. Associated medical problems commonly exist and must be treated. Among these are hyperpyrexia, infection, hypotension, hypovolemia, dysrhythmia, hypokalemia, hypomagnesemia, and hypophosphatemia. Admission to a critical care unit is necessary.

Nursing diagnoses. Nursing diagnoses for patients with

Table 39-2   Medications used in treatment of alcohol withdrawal

Medication	Indication	Usual dose and route	Special considerations
Atenolol (Tenormin)	Minor withdrawal	50-100 mg orally	Provides symptomatic relief; contraindicated in congestive heart failure, diabetes mellitus, bronchospasm
Chlordiazepoxide (Librium)	Minor withdrawal; anticonvulsant	25-100 mg orally	Titrate dose to achieve sedation
Clonidine (Catapres)	Minor withdrawal	0.1-0.4 mg orally	Provides symptomatic relief
Diazepam (Valium)	Delirium tremens; anticonvulsant	5-10 mg IV; sample regimen: 10 mg IV, then 5 mg IV every 5 min until patient is sedated	Titrate dose to achieve sedation; may be necessary to repeat frequently; large doses are necessary; watch for respiratory depression; IV rate is 5 mg/min
Lorazepam (Ativan)	Delirium tremens; minor withdrawal	1-5 mg intramuscularly or orally	Recommended for elderly patients or patients with liver disease
Paraldehyde	Delirium tremens	5-30 ml rectally or orally	Obsolete
Phenytoin (Dilantin)	Anticonvulsant	100-300 mg orally; 500-1000 mg IV, loading dose	Not usually needed for simple alcohol-related seizures; IV rate ≤ 50 mg/min; do not mix with other drugs or solutions; flush with normal saline solution after IV administration; with IV use, monitor heart rate and rhythm, blood pressure, respiratory rate, and central nervous system

delirium tremens include hyperthermia, high risk for injury, high risk for violence: self-directed or directed at others, altered thought processes, altered nutrition: less than body requirements, fluid volume deficit (1) and (2), and high risk for infection.

Wernicke-Korsakoff syndrome. Wernicke's encephalopathy and Korsakoff's psychosis are each aspects of Wernicke-Korsakoff syndrome, caused by thiamine (vitamin B_1) deficiency. Individuals with alcoholism are particularly at risk because they tend to have nutritional deficits and because alcohol reduces intestinal absorption of thiamine. Along with the thiamine deficiency, there may be an inherited inability to utilize thiamine. Untreated Wernicke's encephalopathy progresses to the degenerative brain lesions of Korsakoff's psychosis. Classically, Wernicke's encephalopathy is demonstrated by the triad of (1) global confusional state, (2) ophthalmoplegia and nystagmus, and (3) ataxia; in practice, stupor and coma may be more common findings. Likewise, Korsakoff's psychosis has traditionally been defined as the triad of (1) memory loss, (2) learning deficits, and (3) confabulation, but it now seems that dementia may be the dominant presentation. Research has shown that Wernicke-Korsakoff syndrome may have an incidence as high as 12% but is seldom accurately diagnosed before death.[13]

Because Wernicke-Korsakoff syndrome is apparently missed frequently in clinical assessment and has devastating consequences and because there are no contraindications or complications associated with thiamine administration, some experts recommend administering thiamine to all intoxicated patients, all patients known to have alcoholism, all seriously malnourished patients, and all those with an altered mental status. It is particularly important to think of thiamine administration whenever a 50% dextrose solution is being given, because glucose is liable to totally deplete thiamine in individuals with thiamine deficiency and precipitate an acute Wernicke's encephalopathy. The dose is 100 mg IV or intramuscularly, depending on the acuity of the situation.

Disulfiram (Antabuse) reactions. Disulfiram (Antabuse) is prescribed to assist individuals during alcohol treatment programs. The drug action primarily depends on its production of unpleasant side effects when combined with alcohol in any form, including alcohol-based cough syrups, fermented vinegar, and sauces or other foods cooked or combined with alcohol. Metronidazole (Flagyl) and certain oral hypoglycemics can produce a similar response, although usually less severe. Particularly sensitive individuals may have a reaction even to external use of alcohol, such as rubbing alcohol or shaving lotion. Symptoms appear within 90 minutes but usually within 5 to 15 minutes after ingestion of alcohol. It is important that recipients understand that disulfiram effects continue for as long as 6 to 12 days after ingestion.

Signs and symptoms include bright red flushing of the face, neck, and upper thorax; sweating; throbbing headache; hyperventilation; tachycardia; hypotension; nausea and vomiting; decreased level of consciousness or coma; and reddened conjunctiva. The nurse should look for a patient's Antabuse card because mild reactions may be confused with other drug reactions.

Emergency management
1. Ask the patient to lie down, and provide reassurance about what is happening. Position the patient on the side if possible, since vomiting is likely. Determine how much alcohol has been ingested. (Ingestion of more than 2 to 3 ounces is cause for alarm, because shock and coma are likely.)
2. Elevate the legs.
3. Initiate an IV infusion of normal saline solution.
4. Administer, depending on local protocol, 500 mg ascorbic acid, 12 mg chlorpheniramine (Chlor-Trimeton), 50 mg diphenhydramine (Benadryl), or 25 mg pyribenzamine.
5. A nasogastric tube may be indicated if there is a decreased level of consciousness.
6. Administration of oxygen by nasal cannula may be useful if acute respiratory distress is not relieved by antihistamines.
7. Continue to monitor the electrocardiographic readings and vital signs.
8. Report the incident to the alcohol treatment center or physician who dispensed the disulfuram.

Nursing Diagnoses in Alcohol-Related Conditions

Nursing diagnoses in patients with alcohol-related conditions are as numerous as the associated medical diagnoses. They include substance abuse, high risk for infection, altered nutrition: less than body requirements, sleep pattern disturbance, altered sexuality patterns, high risk for injury, lowered self-concept, high risk for violence: self-directed or directed at others, altered family processes, altered thought processes, diversional activity deficit, noncompliance, ineffective denial, ineffective breathing pattern, ineffective airway clearance, and sensory-perceptual alterations.

Working with patients who have alcoholism is one of the most difficult challenges in emergency nursing. Viewing the aftereffects of alcohol abuse daily is extremely demoralizing. Many nurses have found participating in prevention programs to be an effective antidote and outlet for their negative experiences.[7]

DIABETES-RELATED EMERGENCIES
Diabetic Ketoacidosis

Diabetic ketoacidosis (DKA) is a metabolic disturbance in patients with diabetes mellitus (DM) caused primarily by insulin depletion. Mortality is 6% to 10%. Since many deaths are potentially preventable—those resulting from metabolic imbalances, underlying illnesses, or inappropriate therapy—the emergency nurse must become familiar with recommended therapy.

Pathogenesis. DKA results from an inadequate endogenous or exogenous insulin supply. There may be noncompliance with prescribed insulin regimen, or a malfunctioning insulin pump or stress may create an increased demand. Infection, surgery, trauma, myocardial infarction, cerebrovascular accident, pregnancy, pancreatitis, certain drugs, or even emotional stress may provoke DKA.

DKA is distinguished by hyperglycemia, ketonemia, and acidosis. The early phenomenon in pathogenesis is hyperglycemia. Since sugar acts like an osmotic diuretic, there is an excessive loss of water, sodium, and potassium. Hypovolemia with severe electrolyte imbalance ensues. As metabolic aberrations continue, protein and fat are broken down to meet the body's energy requirements, yielding increased plasma aminoacid levels and fatty acid oxidation, respectively, and giving rise to the acidotic state. To make matters worse, hepatic glucose production is triggered, which aggravates the preexisting hyperglycemic state (Fig. 39-4).

Assessment. DKA usually develops over a period of 2 to 3 days. It is seen more frequently in young adults than in other age-groups. It may be the first sign of undiagnosed diabetes mellitus or a complication of known diabetes mellitus. Patients have symptoms of nausea and vomiting, abdominal pain, thirst, polyuria, and drowsiness. In patients with known diabetes, medication compliance and pressure of stressors should be assessed.

Physical findings typically include tachypnea and hyperventilation (Kussmaul breathing, an attempt at respiratory compensation for the metabolic acidosis), tachycardia, flushed, dry skin, and abdominal tenderness. The nurse should be attuned for dehydration in the presence of good urine output, which is suggestive of DKA. Patients may appear dehydrated or hypovolemic, may have an altered level of consciousness, and may have an acetone odor to their breath. The abdominal symptoms may resemble an acute condition of the abdomen.

Rapid determination of blood glucose level in the ED provides an early diagnostic clue. Laboratory data usually demonstrate a blood glucose level greater than 300 mg/dl, pH concentration of less than 7.30, bicarbonate level of less than 14 mEq/L, and ketonemia. In the differential diagnosis, other causes of ketosis and acidosis should be explored. Hyperosmolar hyperglycemic nonketotic coma, alcoholic ketoacidosis, uremia, lactic acidosis, and toxins are other possibilities.

Multiple laboratory studies and diagnostic tests are indicated to evaluate the correct diagnosis, the severity of illness, and the presence of other underlying illness. Bloodwork should include, at minimum, a complete blood cell count and evaluation of blood glucose, electrolyte, blood urea nitrogen, creatinine, and arterial blood gas levels. Other diagnostic tests that should be performed are an electrocardiogram, urinalysis, and radiographs of the chest.

Management. Treatment encompasses volume resuscitation, insulin therapy, correction of electrolyte imbalances, and management of precipitating events. If an insulin pump is being used (Fig. 39-5) it should be turned off.

Fluid volume is usually depleted, and patients require rapid infusion of normal saline solution. The fluid deficit may be several liters, and infusion of 1 L per hour for the first 2 to 3 hours may be necessary. The solution is changed to dextrose 5% and water and half normal saline solution after hypovolemia and hyperglycemia have been addressed.

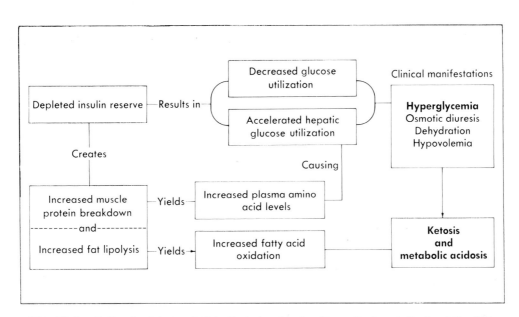

Fig. 39-4 Pathophysiology of diabetic ketoacidosis. (From Barber J, Budassi S: *JEN* 3[3]:9, 1977.)

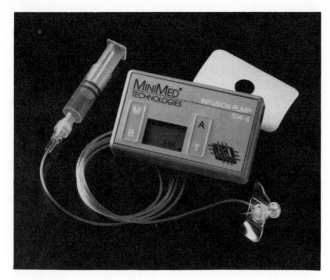

Fig. 39-5 Insulin pump. (From MiniMed Technologies, Inc., Sylmar, Calif.)

Patients must be carefully monitored to determine when hypovolemia has been corrected; urine output, postural vital signs, mental status, pulmonary status, neck veins, and general appearance must be considered. Compromised patients may require central venous pressure or pulmonary artery monitoring.

After fluid replacement has begun, insulin therapy is the next priority. Several alternatives have been proposed to achieve optimum control without complications. The most common approach today is 5 to 10 U regular insulin given IV push (not always used), followed by a continuous infusion of 5 to 10 U/hr regulated by infusion pump. Concentration may vary from 100 U/100 ml to 50 U/500 ml of normal saline solution, depending on hospital policy. Plastic tends to absorb insulin, so it is recommended that the tubing be flushed with the first 50 ml of solution to bind all available sites before starting the infusion. Glucose levels are monitored every hour or two, and the rate of administration is slowed when they approach 200 to 300 mg/dl. Patients should be watched for signs of impending hypoglycemia. Blood glucose levels fall about 75 to 100 mg/dl per hour. Electrolyte values and arterial blood gas levels are also watched closely. Urine samples are tested for sugar and acetone.

Although initial potassium measurements may be high, low, or normal, most patients can be expected to have a deficit. Several factors are influencing potassium levels in DKA. Acidosis drives potassium out of the cell into the extracellular fluid, which may artificially inflate the serum potassium level. However, osmotic diuresis and insulin deficiency result in potassium excretion. As these factors are corrected, the reverse occurs, and profound deficiency is possible unless anticipated. Whenever initial potassium levels are low or normal, replacement should begin as soon as the urine output has been documented. Careful electrocardiographic monitoring should be conducted throughout the period of therapeutic intervention, especially during the first several hours; periodic strips should be saved so that electrocardiographic evidence of hypokalemia or hyperkalemia may be tracked. Potassium levels are also monitored. Low serum sodium, phosphate, or bicarbonate levels may be present, but specific treatment is not generally recommended. The exception is profound metabolic acidosis.

Accurate fluid intake and output measurement is important. If a urinary catheter is needed, it should be removed as soon as possible, since there is high risk for infection. A nasogastric tube may be necessary for some patients. Use of a flowsheet is recommended to facilitate assessment of the multiple physiologic factors that must be assessed over time.

In children it is particularly important to watch mental status, because they are most likely to have the complication of cerebral edema. Cerebral edema develops suddenly 6 to 10 hours after therapy has begun, with rapid deterioration, coma, and respiratory arrest. As yet, there is no effective prevention or treatment, and mortality is about 90%.

Nursing diagnoses. Nursing assessment of these patients may reveal serious problems requiring nursing interventions. Nursing diagnoses include fluid volume deficit, noncompliance, knowledge deficit, pain, and high risk for infection.

Hyperosmolar Hyperglycemic Nonketotic Coma

Hyperosmolar hyperglycemic nonketotic coma (HHNC) is a syndrome caused by combined pancreatic and renal insufficiency in the patient with diabetes. Mortality is high, from 40% to 70%, resulting perhaps from delayed diagnosis, inadequate therapy, or serious associated illnesses.

Pathogenesis. The difference between HHNC and DKA has not been completely established. Systemic stressors seem to trigger HHNC. It may be that more circulating insulin in HHNC inhibits lipolysis, therefore the ketosis seen in DKA, although some HHNC patients are mildly ketotic. Renal insufficiency impairs the ability to excrete glucose, thus causing extremely high glucose levels. Fig. 39-6 delineates the pathophysiology of HHNC.

Common associated conditions include cardiovascular or renal disease, pneumonia, sepsis, gastrointestinal hemorrhage, certain drugs, and stress.

Assessment. HHNC tends to affect older individuals with mild or unknown diabetes mellitus, often those receiving oral hypoglycemic agents. The syndrome develops gradually over 1 to 2 weeks, with polyuria, polydipsia, and dehydration.

Unresponsiveness may be the most frequent reason for transport to an ED, although some patients may be alert or

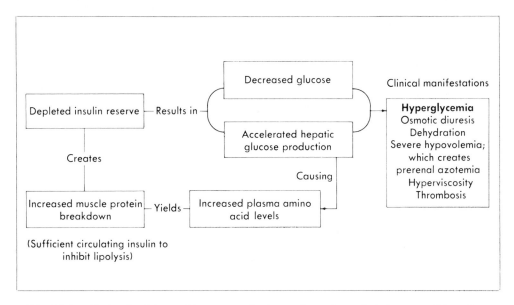

Fig. 39-6 Pathophysiology of hyperosmolar hyperglycemic nonketotic coma. (From Barber J, Budassi S: *JEN* 3[1]:16,1977.)

only mildly confused. Patients may display seizure activity or other neurologic deficits. Respirations are shallow. Dehydration is present but may be difficult to identify on clinical examination in elderly patients.

Laboratory data generally reveal extremely elevated blood glucose levels (greater than 600 mg/dl and up to 2800 mg/dl), plasma osmolarity greater than 350 mOsm/kg, increased sodium, BUN, and creatinine levels, mild ketonemia, and hypokalemia.

Management. In practice the distinction between DKA and HHNC may be difficult to make, but the treatment in any event is quite similar. The goals are fluid volume replacement, correction of the hyperosmolar state and electrolyte imbalances, and management of underlying illnesses.

Treatment of HHNC is begun with normal saline fluid resuscitation. The fluid deficit is usually more severe than in DKA, up to 12 L. Potassium must almost always be replaced, as in DKA. Insulin therapy is less aggressive, and at times insulin may not be necessary.

It is important to identify underlying illness with a workup that includes white blood cell count, radiographic examination of the chest, electrocardiogram, blood and urine cultures, evaluation of serum amylase and liver enzymes, coagulation studies, and cardiac enzyme evaluation as indicated.

Hypoglycemia

Hypoglycemia is the most common cause of coma in patients with diabetes.

Pathogenesis. Glucose intake stimulates the release of insulin from the pancreas to promote glucose utilization and storage. Glycogenolysis and gluconeogenesis supply glucose between meals. Several hormones act to bolster the glucose supply: glucagon and epinephrine act quickly, cortisol and growth hormone more slowly.

Hypoglycemia may be classified into fasting or reactive. Fasting hypoglycemia (4 or more hours after a meal) is the type most seen in emergency care. It results from oversupply of insulin, underproduction of glucose, or the effect of various drugs. The most common cause is insulin induced in the patient with diabetes. Other etiologic factors include misdosage of oral hypoglycemic agents, suicide attempts, alcohol consumption, adrenal insufficiency, hypopituitarism, and surreptitious use to simulate illness. Hypoglycemia may be precipitated by continuing to take one's usual diabetic medication in the face of decreased food intake, increased activity, or illness. Drugs that have been implicated in hypoglycemia include nonsteroidal antiinflammatory agents, clofibrate, salicylates, sulfonamides, phenytoin, rifampin, anabolic steroids, thyroid hormone, probenecid, and propranolol. Infants and children have proportionately smaller glucose stores and are at risk for hypoglycemia.

Assessment. Initial history should concentrate on the diagnosis of diabetes, when the last meal was eaten, dose and time of diabetic medication, recent activities, concurrent illness, and other medications. If the patient is not able to give history, family members, medical records, or a search of patient belongings for medicines or health alerts may provide the missing data. Recognizing hypoglycemia rapidly is important because glucose is necessary for normal central nervous system metabolism: lack of glucose can result in permanent brain damage.

Signs and symptoms may be attributed to the hormonal

responses mobilizing glucose or the central nervous system effects of glycopenia. The sympathetic response created by epinephrine occurs first and causes sweating, tachycardia, restlessness, hunger, and tremulousness. Although persons with diabetes are usually sensitive to these signals, they may be blunted in patients with neuropathy or patients receiving beta-blocking agents. Neuroglycopenic indicators are headache, visual disturbances, psychiatric symptoms, confusion, stupor, coma, seizures, and focal neurologic findings. Hypoglycemia is a great imitator: patients may appear drunk, crazy, or as if they have had a stroke. In infants or children, irritability and lethargy are the most common symptoms.

The diagnosis is made by recognizing the typical clinical symptoms, seeing improvement after glucose administration, and documenting the hypoglycemia. (Diagnostic levels vary, but a guide is less than 35 mg/dl in women and 55 mg/dl in men.)

Management. Many cases of hypoglycemia are managed by paramedics, who administer a dextrose 50% bolus before the patients reach the ED, and patients are already recovering from the crisis. Patients with insulin pumps (Fig. 39-5) should have the pump stopped immediately. Mild symptoms may be managed by oral glucose administration. More serious cases require the establishment of an IV line, and patients receive glucose in the form of 50 ml of 50% dextrose solution given by slow IV push, followed by a continuous infusion. Children are given 25% dextrose solution; neonates, 10% solution. Dextrose can sclerose subcutaneous tissues, so the nurse must be sure that the IV catheter remains in the vein. When possible, before the dextrose is given, blood should be obtained for a rapid blood glucose determination and evaluation of the serum glucose level. Glucagon 1 mg administered intramuscularly is an alternative therapy for some situations. Patients with adrenal insufficiency or those who do not respond well should receive 100 mg of intravenous hydrocortisone.

Because of the risk of brain damage, all patients with altered mental status of unknown cause should have a rapid blood glucose estimate as part of the initial resuscitation. Since recent data indicate that hyperglycemia may also be harmful, dextrose should be reserved for documented hypoglycemia or when rapid blood glucose testing is impossible. Fig. 39-2 outlines management of the comatose patient.

The cause of the episode must be identified, so that a recurrence can be prevented if possible. Interventions include treatment of underlying illness, medication adjustments, life-style adjustments, and patient teaching.

Patients can be discharged after observation if they recover adequately, have a documented normal blood glucose level after discontinuing intravenous glucose therapy, and have eaten a meal and if the cause can be identified. Patients

Table 39-3 Administration and actions of insulins

Type of insulin	Time and route of administration	Time of onset (hours after administration)	Peak action (hours after administration)	Duration of action (hours)
Crystalline zinc* (pH 3-3.5; Zn 0.02-0.04 mg/100 units) (regular)	IV (emergency); subcutaneously (sc) 15-20 min before meals	Rapid, within 1 hour	2-4	6-8
Semilente* (amorphous zinc) (pH 7.2 Zn 0.2-0.25 mg/100 units)	½ to ¾ hour before breakfast; deep sc; never IV	Rapid, within 1 hour	2-4	8-10
Globin zinc (pH 3.4-3.8; Zn 0.25-0.35 mg/100 units)	½ to 1 hour before breakfast; sc	Intermediate rapidity of onset; increases with dose; within 1 to 2 hours	6-8	12-14; also increases with dose
Lente* (combination of 30% Semilente and 70% Ultralente) (pH 7.1-7.4; Zn 0.2-0.25 mg/100 units)	1 hour before breakfast; deep sc; never IV	Intermediate, within 1 to 2 hours	6-8	14-16
NPH (neutral-protamine-Hagedorn) (isophane) (pH 7.1-7.4; Zn 0.016-0.04 mg/100 units)	1 hour before breakfast; sc	Intermediate, within 1 to 2 hours	6-8	12-14
Protamine zinc (pH 7.4; Zn 0.2-0.25 mg/100 units)	1 hour before breakfast; sc	Slow-acting, within 4 to 6 hours	16-20	36-72
Ultralente* (pH 4.8-5.7; Zn 0.2-0.25 mg/100 units)	1 hour before breakfast; deep sc; never IV	Slow-acting, within 4 to 6 hours	8-12	24-36

*Contains no modifying protein (protamine or globin).

with hemodynamic compromise, significant associated illness, new neurologic deficit, intentional overdoses, and oral hypoglycemic overdoses need to be admitted to the hospital. Duration of action of oral hypoglycemic agents ranges from 6 to 72 hours or longer.

Nursing diagnoses. Nursing diagnoses that may be applicable to hypoglycemic patients include high risk for injury, knowledge deficit, noncompliance, altered thought processes, altered cerebral tissue perfusion, and altered nutrition: less than body requirements. Patient education is always indicated, since many patients with diabetes have been shown to have inadequate knowledge about their disease. Table 39-3 reviews the administration and actions of the various insulin products to assist in tailoring teaching to individual patients.

ADRENAL EMERGENCIES
Acute Adrenal Crisis (Insufficiency)

The adrenal hormones are crucial to the maintenance of homeostasis. Acute adrenal crisis, also known as acute adrenal insufficiency or addisonian crisis, presents the emergency care provider with a hemodynamically unstable patient, often without a clearly apparent cause.

Pathogenesis. The adrenal cortex produces two major hormones: cortisol (glucocorticoid) and aldosterone (mineralocorticoid). When the body senses a cortisol deficiency, the hypothalamus secretes corticotropin-releasing factor, stimulating the anterior pituitary gland to secrete adrenocorticotropic hormone (ACTH), which in turn causes the adrenal cortex to produce cortisol. Cortisol enables the body to cope with stress by sustaining the blood glucose level, interacting with catecholamines to strengthen pressor effects in cardiac muscle and arterioles, and enhancing resistance to inflammation, allergy, and toxins. Aldosterone is one component of the renin-angiotensin system. Vasoconstriction causes the kidneys to secrete renin, which is converted to angiotensin I, then angiotensin II, which stimulates the release of aldosterone. Aldosterone acts to preserve fluid volume by promoting kidney conservation of sodium and water; aldosterone secretion also causes potassium excretion and intracellular sequestration.

Adrenal insufficiency may be acute or chronic, primary, secondary, or iatrogenic. Chronic primary adrenal insufficiency, classic Addison's disease, is a result of disease or destruction of the adrenal cortex; both cortisol and aldosterone supplies are inadequate. Most commonly the cause is an idiopathic autoimmune adrenalitis, but other causes include invasion (tumor), infiltration (sarcoidosis, amyloidosis), infection (notably tuberculosis), hemorrhage (sometimes associated with anticoagulant therapy), bilateral adrenalectomies, and certain drugs (mitotane, metyrapone, aminoglutethimide, ketoconazole, and rifampin). Adrenal apoplexy, or bilateral adrenal gland hemorrhage, is seen with septicemia and in newborns. Iatrogenic insufficiency results from the sudden discontinuation of replacement steroid therapy. Finally, adrenal insufficiency may occur subsequent to recent corticosteroid therapy or with known insufficiency and overwhelming stress. Secondary adrenal insufficiency results from impaired functioning of the hypothalamus or pituitary gland, thus reduced secretion of ACTH, thus reduced cortisol secretion. Aldosterone is unaffected. Adrenal crisis refers to the rapid development of signs and symptoms of acute insufficiency. Adrenal crisis may be life threatening, and it should be treated as soon as it is suspected, without waiting for laboratory confirmation.

Assessment. Suggestive historical data include preexisting chronic adrenal insufficiency or present or recent (within the last year) corticosteroid replacement therapy. Crisis precipitants include increased physical or emotional stressors such as infection, trauma, burns, surgery, pregnancy, alcohol withdrawal, myocardial infarction, hypermetabolic states (hyperthyroidism), and certain drugs (hypnotics and general anesthetics).

Objectively the clinical symptoms of adrenal crisis are hypotension, hypovolemia, hyponatremia, hypoglycemia, hyperkalemia, postural responses, shock, fever, abdominal pain, nausea, vomiting, diarrhea, fatigue, and weakness. There may also be evidence of chronic adrenal insufficiency: patients with long-term Addison's disease may exhibit classic mucocutaneous pigmentation on extensor surfaces such as the elbows, knees, and knuckles. These darkened areas may also be noted on the lips, buccal mucosa, and scars. Vitiligo (depigmented skin patches) may be observed. Electrocardiographic abnormalities may include sinus bradycardia or tachycardia, low voltage, low or inverted T waves, prolonged QT interval, or hyperkalemic changes.

Management. Treatment for suspected adrenal crisis should be quickly initiated for all those with obvious risk factors or suggestive clinical symptoms. It should also be routinely considered in those with unexplained or unresponsive hypotension, shock, or sepsis.

Emergency interventions consist of fluid resuscitation and cortisol replacement. While IV lines are being started, blood samples should be drawn for determination of cortisol levels, complete blood cell count, and electrolyte and blood sugar levels. Rapid fluid replacement—up to 3 L in the first few hours—is carried out with the administration of dextrose 5% and normal saline solution, while the patient's response is being monitored carefully. Short-term vasopressor therapy may be needed.

Cortisol is generally replaced in the form of hydrocortisone, first by IV bolus, then by intermittent or continuous infusion. Most of the metabolic and electrolyte abnormalities resolve without further treatment. Aldosterone replacement is not usually necessary immediately, since high-dose cortisol exerts a mineralocorticoid effect. Therapy requires admission to the hospital, usually to an intensive care unit, so that stabilization can be achieved while the search continues for the underlying cause of the crisis.

During treatment of adrenal crisis, patients require close nursing surveillance. Monitoring vital signs and cardiac and hemodynamic monitoring are usually necessary to adequately evaluate the therapeutic response. Fluid intake, urine output, and laboratory values should be carefully monitored.

Nursing diagnoses. In adrenal crisis, the nursing diagnosis of concern is fluid volume deficit (1) and (2) related to abnormal fluid loss. The extracellular fluid volume may be depleted by up to 20% as a result of increased urine output, vomiting, and diarrhea. Fluid replacement is a collaborative intervention.

Patients receiving corticosteroid replacement therapy may have a related knowledge deficit. Patient teaching focuses on the need to take corticosteroids religiously, the importance of tapering when drug use is being discontinued, possible need for additional medication or restarting the drug when the patient is under stress, informing health care providers of past or present treatment, wearing an identifying MedicAlert bracelet or carrying a wallet card, and possibly the use of an emergency corticosteroid injection kit.

THYROID EMERGENCIES

Thyroid emergencies are rare but challenging. Because the thyroid gland controls the body's metabolic rate, thyroid emergencies are characterized by their multisystem manifestations and management approach.

Thyroid activity is initiated by the hypothalamus, which secretes thyrotropin-releasing hormone (TRH). TRH causes the anterior pituitary gland to secrete thyrotropin (TSH) and TSH evokes the release of thyroid hormones from the thyroid gland. Thyroxine is later converted to the bioactive triiodothyronine.

Thyroid disturbances may result in either hyperthyroidism or hypothyroidism. Table 39-4 summarizes the common signs and symptoms of these two entities. The remainder of this section focuses on the emergencies at either end of the spectrum: thyroid storm and myxedema coma.

Thyroid Storm

Thyroid storm is a state of hypermetabolic decompensation that has been described as "a dramatic constellation of symptoms . . . with fever sometimes to hyperthermic levels, severe agitation often with a psychotic component, and tachyarrhythmia sometimes with high-output congestive heart failure."[2] Thyroid storm occurs in a subset of hyperthyroid thyrotoxic patients.

Pathogenesis. There are three major types of hyperthyroidism. The first, true hyperthyroidism, is characterized by an overactive thyroid gland and overproduction of thyroid hormones. In Graves' disease, the most common cause of true hyperthyroidism, thyroid-stimulating immunoglobulins circulate. Other causes include certain tumors and thyroid nodules. In the second type, actually a thyrotoxicosis, there is an increased amount of circulating hormone without over-

activity, which occurs primarily with thyroiditis and with the ingestion of thyroid hormone, either intentionally or unintentionally. Third, drugs, particularly iodine and iodine-containing agents such as amiodarone and lithium, can induce hyperthyroidism.

Thyrotoxicosis does not progress to thyroid storm at a predictable hormone level. More research is needed to establish the true mechanism of thyroid storm, but certain precipitating factors superimposed on preexisting thyrotoxicosis seem to be associated with its onset. These include hospitalization, surgery, trauma, aggressive thyroid gland palpation, thyroid surgery, iodine ingestion, discontinuation of antithyroid medication, stress, pulmonary embolism, cardiovascular accident, infection, DKA, hypoglycemia, toxemia, childbirth, congestive heart failure, and bowel infarction.

Assessment. History-taking should be concentrated on the existence of hyperthyroidism, symptoms suggestive of hyperthyroidism (Table 39-5), precipitating events, and medications.

Development of the storm state is rapid. Signs include a temperature higher than 37.8° C (100° F), disproportionately rapid tachycardia rate for the temperature, central nervous system, cardiovascular, or gastrointestinal system dysfunctions, and other evidence of thyrotoxicosis. The fever may be as high as 41° C (105.8° F); the heart rate in tachycardia may be as rapid as 200 to 300 beats per minute. Central nervous system manifestations include fine tremors, restlessness, anxiety, agitation, labile mood, manic behavior, and psychosis. In addition to the tachycardia, cardiovascular effects include increased stroke volume, systolic blood pressure, and cardiac output; dysrhythmias, including atrial fibrillation and premature ventricular beats; and congestive heart failure. Gastrointestinal disturbances are diarrhea, nausea, vomiting, abdominal cramps, and jaundice.

The diagnosis of thyroid storm is a clinical diagnosis. Laboratory data are not helpful because thyroid hormone levels take too long to be of use to the emergency care provider, and the levels do not differentiate thyroid storm from thyrotoxicosis. Although the condition of this patient is difficult to overlook, it is easy to naively conclude that the individual is a "psych case" from the appearance, behavior, and admixture of complaints if the nurse is not thinking critically about endocrine causes of such symptoms.

Management. Rapid, aggressive therapy is essential. Interventions are directed at fluid resuscitation, reduction of thyroid hormone levels, management of hormone effects, supportive care, and identification of precipitants.

As always, the first priorities in assessment and management are oxygenation and perfusion. Oxygen should be administered and intravenous fluid replacement provided. Hemodynamically significant tachydysrhythmias are usually managed with propranolol. Digoxin and diuretics may be used for cardiac failure.

Table 39-4   Hyperthyroidism and hypothyroidism

Assessment	Subjective	Objective
Hyperthyroidism		
General	Low energy level, labile emotions, weight loss, increased appetite, heat intolerance, insomnia	Cachexia
Skin	Increased sweating	Moist, warm, soft, thin skin; oily, fine, abundant hair; loss of hair at temples; clubbed nails; fingernail separated from base; pretibial myxedema
Neurologic	Restlessness, irritability	Fine tremor of extended fingers and tongue; hyperactive deep tendon reflexes; accelerated speech
Eye, ear, nose, and throat	Diplopia, blurred vision, burning or dry eyes, photophobia, difficulty swallowing	Proptosis; stare; periorbital edema; lid lag; paralysis EOMs; conjunctivitis; corneal ulcerations; diffuse goiter; bruits
Cardiovascular	Palpitations, angina, dyspnea	Tachycardia, PVCs, widened pulse pressure, sharp heart sounds, accentuated precordial thrust, congestive heart failure
Gastrointestinal and genitourinary	Frequent defecation, diarrhea, amenorrhea, shorter menstrual cycle	
Musculoskeletal	Weakness	Decreased muscle strength, especially at shoulders and quadriceps
Hypothyroidism		
General	No energy; weight gain, cold intolerance, sleepiness	Slow speech, obesity, hypothermia, lethargy, puffy appearance
Skin	Rough skin, hair loss	Dry, rough, scaly skin, yellowish skin on palms; dry coarse hair; hair loss, including lateral third of eyebrow; dry, brittle, ridged nails; nonpitting pretibial edema
Neurologic	Personality changes	Nystagmus, delayed deep tendon reflex return phase, slow mentation, ataxia
Eye, ear, nose, and throat	Blurred vision	Hoarse voice, eyelid edema, thick tongue
Cardiovascular	Dyspnea, edema	Enlarged heart, bradycardia, hypertension, pleural or pericardial effusion
Gastrointestinal and genitourinary	Constipation, bloated feeling, menorrhagia, symptoms of urinary tract infection	Megacolon, bladder atony
Musculoskeletal	Cramps	Hypotonia of large muscles, carpal tunnel syndrome

Reduction of thyroid hormone levels is accomplished in the following ways:

1. Antithyroid drugs block the synthesis of thyroid hormones. Propylthiouracil or methimazole (Tapazole) is given orally or via nasogastric tube. Onset of action is within 1 hour; however, enough hormone is stored within the gland to last several weeks.
2. Iodide prevents the release of stored hormones from the thyroid gland. Iodide may be given orally (Lugol's solution) or sodium iodide (1 to 2 g) may be administered by slow IV infusion. Iodide cannot be given until 1 hour after the antithyroid drugs are initiated because unless the antithyroid effect has begun, the iodide may be used to synthesize new hormones.
3. Thyroxine conversion to bioactive triiodothyronine is blocked by the use of propylthiouracil, propranolol, and dexamethasone.

4. In patients who are refractory to the usual treatment, thyroid hormone may be directly removed from the body by peritoneal dialysis, plasmapheresis, or charcoal hemodialysis.

Beta-adrenergic blockade is used to counteract the many thyroid hormone effects, which resemble sympathetic hyperactivity. Propranolol is favored because it also inhibits conversion of thyroxine to bioactive triiodothyronine. A typical regimen is 1 mg/min by slow IV bolus, with 1 to 2 mg repeated every 15 minutes as necessary to a maximum dose of 10 mg every 3 to 4 hours. Careful nursing observation of the therapeutic response is necessary. Alternative drugs include guanethidine, reserpine, atenolol, metoprolol, or esmolol.

Supportive care emphasizes fever control. Acetaminophen may be used, but aspirin is contraindicated (because it increases thyroxine levels). High temperatures should be managed aggressively by use of a cooling blanket or a fan directed at the patient's dampened skin. The patient's nutritional status should be supported by administration of glucose and vitamins. Sedatives should be avoided or used with extreme caution because they mask the patient's mental status and may cause hypoventilation. Patients require critical care after admission.

During ED evaluation and treatment, the existence of a precipitating factor should be carefully explored through history, laboratory data, radiographic evaluation, and physician examination.

Nursing diagnoses. The patient with thyroid storm may demonstrate symptoms that suggest many nursing diagnoses. Nurses should be alert to the possibility of diarrhea, high risk for infection, altered nutrition: less than body requirements, fluid volume deficit (1) and (2), hyperthermia, anxiety, sleep pattern disturbance, altered thought processes, and decreased cardiac output.

Myxedema Coma

Myxedema coma is an extreme version of hypothyroidism that occurs when the body's metabolic rate slows practically to a stop. Although this process may seem innocuous, mortality is as high as 50%.

Pathogenesis. Hypothyroidism may be primary, secondary, or tertiary. Primary failure results from failure of the thyroid gland. Of all patients with hypothyroidism, 95% have primary failure. One common cause is, ironically, the outcome of treatment for Graves' disease with either radioactive iodine or subtotal thyroidectomy, when remaining thyroid tissue atrophies. Another common cause is autoimmune thyroiditis; less common causes are antithyroid drugs (lithium and phenylbutazone), radiation therapy, and infiltrative involvement (tumor, sarcoid, amyloid, or tuberculosis). Secondary disorders refer to pituitary dysfunction resulting in inadequate release of thyroid-stimulating hormone, and tertiary failure occurs when the hypothalamus secretes inadequate thyrotropin-releasing hormone.

Untreated hypothyroidism tends to progress slowly and gradually. Myxedema coma seems to develop when the untreated or undertreated hypothyroid patient is subjected to stress. Precipitants that have been identified are exposure to cold, infection, surgery, trauma, gastrointestinal bleeding, congestive heart failure, cerebrovascular accident, and certain drugs (phenothiazines, narcotics, hypnosedatives, phenytoin, and propranolol).

Assessment. It may be necessary to acquire a history from relatives, friends, medical records, or prehospital providers. Historical clues are symptoms of hypothyroidism (Table 31-5), diagnosed hypothyroidism, previous treatment or surgery for hyperthyroidism, and precipitating factors.

The clinical presentation is captured by the "*hypo*active nine" signs: *hypo*responsiveness, *hypo*ventilation, *hypo*tension, *hypo*(brady)cardia, *hypo*thermia, *hypo*tonia, *hypo*natremia, *hypo*glycemia, and *hypo*adrenalism. Although coma

is the classic presentation, a seizure has been known to herald myxedema crisis. Respiratory failure is a major cause of death; patients are both hypoxemic and hypercarbic. Myocardial contractility, plasma volume, and cardiac output all may be decreased. The most frequent dysrhythmia is sinus bradycardia, but heart block and junctional rhythms may also occur. Electrocardiographic changes may include a low-voltage pattern, widespread ST-T wave changes, or Q-T prolongation. A pericardial effusion, seldom resulting in tamponade, may be present. Patients may be markedly hypothermic; hypothermia is associated with a poor prognosis. Hypotonic gastrointestinal and urinary tracts may be evidenced by ascites, paralytic ileus, megacolon, or urinary retention. Serum sodium levels as low as 110 mEq/L have been reported. Hypoglycemia is rare and tends to signal a secondary hypothyroidism. Both primary and secondary hypothyroidism may be associated with adrenal insufficiency. A thorough head-to-toe examination should be directed at identifying a thyroidectomy scar, signs of hypothyroidism (Table 39-4), or evidence of precipitating factors.

Only tests of thyroid function can confirm the diagnosis of hypothyroidism, but these results are not available in the ED. The diagnosis must be made clinically and should be considered in all patients with unexplained stupor or coma, particularly with associated hypothermia.

Management. The treatment plan incorporates resuscitation, hormone replacement, supportive therapy, and precipitant identification as follows.

Resuscitation. Resuscitation includes intubation, ventilation, oxygenation, and IV volume replacement with crystalloids or colloids or both.

Hormone replacement. Although the choice of hormone is somewhat controversial, many authorities recommend IV thyroxine for immediate treatment of myxedema coma. A dose of 100 to 500 μg is administered slowly. Onset of action occurs in 6 hours. The alternative drug is triiodothyronine.

Supportive therapy. Supportive therapy includes passive rewarming, administration of hydrocortisone, and placement of a nasogastric tube and urinary catheter. Absorption is unpredictable, so all medications should be given IV. Many drugs are metabolized or excreted slowly. Patients may be unresponsive to catecholamines, and pressors may cause dysrhythmias. Hypoglycemia may necessitate dextrose administration. Hyponatremia usually resolves spontaneously.

Search for precipitants. The possibility of infection or other precipitants should be carefully explored, since some of the usual signs (for example, fever, tachypnea, and dysuria) may be obscured in the patient with myxedema.

Evaluation of therapy includes frequent assessment of vital signs, including temperature readings, cardiac monitoring, measurement of arterial blood gases and electrolyte levels, intake and output calculation, and central venous pressure and hemodynamic monitoring.

PHEOCHROMOCYTOMA

Pathogenesis

Pheochromocytoma is caused by catecholamine-secreting tumors. Norepinephrine is more commonly secreted than epinephrine. About 90% of cases of pheochromocytoma occur within the adrenal medulla; 98% are located in the abdomen. Tumors are usually benign, but may be malignant and may metastasize. ED visits are related to signs and symptoms of catecholamine excess.

Clinical signs and symptoms

The combination of hypertension (may be severe, sustained, paroxysmal, or a combination of these) with excessive perspiration, palpitations, and headache is present in virtually all patients. Electrocardiographic abnormalities include sinus tachycardia, premature ventricular contractions, other dysrhythmias, and changes suggestive of ischemia or infarction. Epinephrine-secreting tumors are characterized by hypotension and hypermetabolism. Tumors may appear on a computed tomography scan. Attacks may occur spontaneously or be triggered by trauma, stress, exertion, tyramine-containing foods, or monoamine oxidase–inhibiting drugs.

Therapy

Urgent cases of hypertension are managed by the administration of sodium nitroprusside in a continuous intravenous infusion, with dose titrated to effect. The administration of phentolamine (Regitine) is an alternative: a 1 to 5 mg IV bolus is followed by continuous infusion. Elevate the head of the bed 45 degrees to enhance orthostatic blood pressure reduction. Avoid palpation of the abdomen, which may cause increased catecholamine release. After stabilization, admission, and workup the definitive treatment is usually surgical removal of the tumor.

ACUTE INTERMITTENT PORPHYRIA

Pathogenesis

The porphyrias are a group of inherited metabolic disorders of heme biosynthesis caused by various enzyme defects. Heme precursors, porphyrins, accumulate in the body, especially when accelerated by certain factors. The most common porphyria is acute intermittent porphyria. Acute lead intoxication also produces an acute porphyria.

Clinical signs and symptoms

Acute intermittent porphyria is more common in women and girls and patients of Scandinavian, Anglo-Saxon, and German descent and is characterized by intermittent acute attacks. Precipitants include drugs (barbiturates, chlordiazepoxide, griseofulvin, phenytoin, sulfonamides, sulfonylureas, nonbarbiturate tranquilizers, and probably others), hormones (association with menstruation, oral contraceptives, and pregnancy), infection, and malnutrition. The disturbance has been called "the little imitator."[15] The clinical picture includes abdominal, neurologic, and psychiatric components. Patients may be tachycardic and either hypotensive or hypertensive. The most common symptom is abdominal pain, which may be accompanied by nausea, vomiting, constipation, dilated bowel, fecal impaction, and bladder distention (may mimic an acute abdominal condition). Neurologic abnormalities include muscle weakness, myopathy, cramps, pain, visual disturbances, paresthesias, and seizures. Psychiatric symptoms may further confuse the differential diagnosis. Leukocytosis, hyponatremia, and hypomagnesemia may be present. Urine may appear dark. The result of a Watson-Schwartz test of urine is positive.

Therapy

1. Remove or resolve the precipitant.
2. Manage symptoms with the administration of chlorpromazine, propranolol, pain medication, or a combination of these.
3. Manage seizure with the administration of diazepam.
4. Initiate reversal of aminolevulinic acid synthetase activity with glucose administration.
5. Manage known cases of porphyria with caution and consultation to avoid inducing an attack.

Nursing diagnoses. Nursing diagnoses for patients with myxedema coma may include constipation, urinary retention, high risk for injury, hypothermia, impaired breathing pattern, and decreased cardiac output.

OTHER ENDOCRINE AND METABOLIC DISTURBANCES

The boxes above describe the rare disturbances pheochromocytoma and porphyria.

FLUID AND ELECTROLYTE DISTURBANCES

Fluid and electrolyte disturbances are numerous and complex. While reading the following section, the nurse should keep in mind the following guidelines for management:

1. Maintenance of airway, intravascular volume, and tissue perfusion are always the first priorities in treatment.
2. Clinical assessments must correlate with laboratory findings. When in doubt, perform the test again.
3. Remember that serum levels measure only concentration in intravascular fluid; they are not an absolute measure, and they do not reflect the status of intracellular spaces.
4. In general, treat imbalances at the approximate rate of development.
5. Refer to Table 39-5 for an overview of the often confusing neuromuscular manifestations of electrolyte abnormalities.

Table 39-5 Neuromuscular manifestations of electrolyte abnormalities

	Hypo-kalemia	Hyper-kalemia	Hypo-phospha-temia	Hypo-magne-semia	Hyper-magne-semia	Hypo-calcemia	Hyper-calcemia	Hypo-natremia	Hyper-natremia
Weakness	+ +	+	+ +	+	+	+	+ +	+	+
Paralysis	+	+	−	−	+	−	−	−	−
Myalgias	+	−	+	+	−	+	−	−	+
Fasciculations	+	+	+	+	−	+	−	+	−
Cramps	+	−	−	+	−	+	−	+	+
Restless legs	+	−	−	−	−	−	−	−	−
Tetany	−	−	−	+ *		+	−	−	−
Myotonia	−	+ †	−	−					
Areflexia	+	+	+	−		−	−	−	−
Hyperreflexia	−	+	−	+		+	+	+	+
Choreoathetosis	−	−	−	+		−	−	−	−
Rhabdomyolysis	+	−	+	+ ‡		−	−	+ ¶	+

*Indefinite, may be due to associated hypocalcemia.
†Myotonia may occur in familial hyperkalemic periodic paralysis.
‡Experimental animals (dog, rat) only.
¶Biochemical evidence only (CPK increase, creatinuria).
From Knochel JP: Neuromuscular manifestions of electrolyte disorders, *Am J Med* 72:521, 1982.

Sodium Imbalances

When thinking of sodium imbalances, the old saying, "Where goes sodium, goes water," comes to mind, but this particular reminder is not necessarily true when the body is not functioning normally. It *is* true that sodium imbalances are usually actually water imbalances, but it is *not* true that low fluid volume states are equivalent to low sodium states or vice versa.

Sodium is the major cation in the extracellular fluid and is primarily responsible for the extracellular fluid's osmotic pressure. Normal sodium concentration is approximately 135 to 145 mEq/L. It is important to emphasize that this number represents only the concentration of sodium in plasma: we do not have a measure of the actual amount of sodium in all blood products.

Fluid volume is regulated by the amount of sodium excreted by the kidney. Fluid concentration, on the other hand, is regulated by the amount of water excreted by the kidney. Two hormones are key. Aldosterone causes sodium and water conservation. Antidiuretic hormone (ADH), produced in the hypothalamus and secreted by the pituitary gland, causes water retention. In the absence of resorption stimuli, a dilute urine is excreted. Urine can be excreted with an osmolality ranging from 40 to 1200 mOsm to maintain plasma osmolality within a narrow range.

Sodium is also essential to the "sodium pump," actually the sodium-potassium pump. During depolarization, neuromuscular cell membranes become temporarily permeable and sodium moves into cells, whereas potassium moves out. The sodium pump moves both sodium and potassium back to their original positions during repolarization.

Hyponatremia. Hyponatremia is probably the most common clinical electrolyte abnormality, although it seldom requires emergency management.

Pathogenesis. Hyponatremia is almost always the result of the kidneys failing to excrete sufficient quantities of dilute urine: when water is retained, the relative concentration of sodium decreases and hyponatremia results. This situation may occur during hypovolemic, euvolemic, or hypervolemic fluid states.

A fluid volume deficit may cause the kidney to conserve more water than sodium; fluid losses may be renal (diuretics, glycosuria, mineralocorticoid deficiency, renal disease), extrarenal (gastrointestinal, third space [pancreatitis or peritonitis], or skin [burns or increased sweating]). Excess total body water is the most common cause and most commonly results from the syndrome of inappropriate secretion of ADH (SIADH). In this syndrome ADH is secreted unnecessarily, concentrated urine is excreted, water is conserved, and sodium concentration decreases. SIADH is associated with malignancies, pulmonary disease, and central nervous system disorders. Other causes of total body water excess are hypothyroidism, adrenal insufficiency, psychogenic polydipsia, even, rarely, the ingestion of large quantities of beer (beer potomania).[8] The volume excess may be limited to the extracellular fluid. Edema may be caused by kidney disease, cardiac failure, or cirrhosis. Fluid is sequestered in the interstitial spaces and venous system, the kidneys receive a decreased volume to filter, and they respond to this apparent volume deficit by conserving water. Last, osmotically active substances such as glucose, mannitol, sorbitol, ethanol, and glycerol may draw water from the cells into the intravascular space.

Assessment. Signs and symptoms of hyponatremia are vague, so the diagnosis can seldom be made on clinical examination. Clinical manifestations seem to result from decreased osmolarity and cerebral edema. At serum sodium levels below 120 mEq/L, patients may evidence anorexia, nausea, weakness, confusion, agitation, and disorientation. At levels below 110 mEq/L, seizure activity, coma, or death may result.

Patients should also be assessed for information concerning the causes of the hyponatremia. Health history and medication use are elicited. Edema or hypovolemia may be obvious. Intake and output assessment should be instituted. Laboratory data may supply the diagnosis, as well as the cause. In addition to the measurement of serum sodium levels, blood tests that should be collected include evaluations of other electrolytes, blood urea nitrogen, creatinine, glucose, and osmolality. Routine urinalysis and urine electrolyte and urine osmolality values should also be obtained.

Management. Mild hyponatremia does not require treatment. Treatment plans for symptomatic states are based on each patient's condition and fluid volume status, and the cause. In most cases the treatment is to correct the water imbalance, not to replace sodium. Hypovolemia is managed with the intravenous administration of normal saline solution. Patients with fluid volume excess are placed on a regimen of fluid restrictions.

Only in severe symptomatic hyponatremia is sodium replacement recommended. The best method of replacing sodium has yet to be established. Drawbacks of treatment include overreplacement, fluid volume overload, and the development of central pontine myelinolysis. Hypertonic (3%) saline solution is administered cautiously, and the patient is monitored carefully. An infusion pump should be used, and small volumes only should be hung. Furosemide (Lasix) may be administered to reduce the likelihood of overload. Resulting potassium losses must be replaced. Sodium concentration must be checked hourly. Patients must be admitted to an intensive care unit.

Nursing diagnoses. Patients with hyponatremia may have fluid volume deficit (1) and (2), fluid volume excess, high risk for injury, or altered thought processes.

Hypernatremia

Pathogenesis. Infants, elderly individuals, and debilitated patients are at risk for hypernatremia. The imbalance results from inadequate intake of water or occasionally from excessive sodium intake. Risk groups are unable to independently replace lost fluids. As with hyponatremia, patients may be hypovolemic, euvolemic, or hypervolemic. In certain hypovolemic states, sodium is lost but water loss is greater. These patients may have renal losses via osmotic diuresis (mannitol, glucose, or urea) or extrarenal losses sustained by excess sweating or diarrhea in children. The use of activated charcoal and cathartics for drug overdose has also been reported to result in hypovolemic hypernatremia.[4] In other cases patients may initially be euvolemic, but unreplaced water loss causes hypernatremia. Extrarenal losses include respiratory and skin losses exaggerated by fever, infection, burns, or skin diseases. Renal losses are often caused by diabetes insipidus, in which there is an absence of ADH secretion or the kidney fails to respond to ADH, and large volumes of dilute urine are excreted. The only category in which sodium is actually increased is hypervolemic hypernatremia. In response to increased sodium, the extracellular fluid volume expands and the intracellular volume is reduced. This situation is usually a result of exogenous sodium intake, for example, the overadministration of sodium bicarbonate during resuscitations after cardiac arrest.

Assessment. Signs and symptoms may be similar to those of hyponatremia, although in this case they are caused by hyperosmolarity and cellular dehydration. History of health problems, recent illnesses, fluid intake, and medications should be obtained. Patients are usually thirsty and may appear dehydrated. Early symptoms include anorexia, nausea, and vomiting. When the sodium concentration rises to 160 mEq/L, neurologic symptoms predominate. Agitation, irritability, lethargy, coma, muscle twitching, and hyperreflexia may occur. Intracranial hemorrhages may result from shrunken brain tissue volume or engorged vasculature.

Because the clinical signs and symptoms are so nonspecific, the diagnosis often depends on the return of laboratory data. Laboratory tests should include determinations of electrolyte levels, renal function, glucose levels, urine electrolyte levels, and urine osmolality.

Management. Treatment is focused on restoring a normal body balance of fluid volume and osmolarity and correcting the underlying cause. Fluid replacement is the rule. Patients with unstable hypovolemia initially require the administration of normal saline solution in spite of their hypernatremia, followed by the administration of 0.45 saline solution. Patients with pure water loss receive either oral hydration or intravenous replacement with D_5W or hypotonic saline. Patients with sodium excess receive D_5W and furosemide (Lasix). In all cases slow correction of the imbalance is the goal, since rapid correction may result in neurologic deterioration, cerebral edema, and seizures.

Frequent surveillance of fluid intake and output, sodium values, specific gravity of urine, and mental status is important for these potentially critically ill patients, in whom the mortality may be as high as 75%.

Nursing diagnoses. Nursing diagnoses that may be identified include diarrhea, impaired physical mobility, altered nutrition: less than body requirements, high risk for injury, fluid volume deficit (1) and (2), and high risk for fluid volume deficit, fluid volume excess, impaired skin integrity, and knowledge deficit. Since hypernatremia is almost always preventable, patient and family teaching and attention to adequate fluid intake are especially important interventions.

Potassium Imbalances

Potassium is the most abundant cation in the body and in the intracellular fluid. Potassium is located almost entirely (98%) within the cells; only 2% is contained in the extracellular fluid. A serum potassium value (normal is approximately 3.5 to 5 mEq/L) measures only the extracellular 2% and does not necessarily reflect the potassium supply within the cell. However, it is the ratio between the intracellular and extracellular potassium that is most important, rather than any single number. Changes in extracellular fluid levels have the greatest effect on the ratio.

Potassium is the chief determinant of cell membrane potential and the counterpart to sodium in the sodium-potassium pump. Potassium also governs cell osmolality and cell volume. Potassium imbalances are most obvious when they affect electrically excitable nerve and muscle cells.

Potassium is subject to multiple influences within the body. Alkalosis, aldosterone, insulin, and beta-2 agonists all act to drive potassium from the extracellular fluid into the cell. Acidotic and hyperosmolar states cause potassium to leave the cell. Alkalosis, aldosterone, and hyperosmolarity cause increased renal excretion. When aldosterone causes sodium conservation, potassium is excreted instead, resulting in the common association between hypernatremia and hypokalemia.

Hypokalemia. In general a serum potassium value between 3.5 and 3 mEq/L is considered indicative of mild hypokalemia. The serum potassium value in moderate hypokalemia ranges from 2.5 to 3 mEq/L. Severe, life-threatening levels are those below 2.5 mEq/L or any level accompanied by pronounced clinical effects.

Pathogenesis. Hypokalemia usually results from either increased potassium losses from the body or shifts of potassium from the extracellular fluid into the cells. Sources of increased loss include the skin, gastrointestinal tract, and kidneys. Losses from the skin are increased with burns and increased sweating (sweat may contain up to 9 mEq/L potassium). Gastrointestinal losses are a common cause of potassium depletion: vomiting, nasogastric suction, diarrhea, ileostomy, malabsorption, and laxative abuse have all been implicated. Renal losses have many possible precipitants, including the single most common cause, diuretics. Other precipitants are hyperaldosteronism, osmotic diuretics, drug-induced potassium wasting, and renal disease. Cellular shifts may occur in response to alkalosis, insulin, and beta-2 agonists. Beta-2 agonists number endogenous and exogenous catecholamines, including epinephrine, albuterol, and terbutaline.

Assessment. The routine triage history may uncover many clues suggestive of hypokalemia. Patients who take diuretics or have a gastrointestinal disturbance and are feeling "weak" should inspire electrolyte testing.

The most common manifestations of hypokalemia are neuromuscular. Muscular weakness is seen and is usually more pronounced in lower extremities and proximal muscle groups. Respiratory muscle weakness may cause respiratory failure, even arrest. Postural hypotension and ileus may be present. Patients may also have tetany, cramps, myalgias, paresthesias, "restless legs," and rhabdomyolysis.

Electrocardiographic changes, dysrhythmias, and conduction defects occur, although they are not well correlated with the degree of deficit. Classic changes are U waves, flattened or inverted T waves, and depressed ST segments (Fig. 39-7). Ventricular ectopy is the most common dysrhythmia, and patients often report "palpitations."

Management. Hypokalemia is treated by replacing the depleted potassium supply in a manner consistent with the severity of the deficit. Potassium chloride is usually the preparation of choice. Mild deficits are replaced orally. More severe deficits, symptomatic deficits, or patients on a regimen of digitalis who have angina, myocardial infarction, DKA, or liver failure are treated with IV replacement. Depending on the patient's clinical situation and hospital protocols the rate of replacement may range from 5 to 20 mEq/

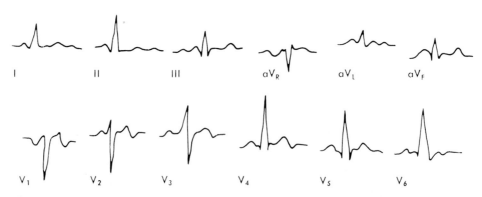

Fig. 39-7   Patient with serum potassium level of 2.7 mEq/L. Hypokalemia is characterized by broadened T waves in limb leads with U waves most prominent in anterior precordial leads. (From *Principles and techniques of critical care,* Kalamazoo, Mich, 1976, The Upjohn Co.)

hr for mild to moderate cases, and from 20 to 60 mEq/hr for severe to life-threatening situations.

Extreme caution and continuous cardiac monitoring with sequential electrocardiogram strips are necessary for replacement rates above 20 mEq/hr. An infusion pump should be used, and a small amount of potassium (no more than 80 mEq) should be mixed at one time. Because of the danger of converting hypokalemia to hyperkalemia, potassium levels should be monitored every hour or two. As a rough guide, keep in mind that 40 mEq raises the serum potassium approximately 1 mEq/L.

Since potassium can be irritating to veins, the concentration for peripheral IV lines should be no higher than 80 mEq/250 ml and the rate of administration no faster than 40 mEq/hr.

Nursing diagnoses. Nursing assessment of hypokalemic patients may reveal diarrhea, noncompliance or knowledge deficit related to use of potassium supplements, impaired skin integrity, or impaired breathing pattern.

Hyperkalemia. Hyperkalemia is considered mild when the levels are between 5 and 6.5 mEq/L and electrocardiographic changes are minimal. Severe, life-threatening hyperkalemia is present when levels are above 7 mEq/L or marked clinical manifestations exist.

Pathogenesis. Hyperkalemia results from increased fluid intake, decreased excretion, or shifts of potassium from the cell into the ECF. Drugs, especially potassium supplements, potassium-sparing diuretics, and iatrogenic potassium overinfusion, may account for up to one third of all hyperkalemic episodes. Decreased excretion is usually caused by renal disease or mineralocorticoid deficiency. Transcellular shifts may result from tissue injury (burns or crush injuries, rhabdomyolysis, hemolysis, or tumor lysis), acidosis, hyperosmolarity, or drug effects (succinylcholine, alpha-adrenergic agents, or digitalis toxicity).

Assessment. The diagnosis of hyperkalemia is most likely to be made by recognition of typical electrocardiographic changes or return of laboratory data. As with hypokalemia, patients have both cardiac and neuromuscular symptomatology but in this instance the cardiac manifestations are more prominent. Electrocardiographic changes (Fig. 39-8) correlate fairly well with severity. Changes progress from the classic, tall, peaked T waves (around 7 mEq/L), through widened QRS complexes, prolonged PR intervals, disappearance of P waves, and distinctive "sine wave" or biphasic tracing (about 9 to 10 mEq/L), and culminate in ventricular fibrillation. Dysrhythmias include sinus bradycardia, sinus arrest, first-degree heart block, nodal rhythm, idioventricular rhythm, and ventricular fibrillation. Rarely, asystole may be the first dramatic presentation.

Neuromuscular symptoms tend to emerge above a level of 6.5 mEq/L and are similar to those that occur with hypokalemia.

Management. Therapeutic interventions are selected according to the severity of the imbalance.

In less severe cases (unsymptomatic or demonstrating only peaked T waves, potassium level less than 7 mEq/L) therapeutic intervention includes the following:

1. Stop the use of potassium-containing substances or drugs that inhibit excretion; restrict dietary potassium.
2. Administer diuretics to increase excretion.
3. Administer sodium polystyrene sulfonate (Kayexalate) cation exchange resin, which removes potassium by exchange with sodium, lowers potassium approximately 1 mEq per gram administered, and takes 1 to 2 hours to act.

In more severe cases, one or all of the following more aggressive interventions may be added:

1. Administer calcium gluconate, which stabilizes the cell membrane: administer 5 to 10 ml of 10% solution IV push over a period of 1 to 2 minutes; may repeat at 2- to 5-minute intervals up to three doses; give in separate IV line from sodium bicarbonate; most rapid onset occurs at 1 to 2 minutes; lasts only 30 to 60

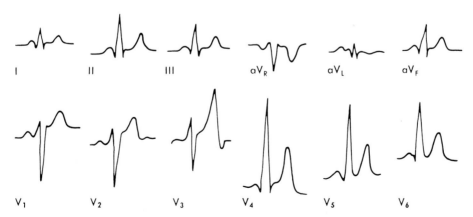

Fig. 39-8   Patient with serum potassium level of 7.5 mEq/L. Hyperkalemia is characterized by tall, peaked T waves, seen best in precordial leads. (From *Principles and techniques of critical care,* Kalamazoo, Mich, 1976, The Upjohn Co.)

minutes; use with extreme caution in digitalized patients.

2. Administer sodium bicarbonate, which drives potassium into cells: administer 50 mEq (1 ampule) IV push over a period of 5 minutes, may repeat once, may follow with infusion; give in separate IV line from calcium gluconate; onset occurs at 5 minutes; duration is 1 to 2 hours.

3. Administer insulin and glucose: insulin drives potassium into cells; glucose prevents hypoglycemia; may give 50% dextrose (50 to 100 ml) and regular insulin (5 to 20 U) IV push or regular insulin (10 to 20 U) in $D_{10}W$ 500 ml by infusion pump over a period of 1 hour; onset occurs in 30 minutes; duration is 4 to 6 hours.

4. Administer albuterol, which drives potassium into cells; new therapy[1]; useful with renal dialysis patients or when fluid limitations are operative; give 10 to 20 mg via nebulizer; onset occurs in 30 minutes; duration is 2 hours.

5. Hemodialysis is used in cases of renal failure and in extremely severe cases.

6. Pacemakers provide external or transvenous pacing for bradydysrhythmias unresponsive to pharmacologic treatment.

7. Administer hydrocortisone for Addison's disease; suspect Addison's disease if postural hypotension is present; administer 100 mg IV push combined with fluid resuscitation.

Obviously, patients must be continually monitored during the period of acute intervention. Electrocardiograms, vital signs, drug and IV fluid administration, and potassium levels must all be attended to vigilantly.

Nursing diagnoses. Impaired skin integrity, decreased cardiac output, anxiety, and altered patterns of urinary elimination are examples of nursing diagnoses that may be appropriate for particular patients with hyperkalemia.

Calcium Imbalances

The more that is learned about calcium, the more pivotal appears its role in regulating cellular activities. Calcium is essential to membrane polarization and depolarization, action potential generation, neurotransmission, and muscle contraction. The so-called calcium channel exists in myocardial cells and allows for transmembrane transport of calcium.

After calcium is ingested in the diet, 99% of it is stored in bone and the remaining 1% circulates in the intracellular and extracellular fluid. Bone serves as a calcium reservoir; when necessary, parathyroid hormone is secreted by the parathyroid glands to increase calcium release from the skeleton. Parathyroid hormone also enhances calcium reabsorption in the kidney and facilitates calcitriol production. Calcitriol, the active form of vitamin D, fosters calcium absorption in the gut and osteoclastic activity. Calcitonin,

a hormone produced in the thyroid gland, causes increased calcium to be deposited in the bone.

Plasma calcium exists in three forms: protein-bound, complexed, and ionized. Total serum calcium concentration is normally 8.5 to 10.5 mg/dl. Ionized calcium is the only physiologically active form and should be measured whenever possible; its normal range is 4.2 to 4.8 mg/dl. A given calcium value must always be considered in association with a patient's albumin value; since protein binds calcium, hypoalbuminemia will result in less protein-bound calcium and a higher serum calcium concentration and vice versa.

Hypocalcemia

Pathogenesis. Hypocalcemia generally results from a lack of parathyroid hormone or vitamin D. Specific causes are many; they include parathyroid or thyroid disorders, magnesium deficiency, multiple blood transfusions, alkalosis, pancreatitis, gastrointestinal or nutritional dysfunction, kidney disease, trauma, shock, sepsis, and certain drugs. In hypocalcemia the nervous system becomes increasingly excitable. Peripheral nerve fibers begin to discharge spontaneously, eliciting skeletal muscle contraction (tetany). Only clinically significant ionized calcium deficiency requires emergency treatment.

Assessment. Subjective data collection for this patient should include the existence of any of the conditions likely to result in hypocalcemia.

Signs of neuromuscular irritability are apparent. The most specific is a positive Trousseau's sign, carpopedal spasm within 3 minutes after inflation of a blood pressure cuff to a level between systolic and diastolic pressure. A positive Chvostek's sign may also be present (muscle contraction when the facial nerve is tapped immediately anterior to the ear). Other manifestations include muscle twitching and cramping; facial grimacing; numbness and tingling of fingers, toes, nose, lips, and earlobes; hyperactive deep tendon reflexes; and abdominal pain. The electrocardiogram may demonstrate a prolonged QT interval (Fig. 39-9), although this result does not correlate well with severity. More serious symptoms include laryngospasm, bronchospasm, seizures, and cardiac failure. Patients may appear anxious, irritable, or even psychotic. A neck surgery scar is helpful in suggesting the possibility of hypocalcemia.

Management. Emergency intervention is easily managed by IV calcium replacement. One to two ampules of 10% calcium gluconate mixed in D_5W is administered over a period of 10 to 20 minutes. With severe deficits, a continuous IV infusion may be necessary after this intervention. Calcium levels, cardiac rhythm, and blood pressure must be carefully monitored while calcium is being administered. An associated magnesium deficiency is possible and should be corrected.

Nursing diagnoses. Nursing diagnoses that may be applicable to these patients include decreased cardiac output, anxiety, high risk for injury, and impaired physical mobility.

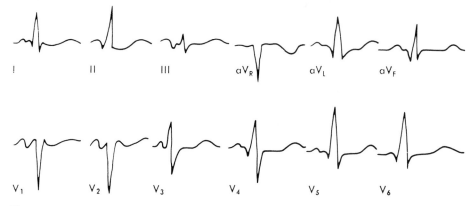

Fig. 39-9 Hypocalcemia. Lengthened QT interval is evident. (From *Principles and techniques of critical care,* Kalamazoo, Mich, 1976, The Upjohn Co.)

Hypercalcemia

Pathogenesis. Hypercalcemia results when calcium accumulates in the blood faster than it can be excreted by the kidneys and results from increased bone resorption, increased calcium absorption, or decreased calcium excretion. Four conditions are most likely to put patients at risk for hypercalcemia: malignancy, primary hyperparathyroidism, immobility, and thiazide diuretic use. Cancer, particularly breast and lung cancer, may precipitate hypercalcemia either through metastases invading bone, ectopic parathyroid hormone production, or secretion of a bone-resorbing substance. Primary hyperparathyroidism is usually caused by an adenoma of the parathyroid glands. Immobility predisposes patients to an increased rate of bone breakdown. Thiazide diuretics have a direct hypercalcemic effect and also potentiate parathyroid hormone. Rarely hypercalcemia may be unintentionally self-induced via ingestion of calcium-containing antacids (milk alkali syndrome).[11]

High ionized calcium levels stabilize cell membranes and suppress nerve conduction. These effects result in depressed functioning of the nervous system. The renal, gastrointestinal, and cardiovascular systems are also affected.

Assessment. Health history and use of medications may be indicative of the causes of hypercalcemia. Symptoms are nonspecific. Patients may have headache, irritability, fatigue, malaise, difficulty concentrating, anorexia, nausea, vomiting, and constipation.

The objective data may be no more helpful; consequently hypercalcemia is often diagnosed as a result of laboratory tests. The neurologic effects are often the primary symptoms. They include lethargy, confusion, and a depressed level of consciousness. Deep tendon reflexes may be depressed. At times the QT interval on the electrocardiogram will be shortened. Patients demonstrate polyuria and polydipsia and may be dehydrated. Ileus may develop. A mastectomy scar or other evidence of malignancy may be apparent.

Chronic hypercalcemia may be associated with renal lithi-asis, peptic ulcers, and pancreatitis. Patients may display band keratopathy and calcium deposits located at the junction of the sclera and the cornea that resemble parentheses.

Management. When serum calcium concentration exceeds 14 to 15 mg/dl, hypocalcemia must be treated as a medical emergency. The most common intervention in the emergency setting is fluid volume expansion and saline diuresis. First, patients are rehydrated with 1 to 2 L of normal saline solution (increases glomerular filtration rate and decreases calcium reabsorption). Continued rapid infusion of saline solution is then combined with IV furosemide administration to achieve a vigorous diuresis of at least 200 ml/hr (increases excretion, blocks reabsorption). The obvious risks of this treatment are fluid overload and congestive heart failure. Patients should be carefully evaluated before therapy is initiated, and they must be monitored intensively during treatment. Central venous pressure monitoring or invasive monitoring is needed. Fluid intake and output must be meticulously managed. Hypomagnesemia and hypokalemia are likely to result and should be treated.

Depending on the clinical situation, other therapeutic options are available. They include the following:

1. Administration of glucocorticoids, which decrease intestinal calcium absorption and increase urinary excretion; used in conjunction with other therapies; effects take days
2. Administration of mithramycin or plicamycin, which inhibits bone resorption; may be toxic; effects take 48 hours
3. Administration of calcitonin, which inhibits bone resorption; mild hypocalcemic; resistance develops
4. Administration of phosphate, which inhibits bone resorption; administered orally
5. Administration of diphosphonates, which inhibit bone resorption; alternative drugs for malignancy-related hypercalcemia
6. Administration of ethylenediamine tetraacetic acid

Table 39-6 Magnesium imbalances*

Imbalance	Factors that increase risk	Clinical signs and symptoms	Therapy
Hypomagnesemia	Alcoholism; chronic diarrhea; diuretic therapy; digoxin therapy; ketoacidosis	Chvostek's sign; hyperactive deep tendon reflexes; tetany; seizures; dysrhythmias; digoxin toxicity (increased susceptibility); hypokalemia; hypocalcemia Magnesium deficiency may be present even when magnesium level is normal.	Depends on severity of symptoms; MgSO$_4$ 2-3 g (10-15 ml of 20% solution) IV over a period of 1 min if needed, followed by continuous infusion; assess respiratory rate, cardiac rhythm, deep tendon reflexes, fluid intake and output, and serum magnesium concentration; absence of patellar reflex is early warning of toxicity
Hypermagnesemia	Acute renal failure; renal insufficiency combined with increased magnesium intake; massive ingestion; iatrogenic factors	Hypotension; asystole; heart block; respiratory failure; muscular weakness or paralysis; loss of deep tendon reflexes; lethargy; hypocalcemia	Depends on severity of symptoms; maintain ventilation and perfusion; administer CaCl 100-200 mg every 3-5 min until symptoms are reversed, followed by continuous infusion; saline diuresis and furosemide may also be used; hemodialysis in most severe cases; monitor vital signs, serum magnesium concentration, deep tendon reflexes

*Normal serum magnesium concentration is approximately 1.4 to 2 mEq/L or 0.6 to 1.2 mmol/L.

Table 39-7 Fluid imbalances

Imbalance	Clinical signs and symptoms	Therapy	Precursors
Dehydration	Thirst, anxiety, weight loss, poor skin turgor, slow vein filling, elevated temperature, tachycardia, dry mucous membranes, decreased level of consciousness, increased hematocrit, increased level of blood urea nitrogen, increased red blood cell concentration	Volume replacement	Any condition in which water output exceeds intake; vomiting, diarrhea
Edema	Weight gain exceeding 5%; rales; dyspnea; puffy eyelids, swollen ankles, and so on; bounding pulse	Salt-poor albumin, exchange resins, diuretics	Protein deficiency, venous obstruction, heart failure, obstructed lymphatic system, toxin ingestion, liver disease, renal disease
Third space syndrome	Hypotension, tachycardia, peripheral vasoconstriction, oliguria, no weight loss, increased hematocrit with no evidence of fluid loss	Plasma, salts, water replacement, diuretics, paracentesis, thoracentesis	Ascites, cellulitis, crush injuries, vascular occlusion, intestinal obstructions

(EDTA), which chelates ionized calcium; used only for life-threatening states; may produce renal damage
7. Dialysis; used as a temporizing measure
8. Surgery; used for parathyroid adenoma or carcinoma

Nursing diagnoses. Nursing diagnoses associated with the medical diagnosis of hypercalcemia may be fluid volume deficit (1) and (2), altered thought processes, constipation, and fatigue.

OTHER FLUID AND ELECTROLYTE IMBALANCES

See Table 39-6 for an overview of magnesium imbalances. Table 39-7 reviews the fluid imbalances of dehydration, edema, and third space syndrome.

REFERENCES

1. Allon M, Dunlay R, and Copkney C: Nebulized albuterol for acute hyperkalemia in patients on hemodialysis, *Ann Intern Med* 110:426, 1989.

2. Bagdade JD: Endocrine emergencies, *Med Clin North Am* 70:1111, 1986.

3. Browning RG et al: 50% dextrose: antidote or toxin? *J Emerg Nurs* 16:342, 1990.

4. Caldwell JW, Nava AJ, de Haas DD: Hypernatremia associated with cathartics in overdose management, *West J Med* 147:593, 1987.

5. Cyr MG, Wartman SA: The effectiveness of routine screening questions in the detection of alcoholism, *JAMA* 259:51, 1988.

6. Gerberich SG et al: Analyses of the relationship between blood alcohol and nasal breath alcohol concentrations: implications for assessment of trauma cases, *J Trauma* 29:338, 1989.

7. Jezierski M: Drunk driving fatalities for teenagers: emergency nurses do something besides talk about it, *J Emerg Nurs* 16:172, 1990.

8. Joyce SM, Potter R: Beer potomania: an unusual cause of symptomatic hyponatremia, *Ann Emerg Med* 15:745, 1986.

9. Lenehan GP, Gastfriend DR, Stetler C: Use of haloperidol in the management of agitated or violent, alcohol intoxicated patients in the emergency department: a pilot study, *J Emerg Nurs* 11:72, 1985.

10. Mayfield D, McLeod D, Hall P: The CAGE questionnaire: validation of a new alcoholism screening instrument, *Am J Psychiatry* 131:1121, 1974.

11. Orwoll ES: The milk-alkali syndrome: current concepts, *Ann Intern Med* 97:242, 1982.

12. Simel DL, Feussner JR: Blood alcohol measurements in the emergency department: who needs them? *Am J Pub Health* 78:1478, 1988.

13. Torvik A et al: Brain lesions in alcoholics: a neuropathological study with clinical correlation, *J Neurol Sci* 56:233, 1982.

14. Tweed SH: Identifying the alcoholic client, *Nurs Clin North Am* 24(1):13, 1989.

15. Waldenstrom J: Neurological symptoms caused by so-called acute porphyria, *Acta Psychiatr Scand* 14:375, 1939.

16. Walsh ME, Macleod DAD: Breath alcohol analysis in the accident and emergency department, *Injury* 15:62, 1983.

17. West LJ, moderator: Alcoholism, *Ann Intern Med* 100:405, 1984.

SUGGESTED READINGS

Ansbaugh P: Emergency management of intoxicated patients with head injuries, *J Emerg Nurs* 3(3):9, 1977.

Bidani A: Electrolyte and acid-base disorders, *Med Clin North Am* 70:1013, 1986.

Budassi SA: Wernicke's encephalopathy and Korsakoff's psychosis, *J Emerg Nurs* 8:295, 1982.

Camuñas C: Pheochromocytoma, *Am J Nurs* 83:887, 1983.

Chambers J, ed: Common fluid and electrolyte disorders, *Nurs Clin North Am* 22:749, 1987.

Daniels GH: Metabolic and endocrine emergencies, In Wilkins EW, ed: *Emergency medicine,* ed 3, Baltimore, 1989, Williams & Wilkins.

Estes NJ, Smith-DiJulio K, Heinemann ME: *Nursing diagnosis of the alcoholic person,* St Louis, 1980, Mosby–Year Book.

Franaszek J, ed: Fluid and electrolytes in trauma, *Trauma Quart* 2(3):1, 1983.

George JE, Quattrone MS: The intoxicated ED patient: a case report, *J Emerg Nurs* 15:444, 1989.

Gerard SK, Hernandez C, Khayam-Bashi H: Extreme hypermagnesemia caused by an overdose of magnesium-containing cathartics, *Ann Emerg Med* 17:728, 1988.

Goldfinger TM, Schaber D: A comparison of blood alcohol concentration using non-alcohol- and alcohol-containing skin antiseptics, *Ann Emerg Med* 11:665, 1982.

Guthrie SK: The treatment of alcohol withdrawal, *Pharmacotherapy* 9:131, 1989.

Halpern AA: Calcium supplements, *J Emerg Nurs* 12:313, 1986.

Halpern JS: Effects of ethanol in trauma, *J Emerg Nurs* 8:261, 1982.

Halpern JS, Davis JW: Use and abuse of alcohol: further perspectives, *J Emerg Nurs* 9:49, 1983.

Hamburger S, Rush D: Endocrine and metabolic emergencies, Bowie, Md, 1984, Robert J Brady.

Hurxthal K: Quick! Teach this patient about insulin, *Am J Nurs* 88:1097, 1988.

Isley WL, Hamburger SC, eds: Endocrine and metabolic crises, *Crit Care Nurs Quart* 13(3):1, 1990.

Jones J et al: Cathartic-induced magnesium toxicity during overdose management, *Ann Emerg Med* 15:1214, 1986.

Jordan RM, Kammer H, Riddle MR: Sulfonylurea-induced factitious hypoglycemia, *Arch Intern Med* 137:390, 1977.

Kent RA: An adult diabetic man with a depressed sensorium, *J Emerg Nurs* 13:186, 1987.

Kirk E, Bradford LT: Effects of alcohol on the central nervous system: implications for the neuroscience nurse, *J Neurosci Nurs* 19:326, 1987.

Knochel JP: Neuromuscular manifestations of electrolyte disorders, *Am J Med* 72:521, 1982.

Marx JA, ed: Alcoholic emergencies, *Top Emerg Med* 6(2):1, 1984.

McElmeel EF, DiDente P: Alcohol withdrawal, *Nurse Pract* 5(1):18, 1980.

McElroy C: Alcohol withdrawal syndromes, *J Emerg Nurs* 7:195, 1981.

McFadden EA, Zaloga GP, Chernow B: Hypocalcemia: a medical emergency, *Am J Nurs* 83:227, 1983.

O'Connor LJ: Acute intermittent porphyria, *Am J Nurs* 81:1184, 1981.

Pointer JE: Glucose analysis: indications for ordering and alternatives to the laboratory, *Ann Emerg Med* 15:372, 1986.

Ragland G: Endocrine emergencies. In Tintinalli JE, Rothstein RJ, Krome RL, eds: *Emergency medicine,* New York, 1985, McGraw-Hill.

Ripley JB: A 39-year-old man with fatal alcohol withdrawal seizures, *J Emerg Nurs* 16:67, 1990.

Roberge R et al: Psychogenic polydipsia: an unusual cause of hyponatremic coma and seizure, *Ann Emerg Med* 13:274, 1984.

Schwartz MW: Potassium imbalances, *Am J Nurs* 87:1292, 1987.

Sheehy SB: Metabolic and endocrine emergencies, *J Emerg Nurs* 11:49, 1985.

Stapczynski JS, Haskell RJ: Duration of hypoglycemia and need for intravenous glucose following intentional overdoses of insulin, *Ann Emerg Med* 13:505, 1984.

Surawicz B, Mangiardi ML: Electrocardiogram in endocrine and metabolic disorders, *Cardiovasc Clin* 8(3):243, 1977.

Tomky D: Tapping the full power of insulin pumps, *RN* 52(6):46, 1989.

Turner RC et al: Alcohol withdrawal syndromes, *J Gen Intern Med* 4:432, 1989.

Werman HA, Davis EA, Rund DA: Abdominal pain and seizures in a young man, *Ann Emerg Med* 16:425, 1987.

Wolfson AB, ed: Endocrine and metabolic emergencies, *Emerg Med Clin North Am* 7:749, 1989.

Daniel J. Cobaugh

Clinical toxicology can be defined as the coordinated delivery of care to a patient who has been exposed to a toxic substance. Exposure to a toxic substance includes accidental ingestion, ocular and dermal contact with such a substance, intentional suicidal attempts, substance abuse, and occupational and environmental exposures.

The multidisciplinary approach to the management of the patient with an exposure to a toxic substance includes initial and continued hemodynamic stabilization, assessment of the potential for toxicosis, gastric decontamination, the use of special antidotes, and extracorporeal procedures for toxin elimination such as hemodialysis and charcoal hemoperfusion. Professionals who are involved in the care of these patients should include physicians, nurses, paramedics, pharmacists, laboratory technologists, and social workers. The care of these patients presents many challenges to the emergency nurse. This chapter focuses on gastric decontamination, extracorporeal elimination, and the management of several common toxicologic emergencies.

EPIDEMIOLOGY

In 1989 the American Association of Poison Control Centers (AAPCC) reported 1,581,540 exposures to toxic substances. Of these exposures, 88.3% were accidental, 9.7% were classified as intentional, 1.5% were reactions to a food or drug, and 0.5% were not classified. Children less than 5 years of age accounted for 61.1% of the exposures. Possible reasons for the high incidence of exposure in this population include children's natural curiosity, increased hand-to-mouth activity, and imitation of adult behaviors. The data reported by the AAPCC represent data collected from 70 participating poison centers. Therefore these data do not reflect the total incidence of exposure to toxic substances in the United States.

POISON CONTROL CENTERS

Regional poison control centers should be regarded as constant sources of information concerning toxicosis. In the United States there are 35 AAPCC-designated regional poison control centers. These centers are staffed by nurses,

pharmacists, and physicians who have been certified as specialists in poison information by the AAPCC or who are board certified in toxicology by the American Board of Medical Toxicology or the American Board of Applied Toxicology. Regional poison control centers offer 24-hour telephone access to population bases of at least 1 million persons. Most often it is the poison control center that initially assesses the potential for toxicity and determines the need for evaluation in the ED. In addition to the expertise of the staff, the regional poison control center possesses a comprehensive group of references to assist in patient assessment.

INITIAL STABILIZATION

In addition to determination of the extent of toxicity, stabilization of the patient must be the first priority of the ED staff. Stabilization includes airway management and cardiac, hemodynamic, and neurologic monitoring. Some antidotes such as naloxone and digoxin-immune Fab (Digibind) should be considered for use during initial stabilization of the patient. After the patient has been stabilized, gastric decontamination should usually be initiated. After this initial care has been delivered, the use of extracorporeal measures such as hemodialysis and charcoal hemoperfusion should be considered.

ASSESSMENT

Assessment of the patient and the potential for toxicosis necessitates a detailed history. Questions aimed at describing the exposure should include: What substance was involved? (If possible have the prehospital care providers or the patient's family bring the product or container to the ED. Often a product is misidentified; for example, the family may state that the patient ingested aspirin when he or she actually ingested acetaminophen.) How long ago did the exposure occur? (Length of time since exposure often indicates which type of gastric decontamination should be used.) Is this an acute exposure or a long-term exposure? (Acute exposures are often managed differently than are long-term exposures.) What amount of the toxic substance was involved? What is the patient's age? What is the patient's weight? (The toxicities of substances such as acetaminophen and aspirin are determined on the basis of milligrams per kilogram.) Does the patient have any clinical effects? When did these symptoms appear in relation to exposure to the toxic substance? What treatment has been delivered before arrival at the ED? Frequently, family members may administer some treatment before the prehospital personnel arrive or before the patient is transported to the ED. These treatments may be inappropriate and may be associated with negative outcomes.

DERMAL DECONTAMINATION

Dermal exposure to toxic substances can often lead to systemic absorption and systemic toxic effects. Areas of dermal exposure should be irrigated as soon as possible. Before irrigation, any exposed clothing should be removed. The emergency nurse should first protect himself or herself to avoid secondary exposure to the toxin. Protection should include wearing protective gloves and gowns when treating a patient whose skin has been exposed to a toxic substance. The exposed area should be copiously irrigated for 10 to 15 minutes with saline solution or water. Neutralizing substances should not be used.

OCULAR DECONTAMINATION

After the eye area has been exposed to a toxic substance, irrigation of the affected eye should occur as soon as possible. Irrigation can often be performed at home after consultation with and instruction from the poison control center. Irrigation should be performed with copious amounts of saline solution or water and should continue for 10 to 15 minutes. Prolonged irrigation may be necessary in cases of exposure to caustic substances. Neutralizing substances should not be administered. If ocular effects persist after irrigation, an ophthalmologist should be consulted. (If any part of the face has been exposed to a toxic substance, check the patient's eyes carefully and follow the same procedures if eyes appear to be affected.)

GASTRIC DECONTAMINATION
Syrup of Ipecac

The plant alkaloids in syrup of ipecac, emetine and cephalin, are responsible for its emetic effects. The emetic effects of ipecac result from a local gastric irritation and a central stimulation of the chemoreceptor trigger zone. Ipecac is an effective emetic in awake and alert patients who require gastric emptying. The use of syrup of ipecac depends on the substance ingested, ingestion of other substances, time since ingestion, and neurologic status of the patient.

Standard doses of ipecac are 15 ml for children less than 12 years of age and 30 ml for older patients. Some poison control centers recommended 30 ml of ipecac for any patient over 1 year of age. These centers state that the time to emesis and the failure rate decrease with increased doses of ipecac. Increased doses result in less time for absorption into the systemic circulation. After administration of syrup of ipecac, 240 to 480 ml of clear fluids should be administered. Fluid administration enhances the gastric emptying associated with ipecac. Ipecac failure is often the result of lack of adequate fluid administration. Emesis after ingestion of ipecac should occur in approximately 15 to 20 minutes. If emesis does not occur within 30 minutes after ipecac administration, reasons for failure should be assessed. After emesis the patient should receive nothing by mouth for 1 hour, and diet should then be advanced as tolerated. Children often sleep after vomiting from ipecac. If the child sleeps, place him or her in a prone position and continue to monitor the child to prevent aspiration.

Adverse effects associated with the acute administration of syrup of ipecac are limited. Protracted vomiting and diarrhea have been reported. Individuals with a preexisting history of Mallory-Weiss syndrome are at increased risk for esophageal perforation during vomiting. Long-term abuse of ipecac in individuals with eating disorders can lead to neuropathies and cardiomyopathies as a result of accumulation of the alkaloids emetine and cephalin.

Use of syrup of ipecac to induce vomiting in patients is contraindicated in the following instances:
1. When the gag reflex is absent
2. When the level of consciousness is decreased
3. After ingestion of an agent that can cause a rapid decrease in level of consciousness (for example, a cyclic antidepressant)
4. When seizure activity is present
5. After a stroke or an acute epileptic seizure has occurred (postictal state)
6. After ingestion of a hydrocarbon or a caustic agent

Gastric Lavage

Gastric lavage should be used in situations in which ipecac-induced emesis is contraindicated or has failed. Like emesis induced by syrup of ipecac, gastric lavage should occur as soon as possible after ingestion for best results. Endotracheal intubation should precede lavage to ensure airway protection. The patient should be placed in a left lateral Trendelenburg ("swimmer's") position. A large diameter orogastric lavage tube (24- to 28-gauge French in pediatric patients and 36- to 40-gauge French in adult patients) should be inserted. In adult patients, 200 to 250 ml aliquots of tap water or saline solution should be administered. In pediatric patients 10 to 15 ml/kg lavage of normal saline solution should be administered in 50 ml aliquots. Gastric lavage should continue until lavage returns are clear. Ideal lavage in an adult involves the use of 5 to 10 L of fluid. In pediatric patients, total lavage volume should be approximately 500 ml. Often gastric lavage returns appear clear when complete gastric emptying has not occurred. To avoid incomplete emptying, the lavage tube should be repositioned. Tube repositioning often leads to further tablet fragment return. Other measures to promote gastric emptying include repositioning of the patient and massaging the patient's epigastric area. Lavage should not be performed in the patient who has ingested a caustic substance, in a patient who has swallowed a sharp object, in an awake patient who has not ingested a substance that will lead to a rapid change in level of consciousness. Adverse effects associated with lavage include esophageal perforation, fluid and electrolyte imbalances in pediatric patients if a hypotonic solution such as water is administered, and epistaxis if nasogastric tubes are used.

Activated Charcoal

Activated charcoal is the product of wood materials that have been chemically treated and then heated to extremely high temperatures. These processes give charcoal the characteristic surface area that enables it to adsorb toxins. Activated charcoal adsorbs toxins with molecular weights 100 and 1000 such as benzodiazepines, theophylline, and cyclic antidepressants. Toxins that are not readily adsorbed by charcoal include lithium, iron, and the toxic alcohols. Adsorption to the surface of activated charcoal in the gastrointestinal tract prevents the absorption of the toxin into the systemic circulation.

Activated charcoal can also decrease serum concentration of toxins such as phenobarbital, theophylline-aminophylline, salicylates, and carbamazepine. This decrease in serum concentration is the result of gastrointestinal dialysis. A concentration gradient is set at the area of the gastric lumen. Toxin is transported from an area of higher concentration (blood) to an area of lower concentration (gastrointestinal tract) where it is adsorbed to charcoal. After the adsorption process is completed, the charcoal-toxin complex is eliminated in the feces. Activated charcoal is indicated for the management of ingestions that involve agents that are not readily adsorbed to its surface.

The pediatric dose of activated charcoal is 1 g/kg, and the adult dose is 50 to 100 g. In most situations, activated charcoal is administered once, after gastric emptying has been achieved with either ipecac or gastric lavage. Multiple doses of activated charcoal are administered when the gastrointestinal dialysis effects of charcoal are desired (that is, charcoal 50 g administered orally or through a nasogastric tube every 4 hours) until theophylline serum concentrations decrease to the therapeutic range. Some authors have suggested that activated charcoal can be administered without previous gastric emptying with syrup of ipecac or gastric lavage, especially when more than 2 hours has elapsed since ingestion. After a prolonged period, gastric emptying will probably be ineffective, whereas activated charcoal can still adsorb toxins in the intestines.

Adverse effects associated with the use of activated charcoal include nausea and vomiting, gastrointestinal obstruction, and pulmonary aspiration. Activated charcoal is contraindicated when the toxin is known not to adsorb to charcoal or when a patient has diminished bowel sounds or ileus.

TOXICOKINETICS

The pharmacokinetic characteristics of numerous drugs have been described at length in the literature and include absorption, distribution, metabolism, elimination, and half-life. In cases of toxicosis, these characteristics often become altered. Toxicokinetics describes the pharmacokinetic characteristics of a drug at toxic serum concentrations.

Absorption

Absorption factors describe how readily a substance is absorbed into the systemic circulation from the gastrointestinal tract or from some other nonintravenous site of administration. Absorption characteristics are useful in determining the period of time after ingestion for which gastric emptying will be effective. Toxins such as liquids that are quickly absorbed into the systemic circulation cannot be readily retrieved by means of emesis or lavage if more than 1 hour has elapsed since ingestion. Anticholinergic substances such as cyclic antidepressants and atropine decrease gastrointestinal motility and therefore prolong absorption time. Therefore, gastric emptying may be more effective with these agents, even if more than 1 hour has elapsed since ingestion. Also, if a substance is readily absorbed, clinical effects from this substance, such as drowsiness, can be expected much sooner.

Distribution

Distribution describes the degree to which a substance travels from the central circulation and is transported to target organs and peripheral-tissue storage sites. This transport includes distribution to cerebral and cardiac tissue and distribution to bone and lipid stores. It is necessary to know a drug's distribution characteristics to determine whether extracorporeal methods of elimination such as hemodialysis or charcoal hemoperfusion will be effective. If the volume of distribution is moderate to high, extracorporeal methods will probably not be effective.

Metabolism

Metabolism, in the context of this chapter, refers to the process by which a drug is biotransformed to a more polar, ionic, water-soluble substance that is eliminated more readily. Metabolism also results in the production of metabolites that have pharmacologic effects, toxicologic effects, or both. The hepatotoxicity associated with acetaminophen is due to the production of a toxic metabolite. When a patient with toxicosis is assessed, the presence of active metabolites must be considered.

Elimination

Elimination refers to the process by which substances are removed through renal and gastrointestinal systems. The route of elimination can have dramatic effects on the potential for toxicosis. An example is the toxic reaction to an excess of digoxin. Digoxin is eliminated by the kidneys.

The elderly patient who has diminished renal function has an increased risk for digoxin toxicity as a result of accumulation.

Half-Life

Half-life is the time necessary for the serum concentration of a substance to decrease to one half of the original concentration. In an overdose, half-life is often prolonged because of the saturation of metabolic and elimination pathways.

CYCLIC ANTIDEPRESSANTS

Cyclic antidepressants such as amitriptyline, imipramine, and desipramine are the most common cause of death resulting from overdose reported to the AAPCC data collection system. These agents are often combined in overdose with other medications that also have serious cardiovascular and neurologic effects. Table 40-1 lists different classes of cyclic antidepressants.

Toxic Dose

Toxicity with these agents cannot be well correlated with a milligram per kilogram amount of antidepressant. Serum concentrations do not correlate well with clinical effects.

Laboratory Tests

The presence of cyclic antidepressants on a quantitative or qualitative laboratory screen confirms that the patient has ingested these agents. Clinical effects do not correlate well with qualitative laboratory measurements. Treatment should be based on the patient's clinical presentation rather than on measurements of serum concentrations.

Mechanism of Toxicosis

Cyclic antidepressants have profound effects on the autonomic nervous system, which result in effects on multiple organ systems. These effects include depletion of catecholamines at the neuromuscular junction, anticholinergic activity, peripheral α_1 blockade, and stimulation of the central adrenergic system. These drugs also have a quinidine-like, membrane-stabilizing effect on cardiac tissue. Cardiovascular and neurologic effects are most prominent immediately after ingestion of these agents.

Clinical Effects

Cardiac. Sinus tachycardia that is caused by the anticholinergic effects of these agents is common. Numerous dysrhythmias are associated with cyclic antidepressants and include supraventricular dysrhythmias, conduction disturbances, ventricular tachycardia, and ventricular fibrillation. The mechanism for these dysrhythmias is similar to the sodium channel–blocking antiarrhythmic effects of quinidine. Cyclic antidepressants cause widening of the QRS complex and prolongation of the PR interval.

Hemodynamic. In addition to decreases in cardiac output associated with dysrhythmias, cyclic antidepressants have direct effects on blood pressure. The therapeutic effects of cyclic antidepressants result from interference with reuptake of the catecholamines, norepinephrine and serotonin. In an overdose, this blockade is profound, and depletion of norepinephrine and serotonin. Norepinephrine depletion results in severe hypotension. Cyclic antidepressants may also have an α_1-blocking effect peripherally, which leads to a decrease in total peripheral resistance and therefore to a decrease in blood pressure.

Neurologic. The neurologic effects associated with an overdose of cyclic antidepressants include rapid decreases in level of consciousness and sudden onset of seizure activity. Seizure activity is thought to be caused by excessive catecholamine stimulation in the brain. Since these changes can be rapid, a patient can be awake and alert one moment, yet proceed quickly to seizure activity and coma.

Anticholinergic. Other toxic effects associated with cyclic antidepressants are related to their anticholinergic effects; these include dilated pupils, dry mouth, urinary retention, and decreases in gastric motility.

Treatment

Cardiac. Cardiac monitoring is imperative in all significant ingestions of cyclic antidepressants. Sinus tachycardia occurs as a result of the anticholinergic effects of these agents. Widening of the QRS complex may indicate serious toxicosis that includes ventricular dysrhythmias, conduction disturbances, and seizures.

Alkalinization. Systemic alkalinization of the serum with sodium bicarbonate has reversed several of the life-threatening conduction disturbances and ventricular dysrhythmias associated with cyclic antidepressants. Sodium bicarbonate (1 mEq/kg) should be administered as an initial dose. The end point of therapy is the maintenance of a systemic pH of 7.5. If no positive effects are observed after the initial

Table 40-1 Classes of cyclic antidepressants

Generic name	Brand name	Chemical class
Amitriptyline	Elavil	Tricyclic
	Endep	
Amoxapine	Asendin	Dibenzoxazepine
Desipramine	Norpramin	Tricyclic
Doxepin	Sinequan	Tricyclic
	Adapin	
Fluoxetine	Prozac	Bicyclic
Imipramine	Tofranil	Tricyclic
Maprotiline	Ludiomil	Tetracyclic
Nortriptyline	Aventyl	Tricyclic
	Pamelor	
Protriptyline	Vivactil	Tricyclic
Trazodone	Desyrel	Noncyclic
Trimipramine	Surmontil	Tricyclic

dose of sodium bicarbonate, a second dose can be administered in 10 minutes. Further doses of bicarbonate should be administered on the basis of arterial blood gas values.

Antiarrhythmic agents. The use of class 1A antidysrhythmics such as procainamide and class 1C antidysrhythmics should be avoided in these patients because of the effects of these antidysrhythmics on sodium channels. Ventricular dysrhythmias respond to lidocaine and phenytoin. Bretylium should be used with caution because of its effects on blood pressure. The mechanism for bretylium-induced hypotension is similar to that for cyclic antidepressant-induced hypotension.

Pacemakers. Mobitz type II block and third-degree heart block may respond to the use of an external pacemaker. Limited clinical data are available to substantiate the efficacy of the use of an external pacemaker in cases of overdose from cyclic antidepressants.

Hemodynamic. Hypotension that follows cyclic antidepressant overdose should be treated initially with a fluid challenge. Hypotension that does not respond to the administration of fluids should be managed with vasopressors. Dopamine may be used as an initial vasopressor. However, patients may respond better to a direct-acting vasopressor such as norepinephrine or phenylephrine. The more positive response results from the catecholamine depletion that is associated with cyclic antidepressants. If norepinephrine is depleted, dopamine may not be effective, since its effects are due in part to stimulation of norepinephrine release.

Neurologic. Seizures should be initially treated with diazepam. Therapy with phenytoin can be initiated with a loading dose and subsequent maintenance doses. Because of the length of time that is necessary to administer phenytoin (25 to 50 mg/min), it is beneficial to the patient to initially treat seizures with a short-acting benzodiazepine such as diazepam.

Gastrointestinal decontamination

Emesis. Syrup of ipecac is contraindicated in overdoses of cyclic antidepressants because of the rapid decrease in level of consciousness associated with overdoses of these agents.

Gastric lavage. Patients who have ingested cyclic antidepressants should receive aggressive gastric lavage with large volumes of fluids.

Activated charcoal. A dose of activated charcoal can be administered before and after gastric lavage. Multiple doses of activated charcoal are not indicated for overdoses of cyclic antidepressants. Serum concentrations of cyclic antidepressants are not significantly decreased with multiple doses of activated charcoal. Also, patients who have ingested overdoses of cyclic antidepressants are at risk for gastrointestinal obstruction because of the decreases in gastrointestinal motility associated with these agents. Close attention should be paid to bowel sounds, if multiple doses of charcoal are administered.

Extracorporeal elimination. Hemodialysis and charcoal hemoperfusion are not effective in the removal of cyclic antidepressants.

ACETAMINOPHEN

Overdoses of acetaminophen can be the result of accidental ingestion in the pediatric patient or intentional ingestion in the adult. Acetaminophen is often included in products that combine cold medicines with analgesic agents. Acetaminophen overdose can cause life-threatening hepatic toxicosis if it is not managed within 12 hours of ingestion.

Toxic Dose

Toxicosis that results from acetaminophen overdose most commonly occurs when doses of 140 mg/kg or greater have been ingested during a short period of time. Remember that it is difficult to determine a milligram per kilogram toxic dose in chronic acetaminophen toxicosis.

Laboratory Tests

Acetaminophen serum concentrations should be drawn 4 hours after an acute ingestion. Any level that is drawn before 4 hours after ingestion cannot be used to accurately predict toxicosis or levels of toxicity. A 4-hour acetaminophen level of greater than 15 µg/ml may indicate hepatotoxicity. Serum concentrations should be plotted on the Rumack-Matthew nomogram (Fig. 40-1) to determine degree of toxicity.

Mechanism of Toxicosis

The life-threatening toxicities that are associated with acetaminophen are due to the formation of a hepatotoxic intermediate metabolite. After therapeutic doses of acet-

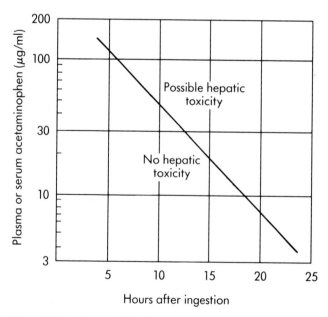

Fig. 40-1 Rumack-Matthew nomogram. (From American Academy of Pediatrics: *Pediatrics* 55:871, 1975.)

aminophen have been given, metabolism occurs by three pathways: sulfate conjugation, glucuronide conjugation, and cytochrome P-450 mixed function oxidase metabolism. Approximately 90% of acetaminophen is metabolized by sulfates and glucuronide. Five percent is metabolized by the P-450 system, and 5% is eliminated unchanged. The P-450 metabolite is the hepatotoxic intermediate. After the administration of therapeutic doses, this toxic intermediate is rapidly detoxified by glutathione. In toxicosis, the sulfate and glucuronide pathways are saturated and greater amounts of acetaminophen are metabolized by the P-450 system. Because of increased production of this toxic intermediate, glutathione stores become depleted and large amounts of this intermediate are available for hepatotoxic effects.

Clinical Effects

The toxic effects that are seen after acute acetaminophen ingestion are traditionally classified in four stages.

Stage I (0 to 24 hours)	Mild gastrointestinal effects such as nausea and vomiting occur.
Stage II (24 to 48 hours)	No signs or symptoms are apparent. Mild increases in hepatic enzymes may be seen in this phase.
Stage III (48 hours)	Fulminant hepatotoxicity occurs with significant increases in hepatic enzymes (ALT and AST), bilirubin, and prothrombin time. The patient may have vomiting, lethargy, right-quadrant tenderness; he or she may appear jaundiced. Bleeding may occur as a result of effects on prothrombin time. Hypoglycemia has also been reported. The patient can progress to complete hepatic coma. Cardiac effects, including dysrhythmias, may occur and are probably due to the hepatotoxicity rather than to a direct cardiac toxicity.
Stage IV (recovery)	Patients begin to recover after an acute insult to the liver about 5 days after ingestion. Permanent hepatic effects are uncommon in patients who recover.

Treatment

Supportive Care

1. Provide respiratory, cardiac, and hemodynamic support in patients who are critically ill.
2. Baseline laboratory work should include an acetaminophen level (at least 4 hours after ingestion), complete blood count, hepatic enzymes, bilirubin, prothrombin time, electrolytes, serum creatinine, and a blood urea nitrogen level.
3. Vomiting can be treated with antiemetic drugs such as prochlorperazine and metoclopramide.

Gastrointestinal decontamination

1. Emesis. Syrup of ipecac can be used to induce emesis in an awake and alert patient after a recent (within 1 hour) acetaminophen ingestion.
2. Gastric lavage. If coingestants that may affect level of consciousness are involved or if a massive amount of acetaminophen has been ingested, gastric lavage should be used.
3. Activated charcoal. Activated charcoal effectively ad-

sorbs acetaminophen in the gastrointestinal tract. Multiple doses of charcoal will not decrease serum concentrations of acetaminophen.

N-Acetylcysteine (Mucomyst)

All patients with an acetaminophen level that is toxic after being plotted on the Rumack-Matthew nomogram should be treated with *N*-acetylcysteine (NAC).

Dosage

1. Loading dose is 140 mg/kg of 20% NAC diluted to a 5% solution with water, cola, or fruit juice.
2. Maintenance dose is 70 mg/kg of 20% NAC diluted to a 5% solution with water, cola, or fruit juice; doses are repeated 17 times.

Administration

Because NAC has a strong, unpleasant smell, the solution should be diluted with fruit juice or cola. Administer the diluted NAC solution in a covered cup through a straw. If the patient cannot tolerate oral administration, consider use of a nasogastric or duodenal tube. If the patient has nausea and vomiting, consider the use of antiemetics.

Extracorporeal elimination

Hemodialysis and charcoal hemoperfusion are of limited use in cases of acetaminophen overdose.

SALICYLATES

Incidence of acute ingestions of aspirin has decreased in the United States over the last two decades. This is probably because of increased use of acetaminophen as an antipyretic analgesic. Use of aspirin has also decreased because of the associated risks of Reye's syndrome. Along with acute ingestions, the practitioner must assess for the possibility of chronic salicylism. Also, other sources of salicylate such as methyl salicylate (Ben-Gay) and bismuth subsalicylate (Pepto-Bismol) should be considered.

Toxic Dosage

Acute ingestions of more than 150 mg/kg are associated with the development of toxic clinical effects.

Laboratory Tests

Salicylate levels should be obtained 6 hours after acute ingestion. A 6-hour salicylate level of more than 40 mg/dl after a single ingestion indicates the potential for toxicosis. After long-term use of salicylates, it is more difficult to use levels to predict degree of toxicity.

Mechanism of Toxicosis

Salicylates have several cellular metabolic effects that are responsible for toxicosis. These effects include direct stimulation of the respiratory centers in the brain, uncoupling of oxidative phosphorylation, and interference with the Krebs' cycle.

Clinical Effects

Respiratory. Hyperventilation occurs as a result of increased carbon dioxide production and direct central respiratory stimulation. Hyperventilation results in development of a respiratory alkalosis. Since children do not have a respiratory drive like that of adults, they often do not develop a respiratory alkalosis.

Gastrointestinal. Salicylates have irritant effects on the gastric mucosa, which leads to nausea, vomiting, and hematemesis.

Metabolic. Metabolic acidosis is common. Uncoupling of oxidative phosphorylation leads to increases in metabolic rate, which result in hyperthermia and hypoglycemia. Hypokalemia and hypocalcemia also occur. Interference with the Krebs' cycle can lead to hypoglycemia.

Neurologic. Mild neurologic effects such as tinnitus and lethargy are common. Massive toxicosis may result in hallucinations, seizures, and coma.

Pulmonary. Noncardiogenic pulmonary edema has been associated with salicylate toxicosis.

Treatment

Administration of fluids and electrolytes. Patients with a history of salicylate ingestion should be hydrated with intravenous fluids. If the patient is hypokalemic, potassium should be replaced.

Hypoglycemia. Any patient who has a decreased level of consciousness should receive 50% dextrose to treat possible hypoglycemia.

Acidosis. Metabolic acidosis should be corrected with sodium bicarbonate. Acidosis can lead to increased absorption of salicylate in the brain.

Seizures. Intravenous diazepam should be used to treat seizures associated with salicylates.

Gastrointestinal decontamination

Emesis. Emesis that is induced by syrup of ipecac can be effective in the treatment of recent salicylate ingestions. Ipecac should not be used if the patient has changes in level of consciousness or seizures.

Lavage. Patients who have ingested massive amounts of salicylate or more than one substance or those who have changes in level of consciousness, seizures, or both should be treated by means of gastric lavage.

Activated charcoal. Activated charcoal is effective in decreasing absorption of salicylates from the gastrointestinal tract. Some authors suggest that multiple doses of activated charcoal may decrease serum concentrations of activated charcoal through gastrointestinal dialysis.

Extracorporeal elimination. Hemodialysis effectively removes salicylates and provides for fluid and electrolyte replacement. Charcoal hemoperfusion removes salicylates but does not provide fluid and electrolyte replacement. Hemodialysis should be considered for patients who have significant levels of salicylate but do not respond to supportive measures.

BENZODIAZEPINES

The benzodiazepines such as diazepam, lorazepam, and triazolam are commonly prescribed as anxiolytics and sedative hypnotics. The levels of toxicity associated with these agents are often very mild. These agents are often ingested along with other central nervous system (CNS) depressants including alcohol, cyclic antidepressants, and barbiturates. When combined with other CNS depressants, the benzodiazepines can have more severe toxic effects.

Toxic Dose

Toxic doses of these agents vary from patient to patient. A milligram per kilogram toxic dose for the benzodiazepines has not been established.

Laboratory Tests

Qualitative and quantitative benzodiazepine serum concentrations confirm the presence of these agents; however, these levels should not serve as guidelines for therapy. Therapy should be based on the clinical status of the patient.

Mechanism of Toxicosis

The toxicity of the benzodiazepines is an extension of their pharmacologic effects. Benzodiazepines potentiate the effects of the inhibitory neurotransmitter γ-aminobutyric acid (GABA). They are not activated by GABA and they do not stimulate release of further GABA.

Clinical Effects

Neurologic. Benzodiazepines may cause drowsiness, lethargy, ataxia, and grade 0 or grade 1 coma. A coma of grade 2, 3, or 4 suggests the involvement of other CNS-depressant toxins.

Hemodynamic. Circulatory changes after ingestion of a benzodiazepine alone are rare. Hypotension has been associated with rapid administration of diazepam because it has a propylene glycol base.

Respiratory. Respiratory depression is rare in cases of pure benzodiazepine ingestion. Respiratory depression has been associated with high doses of and rapid administration of midazolam.

Treatment

Stabilization. Before gastric decontamination is performed, supportive respiratory and cardiovascular care should be provided.

Gastrointestinal decontamination

Emesis. Emesis that is induced by syrup of ipecac can be used in cases of recent ingestion in which level of consciousness has not changed. If coingestants are involved, gastric lavage should be used.

Gastric lavage. Gastric lavage is indicated when large amounts of benzodiazepines have been ingested, when coingestants are involved, or when the patient has a decreased level of consciousness.

Activated charcoal. A single dose of activated charcoal can be effective in adsorbing benzodiazepines from the gastrointestinal tract. Gastrointestinal dialysis with multiple doses of activated charcoal, however, is not an effective treatment for toxicosis caused by these agents.

Benzodiazepine antagonist. Flumazenil is currently under investigation as a benzodiazepine antagonist. This drug competes directly with the benzodiazepine at the benzodiazepine receptor site. Administration of flumazenil results in rapid changes in level of consciousness in patients who have toxicosis caused by benzodiazepines. Flumazenil can be used to rule out the presence of benzodiazepines in a manner that is similar to the use of naloxone for ruling out the presence of opiates.

Extracorporeal elimination. Hemodialysis and charcoal hemoperfusion are of little benefit in cases of benzodiazepine overdose.

OPIATES AND OPIOIDS

Narcotic toxicosis is often associated with intravenous abuse of these agents. In the last decade, many deaths that resulted from abuse of the synthetic fentanyl derivatives or so-called "designer" drugs have been reported. Young children are sensitive to the toxic effects of this group of drugs.

Toxic Dose

A milligram per kilogram toxic dose has not been identified for each individual narcotic. Children are more sensitive to smaller doses of narcotics. In adults, variances are based on levels of dependence. Also, in the case of narcotic abuse, the potency of available street narcotics is variable.

Laboratory Tests

Qualitative and quantitative laboratory values confirm the presence of narcotics. These levels are not clinically useful. The patient's clinical status should be used to guide therapy.

Clinical Effects

Neurologic. Lethargy, somnolence, ataxia, and coma are associated with narcotic toxicosis.

Respiratory. Respiratory depression is one of the most common toxic effects of the narcotics. Noncardiogenic pulmonary edema has also been associated with the opiates.

Cardiovascular. Hypotension can be profound and can lead to circulatory collapse.

Gastrointestinal. In therapeutic doses and in cases of toxicosis, gastric motility is decreased with opiates and opioids. Therefore, activated charcoal must be used judiciously.

Treatment

Stabilization. Before gastric decontamination is performed, cardiovascular and respiratory functions should be stabilized.

Narcotic antagonist. Naloxone is a specific narcotic antagonist that competes directly with opiates at opiate receptors. After the administration of naloxone, dramatic reversal of the toxic opiate effects often occurs.

Dosage. Initial adult and pediatric dosage is 2 mg by direct intravenous administration. Repeat doses should be administered if no effect is observed after this initial dose. If no effect is seen after a total dose of 10 mg, other causes of toxicosis should be considered. If a patient has ingested a long-acting opiate, such as methadone, a continuous infusion of naloxone may be necessary to maintain level of consciousness, respirations, and hemodynamic status. Two thirds of the total loading dose should be administered on an hourly basis. Determine total loading dose, add 10 times this amount to 1000 ml of intravenous fluids, and infuse at 100 ml/hr. Fifteen minutes after initiation of the continuous infusion, administer one half of the initial loading dose to maintain level of consciousness, normal respirations, and normal hemodynamic status.

Gastrointestinal decontamination

Emesis. Emesis induced by syrup of ipecac can be used for gastric emptying in cases of recent ingestion in which no change in level of consciousness has occurred.

Lavage. Patients who have a decreased level of consciousness, respiratory depression, or significant hypotension should receive gastric lavage.

Activated charcoal. Activated charcoal is effective in adsorbing opiates and opioids in the gastrointestinal tract and in preventing their absorption into the systemic circulation. Activated charcoal does not decrease serum concentrations of opiates through gastrointestinal dialysis. Presence of bowel sounds should be determined, since narcotics can delay gastrointestinal motility.

CLONIDINE

An ingestion of even a small amount of clonidine should be considered a life-threatening emergency in the pediatric patient.

Mechanism of Toxicosis

The clinical effects that occur after a clonidine overdose are similar to those that result from a narcotic overdose. Clonidine is an imidazoline antihypertensive agent. Clonidine acts as a central α_2-agonist. This agonism causes decreased amounts of catecholamine release from the central nervous system. Clonidine may also stimulate the production of an opiate-like substance that gives it its opiate characteristics.

Toxic Dosage

As little as 0.1 mg can be toxic in the pediatric patient. Children have survived after ingestion of up to 10 mg, and adults have survived after ingestion of up to 100 mg.

Laboratory Tests

Laboratory values are not clinically significant. Although laboratory values do confirm that clonidine ingestion has occurred, clinical effects should guide therapy.

Clinical Effects

Neurologic. Lethargy, ataxia, confusion, and coma have been associated with overdoses of clonidine.

Respiratory. Respiratory depression similar to that which is caused by narcotics can occur.

Cardiovascular. Bradycardia and hypotension are common after an overdose of clonidine. A paradoxical hypertension has also been reported, which is probably due to loss of α_2 specificity that leads to α_1 stimulation and results in increases in total peripheral resistance.

Treatment

Supportive care. Respiratory and cardiovascular functions must be stabilized before gastric decontamination is performed.

Naloxone. Naloxone is effective in reversing the effects of clonidine toxicosis. Doses of 2 to 10 mg may be necessary as in the case of an overdose of narcotics. A need for high doses of naloxone is common in cases of clonidine toxicosis. Continuous infusions of naloxone are effective in preventing recurrence of symptoms.

Gastrointestinal decontamination

Emesis. Emesis induced by syrup of ipecac is contraindicated in the case of a clonidine overdose because of the rapid absorption of the drug from the gastrointestinal tract and the rapid onset of clinical effects.

Lavage. Gastric lavage should be performed in suspected cases of clonidine toxicosis.

Activated charcoal. Activated charcoal prevents the absorption of clonidine into the systemic circulation by adsorbing clonidine onto its surface. Clonidine does not undergo gastrointestinal dialysis, and therefore, multiple doses of activated charcoal are not required.

DIGITALIS GLYCOSIDES

Sources of digitalis glycoside toxicosis include pharmaceutical preparations such as digoxin and digitoxin. Several plants also contain digitalis glycosides; these include foxglove, lily of the valley, and oleander. A human or animal who ingests a significant amount of these plants may be at risk for digitalis toxicosis.

Mechanism of Toxicosis

Digitalis glycosides block the sodium-potassium-adenosine triphosphatase pump at both therapeutic and toxic doses. Increases in vagal and sympathetic tone are also observed with high serum concentrations of these agents.

Toxic Dose

Clinical effects can occur at various doses. The manufacturer of digoxin-immune Fab lists a dose of 4 mg in a child and a dose of 10 mg in an adult as indications for therapy with Digibind.

Laboratory Tests

Serum concentrations of digoxin can be useful in assessing the degree of toxicity. A serum concentration of greater than 10 ng/ml is an indication for treatment with Digibind. Toxicosis can occur at various serum concentrations; therefore, clinical effects and patient status should guide therapy. Distribution of digoxin to tissue sites requires at least a 12-hour period. Therefore, digoxin serum concentrations that are drawn at a time before 12 hours have passed after ingestion may not reflect equilibrium between blood and tissue concentrations.

Clinical Effects

Neurologic. Drowsiness, lethargy, and coma may occur after an overdose of digitalis glycoside.

Cardiovascular. Multiple arrhythmias including conduction disturbances such as first-degree, second-degree, and third-degree heart block may occur. Ventricular dysrhythmias including ventricular tachycardia and ventricular fibrillation are possible. Asystole has been reported. Patients with such arrhythmias can become profoundly hypotensive.

Ocular. Some patients report visual changes that include the appearance of green halos around objects.

Gastrointestinal. Anorexia, nausea, and vomiting occur, especially in cases of chronic toxicosis.

Treatment

Supportive care. Respiratory and cardiovascular stabilization must occur before gastric decontamination is performed.

Gastrointestinal decontamination

Emesis. Emesis induced by syrup of ipecac can be used for gastric emptying in cases of recent ingestion when patients are free of symptoms.

Lavage. Gastric lavage is indicated in children who have symptoms of toxicosis and in adults who have taken overdoses intentionally. Since placement of the lavage tube may further increase vagal tone, atropine should be available if bradycardia occurs after the lavage tube has been placed.

Activated charcoal. Activated charcoal adsorbs digitalis glycosides in the gastrointestinal tract and therefore decreases systemic absorption of these agents. Multiple doses of activated charcoal have been suggested as treatment for both digoxin and digitoxin toxicosis. Limited clinical experience with this treatment has been reported.

Digoxin immune FAB (Digibind). Digoxin immune FAB is an ovine-derived antibody to digitalis glycosides. Digibind binds to digitalis glycosides and renders them inactive. Indications for use are the presence of two of the following: life-threatening dysrhythmias, serum potassium levels greater than 5 mEq/L, or serum digoxin concentrations greater than 10 ng/ml. The manufacturer also suggests administration of Digibind if more than 4 mg has been ingested by a child or more than 10 mg has been ingested by an adult. Dosage is determined on the basis of pharmacokinetic determination of total digoxin/digitoxin body load.

COCAINE

Recreational use and abuse of cocaine continues to become more common in the United States. Cocaine is abused by inhalation, smoking, and intravenous administration. Such abuse often leads to development of toxic effects. Several deaths that followed vaginal application of cocaine to increase stimulation during sexual intercourse have also been reported.

Mechanism of Toxicosis

Cocaine toxicosis is due to its potentiation of the neurotransmitters, epinephrine and norepinephrine, which leads to a storm (or crisis) of the sympathetic nervous system.

Toxic Dosage

The maximum safe intranasal dose of cocaine for adults has been reported as 200 mg, yet toxic effects can occur at various doses.

Laboratory Tests

Blood concentrations of cocaine should not guide therapy. A qualitative urine screen for cocaine can confirm its presence.

Clinical Effects

Early stimulation phase
Neurologic. Early central nervous system effects are consistent with hyperexcitability and include euphoria, muscle twitching, irritability, headache, and hallucinations. Central nervous system stimulation also results in emesis.

Cardiovascular. Bradycardia, tachycardia, and hypertension can be observed.

Respiratory. During this phase, rate and depth of respiration are increased.

Advanced stimulation phase
Neurologic. Seizure activity that may advance to status epilepticus is observed during this phase.

Cardiovascular. Profound tachycardia and hypertension are observed during this phase. Hypotension can develop after the initial hypertensive period. Hyperthermia is also common during this phase.

Respiratory. Respiratory depression, as evidenced by dyspnea, tachypnea, and cyanosis, occurs. Complete respiratory arrest may occur. Pulmonary edema is possible.

Depression phase
Neurologic. Hyporeflexia and muscle paralysis, which lead to death, can occur in the depression phase.

Treatment

Supportive care. Often supportive care of the patient who has cocaine toxicosis is the mainstay of therapy.

Seizures. Seizure activity should be treated with diazepam. When a patient has seizures that are refractory to diazepam, phenytoin, phenobarbital, and pharmacologically induced paralysis should be considered.

Hyperthermia. External cooling measures such as cooling blankets, ice packs, and ice baths are recommended if core temperature is greater than 105° F. A fever of a lower grade can be treated less aggressively by removing the patient's clothing, placing him or her in a cool room, and providing sponge baths.

Hypertension. The hypertensive phase is often transient and does not require treatment. If treatment is required, propranolol can be administered. Propranolol *may* exacerbate existing hypertension. With the β-blockade that is induced by propranolol, there may be unopposed α_1 stimulation that leads to hypertension. In this case, sodium nitroprusside is indicated because of its vasodilatory effects.

Dysrhythmias. Propranolol can be effective in the control of tachycardia that requires treatment. Ventricular tachycardia and ventricular fibrillation should be treated with lidocaine.

Hypotension. Hypotension should be treated initially by positioning the patient appropriately and administering fluids. If these measures are ineffective, the use of vasopressors such as dopamine and norepinephrine must be considered.

Gastrointestinal decontamination. Since cocaine is most often abused by means of inhalation and intravenous injection, gastric decontamination is often not necessary. The exception to this is the case of the individual who is a body packer or a body stuffer. The body packer has ingested bags of cocaine as a means of transporting the drug. These bags are usually of high quality and difficult to break. A body packer is a person who swallows a bag of cocaine to rid himself or herself of evidence. These bags are often thin and prone to breakage.

Activated charcoal. Activated charcoal should be administered to both a body packer and a body stuffer. In the case of bag breakage, the charcoal will adsorb cocaine in the gastrointestinal tract.

Whole-bowel irrigation. Irrigation and cleansing of the gastrointestinal tract enhances the elimination of bags of cocaine. Isotonic polyethylene glycol and electrolyte solutions, such as Golytely, are used for this purpose.

SUMMARY

Toxicologic emergencies are common events in the emergency care setting. This chapter highlights some of the more commonly available toxic agents. The reader is referred to the several useful texts, microfiche, and computerized programs for further information.

SUGGESTED READINGS

Anderson BA, Manoguerra AS: Counteraction to poison, *Emergency* 23(1):49, 1991.

Buchanan JF: Cocaine intoxication: presentation and management of medical complications, *Physician Assist* 13(11):87, 91, 94, 1989.

Carlton FB Jr: General management of the poisoned patient, *Emerg Care Q* 6(3):1, 1990.

Cooper K: Drug overdose, *Am J Nurs* 89(9):1146, 1989.

Dinolfo J: Coping with salicylate intoxication, *Patient Care* 19(10):80, 87, 90, 1985.

Edwards N: A female patient with cocaine toxicity, AIDS and DIC, *JEN* 17(2):70, 1991.

Flomenbaum NE, Hoffman R: GI evacuation: is it still worthwhile? *Emerg Med* 22(2):80, 87, 91, 1990.

Goldfrank LR et al: *Goldfrank's toxicologic emergencies,* ed 3, New York, 1986, Appleton & Lange.

Goodrich PM: Naloxone hydrochloride: a review, *AANA J* 58(1):14, 1990.

Johnson RB, Steiner JF: Tricyclic antidepressant overdose: a toxicologic emergency, *J Am Acad Physicians Assist* 2(1):16, 1989.

Joy ME, Higbee MD: Extracardiac manifestations of digitalis toxicity in the elderly, *Hosp Formul* 20(9):1015, 1985.

Kearney TE: Salicylate poisoning: recognition and management, *Emerg Med Serv* 18(5):39, 1989.

Leoni MP: Management of acetaminophen overdose: *N*-acetylcysteine, *Crit Care Nurs* 5(4):44, 1985.

Levy DB: Narcotic review, *Emergency* 20(1):16, 1988.

Levy DB: The silent killer: the toxic potential of acetaminophen, *Emergency* 21(7):17, 1989.

Levy DB: Syrup of ipecac review, *Emergency* 21(12):20, 1989.

Levy DB: Naloxone: negating narcotics, *Emergency* 22(7):16, 1990.

Manoguerra AS: Activated charcoal, *Emergency* 15(3):46, 1983.

Manoguerra AS: Ipecac syrup, *Emergency* 19(11):16, 1987.

Miller K: Naloxone: uptown and downtown, *Emergency* 19(4):50, 1987.

Parks BR, Fischer RG: Misuse of syrup of ipecac, *Pediatr Nurs* 13(4):261, 1987.

Riddle K, Lee AJ: Digibind: emergency treatment for digitalis toxicity, *JEN* 15(3):288, 1989.

Schauben JL: Benzodiazepines, *Top Emerg Med* 7(3):39, 1985.

Sketris IS, Wilmhurst D, Anderson JP: Community awareness of the poison control centre and ipecac syrup, *Can J Public Health* 74(2):13, 1983.

Thomas DO: A lethargic 2-year-old child, *JEN* 15(2):123, 1989.

Thurkauf GE: Acetaminophen overdose, *Crit Care Nurs* 7(1):20, 1987.

Wall C: The real risk of acetaminophen overdose, *RN* 48(8):35, 1985.

Westlake C, Funkhauser SW: Cardiovascular effects of recreational cocaine abuse, *ACCN Clin Issues Crit Care Nurs* 1(1):65, 1990.

Hematologic Emergencies

Susan Budassi Sheehy

There are numerous types of hematologic emergencies. Some of the more common ones are discussed in this chapter.

ANEMIA

Anemia, by definition, is a decrease or deficiency of circulating red blood cells. In children the normal level is 4.4 to 5.0 $\times$ 10^6, in adult men the level is 4.4 to 5.9 $\times$ 10^6, and in adult women the level is 3.8 to 5.2 $\times$ 10^6. Anemia can be categorized as acute, which may be life threatening, and chronic, when the patient is not in grave danger of death.

There are three components of oxygen transport: hemoglobin level, hemoglobin's affinity for oxygen, and the amount of blood that is flowing. A decrease in any of these components may trigger a compensation by the other two components. The severity of anemia depends on the patient's ability to compensate for the red blood cell loss. The most common cause of anemia is blood loss. The patient with acute blood loss demonstrates signs and symptoms that include tachycardia, cool clammy skin, decreased blood pressure, and tachypnea. He or she may be cold and thirsty and have a decreased level of consciousness. Response to blood loss depends on the patient's age and general physical condition and the rapidity of blood loss.

Although trauma is a cause of acute anemia, there are many other causes, such as sickle cell disease, in which anemia develops as a result of a viral infection that causes an aplastic condition. Another acute cause is carbon monoxide poisoning, in which hemoglobin molecules take on carbon monoxide molecules instead of oxygen molecules.

Patients with chronic or non–life-threatening anemia usually have the chief complaint of fatigue, headache, irritability, dizziness, and shortness of breath and become tired easily. Diagnosis is made by clinical observation and history, and by laboratory analysis, including a complete blood cell count with a leukocyte differential, red blood cell indices, peripheral smear, and reticulocyte count.

Patients can usually be treated on an outpatient basis. However, if acute shortness of breath, chest pain, or severe dizziness or alteration of level of consciousness develops, it is wise to admit the patient for observation, further diagnostic studies, and therapeutic intervention.

Diseases caused by a diminished red blood cell production are iron deficiency anemia, thalassemia, lead poisoning, vitamin B_{12} deficiency, folate deficiency, chronic liver disease, and hypothyroidism. Aplastic anemia is caused by bone marrow production deficiency, and anemia may be caused by other diseases such as thyroid or adrenal problems, uremia, or liver disease.

Some anemias are caused by an increased destruction of red blood cells that may be caused by enzyme defects, abnormalities of the membranes, or abnormalities of the hemoglobin molecule such as occurs with sickle cell disease. Anemia may also be caused by immunologic factors and by external factors such as infections, drugs, toxins, or heat.

SICKLE CELL DISEASE AND ANEMIA

Sickle cell disease is an inherited disorder that occurs in about 7% of West African and African-American blacks. It is an autosomal recessive disease in which the hemoglobin molecule is altered. A person can have sickle cell *trait*, that is, one sickle cell gene is present, without having the disease. A person with sickle cell *disease* has two sickle cell genes: this person rarely lives to adulthood.

Sickle cells carry a normal amount of hemoglobin, but the cells have a tendency to clump together because of their sickle shape. When this occurs, oxygen and other products do not reach capillaries and ischemia occurs. This result is known as sickle cell crisis. It may be precipitated by exposure to cold, infection, or metabolic or respiratory acidosis. For unknown reasons it also occurs more frequently at night. If the ischemia is prolonged, local tissue necrosis occurs.

Common areas for sickle cell crisis pain in children are the hands and feet and the abdomen, where the crisis may mimic appendicitis. In young adults pain commonly occurs in the long bones, large joints, and the spine. Common signs and symptoms of sickle cell crisis are pain, a history of sickle cell crisis and disease, weakness, and pallor.

Therapeutic intervention includes analgesia (usually with acetaminophen, propoxyphene, meperidine, hydromorphone, or morphine sulfate), compassion, oxygen, hydration with D_5W or D_5 half-normal saline solution, treatment of the infection, and local heat. Recently hyperbaric oxygen therapy has been used with success.[1] Complications include recurrent sickle cell crisis, hemolytic anemia, transient aplastic crisis, cholelithiasis and cholecystitis, delayed sexual maturation, priapism, renal disease, bone disease (infarction leading to avascular necrosis of femoral heads), high output cardiac failure, and autosplenectomy. In addition, a high risk for pneumonia, meningitis, salmonellosis, osteomyelitis, pulmonary emboli, cor pulmonale, and chronic skin ulcers and high incidences of spontaneous abortion, perinatal mortality, and maternal mortality are associated with the disease. These patients also have hepatomegaly, hepatic infarctions, and jaundice.

HEMOPHILIA

Hemophilia is an inherited, sex-linked disorder that occurs in men and boys but is carried by women. This bleeding disorder can range from mild to severe. Fig. 41-1 schematically depicts the primary clotting mechanism. Each factor is a protein or glycoprotein that circulates in human plasma. Clotting factors circulate in an inactive form. Activation of clotting factors requires an initiating mechanism; initiation occurs when a cut or bruise is sustained. The clotting factors are activated in dominolike fashion. The initial activation of Factor XII causes the activation of Factor XI and other clotting factors until fibrinogen becomes fibrin and a clot is formed. If any one of these factors is removed from the sequence, clotting does not occur.

Simply stated, hemophilia can be viewed as a bleeding disorder caused by the absence of a clotting factor. The term *hemophilia* is actually a catchall term for a number of different clotting disorders. Most patients with hemophilia have classic, or type A, hemophilia, which results from a Factor VII disorder. In the majority of patients, Factor VII is not missing and may even be present in excess, but it

may not function or may function less than normally. The degree of severity of the bleeding disorder varies with the actual functional activity of the factor in each patient.

Because hemophilia is a genetic disorder, there is no definitive therapeutic intervention; currently we are able to offer only palliative measures.

Christmas disease is a less common type of hemophilia, also known as type B hemophilia. It is caused by an absence or a functional deficiency of Factor IX. Type A and type B hemophilias have similar clinical presentations. Hemophilia is usually first manifested in infancy and may be evident during circumcision, by bleeding gums, or as epistaxis. The possibilities of lacerations and major trauma aside, one of the worst features of hemophilia is hemarthrosis—bleeding into the joints. Hemarthrosis usually begins in adolescence and involves primarily the knees, ankles, and elbows. Pain accompanies this process, and improperly managed hemarthrosis may lead to arthritis and ultimately to joint destruction. When a patient has hemophilia, even minor trauma can cause major bruises, visceral bleeding, and subdural hematomas.

Because this disorder is usually evident during infancy, a person with hemophilia who comes to the ED because of bleeding is usually able to describe or name the disorder. A bleeding history should be obtained from all patients who have abnormal bleeding. One should also consider obtaining results of a screening coagulation panel test that includes prothrombin time and partial thromboplastin time.

Remember that platelet-mediated hemostasis does not depend on Factor VIII or Factor IX. It is therefore imperative that the bleeding body part be elevated whenever possible and that gentle pressure be applied for 5 to 10 minutes.

In a person with type A hemophilia the functional level of Factor VIII can be augmented by transfusion with fresh frozen plasma, cryoprecipitate from pooled plasma, or glycine-precipitated antihemophilic factor (Table 41-1). The amount of Factor VIII in fresh frozen plasma is small. The volume of platelets required for the patient to receive enough Factor VII from platelet infusion would place the patient at risk of circulatory overload. Cryoprecipitate is given 1 to 2 units per 4 kg body weight, a much smaller volume, but it carries a high risk of hepatitis. Cryoprecipitate still remains the treatment of choice and can actually be administered at home by the motivated and educated family of the patient with hemophilia.

Episodes of hemarthrosis are usually self-limited by the inability of the joint capsule to distend beyond its limits. This inability to continue to distend eventually tamponades the bleeding. The joint should be immobilized, a light pressure dressing placed, and ice applied, and the limb should be elevated. After Factor VIII is administered to correct the coagulation problem, blood in the joint should be aspirated. Weight bearing should be limited, and the patient should be referred to a physical therapist for range-of-motion exercises

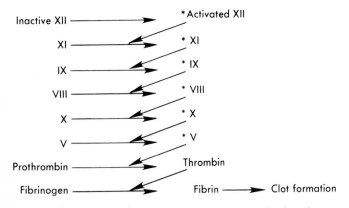

Fig. 41-1 Clotting factors (intrinsic mechanisms).

Table 41-1   Recommended Factor VIII therapy for specific problems in hemophilia

Type of bleeding	Initial dose	Duration	Comment
Skin			
Abrasion	None	None	Treat with local pressure and topical thrombin
Laceration			
Superficial	Usually none; if necessary treat as minor	None	Local pressure and anesthetic with epinephrine may benefit; watch 4 hours after suturing, reexamine in 24 hours
Deep	Minor bleed (12.5 mg/kg)	Single dose coverage	May need hospitalization for observation; repeat may be necessary for suture removal
Nasal epistaxis			
Spontaneous	Usually none; may need to be treated as mild bleed	None	Uncommon; consider platelet inhibition; treat in usual manner
Traumatic	Moderate bleed (25 mg/kg)	Up to 5 to 7 days	Trauma-related bleed can be significant
Oral			
Mucosa or tongue bites	Usually none; treat as minor if persists	Single dose	Commonly seen
Traumatic (laceration) or dental extraction	Moderate (25 U/kg) to severe (50 U/kg)	Single dose; may need more	Saliva rich in fibrin lytic activity; oral ϵ-aminocaproic acid (Amicar) may be given 100 mg every 6 hours for 7 days to block fibrinolysis; check contraindications; hospitalize patients with severe bleeds
Soft tissue and muscle hematomas	Moderate (25 U/kg) to severe (50 U/kg)	2 to 5 days	May be complicated by local pressure on nerves or vessels (e.g., iliopsoas, forearm, calf)
Hemarthrosis			
Early	Mild (12.5 U/kg)	Single dose	Treat at earliest symptom (pain); knee, elbow, ankle most common
Late or unresponsive early cases	Mild to moderate (25 U/kg)	3 to 4 days	Arthrocentesis rarely necessary and only with 50% level coverage; immobilization is critical point of therapy
Hematuria	Mild (12.5 U/kg)	2 to 3 days	Urokinase (fibrinolytic enzyme) is in urine; with persistent hematuria organic cause should be ruled out
Major bleeding			
Gastrointestinal severe bleeding Neck and sublingual Retroperitoneal Intraabdominal Major trauma Head injury Central nervous system bleed Surgical procedure	Major bleed (50 U/kg)	7 to 10 days or 3 to 5 days after bleeding ceases	In head trauma, therapy should be given prophylactically; in severe head trauma or with associated neurologic signs, early computed tomographic scanning recommended

From Rosen P et al: *Emergency medicine: concepts and clinical practice*, ed 2, St Louis, 1987, Mosby–Year Book.

and for close hematologic and orthopedic follow-ups.

Type B hemophilia is relatively rare. It presents us with much greater management problems. Treatment is thus far limited to less than satisfactory administration of fresh frozen plasma. All other treatment modalities are the same as those for patients with type A hemophilia.

LEUKEMIA

There are primarily two types of leukemia, acute and chronic. These types were named for the period of time a person was expected to survive after the diagnosis. Chronic leukocytic leukemia is seen primarily in people more than 50 years of age. The chief complaint is fatigue, frequent infections, easy bruising, weight loss, and skin rashes. Clinically, enlarged lymph nodes and splenic and liver enlargement may be present. A white blood cell count of greater than 5000 cells/mm^3 may be diagnostic.

In acute lymphoblastic leukemia the white cell count is greater than 50,000 cells/mm^3. The appropriate therapeutic intervention depends on the stage of the disease. Making the differential diagnosis includes ruling out infection, tumors, or trauma. The completion of diagnosis usually involves hospitalization to perform in-depth diagnostic studies, including bone marrow evaluation. Once again, therapeutic intervention depends on the stage of the disease and probably includes chemotherapy and radiation therapy.

SUMMARY

Some of the many hematologic disorders for which patients may be seen in the ED have been discussed. The reader is referred to one of many texts listed in the references for this chapter for more detailed information concerning these and other hematologic disorders.

REFERENCE

1. Unger H: Hyperbaric oxygen. Lecture, Symposium Medicus, Cancun, Mexico, Jan 1991.

SUGGESTED READINGS

Alavi JB: Sickle cell anemia, *Med Clin North Am* 68:545, 1984.

Bennett JS: Blood coagulation and coagulation tests, *Med Clin North Am* 68:557, 1984.

Gill FM: Congenital bleeding disorders: hemophilia and von Willebrand's disease, *Med Clin North Am* 68:608, 1984.

Gradisch RE: Priapism in sickle cell disease, *Ann Emerg Med* 12:510, 1983.

Kellermeyer RW: General principles of the evaluation and therapy of anemias, *Med Clin North Am* 68:533, 1984.

Maslow WE et al: The diagnosis of anemia. In Maslow WC et al, eds: *Hematological disease: practical diagnosis,* Boston, 1980, Houghton Mifflin.

Roberts WC, Speicher CE: *The medical laboratory and the emergency department,* Norwalk, Conn, 1984, Appleton-Century-Crofts.

Thompson AR, Harker LA: *Manual of hemostasis & thrombosis,* ed 3, Philadelphia, 1983, FA Davis.

Warth JA, Ruchnagel DA: The increasing complexity of sickle cell anemia, *Prog Hematol* 13:25, 1984.

CHAPTER
42 Infection Control

Molly Strout

Infection occurs when there is an interaction or contact between an infectious agent and a susceptible host. This interaction is called *transmission*. Three factors represent the chain of infection: agent, transmission, and host.

PREVENTION OF INFECTION

The agent or microorganism can be a bacterium, virus, fungus, or parasite. Pathogenicity is the ability of the agent to cause disease. Some agents are highly pathogenic and almost always produce disease in a host. Other agents multiply without causing invasion (colonization) and rarely cause clinical disease.

The major modes of transmission involved in the chain of infection include contact (direct, indirect, and droplet), common vehicle, airborne spread, and vectorborne spread.

A susceptible host is someone who lacks effective resistance to a pathogenic agent. Some characteristics that influence susceptibility include age, sex, disease history, underlying disease, life-style, nutrition, immunization, medications, and trauma.

Direct contact transmission of an agent occurs when there is person-to-person contact between an infected or colonized source and a susceptible host. An indirect transmission occurs when the susceptible host has come in contact with an intermediate object, such as contaminated patient care equipment. Droplet contact transmission involves an infected source and a susceptible host, who must be in close proximity. The infected source, through coughing or sneezing, briefly transmits large infectious particles through the air.

Within the hospital environment the most common mode of transmission of an infectious agent to a susceptible host occurs by direct, indirect, or droplet contact.

Less frequently seen in the hospital environment is the airborne spread of infectious agents. Diseases such as tuberculosis, chickenpox, and measles are transmitted via the airborne mode. With these diseases the infectious agent is suspended in the air for longer periods; thus susceptible hosts may breathe them into their respiratory systems.

Handwashing is considered the single most important pro-

cedure in breaking this chain of infection. In the absence of a true emergency, personnel should always wash their hands at the following times[3]:
1. Before performing invasive procedures
2. Before taking care of particularly susceptible patients, such as those who are severely immunocompromised and newborns
3. Before and *after* touching wounds, whether surgical, traumatic, or associated with an invasive device
4. After situations during which microbial contamination of hands is likely to occur, especially those involving contact with mucous membranes, blood or body fluids, secretions, or excretions
5. After touching inanimate sources that are likely to be contaminated with virulent or epidemiologically important microorganisms; these sources include urine-measuring devices or secretion-collecting apparatus
6. After taking care of an infected patient or one who is likely to be colonized with microorganisms of special clinical or epidemiologic significance, for example, multiply resistant bacteria
7. Between contacts with certain patients in high-risk units

Products containing antimicrobial agents that do not require water for use, such as foams or rinses, can be used in areas where no sinks are available.[3]

There will always be patients in the emergency department (ED) with infections or infectious diseases. Patients who have respiratory infections reflect community and seasonal incidence. Risk to the ED staff of these types of infections, which are usually viral, is probably no greater than the risk to people in nonhospital settings such as schools, offices, or stores.

ED personnel are at greater risk of exposure to bloodborne pathogens, such as hepatitis B virus (HBV) and human immunodeficiency virus (HIV) because of frequent exposure to blood and the unknown status of patients. It is of utmost importance for ED personnel to follow universal precautions, treating *all* patients' blood and certain body fluids as though they are infectious.

The following guidelines are provided to help the emergency care provider maintain minimal risk of HIV infection while caring for many unknown or diagnosed individuals during lifesaving procedures[4]:

I. Health care workers with open skin lesions (exudative, or weeping, dermatitis) should not perform direct patient care or handle contaminated equipment until the condition resolves. Although pregnant health care workers are not known to be at greater risk of contracting HIV infections than nonpregnant workers, the consequences of acquiring an infection should cause one to use special caution when working with suspected patients or contaminated equipment, supplies, or materials.

II. Nurses providing direct patient care should take the following precautions.
   A. Disposable gloves should be worn.
      1. When touching mucous membranes or nonintact skin of all patients, including during dressing changes, during oral, nasal, or endotracheal suctioning, while inserting nasogastric tubes, or while providing oral care or handling reusable thermometers
      2. When performing arterial or venous punctures; when aspirating blood from arterial infusion lines, Swan-Ganz or Hickman catheters, or other vascular access devices; or when handling blood or body fluid specimens, whether for laboratory study or bedside analysis
      3. When changing perineal pads used for vaginal bleeding or discharge or for incontinence
      4. When hanging or changing units of blood or blood products and administration tubing
      5. When bedpans, urinals, and emesis basins are emptied and when stomal care is given
   B. If a glove is torn or punctured, it should be removed, hands should be washed, and new gloves should be used.
   C. Wash hands immediately if contaminated with blood or body fluids, between patient contacts, after touching contaminated inanimate objects, and after removal of gloves.
   D. Wear additional appropriate barrier precautions (for example, masks, gowns, or eye coverings) when the possibility of extensive exposure to blood or other body fluids is present.
      1. During resuscitation of trauma patients, with or without multiple transfusions
      2. During emergency deliveries, especially while handling the placenta and infant, until all blood and amniotic fluid have been removed from the baby
   E. If clothing is soiled with blood or body fluids, it may be washed in a regular laundry cycle.
   F. Use artificial airway and resuscitation devices rather than mouth-to-mouth rescue breathing. Although the risk of transmission in saliva is only theoretical, this precaution also helps prevent other forms of infection.
   G. Needles should not be recapped, bent, or broken, since these actions increase the risk of unintentional needle-stick injury. During emergency procedures, take extra care to place needles directly in puncture-proof containers. A conscious effort must be made to avoid setting needles on the bed or the bed linen or dropping them on the floor, especially when one is working with catheters that require withdrawing a needle before attaching the intravenous tubing.

III. Nurses giving indirect patient care should take precautions.
   A. Nondisposable sharp instruments should be carried in a puncture-resistant container to the area where they can be cleaned; they should not be carried on one's hand.
   B. Reusable equipment should be scrubbed of all debris and blood, then disinfected; rinsing with water is not sufficient. Persons who are doing the cleaning should wear gloves. Boxes of disposable gloves and plastic bags should be kept in nonsterile utility rooms and in patient bathrooms to encourage the use of the gloves and bags during handling of contaminated items.
   C. Work areas, countertops, emergency stretchers, specimen analysis kits, and monitoring equipment that have been contaminated with blood or body fluids should be wiped with absorbent toweling to remove excess materials and then washed with isopropyl alcohol, a 1:10 dilution of sodium hypochlorite (household bleach), or other suitable germicide approved by the Environmental Protection Agency. One should be cautious with sodium hypochlorite because it is corrosive to metals, especially aluminum.
   D. Disposal of wastes should be carried out properly.
      1. Blood, body fluid drainage, or other contaminated liquids should be carefully poured into a drain and flushed into the sewer system.
      2. Solid contaminated items should be placed in sturdy plastic bags, labeled, and disposed of according to hospital policy for contaminated items.

IV. The Centers for Disease Control (CDC) published the following suggested protocol for managing HIV exposure (although each institution develops its own specific policies and procedures).
   A. Significant exposure is suspected if a person is inoculated with contaminated blood or body fluid parenterally, is splashed with blood or fluid on the mucous membranes of the eyes or mouth, or has extensive cutaneous exposure to open skin lesions.

B. The person considered to be the source of HIV should be assessed by clinical and epidemiologic examination to determine the relative likelihood of HIV infection. If the assessment suggests that the patient is infected, he or she should be informed of the incident and requested to have serologic testing.

C. The person possibly exposed to HIV infection should have serologic testing as soon as possible if the source person has AIDS, has evidence of HIV infection, or has declined to be tested.

1. If tests of the newly exposed person have seronegative results, he or she should be retested in 6 weeks and subsequently on a periodic basis (that is, at 3, 6, and 12 months) to determine whether transmission has occurred. Most infected individuals show seroconversion during the first 6 to 12 weeks.

2. During the follow-up period, especially the first 6 to 12 weeks, the newly exposed individual should observe the U.S. Public Health Service recommendations for the prevention of transmission of AIDS.

Blood is the single most important source of HIV, HBV, and other bloodborne pathogens in the occupational setting. Infection control efforts for HIV, HBV, and other bloodborne pathogens must focus on preventing exposures to blood and delivery of HBV immunization.[9]

Table 42-1   Body fluids and tissues from which HIV has been isolated or transmission documented

Body fluid or tissue	Isolated	Transmission documented	Occupational transmission documented
Blood	X	X	X
Serum	X		
Vaginal secretions	X	X	
Semen	X	X	
Breast milk	X	X	
In utero		X	
Pleural fluid		X	X
Alveolar fluid	X		
Saliva	X		
Tears	X		
Urine	X		
Cerebrospinal fluid	X		
Synovial fluid	X		
Amniotic fluid	X		
Brain	X		
Marrow	X		
Transplanted kidney		X	
Transplanted bone		X	
Transplanted liver		X	

From Kelen GD: Human immunodeficiency virus and the emergency department: risks and risk protection for health care providers, *Ann Emerg Med* 19(3):243, 1990.

Universal precautions also apply to semen and vaginal secretions, although these body fluids have been implicated in sexual transmission rather than occupational transmission.[9]

Universal precautions also apply to tissues and the following fluids: cerebrospinal fluid (CSF) and synovial, pleural, peritoneal, pericardial, and amniotic fluid. The risk from these fluids is unknown.[9]

Universal precautions do not apply to feces, nasal secretions, sputum, sweat, tears, urine, or vomitus unless these contain visible blood. The risk of transmission of HIV and HBV from these fluids and materials is extremely low or nonexistent.[9]

Table 42-1 summarizes body fluids and tissues from which HIV has been isolated or transmission documented.

Hospital infection control practitioners (ICP) usually have responsibility for infection control in the ED. Responsibilities include education about reducing risk of infection, isolation precautions, management of employee exposures, and orientation for new employees. The ICP would also act as a consultant to the ED for development of policies and procedures.

Some infectious diseases must be reported according to state and local regulations. Reporting is usually the responsibility of the ICP. It is important in the ED to be familiar with what diseases are reportable and to follow hospital policy in notifying the appropriate person or agency.

SPECIFIC TYPES OF INFECTIOUS DISEASES
Acquired Immunodeficiency Syndrome

Acquired immunodeficiency syndrome (AIDS) is an infection caused by the human immunodeficiency virus (HIV). It is transmitted by sexual contact or contaminated blood contact (sharing syringes among intravenous drug users or receiving contaminated blood products), or from an infected woman to her unborn baby. HIV infection may not always progress to AIDS and may remain asymptomatic for many years.

People with AIDS are most likely to come to the ED because of an opportunistic infection such as *Pneumocystis carinii* pneumonia, cryptococcal meningitis, or cerebral toxoplasmosis. They might also have granulocytopenia, thrombocytopenia, or intracerebral cancer. An example of a nonemergency infection that may be seen in the emergency department is oral thrush.[5]

Bloodstream Infection or Septic Shock

Infection must be suspected and actively sought in any acutely ill patient who arrives at the ED with no other obvious cause of illness. Patients who are especially susceptible to infections include immunocompromised individuals and those whose natural mechanical barriers of defense have been breached or manipulated through injury or surgery. Examples of the latter include those who have temporary or indwelling intravenous catheters (for example,

Hickman catheter) or who have had trauma or surgery.[5] (See Chapter 14 for a full discussion of signs and symptoms or therapeutic intervention for septic shock.)

Cellulitis (anaerobic). Anaerobic cellulitis can be caused by *Clostridium perfringens* or other nonclostridial anaerobic bacteria. This condition occurs in devitalized subcutaneous tissue and often causes gas formation.

Signs and symptoms of cellulitis are a dirty wound that develops an erythematous area. An exudate forms that is foul smelling, and crepitus is evident. Other than the pain associated with separation of muscle groups, there is minimal pain, and the patient apears otherwise healthy.

Therapeutic intervention includes a fasciotomy, if the vascular system is compromised, incision and drainage, the administration of antibiotics, and possibly, hyperbaric oxygen treatment.

Chancroids. Chancroids are a sexually transmitted disease (STD) caused by the gram-negative coccobacillus *Haemophilus ducreyi*. Signs and symptoms include lesions in the genital-perineal area. Typically a lesion begins as an erythematous papule, which becomes a pustular papule, then a painful, sharply demarcated, nonindurated ulcer. The ulcer may be necrotic. Usually, inguinal lymph node tenderness is unilateral.

Complications can include secondary infections, necrosis, groin fistulas, paraphimosis, or phimosis.

Therapeutic intervention includes administration of erythromycin, ceftriaxone, or trimethoprim-sulfamethoxazole. Enlarged glands may be aspirated. Incision and drainage are contraindicated.

Chlamydia. *Chlamydia trachomatis* is a bacterial pathogen transmitted sexually. It is the most prevalent STD caused by bacteria in the United States. It has been isolated from 30% to 50% of patients with nongonococcal urethritis (NGU). Other sexually transmitted agents found in NGU include *Ureaplasma urealyticum, Trichomonas vaginalis, Candida albicans,* and herpes simplex virus.

Signs and symptoms of NGU in a man include itching, dysuria, urethral discharge, and meatal erythema. Complications can include proctitis, epididymitis, prostatitis, and urethral strictures.

When chlamydial NGU is sexually transmitted to women, it can cause mucopurulent endocervicitis and pelvic inflammatory disease. Women may be asymptomatic. When symptoms are present, they include a yellow, mucopurulent endocervical exudate and cervical friability. Complications can include endometritis, salpingitis, and infertility. During pregnancy the infection can ascend, causing puerperal infection in the mother and conjunctivitis or pneumonia in the baby.

Therapeutic intervention includes treatment with appropriate antimicrobial agents. All sexual partners exposed to *Chlamydia trachomatis* should also be examined and treated with antibiotics.

Condylomata acuminata (genital and anal warts). Genital and anal warts are sexually transmitted and caused by the human papilloma virus. Lesions are evident as single or multiple fleshy, soft, painless growths around the anus, vulvovaginal area, penis, urethra, perineum, or oral cavity. Complications include enlargement and tissue destruction.

Therapeutic intervention includes cryotherapy or carbon dioxide therapy, or the administration of podophyllin 10% in compound tincture of benzoin. Oral warts should be treated with cryotherapy, electrosurgery, or surgical removal.

Diphtheria. Diphtheria is an acute bacterial disease of the tonsils, pharynx, larynx, nose, and occasionally, other mucous membranes and skin. Diphtheria is caused by the organism *Corynebacterium diphtheriae*.

Signs and symptoms include a moderately severe sore throat and enlarged and tender cervical lymph nodes. In severe cases, edema of the neck can cause airway obstruction. A cytotoxin released from the bacteria causes a characteristic patch or patches of a grayish membrane surrounded by inflammation. Late effects of absorption of toxin can include cardiac and neurologic involvement.[1]

Therapeutic intervention includes ensurance of airway, breathing, and circulation (ABCs); administration of antitoxin; and antibiotic therapy. Special efforts should be made to ensure that health care workers in the ED are fully immunized and receive booster doses of diphtheria toxoid every 10 years.[1]

Epiglottitis. Epiglottitis is a disease caused by a bacterial infection; the causative organism is usually *Haemophilus influenzae* type b. When the epiglottis enlarges, airway obstruction occurs. Epiglottitis may be a life-threatening condition. The most commonly affected age-group is 2- to 7-year-olds. Epiglottitis is occasionally seen in adult patients.

Signs and symptoms include rapid onset, sore throat, progressive dysphagia, drooling, and a low-grade fever. The patient also has a muffled voice and respiratory stridor, with difficulty breathing and periorbital cyanosis.

Therapeutic intervention is to maintain an open airway and ensure ventilation by administering 100% oxygen and considering endotracheal intubation or cricothyrotomy or both. An IV line should be initiated, and antibiotics administered.

Gas gangrene (clostridial myonecrosis). Gas gangrene is a necrotizing anaerobic infection of fascia and muscle. The causative organism is usually *Clostridium perfringens*. This infection occurs most frequently in postsurgical or contaminated wounds. Risk factors include diabetes, peripheral vascular disease, and cancer.

Signs and symptoms include swelling and local pain and tenderness over the infected area. There may be an oozing fluid that is usually serosanguineous and initially brown or red and sweet smelling, later turning green or black. The patient is diaphoretic, demonstrates pallor, has a low-grade fever, delirium, and blebs, and is unable to contract the muscle.

Therapeutic intervention must include prompt, complete

excision of necrotic muscle. Administration of penicillin G or chloramphenicol is recommended. Hyperbaric oxygen therapy may be useful, but would never be a substitute for immediate surgery.

Gastroenteritis (infectious diarrhea). Diarrhea accompanied by fever indicates infectious diarrhea until the possibility is ruled out. It is important to obtain a good history to determine onset of diarrhea and possible precipitating factors.

Etiologic agents can be bacterial, viral, or parasitic. The box below lists common agents.[10]

Therapeutic intervention includes supportive therapy, especially administration of fluids and electrolytes. Antimotility agents may worsen the disease.

Gonorrhea. Gonorrhea is an STD caused by the bacteria *Neisseria gonorrhoeae*. The highest incidence occurs in the 20- to 24-year-old age-group. Infections depend on the involved body sites and can be genital, anorectal, or pharyngeal. Most men with gonorrhea (>90%) are symptomatic and have dysuria, frequency, and purulent urethral discharge. Women are often asymptomatic. When symptoms in women are present, they can include abnormal vaginal discharge, abnormal menses, or dysuria.

Complications can include pelvic inflammatory disease and infertility in women and epididymitis, urethral stricture, and prostatitis in men. Babies born to infected mothers can exhibit ophthalmia neonatorum, scalp abscesses at fetal monitor sites, rhinitis, pneumonia, or anorectal infections. All infected individuals are at risk of disseminated gonococcal infection, which can include septicemia, arthritis, dermatitis, meningitis, endocarditis, and perihepatitis.[2]

Therapeutic intervention includes treatment with appropriate antimicrobial agents and prophylactic treatment of sexual partners. In various parts of the country a penicillinase-producing *Neisseria gonorrhoeae* is prevalent. Patients who are proven to be infected with this organism or who live in a geographic area where incidence is high must be treated accordingly.

Granuloma inguinale. The gram-negative coccobacillus *Donovania granulomatis* causes granuloma inguinale. Although it rarely occurs in the United States, when seen, it is most commonly seen in men from the southern states.

COMMON ETIOLOGIC AGENTS FOR INFECTIOUS DIARRHEA

Bacterial	Viral	Parasitic
Escherichia coli	Rotavirus	*Entamoeba histolytica*
Salmonella	Parvovirus	*Giardia*
Shigella	Enterovirus	*Strongyloides*
Campylobacter	Adenovirus	
Vibrio		
Yersinia		
Clostridium		

The cardinal sign is painless, granulating red lesions. Therapeutic intervention is administration of antibiotics. Complications include urethral strictures, engorged pelvic glands, and rarely, elephantiasis.

Hepatitis A virus. Hepatitis A virus has many characteristics of enteroviruses. It is not related to hepatitis B virus in any way, except that both cause liver inflammation.

Most transmission occurs in the United States in day care centers, among male homosexuals, and among household contacts of persons with acute cases. It is spread via the fecal-oral route. Occasionally an outbreak occurs because of contaminated food or improper sewage treatment.

Signs and symptoms (after an incubation period of 15 to 45 days) include fever, malaise, nausea, vomiting, anorexia, dark urine, and light-colored stools.

Therapeutic intervention includes administering postexposure immune globulin (Ig) in the early incubation period. When given early, Ig can prevent 80% to 90% of cases. If given more than 2 weeks after exposure, Ig will probably not be effective.[11]

Hepatitis B. Hepatitis B is an infection of the liver caused by HBV. It is transmitted by sexual contact or contaminated blood contact (sharing syringes among intravenous drug users or receiving contaminated blood products) or from an infected woman to her unborn baby.

Five percent to 10% of Americans have had HBV infections. Much higher rates of infection are seen in populations of Third World nations, particularly parts of Africa, Southeast Asia, and Oceania. Approximately 10% of those infected with HBV become chronic carriers.[10]

Signs and symptoms include an insidious onset, rash, urticaria, arthralgia, severe illness, even death (1% of all cases). Chronic active HBV infections develop in 25% of carriers. Such infection puts carriers at risk for liver cancer or cirrhosis.

Therapeutic intervention includes treatment of symptoms. After an exposure to HBV it is appropriate to administer hepatitis B immune globulin (HBIg) and hepatitis B vaccine. This type of preventive treatment is also recommended for infants born to infected mothers. It is important for ED staff to receive HBV vaccine as part of universal precautions.

Herpes genitalis (genital herpes). Herpes simplex virus (HSV) is spread by direct mucous membrane contact with infected secretions. Urogenital herpesvirus infections can be caused by HSV-1 through contact with infectious oral secretions. Most infections (70% to 90%) are caused by HSV-2 through contact with infectious genital secretions.[2]

Signs and symptoms include single or multiple vesicles anywhere on the genitalia. These vesicles may rupture, forming shallow ulcers. With the first or primary infection, symptoms are severe and include fever, malaise, anorexia, and bilaterally tender inguinal lymph nodes. The lesions from a primary infection last longer than subsequent recurrences, up to several weeks. Recurrent infections are often preceded by tingling, pain, burning, or itching.

Complications can include neuralgia, meningitis, ascending myelitis, urethral stricture, urinary retention, and secondary bacterial infection. A neonate born to a mother with an active genital infection can become infected during vaginal delivery. Symptoms in the neonate range from mild, limited infection to a fatal, disseminated one.

Therapeutic intervention includes administration of acyclovir, an antiviral agent. Antibiotics are indicated only if there is a secondary bacterial infection.

Herpes labialis (oral herpes). Oral herpes is caused by HSV-1 and appears as small, fluid-filled blisters that form on the facial area, especially around the mouth and nose. Primary infection or the first attack is usually the most severe.

Signs and symptoms are burning and itching around the infected area, low-grade fever, and cervical lymphadenopathy.

Therapeutic intervention can include administration of the antiviral agent, acyclovir. Antibiotics are indicated only if there is a secondary bacterial infection.

Histoplasmosis. Histoplasmosis is a pulmonary infection caused by inhalation of the fungus *Histoplasma capsulatum*. This fungus is found in the excrement of birds and bats.

Signs and symptoms are variable and nonspecific. Fever and headache occur in almost all cases; chills, cough, and chest pain occur in two thirds of cases; and less frequently, weakness, weight loss, myalgia, and fatigue are present.[8]

Disseminated histoplasmosis has been included by the CDC as one of the defining infections in AIDS.

Therapeutic intervention includes administration of an antifungal agent.

Influenza. Influenza is a viral, respiratory illness that usually causes epidemics during the winter. Epidemics are usually caused by influenza type A.

Signs and symptoms can range from mild, nonspecific malaise to full-blown illness consisting of sudden onset of headache, diffuse myalgia, and fever followed by severe malaise and respiratory symptoms. Complications can include pneumonia or a secondary bacterial infection.

Treatment includes primary prevention by the administration of influenza vaccine. Influenza vaccine is recommended for the following[2]:

1. Children and adults with chronic cardiopulmonary diseases requiring hospitalization or regular ambulatory care within the preceding year
2. Residents of nursing homes and other extended care facilities
3. Physicians, nurses, medical students, and other health care workers
4. Adults 65 years of age and older
5. Persons with chronic metabolic diseases, renal abnormalities, anemia, immunosuppression, cystic fibrosis, or asthma
6. Providers of essential community services

Influenza vaccine is contraindicated for individuals with anaphylactic hypersensitivity to eggs.[2]

Legionella pneumophila (Legionnaires' disease). Legionnaires' disease is a pneumonia caused by the gram-negative bacillus *Legionella pneumophila*. The disease was recognized after the 1976 outbreak of pneumonia at an American Legion convention in Philadelphia.

Transmission of this organism occurs as a result of airborne spread from environmental sources. Several outbreaks have been linked to air from air conditioning systems or aerosolized water from colonized shower heads.

Signs and symptoms include high fever, bradycardia, gastrointestinal symptoms (diarrhea), changes in mental status, and nonproductive cough.

Therapeutic intervention includes administration of erythromycin or rifampin.

Lyme disease. Lyme disease is a tick-borne illness caused by a spirochete, *Borrelia burgdorferi*. This organism has been isolated from the tick *I. dammini*. Lyme disease is seen primarily in three geographic areas of the United States: the northeastern coastal region; Minnesota and Wisconsin; and areas of northern California, southern Oregon, and western Nevada. The distribution of Lyme disease appears to be widening, however.[2]

Lyme disease follows the pattern of many other spirochetal infections in exhibiting distinct stages and periods of remission. Clinical presentation of stage 1 includes a rash called erythema chronicum migrans, often associated with fever, fatigue, lethargy, headache, and stiff neck. Stage 2 may follow within days or months and includes neurologic and cardiac involvement. Stage 3 can occur within days to years and is characterized by development of arthritis.

Therapeutic intervention includes early diagnosis and appropriate antibiotic therapy.

Meningitis. Meningitis is an inflammation of the meninges of the brain. The infectious agent can be bacterial, viral, or fungal. Common bacterial agents include *Streptococcus pneumoniae*, *Neisseria meningitidis*, *Haemophilus influenzae*, group B streptococci, and *Listeria monocytogenes*. Acute bacterial meningitis is a life-threatening medical emergency. Currently mortality is 10% to 30%.

Signs and symptoms include fever, headache, nuchal rigidity, and mental dysfunction.

Therapeutic intervention includes immediate administration of appropriate antibiotics, anticonvulsants, antipyretics, and general supportive care (maintaining ABCs). Lumbar punctures are performed *except* in patients who are suspected of having a brain abscess. In these patients herniation of the brain can occur if a lumbar puncture is performed.[5]

Mononucleosis. Infectious mononucleosis ("mono") is a viral illness caused by the Epstein-Barr virus of the herpesvirus group. Its mode of transmission is primarily via transfer of oropharyngeal secretions. It is most commonly seen in teenagers and young adults. In the United States, by adulthood 95% of persons have antibodies to Epstein-Barr virus.[2]

Signs and symptoms are fever, sore throat, lymphadenopathy (especially in the cortical area), splenomegaly, hepatomegaly, and extreme fatigue.

Therapeutic intervention is to treat the symptoms and includes rest, fluids, analgesics, and warm saline gargles.

Mycoplasma infection. Mycoplasma are minute bacteria that can cause a number of symptoms, such as pneumonia, tracheobronchitis, pharyngitis, and myringitis. Mycoplasmal pneumonia usually occurs in children and young adults. Many complications can occur, such as sinusitis, myocarditis, polyneuritis, and Stevens-Johnson syndrome.

Signs and symptoms include respiratory tract infection, a dry cough, weakness, fever, pulmonary infiltrates, inspiratory rales, and decreased breath sounds. Therapeutic intervention is to administer antibiotics and provide bed rest, fluids, and a high-protein diet.

Necrotizing fasciitis. Necrotizing fasciitis is a mixed aerobic and anaerobic infection that rapidly dissects deep fascial planes and produces severe toxicity associated with high mortality. It most commonly occurs on the extremities but can also occur on the abdomen, scrotum, or perineum, particularly in persons with diabetes. About half of cases are caused by group A streptococci alone and the rest are caused by mixed aerobic and anaerobic bacteria.[5]

Signs and symptoms include fever, erythema, swelling, pain, bullae, and subcutaneous gas.

Therapeutic intervention must include prompt surgical removal of necrotic tissue and administration of antibiotics.

Pediculosis pubis (crabs). Pediculosis publis is an infestation caused by *Phthirus pubis* (crab or pubic louse). The infestation is transmitted by direct contact with contaminated clothes or bedding or by sexual contact with an infested person.

Symptoms range from slight discomfort to severe itching. Erythematous papules and nits or adult lice or both are present and cling to pubic, perineal, or perianal hairs. Pubic lice can also infest the eyelashes, axilla, scalp, or other body hairs.[2]

Therapeutic intervention includes application of lindane 1% to infested areas. Retreatment in 7 days is recommended if lice are found or if eggs are seen at the hair-skin junction. Sexual partners should also be treated. Contaminated clothing or bed linen should be washed and dried by machine (hot cycle) or dry cleaned.

Pertussis (whooping cough). Pertussis (whooping cough) is caused by *Bordetella pertussis,* a tiny gram-negative coccobacillus. Pertussis is highly infectious, and most cases occur in children. Fifty percent of all reported cases occur in children under 1 year of age.[10]

Pertussis begins with symptoms that mimic the common cold. After 7 to 14 days the disease may develop into the paroxysmal stage, during which the characteristic "whoop" is heard at the end of severe coughing. Complications can include bronchiectasis, otitis media, pneumonia, seizures, and rib fractures from severe coughing.[10]

Therapeutic intervention includes primary prevention by administration of vaccine to all children as recommended. Immunization is not recommended for adults because of the toxicity of the vaccine, even though most adults are susceptible to pertussis (even if they were immunized as children). Illness is less severe in older children and adults.[10]

Therapeutic intervention includes respiratory isolation to stop further spread, maintenance of ABCs, maintenance of fluid and electrolytes, and administration of antibiotics.

Poliomyelitis. Poliomyelitis is a disease caused by poliovirus, which is an enterovirus. Transmission occurs via the fecal-oral route.

Since the introduction of poliovirus vaccines, polio cases in the United States have decreased to about 10 per year. Ninety-five percent of infections are asymptomatic. Symptomatic infections are mostly nonspecific and can include fever, general malaise, headache, nausea and vomiting, abdominal pain, or neck pain. A minority of symptomatic cases result in meningeal irritation and paralysis.[10]

Therapeutic intervention includes primary prevention by administration of vaccine as recommended. In an infected individual treatment would include maintenance of the ABCs.

Rabies. Rabies is a viral illness usually transmitted to humans from bites of infected skunks, foxes, raccoons, bobcats, coyotes, dogs, cats, or bats. Aerosol transmission in bat caves can occur.[10]

Signs and symptoms include viral encephalitis, hydrophobia, or excessive salivation in a patient with a history of an unprovoked animal bite or exposure to bat caves.[10]

Therapeutic intervention for patients at high risk for rabies infection includes prompt administration of tetanus prophylaxis, rabies Ig, and rabies vaccine.

Rheumatic fever. Acute rheumatic fever may occur as a nonsuppurative complication after an upper respiratory infection caused by group A streptococci. Rheumatic fever is a relatively rare but serious complication. When the preceding streptococcal infection is treated with appropriate antibiotic therapy, the incidence of rheumatic fever is reduced to less than 1%.

Signs and symptoms of rheumatic fever include fever, polyarthritis, and carditis; these occur 7 or more days after the onset of the streptococcal infection. Rheumatic fever can be a complication of a mild infection or a severe infection. Recurrent attacks of rheumatic fever can occur, but most of these can be prevented by prophylactic penicillin therapy.

Therapeutic intervention includes prevention by promptly identifying and treating group A streptococcal infections. If rheumatic fever does occur as a complication of a group A streptococcal infection, intervention includes administration of antibiotics and analgesics, fluid and electrolyte replacement, and bed rest.

Rocky Mountain spotted fever. Rocky Mountain spotted fever is a tick-borne disease that occurs in temperate climates in the United States and other areas of North and South

America. The causative bacterium is *Rickettsia rickettsii*.

Signs and symptoms are sudden onset of fever that persists for 2 to 3 weeks, malaise, deep muscle pain, severe headache, chills, and conjunctival infection. A maculopapular rash appears on approximately the third day, occurs on the palms of the hands and soles of the feet, and can spread rapidly to most of the body. Petechiae and hemorrhages are common.[1]

Death is uncommon if this disease is promptly identified and treated with appropriate antibiotic therapy. Therapeutic intervention includes treatment with tetracycline or chloramphenicol.

Rubella (German measles). Rubella is a viral illness spread via the respiratory route. The incubation period for rubella ranges from 14 to 21 days. Since 1941 a great deal of interest has been focused on rubella because of the association between infection during early pregnancy and an increased incidence of congenital malformations (congenital rubella syndrome).

In children there is a minimal prodromal period, and the illness is characterized by rash, lymph node enlargement, and sometimes, conjunctivitis and coryza. In adolescents or adults there is a 1- to 5-day prodromal period characterized by low-grade fever, malaise, anorexia, headache, conjunctivitis, coryza, sore throat, cough, and enlarged lymph nodes. These symptoms subside after the onset of the rash.

Therapeutic intervention includes general supportive care. Immunization programs are the most effective means of preventing fetal infection and congenital rubella syndrome. Live rubella vaccine is recommended for all children 12 months of age or older. Women should not be given the vaccine within 3 months of becoming pregnant or during pregnancy.

Rubeola (old-fashioned measles). Rubeola is a highly infectious viral illness spread via the respiratory route. The incubation period ranges from 8 to 21 days. The infectious period is from 3 to 5 days before onset of the rash until 4 days after the rash onset.

During 1988 and 1989 there was an increase in reported cases of measles. Two factors have contributed to this increase: (1) failure to vaccinate preschool children, and (2) vaccine failure in vaccinated individuals. In 1989, 18,000 cases were reported, and 41 deaths occurred. Measles transmission in hospitals can contribute to and sustain community outbreaks, particularly from ED settings. Any patient suspected of having measles must be isolated in a separate examination room. Susceptible patients or staff should not be placed in this examination room for at least 1 hour (preferably 2 hours) after the patient has left the room.[6]

Signs and symptoms of the classic presentation include a maculopapular rash that lasts 3 days or more, beginning centrally and extending out to the arms and legs, fever, and one or more of the following: cough, conjunctivitis, and coryza.

Therapeutic intervention includes supportive care. The Immunization Practices Advisory Committee of the CDC recommends a two-dose measles vaccine schedule in prevention efforts. All ED staff should be immunized against measles.

Scabies. Scabies is a parasitic infection caused by the mite *Sarcoptes scabiei*. The female mite burrows under the skin to deposit eggs. Transmission occurs by intimate personal contact, often sexual, but transmission can also occur through casual contact. Less frequently, transmission can occur by contact with infested clothing or bedding.

Signs and symptoms include intense itching and the presence of burrows that are 1 to 10 ml long with small, red papules at the end of the burrow. The burrows are most often located on the penis, hands, wrists, elbows, armpits, webs of fingers, knees, outer surfaces of feet, buttocks, and waist.

Therapeutic intervention includes application, as directed, of gamma benzene hexachloride (lindane, Kwell) or crotamiton (Eurax) to all body areas from the neck down.

Scarlet fever (scarlatina). Scarlet fever is a complication of a group A streptococcal infection and occurs when the infecting strain of streptococcus is a toxin producer. Scarlet fever can be associated with a streptococcal pharyngitis or a group A streptococcal infection at any site (wound, skin, and so on).

Signs and symptoms of scarlet fever are a fine rash located mostly on the neck and chest, in the folds of the axillae, elbow, and groin, and on inner surfaces of the thighs. Usually the rash does not involve the face. With severe infections, high fever, nausea, and vomiting may be present.

Therapeutic intervention includes supportive care and administration of antibiotics to treat the streptococcal infection.

Syphilis. Syphilis is an STD caused by the organism *Treponema pallidum*. Syphilis appears in various stages during a number of years. The organism is a spirochete and is able to pass through a human placenta, causing congenital syphilis.

Signs and symptoms depend on the stage of the disease. In primary syphilis the patient has a painless chancre sore that may be either single or multiple. It surfaces on the genitalia and may also appear in other areas. This patient also develops lymphadenopathy. These symptoms occur 10 to 90 days after exposure. The fluid from the chancre contains many spirochetes, which makes the disease highly contagious. These sores usually heal in 10 to 40 days, and the patient believes he or she is cured.

The second stage, also known as secondary syphilis, occurs about 2 months after the initial infection. At this stage the spirochete has spread throughout the body. Signs and symptoms are general malaise, nausea, anorexia, fever, alopecia, joint and bone pain, and a rash that does not itch. Flat white sores develop in the mouth. Papules erupt on the moist areas of the body. At this time the disease is highly contagious and can be spread by mucous membranes coming into contact with one another, such as during kissing. These symptoms continue for 3 weeks to 2 years.

The third stage, also known as tertiary syphilis, may take 2 to 15 years to develop. In this soft and rubbery stage, tumors known as gummas form. They eventually heal and leave scars. These tumors may form anywhere in the body and are most often seen in the stomach, reproductive organs, liver, lungs, and eyes. The patient may be free of pain or may have severe burrowing pain. The gummas may cause erosion of the palate, the nasal septum, or the larynx and may invade the central nervous system, the heart, and other areas of the body. In the heart the myocardium and valves may be damaged.

Table 42-2 lists the stages and typical evolution of syphilis.

Congenital syphilis occurs when the fetus is infected from the mother. The infant may be deformed or blind. This infection may not be evident for several weeks, when the infant begins to show signs of a purulent discharge from the nose and lesions form on the palms of the hands and the soles of the feet. These children may also have vision problems, and progeria may develop.

Diagnosis is made by dark-field microscopic examination of fluid from a lesion. The infection may also be evident in venous blood and cerebrospinal fluid. A Wassermann test of the serum may not demonstrate the disease until several months after the exposure of the victim.

Therapeutic intervention includes administration of benzathine penicillin in various doses, depending on the stage

Table 42-2   Evolution of a typical case of syphilis

Stage	Duration	Clinical disease	Activity of *Treponema pallidum*	Diagnosis	Tissue change
Incubation	2-6 weeks (most often 3-4 weeks)	None	Spirochetes actively proliferate at entry site, spread over body	Identification of *Treponema pallidum:* a. Dark-field microscopy b. Fluorescent antibody technique	Chancre appears at inoculation site
Primary	8-12 weeks	1. Chancre present at inoculation site 2. Regional lymphadenopathy	Chancre teeming with them	1. Dark-field microscopy of chancre 2. STS become positive	Chancre present
Primary latent	4-8 weeks	None	Inconspicuous	STS positive	None demonstrable; chancre has healed with little scarring
Secondary	Variable over period of 5 years (latent periods with recurrences)	1. Skin and mucosal lesions ("mucous patches") 2. Generalized lymphadenopathy	Skin and mucosal lesions rich in spirochetes (highly infectious)	1. Dark-field microscopy of lesions 2. STS positive	1. Infection active: a. Vascular changes b. Cuffs of inflammatory round cells about small blood vessels 2. Resolution spontaneous—little scarring
Latent	Few months to a life time (average 6-7 years)	None	Inconspicuous	STS positive (can be negative)	
Tertiary	Variable—rest of patient's life	Related to organ system diseased and the incapacity thereof	Paucity of spirochetes in classic lesions	1. STS positive or negative 2. Special silver stains of tissue lesions may show spirochetes	1. Gumma 2. Definite predilection to heal in lesions 3. Scarring 4. Tissue distortion and abnormal function

From Mosby's medical and nursing dictionary, St Louis, 1983, Mosby–Year Book.
STS, Serologic tests for syphilis.

of the disease. The patient's sexual partner should also be treated.

Tetanus (lockjaw). Tetanus is an acute illness caused by an exotoxin of the tetanus bacillus or *Clostridium tetani*. This organism grows anaerobically at the site of an injury. The tetanus bacillus can be present in soil, human and animal excrement, and street dust. The organism remains in spore form until conditions are favorable. When favorable conditions occur, the spores germinate and infect the injured soft tissue. This agent secretes a neurotoxin that is rapidly absorbed into the circulation, affecting the central nervous system. The incubation period is variable, ranging from 3 days to several months; 3 to 10 days is the average length. Tetanus cases in the United States are rare because of the high immunization rate. Mortality, however, is high. Information on tetanus prophylaxis can be found in Chapter 18.

Signs and symptoms include a history of a penetrating injury or burn, general malaise, muscle rigidity, a low-grade fever, headache, trismus (lockjaw), and the inability to swallow. The patient also has distortion of facial muscles, risus sardonicus (a sardonic grin), opisthotonos, seizures, and respiratory arrest. *Clostridium tetani* can be cultured from the wound.

Therapeutic intervention includes administration of tetanus immune globulin (TIg). If TIg is not available, tetanus antitoxin (equine origin) should be given. Antibiotics must be administered, and the wound should be debrided if possible. Supportive care must be provided with special attention toward maintenance of the ABCs. It may be necessary to perform a tracheostomy to maintain the airway and administer sedatives and muscle relaxants. Active immunization should also be initiated.

Toxic shock syndrome. Toxic shock syndrome (TSS) is associated with an infection from *Staphylococcus aureus* that produces toxins. TSS has been associated with menstruating women who used tampons, particularly the superabsorbent type. Thirteen percent of cases are *not* associated with menstruation.

Clinical presentation includes acute onset of fever, hypotension, and a diffuse erythematous or scarlatiniform rash that desquamates in 1 to 2 weeks. TSS is associated with multisystem involvement that usually includes three of the following: mucous membrane hyperemia, vomiting or diarrhea, renal failure or pyuria, hepatic enzyme elevation or jaundice, thrombocytopenia, central nervous system disorientation or change in level of consciousness unrelated to fever, and shock.[2]

Intervention includes treating symptoms of shock with fluid replacement and vasopressors and administering appropriate antibiotic therapy. It is essential to drain any collection of *S. aureus* by removal of the tampon or debridement of any infected wounds.

Trichomoniasis. Trichomoniasis is a sexually transmitted vaginal infection caused by the organism *Trichomonas vaginalis*.

Signs and symptoms are erythema and edema of the external genitalia and a vaginal discharge that is pale yellow to greenish gray, frothy, and foul smelling. Men may develop trichomoniasis that manifests as urethritis.

Therapeutic intervention is administration of metronidazole (Flagyl). Because of the disulfuram (Antabuse) effect of metronidazole, consumption of alcohol while taking metronidazole is contraindicated. Contacts must be treated, or reinfection can occur.

Tuberculosis. Tuberculosis (TB) is caused by the bacterium *Mycobacterium tuberculosis* and usually infects the lungs or respiratory system. TB can spread to other foci in the body, such as the kidneys, meninges, and growing bone tissue in children. It is spread by airborne droplets.

The possibility of TB should be considered when a person is initially seen with respiratory symptoms, but especially if the person has spent much time in an underdeveloped nation or has had limited access to health care in this country. Two thirds of TB cases in the United States are in Hispanics, Blacks, American Indians, and Asians. Homeless people are at high risk.[7]

A person's general immune status affects the risk of TB infection. Advanced age, corticosteroid medication, cancer chemotherapy, HIV infection, malnutrition, or chronic illness can reduce a person's immunity and place him or her at risk for TB infection.

Signs and symptoms include fatigue, weight loss, fever, cough, chest pain, hemoptysis, and hoarseness. Diagnosis is confirmed by recovery of *M. tuberculosis* from a sputum sample, positive results from a radiograph, and a positive result from a tuberculin skin test.

Therapeutic interventions include respiratory isolation to prevent spread, administration of antituberculin drugs, and supportive care.

Typhoid fever. Typhoid fever is caused by the bacterium *Salmonella typhosa*. It can be found in contaminated food, water, or milk and carries a high mortality. Complications include intestinal hemorrhage and thrombophlebitis. Signs and symptoms are headache, cough, fever, maculopapular rash, diarrhea, and splenomegaly. Therapeutic intervention is the administration of antibiotics and antipyretics, cool sponging, and prevention by vaccination.

Vaginitis. Vaginitis is associated with three main clinical entities: trichomoniasis, vulvovaginal candidiasis, and bacterial vaginosis. Trichomoniasis is sexually transmitted, whereas candidiasis is not. The significance of sexual transmission is unknown in bacterial vaginosis. There is no single bacterial agent that causes bacterial vaginosis.[2]

Signs and symptoms of vulvovaginal candidiasis include marked pruritus and a cottage cheese–like vaginal discharge. Therapeutic intervention involves local treatment with an antifungal agent.

Signs and symptoms of bacterial vaginosis include a mild to moderate vaginal discharge. Therapeutic intervention is usually administration of metronidazole by mouth.

Varicella-zoster virus. Varicella-zoster virus (V-ZV) is a virus belonging to the herpesvirus family. A first exposure to V-ZV causes varicella or chickenpox. Varicella is a highly contagious illness occurring mostly in childhood. Transmission of varicella is via the respiratory route or by direct contact with lesions. Zoster, or herpes zoster, occurs in individuals who have previously had chickenpox. Zoster occurs mostly in people who have cancer or are immunosuppressed.

Signs and symptoms of varicella are a generalized vesicular skin eruption, urticaria, fever, headache, anorexia, and general malaise. In an immunosuppressed individual varicella may progress to pneumonia, meningoencephalitis, and death.

Localized zoster may begin with pain followed by vesicular skin eruptions, usually unilateral and confined to a small area. Localized zoster can progress to disseminated zoster and can cause severe systemic infection or pneumonia.

Therapeutic intervention includes supportive care and administration of acyclovir to high-risk immunocompromised or immunosuppressed individuals. Varicella zoster immune globulin (VZIg) can be given to high-risk individuals after exposure, such as high-risk neonates, nonimmune children with immunodeficiencies, or nonimmune children with cancer.[2]

SUMMARY

The recognition of the potential for the presence of an infectious disease is paramount in the care of any patient in the ED. In this age of prevalence of life-threatening infectious diseases, one must assume that any patient may be a potential source of the infection; one must employ universal precautions whenever a potential for exposure exists. Careful attention to this matter reduces the spread of infection and contamination.

REFERENCES

1. Bensenson A: *Control of communicable diseases in man*, ed 14, Washington, DC, 1985, The American Public Health Association.
2. Berg R, ed: *The APIC curriculum for infection control practice*, vol III, Dubuque, Iowa, 1988, Kendall/Hunt.
3. Garner, Favero: CDC guidelines for handwashing and hospital environmental control, *Infection Control* 7(4):231, 1986.
4. Halpern J: Precautions to prevent transmission of human immunodeficiency virus infections in emergency settings, *J Emerg Nurs* 13(5):298, 1987.
5. Ho M, Saunders C: *Current emergency diagnosis and treatment*, ed 3, Norwalk, Conn, 1990, Appleton-Lange.
6. Lett S: Measles and nosocomial measles control. Talk presented at APIC 17th Annual Education Conference, June 7, 1990, Washington, DC.
7. Madsen L: Tuberculosis today, *RN* p 45-46, March 1990.
8. Mandell G, Douglas R, Bennett J, ed: *Principles and practices of infectious diseases*, ed 3, New York, 1990, Churchill Livingstone.
9. Morbidity and Mortality Weekly Report, June 1988.
10. Soule B, ed: *The APIC curriculum for infection control practice*, vol I, Dubuque, Iowa, 1983, Kendall/Hunt.
11. Soule B, ed: *The APIC curriculum for infection control practice*, vol II, Dubuque, Iowa, 1983, Kendall/Hunt.

SUGGESTED READINGS

Bennett J, Brachman, P, eds: *Hospital infections*, ed 2, Boston, 1986, Little, Brown.
Krugman S et al: *Infectious diseases in children*, ed 8, St Louis, 1985, Mosby–Year Book.

Psychosocial and Mental Health Assessment

Teresa Willett Steele and Nancy Hogan Grover

Emergency departments (EDs) provide care by means of quick assessment of data, determination of a diagnosis, plan of care, intervention, and immediate evaluation of care provided. However, the condition of the patient who comes to the ED with a psychiatric or psychosocial disorder often does not allow for following this protocol. The patient who comes to the ED often requires a complex assessment resulting in more than one diagnosis. The patient may or may not respond to the planned intervention; thus evaluation cannot be immediate. Keeping these patients' care and management brief is often not possible. The patient's support system must often be involved, discharge planning is more elaborate, and interventions often require time-consuming personal involvement of the caregiver.

These patients present a challenge that is not always welcomed in the ED. However, successful intervention in a crisis or psychiatric situation can be a rewarding experience—one that allows the nurse to practice primary nursing in its purest form.

The patient with a psychiatric emergency arrives at the ED with a severe dysfunction of behavior, mood, thinking, or perception that could, without intervention, create a threat to life, adequate functioning, or psychologic integrity. The term *psychosocial* usually denotes the understanding that both internal (psychologic) and interpersonal (social) factors come into play in determining a person's emotional state. When referring to emergency situations the term *psychosocial* is frequently used to describe conditions that arise from situational causes, whereas the term *psychiatric* is used to describe conditions attributed to the presence of mental illness. The severity of the emergency is related to the patient's ability to function and adapt and to his or her available support system, regardless of the presence or absence of mental illness.[11]

Working with this type of patient requires many skills. Three approaches may be used for a comprehensive assessment of any patient who has a psychiatric emergency.

Aguilera and Messick[1] present a model of the assessment of crisis (a situation that cannot be resolved by an individual's normal repertoire of coping strategies) and a model of *intervention* for resolution of a crisis. The *stress-adaptation* approach emphasizes the role of stress in the increased incidence of illness. Illness is viewed as a pattern of human reactions to stress or as maladaptation. The *human needs* theory is basic to the nursing process. When an individual is unable to meet a need, a problem exists. Maslow[19] outlined the individual's basic needs in a hierarchy that should be familiar to all nurses.

CRISIS INTERVENTION MODEL

Patients who enter the ED in a state of crisis exhibit many behavioral problems. The nurse needs to adapt to change readily and at the same time view each patient as a unique individual with special immediate needs. Therefore it is imperative that emergency nurses have a workable practice model available to correctly assess each patient's immediate problems.

A model that focuses on crisis intervention and incorporates the problem-solving approach has been designed by Aguilera and Messick.[1] This model views human beings as organisms that exist in a state of equilibrium until a stressful

---

CASE STUDY 43-1

EMERGENCY SITUATION MODEL

John Black, a 19-year-old college student, is brought to the ED by two roommates. One of his roommates is holding a cloth over John's bleeding wrist. A pronounced odor of alcohol is present. Using the crisis intervention model, the nurse assesses the following factors:

1. Perception of the problem—John verbally states that he believes life is not worth living because a girlfriend recently broke up with him.
2. Situational support—John states that he is upset that his friends brought him into the emergency room. He does not wish to notify his parents. He says that his only support was his girlfriend.
3. Coping style—John reveals that he believes that the only solution to his problem is to end his life.

event occurs. This stressful event changes a human being's state to one of disequilibrium, and a subsequent need to restore equilibrium occurs. For the problem to be resolved, the following balancing factors must be present: (1) a realistic perception of the event by the patient, (2) the availability of an adequate situational support, and (3) adequate coping skills with which to address the problems. If these three balancing factors are present, there is potential for resolution of the problem, which permits the return to the equilibrium state and prevention of a crisis. Additionally,

this model postulates that when one or more of these balancing factors is absent, the consequence is that the problem is unresolved, disequilibrium increases, and a crisis occurs or is imminent (Fig. 43-1). The scenario presented in the case study on p. 583 is an example of an application of this model in an emergency situation.

The nurse assessed that John had a distorted perception of the event. He did not seek available situational support and he had used maladaptive coping skills. The three balancing factors were absent, which resulted in continued

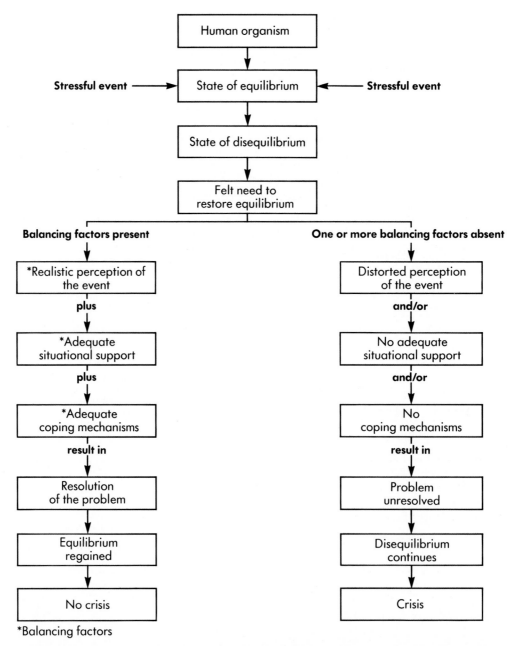

Fig. 43-1 Paradigm: effect of balancing factors in stressful event. (From Aguilera DC, Messick JM: *Crisis intervention: theory and methodology*, ed 6, St Louis, 1990, Mosby–Year Book.)

disequilibrium, a crisis situation, and a suicide attempt (Fig. 43-2).

The steps in the crisis intervention model correlate with the first step in the nursing process, the assessment of the crisis and the identification of the problem. This assessment gives the nurse direction for use of measures that include (1) planning and therapeutic intervention to prevent increased maladaptive behaviors and (2) evaluation and anticipatory planning for admission, discharge, or referral.

Resolution of a crisis usually occurs within 6 weeks and may result in either adaptive or maladaptive behaviors. The immediate action taken by the emergency nurse is imperative. This is a time of increased vulnerability for the patient, and crisis intervention may have the following results: (1) a return to the original level of functioning, (2) increased personal growth, or (3) a less effective level of functioning.[4]

Two additional models that assist the nurse in further assessment, planning, intervention, and evaluation follow.

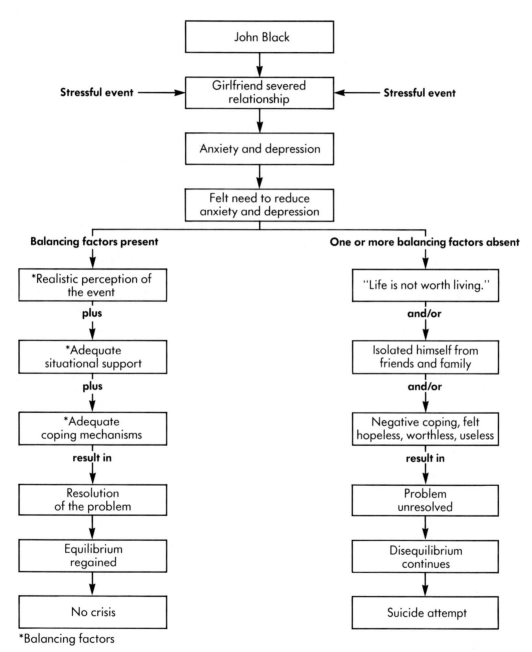

Fig. 43-2   Paradigm: effect of balancing factors in stressful event. (From Aguilera DC, Messick JM: *Crisis intervention: theory and methodology,* ed 6, St Louis, 1990, Mosby–Year Book.)

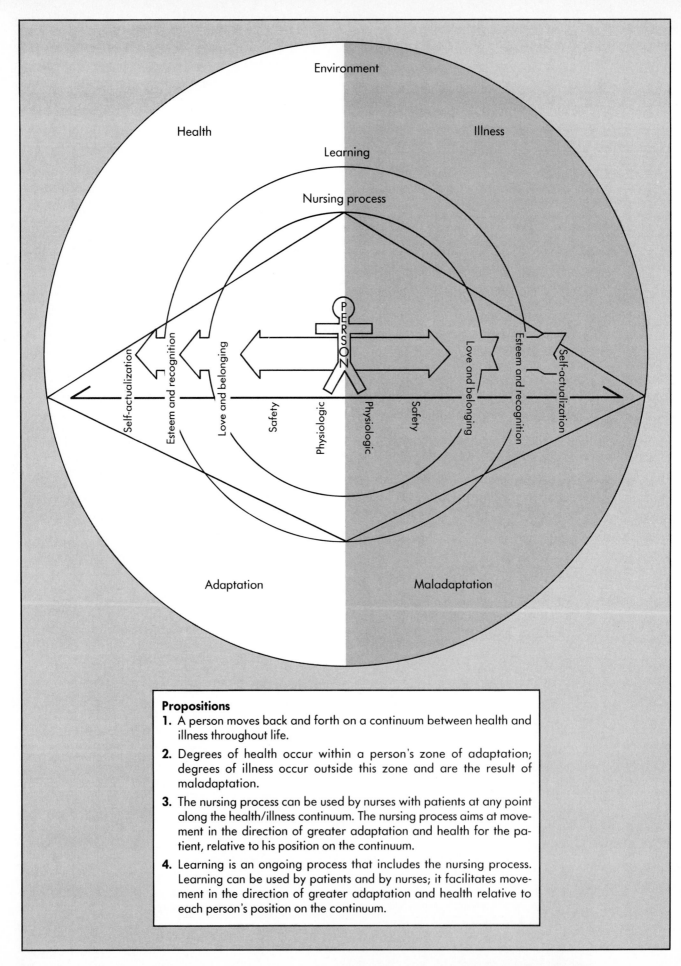

Propositions

1. A person moves back and forth on a continuum between health and illness throughout life.

2. Degrees of health occur within a person's zone of adaptation; degrees of illness occur outside this zone and are the result of maladaptation.

3. The nursing process can be used by nurses with patients at any point along the health/illness continuum. The nursing process aims at movement in the direction of greater adaptation and health for the patient, relative to his position on the continuum.

4. Learning is an ongoing process that includes the nursing process. Learning can be used by patients and by nurses; it facilitates movement in the direction of greater adaptation and health relative to each person's position on the continuum.

Fig. 43-3 Model demonstrates adaptive and maladaptive routes for coping with stress. (Adapted from Husson College and Eastern Maine Medical Center Baccalaureate Nursing Program.)

Stress-Adaptation

Emotions can cause physical changes; for example, in response to rage or fear, the body prepares for flight or aggression (flight or fight response). Swanson[23] identified stress as an actual cause of physical disorders. Emotional arousal triggers the sympathetic branch of the autonomic nervous system and the endocrine system. The physiologic response to stress is more predictable than the behavioral responses.[17] The response remains the same whether the stress is physical, psychologic, or social. When the flight or fight response is sustained, pathophysiologic changes may ensue, for example, high blood pressure, ulcers, or cardiac problems.

The opposite of the flight or fight response is the relaxation response,[3] which is synonymous with the functioning of the parasympathetic branch of the nervous system. This response has a stabilizing effect on the nervous system, which is directly opposite to the disordering effects of flight or fight response. Selye[22] further demonstrated the body's organized response to stress. In his theory, the General Adaptation syndrome, the response progresses through three stages: the stage of alarm, the stage of resistance, and the stage of exhaustion.

The alarm stage is the immediate life-preserving reaction of the sympathetic branch of the autonomic nervous system. During this stage the flight or fight response is activated, increasing secretions of epinephrine and norepinephrine.

The resistance stage occurs when the body adapts through changes in the adrenocortical response to sustain the body's fight for preservation. If the body adapts psychologically, physiologically, or behaviorally, or if the stressors have decreased, the body returns to a normal level of function. However, if the stressors continue over time, exhaustion occurs.

When a person's physical, emotional, and social resources are depleted (exhaustion), physical or emotional disorders ensue, even to the point of death.

Fig. 43-3 and Table 43-1 demonstrate the intermingling of the stress-adaptation and human needs theories in assessment of a patient who comes into the ED with a stress-related or psychiatric complaint. Table 43-1 outlines the three stages of adaptation and the physical and psychologic changes that occur in each, as outlined in Selye's model of the General Adaptation syndrome. Fig. 43-4 demonstrates both the adaptive and maladaptive routes for coping with stress.

Abraham Maslow's hierarchy of needs theory[19] is one of the most popular and widely known theories of motivation. According to Maslow, individuals are motivated to satisfy the following categories of needs:

1. Physiologic needs, including the needs for food, water, air, and sex
2. Safety and security needs, including the needs for stability, self-preservation, and freedom from fear of threat
3. Social needs, including the needs for friendship, affection, acceptance, and interaction with others—"belongingness" and love

---

Table 43-1 General adaptation syndrome

Stage	Physical changes	Psychologic changes
STAGE I Alarm reaction: immobilization of the body's defense forces and activation of the fight or flight mechanism	Norepinephrine and epinephrine are released, causing vasoconstriction, increased blood pressure, and increased rate and force of cardiac contractions	Level of alertness is increased
STAGE II Stage of resistance: optimal adaptation to stress within the person's capabilities	Hormone levels readjust; activity and size of adrenal cortex are reduced; lymph glands return to normal size; weight returns to normal	Use of coping mechanisms is increased and intensified; patient has tendency to rely on defense-oriented behavior
STAGE III Stage of exhaustion: loss of ability to resist stress because of depletion of body resources	Immune response is decreased with suppression of T cells and atrophy of thymus; production of hormones by adrenal glands is depleted; weight loss, enlargement of lymph nodes, and dysfunction of lymphatic system occur; if exposure to the stressor continues, cardiac failure, renal failure, or death may occur	Defense-oriented behaviors become exaggerated; disorganization of thinking and disorganization of personality are apparent; sensory stimuli may be misperceived with appearance of illusions; reality contact may be reduced with appearance of delusions or hallucinations; if exposure to the stressor continues, stupor or violence may occur

Adapted from Kneisl CR, Ames SW: *Adult health nursing: a biopsychosocial approach,* Menlo Park, Calif, 1986, Addison-Wesley.

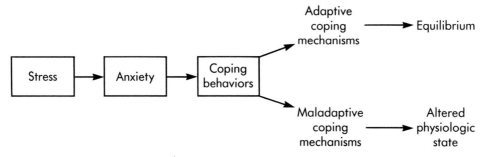

Fig. 43-4 Model of stress continuum. (Adapted from Swanson, AR: Psychophysiological disorders. In Varcarolis EM, ed: *Foundations of psychiatric mental health nursing,* Philadelphia, 1990, WB Saunders.)

4. Esteem needs, including both a need for personal feelings of achievement and self-respect and a need for respect and recognition from others
5. Self-actualization needs, including a sense of self-fulfillment or of reaching one's potential

Maslow[19] believed that these needs were arranged in a hierarchy of ascending importance with the lower-level needs being satisfied before the next higher level could motivate behavior. A person can descend as well as ascend the hierarchy; for example, if an individual's life were threatened, the need for safety would become the dominant need in a person's motivational system, replacing the need for personal recognition.

For patients who come to the ED in states of crisis, recognition of unmet needs is made evident from information that the nurse gathers during the assessment. An unmet need constitutes a problem. Problems are formulated into nursing diagnoses and prioritized, and an acceptable alternative for dealing with the unmet need is found by means of assessment, planning, interventions, and evaluation.

By using these three straightforward approaches, nurses can assess crisis states and levels of stress and adaptation, as well as unmet needs. With such comprehensive data nurses can plan and prioritize interventions for any individual who arrives at the ED with psychiatric or psychosocial concerns.

ASSESSMENT OF PATIENTS WITH PSYCHOSOCIAL STRESSORS

Five to fifteen percent of patient who seek emergency care have a primary psychiatric diagnosis and 33% have a psychologic problem in addition to a physical problem.[26] However, these statistics may not reflect the current pattern. The holistic view of a patient as a biopsychosocial interactive system reinforces the belief that any insult to the patient's overall system has the potential to cause psychosocial as well as biologic problems. Therefore trauma patients who are admitted to the ED need interventions for psychologic stressors as well as for biologic stressors.

Additionally the increasing number of mentally ill patients who live in the community and the accelerating number of young, unemployed homeless persons who have emotional problems make the ED the primary "port of entry" for health care problems of this patient population.

When a patient with psychosocial stressors enters the ED for help, it is important for the practitioner to be aware that the patient is usually extremely anxious because of maladaptive responses to stressors or to a crisis situation.

The nursing process, an interactive, systematic, problem-solving approach, gives the ED practitioner direction in facilitating the patient's speedy return to a state of equilibrium. An accurate assessment, which is the first step of the nursing process, is essential for determining the patient's problem. The assessment of the psychiatric patient involves an in-depth multidimensional interview. The psychiatric interview is an important means of collecting pertinent data from the patient and his or her significant others. The interview should be structured and goal oriented so that both the practitioner and the patient feel comfortable. The interview is conducted to answer three questions: (1) Is something wrong? (2) How urgent is the situation? and (3) Must I, as the practitioner, take action? Table 43-2 identifies nursing actions and theoretic rationale for the interview.[25]

For the interview to progress in a proficient, concise manner, the practitioner must apply specific principles and skills. The most important initial step is to establish rapport and trust. The nurse needs to be aware of his or her own thoughts and feelings regarding mental health patients and to use effective communication skills. A quiet, safe environment for the patient and nurse facilitates open communication and exploration of the precipitating event. When possible, the nurse should obtain information from the family and available members of the patient's support system after the initial interview with the patient. Additional data that should be collected include developmental stage, medical history, medication assessment, mental status examination, life changes, and risk for suicide or homicide. After the data have been collected and analyzed, the nurse formulates a nursing diagnosis. Table 43-3 identifies the necessary assessment skills with corresponding examples of a verbal

Table 43-2 Nursing actions and theoretic rationale when interviewing

Nursing action	Theoretic rationale
The nurse introduces herself or himself by name, title, and role. The nurse addresses the patient by name and asks how he or she prefers to be addressed.	Addressing the client by name and introducing herself or himself by name and title is a way for the nurse to convey respect for the patient.
The nurse provides an interview room that is private and quiet, and does not contain distracting objects. When a room is unavailable, as in the cardiac care unit (CCU), some measure of privacy is provided by use of curtains and screens. Interruptions and interference by other staff members are kept to a minimum.	Privacy encourages the reticent, embarrassed patient to disclose his or her personal problems and feelings. It also eliminates some of the patient's concerns about confidentiality. Distracting objects may prove disturbing to a confused, disoriented, or psychotic patient. The psychiatric interview is demanding of both the patient and the nurse and requires concentration.
The nurse provides two chairs of equal size and comfort and a choice of seating. Additional seating should be available for family interviews and consultations.	The choice of where he or she sits provides clues to the patient's need for personal space, fears of interpersonal closeness, and possible suspiciousness.
The nurse makes prior arrangements and establishes a protocol to provide for safety and security for the patient and herself or himself. This is particularly important in the emergency room or other medical treatment settings.	Medical paraphernalia is potentially dangerous and may also frighten the patient. Help is sometimes needed to manage the confused, assaultive, or suicidal patient. Prior arrangement for this help will allay the nurse's anxiety. Limit setting is also reassuring to the disturbed or impulsive client.
The nurse begins with an open-ended question (a question that indicates a general inquiry, defines an area of interest, but leaves a wide range of interpretation possible). Example: "What brought you here today?"	The open-ended question is broad and allows the patient to verbalize his or her views, thoughts, and feelings. The closed question tends to elicit facts only. Direct, more specific questions are asked (to get additional information) after the patient has told his or her story. This response is nonrestrictive and does not sharply define the answer for the patient, but rather elicits spontaneous and individualistic responses that describe how he sees his problem.
The nurse uses the kind of response, verbal or nonverbal, that encourages the patient to say more. The response may be anything from an expectant look to a request to "tell me more about that."	
The nurse communicates with the patient by the use of silences. Silences, on the part of both the patient and the nurse, are accompanied by facial and bodily expression, gestures, or postures that convey meaning. If, for example, the patient transmits a feeling of anger, the nurse might state something about the anger and ask the patient to put it into words.	The nurse's silence can convey concern and interest, and can facilitate continued communication. The nurse can determine the possible meaning of the patient's silences by observing nonverbal communication and by examining his or her own empathic response.
The nurse uses responses that convey support, empathy, and understanding. Example: "You seem to feel guilty about being unable to work."	This type of response affirms that the nurse accepts the feelings and information the client has offered with concern but without criticism.
The nurse uses confrontation and interpretation to make explicit a connection between a feeling or symptom and the patient's interpersonal or intrapsychic life. Example: "You seem to have these headaches at times when you are most angry."	This encourages the patient to make his or her own additional connections and to explore matters further.
The nurse pays attention to the interview content (words spoken), as well as to the process (what is happening) between the patient and the nurse. Example: The patient states that he or she feels relaxed but fidgets in his or her chair and cannot make eye contact.	By attending to the two levels of a message, the content and the process, the nurse may more accurately assess the patient, what is occurring in the interview, and what may be occurring in the patient's life.

Adapted from Webster M: Psychiatric nursing assessment. In Lego S, ed: *The American handbook of psychiatric nursing,* Philadelphia, 1984, JB Lippincott.

statement or query used to elicit information from the patient.

Self-Awareness (Autognosis)

"What are my thoughts and feelings?" The societal stereotypes of the mentally ill have caused the psychiatric patient to be rejected by others. In addition, the ED staff may exhibit behaviors that reflect a negative view of this population, which increases the challenges of interacting with the patient who has a psychiatric emergency.

Many thoughts and feelings are generated when the nurse is confronted with a patient who has extreme psychosocial stressors. Thus the emergency nurse needs to be aware of his or her inner feelings and needs to acknowledge them.

Table 43-3 Psychiatric and mental health nursing skills necessary in the ED

Skill	Communication
Determine self-awareness (autognosis)	"What are my thoughts and feelings?"
Maintain safe environment	"Let's sit in this safe, quiet place."
Establish rapport; build trust	"I want to help you."
Explore precipitating event	"Tell me about the present problem."
Observe and validate patient's feelings (verbal and nonverbal cues)	"You look sad; tell me how you're feeling."
Set priorities (determine risk for suicide or homicide)	"Have you considered harming yourself or others?"
Assess developmental stage	"Tell me some important events that have occurred during your life."
Explore life changes	"What changes have you had recently? What changes have occurred within the past year?"
Assess health history (medication assessment)	"Has anything like this happened to you in the past? What medications have you taken?"
Mental status examination	"Tell me the meaning of this proverb: A rolling stone gathers no moss."
Collect data from support system	"How does this problem affect the whole family?"
Formulate nursing diagnosis	Risk for self-directed violence related to depressed mood.

Autognosis, a self-diagnosis process that enables the nurse to diagnose thoughts and feelings before initiating actions, is a powerful tool for nurses. By using this process, the nurse identifies thoughts and feelings, make a concerted effort to reframe the negative thoughts and to replace them with positive thoughts, and thereby develops a nonjudgmental acceptance of the patient as a worthwhile person with specific needs. This process enables the nurse to exhibit unconditional positive regard for the patient and is an effective step in establishing rapport.

The nurse must also show respect for the patient, which includes viewing the patient as a unique individual with specific feelings, beliefs, and experiences. It must be understood that there is a reason for all behavior and that "we are all more alike than different." However, if the nurse is unable to cope with specific personal thoughts and feelings and if he or she views mental health patients as "weird" or "repulsive," a detrimental effect on the nurse-patient relationship can result. When these situations arise, it is imperative that the nurse seek consultation or supervision to understand the basis for his or her negative response.

McFarland and Wasli[20] have identified strategies to develop and improve self-awareness and interventions that demonstrate unconditional positive regard and acceptance of the patient's uniqueness. These strategies and interventions are listed in the boxes on the next page.

Safe Environment, Rapport, and Trust Development

"Let's sit in a safe, quiet place"; "I want to help you." An overwhelming sense of impending danger, expressed as feelings of anxiety and fear, is the common internal sensation of patients who enter ED. Anxiety is a sensation that may be picked up by others in the environment, especially by family members and by members of the ED staff. Therefore the practitioner initially must establish rapport and take measures to reduce the external environmental stimuli. Rapport may be facilitated by providing a quiet, attractive interview environment that is professional, safe, and free from interruptions. When several family members or other members of the support system accompany the patient, the nurse, mindful of maintaining confidentiality, should interview the patient alone before talking to the others. This measure demonstrates respect and enables the patient to have a sense of control during this stressful time. It is imperative that the nurse communicate that help is available in a caring manner. A nonthreatening environment enables the patient to (1) trust the ED personnel, (2) share personal information, and (3) be open to future use of health care resources.

Explore Precipitating Event; Observe and Validate

"Tell me about the present problem"; "You look sad; tell me how you're feeling." The self-aware nurse, who has arranged a safe environment for the patient, now needs to focus on the patient's reason for seeking help. An important initial step is to ascertain the precipitating event. The patient may be in such an intense state of anxiety that he or she cannot focus on the problem. Therefore the nurse, through the use of effective communication skills that include observation and validation, needs to explore with the patient what brought him or her to the ED for assistance.

The Aguilera and Messick intervention model[1] gives the nurse direction in three major areas of assessment. Using this model, the nurse should seek responses to the following kinds of questions:

1. Perception of the problem should include the patient's description of the problem in his or her own words. "What is the problem? When did this problem begin? When did you last feel well? How does this problem affect you as a person? What is the meaning of this

STRATEGIES TO HELP THE NURSE DEVELOP AND IMPROVE SELF-AWARENESS

1. Develop awareness of your own verbal and nonverbal communication patterns.
2. Recognize, explore origin of, and attempt to work through stereotypes, prejudices, and negative attitudes.
3. Develop awareness of your own cultural and subcultural values and customs and their influence on personal behavior and awareness of your perception and interpretation of another's behavior.
4. Identify common personal stressors and typical behavioral responses.
5. Identify and increase your own adaptive coping patterns in response to stress.
6. Identify and develop constructive personal ethical values in relation to care of the adult psychiatric patient and to health care in general.
7. Validate perceptions and interpretations of patient's behavior with patient or with professional colleague, as indicated.
8. Examine your own motives, feelings, and behavior.
    Develop self-acceptance, self-esteem, and self-respect.
    Develop ability to differentiate clearly between your own feelings and those that belong to the patient.
9. Seek qualified supervision as needed, especially when providing one-to-one therapy.
10. Act in response to facts, not assumptions or possible misperceptions.
11. Identify the awareness of anxiety developing within you during a nurse-patient interaction, and seek to gain information about the patient's anxiety level by using your anxiety level as guide.

INTERVENTIONS THAT DEMONSTRATE UNCONDITIONAL POSITIVE REGARD AND ACCEPTANCE OF THE PATIENT'S UNIQUENESS

1. Communicate value of the patient's being and potential.
    Preserve patient's individuality, opinions, uniqueness, and feelings.
    Be nonevaluative and nonjudgmental.
    Avoid reducing self-esteem of patient.
2. Demonstrate sincere and nonpossessive caring and concern.
3. Communicate openness and willingness to engage in a therapeutic nurse-patient relationship.
4. Convey acceptance of patient's uniqueness, but do not show approval of inappropriate behavior.
5. Remain objective in observing and identifying reasons for patient's behavior.
6. Make yourself available.
    Do not communicate indifference or rejection.
    Offer presence and spend time with patient.
    Demonstrate concern, understanding, and interest.
7. Develop and use open-minded, accurate, and flexible interpersonal perceptions.
8. Do not attempt to negate patient's perception of an experience by comments such as, "Oh, it can't be *that* bad."
9. Demonstrate availability to patient by taking time to assist him or her therapeutically.
10. Attempt to understand the patient's perspective and feelings.
11. Demonstrate awareness and understanding of differences in cultural and subcultural values and customs.
12. Demonstrate flexibility, that is, a responsiveness to change in conditions.

crisis? What is the worst thing that could happen right now?"

2. Support system and current changes in biopsychosocial supports should be assessed. "What physical changes are present? Have you had sleep disturbances, or a change in appetite or weight? Do you feel physically healthy? What psychologic changes are present? Depression? Anxiety? Are you feeling angry? Depressed? What social changes have occurred? Inter-personal conflicts? Recent losses? From whom do you usually seek help?"

3. Coping mechanisms should be determined; to decrease the painful emotional stress, patients may use positive or negative coping skills. "What is your usual way of coping with stress? What have you done recently to help you cope? Does this help?"

Throughout the interview, the nurse should be aware of congruent and incongruent communication and should use effective observation skills. Active listening, direct questioning, and validation of verbal and nonverbal behaviors enable the practitioner to identify the presenting problem more clearly.

Priority Setting: Risk for Suicide or Homicide

"Have you considered harming yourself or others?" During the interview process with a patient in crisis, the nurse needs to place priority on assessing the client's motivation toward harm of self or others. In spite of popular beliefs to the contrary, the capacity for self-destruction is universal. Suicidal thoughts are ubiquitous, from those of the child who daydreams of how sorry her mother would be for punishing her if she were dead to those of the older person who thinks at times of freeing his children of the burden he has become. To complicate the picture, the lethality of suicidal behavior seems to exist on a continuum, not as an "either/or" dichotomy. At one end of this continuum is the person who rides a fast motorcycle or the somewhat depressed person who, seemingly preoccupied, crosses the street without looking carefully. At the other end of the continuum is the person who takes what he or she knows is a lethal dose of drugs when he or she knows no one will find him or her. Suicidal behavior is described by many as a sort of gamble. Some individuals may perpetrate suicidal behavior that may or may not be lethal and allow the deciding factor to be fate, God, or their loved ones.

The importance of accepting the responsibility for exploring a patient's risk for suicide is underscored by the fact that in a group of seriously suicidal persons, two thirds had communicated their intentions to someone, and more than half of them had sought professional help within 1 month of the act. Because psychiatric and medical emergencies often occur "after hours" and because EDs are chosen for expedient care by many who are unable or unwilling to wade through the quagmire of red tape that often precedes obtaining psychiatric help, EDs are frequently (willingly or unwillingly) left with the enormous task of deciding whether someone is suicidal. The answer is never clear-cut.

Many professionals are reluctant to ask a person if he or she tried to kill himself or herself, even after the most serious attempts, because the professionals fear that they would be intruding. Direct questioning will not precipitate a suicide attempt; to the contrary, a patient who can bring himself or herself to talk about suicide in a therapeutic setting is under significantly less internal pressure to act on thoughts of suicide. The sharing of a painful problem can reduce its intensity. Patients probably often wonder why the ED staff does not ask whether they are having suicidal thoughts, given the sometimes obvious circumstances: "Is it that the staff does not care? Or do staff members believe that the situation is hopeless?"

The nurse should ask questions in a natural and relaxed manner that gives the patient complete permission to discuss feelings, plans, and so on. The nurse might ask what led to an attempt: "What's been happening? It must be pretty awful." After a suicide attempt, the nurse needs to know whether the attempt has changed things in any way. The nurse might ask the patient what his or her significant others think about the attempt. Has a husband who was threatening to leave decided to stay and be supportive? How does the patient feel about the attempt in retrospect? Are there significant others who can care for the patient? Does the patient have plans for and concerns about the future? The patient should be asked whether he or she perceives "any way out, any hope."[11] ED staff need to have a readily available method to help them in the evaluation of suicidal risk. A simple, concise guide, which was developed by Patterson,[21] employs the acronym *SAD PERSONS* to assess the patient who is at high risk for suicide; the guide is shown in the box below.

SAD PERSONS ASSESSMENT

S (sex)
Women attempt suicide three times more often than men. Men kill themselves more than three times as often as women.

A (age)
Bimodal distribution: 19 years or younger; 45 years or older

D (depression)
The diagnosis of depression is a good predictor of suicidal risk.

P (previous attempts)
A previous suicide attempt increases the future risk, especially in the year after the attempt.

E (ETOH [ethanol])
Fifteen percent of all alcoholics and heavy drug users commit suicide.

R (rational thinking loss)
Psychotic persons with irrational thoughts and impaired judgment have increased incidence of suicide.

S (social supports lacking)
Recent loss of social support and cumulative losses of significant others, employment, or religious supports.

O (organized plan)
The person with a specific lethal plan is at a high risk for suicide.

N (no spouse)
Divorced, widowed, separated, or single persons, especially those with no children are more likely to be in the high-risk category.

S (sickness)
Patients with chronic, debilitating, and severe illness often seek medical attention before a suicide attempt.

Table 43-4   Guidelines for action

Total points	Proposed clinical action
0 to 2	Send home with agreement to seek follow-up care.
3 to 4	Follow up closely; consider hospitalization.
5 to 6	Strongly consider hospitalization, depending on confidence in the follow-up arrangement.
7 to 10	Hospitalization or psychiatric commitment.

With this tool one point is scored for each factor that is present in the patient. The total score ranges from 0 (little risk) to 10 (high risk). Patterson and others[21] identified some important guidelines for the practitioner who uses this assessment tool (Table 43-4).

Hoff[12] described signs that help predict suicide risk (Table 43-5) by comparing persons who complete or attempt suicide with the general population. Four signs that place a person at an extremely high risk for suicide are (1) suicide plan, (2) history of suicide attempts, (3) limited psychologic and social resources, and (4) ineffective communication.

After the patient has been assessed for suicide risk, if the nurse determines that the patient has an organized plan to commit suicide, the next step is to assess the lethality. Hoff[12] developed a lethality assessment scale with typical indicators (Table 43-6).

Along with skill in assessing the suicide patient, the ED staff need to have criteria to recognize the assaultive or homicidal patient. Hoff[12] identified the following guidelines with which to assess the risk for assault or homicide:
1. History of homicidal threat
2. History of assault
3. Current homicidal threats and plans
4. Possession of lethal weapons
5. Use or abuse of alcohol or other drugs
6. Conflict in significant social relationships, such as infidelity or threat of divorce
7. Threats of suicide following homicide

The astute practitioner is alert to signs of extreme depression or rage directed toward the self or others and uses assessment skills to identify these high-risk patients.

Assessment of Developmental Stage

"Tell me some important events that have occurred during your life." Nurses need in-depth knowledge of normal growth and development. Developmental stages are universally experienced series of biologic, social, and psychologic events that occur on a timetable and include specific tasks or challenges to be met.[14] Erikson[6] described the "eight stages of man" as developmental stages with two opposing energies—a negative and a positive force—which have the potential for growth or stagnation when tasks are fulfilled or unfulfilled. Developmental tasks may be fulfilled positively when a person has the necessary coping skills, resources, and supports. However, when a person's coping patterns, resources, and supports are maladaptive, extreme stress may develop, and a negative developmental crisis may occur. When this developmental crisis occurs, there is a potential for the patient to be "stuck" in a stage of psychosocial development, thereby preventing positive growth and fulfillment of future tasks. During the interview process, the nurse should be continuously observant for cues that identify specific crises that would have a negative developmental effect.

Erikson's eight stages of development[6] with corresponding tasks and areas of resolution, as well as concepts and basic attitudes for each stage of development, can be found in Table 43-7.

Explore Life Change Units

"What changes have you had recently?" "What changes have you had within the past year?" When a patient seeks help from the ED, the nurse is initially unaware of the "real problem"; however, he or she makes the assumption that the patient has experienced a change or a recent stressful life event. Stressful life events require that the patient initiate coping mechanisms to maintain the equilibrium of the body system. The amount of coping needed depends on the individual and the type and number of stressors present. How does the nurse assess stressful life events? Holmes and Rahe[13] conducted research on life changes, (including desirable changes), and the amount of social readjustment required to cope with these changes. They developed a social readjustment rating scale (Table 43-8) and ranked 43 important life events by assigning a specific life change unit (LCU) to each life event on the basis of the amount of coping behavior needed by the individual to deal with the event. Events such as death of a spouse rated highest, at 100 LCUs, and minor violations of the law rated lowest, at 11 LCUs. The researchers used the 43-item questionnaire to assess the significant events and stressors that had occurred in an individual's life during the previous 12 months.

The research demonstrated that the higher the LCU score is, the more likely it is that a change in health will occur (Table 43-9). Additionally, persons with high scores in life changes are more apt to have accidents and injuries.[9]

This tool is a quick, objective assessment method that assists the nurse in identifying life changes. The use of this questionnaire during the psychiatric interview gives a comprehensive view of the multiple stressors that the patient has been coping with during the past year. The nurse must be alert to the risk for the development of physical or psychiatric illness or both, when the score approaches 200 or more LCUs within 1 year.[25]

Table 43-5   Signs that help predict suicide risk: comparison of persons who complete or attempt suicide with the general population

Signs	Suicide	Suicide attempt	General population
Suicide plan*	Specific, with available, highly lethal method; does not include possibility of rescue	Less lethal method, including plan for rescue; risk increases if lethality of method increases	None or vague ideas only
History of suicide attempts*	65% have history of highly lethal attempts; if rescued, it was probably accidental	Previous attempts are usually low lethal; rescue plan included; risk increases if there is a change from many attempts that are low lethal attempts to one that is highly lethal	None or low lethal with definite rescue plan
Resources* (psychologic, social)	Very limited or nonexistent; or, person *perceives* self as having no resources	Moderate, or in psychological and/or social turmoil	Either intact or able to restore them through nonsuicidal means
Communication*	Feels cut off from resources and unable to communicate effectively	Ambiguously attached to resources; may use self-injury as a method of communicating with significant others when other methods fail	Able to communicate need fulfillment directly and nondestructively
Recent loss	Increases risk	May increase risk	Is widespread but is resolved nonsuicidally through grief work, etc.
Physical illness	Increases risk	May increase risk	Is common but responded to through effective crisis management (natural and/or formal)
Drinking and other drug abuse	Increases risk	May increase risk	Is widespread but does not lead to suicide of itself
Isolation	Increases risk	May increase risk	Many well-adjusted persons live alone; they handle physical isolation through satisfactory social contacts
Unexplained change in behavior	A possible clue to suicidal intent, especially in teenagers	A cry for help and possible clue to suicidal ideas	Does not apply in absence of other predictive signs
Depression	65% have a history of depression	A large percentage are depressed	A large percentage are depressed
Social factors or problems	May be present	Often are present	Widespread but do not of themselves lead to suicide
Mental illness	May be present	May be present	May be present
Age, sex, race, marital status	These are statistical pedictors that are most useful for indentifying whether an individual belongs to a high-risk group, not for clinical assessment of individuals	May be present	May be present

*If all four of these signs exist in a particular person, the risk for suicide is very high, regardless of all other factors. If other signs also apply, the risk is further increased.

From Hoff LS: *People in crisis*, ed 3, Redwood City, Calif, 1989, Addison-Wesley.

Table 43-6   Lethality assessment scale*

Key to scale	Danger to self	Typical indicators
1	No predictable risk of immediate suicide	Has no notion of suicide or history of attempts, has satisfactory social support network, and is in close contact with significant others
2	Low risk of immediate suicide	Has considered suicide with low lethal method; has no history of attempts or recent serious loss; has satisfactory support network; has no problems with alcohol; basically wants to live
3	Moderate risk of immediate suicide	Has considered suicide with highly lethal method but has made no specific plan or threats; or, has plan with low lethal method, history of low lethal attempts, with tumultuous family history and reliance on Valium or other drugs for stress relief; is weighing the odds between life and death
4	High risk of immediate suicide	Has current highly lethal plan, obtainable means, or history of previous attempts; has a close friend but is unable to communicate with him or her; has a problem with alcohol; is depressed and wants to die
5	Very high risk of immediate suicide	Has current, highly lethal plan with available means or history of highly lethal suicide attempts; is cut off from resources; is depressed and uses alcohol to excess; is threatened with a serious loss such as unemployment, divorce, or failure in school

*From Hoff LA: *People in crisis,* ed 3, Redwood City, Calif, 1989, Addison-Wesley.

Table 43-7   Erikson's eight stages of development*

Age	Stage of development	Task and area of resolution	Concepts and basic attitudes
Birth to 18 months	Infancy	Trust versus mistrust	Ability to trust others and a sense of one's own trustworthiness; a sense of hope
18 months to 3 years	Early childhood	Autonomy versus shame and doubt	Self-control without loss of self-esteem; ability to cooperate and express one's self
3 to 5 years	Late childhood	Initiative versus guilt	Realistic sense of purpose; some ability to evaluate one's own behavior versus self-denial and self-restriction
6 to 12 years	School age	Industry versus inferiority	Realization of competence; perseverance versus feeling that one will never be "any good"; withdrawal from school and peers
12 to 20 years	Adolescence	Identity versus role diffusion	Coherent sense of self; plans to actualize one's abilities versus feelings of confusion, indecisiveness, possibly antisocial behavior
18 to 25 years	Young adulthood	Intimacy versus isolation	Capacity for love as mutual devotion; commitment to work and relationships versus impersonal relationships, prejudice
25 to 65 years	Adulthood	Generativity versus stagnation	Creativity, productivity, concern for others versus self-indulgence, impoverishment of self
65 years to death	Old age	Integrity versus despair	Acceptance of the worth and uniqueness of one's life versus sense of loss, contempt for others

*Erikson E: *Childhood and Society,* ed 2, 1963, WW Norton.
From Wilson H, Kneisl C: *Psychiatric nursing,* ed 3, Menlo Park, Calif, 1988, Addison-Wesley.

Table 43-8 Holmes and Rahe social readjustment rating scale

Rank	Life event	Life change units
1.	Death of spouse	100
2.	Divorce	73
3.	Marital separation	65
4.	Jail term	63
5.	Death of close family member	63
6.	Personal injury or illness	53
7.	Marriage	50
8.	Fired at work	47
9.	Marital reconciliation	45
10.	Retirement	45
11.	Change in health of family member	44
12.	Pregnancy	40
13.	Sex difficulties	39
14.	Gain of new family member	39
15.	Business readjustment	39
16.	Change in financial state	38
17.	Death of close friend	37
18.	Change to different line of work	36
19.	Change in number of arguments with spouse	35
20.	Mortgage of $10,000	31
21.	Foreclosure of mortgage or loan	30
22.	Change in responsibilities at work	29
23.	Son or daughter leaves home	29
24.	Trouble with in-laws	29
25.	Outstanding personal achievement	28
26.	Spouse begins or stops work	26
27.	Begin or end school	25
28.	Change in living conditions	25
29.	Revision of personal habits	24
30.	Trouble with boss	23
31.	Change in work hours or conditions	20
32.	Change in residence	20
33.	Change in schools	20
34.	Change in recreation	19
35.	Change in church activities	19
36.	Change in social activities	18
37.	Mortgage or loan of less than $10,000	17
38.	Change in sleeping habits	16
39.	Change in number of family get-togethers	15
40.	Change in eating habits	15
41.	Vacation	13
42.	Christmas	12
43.	Minor violations of the law	11

From Holmes T, Rahe R: The social readjustment rating scale, *J Psychosom Res* 11:216, 1967.

Table 43-9 Life change unit assessment method

Scoring	LCU in 1 year	Physical symptoms
0 to 149	No life crisis	No significant problems
150 to 199	Mild life crisis	30% chance of physical symptoms
200 to 299	Moderate life crisis	50% chance of physical symptoms
300 +	Major life crisis	80% chance of major illness within 2 years

Assess Health History

"Has anything like this happened to you in the past?" **"What medications have you taken?"** Assessment of the health history includes the medical history, family history, and psychiatric history. Important questions to ask include the following[25]:

Medical history
1. Has the patient experienced any significant illness, injury, or surgery?
2. Did he or she require hospitalization?
3. How did he or she react to the illness or hospitalization?
4. Is he or she taking any prescribed or illicit drugs?
5. Does he or she have any allergies?
6. Has he or she experienced any significant side effect of psychotropic medication?

Family history
1. Who constitutes the patient's nuclear family, extended family, and family of origin?
2. Was he or she an only child, the youngest, or the oldest child?
3. Were there breakdowns in the family unit because of separation, divorce, or death?
4. Is there a history of physical or psychiatric illness in other family members?
5. Is there a history of suicide attempts or completed suicide, alcoholism, or child abuse?

Psychiatric history
1. Has the patient received any psychiatric treatment in the past?
2. Has he or she been hospitalized for this treatment?
3. What medications were prescribed?
4. Did he or she receive electroconvulsive therapy?
5. What were the results of any treatment modality?

The nurse must assess for alcohol and illicit drug habits. If the nurse is hesitant to query the patient about chemical dependency, the patient may in turn avoid revealing this data. A direct, nonjudgmental approach usually facilitates a truthful response from the patient. If the patient replies affirmatively that alcohol or drugs are a part of his or her life, answers to the following questions will be necessary: (1) What is the substance? (2) How much of the substance is usually taken? (3) When was the last time he or she took this substance? and (4) What is the usual pattern of taking this substance and the usual route of administration?

Patients may be hesitant to reveal their use of alcohol and illicit drugs, which necessitates additional observation skills, including observation for needle marks, watery red eyes, change in pupil size (dilated or constricted), tremors, flushed appearance, inflamed mucous membranes, and the odor of drugs or ethanol.

A medication and drug assessment should include psychiatric, nonpsychiatric, and over-the-counter medications along with alcohol and street drugs. The following is a comprehensive assessment tool.[16]

Medication and Drug Assessment

Psychiatric medications. Concerning each medication ever taken by the patient, obtain the following information:
1. Name of drug
2. Reason prescribed
3. Date started
4. Length of time taken
5. Highest daily dose
6. Prescribed by whom
7. Summary of effects
8. Side effects or adverse reactions
9. Was it taken as prescribed? If not, explain.
10. Were other family members prescribed this drug?
11. If so, reason prescribed and effectiveness

Prescription (nonpsychiatric) medications. Concerning each medication taken by the patient in the past 6 months and for major illness that occurred more than 6 months ago, obtain the following information:
1. Name of drug
2. Reason prescribed
3. Date started
4. Highest daily dose
5. Prescribed by whom
6. Summary of effects
7. Side effects or adverse reactions
8. Was it taken as prescribed? If not, explain.

Over-the-counter (nonprescription) medications. Concerning each medication taken by the patient in the past 6 months, obtain the following information:
1. Name of drug
2. Reason taken
3. Date started
4. Frequency of use
5. Summary of effects
6. Side effects or adverse reactions

Alcohol and street drugs
1. Name of substance
2. Date of first use
3. Frequency of use
4. Summary of effects
5. Adverse reactions

There are many risk factors for the development of drug interactions. After a comprehensive history and drug data have been gathered, the nurse assesses for the following[16]:
1. Polypharmacy
2. High drug doses
3. Special needs of geriatric patients
4. Debilitation or dehydration
5. Concurrent illness
6. Compromised organ system function
7. Inadequate patient education
8. History of noncompliance
9. Failure to include patient in treatment plan

MENTAL STATUS EXAMINATION
"Tell me the meaning of this proverb: A rolling stone gathers no moss."

Up to this point in the interview, the nurse has been collecting data about the present problem, stage of development, life changes, and health history. While gathering this data, the nurse has been attending to the patient's behavioral and emotional responses; thus, mental functioning has been measured indirectly. The mental status examination assesses the patient's emotional state and level of mental functioning. Malasanos and others[18] have designed a concise health history and mental status examination format that addresses present status, history, associated conditions, and family history. An affirmative response to any of the questions warrants further investigation.

Health history and mental status examination. A yes response to any of the following questions must be further investigated. Use the following indicators throughout the assessment: (1) onset (specific date, sudden or gradual, (2) duration, (3) frequency, (4) precipitating factors, (5) aggravating or alleviating factors, (6) treatment received, and (7) outcome.

Present status
1. What are your concerns or symptoms?
   Description: fear, sadness, guilt, shame, anxiety, powerlessness, or loss of self-esteem
2. Have you noticed recent changes in yourself?
   Description: anxiety, weight loss or gain, irritability, passivity, discouragement, guilt, indecision, rapid speech, pain, dyspnea, anorexia, insomnia, hypersomnia, restlessness, decreased sexual activity, faintness, headache, tremors, nausea, vomiting, or diarrhea
3. Do you currently use or abuse illicit or prescription drugs or alcohol?
   Type
   Amount
   Reasons
4. Do you feel you are able to adequately care for yourself?
   Hygiene or activities of daily living
   Financial transactions
   General communications

5. Are you employed?
   Type of work
   Number of absences in last year
   Reasons for absences
6. Do you have difficulty fulfilling work expectations?
   Description of difficulties

History

1. Have you used or abused illicit or prescription drugs or alcohol in the past?
   Type
   Amount
   Reasons
2. Has your relationship with your family changed?
   Description: discord, withdrawal, physically abusive or abused, estrangement, separation, or divorce
3. Have you ever considered harming yourself or others?
   Description: who, when, how, and where
4. Have you had electroconvulsive therapy?
   Description: when and how many treatments?

Associated conditions

1. Have you had trauma to your head?
   Type
   When
   Causative factor
   Change in consciousness
   Residual effects
2. Have you had brain surgery?
   Type
   When
   Residual effects

Family history

1. Does anyone in your family have a diagnosed psychiatric disorder?

A sample assessment record is shown in the case study below.

The caregiver must know that altered mental status may be caused by a primary physiologic problem. Therefore the patient needs a complete physical examination along with a mental status examination. In addition, the following data are necessary: vital signs, allergy history, medical history, family history, and results of diagnostic tests. The multiple causes of altered mental status may be remembered by referring to the mnemonic, *TIPS,* and to the vowels, *AEIOU* as developed by Henry.[10] The mnemonic and vowels are shown in the box below.

A more in-depth mental status examination is warranted when a definite psychologic problem is identified. Mental functions to assess include attitude, affect, speech, thought processes, sensorium and reasoning, risk for danger, and psychologic assets.[8]

Attitude. What is the general overall presentation of the patient's behavior. How cooperative is he or she? Does he or she engage in solitary activity? Parallel activity? Group activity? What is the extent of his or her participation in interpersonal relationships?

Affect and mood. Affect is the emotional state of the patient—the way he or she appears to others. Mood is what the patient says in regard to how he or she is feeling—happy, sad, and so on. Is the patient's affect appropriate to the situation? For example, a patient who walked about with a constant grin would be displaying inappropriate affect and would not be experiencing his or her total environment. Appearance may belie feelings. When this happens, as when the patient feigns cheerfulness when he or she actually feels depressed, the affect and mood are in disharmony. Are mood

---

CASE STUDY 43-2

Sample Assessment Record

Patient states that his wife died 3 months ago after a short illness and that since then he has felt sad and lonely. Admits to insomnia since her death. He falls asleep easily but awakens after an hour or two, then sleeps only intermittently and finally arises at dawn. He feels tired and listless all day. Has gained 10 pounds as a result of increased intake of junk food and fast foods because he does not cook for himself. Also admits to drinking five to seven beers daily for the past 3 months but denies ever using or abusing drugs. Patient does not socialize with old friends because he feels he cannot fit in anymore. Works on an assembly line and has had no absences in last 5 years. Is able to meet work requirements. Denies past episodes of mental illness and has no suicidal ideation. Denies having had head trauma and brain surgery.

MNEMONICS FOR CAUSES OF ALTERED MENTAL STATUS

Tips
T Trauma, temperature changes
I Infection, both neurologic and systemic
P Psychiatric, porphyria
S Space-occupying lesions, stroke, subarachnoid hemorrhage, shock

Vowels
A Alcohol and ingested drugs and toxins
E Endocrine; exocrine, particularly liver, electrolytes
I Insulin: diabetes mellitus
O Oxygen, opiates
U Uremia, renal causes including hypertensive problems

From Henry G: Neurologic emergencies, *Emerg Med,* p 22, 1989.

swings present; does the patient cry one minute and laugh the next?

Speech characteristics. Does the patient's speech include circumstantiality, scattering, a loosening of thought associations, a degree of vagueness, a tendency to overgeneralize, the use of global pronouns lacking specific referents (terms such as "they" and "them")? Is the patient unable to describe participation in an experience? These are some of the characteristics of speech that help the nurse to detect the presence or absence of difficulties with thought processes.

Thought processes. Does the patient's conversation flow in a logical sequence? Does his or her conversation make sense? How does the patient experience the world around him or her? Is he or she in contact with reality? Does the patient experience hallucinations (sensory impressions that lack external stimuli)? Does he or she experience delusions (false beliefs not based on fact)? Can the patient interpret a proverb abstractly (e.g., "A rolling stone gathers no moss.")?

Sensorium and reasoning. Is the patient aware of his or her immediate situation? Is he or she alert? Is the patient oriented to time, place, and person? Do his or her recent and remote memories appear to be intact? Is the patient able to perform simple calculations? Is he or she able to conceptualize and make appropriate judgments? Does the patient understand his or her condition and the present situation? Does he or she know things that would be considered common knowledge?

Risk for danger. Does the patient display a positive self-concept? Has he or she ever thought about harming or has he or she actually harmed himself or herself or others? Does the patient have a history of uncontrollable temper? Has he or she ever been in trouble with the law? Is the patient able to cope with situations that are not to his or her liking? What life stresses has the patient experienced? How has he or she handled or responded to these?

Psychologic assets. The outcome of an illness depends as much on the patient's assets as on the nature of the pathologic condition. Does the patient have: a positive self-image? A repertoire of coping mechanisms? Interested and supportive significant others? Financial stability? Satisfying interests and hobbies? The ability to get along with others?

Checklists for mental health assessment. After the seven mental functions have been assessed, the nurse needs to analyze the data. By compiling the data acquired from appearance, behavior, conversation, or the "ABC approach," the nurse may gain insight into the patient's mental functioning. The following three checklists present a range of signs and symptoms that may suggest a psychologic dysfunction in appearance, behavior, or conversation.[8] They are not in themselves necessarily reflective of mental illness, nor are they all necessarily confined to one of the areas; signs and symptoms may overlap with all three areas.

Appearance

Mental functions and appearance	Examples

1. Attitude
  a. Cooperativeness
  b. Interpersonal relationships
	Patient is aloof, unclean, disheveled, indifferent

2. Affect and mood
  a. Appropriate
  b. Harmony
  c. Swings
	Patient has masklike face; is apathetic, flat, rigid, labile, euphoric, depressed, suspicious, hostile; displays inappropriate affect; shows physical signs of anxiety (flushing, sweating, tremors, respirations)

3. Speech characteristics
  a. Description
  b. Speed
  c. Quantity
	Patient is soft-spoken, loud, boisterous; has monotonous, slow, or rapid speech

4. Thought processes
  a. Logical
  b. Coherent
  c. Perceptual
	Patient is inattentive, easily distracted, or preoccupied

5. Sensorium and reasoning
  a. Levels of consciousness
  b. Orientation
  c. Memory (recent, remote)
  d. Calculation
  e. Abstract thinking
  f. Judgment and insight
  g. Intelligence
	Patient displays decreased or absent physiologic reflexes, disinterest, peculiarity of dress, bewilderment

6. Risk for danger
  a. Self-concept
  b. Harm to self or others
	Patient is docile, sad, hostile, angry, apathetic

7. Psychologic assets	Few or no physical assets

Behavior

Mental functions and behavior	Examples

1. Attitude
  a. Cooperativeness
  b. Interpersonal relationships
	Patient is negativistic, uncooperative, hostile, belligerent, passive, drooping, withdrawn, impulsive; has slow gait

2. Affect and mood
  a. Appropriate
  b. Harmony
  c. Swings
	Patient is overactive or underactive, cries or laughs easily, wrings hands, paces floor, strikes head with hands, holds fixed posture for prolonged periods, has silly smile

3. Speech characteristics
  a. Description
  b. Speed
  c. Quantity
	Patient grimaces, stammers, stutters; displays uncoordinated or exaggerated movement, mutism, echolalia

4. Thought processes
  a. Logical
  b. Coherent
  c. Perceptual
	Patient avoids anxiety; displays phobic behavior, compulsiveness, echopraxia

5. Sensorium and reasoning
  a. Levels of consciousness
  b. Orientation
  c. Memory (recent, remote)
  d. Calculation
  e. Abstract thinking
  f. Judgment and insight
  g. Intelligence
	Patient displays stupor, lethargy, coma, confusion, agitation, delirium, panic, twilight state, behavior problems, conduct disorder

Mental functions and behavior	Examples

6. Risk for danger
  a. Self-concept
  b. Harm to self or others
	Patient has made suicide attempts; is malingering, withdrawn, assaultive, combative, violent, lacks temper control; displays antisocial or criminal behavior (history of arrests), irritability, explosiveness, excitability, maladaptive coping

7. Psychologic assets	Few or no behavioral assets

Conversation

Mental functions and conversation	Examples

1. Attitude
  a. Cooperativeness
  b. Interpersonal relationships
	Patient avoids certain topics, is pessimistic

2. Affect and mood
  a. Appropriate
  b. Harmony
  c. Swings
	Patient displays disharmony in thought processes; talks of guilt, sin, or unworthiness

3. Speech characteristics a. Description	Patient displays exaggeration, confabulation, blocking of thought,

Mental functions and conversation	Examples
b. Speed c. Quantity	circumstantiality, tangentiality, autistic speech, incoherence, flight of ideas; is overtalkative; uses neologisms

4. Thought processes
  a. Logical
  b. Coherent
  c. Perceptual
	Patient displays phobias, obsessions, paranoid ideas, illogical flow; expresses feelings of strangeness, depersonalization; has hallucinations or delusions (somatic, grandeur, persecution, alien control)

5. Sensorium and reasoning
  a. Levels of consciousness
  b. Orientation
  c. Memory (recent, remote)
  d. Calculation
  e. Abstract thinking
  f. Judgment and insight
  g. Intelligence
	Patient displays aphasia, memory defect, disorientation, poor judgment, lack of insight, inability to think abstractly or perform calculations

6. Potential for danger
  a. Self-concept
  b. Harm to self or others
	Patient has ideas of self-accusation and condemnation, self-deprecation, suicidal ideation

7. Patient's psychologic assets	Few or no conversational skills

---

INSTRUCTIONS FOR ADMINISTERING MINI-MENTAL STATE EXAMINATION*

Orientation

1. Ask for the date. Then ask specifically for parts omitted (e.g., "Can you also tell me what season it is?") One point is scored for each correct answer.
2. Ask in turn "Can you tell me the name of this hospital (town, county, etc.)?" One point is scored for each correct answer.

Registration

Ask the patient if you may test his or her memory. Then say the names of three unrelated objects (e.g., car, house, book) clearly and slowly, allowing about 1 second for each. After you have said all three words, ask the patient to repeat them. This first repetition determines his or her score (0 to 3), but keep saying the words until he or she can repeat all three in up to six trials. If he or she does not eventually learn all three words, recall cannot be meaningfully tested.

Attention and calculation

Ask the patient to begin with 100 and count backwards by sevens. Stop after five subtractions (93, 86, 79, 72, 65). Score the total number of correct answers.

If the patient cannot or will not perform this task, ask him or her to spell the word *world* backwards. The score is the number of letters in correct order (e.g., dlrow = 5, dlorw = 3).

Recall

Ask the patient if he or she can recall the three words you previously asked him or her to remember. Score 0 to 3 points.

Language

1. Naming. Show the patient a wristwatch and ask him or her what it is. Repeat this procedure with a pencil. Score 0 to 2 points.
2. Repetition. Ask the patient to repeat a sentence after you. Allow only one trial. Score 0 to 1 points.
3. Three-stage command. Give the patient a piece of plain, blank paper and repeat the command. Score 1 point for each part correctly executed.
4. Reading. On a blank piece of paper print the sentence "Close your eyes" in letters large enough for the patient to see clearly. Ask him or her to read it and do what it says. Score 2 points only if he or she actually closes his or her eyes.
5. Writing. Give the patient a blank piece of paper and ask him or her to write a sentence for you. Do not dictate a sentence; it is to be written spontaneously. The sentence must contain a subject and verb and be sensible. Correct grammar and punctuation are not necessary.
6. Copying. On a clean piece of paper, draw intersecting pentagons, each side about 1 inch in length, and ask the patient to copy the drawing exactly as it is. All 10 angles must be present and two must intersect for the patient to score 1 point. Tremor and rotation are ignored.

Sensorium

Estimate the patient's level of sensorium along a continuum, from alert on the left to coma on the right.

---

*Adapted from Folstein M et al: Mini-mental state: a method for grading the cognitive state of patients for clinicians. *J Psychiatr Res* 12:189, 1975.

Mini-mental state examination. An additional evaluation tool may be necessary when the nurse assesses that the patient is disoriented. The mini-mental state examination developed by Folstein and others[7] estimates the severity of cognitive impairment. This is an 11-question instrument and requires only 5 to 10 minutes to administer, which makes the tool valuable for use with the elderly patient whose cognitive impairment allows him or her to cooperate for only a short time. The instrument is divided into two parts. The first part requires vocal responses only, and the maximum score is 21. The second part involves reading and writing, and the maximum score is 9. The maximum total score is 30. The test is not timed but is scored immediately. Patients who score 24 or less are considered to have cog-

nitive disorders. A score of 20 or less is usually found in patients with dementia, delirium, schizophrenia, or affective disorders, not in normal elderly persons or in patients with a primary diagnosis of neurosis or personality disorder.[25] The examination is shown in the box on the preceding page. Fig. 43-5 illustrates the score sheet.

Collect Family and Support System Data

"How does this problem affect the whole family?" Assessment of the patient's family or support system or both is an important task of the emergency nurse. When a family member or significant other accompanies a patient to the ED, the nurse needs to quickly assess the strengths or weaknesses of this support system. Additionally, the nurse needs

---

Name _____ Unit _____

Date _____

Maximum Score	Score	
		Orientation
5	( )	What is the year (season, day, month)?
5	( )	Where are we: (state, county, town, hospital, floor)?
		Registration
3	( )	Name 3 objects: 1 second to say each. Then ask the patient all 3 after you have said them. Give 1 point for each correct answer. Then repeat words until he or she learns all three. Count trials and record. Trials:
		Attention and Calculation
5	( )	Serial sevens. 1 point for each correct answer. Stop after five answers. Alternatively, spell "world" backwards.
		Recall
3	( )	Ask for the three objects repeated above. Give 1 point for each correct.
		Language
9	( )	Name a pencil and a watch (2 points). Repeat the following: "No ifs, ands, or buts" (1 point)
		Follow a three-stage command: "Take a paper in your right hand, fold it in half, and put it on the floor" (3 points)
		Read and obey the following:
		Close your eyes. (1 point)
		Write a sentence. (1 point)
		Copy the design. (1 point)
		Total score
		Assess level of consciousness along a continuum

    Alert   Drowsy   Stupor   Coma

    Examiner _____

Fig. 43-5 Score sheet for mini-mental state examination. (Adapted from Folstein M et al: Mini-mental state: a method for grading the cognitive state of patients for clinicians, *J Psychiatr Res* 12:189, 1975.)

to be aware that each member of the family may be experiencing various degrees of stress depending on his or her coping style.

The simple analogy of a mobile and correlation of this mobile to a family system may give the practitioner a clearer view of the effects of change within a family system. When there is a change in one piece of the mobile, there is a change in the direction of movement of the entire mobile; likewise, a change in one member of a family affects the balance or equilibrium of the whole family. The collection of date from family members is facilitated by use of the intervention model created by Aguilera and Messick.[1] Therefore an assessment of the family system and the direction of the balancing factors that will best effect the family's return to equilibrium is of utmost importance. The following general areas are assessed:

1. Realistic perception of the event by the family. The goal is to clarify the problem and to encourage the family to focus on the immediate situation. By using the direct questioning approach, the nurse could ask the following questions: What does this mean to you? How does it affect you right now? What meaning does this have for the future?

2. Identification of adequate family coping mechanisms. The goal is to obtain clear delineation of methods used to decrease anxiety and enhance positive coping. Responses to the following questions give the nurse an overall view of family coping styles: Have you ever experienced anything like this before? How have you coped with high anxiety situations in the past? What did you try? What worked? What didn't? What do you usually do when you feel like this?

3. Identification of situational supports available to the family. The goal is to identify family resources, including emotional, physical, social, and spiritual support that may be tapped during this crisis. The following questions are useful during assessment of situational supports: Are there persons in your family or community that you can call on for help right now? Who are they? Should they be contacted? Whom can you trust? With whom do you have the closest ties?

An analysis of this data gives the practitioner direction for the following interventive strategies:

1. If the perception of the problem is realistic, the nurse validates this perception; conversely, if the perception is distorted, the nurse points out the distortions.

2. The nurse assists the family in identifying and establishing positive coping skills in response to this crisis.

3. The nurse connects the family with effective, available resources and encourages the ongoing use of this support.[15]

Formulate a Nursing Diagnosis

Potential for self-directed violence related to depressed mood. During the interview process, the nurse obtains subjective and objective data that are necessary for completing the first step of the nursing process, the assessment step. After analysis of this data, a nursing diagnosis is formulated. Carpenito[5] defines nursing diagnosis as "a statement that describes a health state or an actual or potential alteration in one's life processes (physiological, psychological, sociocultural, development and spiritual). The nurse uses the nursing process to identify and synthesize clinical data and to order nursing interventions to reduce, eliminate, or prevent (health promotion) health alterations which are in the legal and educational domain of nursing."

The purposes served by nursing diagnosis include the following[24]:

1. Help define the practice of nursing
2. Provide nurses with a common frame of reference
3. Improve communications among staff members and between facilities
4. Help define a body of unique nursing knowledge
5. Differentiate nursing from medicine
6. Facilitate intraprofessional and interprofessional communications
7. Make nurses more accountable for care
8. Assist nurse educators and students in focusing on nursing phenomena rather than on medical phenomena

The American Nurses' Association Division of Psychiatric and Mental Health Nursing Practice[2] states that the nursing diagnosis is related to actual or potential health problems in regard to the following:

1. Self-care limitations or impaired functioning, the general causes of which are mental and emotional distress, deficits in the ways significant systems are functioning, and internal psychic or developmental issues
2. Emotional stress or crisis components of illness, pain, self-concept changes, and life-process changes
3. Emotional problems related to daily experiences such as anxiety, aggression, loss, loneliness, and grief
4. Physical symptoms that occur simultaneously with altered psychic functioning, such as altered intestinal functioning or anorexia
5. Alteration in thinking, perceiving, symbolizing, communicating, and decision-making abilities
6. Impaired abilities to relate to others
7. Behaviors and mental states that indicate the client is a danger to self or others or is gravely disabled

An example of an approach to determine a nursing diagnosis follows.

During the interview process, the nurse collected from the patient the following data: depressed mood, feelings of worthlessness, anger turned inward, multiple recent losses, and irrational feelings of guilt; additionally, the client stated that he or she had thoughts of killing himself or herself (suicidal ideation). After an analysis of these data, a nursing diagnosis was formulated—risk for self-directed violence related to depressed mood, multiple losses, anger turned inward, and feelings of worthlessness and guilt.

SUMMARY

The preceding nursing skills, including self-awareness, maintaining a safe environment, establishing rapport and building trust, exploring the precipitating event, observing, validating and setting priorities, and the assessment of health history LCUs, developmental state, mental status, and support systems are vital for a comprehensive psychiatric interview. The interview is the main tool by which the practitioner gains knowledge of the patient, interprets what is wrong, and identifies a nursing diagnosis. This process facilitates the establishment of a therapeutic alliance that allows for effective interventions leading to adaptive coping behaviors and resolution of the crisis or problem.

REFERENCES

1. Aguilera DC, Messick JM: *Crisis intervention: theory and methodology,* ed 5, St Louis, 1986, Mosby–Year Book.
2. American Nurses' Association Division on Psychiatric and Mental Health Nursing Practice: *Standards of psychiatric and mental health nursing practice,* Kansas City, Mo, 1982, The Association.
3. Benson H: *The relaxation response,* New York, 1975, William Morrow.
4. Benter SE: Crisis intervention. In Stuart GW, Sundeen SJ, eds: *Principles and practice of psychiatric nursing,* ed 3, St Louis, 1987, Mosby–Year Book.
5. Carpenito LJ: *Nursing diagnosis: applications to clinical practice,* ed 2, Philadelphia, 1987, JB Lippincott.
6. Erikson E: *Childhood and society,* ed 2, New York, 1963, WW Norton.
7. Folstein M et al: Mini-mental state: a method for grading the cognitive state of patients for clinicians, *J Psychiatr Res* 12:189, 1975.
8. Grimes J, Burns E: Mental health assessment. In *Health assessment in nursing practice,* ed 2, Boston, 1987, Jones and Bartlett.
9. Hansen PA, Rhode JM, Wolf-Wilets V: Stress management. In McFarland GK, Thomas MD, eds: *Psychiatric mental health nursing,* Philadelphia, 1991, JB Lippincott.
10. Henry G: Neurologic emergencies, *Emerg Med Clin North Am,* 209(5):22, 1988.
11. Herman S: *Handbook of emergency nursing: the nursing process approach,* Norwalk, Conn, 1988, Appleton-Lange.
12. Hoff LE: *People in crisis,* ed 3, Menlo Park, Calif, 1989, Addison-Wesley.
13. Holmes TH, Rahe RH: The social readjustment rating scale, *J Psychosom Res* 11(8):213, 1967.
14. Horowitz JA: Human growth and development across the life span. In Wilson HS, Kneisl CR, eds: *Psychiatric nursing,* ed 3, Menlo Park, Calif, 1988, Addison-Wesley.
15. Kleeman KM: Family systems adaptation. In Cardona VD et al, eds: *Trauma nursing from resuscitation through rehabilitation,* Philadelphia, 1988, WB Saunders.
16. Laraia MT: Psychopharmacology. In Stuart GW, Sundeen SJ, eds: *Principles and practice of psychiatric nursing,* ed 3, St Louis, 1987, Mosby–Year Book.
17. Lesse S: Relationship of anxiety to depression, *J Psychother* 36:332, 1982.
18. Malasanos L, Barkauskas V, Stoltenberg-Allen K: Assessment of mental status. In *Health assessment,* ed 4, St Louis, 1990, Mosby–Year Book.
19. Maslow AH: *Toward a psychology of being,* ed 2, New York, 1982, D. Van Nostrand.
20. McFarland, GK, Wasli EL: *Nursing diagnoses and process in psychiatric mental health nursing,* Philadelphia, 1986, JB Lippincott.
21. Patterson WM et al: Evaluation of suicidal patients: the SAD persons scale, *Psychosomatics* 24:343, 1983.
22. Selye H: *Stress without distress,* New York, 1974, JB Lippincott.
23. Swanson AR: Psychophysiological disorders. In Varcarolis EM, ed: *Foundations of psychiatric nursing,* ed 1, Philadelphia, 1990, WB Saunders.
24. Varcarolis EM: The nursing process in psychiatric settings. In Varcarolis EM, ed: *Foundations of psychiatric mental health nursing,* Philadelphia, 1990, WB Saunders.
25. Webster M: Psychiatric nursing assessment. In Lego S, ed: *The American handbook of psychiatric nursing,* Philadelphia, 1984, JB Lippincott.
26. Yoder L, Jones SL: Changing emergency department use: nurses' perception and attitudes, *JEN* 7:156, 1986.

Psychiatric Emergencies: Biopsychosocial Stressors

Nancy Hogan Grover and **Teresa Willett Steele**

$\mathbf{P}$atients may arrive at the emergency department (ED) with a variety of biopsychosocial stressors, which result in conditions that can be classified under one of many available psychiatric and mental-health diagnoses. In this chapter the more common diagnoses are reviewed.

ABUSE

Many theories trace the origins of abusive and violent behavior patterns to physiologic, psychologic, and sociocultural influences, as well as to the developmental processes of early childhood. Reenactment of abusive and violent behavior in an adult may be the legacy of adults who were traumatized by violence and abuse as children, those who are biologically predisposed to such behavior, or those whose sociocultural environment fosters aggressor-and-victim behavior.

Abuse of the Elderly

Elder abuse may take the form of physical or psychologic abuse or both. Physical indications of abuse occur more commonly in clusters of symptoms than as a single symptom. Assess for the presence of two or more of the following: bruises, welts, lacerations, puncture wounds, dehydration, malnutrition, fractures, signs of overmedication, burns, poor hygiene, or lack of needed medical attention. Also assess for any signs of sexual assault. Psychologic abuse is less obvious, therefore more difficult to assess. It often consists of insults, ridicule, humiliating verbal assaults and threats, provocation of fear, and isolation of the individual from the rest of the family or from the community (for example, in a nursing home).

Assessment of the day-to-day living situation and the family's method and level of functioning can often best be done by asking the patient to enumerate daily activities, relationships, and socialization within the family. This information can also be helpful in appraising the elderly individual's mental status. Understanding the support system and the coping mechanisms of the victim is crucial to the plan of care. Interventions should center around identifying the stressors and working to alleviate or diminish them.

Sexual Abuse and Rape

Sexual assault encompasses any forced and violent vaginal, anal, or oral-genital contact or penetration or any sexual contact that is against the victim's will and without the victim's consent. Sexual abuse is one of the most traumatic crises; such abuse escalates anxiety to high levels and states of panic and engulfs its victims in the fear of death. The victim of sexual assault carries the burden of shame, guilt, and embarrassment; sexual assault is an act of violence, and sex is the weapon used by the aggressor.[6]

On the basis of a landmark study of 92 rape victims, Burgess and Holstrom[6] documented the existence of the rape-trauma syndrome. The rape-trauma syndrome comprises (1) the acute phase as outlined in Table 44-1 and (2) the long-term reorganization process, which occurs after an actual or attempted sexual assault. Each phase has its separate symptoms. The acute phase includes (1) immediate impact reaction, (2) physical reactions, and (3) emotional reaction to a life-threatening situation. The long-term process includes (1) reorganization of a disrupted life-style, (2) dreams and nightmares, and (3) phobic reactions. The physical, emotional, and behavioral stress reactions result from the person being faced with a life-threatening situation.

Two variations of the rape-trauma syndrome are compounded reaction, in which the victim has symptoms related to assault or abuse and a reactivation of symptoms of previously existing conditions, and silent reaction, in which various symptoms occur but the victim never mentions that a rape has occurred.

Crisis counseling is effective with victims who have the typical rape-trauma syndrome. Additional professional help is needed for victims with compounded reactions. The silent reaction to rape means that counselors must be alert to certain clues that indicate the possibility of rape, even when a person never initiates mention of the attack. Some important therapeutic techniques are outlined in Table 44-2.

ED protocol for physical injury and evidence should be followed, but keep in mind throughout interventions that some victims see the hospital as a safe place and others see it as an impersonal place.

Table 44-1 Acute phase of rape-trauma syndrome

Impact reaction	Somatic reaction	Emotional reaction
EXPRESSED STYLE		
Overt behavior such as crying, sobbing, smiling, restlessness, agitation, hysteria, volatility, anger, tenseness	Evidenced within the first several weeks after a rape Physical trauma: bruises (breasts, throat, back), soreness, skeletal muscle tension	Fear of physical violence and death; denial, anxiety, shock, humiliation, fatigue, embarrassment, desire for revenge, self-blame, lowered self-esteem, shame, guilt
CONTROLLED STYLE		
More covert behavior: masked facies, appears calm, may appear shocked, numb, confused, disbelieving; easily distracted; has difficulty making decisions	Headaches, sleep disturbances, grimaces, twitches Gastrointestinal: stomach pains, nausea, poor appetite, diarrhea Genitourinary: vaginal itching, vaginal discharge, pain, discomfort	

From Burgess A, Holstrom L: Rape: victims of crisis, ed 1, Bowie, Md, 1975, Prentice-Hall.

Table 44-2 Key therapeutic techniques used with victims of rape

Intervention	Rationale
Do not leave person alone.	Prevents increase in isolation, escalation of anxiety
Maintain neutral behavior.	Decreases emotional burden
Provide nonjudgmental care.	Lessens feelings of shame and embarrassment
Maximize emotional support; stay with victim; show concern for victim's needs; encourage problem solving whenever possible.	Prevents further disorganization; decreases potential for escalation of anxiety; validates person's worth; increases person's sense of control
Ensure confidentiality.	Encourages person to share feelings about event; protects a person's self-concept and sense of control
Encourage person to talk.	Helps person sort out thoughts and feelings; lowers anxiety by decreasing feelings of isolation
Allow expression of negative affect and "behavioral self-blame."	Helps person to gain a sense of control
Engage support system (family, friends) when appropriate.	Provides warmth and feelings of safety when shock wears off and acute disorganization phase begins
Emphasize that the person did the right thing in attempting to save his or her life.	Helps reduce guilt and maintain self-esteem

From Burgess A, Holstrom L: Rape: victims of crisis, ed 1, Bowie, Md, 1975, Prentice-Hall.

Sexual abuse that occurs in children produces clear patterns of immediate effects, but it is far more difficult to draw a definite connection between such abuse and later psychologic problems.

A significant degree of overlap has been found between victims of abuse and those who suffer from borderline personality disorder—persons whose relationships, emotions, and sense of self are all unstable and who often become inappropriately angry or injure themselves.

Some female victims of abuse "space out" or feel as if they are outside their own bodies and times (dissociation); some have physical complaints without any apparent medical cause (somatization). Both of these manifestations resemble the hysteria that Freud described.

Some therapists believe that post-traumatic stress disorder (PTSD), a diagnosis which has most often been applied to veterans of combat, may also be an appropriate diagnosis for some of those who have been sexually abused. Symptoms include flashbacks to the traumatic event or events, recurring dreams about it or them, a feeling of estrangement from others, and a general sense of numbness.[11]

Domestic Violence

Spouse abuse is described by Martin[12] as "an act carried out with the intention of, or perceived intention of, physically injuring one's spouse." Any person who is physically abused by his or her spouse is also psychologically abused. This abuse includes not only physical battering but also sexual abuse, social isolation, home imprisonment, economic deprivation, and verbal harassment.[9] An estimated 5 million women are abused by their mates each year, but there are no reliable estimates of the number of men who are battered.

Men and women who batter others are found in all socioeconomic, educational, age, and racial groups. Their violence is learned behavior that is used to control their mates. Men who batter believe in male supremacy and being in control; they dominate others and act out the dominant male sex role within the family because the family has traditionally been a safe place to do so. Battering bolsters their low self-esteem and insecurity by making them feel more in control, powerful, and masculine. These men cannot control their aggression, have no guilt about expressing it, and feel that it should not have negative consequences. Extreme jealousy of the mate is often a characteristic of men who batter, and violence is more likely to occur when alcohol or some other mind-altering substance has been used.

Coping mechanisms used by many battered women who are living in terrifying situations prevent the dissolution of their marriages. Coping mechanisms take the form of beliefs or myths that reinforce the denial and protect the marriage.[8] Some of the more common beliefs are (1) "I'm staying for the sake of the children," (2) "I can't survive without him," (3) "He will change—he doesn't really mean it," (4) "I did something to deserve the battering—I provoked it," and (5) "If I did things right, the beatings wouldn't occur."

Walker[18] developed a cycle theory of domestic violence. The cycle of violence consists of the following stages: (1) the tension-building stage, characterized by minor incidents such as pushing, shoving, and verbal abuse, (2) the acute battering stage, during which the batterer releases built-up tension by brutal and uncontrollable beatings, and (3) the honeymoon stage, characterized by kindness and loving behaviors.

In the honeymoon stage, which occurs after the beatings, both persons are in shock, and the woman may contemplate leaving or initiating legal action at this time. The man feels remorseful and is apologetic; the woman believes his promises and drops her plans to leave or take legal action. At this point the victimization is complete, and without intervention the cycle will repeat itself. Violence never diminishes but always escalates in frequency and intensity with each episode. The woman's self-esteem decreases, leading to depression, hopelessness, and immobilization.

Victims of domestic violence often come to the ED for treatment of their injuries but not for treatment of the underlying problem. However, without social, moral, and psychologic support, it is almost impossible for a woman to free herself from a violent domestic situation.

Some types of injuries that indicate domestic violence and are dealt with in the ED[16] and in clinical settings are described in the box above, right. Physical symptoms of domestic violence are listed in the box at right.

Awareness on the part of the emergency nurse of his or her reactions to domestic violence is essential in the assessment process. Table 44-3 outlines common responses of health care professionals to domestic violence.

The nursing assessment of a woman or man who has signs of possible domestic abuse should include assessment

---

TYPES OF INJURIES DEALT WITH IN THE ED AND IN CLINICAL SETTINGS

Emergency department

Bleeding injuries, especially to the head and face

Internal injuries, concussions, perforated eardrums, abdominal injuries, severe bruising, eye injuries, and strangulation marks on the neck

Back injuries

Broken or fractured jaws, arms, pelvis, ribs, clavicle, and legs

Burns from cigarettes, appliances, scalding liquids, or acids

Psychologic trauma, anxiety, attacks of hyperventilation, heart palpitations, severe crying spells, and suicidal tendencies

Miscarriages

Clinic or office

Perforated ear drums, twisted or stiff neck and shoulder muscles, headache(s)

Depression, stress-related conditions (for example, insomnia, violent nightmares, anxiety, extreme fatigue, eczema, or hair loss)

Talk of having "problems" with the spouse, description of him or her as very jealous or impulsive or as an alcohol or drug abuser

Repeated visits with new complaints

Both settings

Observe children for signs of stress caused by family violence, for example, emotional, behavioral, school, or sleep problems or increased aggressive behavior.

PHYSICAL SYMPTOMS INDICATING POSSIBLE SPOUSE ABUSE

Chief complaints without physical cause

Headache

Abdominal pain

Insomnia

Choking sensation

Chest pain

Back pain

Dizziness

"Accidents"

Presenting problems (signs of high anxiety and chronic stress)

Agitation

Hyperventilation

Panic attacks

Gastrointestinal disturbances

Hypertension

Physical injuries

From Swanson RW: Battered wife syndrome, *Can Med Assoc J* 130:709, 1984.

Table 44-3 Common responses of health care professionals to spouse abuse

Feeling	Source
Anger	Feelings of anger are usually directed toward the man who abused his spouse, toward the woman who allowed the abuse to happen, and toward society for condoning the occurrence of abuse through attitudes, traditions, and laws.
Embarrassment	The battered woman is a symbol of something close to home—the stress and strain of family life unleashed in the form of uncontrolled anger.
Confusion	The battered woman challenges our cherished view of the family as a haven of safety and privacy.
Fear	A small percentage of batterers are dangerous to others.
Anguish	The nurse may have experienced family violence as a victim or as a relative of a victim.
Helplessness	The nurse wants to do more to eliminate the problem, to cure it.
Discouragement	If the woman chooses not to prosecute or not to leave, the nurse may believe that he or she has failed to help the patient.

Adapted from Swanson RW: Battered wife syndrome, *Can Med Assoc J* 130:709, 1984.

---

of the level of anxiety, support systems, actual physical abuse, suicide risk, and drug and alcohol use.

When women do seek treatment for injuries that were caused by domestic violence, two stages occur: the *crisis stage* and the stage of *internal change and rebuilding*.[19] Interventions during the crisis stage should include (1) providing a safe atmosphere for reducing posttraumatic injury, (2) encouraging decision making, (3) supplying referral information, and (4) maintaining concise, accurate records.

The stage of internal change and rebuilding focuses on rebuilding lives, eliminating destructive ways of relating to others, and increasing self-esteem. Interventions during the crisis stage, particularly referral for psychotherapy, support that change. Therapy is most effective after crisis intervention, when the life of the woman is less chaotic and many modalities of support are available, including individual, couple, family, and group therapy.

PSYCHOPHYSIOLOGIC RESPONSE TO STRESS

John Tenser, in the case study above, is having a psychophysiologic response to stress. The term *psychophysiologic disease* was adopted in the 1968 *Diagnostic and Statistical Manual (DSM) II*[1] and referred to all physical symptoms in which psychic elements played a significant role in initiating or maintaining chemical, physiologic, or

---

---

structural alterations responsible for a patient's complaint. Presently *DSM III-R*[2] refers to physical conditions affected by psychologic factors such as those disorders with psychogenic components or "any physical conditions to which psychologic factors are judged contributory."

In the earlier half of this century, the specific disorders first classified as *psychosomatic* were ulcerative colitis, rheumatoid arthritis, hyperthyroidism, hypertension, peptic ulcer, bronchial asthma, and neurodermatitis. These were known as Alexander's Seven, after the clinician who studied these disorders and identified emotional components of each.[11] Today there are many more conditions recognized as having psychogenic components. These conditions include, as classified by the system affected, gastrointestinal (gastric and duodenal ulcer, ulcerative colitis, and irritable bowel syndrome); cardiovascular (hypertension, angina pectoris, acute myocardial infarction, and migraine headaches); respiratory (asthma and hyperventilation); skin (psoriasis, urticaria, and acne); and musculoskeletal (tension headaches and rheumatoid arthritis). Additional conditions presently considered psychogenic include chronic pain, menstrual disorder, insomnia, sexual dysfunction, obesity, and cancer. Siegal[14] refers to all disease processes as having psychogenic bases and he postulates that patients may have an impact on their progress toward health when they take control of their minds and bodies.

In *DSM III-R*,[2] the diagnostic criteria for psychologic factors affecting physical condition include the following:

1. Psychologically meaningful environmental stimuli are temporally related to the initiation or exacerbation of a specific physical condition or disorder.
2. The physical condition has either demonstrable or-

ganic causes (for example, rheumatoid arthritis) or a known pathophysiologic process (for example, migraine headaches).

3. The condition does not meet the criteria for a somatoform disorder.

In other words, for a diagnosis of a psychophysiologic disorder, a psychologic stimulus related to the exacerbation of a physical condition and a physical condition with an organic cause or a pathophysiologic process must be present. Thus it can be assumed that patients with psychophysiologic problems unconsciously repress stressful feelings and that such emotional stress is expressed in physical conditions.

John Tenser, described in the case study on p. 608, is a perfect example of how this process works: rather than seeking relief from the personal and professional stress in his life, he coped maladaptively by using the defense mechanism of denial, and he ignored the "strange" physical sensations. He continued to increase his workload until a crisis occurred, which necessitated a sudden visit to the ED. ED staff members are usually proficient at taking care of priority problems. The ED physician initiates immediate interventions, conducts a physical examination, orders the necessary laboratory tests, and formulates a preliminary physical diagnosis. The nurse complements the physician's medical assessment by eliciting information that is not obtained by the physician. In the nursing process a scientific problem-solving approach gives the nurse a framework with which to assess the patient, plan interventions, and evaluate the patient's response to biopsychosocial stressors.

Assessment

Through the interview process, the nurse identifies the patient's specific needs and gathers information on the client's current life situation, recent life changes, a psychosocial history, and present emotional status. The use of the following models, Maslow's Hierarchy of Needs and the Crisis Intervention Model, along with assessment of John's life change units (see Chapter 43) assist the nurse in gathering pertinent data.

Maslow's Hierarchy of Needs

The need that motivated John to seek help from the ED was his response to a physiologic problem. His most basic needs, for oxygen, for rest, and ultimately for survival, were unfulfilled. With an acute myocardial infarction, John's chances for survival decreased the longer he waited to enter the health care system. Oxygen is usually necessary because of the compromised heart muscle, and rest is a definite need for John because of his extremely long hours of physical work and overall continued psychologic stress.

Thus priority needs were the physiologic needs, and interventions should focus on the fulfillment of these basic

---

NURSING CARE PLAN

Goal

The patient will achieve a realistic perception of the precipitating event and subsequent experiences.

Interventions

1. Ask the patient to describe the sequence of events in a process of adjusting to stressors.
2. Clarify experiences by restating previously unconnected facts.
3. Clearly define the problem with the patient.
4. Help the patient to gain an understanding of the crisis by discussing effects of present stressor(s), and link present problem to past behaviors.
5. Focus on changing the present.

Goal

To assist the patient in perceiving himself or herself as able to cope with stress.

Interventions

1. Convey trust in the patient's ability to act.
2. Provide direction and assistance in areas in which the patient needs help.
3. Assist the patient in understanding the coping process.
4. Give empathetic responses to the patient's expression of feelings.
5. Encourage the patient to accept feelings.

Goal

To develop coping responses to the emotional reactions to stress, a specific event, or illness.

Interventions

1. Teach the patient skills relevant to problem solving, relaxation, use of imagery, and assertive communication.
2. Assist the patient in working through denial and in understanding and accepting that denial may be a coping response that can be useful at a particular time.
3. Assist the patient in identifying and making changes in health-related behaviors.

Evaluation and outcome criteria

1. Patient can accurately appraise stress.
2. Patient uses adequate coping resources.
3. Patient resolves the stress-producing episode.

needs. Initial interventions should focus on correcting the maladaptive physiologic stressors, relief of pain, and administration of medications and oxygen as necessary.

Crisis Intervention Model

The stressful event that caused John to develop a state of disequilibrium and initiated his entry into the health care system was the "severe, crushing chest pain." When he felt a need to restore equilibrium, he sought help from the ED. The following balancing factors were absent: (1) John's perception of "the event" was originally ignored. He did not seek help when he initially had the "strange feelings" in his chest. (2) Situational support was absent; John believed he was "tough" and "indestructible." Therefore he did not seek help before his entry into the ED. (3) Coping mechanisms were inadequate; John used denial and additional maladaptive coping mechanisms, including smoking, alcohol consumption, overeating, and workaholic behaviors. Because these three balancing factors were absent, John's problem was unresolved, disequilibrium continued, and the crisis that motivated John to enter the ED for help developed.

Stressful life events that John had experienced during the past year, with the numeric value of life change units (see Chapter 43), included loss of both parents (126), business readjustment (39), son's problem with the law (63), change in responsibility at work (29), trouble with boss (23), change in work hours or conditions (20), mortgage over $10,000 (31), change in sleeping habits (16), and change in eating habits (15). The total value of the life change units for John is 359. This score reflects that John was a major risk for developing a physical illness in response to stressful life events. The data gathered from the use of this model validate John's present status. A crisis developed as a result of maladaptation to multiple stressors or a psychophysiologic disease.

After analysis of the assessment data, a nursing diagnosis for John is established as ineffective individual coping related to situational crisis, continued stress during 1 year, and inadequate psychologic resources.

The goals and interventions outlined in the box on the preceding page may facilitate John's change from maladaptive to adaptive responses to stress. While the patient is in the ED, the immediate psychosocial interventions should focus on displaying empathy, using effective communication skills, encouraging the expression of feelings, using imagery and relaxation exercises, giving emotional support, and initiating health-related teaching. As John progresses in his recovery, counseling should be directed toward reducing competitiveness and time-urgency and creating life-style changes.

Like John, who entered the ED for assistance, patients who exhibit extreme psychophysiologic responses to stress are seen more frequently in EDs than in psychiatric clinics. Therefore the emergency nurse must understand the mind-body interaction process and use the nursing process or a scientific problem-solving approach for patients with psychophysiologic disorders.

COPING WITH SEVERE STATES OF ANXIETY

Health care providers need an understanding of the various human responses to stress. Some individuals may view stress as a challenge and are able to cope positively by learning adaptive behaviors, thus reducing stress to a manageable level. Others view common, everyday exercises as negative, stressful events, use maladaptive coping mechanisms, and have ongoing, unrelenting anxiety. This state of overwhelming anxiety may cause functional impairments and subjective distress; over time a pathologic neurotic disorder may develop in the anxious person.

The conditions that result when anxiety is not relieved by ordinary use of defense mechanisms are classified as (1) anxiety disorders, (2) somatoform disorders, and (3) dissociative disorders.

Common behaviors and symptoms observed in persons with these disorders include (1) overt anxiety, (2) phobias, (3) obsessions, (4) compulsions, (5) changes in consciousness, and (6) alterations in identity.[7]

Anxiety Disorders

"I feel like something terrible is going to happen!" The preceding statement expresses the feeling of a person with an anxiety disorder. The anxiety disorders, which were originally called neurotic diseases, are now considered some of the most common psychiatric problems that cause a patient to seek help from health care professionals. The person with an anxiety disorder responds maladaptively to stressors that do not ordinarily cause discomfort for the average person. Anxiety disorders include panic disorder, phobias, generalized anxiety, and somatoform disorders.

Panic disorder. Panic disorders are recurrent attacks of severe anxiety. Panic attacks (see the case study below) are characterized by sudden onset with intense, apprehensive dread and at least four of the following symptoms: dyspnea,

---

CASE STUDY 44-2

Anxiety Disorder

Ernie Fear, a 49-year-old salesman, was traveling along a remote rural highway when he felt a sudden onset of intense terror. His heart was pounding, and he felt a tight sensation, "like a band" around his chest. He was short of breath, felt numb, had tingling sensations in his hands, and feared that he was going to die. He drove haphazardly to a hospital and entered the ED.

Diagnosis

Panic attack, an anxiety disorder, a maladaptive response to stress

palpitations, chest discomfort, syncope or dizziness, trembling or shaking, sweating, choking, nausea or abdominal distress, depersonalization, numbness or tingling sensations, flushes (hot flashes) or chills, fear of dying, and fear of going crazy or losing control.[2]

Panic attacks usually last only for several minutes; however, persons with panic disorders are typically plagued by anticipatory anxiety or a constant dread of the next attack. Because the psychologic terror experienced during a panic attack can be so compelling, many people begin to doubt their sanity. A person who has had panic attacks for a long time may develop symptoms of agoraphobia.

Phobias or phobic disorders. A phobia is an irrational, persistent fear related to one or several specific objects in the environment. Phobias are divided into three categories, agoraphobia, simple phobia, and social phobia.

Agoraphobia. Agoraphobia is a fear of becoming terrified in situations from which there is no easy escape or in which no help can be found. Persons with agoraphobia may be fearful in any situation away from their homes and may become homebound. Others may avoid open spaces, standing in a line, or being in a crowd. Many people with agoraphobia also have a panic disorder.

Simple phobia. Simple phobia is a fear of becoming terrified and needing to escape from a single, specific situation such as driving on bridges or through tunnels; other such situations include fear of flying, elevators, closed spaces, or heights.

Social phobia. Social phobia is the fear of embarrassing oneself in public (for example, eating in public). The person with social phobia may become preoccupied with the risk of choking on food and vomiting in front of others or with the fear of public speaking. Extreme shyness is a generalized form of social phobia.

Generalized anxiety. Unrealistic or excessive anxiety and worry that persists for 6 months characterizes generalized anxiety. At least six of the following 18 symptoms are present. Symptoms of *motor tension* include trembling, twitching, or feeling shaky; muscle tension, aches, or soreness; restlessness; and easy fatigability. Symptoms of *autonomic hyperactivity* include shortness of breath or smothering sensations; palpitations or accelerated heart rate; sweating or cold, clammy hands; dry mouth; dizziness or light-headedness; nausea, diarrhea, or other abdominal distress; flushes or chills; frequent urination; and trouble with swallowing. Symptoms of *vigilance and scanning* include feeling "keyed up" or on edge; exaggerated startle response; difficulty concentrating or "mind going blank" because of anxiety; trouble with falling or staying asleep; and irritability.[2]

Obsessive-compulsive disorder consists of preoccupation with persistent, intrusive thoughts that cannot be dismissed (obsessive) or repeated performance of rituals, designed to produce or prevent some event (compulsive).

Posttraumatic stress disorder (PTSD) occurs after a psychologically traumatic event outside the range of usual experience (for example, military combat, rape, natural disasters, or disasters of human origin). The individual with PTSD has experiences such as recurrent dreams or thoughts about the event, feelings of numbness, detachment, or estrangement from the environment or the people in it, and at least two of the following: sleep disturbance, hyperalertness, guilt about surviving, difficulty concentrating, memory impairment, and avoidance of activities that trigger the memory of the event.[2]

Most patients with anxiety disorders do not seek help from the ED; however, the patient with a panic attack does come to the ED and has the anxiety disorder that is most commonly treated there.

A patient who enters the ED with a panic disorder appears agitated and terrified. The patient may have cardiac-related symptoms such as palpitations, precordial pain, and shortness of breath. He or she may have disturbances of respiration, gastrointestinal distress, trembling, diaphoresis, and paresthesias. The characteristic psychologic symptom is a feeling of apprehension that something terrible is going to happen. Attacks may last from a few minutes to a few hours.

Anxiety is a form of fearful reaction that is without a tangible object or reason for fear. Anxiety differs from object-related fear in the following ways:

1. Anxiety is "free floating" and not restricted to definite situations or objects.
2. Anxiety is not accompanied by any degree of insight into its immediate cause.
3. Anxiety is usually experienced in terms of its physical manifestations, although the individual does not recognize them as such.
4. Anxiety is prompted by anticipation of future threats against which current avoidance responses would not be effective.
5. Anxiety is not controlled by specific psychologic defense mechanisms.

Immediate interventions for the patient with extreme stress resulting from a panic attack include the following[4]:

1. Administer medications as ordered. The medications may include alprazolam (a benzodiazepine), imipramine (a tricyclic antidepressant), and phenelzine (a monoamine oxidase inhibitor).
2. Relieve the "fight or flight" symptoms by moving the patient to a quiet, safe space.
3. Communicate in short, single statements. "I will stay with you." "You are safe here."
4. Allow the patient to pace around the room to expend energy.
5. Be aware that touching the patient may cause increased fear and anxiety; however, once rapport and trust are established, touching him or her on the arm, shoulder, or hand may be comforting.
6. Encourage the patient to vent feelings and verbalize fears.

7. Reassure the patient that with time, symptoms will subside.

8. Initiate and teach relaxation and visualization exercises.

9. Encourage the patient to reduce use of caffeine.

10. Identify adaptive coping behaviors and reinforce positive behaviors.

Panic attacks may occur without an identifiable precipitant, or these attacks may develop in response to a sudden loss. Therefore the patient needs to be encouraged to express feelings when losses occur, to reduce the exacerbation of a panic attack. Additional treatment for panic disorders includes drug therapy, supportive therapy, and behavioral therapy.

Somatoform Disorders

Somatoform disorders are a group of disorders characterized by physical symptoms with no apparent organic or physiologic basis. The four distinct diagnostic groups include somatization disorder, conversion disorder, hypochondriasis, and somatoform pain disorders.

In these disorders, anxiety is transformed into physical symptoms that often involve sensory and motor function. Symptoms of these disorders cannot be explained by physical findings but can be linked to psychologic factors such as stress at the time of onset and secondary gain. The physical symptoms are the primary gain, since they provide temporary relief from anxiety. The physical symptoms are experienced as real and are not under the voluntary control of the individual.[5]

Somatization disorder. Somatization disorder is characterized by the expression of an emotional turmoil or conflict through physical symptoms. Patients with somatization disorder have multiple somatic complaints and have 15 or more symptoms persisting for several years. After a medical workup, no physiologic disorder is found. These patients frequently consult with numerous doctors and have exploratory surgery and many diagnostic tests performed. Abuse of alcohol or medications is often associated with this disorder.

Conversion disorder. Conversion disorder, originally known as hysterical neurosis, describes a loss of physical functioning for which no organic basis exists (for example, blindness that occurs without cause). Conversion disorder is the expression of a psychologic conflict or need. One of the following psychologic factors must always be present for this diagnosis. (1) A close relationship exists between the time of onset of the symptoms and the occurrence of a conflict-producing event. (2) The presence of the symptom allows the individual to avoid some activity that is personally unpleasant. (3) The symptom enables the patient to get support from the environment. The primary gain is achieved by avoiding the conflict, and the secondary gain is achieved by avoiding the unpleasant activity and receiving the support from the environment. An important outward appearance that the patient maintains is *la belle indifference*, an attitude

---

CASE STUDY 44-3

Somatoform Disorder

"Oh! I'm so sick!"

Early one November morning, Mary Soma arrived at the ED by ambulance. She had awakened at 5:00 AM, voicing numerous "vague" complaints to her husband. The complaints included pain in her eyes, a sore nose, a dry, sore mouth, feeling "funny" in the head, neck soreness, vague cramplike sensations in her abdomen, burning sensation during urination, loss of appetite, inability to feed herself because of pains in her hands, lameness in her back, and sore feet. Her husband stated that he was eating breakfast when he noticed an ambulance pulling into the driveway. This was the sixth time this month that Mary had called an ambulance. During the past few years, Mary had visited several physicians, including a gastroenterologist, an ophthalmologist, a rheumatologist, a urologist, an ear, nose, and throat specialist, and several general practitioners. Her husband stated that several physicians had recommended that Mary see a psychiatrist; however, Mary refused or cancelled appointments because she said that she was not "crazy." Additionally, her husband brought with him an in-depth list of all the medications that Mary had been taking for the past year. He voiced exasperation regarding Mary's multiple problems and the "unnecessary ambulance trips." Mary did not show signs of stress, and she appeared to "enjoy" the attention she received from the ED staff. A physical examination and diagnostic tests revealed no evidence of physiologic disease. Mary was discharged from the ED, and it was recommended that she make an appointment with a psychiatrist. Mary's case is an example of a long-standing somatoform disorder.

---

of unconcern about the symptom, which reaffirms that the primary gain has been achieved.

Hypochondriasis. Hypochondriasis is a disorder in which the patient has an abnormal preoccupation with the belief that he or she has a serious illness or illnesses. The individual continually seeks medical care for physical signs and vague symptoms. These patients are commonly seen hopping from one physician to another, and they frequently seek care from EDs. They also frequently overuse medications. The symptoms of this disorder serve the purpose of controlling anxiety. Impaired social and occupational functioning is always present.

Somatoform pain disorder. Somatoform pain disorder has as its chief symptom severe and prolonged pain related to psychophysiologic factors. This pain is psychogenic; however, health care providers must be aware that the patient experiences the pain as real. Secondary gain may be prevalent because of the attention received when painful sensations are expressed (see the case study above).

When the patient with a somatoform disorder enters the ED, it is important that the nurse treat the patient with respect and in a caring manner. Health care professionals may have a difficult time being objective with these patients and may think, "There is nothing really wrong because it's all in his or her head." However, extreme anxiety is present but has been repressed by the patient's use of physical problems to "hide" it. Repression is not a conscious process; therefore the nurse needs to help the patient to identify connections between the anxiety and stress and the physical symptoms. A teaching model may be beneficial for explaining the effects of stress on the body. Additionally, urge the patient to verbalize perceived positive and negative feelings, as well as fears and concerns. Decrease the amount of time and attention given to the patient's physical complaints. Discuss the concept of secondary gain with the patient and family; set limits and develop a mutual plan to reduce secondary gains. When the patient does not readily comply, the nurse should not get discouraged because these behaviors usually have been part of this person's life for a long time and change is a difficult process. Maintain a positive, hopeful posture: change can occur.

Dissociative Disorders

Dissociative disorders, like somatoform disorders, provide the patient with a means to avoid anxiety by use of dissociation, a defense mechanism. In the dissociative process, there is a splitting off from awareness of an idea, emotion, or experience that is too difficult to handle. The anxiety-producing material is then repressed and remains in the unconscious where it has a life of its own, separate from what is known to the individual.[17]

Dissociative disorders include psychogenic amnesia, fugue disorder, depersonalization disorder, and multiple personality disorder (see the case study below).

A patient who exhibits characteristics of a dissociative disorder may be brought to the ED by law enforcement officials and may be seeking help for physical problems brought on by abuse, homelessness, or exposure to multiple biopsychosocial stressors.

Psychogenic amnesia. An individual with psychogenic amnesia is unable to remember important personal information; such amnesia usually follows psychologic stress. Examples of stressors include a broken love affair, financial

ruin, extreme marital difficulties, and combat duty in wartime. The patient may appear calm, and all other areas of memory are usually intact, with the exception of this event. The amnesia is adaptive and allows the patient relief from anxiety (primary gain). *La belle indifference,* a relaxed state, may be present. Hypnosis may assist in uncovering repressed information. Brief therapy focuses on building trust and supporting the patient until memory returns and conflicts can be explored.

Fugue disorder. A fugue state is an abrupt, massive amnesia with a sudden temporary alteration in consciousness. A new identity is assumed. During this process, the individual has amnesia about his or her old identity, assumes a new one, and travels away from home or customary place of work. Stress and major disruption of significant relationships are the precipitators. There may be a history of heavy drug or alcohol use before onset of the symptoms of this disorder. Recovery from a fugue state leaves the individual able to remember his or her former life but not the time spent in the fugue state. Therapy focuses on identifying adaptive coping styles after uncovering the conflict.

Depersonalization. In depersonalization an individual's sense of self is altered, and he or she perceives parts of his or her body as increased or decreased in size or altered in form. A sensation of being outside one's own body, as an observer, is a prominent symptom. This process can serve as a defense mechanism, protecting an individual's sense of self through "splitting off." Therapy aims at assisting the patient to recognize anxiety and the role that splitting plays in the avoidance of stressful events. The patient should be assisted in developing new coping strategies for dealing with anxiety.

Multiple personality disorder. The essential feature of multiple personality disorder is the existence within the person of two or more distinct personalities or personality states. Additionally, at least two of these personalities or personality states recurrently take full control of the person's behavior.[2] Physical and emotional abuse and sexual trauma during childhood are common factors in most cases. Transition from one personality to another often occurs during times of extreme stress. Hypnosis is used to explore the existence and characteristics of other personalities. The aim of this long-term therapy is to unite the personalities and form a whole, integrated personality.

Patients with dissociative disorders may enter the ED seeking relief from deep-seated anxiety and expressing feelings of loss of the "real self." A calm, empathetic posture focusing on encouraging the verbalization of anxious feelings assists these patients in maintaining some control in their out-of-control, "split" environment.

PERSONALITY DISORDERS

Personality disorders are a group of psychiatric disorders characterized by life long patterns of maladaptive responses to stress, by problems in developing work behaviors and

---

CASE STUDY 44-4

Dissociative Disorder

"Who am I?" "Where am I?"

Cathy Loss, a young woman, was found in an abandoned car on a desolate road by two hikers. She appeared pale and emaciated; numerous bruises were observed on her extremities. She was unable to recall her full name or address, and no identification was available. After the police were notified, she was brought to the ED. Cathy may have been experiencing a dissociative disorder.

TYPES OF PERSONALITY DISORDERS

Paranoid personality
Characterized by history of mistrust of others

Schizoid personality
Characterized by withdrawal from society

Histrionic personality
Characterized by history of dramatic displays of emotions, including temper tantrums and suicide threats, attention-seeking behaviors, a desire for activity, and brief relationships with others

Antisocial personality
Characterized by history of antisocial behavior involving courts, prisons, and health and welfare agencies

Borderline personality
Characterized by history of instability of affect, impulsivity, periods of intense anger, intense, clinging relationships, and unpredictable, self-destructive acts; involves use of primitive defenses (splitting: people and the world are viewed as good or bad), projective identification, and denial; accounts for only 1% to 5% of cases, but patient is remembered because of management problems and the intense feelings he or she arouses in staff members

Compulsive personality
Characterized by orderliness, obstinateness, parsimony, emotional constriction, rigidity, indecisiveness, devotion to a task; overly concerned with rules and morals

Passive-aggressive personality
Characterized by a history of resistance to most expectations involved in social and work settings and by procrastination, forgetfulness, and inefficiency

Avoidant personality
Characterized by hypersensitivity to potential humiliation, rejection, or shame; unwillingness to develop relationships unless there is a guarantee of uncritical acceptance; usually isolated and low in self-esteem

Schizotypal personality
Characterized by *oddness* in thought, perception, speech, and behavior, but not enough to meet the criteria for schizophrenia; multiple features may be present in this disorder

Narcissistic personality
Characterized by inflated sense of esteem with extreme self-centeredness; the individual shows deficient empathy for others in spite of a wish for their admiration; these individuals feel entitled to special treatment without reciprocity and have little capacity for warmth or mutual interpersonal relationships

Dependent personality
Characterized by passively allowing others to assume responsibility for major areas of his or her life because of lack of self-confidence and an inability to function independently

---

intimate relationship behaviors, and by the capacity to perpetuate interpersonal problems and annoy others, often with little or no anxiety or guilt.[13]

Personality disorders are present in about 15% of the adult population. Not much is known about the cause of these disorders, but a genetic factor is possible, as are disturbances in early childhood. Early childhood disturbances could be faulty or arrested emotional development that interferes with adequate social control or "conscience" (that is, superego) formation; deprivation of basic needs during early childhood; and physical or emotional trauma or both during childhood or adolescence.

General characteristics of personality disorders include the following:

1. Common use of the defense mechanisms of fantasy, isolation, dissociation, projection, somatization, and splitting
2. Perception of self as extremely important and powerful
3. Formation of dependent, demanding, and entangled interpersonal relationships which are used to achieve specific need gratification

4. Low tolerance for frustration and stress without apparent anxiety
5. Help seldom sought by the patient himself or herself
6. Pathologic behavior that is directed toward and against others
7. Frequent confrontations with society's mores, norms, and laws

Generally, a firm, calm, consistent, and quiet approach is most effective and produces the least amount of manipulative or explosive response behavior. Give clear, concise explanations and directions to avoid verbal entanglements with the patient. Consistent application of firm limit-setting offers positive guidance toward establishing self-control and consistent decision making enables the nurse to maintain an objective viewpoint.

Eleven types of personality disorders described by Grimes and Burns[10] are shown in the box above.

Interventions

The nursing care of individuals with personality disorders rests heavily on the nurse's ability to deal with his or her own emotional reactions to the character traits of the patient. Nurses must be able to set firm, consistent limits on the behavior, communicate expectations for a change in behavior to the patient, and maintain a consistent team approach in understanding the dynamics of the behavior.[13]

Treatment is difficult because anxiety is generated in therapists and staff members when a patient responds with anger, defensiveness, and authoritarianism. In addition, patients with these disorders do not perceive themselves as sick.

The key to initial management of demanding patients (including those with personality disorders) is to determine the exact nature of their demands and to find a way to meet the demands or find acceptable substitutes.

Excessive demands are usually symptoms of a person's fears or sense of being overwhelmed by anxiety and other painful feelings. Satisfying the demands reduces the patient's fears and also reduces the chance of use of more primitive behaviors.

Psychotherapy is helpful and can be *long-term,* with the focus on personality change, or *short-term,* with the focus on adaptation—involving support and guidance with problems of living, assistance in limiting contact with situations that provoke problems, and help with developing personal assets. Self-help groups are useful because patients usually require more support than any one person can provide.

Drug therapy involves the use of antianxiety agents, antipsychotics during psychotic episodes, and antidepressants; there is no one specific medication for the treatment of personality disorders.

PSYCHOSES

Psychoses are psychogenic reactions in which severe personality disorganization and disintegration occur, along with marked distortions of perception of reality, thought, affect, and motivation. Types of psychoses are schizophrenia, major affective disorders, and organic acute brain syndrome.

Schizophrenia is characterized by varied symptoms of disordered simple thinking and bizarre social behaviors. The following are types of schizophrenia:

1. Hebephrenic or disorganized, characterized by incoherence, foolishness, and regressive behavior
2. Catatonic, characterized by a stuporous state in which the patient is mute, immobile, and displays waxy flexibility; the patient may retain urine and feces; or characterized by an excited state in which the patient is negative, assaultive, aggressive, hyperactive, or agitated; the patient may complain about or refuse to respond to a request
3. Paranoid, characterized by delusions of persecution and grandeur
4. Schizoaffective, characterized by disturbances in affect and thought association; some autistic and ambivalent behaviors, but not to the degree of severity associated with acute paranoid schizophrenia

5. Chronic undifferentiated, characterized by a variety of symptoms found in several types of psychosis
6. Childhood, occurs in childhood; often described as autism

The major *affective disorders* are the following:

1. Manic-depressive or bipolar disorder, which includes states of both mania and depression
2. Involutional melancholia, also called unipolar disorder; may be accompanied by paranoid states

Organic or acute brain syndrome is most likely caused by a combination of biochemical, social, and psychological factors. Characteristics include major personality disorganization and marked interference with the ability to function personally and interpersonally. Significant discrepancies between thoughts or feelings and behavior are also present. Substitution of fantasy for reality often occurs. Delusional and hallucinatory systems, disorientation, and regression are commonly present.

Dynamics

Dynamics involve loss of ego boundaries, denial of reality, severe regression, threatened security and identity, superficial interpersonal relationships, and failure or inability to trust self or others.

Concepts and Principles for Nursing Care

Attitudes of staff members can make or break the possibility of recovery for the patient with psychosis. Care must be directed toward the maintenance of "reality" relationships. Genuine interest, honesty, warmth, and optimism are essential for establishing contact with persons who have psychoses. Physical and psychologic needs merit equal attention. Familiar routines and familiar persons contribute to security. As a social being, a human being's psychologic equilibrium needs to be maintained through satisfying relationships with others, both individually and in groups.[10]

Psychosis

Psychosis occurs when a person's mental capacity, affective response, and capacity to recognize reality, communicate, and relate to others are impaired enough to interfere with his or her capacity to deal with ordinary daily life. The patient with a psychosis is often brought to the ED by concerned family members or police officers. Occasionally the patient appears alone, with minor, vague, or no complaints. He or she may be or may become out of control to the point of hurting himself or herself or others; such a condition, coupled with the extreme discomfort of the patient with acute psychosis, makes this an emergency that should be treated immediately.

When the disturbed patient is first brought in, he or she should be immediately brought to a quiet, sparsely furnished room, preferably one that includes just a sturdy stretcher and a heavy desk, with perhaps one chair. Nothing should be left in the room that can be thrown or could prove to be dangerous. Police officers and family members should quickly be asked for a brief account of the behavior that preceded the patient's arrival at the hospital, to determine such things as how much protection he or she needs and whether the presence of a family member helps or hinders the patient. Probably the two most dangerous types of patients are the patient with paranoid psychosis and the patient who is in a toxic condition.

When persons are intensely paranoid, they may feel as if they are fighting for their lives, and any behavior is rationalized as self-defense. When patients are in toxic conditions, their emotionality is increased at the same time that their normal inhibitions to aggressive or self-destructive behavior are stripped away.

If there is any reason to think that a patient may be dangerous (for example, if police officers tell the nurse that the patient attacked someone without provocation or that he or she made a determined effort to escape en route to the ED), a locked room or restraints that should be available can be used if necessary. It is necessary to create an environment that is as controlled and safe as possible for the time-consuming tasks of evaluating, treating, and planning and implementing hospitalization or other dispositions for such patients. The patient should be advised of what is being done and any fears should be allayed. Emergency nurses should pay attention to their "gut" reactions to a patient and never underestimate or disregard their intuition. Since a patient can be carrying any number of dangerous objects, from a nail file in a purse to a concealed razor blade, it is a good policy to have all patients undress and get into hospital clothing. Their personal effects should be gathered and put into safekeeping. Patients should be told matter-of-factly that this procedure is hospital policy and that the procedure is followed for all patients so that physicians can examine them. They should be reminded that they are in a hospital and that they are safe. Patients should be told that the restraints (if necessary) are to provide some of the control that they will regain soon. Patients should also be told that as long as they are having difficult, frightening, extremely painful feelings, it is expected that they will be confused about making decisions. Patients should be reminded that staff members are there to help make decisions for them until they can make decisions for themselves. This information is sometimes reassuring and lifts some of the burden of decision making from patients who may feel ambivalent about any decision. Optimally, a family member, aide, or security guard should stand by and watch each patient.

If the legality of detaining a patient against his or her will is a concern, ED staff members should be guided by the knowledge that courts are less concerned with the absolute "right or wrong" of an action than with how justifiable it is. If the nurse can justify such precautions in light of a patient's past or present behavior and the reasonable possibility of harm to himself or herself or others, the action is usually well advised. Nurses might ask themselves if it

would be more difficult to justify why they did not treat the patient and allowed him or her to leave. Safety is the foremost concern for both the patient and others.

Every patient whose behavior seems bizarre deserves to have as complete a medical workup as possible. The patient's unwillingness to cooperate and refusal of treatment are usually symptoms of the illness, not reasons to dispense with the examination or allow the patient to leave: this is the philosophy of most knowledgeable medical practitioners and the courts. The ED has just as much responsibility to treat someone who is not competent to refuse that treatment and who is in need of it as to treat a pleasant, cooperative patient. A psychiatrist or psychiatric clinical nurse specialist should be consulted to assist with both evaluation and treatment of the patient.

As soon as the patient is brought under control and is as comfortable as possible, the diagnostic detective work begins. The first task is to decide whether there is any question that the behavior is organic, that is, caused by chemical or physiologic sources. It is often helpful to gather information before talking to the patient. In this way the nurse is knowledgeable about the patient's situation before speaking with him or her, and if the patient denies any problem, the nurse can gently remind him or her of the reasons that others are concerned. A nurse should ask the patient about how he or she perceives certain events that others have told the nurse about. When patients are unaccompanied or unable to communicate, names and telephone numbers are especially helpful and may be furnished by police officers or ambulance attendants or may be found in the patient's wallet or address book. Neighbors and landlords may help, if relatives are not available. To predict the patient's course, it is important to know how acute the patient's condition is and what the progression of symptoms has been. When no information but a name is available, calling nearby state and private psychiatric hospitals may be helpful. The patient may have left a facility or wandered away from a group of patients on an outing in the area. In the aftermath of "deinstitutionalization," many former patients from the "closed wards" are without structure and may decompensate or wander from ED to ED. Without resources, these patients seem to fall into the cracks between inpatient and outpatient facilities. The nurse should ask about previous hospitalizations and medications and try to learn about the pattern of illness characteristic of this patient. These patients, and others without financial or social supports, may appear in the ED often enough to make a simple, informative "Repeater File" system helpful. Current treatment plans, effective approaches, and names and numbers of those who know the patient may be included in a file.

When any patient is interviewed, there should be only one anxious person in the room. Therefore the nurse should begin by arranging the environment to be as safe and comfortable as possible. The patient may exhibit pressured speech, the content of which may be tangential or "word salad." If the nurse listens well, themes such as fear and vulnerability may become apparent. Patients are often very sensitive and alert to the feelings and actions of others around them and may quickly sense negative feelings or insecurity in staff members. Nurses should appear calm, competent, and genuinely interested. They should not become angry if the patient's behavior is disagreeable. Patients may overreact to perceived anger. The nurse may instead appear disappointed and convey to the patient a respect for him or her and the clue that more is expected from him or her. People often live up to others' expectations; if a patient overhears that he or she is being called crazy, he or she may be more likely to act that way. The nurse should not directly challenge what the delusional patient is saying, should ask more questions about his or her thoughts, and should explore them further in conversation with the patient. If the patient demands to know whether the nurses agree with him or her, nurses can honestly answer by saying that they are trying to understand and are sure that he or she realizes how difficult it is, and ask whether he or she could explain more to them. They may tell the patient that they do believe that he or she would not mislead others intentionally.

Sometimes anxiety may be reduced by offering the patient a cup of coffee, a cigarette, or a drink of water, although this should be done only if the nurse feels comfortable about it. (Matches should be kept, coffee should be cooled, and water and cigarettes may need to be held for the patient.)

Some type of mental status examination should always be performed. The patient should be asked about frightening voices: auditory hallucinations are common in functional psychosis. Men report voices saying that they are homosexual, women say they are being called prostitutes, and both describe voices that tell them to kill themselves or tell them that they are better off dead. The patient with an acute schizophrenic psychosis usually has a flat or shallow affect, accompanied by ambivalent, constricted, and inappropriate responsiveness and loss of empathy with others. He or she may exhibit forced speech, lack of speech, or blocking. Thinking may be disturbed and the patient may misinterpret reality. Disordered thought with clear sensorium is common. The schizophrenic patient commonly says that his or her mind is being controlled, either electronically or in some other way.

The patient may be combative, withdrawn, regressive, or catatonic. The patient may be a late adolescent, a young adult who is having his or her first psychotic episode, or a chronic schizophrenic who is having a stressful experience.

Careful observation of the patient provides clues to his or her history. For example, the nurse may notice that an incoherent male patient, who appears not to have shaved for a few days, has a bank deposit receipt dated 1 week ago. If the person's condition has deteriorated to this extent in 1 week, his condition may be acute.

Acute paranoid schizophrenia is characterized by persecutory or grandiose delusions and sometimes by hallucinations or excessive religiosity. A patient with this type of schizophrenia, as previously noted, is often hostile. A systematized delusion, sometimes built on actual situations but carried to outlandish lengths, may be present. The patient may carry a notebook with handwritten, loosely associated themes. Some patients carry religious objects on their persons. The patient with paranoid psychosis should be managed with the utmost care: he or she presents a high risk for aggression or violence and a difficult challenge.

Hypomania and manic psychosis are occasionally encountered in the ED. Hypomania involves a classic triad of symptoms, elated but unstable mood, incessant speech, and increased motor activity. The patient with hypomania talks easily, humorously, and endlessly. He or she is friendly, then uninvitedly personal. Beneath this thin veneer of well-being, however, is an intolerance for frustration, impulsive, ill-considered actions, and blatant disregard of obvious difficulties.

In acute mania, all of these characteristics are present, but they are more intense and more disturbing. Propriety and discretion are painfully absent. The content of the patient's conversation is frequently sexual and often loud. Manic patients may have recurrent episodes of mood elevation; they may also have periods of depression. Lithium is a specific drug used in the treatment of manic-depressive illness. The manic patient should not be encouraged to talk and should be asked to be succinct in giving a history, in the interest of effecting the best care. Physical restraints are often agitating, and use of them should be avoided. The patient should be given a private room or area in which he or she can pace if he or she feels the need.

Whatever the type of psychosis, an appropriate disposition should be determined. If family is willing, and if the patient is thought to be able, a relatively disturbed person may go home with medication, solid follow-up care, and the option of returning to the ED or a more appropriate place if he or she becomes worse or worries the family. If the patient is clearly unmanageable in another setting, hospitalization must be arranged. The determination of where the patient will be hospitalized depends on such factors as the patient's willingness to be admitted, insurance status, and the availability of beds. If the patient is extremely agitated and self-destructive, even when restrained, some medication may be required. However, if the patient is going to be hospitalized, particularly if the patient is going to be committed to another hospital where the concurrence of the accepting physician determines whether he or she will be admitted, the staff members in the ED should use drugs sparingly, if at all. Ideally, the person at the accepting facility should clearly observe the pathologic condition or trust the judgment of the referring agency. Medication may miraculously "cure" the patient or make him or her so sleepy as to preclude an interview. Family or friends should accompany the patient to enhance the transition and facilitate any further history taking. Even if the patient is willing to go to the hospital, the ED may want to send the patient with a commitment paper, in the event that the patient changes his or her mind en route and ambulance drivers are left without the legal right to restrain the patient.

SCHIZOPHRENIA

Schizophrenia, as discussed earlier, encompasses a group of mental disorders that have varied symptoms of disordered thinking and bizarre social behaviors.

Clinical Manifestations

Early signs of schizophrenia are the following:
1. Blocking or cutting off conversation; not responding as usual to friends; appearing aloof
2. Having blackouts or other spells
3. Expressing various concerns about body symptoms
4. Forgetting and abandoning plans or life goals
5. Disregarding social customs and talking about abstract ideas such as love, creation, equality

Onset

Schizophrenia may occur after an experience involving loss, separation, rejection, or the use of lysergic acid diethylamide (LSD), marijuana, alcohol, or amphetamines.

Acute Phase

Hallucinations, especially auditory hallucinations, and the following characteristics may be present during the acute phase:
1. Voices that are making general comments are heard.
2. Voices may be saying, "You are this . . . You do that"; voices may make obscene and threatening remarks or command the patient to perform a violent act.
3. Tactile and olfactory hallucinations may indicate temporal lobe epilepsy or the presence of a tumor. Cocaine abuse may also cause tactile hallucinations.
4. Visual hallucinations occur in both hysteria and schizophrenia, but they can also be indicators of organic disorders.
5. Patients also have sensory disturbances, especially optical (for example, seeing changing shapes and figures) during the acute phase. In addition they have delusions of persecution, grandeur, or impending destruction.
6. Thinking is autistic and characterized by being highly personal and not logical, with perseveration, blocking, concretization, and loosening of associations.
7. Speech is characterized by incoherence, use of symbols, and concrete responses; also possible are echolalia, flight of ideas, neologisms, and inability or unwillingness to speak.
8. Patients exhibit inappropriate behavior such as grimacing, negativism, anergy (state of inaction), suggestibility, poor personal hygiene, and few social manners.

9. Blunting, ambivalence, and inappropriateness of affect are also indicators of the acute phase.

Residual Phase

Symptoms of flat or blunted affect, rambling speech, poor hygiene and grooming, and distortion of some perceptual experiences may remain.

Relapse Phase or Stage of Decompensation

The nurse can determine that a patient is in the relapse phase when the following indicators are observed:
1. Feelings of being overwhelmed
2. Feelings of boredom and apathy
3. Disinhibition; impulsive expression of feelings
4. Psychotic disorganization with increasing perceptual and cognitive dysfunction, loss of identity, and loss of self-control
5. Psychotic reaction with a decrease in anxiety and a disturbed organization of self

Therapeutic Intervention

The patient's relationship with a therapist is vital. The therapist must be able to understand the patient, offer the patient support and guidance, and engage him or her in a therapeutic relationship and other treatment modalities.

The importance of social relationships in support of the patient during recovery is being recognized. Self-concept is enhanced; approval is given, even after the acute phase of the illness; opportunities for the patient to vent feelings and receive feedback from friends are provided; and material help is given.

Family support and involvement are necessary. Expression of hostility, overinvolvement, and frequent criticism contribute to the recurrence of symptoms in the patient.

Treatment choices are related to the stage of the disease, the amount of regresssion, the availability of reality testing, the motivation for treatment and the patient's stress management skills, available resources, and ability to relate to a therapist.

Long-term treatment of the patient involves programs that assist in many areas: basic needs for food, a place to live, and clothing, assistance with medical problems, development of social and vocational skills, medication needs, and development of a social support system. This treatment requires collaboration among health professionals. Frequently, services are not readily available and patients seek help among themselves: a "ghettoization" of the chronically mentally ill occurs.

A variety of available therapies that are used to meet treatment goals designed for the individual patient include the following:
1. Short hospitalization
2. Day treatment and outpatient treatment
3. Rehabilitation services
4. Milieu therapy

5. Drug therapy with antipsychotic agents
6. Individual psychotherapy
7. Family therapy
8. Group therapy
9. Behavior therapy
10. Electroconvulsive therapy
11. Psychoanalysis

PARANOID DISORDERS

Paranoid disorders represent a group of mental disorders manifested by delusions of jealousy and persecution unexplained by the presence of other psychiatric disorders.

Causes

No specific cause of paranoid disorders is known, but research suggests several factors. The psychodynamic theory postulates that delusions are based on the use of denial and projection as defenses against homosexual wishes. Other possible causes are childhood developmental deficits or failure to develop basic trust, which may be related to physical abuse, single-parent families, unpredictable parental behavior, or other forms of rejection.

Parental expectations of perfection and high achievement and stressful situations involving lowering of self-esteem, increasing distrust, envy, isolation, and other factors may lead to a delusional system that is frightening but partially comforting.

Clinical Manifestations

Paranoia is characterized by a clear, logical, lasting delusional system. Interpersonal relationships are poor because the person with a paranoid disorder mistrusts everyone.

Therapeutic Intervention

Hospitalization is generally not indicated because the person with paranoia seldom seeks treatment, and his or her community develops a tolerance for the odd behaviors. If delusions are causing a person to behave in ways that are dangerous to self or others, hospitalization is indicated. Drug therapy consists of the use of antipsychotic medications. Psychotherapy initially deals with the problem of establishing a trusting relationship and with immediate, concrete problems; later, delusions and the mistrust of others are discussed.

AFFECTIVE DISORDERS

Affective disorders are a group of mental disorders that are characterized by symptoms of mood disturbance and associated changes in thinking and behavior.

Clinical Manifestations of Selected Types

Major depression. The symptoms of major depression include sadness, apathy, feelings of worthlessness, self-blame, thoughts of suicide, desire to escape, avoidance of simple problems, anorexia, weight loss, decreased interest in sex, sleeplessness, and either reduction in activity or ceaseless activity. In infants and older children, symptoms include refusal to eat, listlessness, lack of activity, fear of the death of a parent, and fear of separation from parents. In adolescents, symptoms include social isolation, negative attitude, sulkiness, feelings of being unappreciated, and acting in antisocial ways.

Bipolar disorder. In a bipolar disorder periods of depression alternate with periods of mania. In a manic episode of bipolar disorder, symptoms include hyperactivity, grandiosity, manipulativeness, irritability, euphoria, mood lability, hypersexuality, delusions, aggression, and sleeplessness. In a depressive episode the symptoms are the same as those of major depression.

Dysthymic disorder. Dysthymic disorder is a new diagnostic category for disorders in which a person has a depressed mood for at least 2 years, no pleasure in activities of daily living, an impairment in social skills, and numerous bodily complaints.

Therapeutic Interventions

Therapeutic interventions for affective disorders include the following:
1. Hospitalization
2. Electroconvulsive therapy
3. Drug therapy
4. Psychotherapy
5. Cognitive psychotherapy
6. Behavioral therapy
7. Maintenance of social supports
8. Prevention of suicide
9. Vigorous exercise

ORGANIC MENTAL DISORDERS

Organic mental disorders represent a group of disorders that have a variety of symptoms, especially a disturbance of cognition.

ED personnel tend to view bizarre behavior negatively. Such behavior is often considered functional rather than organic in cause until proved otherwise: "If the patient looks crazy, then he or she is." "If the patient does not want help, then he or she should not be given it." Help may indeed be given reluctantly. In many instances, however, the organic (or functional) illness is such that the patient is not capable of good judgment or decision making. Whether the patient has a history of psychiatric problems or not, he or she deserves to have ED staff members search out, methodically and logically, all possible causes for his or her illness. The patient should be given the benefit of blood testing to determine a complete blood cell count, electrolyte levels, sugar levels, and toxic screening, as well as a neurologic workup and the like. The rationale for a thorough investigation of causes of abnormal behavior is that in many cases, such as acute organic brain syndrome (AOBS), the pathologic condition is transient and reversible.

Acute Organic Brain Syndrome

In AOBS biochemical or structural impairment is usually present. Characteristics include a disturbed level of consciousness and cognition, clouding of sensorium, physical abnormalities that include changes in the pulse rate and focal reflexes, and the presence of delirium. Symptoms include the following:

1. Behavioral changes. Ability to identify behavioral changes depends on knowledge of the premorbid personality (that is, the normally suspicious person becomes paranoid).
2. Vascillating symptomatology may sometimes lead the health professional to think that the patient is "fooling" or that the patient is better and can be released.
3. Appearance. The patient's affect may be vacant. He or she may be disheveled and preoccupied; may exhibit inappropriate and weird responses (for example, laughing at something serious), purposeless movements (picking or itching), general agitation, or lethargy. The patient's eyes may be darting and either glossy or dull.
4. Speech may be slurred; perseveration and echolalia may be present.
5. Affect may be variable, that is, labile.
6. Thought content is a major diagnostic differentiator between organic and functional illness and includes a continuum of wakefulness or somnolence, inability to focus attention, distractibility by exogenous or endogenous things, inability to grasp meanings, and disorientation that depends on the severity and progression of the illness. The patient is disoriented first to time, then to place, then to person. Many patients with AOBS are disoriented.
7. Visual hallucinations are sometimes mere distortions of what the patient actually sees; visual hallucinations are more common than auditory ones.[14]

Probably most common among the AOBSs are those associated with drug or poison intoxication. Other syndromes are associated with the following signs and symptoms:

1. Circulatory disturbances producing cerebrovascular insufficiency
2. Disturbances in metabolism or nutrition such as hypoglycemia or hypokalemia (The latter, for example, may develop as a result of hyperemesis gravidarum and can result in delusional or depressive mental changes.)
3. Brain trauma such as a concussion
4. Infections such as meningitis, syphilis, or hepatitis
5. Intracranial neoplasms: gliomas, metastatic carcinomas, and meningiomas
6. Epilepsy: grand mal, petit mal, and focal seizures

Many cases of AOBS have psychiatric symptomatology. Classic catatonic states are sometimes encountered in patients with AOBS; such states may be produced by frontal lobe lesions, tumors, vascular lesions, encephalitis, and degenerative states of toxicosis. Most often, multiple, possibly interacting etiologic factors influence a particular case of AOBS, and the patient's response depends on the degree of the insult and the person's premorbid ego strengths. Thus, making the differential diagnosis can sometimes be difficult and confusing but certainly worth the effort, given the treatable and potentially harmful nature of the illness. Medical management is dictated by the cause of the symptoms. Nursing management, in general, includes simplifying and familiarizing the patient with the environment. The nurse should attempt to decrease the number of objects or shadows in the room, which can be misinterpreted by the patient, keep the same staff members or family members in the room, orient the patient to reality with simple statements, and keep lights on. Avoiding the use of physical restraints is optimal, if available personnel are able to stay with the patient, since the restraints only increase confusion and agitation. It is often helpful to reassure the patient that this state of confusion is temporary by telling the patient that even though he or she does not remember something at that particular moment, he or she need not worry because the nurse will remember for the patient until his or her memory improves.[4]

Violence

Although violence is not necessarily the product of a particular disorder, it is usually associated with either functional illnesses, such as character disorders and paranoid schizophrenia, or with organic disorders, such as toxicity and temporal lobe epilepsy. Psychodynamically, violent behavior can be seen as a defense mechanism by which the individual protects himself or herself from unbearable and overwhelming feelings of helplessness. Organically, it can be seen as a disorder or either a specific cerebral anatomic structure or an electrical or metabolic function or a combination of these.

If psychologic or functional causes are inducing the behavior, the nurse should look for events, feelings, and conflicts that may help explain outbursts. If the root of the behavior is organic, it may involve such sources as electrical disturbances of the brain (temporal lobe epilepsy) or metabolic abnormalities such as those caused by barbiturate or alcohol use or withdrawal, electrolyte imbalance, or hypoxia.

In the ED, it is often necessary to decide quickly what to do when a patient has, or escalates to, violent behavior. If the patient is so out of control that there seems to be imminent danger to self or others, restraints may be required. Attempts to subdue a patient with an inadequate number of staff members should not be attempted. Usually no fewer than five strong persons should approach the patient, one staff member for each limb, plus one more. The restrainers should plan their actions beforehand and act quickly and decisively. If the patient requires restraints, they should remain on the patient. Staff members may tend to watch a patient less after he or she is restrained (they should actually watch him or her more closely). Experienced ED personnel know that a patient who gets partially or fully out of restraints represents a high-risk situation. If leather or specifically designed restraints are not available, soft material such as Kerlix (Kendall Healthcare Products Co., Mansfield, Mass.) or stockinette may be used and should be knotted as securely as possible without interfering with blood supply and neural pathways. A securely tied restraint defies the quick, easy extrication by determined patients, which often occurs when "loops" are used. (Looping restraints around extremities may be more useful for the senile, mildly disoriented, and combative patient.) If the patient is extremely intoxicated, supine positioning may be considered to guard against aspiration. Side rails should be up and the stretcher should be locked. If possible, the stretcher should be positioned in such a way as to make tipping it over by rocking less likely. Many patients with severe psychosis seem to feel relieved after being restrained, perhaps because they feel that they are being given the control that they lack, and decisions (even the smallest of which are often difficult for these patients) are being made for them. Patients who are restrained should be reassured that it is primarily for their own safety, that no one will harm them in any way, and that the restraints will be used for a short time, until they regain their own control.

Even with the restraints, some patients may still present a significant danger to themselves. Patients may hit their heads or bite or pull dangerously at restraints. In such cases the benefits of chemical intervention may outweigh the risks of confusing the toxicologic picture, potentiating the effects of other drugs, or clouding the clinical picture.

Abusive, Angry Patient

The abusive, angry patient is a more frequent problem in the ED than is the violent patient. Although prevention is the best means to alleviate the problem of the angry patient, the key to secondary prevention is to remain calm and professional. Nurses should refuse to become embroiled in a person struggle. Because nurses are professionals, they should keep the patient focused on the substance of the issues or point out objectively how they see the situation. Nurses should also listen to what the patient is saying and allow him or her to vent angry feelings. Ventilation relieves the pressure of an anger drive. If the patient is not talking but is acting out his or her anger, the nurse should try to understand the need that prompts the behavior, what the patient is trying to express, and how the environment and the nurse may be influencing the patient's behavior. The nurse may explain that it would be more helpful for the patient to explain what he or she needs rather than merely showing anger, since it is impossible for the nurse to know everything a person is feeling and thinking.

The anger being expressed may actually be displaced (misdirected), that is, the object of that anger may not be the ED or the nurse. The patient may be feeling rage at a terminal diagnosis or the tension and frustration of a lifetime. The nurse may ask if it is the ED or the staff toward which the patient's anger is really directed. It is important not to feed into the patient's "angry system" by fueling potential fires. The nurse should do nothing toward which the patient can direct his or her ready anger and should be a "reality tester" for the patient, asking whether his or her anger is really appropriate in its intensity, in spite of the legitimacy of his or her complaint.

PSYCHIATRIC MEDICATIONS

The best advice concerning the use of psychiatric drugs in the ED is to avoid using them. Whenever possible, medicating patients or dispensing prescriptions from such a transient and episodic area as the ED should be avoided. Often, interpersonal intervention can accomplish much more good and do far less harm than drugs. However, medications to manage a condition and afford relief to the severely disturbed patient in the ED are sometimes necessary. When and whether to medicate are often difficult decisions, especially since diagnoses are seldom clear-cut and reliable. If diagnostic certainty is not possible, the risk of medicating the patient must be carefully weighed against the consequences of not medicating the patient.

Haloperidol (Haldol) is, in many ED situations, the drug of choice for attenuation of the common problems of severe agitation, psychomotor hyperactivity, assaultiveness, mania, and the extreme mental anguish that accompany an acute psychosis. Haloperidol seems to be the safest medication for these purposes and is seldom accompanied by instances of hypotension, which are more common occurrences with chlorpromazine (Thorazine), an effective antipsychotic that has a greater sedative effect. Because haloperidol does not cause pronounced sedation, it seems to be less threatening to the patient with paranoid psychosis, who may be afraid of being "put to sleep." Dystonic reactions are infrequent and seem to occur more often and become problematic when the patient is given the lowest oral doses rather than intramuscular doses. If possible, the nurse should check for vital signs, in particular, blood pressure, and determine and report suspicion of any other drugs or alcohol that the patient may have ingested, even days or weeks before admission, giving special attention to any history of use of central nervous system depressants. Blood pressure and general physical condition should be monitored carefully and frequently after administration of medication to any patient but particularly in those patients whose mental or emotional status is compromised.

Patients with compromised mental status may be able neither to give feedback regarding the effect of the medication nor to understand its purpose. The initial intramuscular dose of haloperidol is 0.5 to 5 mg, with subsequent doses in the same range administered every 30 to 60 minutes. A 40-minute interval between doses prevents unnecessary somnolence caused by the rapid administration of additional doses; such an interval should be maintained unless the patient's safety demands that a dose be administered slightly sooner. Infrequent side effects of lowered seizure threshold and cholinergic blocking can occur.

Contraindications to the use of haloperidol are pregnancy, hypersensitivity, narrow-angle glaucoma, central nervous system depression, and severe cardiac disease with dysrhythmia. Haloperidol is commonly used in the ED for acute schizophrenia, alcoholic hallucinosis, and emergency sedation with uncertain diagnosis. Results with patients for whom the drug is appropriately used are often dramatic. Thought disorders improve significantly, and few and minimal side effects occur. The danger involved with this drug is that it often works so well that ED staff members perceive the patient as cured; thus they may be more inclined to discharge a patient who does not have social supports or the ability to continue with the medication on his or her own and who will probably again become sick when the medication wears off.

Two commonly used minor tranquilizers, or antianxiety agents, are *chlordiazepoxide (Librium)* and *diazepam (Valium)*. The initial intramuscular adult dose of chlordiazepoxide is 25 to 50 mg, with subsequent doses of 25 to 100 mg every 1 to 2 hours. Doses given orally range from 5 to 25 mg, with subsequent doses of 5 to 25 mg and total doses of up to 100 mg daily. Initial intramuscular doses of diazepam range from 5 to 10 mg, with doses of 5 to 10 mg every 1 to 2 hours. The oral dosage ranges from 2 to 10 mg, up to 40 mg daily. When chlordiazepoxide or diazepam is used for the management of acute withdrawal from alcohol, higher doses may be required, depending on the severity of the withdrawal. Doses of chlordiazepoxide (50 to 100 mg) may be followed by repeated doses as needed, until agitation is controlled; up to 300 mg per day may be administered. Diazepam 10 mg administered 3 to 4 times daily during the first 24 hours is also recommended. With both medications, drowsiness and ataxia are frequently encountered side effects. Confusion, hypotension, prolonged sedation, and paradoxic excitement are less common. The latter side effect, called "Valium rage" when induced by that drug, is a distinct ED management problem.

Oxazepam (Serax) has been found to be efficacious in the treatment of a wide variety of disorders: anxiety, tension, agitation and irritability, and anxiety associated with depression. An oral medication, oxazepam seems to be safer in terms of tolerance and toxicity than other related compounds such as chlordiazepoxide and diazepam. Dosages of 10 to 30 mg, up to 120 mg per day, are suggested. Oxazepam may be considered when a prescription is being given to a patient in the ED. As with all prescriptions given in the ED, the number of pills should be limited to less than the number that would produce serious consequences if taken at one time. Before the patient is given a sizable prescription, he or she should be asked honestly and with concern if he or she has had any suicidal ideation or if self-destructive behavior is a possibility. The patient should then be referred to a resource that can provide long-term therapy, including further medication and other support, if necessary.

CHEMICAL TOXIC REACTIONS

When a chemical toxic reaction has occurred, a comprehensive history is vital. If the patient is an unreliable historian, gather as much data as possible from a friend or family member who is with the patient.

Alcohol-Related Emergencies

Alcohol-related emergencies are common in most EDs and have become more so as a result of the recognition that alcoholism is a disease rather than as a criminal offense. Police officers in many parts of the country are currently mandated to bring an alcoholic to an emergency care unit or detoxification center rather than to jail. Although alcoholism is considered a psychiatric illness from one vantage point, in the ED it should always be first considered a medical emergency. Acute alcohol intoxication may result in death. An acutely intoxicated person is more likely to sustain a head injury and less likely to relate an accurate history or present a clear-cut diagnostic picture. Chronically intoxicated persons often have chronic illnesses and many medical problems. Nutritional deficiencies with mental sequelae, such as Wernicke-Korsakoff syndrome and Korsakoff's syndrome, seizure disorders, tuberculosis, hepatic coma, alcoholic hallucinosis, and delirium tremens are frequently observed and should be kept in mind.

Obtaining telephone numbers of the patient's relatives, friends, landlord, and so on is particularly helpful. These persons may be able to tell the nurse what and how much the patient drinks, what his or her behavior baseline is, whether he or she has currently stopped drinking, and what his or her behavior is like when he or she drinks, when he or she stops, and when he or she involuntarily withdraws. The occurrence of blackouts (periods during which the patient is drinking and continues to function but later does not recall what he or she did) is particularly indicative of chronic alcoholism. A particularly helpful question is one that asks whether the patient has been "sick" lately. In particular, has he or she been vomiting for the past couple of days, and consequently been unable to keep down the normal amount of liquor? The patient may be in withdrawal, although he or she may deny that the drinking has stopped. The possibility that drugs have been taken in combination with alcohol should always be suspected at the beginning of the patient's visit to the ED, not 5 hours later when the patient is obtunded as a result of a serious overdose that went unconsidered.

While the emergency nurse is assessing the alcohol-affected patient, he or she must consider the possibility that immediate management of potentially disruptive and possibly dangerous behavior may be necessary. Intoxication produces confusion, moroseness, combativeness, regression, and a general lack of inhibitions.

While the patient is being evaluated and detoxified, a safe

environment must be provided. He or she should be positioned on the stomach or the side, especially if restraints are required, to prevent aspiration. The possibility of the patient's vomiting or having a seizure should always be kept in mind. Accordingly, the patient's restraints should be kept loose, to prevent injuries to soft tissue or bones in the event of a seizure.

After an initial evaluation, watchful waiting while the patient ideally has some restorative sleep is the safest and most desirable approach. Caffeine in any form may precipitate seizures, and sedatives may potentiate the effects of alcohol. The patient's behavior may be such that he or she presents an imminent danger to self or others. Occasionally a patient is extremely agitated, suicidal, and self-destructive. Avoid unnecessary active intervention. In the event that the patient does not respond to the structure and intervention of the ED after a reasonable time, a small, almost subtherapeutic dose of haloperidol has been used effectively. With haloperidol, as with other medications, the desired effects must be weighed against the possibilities of respiratory depression and coma in the situation of excessive alcohol intoxication. Haloperidol seems to have much less of an effect on central nervous system depression than other tranquilizers have.

An objective, sympathetic approach should be used with every intoxicated person. A punitive approach is counterproductive and may result in a greater management problem. Nurses' responses to verbal abuse from an intoxicated patient are indicative not only of their maturity, self-confidence, and level of professionalism but also of their understanding of the disease of alcoholism and an appreciation of the alcoholic's past and present psychic pain.

An alcoholic's affect may range from the morose to the euphoric; the latter often belies his or her true feelings.

The nurse should remain kind and supportive, indicating a belief in the patient's basic worthiness and expecting the best behavior possible from him or her. Serious consideration should be given to what the patient says while intoxicated, whether it be suicidal ideation or information about situational stresses. However, it is not productive to spend long periods talking with a patient who is intoxicated. Although he or she may feel uninhibited enough to divulge painful information, the extremely intoxicated individual may not remember what was said and may feel differently when sober. A case in point is the patient who arrives in an agitated, suicidal state lamenting that there is nothing to live for, only to leave 4 hours later wondering what happened and quite surprised when asked if he or she would like to talk to someone about the way he or she is feeling.

Ideally, every intoxicated patient should have at least some evaluation of the circumstances that led to the intoxication and the overall pattern of alcohol use. A good way to begin evaluation with a patient who may dismiss, understate, or deny the incident is to gently, positively, and in the least threatening way say the following:

1. "Although the ED is glad to help you, there may be something that could be done to prevent further such visits."
2. "It is important for you to understand the connection between your drinking and your presence in the ED today."
3. "I'm concerned that during your period of intoxication you could have been seriously hurt, because of all reports I have had of your activity."
4. "This worries me and should worry you."

The person with an alcohol problem may be more likely to return for follow-up treatment to the institution with which he or she has become familiar through the visit to the ED and which he or she sees as "knowing his or her situation" more than another. The first and biggest step for any person with alcoholism is to admit that the problem exists. It may be easier to do this if a foundation and tone of trust and help are set during the ED visit, which may be the patient's only contact with helping professionals.

If what the patient says is at variance with what others have said about his or her drinking, he or she should be confronted, but the nurse should be careful not to engage in a battle about whether the patient had three or four drinks or whether he or she has a problem. This kind of confrontation only puts the patient on the defensive and increases his or her denial. The important message to send is that there is genuine concern on the nurse's part, not an effort to get the patient out of the ED as quickly as possible. (Depending on the patient, referrals to Alcoholics Anonymous, clinics for the treatment of alcoholism, individual therapists, detoxification centers, or halfway houses may be in order. The families of such patients may need support, ventilation, reality testing, and referral for themselves. An alcoholism information and referral source is usually available if making a referral for someone is a problem.)

If there is alcoholism within the patient's family, there is greater likelihood, whether because of genetic or environmental factors, that the patient will have alcoholism. This information should be presented in a matter-of-fact way, much as you would caution a patient with a history of diabetes in his or her family.

Alcohol-induced states that may be confused with psychiatric illness are delirium tremens, alcoholic hallucinosis, alcohol paranoid state, Wernicke-Korsakoff syndrome, and Korsakoff's syndrome.

Delirium tremens is an acute, potentially fatal medical emergency. Although the patient's behavior is psychotic, the differential diagnosis can be made quickly on the basis of history, physical appearance, and behavior. The patient is often anxious, extremely agitated, and diaphoretic; he or she also exhibits fine tremors, visual hallucinations, a "picking motion" of the fingers, and elevated vital signs. The delirium is usually preceded by restlessness, irritability, an aversion to food, tremulousness, and disturbed sleep.

Alcoholic hallucinosis exists on a continuum with delirium tremens. The patient is often oriented to time, place, and person and may not be tremulous. This particular condition may resemble schizophrenia. A differential diagnosis is important, since the patient requires prompt and careful medical evaluation and hospitalization rather than psychiatric hospitalization. A medical admission is necessary because many psychiatric facilities are ill-equipped and unable to deliver medical care, even though many physicians are reluctant to hospitalize someone whom they see as a psychiatric case and who presents many potential management problems. The patient may have threatening auditory hallucinations accompanied by an elaborate delusional system.

The patient is likely to respond to his or her hallucinations and ideas, conversing with and acting on them. The symptoms may wax and wane in the ED, which provides a clue to the intoxication. Wernicke-Korsakoff syndrome and Korsakoff's syndrome are caused by the nutritional deficit, especially of thiamine and niacin, often accompanying alcoholism. Wernicke-Korsakoff syndrome involves brainstem destruction, whereas in Korsakoff's syndrome, degeneration is mainly in the cerebrum and peripheral nerves.

Signs and symptoms of Wernicke-Korsakoff syndrome include ophthalmoplegia, apathy or apprehension, clouding of consciousness, and even coma. Korsakoff's syndrome involves disorientation to time and place and peripheral neuropathy. An especially helpful diagnostic clue in both conditions is the presence of memory impairment (especially recent memory) and confabulation (covering up for memory deficit by "filling in false details").

Drug-Related Problems

The many theories and postulations about drug dependence are beyond the scope of this chapter. In dealing with this type of patient, two important points must be remembered. (1) The patient is usually emotionally needy and vulnerable and has suffered, or feels that he or she has suffered, to the point that the patient feels he or she deserves help and (2) the patient may be emotionally draining or manipulative or both and may evoke mixed feelings from the ED practitioner. The practitioner, therefore, must combine self-confidence with kindness and set reasonable but firm limits with such patients.

Addicted patients commonly seek drugs in the ED, especially in large urban hospitals. Patients may request paregoric for a teething child or mimic the symptoms of kidney stones, even by pricking a finger to drop blood in the urine sample. They may say that they are allergic to codeine and pentazocine (Talwin) and ask specifically for oxycodone (Percodan) or meperidine (Demerol) when being treated for "whiplash." They may be desperate enough to steal prescription blanks from the hospital or change a prescription that is given to them.

ED practitioners should be alert, although not suspicious or punitive, when treating patients with possible drug addictions. Needle marks can be observed while taking blood pressure measurements. (Take these measurements in the arm that the patient does *not* offer.) Yawning, pinpoint or enlarged pupils, sneezing, nervousness, reddened nose from scratching or rubbing, unusual thirst, slurred speech, and a general physically rundown appearance (weight loss, unkempt appearance, dental caries) may point to drug dependence.

Heroin and methadone. With the popularity of heroin and the number of methadone-dependent persons maintained at outpatient clinics, the ED encounters many patients who specifically request relief from withdrawal symptoms or the possibility thereof. It has been the policy of many large hospitals confronted with this problem to be firm in not giving anything but medications to provide relief from symptoms, that is, prochlorperazine (Compazine) for nausea and vomiting, Kaopectate for diarrhea, diazepam (Valium) for agitation, and referral to other facilities for maintenance or detoxification. Often patients may be more afraid of possibly withdrawing than having actual withdrawal symptoms. They may have acute anxiety about their need for drugs. A methadone or heroin user may come to the ED on a weekend evening saying that he or she is on a program in another state and in need of a methadone dose. The following considerations should be kept in mind in such situations:

1. The drug-dependent person did not become dependent overnight; in spite of the urgency and anxiety he or she feels, the patient may not belong in an ED.
2. Most maintenance programs have rules, regulations, and contingency plans (such as planning for a patient to get his or her medication in another state, if he or she is traveling, or in another center in the area if necessary) with which the patient is familiar.
3. Methadone stays in the patient's system for approximately 48 hours. Withdrawal symptoms do not begin until 24 to 36 hours after that time, so there is a sufficient "grace period" to allow a patient to skip a day if unavoidable.

Patients who are taking methadone usually do not know their doses, and the history of how many bags of heroin were used per day is unreliable for many reasons.

In planning for referral or individual or family counseling in the ED, the nurses should keep in mind the individual needs of the particular types of patients. The needs of the young include peer support, a sense of identity, self-esteem, purpose, involvement, a place to go, people to fit in with, and a positive role in society. The needs of the elderly patient may include company, purpose, activity, and better medical care. Women may need the means to obtain a life outside the home and assistance obtaining day care and transportation and in acquiring vocational skills. Homosexuals may need social acceptance, self-understanding, acceptance of their sexual orientation, and perhaps counselor support from a homosexual resource group. Veterans may need help with the social, economic, and mental adjustment of leaving the service or help with an addiction that developed during military service. Referrals and advice, then, differ according to the individuals and their situations.[9] Therefore individual and symptomatic treatments in the ED are best. Patients who are exhibiting withdrawal usually manifest symptoms of pupil dilation, increased blood pressure, pulse rate, and respiration rate (greater than 24 breaths per minute), restlessness, stomach cramps, nausea and vomiting, diaphoresis, low-back pain, yawning, and tearing eyes. If significant withdrawal is present and the need to treat the patient is apparent, it may be best to give methadone rather than meperidine or another such drug. Meperidine or morphine is needed in fairly large doses every 4 hours, whereas methadone may be given in increments of 5 or 10 mg, titrating the medication while closely watching the pupil size become smaller, the vital signs decrease, and the other symptoms abate.

Resources available for drug-addicted persons, or at least a telephone number for a drug referral source, should be listed in the ED. Before making referrals, determine what facilities the patient already knows about or has used and which ones he or she can or cannot use at this time. Members of the drug rehabilitation community may be better informed than the nurse is in many instances, and valuable time spent in making telephone calls may be eliminated by careful interviewing.

Barbiturates. Barbiturate dependence is an increasing problem. Patients with barbiturate intoxication or withdrawal problems are frequently seen in the ED. Long-acting barbiturates such as phenobarbital (Luminal) are generally less toxic and have less dramatic withdrawal effects than the short-acting amobarbital (Amytal), pentobarbital (Nembutal), or secobarbital (Seconal). Other sedatives and so-called "minor tranquilizers" may also produce barbiturate-type dependence to a lesser degree. These include diazepam (Valium), chlordiazepoxide (Librium), meprobamate (Miltown), methyprylon (Noludar), and glutethimide (Doriden). Diminished alertness, confusion, lateral gaze, nystagmus, dysarthria, ataxia, and emotional instability are observed in patients who are barbiturate-intoxicated. The emotional instability of these patients frequently has a paranoid-aggressive character, and their tendency toward destructiveness and combativeness in the ED creates a particularly difficult management problem. The successful control of this type of patient requires a neutral, objective approach to care. Negative verbal and nonverbal communications by ED staff members are countertherapeutic. These drugs have the effect of removing inhibitions and bringing to the surface many intense, unresolved feelings. People who might otherwise glibly and without emotion talk of problems, weep bitterly, exhibit aggression, and vent anger and frustration when they are intoxicated. Barbiturates are one of the most frequently used drugs in suicide attempts and the most common cause of drug fatalities. The ED practitioner should be aware of the potential for abuse when patients are given prescriptions in the ED and should make sure that prescriptions are limited.

Hallucinogens. Lysergic acid diethylamide (LSD) "bad trips" seem to be an increasingly rare phenomenon in EDs today. However, the frightening and dangerous effects of other hallucinogens—mescaline, tetrahydrocannabinol, and combinations including these and others—are not at all uncommon. The patients who have been taking hallucinogens and who come to the ED usually exhibit anxiety, hyperactivity, and the sympathetic nervous system signs of pupil dilation and increased vital signs. Symptoms seem to be a function of dose; low doses produce euphoric responses, and high doses produce a hallucinatory psychosis.

With hallucinatory and other drug-induced psychoses, patients seem more disorganized, have less motor retardation, and are more excited than their counterparts who have schizophrenia. They also show better histories of socialization and more intelligence and have better premorbid work records. These factors should be kept in mind when gathering a history about a patient with a questionable diagnosis. The patient usually has some inclination to help the practitioner. Supportive care in a reassuring environment is helpful. The presence of one familiar person who is unquestionably trusted by the patient and who can stay with the patient continuously is invaluable and lends an aspect of reality testing to the patient's condition. Diazepam (Valium), administered orally, is the medication most generally accepted. Phenothiazine compounds may exaggerate the psychotic reaction in some instances.

Belladonna alkaloids. Drugs of the belladonna group can cause severe delirium and psychotic manifestations. Associated symptoms include blurred vision, dry mouth, and difficulty in urinating. Weakness, hallucinations, acute disturbances of the sensorium, rapid, weak pulse rate, flushing and dryness of skin, widely dilated pupils, and an extremely elevated temperature are signs of toxicosis. As with all toxic reactions to drugs, attempts to sedate the patient with more drugs should always be avoided because of the possibility of potentiating central nervous system depression, causing an idiosyncratic reaction, or clouding the clinical picture. If absolutely necessary, small doses of sedatives should be given. Physostigmine salicylate given intramuscularly is a specific antidote. Suspect belladonna toxicosis when drugs including atropine (Donnatal and Donnagel) or scopolamine (Nytol and Sominex) are involved. Some plants contain belladonna alkaloids and, when ingested, cause atropine-like effects.

The patient should be given fluids, catheterized if necessary, and provided with a quiet atmosphere with minimal stimulation.

Bromide toxicosis. Although an infrequent problem, bromide toxicosis (from potassium, sodium, or ammonium) is a type of toxicosis of which the ED practitioner should be aware. The effects can be similar to psychiatric symptomatology. The sequelae comprise four distinct phenomena, simple bromide intoxication, hallucinosis, delirium, and transitory schizophrenia associated with paranoid symptomatology.

In simple bromide intoxication, although oriented, the patient lacks coordination and seems sluggish, forgetful, and irritable; pupil size is irregular and pupils may be slow to react or be fixed and dilated.

Delirium is the most common manifestation of toxicosis, and it characteristically includes disorientation. Mood disturbances, restlessness, inability to sleep, delusions, and hallucinations may also be present.

Transitory schizophrenia is associated with paranoid symptomatology and disturbed rapport and affect; the patient may have had a schizoid premorbid personality and have taken bromides (regularly) for some neurotic symptom. The patient may or may not be disoriented.

In bromide hallucinosis the patient remains well oriented in spite of his or her hallucinations. Whenever an acute, "unusual" psychiatric presentation is encountered, careful history-taking (well water was the source of the bromide in one particular case) and attention to physical findings and bromide level (150 to 200 mg per 100 ml is considered toxic) are necessary, to afford the patient the benefit of definitive therapy.

Marijuana. The popularity of marijuana is second only to that of alcohol for a sizable portion of our society, and its use is widely condoned; however, its tendency to create psychologic dependence and physiologically negative effects creates a potential for distraction from school, work, and other activities, which cannot be overlooked. Problems that arise from marijuana use are often manifested in the form of anxiety attacks. The patient may have increased vital signs, palpitations, hyperventilation, apprehension, restlessness, and preoccupation with and the feeling of imminent death. These patients are often greatly helped by a nurse or designate who stays with them. They may be given diazepam by mouth and reassurance about physical symptoms. Although the reaction may be immediately precipitated by the use of marijuana, the patient's problems often include currently overwhelming stresses and a predisposition toward anxiety attacks.

Conversely, when a patient enters with what appears to be an anxiety attack, he or she should be questioned about drug use and should be reminded that police will not be given the information. Other drugs (for example, cocaine) may trigger an anxiety reaction in a patient who may be reluctant to mention using it. Without that information, the emergency nurse is unable to reassure the patient that the particular substance will not be lethal, and the patient may remain inexplicably frightened after all of the nurse's calming measures have been exhausted.

Phencyclidine. Phencyclidine (PCP or angel dust) warrants a few words in light of its popularity. (It is the third most widely abused drug in many sections of the United States.) Its attendant dangers are different in quality and quantity from any other widely abused drug.

Originally developed in the late 1950s as an anesthetic for humans, PCP's use was discontinued because of untoward psychologic sequelae, and it is currently used infrequently with animals. On the street the drug soon earned a reputation for bad side-effects, which led to its being passed off as or combined with other drugs such as tetrahydrocannabinol (THC) and mescaline. Differential diagnosis of PCP poisoning in the ED is difficult, since PCP is thought to mimic, precipitate, and exaggerate psychiatric illness. A patient may present a picture of anxiety, psychosis, or toxicosis. The degree of severity varies greatly. Pharmacologically, PCP is an analgesic, with sympathomimetic and central nervous system stimulant and depressant properties. A constellation of signs that is particularly helpful in identifying PCP poisoning includes acute onset of unusual behavior in a young patient who has a history of intermittent drug abuse, elevated systolic and diastolic blood pressure, small pupils, and vertical nystagmus.

In low to moderate doses, signs also include ataxia, increased deep-tendon reflexes, clonus, tremors, amnesia, anxiety or agitation, image distortion, euphoria, increased pulse rate and blood pressure, nausea and vomiting, and increased urine output. In cases of high doses, signs include slurred speech, drowsiness, decreased deep-tendon reflexes, convulsions, opisthotonus, coma, decreased respiratory rate, respiratory arrest, depersonalization, disordered thought processes, hallucinations, psychopathologic conditions, dysrhythmias, decreased blood pressure, and decreased urine output. Deaths seem to be related to seizures and respiratory arrest.

The history of a person who abuses drugs may be consistent with that of someone who is likely to manifest psychiatric problems. PCP may come in many forms—tablet, powder, leaf mixture for making cigarettes, and rock crystal. The patient may think he or she has smoked only marijuana, although it has actually been laced with PCP. In addition, symptoms may appear, and often do, up to many days later. Thus the difficulty of a definite diagnosis becomes apparent.

There is a tendency to treat PCP toxicosis as a bad LSD "trip" is treated; this treatment can be a disservice to the patient. Whereas reassurance may be helpful with someone who is on a bad LSD "trip," persons with PCP poisoning respond better to the least amount of stimulation, visual, auditory, and tactile. One person should be the caretaker; the patient should be placed in a dimly lit room that is as quiet as possible. Constant observation or restraints may be necessary for those who are having significant reactions. LSD users usually report ingesting the drug less than 12 hours before admission and usually follow a predictable course of improvement, recovering within 1 to 2 days. The sequelae of PCP poisoning may culminate in an ED presentation several days after its ingestion. The course of PCP poisoning is unpredictable, and it may manifest itself intermittently for days, weeks, or longer.

Blood and urine (urine is more desirable for detection purposes) should be obtained for toxicologic studies. Calculated blood levels as low as 0.06 mg/100 ml caused toxic psychosis and hallucinations in more than 50% of patients tested in one study.

Phenothiazines (for example, Thorazine) should be avoided because they are chemically similar to PCP, and may potentiate its effect or produce an anticholinergic crisis. However, many practitioners have found haloperidol to be useful. Its composition differs significantly from that of PCP. The response to the drug is often a relief of symptoms so dramatic that the patient may be thought to be cured and may be released, although symptoms are likely to return when the medication wears off. Diazepam is also recommended to control agitation and may be helpful in the control of seizures associated with larger doses of PCP. An emerging concept of PCP management theorizes that because the drug is a weak electrolyte (base) that is readily ionized in an acid medium, there is extensive secretion of gastric acid into the stomach, where it becomes trapped because of the impenetrability of membranes to ions. Management with gastric suction, a saline laxative, and acidification of urine and serum has provided successful results.

The possibility of the need for hospitalization should always be kept in mind in cases of PCP toxicosis.

Remember the opportunity that exists for teaching preventive health care in the ED. The ED practitioner should convey, without condemning drug use, that the PCP chemical is a dangerous choice.

Opiates and related compounds. When subcutaneously administered doses are compared for analgesic activity, the opiates and related compounds are listed, in order of ascending strength, as follows: codeine (Darvon roughly equivalent), meperidine (Demerol), morphine (Dolophine roughly equivalent), heroin, and dihydromorphine (Dilaudid). The effects of these drugs, and of morphine in particular, that are of major clinical interest are those mediated by actions on the central nervous system. Certain side effects are produced by actions on other structures; flushing and itching of the skin are caused by release of histamine, and constipation results from a decrease of propulsive movements of the intestines coupled with spasmogenic actions on contractile movements of the intestinal tract and on the sphincters.

In mild cases, opiate poisoning may be treated by vigorous and continued sensory stimulation and gastric lavage if the drug has recently been taken orally. In more severe cases, airway and respiratory support should be the primary focus. When heroin overdose is strongly suspected in the comatose patient, naloxone (Narcan) is usually the narcotic antagonist of choice because it does not add to the respiratory depression. Naloxone is diagnostic as well as therapeutic because of its often dramatic therapeutic effects on opiate overdoses. Relatively small doses of this and other antagonists to opiates may precipitate violent opiate withdrawal responses.

The seasoned ED practitioner is all too familiar with the scene that transpires when the drug-addicted person who is brought into the ED in a comatose state is given naloxone. Within seconds, the patient is awake and flailing, acutely dysphoric, uncomfortable, and confused; ED personnel must be stationed at each of the patient's extremities. Anticipation of this occurrence and intervention can prevent injuries and an abrupt departure of the patient. Side rails on the stretcher should be raised quickly when the naloxone is given, and personnel should be designated to control the patient. Loose restraints may be used if time permits. As soon as the medication is administered and the patient is alert, the staff should make it clear to the patient that his or her discomfort is understood and that it will be time-limited. Explanation of the way in which the patient got to the hospital and what is being done for him or her is in order. In a person who is taking methadone, naloxone wears off within a few hours and the methadone still in his or her system offers relief. The danger of respiratory depression returning as the naloxone wears off is real, and patients should be kept in the hospital well beyond 4 hours after administration of the antidote. Precipitous departures from the ED should be discouraged with a simple but compelling explanation. If the patient is insistent about leaving the ED, arrangements with friends and relatives should be made. With some show of concern and a few measures of comfort for the patient (a cup of coffee or a supervised cigarette smoke), the patient's cooperation can usually be attained.

Dystonic reactions to phenothiazines. Dystonic reactions can be easily mistaken for tetanus, calcium deficiency, seizures, and a host of other conditions. Most often, however, a dystonic reaction is seen as a hysterical conversion or posturing in the psychiatric patient or as malingering for drugs or other secondary benefit by a drug abuser. The psychiatric patient is often unable to relate an articulate history and symptomatology and may even regress under the stress of the interview and the frightening and painful effects of the antipsychotic medication (for example, haloperidol). Vacillating symptoms are typical but often cause staff members to dismiss the symptoms. For the young person who has bought a pill on the street that he or she believed to be Valium or a hallucinogenic, it may seem unsafe to tell the staff what has happened for fear that his or her family or the police will be notified or he or she may have taken the pill 4 or 5 days before and not even associate the pill with the reaction. In a large percentage of cases, the symptoms do not appear for 4 to 5 days after an oral dose. Thus the history often makes the diagnosis of a relatively clearcut reaction confusing.

It behooves the emergency nurse to learn what the common offenders such as Haldol, Prolixin, Compazine, Stelazine, and Thorazine pills look like and to show patients a *Physicians' Desk Reference* for positive identification, since many patients do not know pills by name. Even if the history is not clear, when the following signs and symptoms are present, treatment should be considered[3]:

Table 44-4   Side effects of antipsychotic drugs

Side effects	Comments
Dry mouth, blurred vision, constipation, urinary hesitance, paralytic ileus	Effects result from the drug's interference with acetylcholine. First three should be treated symptomatically and patient should be reassured. In instances of urinary hesitance and paralytic ileus, medication should be withheld until medical evaluation is obtained.
Orthostatic hypotension	Drug should be used with caution if cardiovascular disease is present and in elderly patients. Patient should be warned about possible occurrences and taught to rise slowly and dangle legs before standing.
Photosensitivity	Protect patient from exposure to ultraviolet light. Have patient use sunscreen. Effect occurs most frequently with chlorpromazine. Examine skin often.
Endocrine changes	Endocrine changes include weight gain, edema, lactation, and menstrual irregularities. Treat symptomatically. Reassure patient.
Extrapyramidal reactions	Such reactions are related to dose and duration. Manage by adjusting dose of drug or adding antiparkinsonian drug.
Pseudoparkinsonism	Typical shuffling gait, masklike facies, tremor, muscular rigidity, slowing of movements, and other symptoms mimicking those seen in Parkinson's disease
Akathisia, dystonia	Continuous restlessness, fidgeting, and pacing occur. Spasm of neck muscles, extensor rigidity of back muscles, carpopedal spasm, swallowing difficulties occur; eyes roll back. Onset is acute, but condition is reversible with appropriate medication. Provide reassurance until symptoms subside.
Akinesia	Lethargy and feelings of fatigue and muscle weakness occur; must be differentiated from withdrawal
Skin reactions	Urticarial, maculopapular, edematous, or petechial responses may occur 1 to 5 weeks after initiation of treatment. Withhold drug until after medical evaluation.
Jaundice	Jaundice develops in about 4% of patients and is a dangerous complication; drug should be discontinued.
Agranulocytosis and leukopenia	Chlorpromazine depresses production of leukocytes. Initial symptoms of sore throat, high temperature, and lesions in mouth indicate that drug should be stopped immediately. Rarely, outcome may be lethal.
Ocular changes	Corneal and lenticular changes and pigmentary retinopathy may occur with high dosages over long periods. Periodic ocular examinations are recommended.
Convulsions	Antipsychotic agents lower seizure threshold, making seizures more likely in seizure-prone persons. Persons with a history of seizures or organic conditions associated with seizures require an increased dosage of anticonvulsant medication if antipsychotics are used.
Tardive dyskinesia	Insidious onset of fine vermicular movements of tongue occurs, which is reversible if drug is discontinued at this time; can progress to rhythmic involuntary movements of the tongue, face, mouth, or jaw, with protrusion of tongue, puffing of cheeks, and chewing movements; no known treatment is available; often irreversible. Prevention is imperative. Women more than 50 years of age who have taken prolonged doses are particularly at risk. Do not withhold drug until after medical evaluation; symptoms will increase.[17]

1. Oculogyric crisis, that is, upward rotation of the eyes into the head
2. Buccolingual crisis, that is, protruding or retracting of the tongue, and facial grimacing; patient feels as though his or her tongue is being pulled back
3. Torticollic crisis, that is, severe contractions of neck muscles, retrocollic or torticollic
4. Opisthotonic crisis, that is, opisthotonic reaction, scoliosis, or lordosis
5. Tortipelvic crisis, that is, spasm of the abdominal wall, abdominal pain, bizarre gait; lordosis, or kyphosis

The first three are often seen in combination.

Results of treatment are usually fast and dramatic; diphenhydramine (Benadryl), benztropine (Cogentin), or trihexyphenidyl (Artane) may be used. Since the half-life of phenothiazines is 24 hours, the patient must be given medication orally to prevent the return of symptoms for the next 2 or 3 days.

Nursing considerations should include reduction of early anxiety to facilitate an accurate initial history. The drug abuser may be reminded that personnel will not divulge his or her story to anyone else. The patient should be assured

Table 44-5   Psychotropic medications: medical contraindications and precautions

Drug group	Contraindications	Precautions
Antipsychotics	Comatose states, central nervous system depression, bone-marrow depression, impaired liver function, epilepsy, and hypersensitivity to these medications	Use cautiously in pregnant patients and in patients with depression, respiratory disease, cardiovascular disease, hypotension, allergy history. Use lower doses in elderly patients.
Antidepressants Tricyclics	Acute myocardial infarction, hypersensitivity to these medications, concurrent administration of a monoamine oxidase inhibitor	Use cautiously in patients with urinary retention, benign prostatic hypertrophy, narrow-angle glaucoma, increased ocular pressure, convulsive disorders, cardiovascular disorders, thyroid disease, and organic mental disorders and in children under 12 years of age, and pregnant patients.
Monoamine oxidase inhibitors	Hypertension, cardiovascular disease, headaches, pheochromocytoma, liver or advanced renal disease, quiescent schizophrenia, concurrent administration of a tricyclic antidepressant	Safe use in pregnancy is not established.
Lithium	Significant renal disease, dietary salt restriction, cardiovascular disease, brain damage	Use cautiously in pregnant patients, children under the age of 12, elderly patients, patients who are breastfeeding, and patients with thyroid disease, mild kidney or heart disease, or epilepsy
Antianxiety medications	Glaucoma, hypersensitivity to these medications	Use cautiously in patients who have a history of allergies, dependency on these drugs, hepatic disorder, or renal impairment. Use lower doses with the elderly patients or breastfeeding mothers.
Carbamazepine	Severe renal disease, cardiovascular disease, liver disease	Use cautiously in patients with cardiovascular disease, renal or liver disease, or blood dyscrasias

Adapted from Birkhimer LJ, DeVane CL: The neuroleptic malignant syndrome: presentation and treatment, *Drug Intel Clin Pharm* 18(6):462, 1989 and Jann MW et al: Alternative drug therapies for mania: a literature review, *Drug Intel Clin Pharm*, 18(7,8):577, 1984.

that the symptoms are easily and completely reversible. The nurse should convey his or her ability to handle the situation and let the patient know that this happens to many people. The symptoms are terrifying, especially to patients who are normally unable to cope and susceptible to delusions. The temptation to tell a psychiatric patient to stop taking the medication should be considered carefully. The particular medication may be the drug of choice for the patient, who may become psychotic without it. Ideally, the patient's physician should be notified and the patient should be told to contact that physician for advice as soon as possible. The patient should be told that his or her medication is a good one with controllable side effects, which many medications have. This information reassures the patient and reinforces the patient's faith in his or her physician and the prescribed medications.

Table 44-4 presents side effects of antipsychotic drugs. Psychotropic medications are presented in Table 44-5.

REFERENCES

1. American Psychiatric Association: *Diagnostic and statistical manual of mental disorders,* ed 2, Washington, DC, 1968, American Psychiatric Association.
2. American Psychiatric Association: *Diagnostic and statistical manual of mental disorders,* ed 3, Washington, DC, 1987, American Psychiatric Association.
3. Baker LJ: Psychophysiological disorders. In Gary F, Kavanaugh CK, eds: *Psychiatric mental health nursing,* Philadelphia, 1991, JB Lippincott.
4. Benfer BA, Schroder PJ: Dissociative disorders. In Gary F, Kavanaugh CK, eds: *Psychiatric mental health nursing,* Philadelphia, 1991, JB Lippincott.
5. Braverman BG: Calming a patient with panic disorder, *Nursing 90* 20(1):32C, 1990.
6. Burgess A, Holstrom L: *Rape: victims of crisis,* Bowie, Md, 1975, Prentice-Hall.
7. Charran HS: Repetitive and ineffective neurotic defenses. In Varcarolis EM, ed: *Foundations of psychiatric mental health nursing,* Philadelphia, 1990, WB Saunders.
8. Gemmill FB: A family approach to the battered woman, *J Psychosoc Nurs Mental Health Services* 20:22, 1982.
9. Germain CP: Sheltering abused women: a nursing perspective, *J Psychosoc Nurs* 22:24, 1984.
10. Grimes J and Burns E: Mental health assessment. In *Health assessment in nursing practice,* ed 2, Boston, 1987, Jones and Bartlett.

11. Kohn AI: Shattered innocence, *Psychology Today,* Feb 1987.

12. Martin D: Overview: scope of the problem. In U.S. Commission on Civil Rights, battered women: issues of public policy, Washington, DC, 1978.

13. McFarland GK, Wasli EL: *Nursing diagnoses and process in psychiatric mental health nursing,* Philadelphia, 1986, JB Lippincott.

14. Siegel BS: *Love, medicine and miracles,* New York, 1986, Harper and Row.

15. Swanson AR. In Varcarolis EM, ed: *Foundations of psychiatric nursing,* ed 1, Philadelphia, 1990, WB Saunders.

16. Swanson RW: Battered wife syndrome, *Can Med Assoc J* 130(6):709, 1984.

17. Taylor M: *Mereness' essentials of psychiatric nursing,* St Louis, 1990, Mosby–Year Book.

18. Walker L: *The battered woman,* New York, 1979, Harper and Row.

19. Weingourt R: Never to be alone: existential therapy with battered women, *J Psychosoc Nurs* 23:24, 1985.

Obstetric and Gynecologic Emergencies

Susan Budassi Sheehy, Peggy McCall, and Patricia Varvel

When a woman comes to the ED for a gynecologic or obstetric problem, she is often uncomfortable both physically and psychologically. She may have pain, vaginal bleeding, or shocklike symptoms; she may have had a traumatic experience; or she may be pregnant, in labor, or in the process of aborting.

The emergency nurse, with a careful and sensitive approach to the individual woman, may help make this experience less frightening, less embarrassing, and less traumatic by following a few basic principles.

Information about the onset of signs and symptoms should be solicited in confidence, and privacy should be afforded for all aspects of the examination, as well as for the discussion of problems among members of the emergency department (ED) team. The nurse can further ensure the comfort of the woman by carefully explaining all procedures, by assisting in appropriate positioning and draping, by instructing the patient in techniques of relaxation, and by providing psychologic support at the time of examination.

Before any procedures are actually begun, the woman should remove her underclothing and any constricting garments. It is important that the nurse carefully fold or place these belongings on hangers, since they are important parts of the woman's identity. Time should be given to allow the patient to void so that the bladder is empty and does not interfere with digital examination of any of the pelvic or abdominal structures. The exception to this is the patient who has been sexually assaulted; she should not void until the examination is completed. When the pelvic examination procedures are completed, it is important for the nurse to help the woman back into a comfortable position, to provide tissue paper or other cleansing agents to remove lubricants and secretion from the perianal area, and to provide time for the woman to regroom before she is ushered back into a waiting or conference area or to prepare for admission as an inpatient.

OBSTETRIC EMERGENCIES
First-Trimester Emergencies

Ectopic pregnancy. Ectopic pregnancy occurs when the fertilized ovum implants anywhere other than in the endo-metrium of the uterine cavity, such as in the fallopian tube, the ovary, the cervix, or the abdominal cavity, and begins to grow and possibly rupture. Rupture usually occurs after the twelfth week of pregnancy. Ninety-five percent of all ectopic pregnancies involve one of the fallopian tubes (Fig. 45-1). Ectopic pregnancy is one of the major causes of maternal death because it involves the rupture of a highly vascularized area. Death is usually the result of hemorrhage. Women with ruptured ectopic pregnancies are often seen in the ED. Predisposing factors include previous tubal infections, adhesions from previous surgery, tubal ligations, and possibly the presence of intrauterine devices. The most common site for tubal implantations is the ampulla, followed by the isthmus. Ectopic pregnancy is a condition that may confuse the best diagnostician. Being the great imitator, it may be mistaken for a ruptured ovarian cyst, appendicitis, pelvic inflammatory disease (PID), or incomplete abortion. Pelvic pain and vaginal bleeding or spotting in a woman of childbearing age should always be treated as an ectopic pregnancy until this possibility is ruled out. Pain, if present, varies from mild to severe in the abdomen, and if the ectopic pregnancy is leaking or has ruptured, includes the classic Kehr's sign—radiating shoulder pain that occurs when the diaphragm is irritated from blood loss in the peritoneum.

Ectopic pregnancies manifest in two forms: acute (or ruptured), with intraperitoneal hemorrhage, acute pain, and shock; and chronic (or unruptured), with less pain and no shock. In either case, vaginal bleeding may be absent, spotty, or profuse. Ruptured ectopic pregnancy is often seen in the ED in a young woman who has severe abdominal pain radiating to one or both shoulders accompanied by slight vaginal spotting and a blood pressure reading that demonstrates severe hypotension. The nurse should place her in Trendelenburg's position, place and inflate the pneumatic antishock garment, start two large-bore intravenous (IV) lines, and run Ringer's lactate solution. Consider a transfusion of O negative blood for severe cases that do not respond to the administration of crystalloids. Draw blood for a complete blood cell count (CBC), determination of sedimentation rate, and typing and cross-matching for possible transfusion. In many larger institutions, it is now pos-

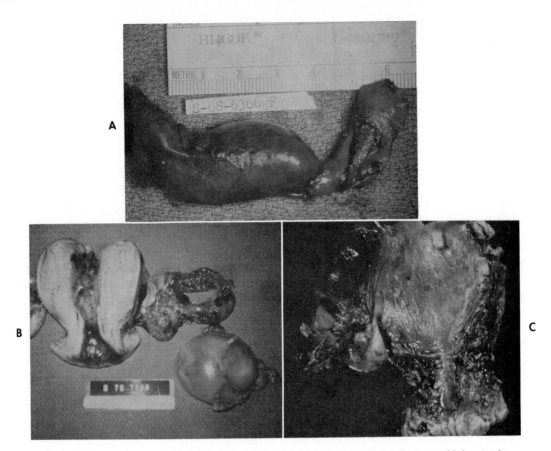

Fig. 45-1 **A,** Ectopic pregnancy. **B,** Ruptured ectopic pregnancy. **C,** Interstitial ectopic pregnancy.

sible to determine pregnancy at early gestation with a blood sample for radioimmunoassay and radioreceptor assay, but for those institutions without facilities to perform this test, the urine is still used for pregnancy testing. It should be remembered, however, that a negative urine test for human chorionic gonadotropin (hCG) is not entirely reliable in ruling out an ectopic pregnancy, since not all ectopic pregnancies are established enough to provide sufficient levels of hCG to give a positive result.

History taking is again of utmost importance for differential diagnosis of septic shock, PID, or ectopic pregnancy; sudden onset of pain, sexual activity, missed or abnormal menstrual periods, and history of tubal infections or surgery are especially indicative of ectopic pregnancy. A normal sedimentation rate and absence of a fever should rule out PID. Pelvic radiographs are not helpful, but the pelvic ultrasonographic study is specific for ectopic pregnancy. In this author's experience, women with ectopic pregnancies often state that they feel as if they need to have a bowel movement. Fifteen percent of patients with ectopic pregnancy are symptomatic before the first missed period.[12] In these cases the patient will not have missed a menstrual period and most likely does not know that she is pregnant.

The patient needs no preparation for ultrasonography, which gives a picture of pelvic structures, other than hydration so that the full bladder can be used as a point of reference for the radiologist.

Although still performed in many areas of the United States, culdocentesis (needle aspiration of the Douglas' cul-de-sac through the vagina) is not recommended, since the procedure is not infallible. Aspiration of blood from the cul-de-sac is diagnostic for intraperitoneal bleeding, but absence of blood does not rule out ectopic pregnancy. The use of laparoscopy as a safe and effective diagnostic tool is the usual course of action. If a tubal pregnancy is found, a salpingectomy is performed. Laparoscopy involves giving a general anesthetic and making a small incision (approximately 1 to 2 inches wide) at the umbilicus through which a slender tube containing a telescopic lens is passed into the peritoneal cavity. This lens permits the gynecologist to examine the ovaries, fallopian tubes, and the outside of the uterus without subjecting the patient to the trauma of the exploratory laparotomy and a prolonged hospital stay. The patient can usually be discharged as soon as she recovers from anesthesia, if no condition requiring surgery is found.

If the patient is in shock, the nurse should stabilize the

condition with fluid or blood replacement as indicated, administer oxygen if blood loss is sufficient to cause respiratory difficulties, and transfer the patient to the operating room if indicated. The nurse must also recognize the patient and family's need for emotional support. The patient may have fear not only for her life but for her future childbearing ability, sadness that the pregnancy is not normal, or guilt if she had not wanted a baby. If single, she may fear that her parents and friends will find out about her sexual activity. The nurse must always keep in mind the patient's right to privacy.

Abortion. Abortion is the number one cause of vaginal bleeding in women of childbearing age. It is estimated that 15% to 20% of all pregnancies result in spontaneous abortion.[5] Abortion should be considered a possibility in any woman of childbearing age who has vaginal bleeding. Abortion is defined as the termination of a pregnancy at any time before the fetus has achieved viability (24 weeks of gestation). Types of abortion are:

1. Threatened abortion. Vaginal bleeding or spotting with mild cramping but with a closed or only slightly opened cervical os indicates a threatened abortion.
2. Inevitable abortion. Bleeding is more profuse, the cervical os is opened, and there is severe cramping. No products of conception have been passed.
3. Habitual abortion. Spontaneous abortions that occur successively with three or more pregnancies are termed habitual abortions.
4. Incomplete abortion. Some of the products of conception have been passed but some are retained. Bleeding is often profuse and cramping is usually present.
5. Complete abortion. All the products of conception have been passed. Uterine cramping will usually stop. Slight bleeding may continue for several days.
6. Missed abortion. The fetus dies in utero and is not expelled. The mother may not be aware that anything is wrong unless she becomes septic when the fetus begins to macerate or unless she notices that there is no fetal movement or growth. The first indication that something is wrong may be when the obstetrician notes a discrepancy in the size of the uterus in relation to the anticipated date of delivery. A definite diagnosis of fetal death is made when the result of a pregnancy test is converted from positive to negative.
7. Septic abortion. A septic abortion occurs as the result of infection, either when with uterine contents are intact (missed) or after the contents have been removed surgically. A woman with a septic abortion can show various signs. The emergency nurse should be alert to this possibility in the woman who has severe, steady, lower abdominal pain, high temperature, chills, and malodorous cervical discharge and who is in shock, possibly with renal or cardiovascular failure, especially if the woman has a history or suspected

history of mechanical attempts to induce abortion. If she does have a septic abortion, speed of diagnosis and treatment can mean the difference between life and death.
8. Therapeutic abortion. The pregnancy is terminated by medical means. Most often women with this type of abortion are seen in the ED because of retained products of conception and continued bleeding.

Assessment for all first-trimester emergencies should include close observation of signs, significant blood loss, and hypovolemia. Palpate the patient's abdomen for the presence of pain, which may be indicative of an ectopic pregnancy. A pelvic examination should be carefully performed to determine the source of bleeding, to look for products of conception, and to determine the dilation or nondilation of the cervical os. In addition, observe for purulent discharge, which may indicate that an infection, such as a septic abortion, is present.

A bimanual examination is performed to palpate the uterus and other reproductive structures. Palpate the cervix for firmness. Determine uterine position and size by palpation. Also note any uterine tenderness. Palpate the adnexa for tenderness and the presence of masses. Consider a pelvic ultrasonographic study to rule out ectopic pregnancy.[4]

Often the diagnosis of a threatened, incomplete, or complete abortion can be determined from clinical findings alone. A serum hCG or urine hCG determination verifies pregnancy.

Therapeutic intervention depends on the type of abortion. Fifty percent of threatened abortions may result in incomplete or complete abortion within a few hours.[3] A patient with a threatened abortion should be observed closely. Document the amount of blood lost and replace blood loss with crystalloid solutions to maintain blood pressure at an adequate level. Give the patient much emotional support and let her know that the main thing she can do is rest in bed. She should, however, avoid douching and intercourse, which may increase bleeding, cramping, or infection if the cervical os is open.

Aftercare instructions for those patients who are being sent home are to rest and to return to the ED if bleeding increases (need for more than one sanitary pad in an hour) or if dry tissue is passed. The patient should also return if chills or fever develops.

If the abortion state becomes inevitable or incomplete, further therapeutic intervention should be started. Diagnosis is made by means of clinical evaluation, observation of an open cervical os, and the presence of heavy bleeding or products of conception. The possibility of ectopic pregnancy should be ruled out before any treatment is started.

Therapeutic intervention begins with determination of the woman's Rh type. If the patient's blood type is Rh negative, test for the presence of antibodies that may have formed as a result of a previous pregnancy or a blood transfusion. Obtain a consultation for the way to handle the Rh situation.

Also obtain a CBC. If there has been significant blood loss, send a blood specimen for typing and cross-matching. Start two large-bore IV lines, and administer Ringer's lactate solution.

Definitive therapeutic intervention for inevitable or incomplete abortion is usually suction curettage in the ED or during surgery and emotional support. Patients also need to be referred for reproductive counseling and grief counseling. Consider antibiotic therapy if the possibility of infection exists.

If suction curettage is performed, whether in the ED or during surgery, the patient should be observed for at least 2 hours afterward. Oxytocin (Pitocin) is usually given intravenously. When vital signs return to normal, bleeding is minimal, and hematocrit is at least 26%, the patient may be discharged. The patient is usually discharged with instructions to take an ergotic preparation to continue uterine contractions. If the patient's hematocrit dropped during the procedure or afterward, she should also be placed on a regimen of oral iron supplements.

If complete abortion has occurred, all products of conception will have been passed from the uterus. It is difficult to determine whether the abortion is complete, even during pelvic examination. In general, the standard of practice is to assume that some products of conception have been retained. Therefore, suction curettage should be performed to avoid the possibility of retained products of conception, continued bleeding, and possible sepsis. Some practitioners agree that if complete abortion is likely, it is reasonable to delay suction curettage for 2 to 3 hours so that the patient can be observed for further bleeding or cramping or both.

Antepartum Emergencies

Prolapsed cord. A prolapsed umbilical cord constitutes an absolute emergency. In this situation the umbilical cord is preceding the fetus through the birth canal and will become entrapped when the fetus passes through the birth canal, causing an obstruction of fetal circulation.

There are three variations of this condition. The first is a situation in which uterine membranes are intact and the cord is being compressed by fetal parts but is not visible externally. This variation should be suspected when there are signs of fetal distress, most prominently bradycardia.[6] This variation is actually called "a cord presentation" rather than a true prolapse.

In the second variation the cord may not be visible but can be felt in the vagina or cervix. In the third and most extreme variation the umbilical cord actually protrudes from the vagina.

Therapeutic intervention is aimed at relieving pressure from the cord and expediting cesarean section. Place the mother in a Trendelenburg's position or in a knee-chest position with buttocks elevated. Both of these positions remove some of the pressure by gravity. Administer oxygen at 6 L/min via a nonrebreather mask. Place a gloved hand in the vagina and manually elevate the presenting part of the cord. In addition, insert a Foley catheter and instill 500 to 700 ml saline solution into the mother's bladder to assist with cord decompression by elevating the uterus.[2]

Placenta previa. Placenta previa is characterized by painless bleeding that usually occurs around the eighth month of pregnancy. The uterus feels soft and flaccid. Placenta previa is caused by the implantation and development of the placenta in the lower uterine segment rather than at the normal implantation site in the upper uterine segment. This implantation causes the placenta to partially or completely cover the internal cervical os. *Previa* means "in front of" or "first," that is, before the presenting fetus. By implanting in the lower uterine segment instead of the higher segment, the placenta is in the zone of effacement (thinning) and dilation. The clinical course and outcome depend on the extent of the placenta's coverage of the internal os.

Types of placenta previa are classified as follows:
1. Total, in which the placenta completely covers the os
2. Partial, in which the placenta partially covers the os
3. Marginal, or low implantation, in which the placenta is adjacent to but does not extend beyond the margin of the os

Although total placenta previa is rare, either marginal or partial placenta previa occurs in one of every 200 pregnancies. Seventy-five percent of cases of placenta previa occur in multiparous women. Multiparity with advancing age and a rapid succession of pregnancies are believed to be among predisposing factors.

The cause of placenta previa is not known, but there are several theories. One is that the ovum implants in the area of the healthy endometrium, which in these patients is found in the lower segment of the uterus. Another theory is that abnormal motility causes the ovum to pass through the uterus quickly and to implant in the lower segment.

Hemorrhage is the first and most commonly seen sign. Because it is not accompanied by contractions, there is no associated pain. Because the cervix begins to dilate and efface in the eighth month, maternal vessels tear when the patient is asleep, and bleeding may cease spontaneously or continue, depending on how large the torn vessels are. After two or three hemorrhages, labor usually begins. Membranes may also rupture prematurely, with the resulting possibility of infection. Premature labor and an abnormal presenting part can further complicate the delivery. In total placenta previa, bleeding occurs earlier and is more profuse. Placenta previa should always be suspected when painless uterine bleeding occurs in the last half of the pregnancy.

Diagnostic studies should include ultrasonography, if available. This is specific in determining the position of the placenta. Radiographic studies are still made in areas where ultrasonography is not available. CBC, typing and cross-matching for several units of blood, and clotting studies should be performed immediately. The nurse should establish a large-bore IV line, administer a crystalloid solution such as Ringer's lactate, and transfer the patient to the labor and delivery unit for monitoring and, if indicated, immediate cesarean section.

Assessment of vital signs should always include assessment of fetal heart rate. Always remember that in the case of a pregnant woman there are two patients to consider. Although most hospitals have fetoscopes, it is also recommended that a Doppler be used, since it is more sensitive in picking up the heart tones of the 20- to 24-week-old fetus. If fetal heart tones are not heard, this finding should be reported immediately. Normal fetal heart rate is 120 to 160 beats/min. Stay with the patient and encourage her to talk. Provide necessary assistance for her husband or significant other with admitting procedures and in calling family. The maternal mortality for placenta previa is approximately 1.5%. Fetal mortality depends on gestational age and the extent of fetal anoxia.

Abruptio placentae. Another major complication of pregnancy in the last trimester is the premature separation of the placenta from the uterus. This is known as abruptio placentae. The primary cause is unknown, but there are several theories. One of these is that abruptio placentae is related to preeclampsia, since 25% to 60% of all abruptions occur in preeclamptic mothers. Another suspected cause is the increased venous pressure that occurs when the vena cava is compressed in the supine position by the gravid uterus. Contributing factors such as advanced maternal age (35 and over), multiparity, a short cord, and trauma also play a large part. A partial separation can occur with either occult or frank hemorrhage. A complete separation occurs with frank hemorrhage. Although frank hemorrhage is always an emergency because of blood loss and because it is associated with hypotension and hypoxia, the more dangerous of the two is occult hemorrhage, since it is not readily detected and since the extent of the bleeding is usually not known unless the patient has symptoms of shock. Occult hemorrhage can occur (1) if the fetal head is engaged, (2) if the placenta is separated at the center but the margins are attached, and (3) if blood breaks through the membranes and effuses into the amniotic cavity.

Preeclampsia and eclampsia. Preeclampsia and eclampsia were formerly thought to be caused by toxins in the bloodstream and thus were referred to as toxemia of pregnancy. It is now known that no "toxins" are present except the body's own breakdown products that result from metabolic processes. Preeclampsia and eclampsia are hypertensive disorders specific to pregnancy and occur in the last trimester, usually after the twentieth week of gestation or soon after delivery. The nonseizure state is called preeclampsia and the seizure state, eclampsia. Both of these states are manifested by hypertension and a combination of other signs and symptoms. Eclampsia is a major cause of maternal morbidity and death. In North America, preeclampsia or eclampsia occurs in 5% to 8% of all pregnancies.[1] Five percent of patients with eclampsia die from this

disease. It is most common in primigravidas less than 20 years old or more than 35 years old. Fetal mortality is high—five times higher than in noneclamptic pregnancy.[11]

Severe preeclamptic states are characterized by the following:

1. Blood pressure greater than 160/110 mm Hg
2. Proteinuria (5 g or more per 24 hours)
3. Oliguria (output) less than 400 ml per 24 hours
4. Headaches
5. Visual disturbances
6. Abdominal pain
7. Pulmonary edema and cyanosis
8. Hyperreflexia
9. Thrombocytopenia
10. Abnormal liver function tests
11. Hemolytic anemia

Symptoms of eclampsia can include all the preceding and seizures or coma or both. The cause of these disorders is unknown. Current theories include the following:

1. Impaired uteroplacental circulation as a result of uterine distension
2. Overstimulation of the adrenal cortex by a hypertrophic anterior pituitary gland or the placenta itself or both
3. Poor dietary habits, particularly diets in low protein
4. Loss of sodium during pregnancy, which causes hypovolemia and vasospasm

---

MAGNESIUM SULFATE USE IN PREECLAMPSIA AND ECLAMPSIA

Loading dose
4 g 10% magnesium sulfate in 250 ml D_5W solution, given IV over a period of 15 minutes

Maintenance dose
1-3 g 10% magnesium sulfate per hour

Therapeutic serum magnesium level
4.8-8.4 ml/dl

Monitoring parameters
Cardiac monitor

Urinary output
At least 30 ml/hr

Deep-tendon reflexes
Loss means toxicity

Cautions
Respiratory rate must be greater than 12 breaths/min
Antidote for decreased respirations is calcium gluconate
1 g (10 ml in 10% solution) given slowly IV

Adapted from Farrel RG, ed: *OB/GYN emergencies: the first 60 minutes,* Rockville, Md, 1986, Aspen.

Management of preeclampsia and eclampsia depends on severity. Mothers who are receiving good prenatal care are probably monitored closely by their physicians and put on a regimen of bed rest at home or in an antepartal unit of the hospital long before they require treatment. For this reason, the mother who is seen in the ED is probably in a severe preeclamptic or eclamptic state. The recommended treatment is to stabilize the mother's condition, place her in a room in which one-to-one nursing is provided, and monitor vital signs and fetal heart tones until the patient can be transferred to the labor and delivery suite, where the mother will be sedated and the baby will be delivered. Magnesium sulfate is used to prevent seizures[7] and to control seizures if they do occur. The use of magnesium sulfate is shown in the box on the preceding page. Systolic and diastolic blood pressure should be slowly reduced to 150/90 mm Hg. The drug of choice is hydralazine (Apresoline). Blood pressure should be reduced to a level at which intracranial bleeding is no longer a threat. Blood pressure must not be reduced too much because there is danger that a greatly reduced blood pressure may reduce blood flow to the placenta and result in fetal distress.

Hydralazine is used because it causes an increase in cardiac output and because it increases both renal and cerebral blood flow while reducing peripheral resistance. Hydralazine should be given carefully, and the patient should be closely observed for hypotension. Close monitoring of intake and output is important, since renal condition is significant. The use of hydralazine is shown in the box at right.

Table 45-1 outlines some major symptoms of obstetric emergencies. When a pregnant woman appears in the ED with any of these symptoms, the nurse who is assessing her should be particularly aware of edema. Complete vital signs, including fetal heart tones, should be obtained. Precautions should be taken for the patient's safety if she has seizures (side rails up, maintenance of an open airway, and suction at hand). An IV line should be established with a large-bore cannula and should be kept open. Blood should be drawn for a CBC and electrolyte, coagulation, and liver studies. A Foley catheter should be placed to determine renal output. Immediate transfer to the labor and delivery unit is rec-

---

HYDRALAZINE (APRESOLINE) USE IN PREECLAMPTIC AND ECLAMPTIC HYPERTENSION

Parameters

Given when systolic blood pressure is greater than 180 mm Hg and/or diastolic blood pressure is greater than 110 mm Hg

Dosage

May be given as a bolus or IV drip

Bolus: 5 mg hydralazine IV, 10 mg given 15 minutes later if blood pressure remains above 150/90-100 mm Hg; 10 mg bolus may be repeated as needed to maintain blood pressure at about 150/90-100 mm Hg

IV drip: 80 mg hydralazine in 500 ml D$_5$W solution infused at 30 to 32 ml/hr (5 mg/hr); increase infusion rate (titrated) every 15 minutes until blood pressure is about 150/90-100 mm Hg

Caution

Pay close attention to hypotension. Remember, hypotension causes a decreased blood flow to the placenta.

Side effects

Flushing, tachycardia

Adapted from Farrel RG, ed: *OB/GYN emergencies: the first 60 minutes*, Rockville, Md, 1986, Aspen.

---

ommended. To allay anxiety, the patient and her family should be kept informed.

External hemorrhage usually accompanies partial separation and is considered more common. Clinical findings in abruptio placentae vary with the degree of separation and bleeding. Blood loss of less than 500 ml is considered mild to moderate. Apparent blood loss of more than 500 ml is considered moderate to severe. A complete abruptio placentae is considered severe and causes severe hypovolemia and shock. The uterus is usually relaxed in mild to moderate cases and rigid in severe ones. Pain is usually mild or localized in partial separation and severe and generalized in a complete separation. Fetal heart tones are normal to slow

---

Table 45-1 Major symptoms of obstetric emergency and differential diagnosis

Clinical causes	Hemorrhage	Shock	Pain	Convulsions	Fetal distress	Differential diagnosis
Placenta previa	X	X			Decreased fetal heart tone	
Abruptio placentae	(usually internal)	X	X		Decreased or absent fetal heart tone	
Ectopic pregnancy		X	X			Positive results of pregnancy test
Eclampsia and preeclampsia			X	X		
Prolapsed cord					Decreased or absent FHT	Visualize fetal cord

in partial separation and irregular to absent in complete separation. There may be excessive fetal movements or none at all.

Therapeutic intervention is prompt replacement of blood, clotting studies, replacement of fibrogen as needed, and delivery of the fetus by cesarean section as soon as possible. Maternal mortality is 1%, unless the pregnancy is accompanied by hypofibrinogenemia. Fetal mortality in a complete abruption is close to 100%, and in partial abruption it is 30% to 60%. Fetal death occurs as a result of anoxia.

Disseminated intravascular coagulation. Disseminated intravascular coagulation, in which the clotting mechanism is activated and accelerated, can occur as a complication of pregnancy. It is most often seen in severe cases of abruptio placentae in the form of hypofibrinogenemia, but it can also occur as a result of excessive blood loss during delivery, after amniotic fluid embolus at delivery, or after fetal death in utero. In this hypercoagulatory state, clotting factors are used up before the liver has time to manufacture and send in replacements. During pregnancy the level of fibrinogen increases to more than 440 mg, whereas the normal fibrinogen level is 200 to 400 mg. When this level falls below 100 mg, blood will not clot. Causes of hypofibrinogenemia in abruptio placentae are not completely understood, but it is thought that the deposition of fibrin at the site of placental separation depletes the amount of circulating fibrinogen. This depletion causes patches of fibrin to detach from the capillary space and reenter the maternal circulation as microemboli, which can cause necrosis of the organs. The kidneys are most often affected, and acute renal failure may occur.

Therapeutic intervention is aimed at correcting the cause. All cases of disseminated intravascular coagulation are not caused by low fibrinogen levels and may be caused by low levels of any of the clotting factors. If possible, consultation with a pathologist is often the wisest and most efficient way to determine the affected factor. Replacement of the factor often reverses the condition. Heparin is occasionally used to neutralize the circulating thromboplastin and to slow down clot formation, thereby slowing the depletion of the clotting factors. Platelets, fresh frozen plasma, and packed red blood cells may all be used in the management of disseminated intravascular coagulation. The kidneys may require support with dialysis. In the case of abruptio placentae, the fetus should be delivered immediately.

DELIVERY

In this time of decreasing access to a dwindling number of obstetricians, the probability of an increasing number of deliveries occurring in prehospital care settings and in the ED is high. If a patient in labor arrives in the ED and time permits, a rapid obstetric examination should be performed and a brief obstetric history should be obtained. It is important to know the mother's gravida and para status as these may help to estimate the amount of time until imminent

delivery is evident. Also, ask about her estimated date of confinement (that is, due date). This information allows for the preparation of the proper equipment and personnel, should delivery occur in the ED.

The first stage of labor is the time from the onset of regular contractions until complete cervical dilation. This is generally the longest of the three stages of labor. The second stage of labor is the time from full cervical dilation until delivery of the baby. The mother may have the urge to push in this stage. The average time for stage two is from 20 minutes to 1 hour. The third stage of labor is from the delivery of the baby until the delivery of the placenta. This stage usually lasts from 5 to 15 minutes. In cases in which the placenta fails to detach from the uterine wall, it may be necessary to manually remove the placenta.

When a woman in labor arrives at the ED, if time permits, a brief physical examination should be performed. First, check fetal heart tones. Normal fetal heart tones are from 120 to 160 beats/min. Prolonged bradycardia or tachycardia may indicate fetal distress. In this case, place the mother on her left side and give her supplemental oxygen at high flow. Arrange for immediate obstetric consultation for a possible emergency delivery, possibly by cesarean section.

Once it has been determined that the fetus is well, one

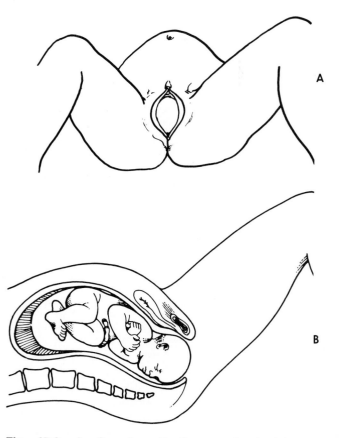

Fig. 45-2 A, Crowning. **B,** Cross-sectional view of crowning.

should then examine the mother's abdomen. Uterine height should be measured. A full-term fetus causes the uterus to be at the xyphoid level. Palpate contractions as they occur, and assist the mother to relax in between contractions. As an emergency nurse involved in the delivery of a baby, remember that the mother will do most of the work. Your basic role is to provide psychologic support and "coaching" to the mother and to ensure that the infant, once it is delivered, is breathing adequately, has a good pulse, and is kept warm.

If crowning (Fig. 45-2) is not present, perform a manual vaginal examination to determine dilation and effacement of the cervix and the station of the fetus. Use sterile technique. If fluid is present, check to see whether it is amniotic fluid. Test the acidity of the fluid. Amniotic fluid is neutral, and normal vaginal secretions are acidic.[9] If the test is equivocal because of the presence of blood, it should be assumed that the membranes have ruptured and that amniotic fluid is present.

A rapid decision should be made as to whether the delivery is imminent and the baby will be delivered in the ED or whether time permits transport to the obstetric area of the hospital. If there is a possibility that the mother will deliver imminently (indicated by crowning), she should be kept in the ED for delivery. In general, if crowning is not present, there is usually time to safely transport the mother to the labor and delivery suite.

Preparing for Delivery

In an emergency situation, place the mother on a stretcher. (The author advises against the use of an obstetric and gy-necologic stretcher that "breaks" in this situation because the caregiver may be inexperienced in assisting with the delivery of a baby and because there is a possibility that the baby may be dropped.) Equipment used for an imminent delivery should be readily available. Sterile disposable delivery kits usually have most of the equipment necessary for the delivery, or you may assemble (ahead of time, of course) your own equipment (Fig. 45-3). Do not place the equipment between the mother's legs but rather on a surface beside the stretcher.

Use one hand covered with a sterile towel or a 4 × 4 inch dressing and apply gentle pressure to the infant's head as it crowns, to prevent an explosive delivery and possible tearing of the perineum. When the head is delivered, quickly suction the infant's mouth and then the nose to prevent aspiration. At this point, check for pressure of the umbilical cord around the infant's neck. If the cord is loose, carefully slip it over the infant's head. If it is tight, clamp it in two places and cut the cord. Once the head is delivered and has rotated, hold it gently in both hands (Fig. 45-4) and apply a gentle downward pressure to assist with the delivery of the anterior shoulder and gentle upward traction to assist with delivery of the posterior shoulder. Carefully support the infant's head (Fig. 45-5). Once the shoulders are delivered, the delivery of the rest of the infant's body usually occurs quite rapidly (Fig. 45-6).

Keep the infant in a head-dependent position at the level of the introitus to prevent aspiration. Once again, suction the mouth and nose. If spontaneous breathing or crying does not occur, gently rub the infant's back with a towel to stimulate breathing.

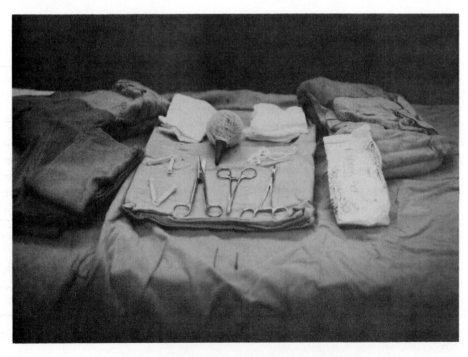

Fig. 45-3 Equipment used for emergency deliveries.

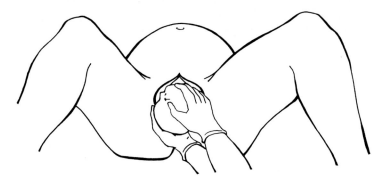

Fig. 45-4   Hold head gently in both hands.

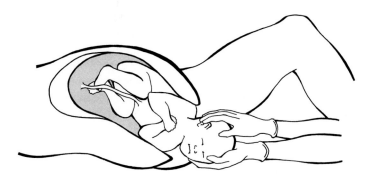

Fig. 45-5   Carefully support infant's head as it is born.

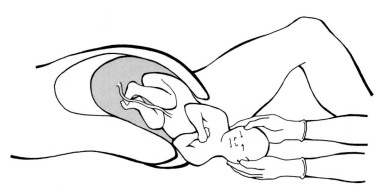

Fig. 45-6   Once anterior shoulder is delivered, remainder of delivery occurs quite rapidly.

The umbilical cord should be clamped in two places, at least 6 inches from the umbilicus, and cut as soon as it is convenient. Cutting usually occurs when the cord has stopped pulsating. Do an Apgar score (Table 45-2) at the time of birth and 5 minutes afterward.

The Apgar score is a system that is used to predict health outcomes by scoring and totalling five key factors that are monitored at the time of delivery and 5 minutes after birth. Each factor is scored from 0 to 2. *Zero* is poor response or absence of the factor that is being measured, *1* indicates some response, and *2* indicates a normal finding. A total high score of 10 is possible. A score of 7 to 10 is considered very good. A score of 4 to 6 indicates a moderately depressed infant, and a score of 0 to 3 indicates a severely depressed infant.

Place the infant on the mother's abdomen, and encourage the mother to nurse the infant. Suckling stimulates the uterus to contract. It also reassures the mother that her infant is okay, and it helps keep the infant warm. Also place a warmed blanket or towel over the infant. Put identification

Table 45-2 Apgar score

	Score		
Factor	0	1	2
A = Appearance (color)	Blue	Blue limbs, pink body	Pink
P = Pulse (heart rate)	Absent	<100	>100
G = Grimace (muscle tone)	Limp	Some flexion	Good flexion
A = Activity (reflexes irritable)	Absent	Some motion	Good motion
R = Respiratory effort	Absent	Weak cry	Strong cry

bands on both the infant's wrist and ankle. If the infant does not cry immediately and have or maintain good skin color, he or she must be resuscitated. A useful mnemonic, provided in the box below, is *TABS* ("to keep tabs on the infant").

For further information on neonatal resuscitation, refer to Chapter 13.

After the delivery of the infant, stage three of labor begins. At this point, if possible, unclamp the cord and obtain laboratory specimens from the cord for determinations of hematocrit, hemoglobin level, blood type, Rh factor, and bilirubin level. Reclamp the cord and palpate the uterus

---

TABS MNEMONIC

T (*temperature*)
Dry and cover the neonate as soon as possible to prevent heat loss. Consider the use of a heated isolette (Fig. 45-7).

A (*airway*)
Suction the mouth first and then the nose. A neonate who has had fetal distress in utero may have meconium present. Early suctioning (at the delivery of the head) with the use of a suction trap, is important. If the airway cannot be cleared, the neonate should be endotracheally intubated and suctioned.

B (*beats [heart rate]*)
If significant bradycardia is present (<80 beats/min) and does not improve with ventilation, chest compressions should be initiated (see Chapter 13). A brachial pulse should be palpable with compressions. Continue ventilating the neonate.
Consider pharmacological support with drugs such as epinephrine, atropine, naloxone, dextrose, and sodium bicarbonate (again, see Chapter 13).

S (*sugar*)
A blood glucose level of <40 mg/100 ml is a critical level in a neonate. If glucose is given, it should be administered in a 25% solution at 0.5 g/kg (or 2 ml/kg of a 25% solution). A 50% solution is too hypertonic for a neonate.

---

through the abdominal wall. Prepare for the delivery of the placenta, which usually occurs 5 to 10 minutes after the infant is born. Usually a sudden gush of blood occurs when the placenta separates from the uterine wall; the uterus rises up in the abdomen, and the umbilical cord that protrudes from the vagina will lengthen. Do not pull on the umbilical cord, since this could cause uterine invasion.

When the placenta has separated, apply slight traction on the umbilical cord and place your hand on the dome of the uterus, pressing it downward slightly toward the suprapubic area. As the placenta enters the vaginal area, continue applying gentle traction to the umbilical cord and carefully remove the placenta.

Unusual Deliveries

Breech delivery. The issue with a breech delivery as opposed to a vertex (head-first) delivery is that the head, the largest fetal body part, is delivered last. It is common for a woman whose fetus is in a breech presentation to be scheduled for a cesarean section. Unfortunately, in the emergency setting, when a woman arrives in labor with delivery imminent, even if the fetus is in a breech position, there may not be time to arrange for a cesarean section, and delivery must be completed in the ED, especially if the fetus has been delivered to the level of the umbilicus.

Categories of breech presentation are (1) a complete breech, in which the fetus has both knees and hips flexed; (2) an incomplete breech, in which one or both feet or knees usually present first; and (3) a front breech, in which the fetus's hips are flexed and the legs extend in front of the fetus.

In the case of any breech presentation, it is usually best to allow the fetus to deliver spontaneously up to the level of the umbilicus. If the fetus is in a front breech presentation, after the buttocks are delivered, one may have to extract the legs down into the introitus. Once the umbilicus can be visualized, gently extract a generous amount of umbilical cord. Then rotate the fetus to align the shoulders in an anterior-posterior position. Place gentle traction on the fetus until you can see the axilla. Then pull upward gently on the feet to allow for delivery of the posterior shoulder. Carefully extract the posterior arm. Then gently pull downward on

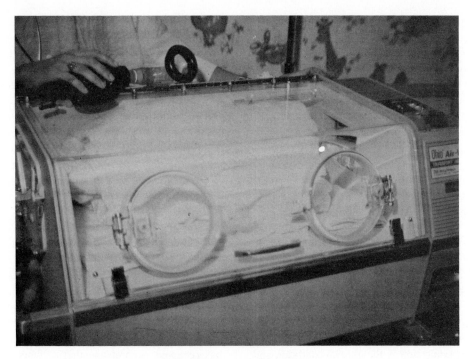

Fig. 45-7 Heated isolette.

the feet to deliver the anterior shoulder. Rotate the fetus' buttocks to the mother's anterior. Using a Mauriceau maneuver, rest the fetus on your arm and place your index and middle finger in the fetus' mouth, gently flexing the head. Do not apply traction with this hand. Grasp the fetus at the base of the neck and tip of the shoulders with your other hand and apply gentle traction. If assistance is available, have the other person apply firm, steady pressure to the top of the fundus towards the suprapubic area. The neonate should then be suctioned and the cord clamped.

Multiple deliveries. In delivery of twins (or more than two infants), there are some additional concerns. Often multiple-birth neonates are premature or have a host of other problems. The initial and most important objective is to ensure the safe delivery of both fetuses. The best advice is to take one at a time "as they come." The first may present either vertex or breech. Follow the information given previously for the type of presentation seen. The second fetus usually has membranes intact. If the second fetus is in the head-first position, you may elect to rupture the membranes and allow the mother to deliver the fetus by pushing when she has a contraction. If the second fetus is breech, the feet should be delivered, then the membranes should be ruptured. Both of the neonates should be suctioned as they are delivered. Both cords should be clamped, and both neonates should be identified with wrist and ankle bands.

Amniotic fluid embolism. Amniotic fluid embolism is a catastrophic event in which maternal mortality may be as high as 85%. An amniotic fluid embolism results when, during either the labor or the delivery phase, amniotic fluid leaks into the mother's venous circulation. This "embolus," which is composed of squamous epithelial cells, lanugo, and vasoactive chemicals, travels to the pulmonary circulation, where it causes sudden, severe obstruction, resulting in respiratory arrest followed by cardiac arrest.

Amniotic fluid emboli are seen more commonly in cases of placenta previa, abruptio placentae, and precipitate labor, in the multiparous woman, and in cases of intrauterine fetal death.[10]

Initially the mother may demonstrate profound hypotension, tachycardia, tachypnea, cyanosis, and hypoxia followed by cardiopulmonary arrest. Coagulopathies are also often seen.[8]

Therapeutic intervention must be rapid and aggressive. Administer oxygen at high flow via nonrebreather mask and consider rapid endotracheal intubation and mechanical ventilation with positive end-expiratory pressure. Crystalloid solutions and blood products should be administered. Consider the use of fresh frozen plasma in anticipation of coagulopathies.

POSTPARTUM EMERGENCIES
Postpartum Hemorrhage

Excessive bleeding in the postpartum period is an emergency. Bleeding can occur immediately after delivery or it can be delayed for 7 to 14 days. The main causes of postpartum bleeding are (1) subinvolution of the uterus, (2) retained secundines (pieces of placenta or membranes present in the uterus), and (3) vaginal or cervical tears incurred during delivery. Postpartum hemorrhage is usually described as blood loss in excess of 1000 ml within 24 hours of delivery.

Subinvolution usually occurs at 7 to 14 days after delivery, when the thrombi detach from the placental sites and the sites begin to bleed. If the involutional process is not progressing as it should in returning the gravid uterus to its nonpregnant state, the bleeding may become excessive. The retention of membranes or placental fragments can also cause sudden hemorrhage, since they interfere with the involutionary process. With the growing popularity of home delivery, the emergency nurse should also be aware of a condition known as placenta accreta, in which the placenta fails to separate from the uterine wall after delivery because it has grown into the uterine muscle itself. If this is the case, immediate surgery is indicated. Cervical tears and vaginal lacerations may become more common if the present trend of home deliveries continues, since home deliveries preclude the use of the episiotomy as a means to deliver a relatively large head through a relatively small vaginal opening.

Assessment. When assessing the patient with postpartum bleeding, the nurse should survey the general condition and note the presence or absence of pain, the color of skin (Is there cyanosis? Is she pale or flushed?), and the patient's posture, gait, motor activity, and facial expression. In obtaining a history of the present problem, the following information should be elicited:

1. Quantity, character, and duration of bleeding. How does it compare with the patient's normal menstrual period? How many pads has she used, and how does it compare with the number she normally requires during a period?
2. Menstrual history. When was the date of her last period? Was it heavier or lighter than usual?
3. Does she have pain? What is the nature of the pain— is it dull, achy, cramping, constant, or radiating? Where is the pain? How long has she had it? Was its onset gradual or sudden?
4. Is there any history of trauma?
5. When did she deliver? Has she ever had any infections of the reproductive system? Has she had previous episodes of bleeding?

Check the pad the patient is wearing to objectively evaluate the amount of bleeding. Note the presence or absence of clots or odor. Examine and save any clots or tissue that the patient may have brought with her for laboratory examination. Note the condition of the abdomen. Is it distended or flat? Is there rebound tenderness? Are there bowel sounds?

Evaluate the patient's condition, and institute appropriate measures for stabilization if necessary. If bleeding is profuse, two IV lines with large-bore needles capable of delivering crystalloids and blood should be established. If respirations are labored, administer oxygen. For all patients, a CBC with sedimentation rate is necessary for evaluation, and a clot should be drawn for type and cross-match studies for blood transfusions, if they should become necessary.

While collecting data and stabilizing the patient, prepare her for a vaginal examination. Explain each procedure and reassure her of your concern for her feelings by allowing her to express them.

Postpartum bleeding generally responds to the administration of IV oxytocin (Pitocin), bed rest, and fundal massage. If bleeding is massive, a gloved hand made into a fist can be placed in the vagina, exerting pressure anterior to the cervix. Use the other hand to compress the posterior wall of the uterus, thereby compressing the fundus between both hands.

Consider intravenous administration of narcotics or the use of an inhalational nitrous oxide and oxygen mixture.

Treatment of retained secundines is removal of the offending piece by dilation and curettage and a thorough exploration of the uterus after the patient has received general anesthesia. Suturing of vaginal lacerations can be performed in the ED, but because of the possibility of damage at the cervix as well, suturing is best performed after the patient has received general anesthesia, when a good pelvic examination can also be performed.

Postpartum Infection

Vaginal lacerations, cervical tears, episiotomy sites, placental implant sites, and retained tissue may be host sites for infection. Patients usually have fevers, abdominal or pelvic pain, and occasionally foul-smelling lochia.

Therapeutic intervention is to culture any drainage and, usually, to treat with antibiotics.

GYNECOLOGIC EMERGENCIES
Ovarian Cyst

Patients with ruptured ovarian cysts can have the same symptoms as those with ectopic pregnancy, except that the pregnancy test result is negative. The *corpus luteum cyst* of the ovary arises as a result of a hemorrhage in a mature corpus luteum, which causes cystic changes in the wall itself. This cyst is clinically significant, since it can become quite large, causing menstrual irregularities. After several cysts have formed, one can rupture and cause additional bleeding and occasionally, massive intraperitoneal hemorrhage. When this hemorrhage occurs, it constitutes a surgical emergency in its own right. Nursing interventions include all of those discussed for ectopic pregnancy.

Dermoid cysts, or benign cystic teratomas, are those that arise in the ovary from all three germ cell layers and most often contain hair and teeth, and sebaceous material but can contain tissue from almost any structure in the body (Fig. 45-8). These cysts represent 20% of all ovarian cysts and usually appear during active reproductive life. Dermoid cysts most commonly manifest as acute abdominal and pelvic pain when they become twisted on their pedicles (torsion) or begin to leak contents into the peritoneal cavity.

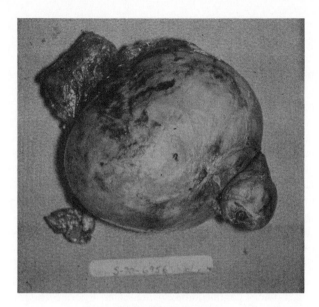

Fig. 45-8 Dermoid cyst.

Ovarian endometriomas or "chocolate cysts" occur when actively growing and functioning endometrial tissue is present in the ovary. The endometrial tissue cyclically bleeds with each menstrual period and forms a cyst that contains blood with blood clots (Fig. 45-9). This situation not only causes menstrual irregularities and chronic pelvic pain but also can become an emergency if the cyst ruptures, causing hemorrhage and shock. Again, the nurse should stabilize the patient, then after evaluation transfer her to the operating room for an emergency laparoscopy.

Ovarian Abscess

A tuboovarian abscess is a complication of untreated PID, and if ruptured, can bring the patient into the ED with gram-negative sepsis and septic shock. In this case, the differential diagnosis from ectopic pregnancy is a clear history of febrile illness, pelvic pain, foul-smelling vaginal discharge, increased white blood cell count, and elevated sedimentation rate.

Culdocentesis is definitely contraindicated, since all treatment is aimed at bringing infection under control before any invasive procedures are attempted, if possible. The rupture of the pus-filled tuboovarian abscess causes peritonitis, and large doses of a combination of antibiotics, usually a combination of penicillin, cephalosporin, clindamycin, kanamycin, or gentamicin, are started by IV infusion immediately. A nasogastric tube is usually placed, since peristalsis is slowed by the bowel irritation. If rupture has occurred, immediate surgery is indicated. If the abscess is unruptured, the patient is admitted to the hospital for at least 48 hours of antibiotic therapy before surgery to remove the abscess is considered.

Pelvic Inflammatory Disease

One of the most common and distressing gynecologic conditions seen in the ED is PID. PID is an acute or chronic infection that may involve the uterus, fallopian tubes, ovaries, and adjacent structures such as the peritoneum and the intestines. The most frequent cause of PID is *Neisseria gonorrhoeae*, but PID can also be caused by staphylococci, streptococci, the tubercle bacillus, or a variety of nonspecific organisms. *Neisseria gonorrhoeae* usually causes acute sal-

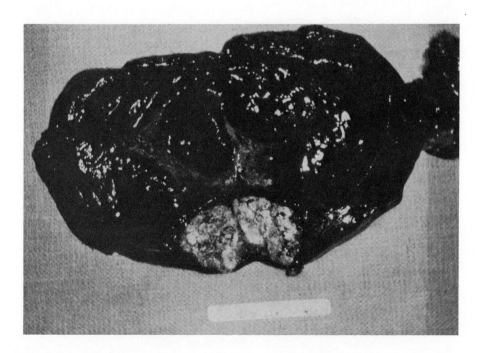

Fig. 45-9 Ovarian endometrioma or "chocolate cyst."

pingitis, which in turn causes the pain that brings the patient into the ED. The transmission of the disease is by sexual contact. The incubation period is 3 to 8 days. The organism primarily infects the urethra, Skene's ducts, and the Bartholin's glands; the fallopian tubes become involved by direct extension. The patient usually comes in after menses; symptoms include the following:

1. Acute, generalized lower abdominal pain
2. Anorexia, nausea, and vomiting
3. Fever and chills
4. Pain during pelvic examination and movement of the cervix
5. A tense abdomen with rebound tenderness
6. Leukocytosis with white blood cell counts of 15,000 to 30,000
7. Purulent vaginal discharge

Diagnostic procedures should include a CBC with sedimentation rate, urinalysis, and cervical smears and cultures for Gram's stain, anaerobes, and aerobes.

Place the patient in a semi-Fowler's position, to facilitate drainage of the discharge, until the ED physician is ready to perform the vaginal examination. See that the blood work is completed and the urine specimen is collected. Explain to the patient what is going to be done, and position her for the vaginal examination, being sure that the speculum, gloves, and proper culture tubes are available. Careful handwashing technique and disposal of tissues and pads are especially important when dealing with a gynecologic infection. In mild cases of PID, treatment requires only a prescription for antibiotics, and the patient can be released to receive follow-up care from a private physician.

Again, it is important for the emergency nurse to be aware that many patients who have symptoms of abdominal pain are incorrectly diagnosed as having early PID, treated with penicillin, and sent home with an unruptured ectopic pregnancy. The nurse should be aware that a normal temperature, normal white blood cell count, and normal sedimentation rate *do not support* the diagnosis of PID. The attitude of the nurse as teacher and provider of support for the patient is of great importance. If the nurse cannot accept the patient as a person of worth who has a disease, the patient may not be receptive to instructions to see her physician for follow-up care and to be sure that her sexual partner is treated. Inadequately treated or untreated PID with salpingitis causes scarring of the fallopian tubes, and the patient may be unable to conceive a child. With early diagnosis and treatment of PID, the prognosis is excellent, provided that the patient's sexual partner is also treated so that reinfection does not occur. Other complications of untreated PID are endometritis, tuboovarian abscess, peritonitis, sepsis, shock, and death.

Bartholin's Gland Abscess

A patient with Bartholin's gland abscess has severe pain in the vulva and obvious swelling (Fig. 45-10). The treatment is incision and drainage of the abscess and administration of antibiotics. The patient is usually hospitalized.

Vaginal Infections

Women with vaginal infections are also seen in the ED when pain becomes intolerable. *Trichomonas vaginitis* causes a thin, watery discharge that is malodorous, burning,

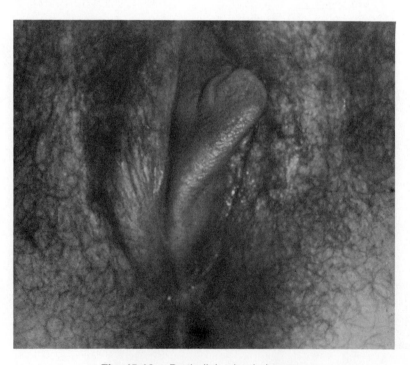

Fig. 45-10 Bartholin's gland abscess.

and itchy and becomes worse after a menstrual period. Diagnosis is confirmed by recognition of the motile, flagellated *Trichomonas vaginalis* on a fresh smear of the discharge. The organism can also be found in the urine in some cases, and it causes symptoms of urinary tract infection. Treatment of choice is the administration of metronidazole (Flagyl) orally to both the patient and her sexual partner. If the patient's sexual partner is not treated, the organism can remain in the male urethra and prostate asymptomatically and the patient will be reinfected with the next contact.

Intense itching with the presence of a thick, cheesy, white discharge and inflamed vaginal mucosa indicates *monilial vaginitis*. It is caused by *Candida albicans* and is frequently associated with diabetes, pregnancy, or broad-spectrum antibiotic therapy. Diagnosis is confirmed by culture or by special examination of a fresh smear of the discharge. Treatment is with nystatin (Mycostatin). This infection does not require treatment of the partner.

In recent years the incidence of *genital herpes* seen in patients in the ED is increasing at an alarming rate. This disease, caused by herpesvirus hominis or herpes simplex 2, is considered to be of venereal transmission. In women, multiple small vesicles appear on the labia, the clitoral prepuce, and along the vagina (Fig. 45-11). In 75% of cases, these vesicles are seen on the cervix as well. The presenting symptom is severe pain in the vulvovaginal area—often so severe that the patient is unable to void, or if able to void, holds urine in an attempt to avoid the scalding pain that occurs when urine passes over the affected area. She may, therefore, have a distended bladder, fever because of dehydration, and a waddling gait. The incubation period is usually 10 days to 2 weeks, and symptoms can occur periodically after the initial infection. A specific diagnosis can be made from recognition of viral inclusion bodies on a smear. The lesions may become infected secondarily with

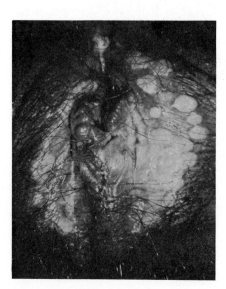

Fig. 45-11   Characteristic lesions of vaginal herpes.

bacteria when scratched, and this secondary infection may further cloud differential diagnosis. There is no specific treatment, and supportive care is given until the disease runs its course. Supportive therapy may include a regimen of analgesics for pain, sitz baths, insertion of a Foley catheter, IV therapy to correct dehydration, and the use of compresses and drying agents. Antibiotics have no effect and should not be used unless there is a secondary infection.

Nursing intervention should include the use of good hand-washing techniques for both the nurse and the patient, the careful disposal and cleaning of used equipment, and emotional support and understanding. This disease tends to be recurrent and is not something that the patient can take lightly, since it can change her life-style. The condition is particularly dangerous when it occurs during pregnancy. Infant mortality for herpes encephalitis is 95%. If active lesions are present at term, most obstetricians perform a cesarean section to prevent exposure of the infant during vaginal delivery.

GYNECOLOGIC TRAUMA

Trauma to genital organs is observed in the ED as vaginal bleeding, as a hematoma of the perineum, or as obvious laceration of the vagina. It can be caused accidentally (most often seen in children) or by sexual abuse. Careful examination of the external genitalia must be performed to assess the extent of the injury. The entire vagina must be visualized to avoid overlooking an associated but separate vaginal injury. In addition to a CBC, a urine screen for hematuria should be obtained to rule out intraperitoneal injury.

If, as is most often the case, the patient is a child, it may be difficult to adequately examine her in the ED. The preferred treatment is admission, a complete examination, and repair after the patient has received general anesthesia. In treating children, a working knowledge of growth and development is essential. It is important to accomplish the following:

1. Gain their confidence
2. Be direct and honest
3. Be aware of age idiosyncrasies
4. Set limits for their behavior
5. Support patients and their families

Emergency nursing interventions include preparing the patient mentally and physically for the examination and providing emotional support for the patient and family by listening attentively and by calmly reassuring them. Be aware that most patients, especially children, are aware of family members' fear; in calming the family, you become much more effective in calming the patient. The nurse should be aware that there is always the possibility of abuse and that discrepancies in history as related to symptoms should be noted. If child abuse is suspected, it must be reported to child welfare authorities; all 50 states now require this by law.

Another clinical condition that is evidenced by trauma or

infection in children is the presence of a foreign body in the vagina (paper, erasers, and so on). The chief symptom is a bloody, watery discharge secondary to vaginitis. Foreign bodies can occasionally be removed in the ED, but more often admission is required for examination after the patient has received anesthesia and for treatment with antibiotics.

SEXUAL ASSAULT

Anyone of either sex, at any age, can be sexually assaulted. Sexual assault is one of the four most violent and frequent crimes occurring in the United States each year, and women and girls are most often the victims. During the assault, victims often fear for their lives and thus may submit to the demands of the assailant. After the assault, victims often have a feeling of disbelief, followed by a period of shock. Victims may also have feelings of guilt or self-blame, fear, extreme vulnerability, helplessness, personal violation, shame, and embarrassment. Victims may cry for no obvious reason. A few days after the assault, the victims may say that they want to forget the disruption in their lives and return to school or work. Later they begin to feel depressed and angry and need to verbalize their feelings.

When a victim of sexual assault arrives at the ED, try to place the patient in an area away from the noisy routines of the department. Try not to leave the victim alone. Ideally, all personnel should be trained as rape counselors. If possible, the person who takes the initial history should be the one to remain with the patient throughout the stay in the ED.

Informed consent is required to treat the victim of sexual assault. If the victim comes to the ED without the police, the police must be notified, as they would be for any violent crime. The victim does, however, have the right to decide whether or not to give them any information. The patient may choose to have only a medical examination and refuse to have specimens collected for forensic tests. Encourage, but do not force, the victim to speak with the police. Let the patient know that the police need whatever information they can get to be able to apprehend the assailant and that this information may prevent an assault on another person. Check to find out whether the hospital bill is covered by an agency in your community that compensates victims of violent crimes, and give the patient this information.

It is not the responsibility of ED personnel to decide whether a person was sexually assaulted; their responsibilities are to ensure the physical well-being of the patient, collect specimens, and provide psychologic support. If the victim wants only medical treatment, a regular consent form is appropriate. If specimens are collected for legal evidence, a special form must also be signed, which indicates that the victim has given consent to release these specimens to the police and a forensic laboratory.

Before the patient leaves the department, locate a family member or a friend with whom the victim can spend the night. Place the victim in immediate contact with a rape crisis or a rape hotline counselor, and arrange for immediate counseling.

History Taking

Explain to the patient that some of the questions you will be asking may be somewhat embarrassing and difficult to answer but that she should make every effort to answer these questions as accurately as possible. Allow the patient to talk openly. With children, you may want to use a puppet or a doll so that they can point to areas on the doll corresponding to where they have been hurt. Record all information accurately and thoroughly, since you may be called on to testify in court much later.

It is essential to collect details such as the date and time of the assault and the place and the surrounding events. Ask whether there was penetration, how many assailants there were, whether the victim can remember any identifying information about the assailant(s). Did the assailant(s) use a condom? Was physical force or a weapon used? Ask her about her menstrual history and about the last time she had intercourse before the sexual assault. Has she ever been pregnant, or is she pregnant now? What did she do after the assault? Did she shower? Douche? Defecate? Was she under the influence of alcohol or drugs during the assault? Ask if the victim has any allergies or any history of gynecologic difficulties or problems.

Physical Examination

Inspect the patient's entire body for bruises, ecchymoses, lacerations, or other injuries. Inspect the external genitalia, perineum, cervix, and vaginal wall. Collect specimens for a wet mount, a dry smear, a fixed smear, and a culture. Be sure not to use a lubricant other than water on the speculum. Collect an oropharyngeal culture if indicated. Send a urine sample to the laboratory for a pregnancy test to determine whether the woman was pregnant at the time of the rape. Note any negative findings or descriptions on the chart. Arrange for psychologic follow-up care. If the use of alcohol or drugs is suspected, check for the presence of these. Collect fingernail scrapings, pubic hairs (combed or clipped), and vaginal smears for slides.

Therapeutic Intervention

Treat the patient for any physical trauma. Protect the patient against pregnancy and venereal disease. The usual course of treatment includes two Ovral tablets given in the ED, followed by two tablets 12 hours later; this medication causes a menstrual period 2 days after administration. Penicillin, 4.8 million units, is given intramuscularly (provided there is no sensitivity to penicillin), and 1 g probenecid is given orally. The patient should have psychologic care within 24 hours, again in 48 hours, and then as often as deemed necessary, usually weekly. (See Chapters 44 and 50 for additional information on psychosocial aspects of sexual assault.)

VAGINAL BLEEDING

It is common for a woman to arrive at the ED with the chief complaint of abnormal vaginal bleeding. The key to appropriate therapeutic intervention is to identify and treat those conditions that may be life threatening and to identify and treat or provide appropriate referral for those that are not. A normal menstrual period occurs when an ovum that has not been fertilized passes through the reproductive system. When the ovum has not been fertilized and implanted, hormonal levels decrease and the superficial layer of the endometrium sloughs off. This sloughing off generally occurs every 27 to 30 days.

Abnormal Vaginal Bleeding

Menorrhagia. If menstrual bleeding is profuse, the term used to describe it is menorrhagia, which is usually the result of anovulation (no ovulation). Menorrhagia occurs because the endometrium continues to thicken and soften in preparation to accommodate a fertilized ovum. Because there is no ovum, the endometrium becomes thicker until normal hormone levels cannot continue to support it. When the much-thickened superficial layer of the endometrium sloughs off and the subsuperficial layer of hemorrhage is released, bleeding is usually profuse.

Systemic causes of vaginal bleeding. Systemic causes of abnormal vaginal bleeding usually include those conditions that produce prolonged clotting time or impair metabolism, such as acute leukemia, hypothyroidism, or cirrhosis of the liver. Other causes may be systemic infections or use of anticoagulants. One should also consider that emotional stressors may affect normal hormonal balance and cause abnormal vaginal bleeding.

Anatomic causes. Abnormal vaginal bleeding may occur during the first trimester of pregnancy. First-trimester bleeding may be the result of spontaneous abortion or ectopic pregnancy, both of which are discussed earlier in this chapter. Antepartum complications include placenta previa and abruptio placentae. These conditions are also discussed earlier in this chapter. Abnormal vaginal bleeding may also occur as a result of lesions, infections, or the presence of foreign bodies.

Foreign bodies may be objects that have been placed in the vaginas of children or the elderly and intrauterine devices, diaphragms, and tampons in women of childbearing age. Regardless of the type of foreign object, if significant bleeding has occurred and the woman is anemic or still hemorrhaging, the foreign body must be removed and repair must be considered.

Lesions that are located in areas from the vulva to the fallopian tubes may be the cause of abnormal vaginal bleeding. Lesions can be caused by perforation and ruptures resulting from trauma, cervicitis, or cancer. The type of lesion is usually confirmed by dilation and curettage, direct visualization, or biopsy.

Hormonal dysfunction. Hormonal dysfunction from whatever origin can cause either anovulatory or ovulatory bleeding. Much of the diagnosis and therapeutic intervention depends on the woman's age and result of diagnostic studies.

Postoperative bleeding. Bleeding that occurs after surgical procedures is relatively easy to diagnose, provided a good history is obtained. Bleeding may occur after dilation and curettage, hysterectomy, abortion, or conization.

Regardless of the cause of vaginal bleeding, it should first be determined whether the amount of blood loss has placed the woman in a life-threatening situation. This can usually be determined by obtaining vital signs, including skin vitals (color, temperature, and moisture). (See Chapter 19.) If vital signs indicate shock or a preshock state, administer supplemental oxygen, start two large-bore IV lines, administer crystalloid solutions or blood products or both, obtain blood specimens for CBC and type and cross-match studies, attempt to control bleeding, and consider preparation for surgery. Concurrently, obtain a good history and perform a physical examination, including a vaginal examination. Consider obtaining a serum hCG or ultrasonographic study or performing a culdocentesis (only if ultrasonography is not available).

Therapeutic intervention may include endometrial biopsy, insertion of a balloon-tipped Foley catheter into the uterine chamber and inflation of the balloon, hormone therapy, or surgery, depending on the nature of the bleeding.

If bleeding is not life threatening, there is usually more time to determine the nature of the bleeding. History should include the date of the last menstrual period, the number of days and the amount of bleeding, possibility of pregnancy, and whether the patient has abnormal pain.

REFERENCES

1. Chesley LC: Hypertension in pregnancy, *Kidney Int* 18:234, 1980.
2. Farrell RG, ed: *OB/GYN emergencies: the first 60 minutes*, Rockville, Md, 1986, Aspen.
3. Funderburk SJ et al: Outcome of pregnancies complicated by early vaginal bleeding, *Br J Obstet Gynaecol* 87:100, 1980.
4. Gleicher N et al: Direct diagnosis of unruptured ectopic pregnancy by real time ultrasonography, *Obstet Gynecol* 61:425, 1983.
5. Jones HW, Jones GS: *Novak's textbook of gynecology*, ed 10, Baltimore, 1981, Williams & Wilkins.
6. Katz K et al: Management of labor with umbilical cord prolapse, *Am J Obstet Gynecol* 142:237, 1982.
7. Knuppel RA, Montenegro R: Preeclampsia-eclampsia: an overview, *J Fla Med Assoc* 70(9):741, 1983.
8. Morgan M: Amniotic fluid embolism, *Anesthesia* 34:20, 1979.
9. Pritchard JA, Macdonald PC, Gant WF, eds: *Williams' obstetrics*, ed 17, New York, 1985, Appleton-Century-Crofts.
10. Sterner S et al: Amniotic fluid embolism, *Am J Emerg Med* 13:343, 1984.
11. Sullivan JM: *The hypertensive diseases of pregnancy and their management*, Chicago, 1982, Mosby–Year Book.
12. Tancer ML et al: A fifteen year experience with ectopic pregnancy, *Surg Gynecol Obstet* 152:179, 1981.

CHAPTER 46

Pain Management

Deborah Trautman and **Paul Paris**

In the practice of emergency nursing an opportunity exists to assist patients in the relief of acute pain. Pain is the most frequent complaint that motivates people to seek emergency medical care. Emergency nurses are challenged to manage acute pain of patients with unique needs in a unique and often chaotic environment. The relief of acute pain and suffering should be a primary goal of treatment of acute painful injury or illness. However, emergency nurses and physicians often fail to achieve or address pain management adequately. Traditionally, prompt management of pain in the ED has been neglected. Although management of the airway, breathing, and circulation is universally accepted as essential in emergency are, frequently the goal of relieving pain is not. Effective pain management may be neglected for several reasons. Generally, however, three prominent reasons emerge. First, emergency nurses and physicians often believe that treating pain early may delay or complicate the workup or examination of the patient. Second, the nurse or physician may not believe or understand the patient's complaint of pain. Third, health care practitioners may be reluctant to use narcotics for fear of inducing addiction or causing uncontrollable life-threatening side effects such as respiratory depression. Therefore, because these practices help to promote continued inadequate pain management in the ED, it is essential that we educate ourselves about these concerns. Emergency nurses have an obligation to advocate effective pain relief for their patients. This advocacy can be facilitated by increasing one's knowledge of pain, emphasizing a more prominent role in helping patients and physicians manage acute pain, and monitoring treatment plans to ensure safe and effective pain management for ED patients.

DEFINITION OF PAIN

Attempts at defining pain vary widely; however, the definition most commonly accepted in nursing is "whatever the experiencing person says it is, existing whenever he or she says it does, including both verbal and nonverbal behavior."[7] Pain is subdivided into two types: acute and chronic. McCaffery[8] defines acute pain as "an episode lasting from a second to less than six months." Chronic pain is usually defined as pain that lasts for 6 months or longer. In addition, acute pain is usually a symptom of an identifiable disease, which persists only as long as the disease itself and responds to adequate pain management. Chronic pain may be associated with chronic tissue disease, may not have an identifiable cause, may last longer than the normal healing period for an acute injury or disease, and may not respond to standard analgesic interventions. Chronic pain management is beyond the scope of emergency care. This chapter focuses exclusively on the management of acute pain.

In understanding acute pain management the nurse must recognize that acute pain has two components: the actual physical stimulus and the patient's cognitive and emotional interpretation of it. Although removal or treatment of the cause, the actual physical stimulus, is of course the most reliable and therapeutic approach to the problem, nursing interventions and the nurse's role in particular can greatly influence the patient's interpretation. A patient's interpretation of pain is influenced by a variety of factors. Among these are culture, religious beliefs, trust and fear about the ED visit, and coping styles. A calm, empathetic nurse can do much to minimize a patient's fears and to facilitate early pain management. In a study of 148 patients, Copp[4] found that patients frequently shared ideas on how nurses and doctors could help them with their pain.[3] These ideas, applicable to the ED, suggest that the nurse should slow down, not be hurried, talk to the patient about his or her pain, not tell patients that they do not have pain, be realistic instead of casual or flip, not ignore patients, not be callous, and not make judgments. These are important points for the nurse to incorporate into his or her role in assisting with pain management. Traditionally, many nurses have considered their role in pain management to be simply the administering of physicians' orders; in the twentieth century this is an antiquated belief and minimizes the nurse's contribution to patient care. The emergency nurse's role is vital to facilitating early relief of pain and suffering. The nurse should assure the patient that the health care team believes the patient and will treat the pain soon and effectively.

ROLE OF THE NURSE IN MANAGING PAIN

Key components of the nurse's role in pain management include the following:

1. Establishing an effective, supportive relationship with the patient
2. Believing, collaborating with, and respecting the patient's response to pain and its management
3. Educating patients about the occurrence, onset, and duration of pain, methods of pain relief, and preventive measures
4. Informing the patient of what he or she is likely to experience while in the ED, to assist in minimizing fear of the unknown
5. Maintaining current knowledge and competencies
6. Monitoring patient response and effectiveness of treatment
7. Communicating frequently and effectively with both the patient and the physician regarding the treatment plan and its effectiveness
8. Ensuring the safety of the patient at all times (Closely monitoring each patient promotes assessment of treatment effectiveness and minimizes the possibility of disastrous side effects.)
9. Maintaining a calm, empathetic manner
10. Researching the multidimensional nature of pain, its assessment and subsequent management, and using this research in practice

Incorporating these 10 components into the nursing role facilitates an effective nursing approach to pain management. Establishing trust and alleviating fear should be primary goals of the nurse. With the establishment of a therapeutic relationship, each patient has an increased probability of successful pain management. The nurse should take caution to avoid letting his or her personal attitudes, beliefs, or values influence perceptions of a patient's pain or the selection of interventions. As Burke and Jerrett[2] found in many instances, tradition, intuition, and stereotypes influence interventions selected for pain management. The researchers studied student nurses' perceptions of the best interventions for people of various ages who were in acute pain. Age was identified as a factor that influenced both the number and type of interventions selected. In this study student nurses selected more interventions for adolescents and adults and fewer interventions for infants, toddlers, preschool-aged children, school-aged children, and elderly individuals. Of the eight possible types of interventions (medication, physical comfort, verbal reassurance, massage, distraction, relaxation techniques, breathing techniques, and imagery) a mean of 3.3 types was selected for infants, 5.0 for adults, and 4.5 for the elderly persons. Although additional research is indicated, nurses must not let personal beliefs negatively influence practice.

HOW PAIN IS TREATED: ASSESSMENT

The management of acute pain begins with the initial nursing assessment. A concise, comprehensive assessment is essential. Not all patients can or will adequately verbalize key components of their pain. Assessment indices must include both subjective and objective measures. Because of the broad scope of nursing literature on patient assessment, the following discussion is limited to a brief summarization of the nursing assessment of pain. For more detailed assessment techniques, see McCaffery and Beebe.[9]

An initial focused assessment should be conducted to collect data about the patient's pain. Carpenito[3] defined a focused assessment as "the acquisition of selected or specific data as determined by the nurse and the client or family or by the condition of the client." Assessment of pain should include location, quality, intensity, onset, duration, and aggravating or alleviating factors.

Techniques such as facilitation (saying "mm-hnnn" or "go on"), reflection, repeating key phrases the patient has stated in question format (such as, "Has it spread?"), and clarification of ambiguous statements facilitates collection of data pertinent to the chief complaint.[1] It is important to avoid prompting the patient by asking leading questions. For example, consider the following scenario, in which a 72-year-old woman with a complaint of chest pain is seen at the ED.

Patient: I want to be seen by a doctor. I have a pain in my chest.
Nurse: Tell me about your pain.
Patient: It hurts.
Nurse: Does it travel to your arms? (incorrect)
Nurse: Tell me where it hurts. (correct)

Adequate assessment of a patient's pain is hampered when the nurse makes inferences about the patient's pain.[8]

Objective data should include but not be limited to a physician's description of the patient, any noted facial expressions, and measurements of pulse rate, blood pressure, and respiratory rate. After the initial assessment is conducted, it is imperative that the emergency nurse ensure an ongoing assessment and evaluation of the patient's pain. This ongoing assessment facilitates determining the efficacy of treatment.

TREATMENT MODALITIES FOR MANAGING PAIN

The following discussion includes both new and traditional methods of treating patients in pain. A brief summary is given of general principles of analgesia, narcotics, nitrous oxide, nonnarcotic drugs, local anesthesia, and noninvasive pain relief methods, and pertinent emergency nursing implications are reviewed.

Analgesia

Although pain management is complex and requires a multidisciplinary approach, the nurse is often the most appropriate member of the health care team to assist and coordinate effective and safe pain management because of the nurse's ability to continuously maintain close contact with the patient. In this capacity the nurse functions as an advocate for the patient. Communicating the patient's complaints of pain to the physician can directly contribute to the physician's selection of therapy to meet the unique needs of each patient and may improve the outcome of treatment.

Because of nursing's key role in effective pain management, eight basic tips should be reviewed:

1. There is no universally superior method of pain management.
2. The goal of pain management is to prevent pain whenever possible. Pain relief is more effective if initiated soon after onset of pain.
3. The underlying cause of pain is an important consideration in selecting analgesia.[12]
4. The calm, quiet patient does not preclude the presence of pain.
5. A patient's refusal to accept pain medication may be related to fear of addiction, sedation, or loss of control or fear of method of administration. Nursing can intervene, discuss the patient's concerns, and ultimately facilitate the patient's ability to make an informed decision regarding consent to treatment.[12]
6. A patient's request for specific pain medication does not automatically imply that he or she is a drug seeker.
7. A patient's tolerance of pain is not directly proportional to the amount of analgesic required to relieve pain.
8. All pain is real; pain is what the patient says it is.

Narcotics

Narcotic analgesics or opiates are effective in the relief of acute pain. Narcotics can be classified as narcotic agonists, narcotic agonist-antagonists, and narcotic antagonists.

Morphine is the prototypical opioid agonist with which all other opioids are compared.[12] Morphine and other narcotic analgesics directly affect the central nervous system, causing analgesia, changes in mood and emotion, respiratory depression, bronchoconstriction, miosis (pupil constriction), nausea, vomiting, and decreased gastric motility. Cardiovascular effects of narcotics are variable and require close monitoring of vital signs. Although morphine does not dramatically alter heart rate and blood pressure when administered in the right dosage, higher doses can decrease heart rate and blood pressure. The efficacy of narcotic agonist-antagonist analgesics depends on proper dosage, rates of administration, and frequency of use (Table 46-1). Narcotic classification is given in the box on p. 652.

Health professionals' fears of inducing addiction result in ineffective pain management. Although physical dependence on narcotic agents may occur, it is rarely life threatening. Close clinical observation minimizes the untoward effects of respiratory depression.

Questions and concerns arise when ED nurses consider narcotic administration for a known substance abuser. Substance abuse does not preclude the option of narcotic analgesia as an appropriate treatment modality. The substance abuse patient or narcotic addict has the right to effective pain management. Nurses should discuss the treatment plan with the patient and physician. The goal is to deliver humane care to a person with pain who happens to be a narcotic addict by (1) relieving the pain and (2) keeping the person out of withdrawal.[9] ED nurses should, however, anticipate the need for larger than usual doses. In the ED environment the primary goal remains relief of acute pain, not rehabilitation.

Nurses should also be aware of mistakes that commonly occur with administration of narcotic analgesics. These include wrong dose, wrong route, wrong frequency of administration, and wrong drug.

Wrong dose. The most important factor in achieving adequate analgesia with a given narcotic is titrating the dose to achieve the desired degree of analgesia. A wide interpatient variability exists in the effective analgesia concentration. The approach of treating all patients with 75 mg of

Table 46-1   Narcotic agonist-antagonist analgesics

Drug	Average oral dose (mg)	Average parenteral dose (mg)	Duration (hr)	Comments	Precaution
Pentazocine (Talwin)	50 to 100	30 to 60	2 to 3	Suppositories available	Increase stroke work; high incidence of psychotomimetic effects
Nalbuphine (Nubain)	40	10 to 15	3 to 4	Minimal if any hemodynamic effects; ceiling on respiratory depression; low abuse potential	Can precipitate withdrawal if dependence on narcotic agonist
Butorphanol (Stadol)	Not available	1 to 4	2½ to 3½		Cardiovascular effects similar to pentazocine; can precipitate withdrawal
Buprenorphine (Buprenex)		0.3 to 0.6	5 to 6	Partial agonist can be given sublingually; long analgesic action	Not completely antagonized by naloxone

NARCOTIC CLASSIFICATION

Agonists
Naturally occurring alkaloids and semisynthetic opiates
   Natural
      Morphine
      Codeine (methylmorphine)
   Semisynthetic
      Oxymorphone (Numorphan)
      Hydromorphone (Dilaudid)
      Hydrocodone (Vicodin, Hycodan)
      Heroin (diacetylmorphine)
      Oxycodone (Percodan, Tylox)
Meperidine and related phenylpiperidines (synthetic)
   Meperidine (Demerol)
   Alphaprodine (Nisentil)
   Diphenoxylate (in Lomotil)
   Fentanyl (Sublimaze)
   Alfentanil
   Sufentanil (Sufenta)
Methadone and related drugs
   Methadone (Dolophine)
   Propoxyphene (Darvon)
Morphinan derivatives
   Levorphanol (Levo-Dromoran)
   Dextromethorphan

Agonist-antagonists
Nalorphine type
   Pentazocine (Talwin)
   Nalbuphine (Nubain)
   Butorphanol (Stadol)
Morphinelike drugs
   Buprenorphine (Buprenex)
   Meptazinol
   Profadol
   Propiram

Antagonists
Allyl-substituted compounds
   Nalorphine (Nalline)
   Naloxone (Narcan)
   Naltrexone (Trexan)
   Nalmefene

meperidine (Demerol) or 10 mg of morphine is ineffective in many patients. Doses should be individualized for each patient.

Wrong route. The most commonly used route for parenteral administration of narcotics is intramuscular injection. This route has several disadvantages and should not be the primary route of choice. The following are disadvantages of intramuscular injections:

1. Painful administration
2. Delayed onset of action
3. Inability to predict effect
4. Inability to easily titrate dose
5. Diurnal variation in level achieved
6. Disease state may affect level achieved
7. Level depends on muscle used

Intravenous (IV) and subcutaneous routes are preferred.

Wrong frequency of administration. The error that commonly occurs is failure to repeat narcotic administration frequently enough. Patient-controlled analgesia is an analgesia administration system designed to enable maintenance of optimal serum analgesic levels throughout a therapeutic course.[5] This system provides the patient with the ability to administer small IV doses without excessive sedation. Although patient-controlled analgesia is not currently widely used in the ED setting, its advantages suggest that its inclusion into practice would be beneficial for some ED patients.

Wrong drug. In general, most narcotics can effectively produce desired degree of analgesia if the proper dose is given. The exceptions to this rule are oral codeine and propoxyphene (Darvon); codeine at any dose is not an extremely potent narcotic, and propoxyphene has little justification for use. Many studies have shown that propoxyphene is no better or only marginally more effective than a placebo.[11] Morphine, meperidine, fentanyl, and midazolam (Versed) are among those considered effective for use in the ED.

Nitrous Oxide

Nitrous oxide, a sedative analgesic agent, is a mixture of 50% nitrous oxide and 50% oxygen (Table 46-2). Nitrous oxide is self-administered through a demand valve. The benefits of use include rapid onset, safety, ease of administration, short duration, effectiveness, and inexpensiveness.[13] A potential side effect may be cardiovascular depression when nitrous oxide is used concomitantly with narcotics. However, research indicates that a 50:50 combination provides a safe, low-risk treatment modality without major side effects.

Contraindications for use include impairment of consciousness, inebriation, inability to understand instructions, dyspnea, cyanosis, presence or suspicion of pneumothorax, decompression sickness or air embolism, severe chronic lung disease, and abdominal pain with distention or suspicion of obstruction.

The primary nursing responsibility is patient teaching. Nurses should instruct patients to breathe normally. Deep or rapid breathing produces hyperventilation, which causes light-headedness and minimizes effective inhalation. The gas should be self-administered. Family or friends must be instructed not to assist the patient. The risk of overdose is minimal if the gas is self-administered: when the patient becomes drowsy, the mask or mouthpiece simply falls away. In addition to patient teaching, the ED nurse should ensure that the equipment is maintained. A daily inspection and cleaning schedule is optimal.

Table 46-2   Studies in the use of self-administered nitrous oxide mixtures

Study (year)	No. of patients	Relief (%)	Side Effects	Conclusions
Baskett (1970)	305	97	20%; none major	Safe, effective
Marsden (1979)	100	92	Not reported	Safe, effective
Flomenbaum (1979)	26	100	7, none major	Useful in minor surgical procedures
Thal (1979)	47	93	Not reported	Safe, effective
Nieto (1980)	124	82	4.9%; mild	Safe, effective; used 70:30 mixture because of ground elevation
Amey (1981)	88	85	48%; mild	Ideal analgesic for prehospital care
McKinnon (1981)	72	95	44%; mild	Safe, effective
Donen (1982)	240	93	29%; mild	Well-suited, safe
Stewart (1983)	1201	90	20%; mild	Safe, effective; emphasized anxiolytic effects

Nonnarcotic Analgesics

Nonnarcotic analgesics (listed in the box below) are used widely in emergency medicine. Unlike the opiates that affect the central nervous system, nonnarcotics affect the peripheral nervous system. Nonnarcotic agents inhibit prostaglandin synthesis. Pain, edema, and inflammation are minimized as a result of the blocking of prostaglandin release.[10] Nonsteroidal antiinflammatory drugs (NSAIDs) are indicated for mild to moderate pain. They are frequently prescribed to treat musculoskeletal injuries, headaches, arthritis, dysmenorrhea, pleuritis, pharyngitis, ureteral colic, and other common painful conditions.[13] Major side effects include gastrointestinal hemorrhage, renal failure, platelet dysfunction, and anaphylaxis. Acute hypersensitivity may also occur. Concomitant use with a narcotic analgesic agent augments pain relief.

Ketorolac (Toradol), a new NSAID available in the United States for short-term management of pain, is one of the first potent injectable analgesic, antiinflammatory, antipyretic agents of the 1990s. Ketorolac inhibits prostaglandin synthesis. Its use is not recommended for obstetric preoperative medication or analgesia. Contraindications include demonstrated hypersensitivity to ketorolac, angioedema, bronchospasm with aspirin or other NSAIDs, and complete or partial syndrome of nasal polyps. The recommended initial dosage is 30 or 60 mg every 6 hours as needed. Lower dosages are recommended for patients who weigh less than 50 kg or patients more than 65 years of age. Side effects are minimal but may include drowsiness, dyspepsia, gastrointestinal pain, nausea, diarrhea, edema, headache, and diaphoresis. Routine use with other NSAIDs is not recommended. However, ketorolac can be used concomitantly with morphine and meperidine without adverse effects.[14]

Local Anesthesia

Local anesthetics are commonly used for minor surgical procedures performed in the ED. Onset of rapid nerve block occurs within minutes and conversely reverses within minutes or hours. Lidocaine, bupivacaine, procaine, and the topical preparation, tetracaine (Pontocaine), are frequently used agents. A comparison of these agents is presented in Table 46-3.

General Considerations

Emergency nurses should monitor blood pressure, pulse rate, and respiration rate during treatment with injectable agents because systemic toxicity may occur if dosage administration is too high. Additionally, lidocaine and bupivacaine with epinephrine should not be used on digits, the penis, ears, or the nose because of vasoconstrictive effects. Patient teaching includes explaining the procedure and informing the patient that pain will be blocked but touch and pressure will remain intact. Pain management is facilitated if the patient is assisted into a comfortable position before initiation of the procedure and if distraction techniques are used. Research has shown that music provides an effective distraction during the procedure.[12] The numbing effects of local anesthetics provide a safe mechanism for pain control in the ED.

COMMONLY PRESCRIBED NONNARCOTIC ANALGESICS

Acetaminophen (Tylenol)
Acetylsalicylic acid (aspirin)
Nonacetylated salicylates (Dolobid, Trilisate)
Acetic acids (indomethacin, sulindac, tolmetin)
Propionic acids (ibuprofen [Motrin, Advil, Nuprin, Medipren], fenoprofen [Nalfon], Ansaid, naproxen [Naprosyn])
Oxicams (Feldene)
Ketorolac tromethamine (Toradol)

Table 46-3 Local anesthetic agents*

Agent	Uses	Dose and rates	Contraindications
Lidocaine	Peripheral nerve block: caudal, epidural, spinal; surgical anesthesia	Dependent on route; 0.5%, 1%, 1.5%, 2% with or without epinephrine; 4% without epinephrine; topical 5%; viscous	Hypersensitivity; children less than 12 years of age, elderly; liver disease
Bupivacaine	Peripheral nerve block: epidural and caudal	Dependent on route; 0.25%, 0.5%, 0.75% with or without epinephrine	Hypersensitivity; children less than 12 years of age, elderly; liver disease
Procaine	Peripheral nerve block: spinal, epidural; perineum, lower extremity infiltration	Dependent on route; 1%, 2%, 10%	Hypersensitivity; children less than 12 years of age, elderly; liver disease
Tetracaine, topical (Pontocaine)	Pruritus, sunburn, toothache, sore throat, oral pain, rectal pain, control of gagging	Apply to affected area; 1 oz for adults; ¼ oz for children; 2% solution aromatic spray; liquid; ointment; gel	Hypersensitivity; infants less than 1 year of age, application to large areas

*Adapted from Skidmore-Roth L: *Mosby's 1991 nursing drug reference,* St Louis, 1991, Mosby–Year Book.

Noninvasive Pain Relief Methods

Cutaneous stimulation, distraction, hypnosis, imagery, and relaxation are psychologic parameters of pain management. These approaches are briefly discussed here.

Cutaneous stimulation. Cutaneous stimulation applies to techniques that stimulate the skin for the purpose of pain relief. Massage, vibration, superficial heat and cold, ice application and massage, methanol application to the skin, and transcutaneous electrical nerve stimulation are techniques that may be used. Effects of cutaneous stimulation are variable; nursing skill and preparation are required before this method is used as a pain management intervention. ED staff nurses should receive an initial orientation and continuing education about these techniques before using this pain management intervention.

Distraction. Distraction facilitates pain management by assisting the patient in focusing on a stimulus other than the pain. Usually distraction minimizes but does not entirely alleviate pain. For distraction to be effective, it must be of interest to the patient. Research indicates that music has beneficial pain relief qualities. In September 1989, a study was conducted to determine whether music significantly reduces the anxiety and pain associated with laceration repair in the ED.[12] Adult patients 18 years of age and older, who were not under the influence of analgesics, alcohol, or other mood-altering substances, were included. Patients were randomly assigned to one of two groups, a control group, who received standard laceration repair with lidocaine only, and a music group, who received standard laceration repair with lidocaine and music. Patients in the music group were permitted to select from a variety of audio cassette tapes and to listen to their choice of music through a headset. Psychologic variables included the state subscale of the Spielberger State-Trait Anxiety Inventory, a visual analog pain-rating scale, and a brief questionnaire. Pain (P) scores were significantly lower ($p < 0.001$) in the music group (mean of 2.04) when compared with the control group (mean of 5.92). The authors concluded that music can be a safe, effective, inexpensive, noninvasive adjunct to pain management in the ED.

Hypnosis, imagery, and relaxation. Hypnosis is rarely used in emergency nursing, because few nurses have the knowledge or skills necessary to induce a trancelike state. However, the nurse functioning in the capacity of patient advocate can assist the patient in pursuing this method of pain management by referring the patient to available community resources for continued pain management. The phenomenon of self-hypnosis is becoming more widely accepted among health care professionals. Nurses interested in courses on hypnosis can obtain information by contacting the American Society of Clinical Hypnosis, 2250 East Devon Avenue, Suite 326, Des Plaines, IL 60018.

Using one's imagination to control pain is a form of distraction that produces relaxation. This technique does not imply that the pain sensation is imaginary. McCaffery and Beebe[9] identified the following types of imagery: (1) subtle or conversational, (2) simple, brief symptom substitution, (3) standardized imagery techniques, and (4) systematically individualized imagery techniques. In all four types the imagination is used to develop images that promote pleasant sensations and diminish pain perceptions. For example, some patients have decreased pain when assisted in imagining that they are on a quiet beach listening to the sound of the waves washing over the sand. Effectiveness depends on the familiarity of the image and its pleasantness to the patient.

Relaxation techniques promote an anxiety-free state. When a patient is relaxed, skeletal muscle tension is minimal. Deep-breathing instructions can promote relaxation. The nurse should instruct the patient to inhale deeply through the nose and to exhale slowly through the mouth. Repeating this exercise several times while concentrating on muscle relaxation is a simple technique that can be taught relatively easily in the ED.[6]

SUMMARY

Pain management in emergency nursing is exciting and challenging. Dunwoody[5] summarizes that "few things we do for patients are more fundamental to the quality of life than relieving pain." Emergency nurses promote the highest quality of services to their patients when continuous aggressive efforts are directed at ensuring relief of pain and suffering for all patients.

REFERENCES

1. Bates B: *A guide to physical examination*, ed 3, Philadelphia, 1983, JB Lippincott.
2. Burke SO, Jerrett M: Pain management across age groups, *West J Nurs Res* 11:164, 1989.
3. Carpenito LJ: *Nursing diagnosis: application to practice*, Philadelphia, 1983, JB Lippincott.
4. Copp LA: The spectrum of suffering, *Am J Nurs* 90(8):35, 1990.
5. Dunwoody CJ: Patient controlled analgesia: rationale, attributes, and essential factors, *Orthop Nurs* 6(5):31, 1987.
6. Fincke MK, Lanros NE: *Emergency nursing: a comprehensive review*, Rockville, Md., 1986, Aspen Publications.
7. McCaffery M: *Cognition, bodily pain and man-environment interactions*, Los Angeles, 1968, University of California.
8. McCaffery M: *Nursing management of the patient with pain*, ed 2, Philadelphia, 1979, JB Lippincott.
9. McCaffery M, Beebe A: *Pain: clinical manual for nursing practice*, St Louis, 1989, Mosby–Year Book.
10. McGuire L: Administering analgesics: which drugs are right for your patient, *Nursing* 20(4):34, 1990.
11. Miller RR et al: Propoxyphene hydrochloride: a critical review, *JAMA* 23:996, 1979.
12. Paris PM et al: Use of music to reduce anxiety and pain associated with laceration repair, *Ann Emerg Med* 20(4), 1991.
13. Paris PM, Stewart RD: *Pain management in emergency medicine*, Norwalk, Conn., 1988, Appleton & Lange.
14. *Product information: Toradol*, Palo Alto, 1990, Syntex Laboratories.

CHAPTER 47

Pediatric Triage and Assessment

Donna Ojanen Thomas

Triage is one of the most important aspects of caring for a child in the emergency department (ED). Recognition of life-threatening or potentially life-threatening conditions is the first step in providing the appropriate treatment.

A sick child in the ED usually makes nurses who are not used to dealing with children uneasy, just as an adult with chest pain causes alarm to a pediatric nurse. Triage of a child in the ED does not require that the nurse be familiar with every childhood disease, medication, and neurologic reflex, nor does it require a bevy of specialized equipment. Pediatric triage does require an understanding of some concepts, including the following:

1. Anatomic, physiologic, and developmental differences
2. Recognition of the critically ill child, based on these differences
3. Recognition of conditions leading to pediatric arrest (hypoxia and shock) and appropriate interventions
4. Dealing with parents
5. "Rules" of pediatric triage

Children are more difficult to evaluate than adults for several reasons, including the following:

1. Symptoms may be less specific, such as fever.
2. Communication is difficult; the nurse must depend on the parent for history.
3. The child's response to illness and injury depends on the current developmental stage.
4. Children can compensate for longer periods of time; thus they may not be outwardly symptomatic even though they have a life-threatening condition: normal vital signs do not always indicate a stable condition.
5. Vital signs may be difficult to obtain, and appropriately sized equipment (such as blood pressure cuffs) must be available.

Because recognition is the first step in prevention, initial triage and assessment of the child are important. This chapter discusses pediatric triage and assessment based on the anatomic, physiologic and developmental differences of the child and the signs and symptoms in the pediatric patient that may indicate serious illness or injury.

SPECIAL CONSIDERATIONS FOR CHILDREN: THE DIFFERENCES

Children are different. Some of these differences are quite obvious (size, dependency, and inability to communicate). Others, although less obvious, are important to keep in mind when performing the triage examination and assigning an urgency to the child's condition (Fig. 47-1).

Airway, Breathing, and Circulation

The most important differences between children and adults lie in the respiratory and circulatory systems, airway, breathing, and circulation (the ABCs). These differences and nursing implications are listed in Table 47-1. Respiratory disorders are the most common cause of illness in infants and children and are the third most common group of diseases that cause death in the 1- to 14-year-old age-

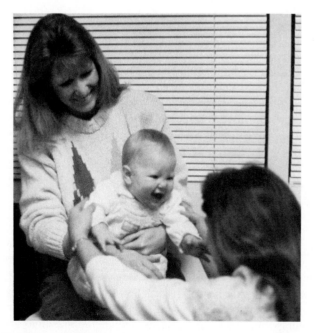

Fig. 47-1 During initial assessment, emergency nurse must take time to gain child's and parent's trust.

Table 47-1 Pediatric triage: differences in airway, breathing, and circulation

Factor	Nursing Considerations
AIRWAY	
Large tongue	Airway can easily become obstructed by tongue; proper positioning is often all that is necessary to open the airway
Smaller diameter of all airways; in 1-year-old child, tracheal diameter is less than child's little finger	Small amounts of mucus or swelling can easily obstruct the airways; child normally has increased airway resistance
Cartilage of larynx is softer than adults	Airway of infant can be compressed if neck is flexed or hyperextended; provides a natural seal for endotracheal tube; cuffed tubes are not necessary in children less than 8 years of age and may damage airway
Cricoid cartilage is narrowest portion of larynx	
BREATHING	
Sternum and ribs are cartilaginous; chest wall is soft; intercostal muscles are poorly developed; infants are obligate nose breathers for first 4 weeks of life; increased metabolic rate (about twice that of an adult); increased respiratory demand for oxygen consumption and carbon dioxide elimination	Infant's chest wall may move inward instead of outward during inspiration (retractions) when lung compliance is decreased; greater intrathoracic pressure is generated during inspiration; anything causing nasal obstruction can produce respiratory distress; respiratory distress increases oxygen demand, as does any condition that increases metabolic rate, such as fever
CIRCULATION	
Child's circulating blood volume is larger per unit of body weight, but absolute volume is relatively small; 70% to 80% of newborn's body weight is water (compared to 50% to 60% of adult body weight); about one half of this volume is extracellular	Blood loss considered minor in an adult may lead to shock in child; decreased fluid intake or increased fluid loss can quickly lead to dehydration
Increased heart rate, decreased stroke volume (cardiac output equals heart rate times stroke volume); cardiac output is higher per unit of body weight	Tachycardia is the child's most efficient method of increasing cardiac output and is the first sign of shock; CO decreases if heart rate is greater than 180 to 200 beats per min

From Hazinski MF: *Nursing care of the critically ill child,* St Louis, 1984, Mosby–Year Book; Holsclaw DS: Early recognition of acute respiratory failure in children, *Pediatr Ann* 6:57, 1977.

group, after cancer and congenital malformations.[5] The triage nurse must be familiar with pediatric anatomic and physiologic differences of the airway and common conditions that may predispose a child to respiratory distress. Respiratory distress is the preceding event in most pediatric cardiac arrests.[6] Hypovolemic shock is another common cause of cardiac arrest in the pediatric patient. Recognition of respiratory distress and shock and early intervention to prevent cardiac arrest are two main objectives of the initial triage assessment.

Types of Complaints

Complaints of children who enter the ED are different from those of adults. For example, cardiac complaints are uncommon in pediatric patients (except for those children with congenital heart disease), but respiratory complaints are common. Because young children have decreased immunity, they have increased susceptibility to infections and have frequent colds, ear infections, and gastrointestinal infections. Unintentional ingestions of poisonous substances

are common in children, whereas ingestions as a suicide gesture are more common in adults. Children are generally a healthy lot and usually come in without histories of chronic conditions or numerous allergies and medications, which makes history taking much easier and certainly briefer.

Childhood injuries are often developmentally related and frequently preventable. For example, motor vehicle accidents, a major cause of death, are often related to lack of safety restraints in young children. As the child becomes more mobile, bicycle, skateboard, and roller blade accidents become more prevalent. Drowning accidents occur because of lack of supervision in younger children and because older children attempt to swim beyond their ability.

Although pediatric complaints in the ED may be different, the goals of triage remain the same: to recognize the emergent situations and to intervene quickly to prevent deterioration. In pediatrics, triage may mean differentiating between the sick child and the obviously seriously ill child. This step is the most important and often the most difficult aspect of triage.

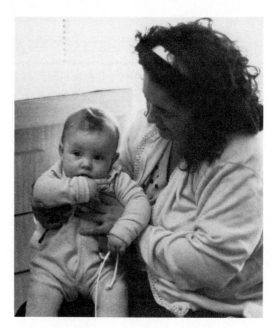

Fig. 47-2 Emergency nurse needs to listen to parent's concerns and assessment of child's condition.

Dealing with Parents

The child is usually accompanied to the ED by someone who knows him or her better than anyone else, a parent or guardian. The triage nurse must depend on this person for the history and symptoms. Often the triage nurse can learn much by asking, "What worries you the most about your child?" Even if the complaint seems trivial, the nurse must try not to be judgmental, since the parent's main concern is the child's welfare. The nurse needs to listen to the parent, since he or she may intuitively know that the child is ill (Fig. 47-2).

"Rules" of Pediatric Triage

The following general, unofficial "rules" may assist the triage nurse in evaluating the child:
1. Parents know their children better than you do: listen to them. The parent's history can give good clues to the cause of the illness or injury and help the triage nurse to determine urgency.
2. The anxiety of the parent may be inversely proportional to the degree of illness or injury of the child. This rule also has exceptions. The corollary to this rule should be to *look* at all children, no matter what the chief complaint may be and no matter how calm the parent is.
3. Remember the ABCs: kids are different. These differences are described in Table 47-1. Do not focus on the obvious, because a subtle, more serious problem can be overlooked.

4. Some kids can talk and walk and still be in shock. You cannot always depend on the appearance of the child. The history and vital signs must be considered, but normal vital signs should not give a false sense of security. Vital signs are discussed later in this chapter.
5. Never tell a parent that his or her child cannot be evaluated in the ED, no matter what the chief complaint is. With the development of preferred provider and health maintenance organizations, authorization for payment may be refused. Remember that you must make sure that the parent realizes that it is the authorization for *payment* that is being denied, not authorization for *care*. A triage assessment still must be performed and documented before referral elsewhere, to evaluate whether immediate care is needed.

THE PEDIATRIC TRIAGE EXAMINATION

Depending on the facility, the triage examination may be brief, involving only taking a chief complaint and looking at the child, or the initial assessment may include obtaining vital signs and providing some treatment such as antipyretics, splinting, or ice packs. Whatever triage protocols exist, the most important aspect is prompt assessment that includes observation and history.

Although only a primary assessment may be performed at the triage area, the secondary assessment is also included in this discussion.

History and Observation

Remember rule no. 2. The history is an important part of the pediatric triage assessment. In small infants, the history may be vague and nonspecific and may be limited by the parent's ability to give it. The "AMPLE" mnemonic (*a*llergies, *m*edications, *p*ast medical history, *l*ast meal, *e*vents surrounding incident) is useful in eliciting a history. Past medical history is important in determining if the child has a prior condition that may affect the assessment (congenital heart disease or a chronic respiratory condition). A good question to ask the parent may be, "What does your child normally look like?" or "Does he or she look normal to you?"

Observation variables (playfulness, eye contact, attention to environment) have been shown to be more important than history in predicting serious illness.[3,9] The triage nurse can usually observe the child while obtaining the history or while performing the assessment. Observation may have to be performed as a separate entity of the examination to allow the child to feel comfortable and may take more time than the busy ED nurse has.

Observation scales and scoring systems have been developed to assist in identifying sick children. These scoring systems are general and do not apply to any organ system but may be a useful tool for the triage nurse. An example of an observation scoring system is shown in Table 47-2.

Table 47-2 Predictive model: six observation items and their scales

Observation item	Normal	Moderate impairment	Severe impairment
Quality of cry	Strong with normal tone; content and not crying	Whimpering or sobbing	Weak, moaning, or high-pitched
Reaction to parenteral stimulation	Cries briefly, then stops; content and not crying	Cries off and on	Continual cry or hardly responds
State variation	If awake, stays awake; if asleep and stimulated, wakes up quickly	Eyes close briefly; awake or awakes after prolonged stimulation	Falls asleep or will not rouse
Skin color	Pink	Pale extremities or acrocyanosis	Pale, cyanotic, mottled, or ashen
Hydration	Skin normal; eyes normal; mucous membranes moist	Skin normal; eyes normal; mouth slightly dry	Skin doughy or tented, dry mucous membranes, sunken eyes
Response (talk, smile) to social overtures	Smiles or alerts (less than or equal to 2 months of age)	Brief smile or alerts briefly (less than or equal to 2 months of age)	No smile; face anxious, dull, expressionless; no alerting (less than or equal to 2 months of age)

From McCarthy PL et al: Predictive values: observation scales to identify serious illness in febrile children, *Pediatrics* 70(5):802, 1982.

Pediatric Primary Assessment

The primary assessment consists of evaluation of the ABCs and the neurologic status and may be the only part of the assessment performed at triage to determine urgency.

Respiratory assessment. Rule no. 3 applies here. Any child with symptoms of respiratory distress requires immediate attention. The triage nurse can use observation variables listed in Table 47-2 and clinical signs and symptoms to help determine the degree of respiratory distress. A child who comes to the ED with respiratory complaints but is running around and looks well is probably not in respiratory distress, whereas one who is listless and pale may be in moderate to severe distress.

Signs and symptoms of increased work of breathing caused by respiratory distress include the following:

1. Retractions, that is, a sinking in of soft tissues relative to the cartilaginous and bony thorax[13]
2. Nasal flaring and use of accessory muscles
3. Tachypnea
4. Adventitious breath sounds: wheezing and grunting are indicative of lower airway obstruction, whereas a barking cough or stridor usually indicates upper airway obstruction.
5. Dysphagia and drooling, which usually indicates upper airway obstruction

Signs and symptoms of severe hypoxia include the following:

1. Bradycardia (Bradycardia in children is almost always caused by hypoxia.)
2. Agitation or decreased level of consciousness
3. Pale skin or cyanosis (Cyanosis is a late sign indicating severe hypoxia.)

4. Head bobbing (an up-and-down movement of the head with each breath)
5. Preference of a child for a certain position
6. Hypoventilation or apnea

Usually the child can remain in the parent's lap during the examination. The child's shirt can be unbuttoned so that the nurse can observe the chest movements and listen to breath sounds. Breath sounds and their significance are summarized in Table 47-3. The oxygen saturation level is also helpful in determining the degree of distress and is easy to evaluate during triage if pulse oximeters are available (Fig. 47-3).

Any child in respiratory distress deserves immediate triage and intervention. The differential diagnosis of respiratory distress is based on the history and clinical signs and symptoms. The box on p. 662 lists some common causes of respiratory distress in children.

Despite the cause of respiratory distress, the treatment is recognition and the administration of oxygen. Oxygen can be administered by cannula or mask or by the "blow by" technique, in which the parent holds the oxygen tubing in front of the infant's nares and mouth.

Other interventions for the child who is in respiratory distress include the following:

1. Allow the child to maintain a position of comfort.
2. Allow the parent to remain with and hold the child.
3. Have the physician see the child as soon as possible.
4. Observe for signs of increasing distress.

The child with symptoms of severe distress needs further intervention, which may include the use of bronchodilators or intubation.

Cardiovascular assessment. The goal of obtaining a car-

Table 47-3   Abnormal breath sounds and their significance in children*

Breath sound	Significance
Stridor, an inspiratory crowing sound	Caused by upper airway obstruction; high-pitched in croup and foreign body aspiration, low-pitched and muffled in epiglottitis
Wheezing (usually inspiratory but may be expiratory)	Caused by lower airway obstructions; bilateral wheezing suggests asthma or bronchiolitis; unilateral wheezing suggests foreign body aspiration
Decreased or unequal breath sounds	Airway obstruction, pneumothorax, pleural effusion
Grunting	Caused by early closure of the glottis during exhalation with active chest wall contraction; increases expiratory airway pressure, preventing airway collapse; creates positive end expiratory pressure (PEEP); seen in diseases with diminished lung compliance such as pulmonary edema; also occurs as a result of pain

*Breath sounds should be assessed over the lateral chest wall and over the anterior chest. Breath sounds heard only over the anterior chest may be misleading, because the child's thin chest wall allows transmission of central airway breath sounds.
From American Academy of Pediatrics and American College of Emergency Physicians: *Advanced pediatric life support*, Elk Grove Village, Ill, and Dallas, 1989, The Academy and College.

diovascular assessment in the child is to recognize shock or conditions that might lead to shock and to intervene to prevent cardiovascular collapse. The history of the illness or injury is important in interpreting signs and symptoms. Observation of the child plays a major role as well. The following elements are important to observe:

1. Color of the child. Pallor may indicate decreased perfusion caused by diminished cardiac output.
2. Capillary refill. Capillary refill is measured by applying pressure to the nail beds or forehead, releasing, and watching for the return of circulation, which should occur in 2 seconds. A delay of 5 seconds or more is abnormal.
3. Level of consciousness. Decreased perfusion to the brain may result in lethargy and confusion.

The triage nurse should also assess the following:

1. Skin turgor. Check mucous membranes for moistness.
2. Anterior fontanel. A bulging fontanel may indicate increased intracranial pressure, whereas a sunken fontanel may indicate dehydration.

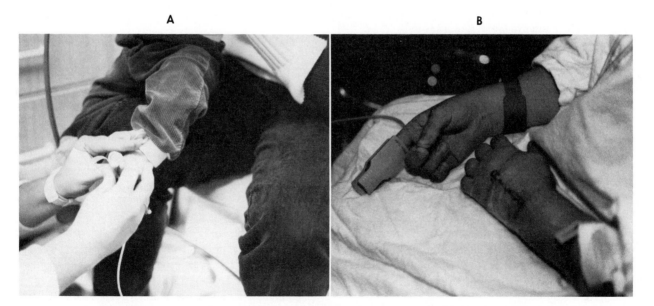

Fig. 47-3   Use of pulse oximeter can help determine degree of respiratory distress. Different probes are available. For infants, **A,** finger or toe probes. For older, more cooperative children, **B,** finger probe.

CAUSES OF RESPIRATORY DISTRESS IN CHILDREN

Upper airway
Croup
Epiglottitis
Foreign body aspiration
Other infections (bacterial tracheitis, retropharyngeal abscesses)
Congenital anomalies

Lower airway
Asthma
Bronchiolitis
Pneumonia
Foreign body
Trauma

---

3. Peripheral pulse rates. Decreased perfusion to extremities results in weak peripheral pulse(s).
4. Vital signs: temperature, pulse rate, respiration rate, and blood pressure. Average vital signs for the pediatric patient are listed in Table 47-4.

Vital signs must be documented as part of the baseline assessment. Remember rule no. 5. Children in early shock, because of their ability to compensate, may have a normal blood pressure reading initially. A dropping blood pressure is a serious sign that warrants immediate intervention. A child can lose a significant amount of blood before the blood pressure decreases. Table 47-4 lists average blood pressures by age. Another method of estimating normal blood pressure is to use the following formula:

$$\text{Systolic pressure} = 80 + (\text{Age in years} \times 2)$$

Tachycardia may be the first sign of shock in a child but is often hard to evaluate, since tachycardia can also be related to fever and anxiety. Tachycardia in a lethargic child could be indicative of early shock. To compensate, the heart rate in a child with decreased cardiac output will increase.

Table 47-4 Average vital signs by age

	Pulse rate (beats/min)	Respiration rate (breaths/min)	Blood pressure
Newborn	120 to 160	40 to 60	80/40
1 year	80 to 140	30 to 40	82/44
3 years	80 to 120	25 to 30	86/50
5 years	70 to 115	20 to 25	90/52
7 years	70 to 115	20 to 25	94/54
10 years	70 to 115	15 to 20	100/60
15 years	70 to 90	15 to 20	110/64

Hypervolemic shock is the most common type of shock in the pediatric patient and is caused by decreased circulating blood volume.[1] As stated in Table 47-1, the child has less total blood volume than an adult has. An infant has approximately 80 mg/kg of circulating blood volume, neonates have about 90 ml/kg, older children have about 70 mg/kg, and adults have 65 to 70 mg/kg.[4,7] Children can become hypovolemic from undetected bleeding more rapidly than adults can. Also, because of the large proportion of total body water contained in the extracellular fluid, a child with decreased fluid intake and increased losses because of vomiting and diarrhea can quickly become dehydrated.

The goals in the treatment of shock are early recognition, maintaining the airway, and supporting the circulation with intravenous fluids. Early recognition is the responsibility of the triage nurse and is the most important factor in the final outcome. The treatment of shock is discussed in greater detail in Chapter 49.

Neurologic assessment. Many scales exist for evaluating the neurologic status of a child. The Glasgow coma scale is a commonly used method and is discussed in Chapter 49.

The two most important parts of the neurologic examination, which are performed in the triage area, are the history and the evaluation of the child's level of consciousness

Table 47-5 AEIOU TIPS mnemonic for evaluating altered level of consciousness

Cause	Comments
*A*lcohol	More common in adolescents than in younger pediatric patients
*E*ncephalopathy	Hypertension, hepatic, Reye's syndrome
*E*ndocrinology	Thyroid, adrenal
*E*lectrolytes	Alterations in sodium, potassium, calcium, or magnesium levels
*I*nsulin	Hypoglycemia or hyperglycemia
*I*ntussusception	Decreased level of conciousness may be the first manifestation of intussusception before abdominal symptoms appear
*O*verdose	Opiates and other toxins, ingested, inhaled, or transferred to the fetus before birth
*U*remia	Hemolytic uremic syndrome, chronic renal impairment
*T*rauma	One of the major causes; usually, head injuries and chest injuries leading to hypoxia
*I*nfection	More common in children than in adults; meningitis, encephalitis, Reye's syndrome and sepsis
*P*sychiatric	Rare in children; should only be considered after other factors are ruled out
*S*eizure	Postictal states, syncope

From American Academy of Pediatrics and American College of Emergency Physicians: Advanced pediatric life support, Elk Grove Village, Ill, and Dallas, 1989, The Academy and College.

(see box below). The AVPU mnemonic (*a*lert, responds to *v*erbal stimuli, responds to *p*ainful stimuli, *u*nresponsive) can be used to evaluate and describe level of consciousness, especially for the preverbal child.

Evaluating the history and the level of consciousness can

MININEUROLOGIC EXAMINATION

History

1. Time and mechanisms of injury
2. Neurologic status when patient is first seen after injury; elapsed time between time of injury and arrival in hospital.
3. Any neurologic change that may have occurred.

Level of consciousness

1. Aware. May be disoriented or confused but still awake
2. Lethargic. Can be aroused to follow commands
3. Stuporous. Cannot be aroused to follow commands; purposeful withdrawal in response to deep painful stimuli
4. Semicomatose. Only reflex responses to pain, that is, decorticate or decerebrate
5. Comatose. No response to pain

Pupils

1. Size. Equal or not equal
2. Reaction to light

Response to pain

1. Purposeful
2. Semipurposeful
3. Decorticate
4. Decerebrate
5. No response

Movement of extremities

1. Spontaneous
2. Response to pain

Plantar responses

1. Upgoing
2. Downgoing
3. Equivocal

Facial movements

Central or peripheral weakness may be present

Fundi

Describe hemorrhages. Rare to see papilledema sooner than 12 to 24 hours after injury

Cerebrospinal fluid otorrhea or rhinorrhea

Usually blood with or without cerebrospinal fluid in acute phase

Vital signs

Obtain baseline; monitor closely

From Matlak M et al: *Initial management of the injured child*, 1980, Salt Lake City, Primary Children's Medical Center.

---

be enough to classify the child's condition as an emergency. An altered level of consciousness in any child is considered an emergency condition.

A commonly used mnemonic, AEIOU TIPS, is useful when causes for altered level of consciousness are being considered (Table 47-5). Intussusception as a cause of altered consciousness in the infant has been added to this mnemonic, since lethargy has been found to be a common symptom of this condition.[8]

Treatment of children who arrive at the ED with an altered level of consciousness includes assessment of airway, breathing, and circulation and assessment for injury or illnesses. The child must be evaluated for symptoms of increased intracranial pressure to prevent central nervous system injury. Laboratory studies may be ordered to detect presence of toxins or electrolyte abnormalities.

Secondary Assessment

The secondary assessment consists of obtaining vital signs and performing a head-to-toe survey. During triage the secondary assessment is usually limited to evaluating the area of the chief complaint; the rest of the examination is performed later, when the patient is taken to a treatment room. The secondary assessment is summarized in Table 47-6.

Things to remember when performing a secondary assessment on a child include the following:

1. Do not focus on the obvious injury. Remember rule no. 3.
2. Do not be fooled by a known patient with a chronic condition. Listen to the parent's concerns (rule no. 1).
3. Consider child abuse in suspect circumstances. Know your responsibility in reporting.
4. Communicate your findings to other personnel, and document your assessment. Parents offer information to the triage nurse, then assume they don't have to mention it again.
5. Practice doing assessments on all children when time permits. This practice will help improve your assessment skills with children.

Vital Signs

All triage systems should include obtaining vital signs in the initial assessment, including temperature, pulse rate, respiration rate, blood pressure, and weight. The weight can be considered the "fifth vital sign" and is necessary because all medications are based on the weight of the child.

Pulse and respiration rates can be obtained while the nurse is evaluating airway and breathing. Temperatures are easily obtained, especially with the availability of thermometers that measure temperature of the tympanic membrane. Blood pressures are often deferred because a cuff of the right size is not available or because the child resists the procedure. Blood pressure cuffs are inexpensive and should be available. The cuff must cover about two thirds of the upper arm; a cuff that is too small will give a falsely high reading,

Table 47-6 Pediatric secondary assessment

Body area	Conditions to be assessed
Head	Presence of injuries; presence of pain or tenderness; anterior fontanel: depressed, flat, bulging (Most infants have an open anterior fontanel until about the age of 18 months.)
Eyes	Pupils: size and reaction; presence of tears; movement of eyes; drainage or periorbital swelling; presence of injuries; visual acuity (if appropriate)
Ears	Drainage; presence of pain; bruising behind ears (may indicate basal skull fracture)
Nose	Nasal flaring: may indicate increased respiratory effort; odor: foul odor may indicate presence of foreign body
Throat. Do not attempt to examine if child is in severe respiratory distress	Swelling or exudates in pharynx; swelling of cervical lymph nodes
Mouth	Color of oral mucosa; presence of lesions; moistness of lips and mucous membranes; odor of breath
Chest	Respiratory status as indicated during primary assessment; presence of rashes or bruising; presence of tenderness
Abdomen	Distention; bowel sounds; tenderness
Genitalia and rectum (may be assessed when rectal temperature is being taken or may be deferred)	Diaper rash; vaginal discharge or irritation; odor; rectal bleeding or tears; discharge from penis; trauma
Skin, extremities, and bilateral comparison	Presence of swelling; examine deformity; pain; movement; sensation; color; pulse rates; presence of rashes or bruising
Vital signs	Temperature, pulse rate, respiration rate, blood pressure, weight

Table 47-7 Some causes of abnormal vital signs in children

Vital sign and variation	Causes and nursing considerations
TEMPERATURE	
Hyperthermia (fever)	Viral infections: most common cause (upper respiratory, gastrointestinal); bacterial infections (pneumonia, otitis media, urinary tract infections, bacteremia); collagen vascular diseases (rheumatic fever, Schönlein-Henoch purpura); drug intoxications (salicylates, atropine, amphetamines); malignancies; because infants localize infections poorly, any infant under 3 months of age with a fever should be evaluated as soon as possible to rule out serious bacterial infection
Hypothermia	Sepsis; shock; exposure; infants have an unstable temperature-regulating mechanism and can become hypothermic as a result of exposure; hypothermia can lead to metabolic acidosis, decreased respiration rates, bradycardia, and cardiopulmonary arrest; every attempt should be made to keep an infant warm
PULSE RATE	
Bradycardia	Most common cause is hypoxia (Bradycardia equals hypoxia until proven otherwise.); other causes include hypotension, acidosis, drug ingestions (narcotics, sedatives); bradycardia in children is always an emergency condition, possibly signalling impending arrest; supplemental oxygen should always be provided immediately, as well as any other interventions to support airway, breathing, and circulation
Tachycardia	Earliest sign of shock; supraventricular tachycardia is the most common dysrhythmia in children[2]; other common causes include anxiety, fever, ingestions (anticholinergics, tricyclic antidepressants)
RESPIRATION RATE	
Tachypnea	"Quiet" tachypnea (occurs with no other signs of respiratory distress): consider diabetes, ketoacidosis, poisonings, or dehydration; other causes of tachypnea include respiratory distress, fever, and congestive heart failure in the child who has congenital heart disease
Bradypnea	Respiratory failure; shock; acidosis; hypothermia; ingestions (narcotics)
BLOOD PRESSURE	
Hypertension	Increased intracranial pressure; renal disease; cardiovascular disease (children with coarctation of the aorta have increased blood pressure in upper extremities, as compared with blood pressure in lower extremities); endocrinologic disorders; drugs (pressor agents, corticosteroids, amphetamines)
Hypotension	Shock (late sign); drug ingestions (tricyclic antidepressants, narcotics, clonidine)

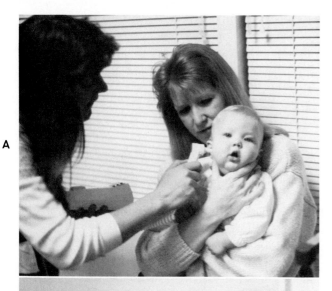

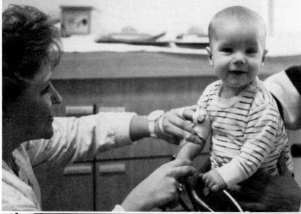

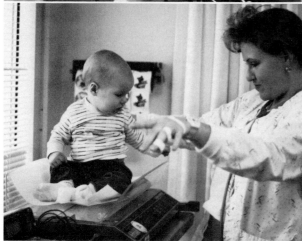

Fig. 47-4 **A,** Tympanic thermometers make taking child's temperature in triage area easy and nontraumatic. **B,** Obtaining measurements of blood pressure should be part of assessment. Cuff must cover about two thirds of upper arm. **C,** Weight should be considered "fifth vital sign" and is necessary for calculating dosages of medications and fluids.

Table 47-8 Triage categories and examples for pediatric patients

Category	Definition and examples
Emergent	Children who have a condition that may result in loss of life or limb if not treated immediately; examples include cardiopulmonary arrest, coma, and uncontrolled bleeding
Urgent	Children who require prompt care but will not be in danger of death or severe impairment if left untreated for a period of time, usually a few hours; examples include lacerations with bleeding controlled and possible nondisplaced fractures without neurologic impairment
Nonurgent	Children with nonurgent complaints require treatment, but time is not a critical factor; examples include sore throats, mild gastroenteritis, and minor sprains

whereas one that is too big will give a falsely low reading (Fig. 47-4).

The weight of the child can be obtained at triage or estimated. Weight is important for calculating medication doses, assessing degree of dehydration, and comparing a child's growth and development to the normal growth and development for that age-group.

The triage nurse needs to be aware that vital signs vary with the age of the child (Table 47-5). Alterations from normal must be viewed along with the child's history and other signs and symptoms. Some causes of alterations in vital signs are listed in Table 47-7.

CLASSIFICATION SYSTEMS FOR PEDIATRIC PATIENTS

The triage codes used in most EDs consist of the terms *emergent, urgent,* and *nonurgent.* This system can be and is used with the pediatric patient. Table 47-8 defines these categories and gives examples of conditions for each.

Classifying conditions into rigid categories is difficult in pediatric emergency nursing. Fever, for example, could be considered a nonurgent condition, but if it exists in an infant under 3 months of age, it becomes an urgent condition.

Use of Algorithms

Using algorithms based on symptoms can be a useful way to determine urgency in pediatrics. These algorithms should serve only as a guideline in establishing urgency and are not the "golden rule." They are helpful when orienting staff to triage and show the thought process that must be involved.

Figs. 47-5 to 47-9 are examples of algorithms for fever, respiratory distress, lethargy, rashes, and vomiting or diarrhea, which are common complaints in the ED.

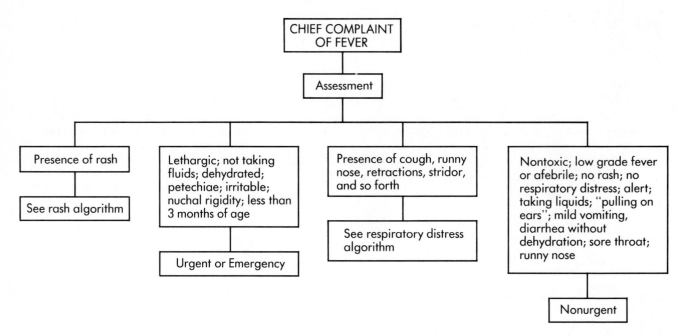

Fig. 47-5 Algorithm for chief complaint of fever. (From Laura S. Cambell.)

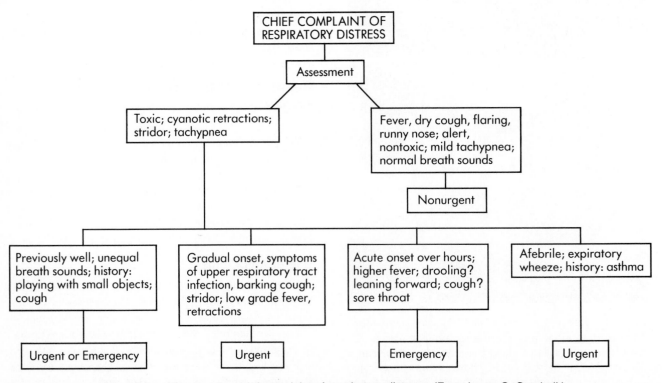

Fig. 47-6 Algorithm for chief complaint of respiratory distress. (From Laura S. Cambell.)

INITIATING TREATMENT IN THE TRIAGE AREA

Treatment can be initiated in the triage area if supporting protocols and policies exist. Initial treatment usually is limited to the following:

1. Administering antipyretics. Fifteen milligrams per kilogram body weight of acetaminophen is the antipyretic of choice. Aspirin is not used to treat fever because of its association with Reye's syndrome.
2. Basic first aid, including ice packs, splinting, and bandages
3. Initiating laboratory or radiologic studies. Protocols should exist to establish which laboratory tests or radiologic examinations can be ordered by the nurse.

Generally the nurse is permitted to order extremity films.

Administering antipyretics seems to be the most common treatment given to children at triage. This treatment helps make the child more comfortable during the wait and allows the physician to better evaluate the child. Of course, any interventions performed during triage should be documented.

LEGAL ISSUES IN PEDIATRIC TRIAGE

Many risk factors exist in triage of the pediatric patient. Most of these are related to a failure to recognize an emergency condition. Errors commonly made include the

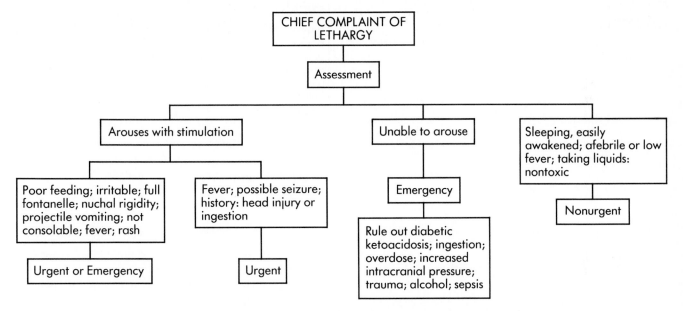

Fig. 47-7 Algorithm for chief complaint of lethargy. (From Laura S. Cambell.)

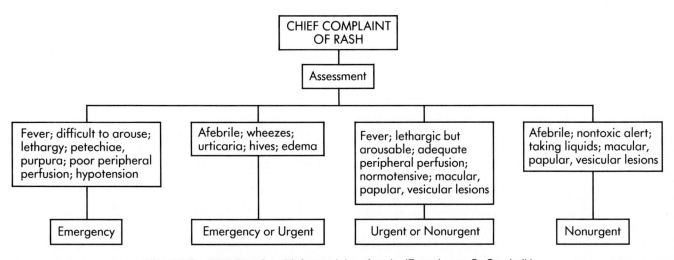

Fig. 47-8 Algorithm for chief complaint of rash. (From Laura S. Cambell.)

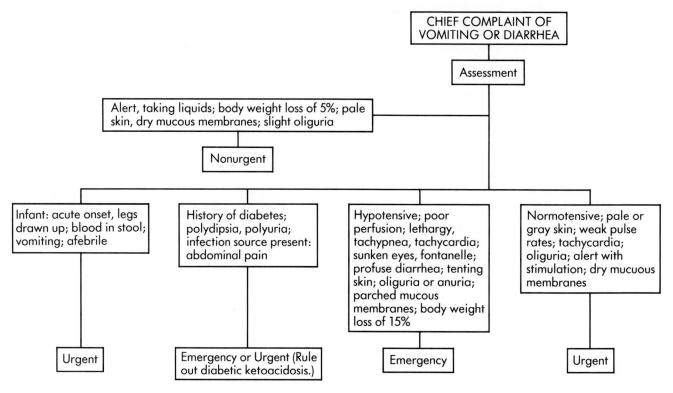

Fig. 47-9   Algorithm for chief complaint of vomiting or diarrhea. (From Laura S. Cambell.)

following[6]:

1. Failure to recognize respiratory distress
2. Failure to recognize shock
3. Failure to recognize a potentially lethal injury

Prompt triage, assessment, and intervention can prevent these situations. Nurses also need to be properly trained in pediatric assessment skills.

Telephone Advice Calls (Nurse Calls)

Emergency department personnel are frequently asked to give medical advice over the telephone. For obvious legal reasons, many EDs are opting not to give this advice. It has been recommended that EDs not give advice unless the situation is an extreme emergency or the patient has been seen recently in the facility.[6] If the child has been seen recently in the ED, additional entry should be made on the chart concerning the telephone call. Other callers should be told, "I'm sorry, I cannot give you any medical advice over the telephone. We would be happy to evaluate your child if you bring your child to the hospital."[10]

Giving advice to parents over the phone is a good public relations program. If a hospital decides to set up such a program, the following criteria should be followed[11,12]:

1. Advice given should be governed by policies and standards of care.
2. A policy should exist stating who will take the calls;

a registered nurse or a physician, not an ED clerk or secretary, should handle all calls.
3. Legal counsel should be obtained to review the policies and standards of care.
4. A quality assurance mechanism should be in place to allow for review of calls and advice given and for updating protocols.
5. All calls should be documented, including the name of the child, age, private physician, problem, advice given, follow-up care provided, and family's phone number.
6. Advice given should be based on symptoms and should not be diagnostic.
7. Parents should always be told that they may be seen in the ED at any time, no matter what the problem is (remember rule no. 5).

Taking advice calls takes nursing staff away from other ED duties. If the hospital decides to develop a program for handling these types of calls, the ED should attempt to obtain designated staff to handle the calls.

SUGGESTED PEDIATRIC TRAINING

Nurses who care for children in adult facilities should have baseline training and frequent updating of their pediatric skills, especially in the area of assessment. Some of this training can be obtained through continuing education and by contacting the nearest pediatric facility to arrange in-service programs.

The American Heart Association and other agencies have developed advanced pediatric life support programs. These are excellent classes that offer lectures and practice sessions in the areas of recognition and intervention. The Emergency Nurses Association and the Emergency Medical Services for Children Project are cooperating in the development of a pediatric emergency nursing course, which will be in the form of self-study modules.

General knowledge requirements should include the following:

1. Pediatric assessment skills, including emphasis on recognition of respiratory distress, shock, other life-threatening situations, and the anatomic and physiologic variables that make children different
2. Advanced pediatric life support, which includes intervention skills
3. Protocols for managing pediatric trauma
4. Equipment necessary to care for the pediatric patient (see Chapter 49)
5. Knowledge of transport protocols, including how to initiate transfer and stabilization before transport

SUMMARY

Pediatric triage involves recognition of life-threatening conditions in children to ensure prompt intervention. Pediatric triage is a blend of good nursing assessment, history, and observation, focusing on the child, not the complaint.

Emergency nurses must always keep in mind the differences in children that make them unique anatomically, physiologically, and socially. Constant practice and necessary education, as well as obeying the "rules" of triage, increase the confidence level of the ED nurse and improve the care of the child.

REFERENCES

1. American Academy of Pediatrics and American College of Emergency Physicians: *Advanced pediatric life support,* Elk Grove Village, Ill, and Dallas, 1989, The Academy and College.
2. Danilowicz D: Dysrhythmias in children. In Zimmerman S, Gildea JH, eds: *Critical care pediatrics,* ed 2, Philadelphia, 1985, WB Saunders.
3. Guraraj VJ et al: To tap or not to tap? What are the best indicators for performing an LP in an outpatient child? *Clin Pediatr* 12:488, 1973.
4. Hazinski MF: *Nursing care of the critically ill child,* St Louis, 1984, Mosby–Year Book.
5. Holsclaw DS: Early recognition of acute respiratory failure in children, *Pediatr Ann* 6:57, 1977.
6. Luten R: *Problems in pediatric emergency medicine,* New York, 1988, Churchill Livingstone.
7. Matlak M et al: *Initial management of the injured child* (booklet), Salt Lake City, 1980, Primary Children's Medical Center.
8. McCabe J et al: Intussusception: a supplement to the mnemonic for coma, *Pediatr Emerg Care* 3:118, 1987.
9. McCarthy P et al: History and observation variables in assessing febrile children, *Pediatrics* 65:6, 1980.
10. Selbst S, Korin J: The telephone in pediatric emergency medicine, *Pediatr Emerg Care* 1:108, 1985.
11. Thomas DO: The ABCs of pediatric triage, *JEN* 14:154, 1988.
12. Verdie V: Emergency department telephone advice, *Ann Emerg Med* 18:278, 1989.
13. Whaley L, Wong D: *Nursing care of infants and children,* ed 3, St Louis, 1986, Mosby–Year Book.

SUGGESTED READINGS

Baldwin G: *Handbook of pediatric emergencies,* Boston, 1989, Little Brown.
Barkin R: *The emergently ill child,* Rockville, Md, 1987, Aspen.
Brown J: *Pediatric telephone medicine: principles, triage, and advice,* Philadelphia, 1989, JB Lippincott.
Eichelberger M, Stossel-Pratsch G: *Pediatric emergencies manual,* Baltimore, 1984, University Park Press.
Fleisher G, Ludwig S: *Textbook of pediatric emergency care,* Baltimore, 1988, Williams & Wilkins.
Katz H: *Telephone manual of pediatric care,* New York, 1982, John Wiley & Sons.
Kelley S: *Pediatric emergency nursing,* Norwalk, Conn, 1988, Appleton & Lange, 1988.
Long S: Approach to the febrile patient with no obvious focus of infection, *Pediatr Rev* 5:305, 1984.
McCarthy P et al: Predictive values: observation scales to identify serious illness in febrile children, *Pediatrics* 70:802, 1982.
McGear R, Simms J: *Telephone triage and management: a nursing approach,* Philadelphia, 1988, WB Saunders.
Perkin R, Levin D: Shock in the pediatric patient. Part I. *J Pediatr* 101:163, 1982.
Perkin R, Levin D: Shock in the pediatric patient. Part II: therapy, *J Pediatr* 101:319, 1982.
Rund D, Rausch T: *Triage,* St Louis, 1981, Mosby–Year Book.
Schmitt B: *Pediatric telephone advice,* Boston, 1980, Little Brown.
Thomas DO: The ABCs of pediatric emergencies, *RN* 49:34, 1986.
Thompson J, Dains J: Comprehensive triage: a manual for developing and implementing a nursing care system, Reston, Va, 1982, Reston.

Pediatric Medical Emergencies

Deborah P. Henderson and **Martha M. Bohner**

Few emergencies cause more anxiety for ED personnel than pediatric illnesses and injuries. From the initial radio call, or on arrival of a frantic caretaker bringing in a sick child, there is a heightened sense of urgency and increased activity in the emergency setting. One reason for the anxiety is a general concern for all young children. Other reasons are that these children need special sizes of equipment, drug dosages measured on a per kilogram basis, and precise fluid administration protocols. Care of the child also requires emergency personnel to draw on less frequently used knowledge of the illnesses and injuries unique to the pediatric age-group.

The admonition that "children are not little adults" may only increase anxiety about caring for pediatric patients. Although it is true that there are differences in some aspects of care, it is more important to remember that the basic principles are the same for children and adults. As with adults, diseases affecting the airway, breathing, and circulation, and the neurologic status of pediatric patients, are of primary concern. For both children and adults, rapid assessment and early intervention are critical when there is airway compromise, cardiovascular instability, or altered mental status. The greatest difference in attending to the needs of children is in early recognition of children's physiologic responses to hypoxia and circulatory problems. Learning the differences in these responses allows intervention before decompensation occurs. Also helpful in caring for children is a general knowledge of the age ranges for, and the signs, symptoms, and treatment of, serious childhood illnesses. These special issues involved in the assessment and care of medical emergencies in children are discussed in this chapter.

RESPIRATORY EMERGENCIES

Recognition of respiratory distress and failure in the pediatric patient is crucial because respiratory arrest is almost always the precursor to cardiac arrest in children. Once a respiratory emergency has been identified, early intervention may halt the otherwise inevitable progression to respiratory failure, poor tissue perfusion (shock), cardiac ar-

rest, and death. To assist in assessment, respiratory emergencies can be roughly divided into upper and lower respiratory tract problems, and a third category comprising nonrespiratory problems that manifest some of the signs and symptoms of respiratory distress.

Assessment: Signs of Respiratory Distress in Children

General appearance. An awake, well child is alert and active, and, if crying, is easily consoled; skin color is normal, not pale, mottled, or cyanotic. Children who *are* sick generally *look* sick. Observe the child's position. A child in respiratory distress finds a position of comfort with the body leaning slightly forward and the head in the "sniffing" position, as if smelling a flower. This position allows maximum airway opening.

Respiratory rate and pattern. The young child's respiratory muscles are not well developed, and the diaphragm plays an important role in breathing. Chest auscultation and observation of the rise and fall of the abdomen are the best methods for assessing respiratory rate in patients less than 2 years of age. Respiratory rates are often irregular in small children, so the rate should be carefully assessed for a full minute.

Normal respiratory rates vary by age. A neonate has a normal respiratory rate ranging from 30 to 40 breaths/min. The rate slows as the child grows older. With respiratory distress the child's respiratory rate increases initially. *A resting respiratory rate faster than 60 breaths/min must be considered a sign of respiratory distress in a child, regardless of age.* As respiratory failure progresses and the child becomes more acidotic, mental status changes are observed, and the respiratory rate slows. Bradypnea is therefore a serious sign in a pediatric patient; an adult respiratory rate (12 to 16 breaths/min) should be considered an unusually slow rate for any preadolescent child.

Abnormal respiratory patterns such as Cheyne-Stokes respirations (respirations gradually increasing in depth, then decreasing, with periods of apnea interspersed) or Kussmaul's respirations (rapid, deep respirations often associated with diabetic ketoacidosis) indicate, as in an adult, critical illness or injury.

Work of breathing. Children in respiratory distress show increased work of breathing and use accessory muscles (intercostal, spinal extensor, and neck muscles) for breathing. As work of breathing increases, intercostal, substernal, and supraclavicular retractions are seen.

Inspiration is an active process in which muscles are used to expand the chest. Exhalation is passive, relying on the elasticity of the lungs and chest wall. Under normal circumstances these two processes are balanced, and expiration takes roughly the same amount of time as inspiration (inspiration/expiration ratio 1:1). When the air passages are narrowed by inflammation or obstruction, time required for inhalation may remain the same with an increase in effort, but exhalation will take substantially longer than inspiration (inspiration/expiration ratio 1:2 or 1:3).

Quality of breathing. The quality of breathing includes both depth and sound of breathing. The child's chest should expand symmetrically. As in an adult, asymmetry or inadequate expansion indicates serious problems such as pneumothorax or hemothorax, foreign body obstruction, or flail chest. When auscultating a child's chest, place the stethoscope at the anterior axillary line, at the level of the second intercostal space on either side. This will help to identify the location of any abnormal breath sounds. The small size of the child's chest and the thinness of the chest wall cause sounds on one side of the chest to be transmitted throughout the thorax (and even into the abdomen), so listening to the anterior and posterior aspects of the chest may not be as useful for assessment as in an adult.

Mental status. Alertness, relation to caretakers, willingness to play, and consolability are important observations in assessing the mental status of children. Irritability is often a sign of hypoxia, but a restless child who becomes progressively quieter should be carefully assessed to make certain that improved oxygenation rather than respiratory failure or exhaustion is causing the restlessness to abate.

Monitoring. Arterial blood gas analysis gives the clearest picture of the respiratory status of a patient. For pediatric patients the value of this precision must be carefully considered, because additional stress brought on by the procedure is likely to cause further deterioration in the patient's condition.

The pulse oximeter is a useful, noninvasive means of continuously measuring oxygen saturation and correlates well with arterial blood gas measurement of this variable. An oxygen saturation of 90% to 93% is the lowest acceptable range in children. The pulse oximeter's major limitation is that it does not provide any indication of carbon dioxide and acid-base balance. Because pulse oximetry relies on analysis of the color of hemoglobin, it may not be useful when extremity perfusion is diminished from trauma, when there is cold ambient temperature or a vasopressor is used, or when the number of erythrocytes is decreased, as in anemia.

Upper Airway Distress

The upper airway includes the trachea, larynx, glottic opening, epiglottis, pharynx, and the nasal and oral cavities. Upper airway distress in children may be from aspiration of a foreign body or from swelling of structures in the upper airway as a result of inflammatory processes such as upper respiratory tract infections, croup (laryngotracheitis), epiglottitis (supraglottitis), retropharyngeal or peritonsillar abscess, and anaphylactic reactions. Sounds of upper respiratory tract obstruction include nasal congestion, gurgling, hoarseness, grunting, stridor, and rhonchi.

Croup. Croup (laryngotracheitis) is an infection causing inflammation of the larynx and subglottic area. Croup affects more boys than girls, and the highest incidence is in the fall and winter months. The child is often brought to the ED by an anxious caretaker, who says that the child has had fever and a cold for a few days and is having difficulty breathing. When examining the patient, auscultate the chest to determine adequacy of air movement and observe mental status serially. A patient with severe croup has stridor at rest or when sleeping, deep sternal retractions, restlessness, and cyanosis. Children with severe croup, those who are unable to take feedings, and those whose caretakers are unable to provide adequate home care will probably require hospitalization. Croup usually responds well to mist treatment, however, and many children improve sufficiently to be taken home. When a child with croup is discharged, the caretakers should be provided with instructions for home care of croup and may also require considerable reassurance. Table 48-1 shows some of the differences between croup and epiglottitis (supraglottitis), together with the emergent treatment of these diseases.

Epiglottitis (supraglottitis). Epiglottitis (inflammation of the area above the glottis) is a relatively rare disease with the dangerous potential of complete airway obstruction; the term *supraglottitis* is used in preference to *epiglottitis* because the former includes swelling in any portion of the region above the vocal cords (glottis). Supraglottitis occurs most often in children less than 6 years of age and should always be considered a possibility when a child arrives in the ED in respiratory distress, appears ill, and has difficulty swallowing. Caretakers usually describe a sudden onset of illness with high fever (>39.4° C [>103° F]).

Allow the child to assume a position of comfort on the caretaker's lap, give oxygen (blow-by if mask is not well tolerated), and prepare for possible endotracheal intubation or surgical airway. A bag-valve-mask device may be necessary if ventilation is inadequate. Most pediatric patients, even with a high degree of obstruction, can be ventilated with a bag-valve-mask device. Whenever possible, specialists should be called immediately on arrival of the patient; if intubation is required, it should be performed by the most experienced personnel available and may require anesthesia. Defer the starting of an IV line, because this can be performed in surgery if necessary and the risk of

Table 48-1   Comparison of epiglottitis and laryngotracheitis (croup)

	Epiglottitis (supraglottitis)	Laryngotracheitis (croup)
Age	1 to 6 years	6 months to 3 years
Onset	Rapid	Several days of upper respiratory infection or cough or both
Usual cause	Bacteria (i.e., *Haemophilus influenzae*)	Parainfluenza or other virus
Fever	High: >39.4° C (103° F)	Varies; often low grade
Clinical assessment	Appears ill; dyspnea, drooling, dysphagia	Upper respiratory infection, barking cough, stridor
Complications	Asphyxia (caused by inflammation and obstruction in supraglottic area)	Asphyxia (caused by inflammation and obstruction in subglottic area)
Field treatment	Oxygen, rapid transport to health care facility	Oxygen, rapid transport to health care facility
ED treatment	Calm environment, oxygen; defer IV line; prepare resuscitation equipment; possible need for ventilatory support with bag-valve-mask device, possible intubation or surgical airway	Varies with severity; oxygen, mist treatment, epinephrine, racemic epinephrine; hospitalization if severe, if racemic epinephrine is given, or if caretakers unable to treat patient at home

upsetting the patient and further obstructing the airway is too great. A lateral neck radiograph is often taken, if the patient is stable, to show the swollen epiglottis. Most patients with severe respiratory distress from supraglottitis go directly to the operating room, if available, for intubation or tracheostomy. Antimicrobial therapy will be used to treat the infection; steroids are not used.

Peritonsillar and retropharyngeal abscesses. Other diseases with signs and symptoms similar to supraglottitis include peritonsillar abscess, which on rare occasions may compromise the child's airway, and retropharyngeal abscess, which has a less abrupt onset than supraglottitis and may also pose substantial risk to airway patency. A child with peritonsillar or retropharyngeal abscess needs attention to and support of respiratory and circulatory function. Retropharyngeal abscesses require drainage in the operating room, but a peritonsillar abscess may sometimes be drained in the ED if there is danger of airway compromise. IV antibiotics are given for both types of abscess.

Foreign body obstruction. Small children spend a good deal of time playing on the floor; and small objects found on the floor are likely to end up in their mouths. A child brought to the ED with sudden onset of breathing difficulty should be suspected of foreign body aspiration if no other cause is apparent. Suspicion of upper airway obstruction increases when stridor, unequal breath sounds or unequal chest rise, and/or a history of playing with small objects is present. When an object fully obstructs the airway, perform the Heimlich maneuver (alternating with back blows for the child less than 2 years of age). Allow the child to assume whatever position is most comfortable if ventilation appears adequate. Unless the object can be easily observed high in the upper airway, the exact location has to be determined by radiograph and bronchoscopy will probably be necessary for removal. Swallowed objects are usually allowed to pass normally through the gastrointestinal tract, except long,

sharp objects, which may perforate the intestine, and nickel-cadmium batteries, which must be removed because of the danger of toxic leakage.

Lower Airway Distress

Asthma. Diseases of the lower airway are familiar to ED personnel: asthma, pneumonia, and bronchiolitis are the most common. Asthma, a recurrent reactive airway disease, affects 5% to 10% of all American children. The most obvious sign of asthma is wheezing, which may range from mild to severe, accompanied by tachycardia, chest retractions, and anxiety. Expiration may be prolonged because of the narrowed airway. Obtaining a thorough history may be useful in trying to determine the cause of the asthma and to assess the severity of the situation. Repeated asthma attacks are a dangerous sign: a child who has been hospitalized recently is likely to be more seriously ill than one who has not had an acute episode for several months or a year.

There are three components to asthma: bronchoconstriction, inflammation, and edema. Current medical regimens attend to all these problems, often including a beta agonist or theophylline to reduce bronchoconstriction and steroids, or cromolyn to reduce inflammation and edema. Recommended therapy for immediate management of asthma in the ED is a controversial topic, and many hospitals have their own specific protocols. Some general recommendations include giving oxygen, using inhaled and oral medication rather than injections whenever possible, and limiting the use of arterial blood gas measurement to patients with impending respiratory failure not responding to treatment. Although used less often in the emergency setting, a good measure of response to therapy is peak flow or forced expiratory volume in 1 second, which is monitored by a simple hand-held device or more sophisticated electronic equipment. Some of the medications used for asthma are shown in Table 48-2. If the child has a fever, a complete blood

Table 48-2 Medications used for asthma

Medication	Dose	Age dosage	Method	Comments
Albuterol 5% solution	0.01-0.03 ml/kg in 2 ml NS (0.05-0.15 mg/kg); maximum 0.5 ml (2.5 mg)	<2 yr, 0.15-0.30 ml; 2-5 yr, 0.3-0.4 ml; 5-10 yr, 0.4 ml	Nebulizer	Peak onset 30-60 min; duration 4-6 hr
Aminophylline	0.9 mg/kg/hr (adjusted for blood level)	Child; 1.1 mg/kg/hr; adolescent; 0.9 mg/kg/hr	IV	If taking theophylline, draw blood level first; toxicity: nausea, vomiting, seizures
Cromolyn		Infant/child dose 10 mg	Nebulizer	
Epinephrine 1:1000 solution	0.01 ml/kg; maximum 0.35 ml		Subcutaneous	May cause tremor, restlessness, tachycardia
Hydrocortisone	4 mg/kg		IV	
Isoproterenol 0.2 mg/ml	0.5 to 5 µg/min 5 ml (1 mg) in 250 ml NS	0.1 µg/kg/min	IV infusion	
Ipratropium bromide	Pediatric dose not established; 2 puffs 4 times daily?	Pediatric dose not established	Nebulizer	Peak onset 1-2 hr; duration 3-4 hr
Isoetharine	0.3 ml/kg up to 0.5 ml (0.03 mg/kg); dilute in 2 ml normal saline solution (NS)		Nebulizer	Peak onset 15-30 min; duration 2-4 hr; contains sulfites
Methylprednisolone	1-2 mg/kg/dose every 6 hr		IV	
Metaproterenol 5% solution (50 mg/ml)	0.01 ml/kg (0.5 mg/kg) in 2.5 ml NS; maximum 0.4 ml/dose	<3 yr, 0.1 ml; 3-7 yr, 0.2 ml; >7 yr, 0.3 ml	Nebulizer	Peak onset 30-60 min; duration 4-6 hr
Epinephrine (Sus-phrine) 5 mg/ml	0.005 ml/kg; maximum 0.015 ml/kg	1 mo-12 yr, 0.005 ml/kg	Subcutaneous	May cause tremor, restlessness, tachycardia
Terbutaline 0.1% solution	0.03-0.5 ml/kg (0.03-0.05 mg/kg); dilute in 2 ml NS	<2 yr, 0.15-0.2 ml; 2-5 yr, 0.3 ml; 5-10 yr, 0.5 ml	Nebulizer	Peak onset 30 min; duration 3-4 hr

cell count (CBC) may be drawn, preferably before the administration of medication, because laboratory tests may be affected by the medication.

Bronchiolitis. Most commonly found in infants less than 18 months of age, bronchiolitis can be a life-threatening illness. An inflammatory process causes edema in the bronchial mucosa with resultant expiratory obstruction and air-trapping. It is characterized by low-grade fever, wheezing, and cough. Bronchiolitis has a broad spectrum of severity. An accurate history helps to assess the severity and predict the course of this illness. Because bronchiolitis is often difficult to differentiate from bronchial asthma, careful evaluation should be made in the ED: arterial blood gases, CBC, and laboratory tests including cultures from the nasopharynx are usually ordered. A chest radiograph may also be taken to demonstrate air-trapping. Hospitalization is necessary for infants who have had an apneic episode and for all infants less than 2 months of age.

Pneumonia. A majority of pneumonias in children are caused by viruses, although bacterial pneumonia, usually caused by group B streptococci and gram-negative bacilli, is more likely to occur in the first few weeks of life. Whether viral or bacterial, pathogens reach the lung and cause an inflammatory response resulting in accumulation of fluid in the lungs, tachypnea, cough, and fever. Bacterial pneumonia tends to have an abrupt onset with a high fever, from 38.5° to 41° C (101.3° to 105.8° F). In viral pneumonia the fever is usually less than 39° C (102.2° F). Management in the ED includes careful assessment of respiratory status, use of oxygen, and diagnostic examinations such as laboratory tests and chest radiograph. Most children with pneumonia who are well hydrated and not in respiratory distress can be discharged and treated with medication on an outpatient basis, but the caretaker's ability to comply with the medical regimen prescribed should be considered.

Additional nonrespiratory problems causing signs of respiratory distress are those resulting in metabolic acidosis, such as metabolic ketoacidosis and ingestion of aspirin and antifreeze, for instance. When a patient has tachypnea or bradypnea and no sign of airway compromise, these causes should be considered. Respiratory syncytial virus is most often the causative agent.

CARDIOVASCULAR EMERGENCIES
Assessment

The blood volume in a child is 80 ml/kg. The total blood volume of a child, however, is much less than in an adult. The loss of 1 cup of blood in a 10 kg child would be equivalent to blood loss of 1 quart in an adult. Children are able to compensate well for volume loss with increased heart rate and peripheral vasoconstriction. Up to one third of blood volume may be lost without a change in blood pressure. As a result, close attention to heart rate, skin signs, and mental status is the key to early recognition of "compensated" shock. Capillary refill time is also often recommended as a sensitive indicator of perfusion in the pediatric patient, and although the use of this means of assessment has not been studied extensively, normal capillary refill time is agreed to be about 2 seconds. More than 3 seconds may be an indication of poor perfusion in a normothermic child.

The causes of cardiovascular emergencies in the pediatric age-group differ from those found in adults, but the three basic categories of cardiovascular compromise are the same. By conceptualizing the heart as a pump, one can roughly group cardiovascular emergencies into three categories related to the functioning of the system: (1) inadequate heart function (pump failure), as in cardiac rhythm disturbances, congestive heart failure (CHF), or congenital heart disease; (2) inadequate volume for circulation (empty pump), caused by dehydration, burns, or trauma; and (3) problems of fluid distribution as in septic shock, anaphylaxis, ingestion, and sickle cell disease.

Inadequate Heart Function (Pump Failure)

Rhythm disturbances. Children have young, strong hearts, so rhythm disturbances are seldom primary events but are most often the result of hypoxia or metabolic disturbances. However, pediatric patients with rhythm disturbances from congenital cardiac problems are seen with increasing frequency in the ED, probably because of increased survival rate through medical advances. The most common congenital problems causing rhythm disturbances are transposition of the great vessels and congenital mitral stenosis. Acquired cardiac diseases such as cardiomyopathies, rheumatic heart disease, and viral myocarditis may also cause rhythm disturbances.

Abnormal rhythms in this age-group can be simply grouped into three categories: fast, slow, and absent, disorganized, or nonperfusing rhythms (Table 48-3). Sinus tachycardia and supraventricular tachycardia are the two major rhythm disturbances found in children. Sinus tachy-cardia in children is considered to be a rate of 140 to 220 beats/min, whereas supraventricular tachycardia is usually a rate higher than 220 beats/min. Bradycardia is an ominous sign in a pediatric patient. Sinus bradycardia is most often caused by hypoxia and should be treated aggressively with ventilation and oxygenation; junctional and idioventricular rhythms are usually terminal rhythms. Absent, disorganized, and nonperfusing rhythms require cardiopulmonary resuscitation and advanced life support procedures.

Congestive heart failure. Congenital heart disease accounts for the majority of children who are seen in the ED with CHF. Preload, afterload, and myocardial contractility are major factors in determining the amount of blood pumped through the circulatory system. When the heart is not able to pump effectively because of chronic disease, rhythm disturbance, pressure on the heart, or excessive fluid volume, fluid backs up in the system, causing signs of overload such as pulmonary edema, jugular vein distension, and enlarged liver. Some of the many signs of CHF are tachycardia, tachypnea, cough, rales, wheezes, rhonchi, cyanosis, pallor, poor appetite, and failure to thrive. The patient who is brought to the ED with CHF requires hospitalization and extensive evaluation and treatment. If the patient is in severe respiratory distress, CHF is managed much the same as in adulthood, with oxygen, furosemide, and respiratory therapy.

Inadequate Fluid Volume (Empty Pump)

The major medical cause of hypovolemia in children is dehydration. A child who has been sick for even a short time with vomiting and diarrhea is at risk, as is a child who has been ill for several days with fever and decreased fluid intake. When output exceeds input over a period of time, dehydration becomes clinically significant and electrolyte imbalances occur. This in turn causes more nausea and vomiting, starting a downward spiral that can be reversed only with medical intervention. A dehydrated child looks sick, with sunken eyes, pale skin, and lethargy. When 5% or more of the child's body mass (weight) is lost, skin and mucous membranes appear dry. In assessing the child it is often helpful to ask the caretaker about intake and output (number of bottles the child has taken and the number of stools or wet diapers per day for small children). Unless fluid volume is replaced and the balance between intake and output is restored, the condition will progress to hypovolemic shock.

Heart rate, skin signs, and capillary refill provide the most useful information about the child's cardiovascular status. If the patient is showing signs of shock, ensure adequate ventilation and oxygenation and give IV fluids (20 ml/kg of normal saline solution, repeated until improvement is seen). If there is difficulty in obtaining venous access in the critically ill child, an intraosseous line may be inserted, with a bone marrow or intraosseous needle. Usual placement of an intraosseous line is in the proximal tibia or distal aspect

Table 48-3   Rhythm disturbances in children

Rhythm	Cause	Characteristics	Treatment
FAST RHYTHMS			
Sinus tachycardia	Fever, anxiety, pain, hypovolemia	Rapid sinus rhythm; rate 140-220 beats/min (bpm)	Treat underlying cause
Supraventricular tachycardia	Reentry mechanism	Paroxysmal sinus rhythm, P waves often undetectable, rate ≥230 bpm	*Unstable:* cardioversion 0.5-1.0 J/kg; *persistent:* 2.0 J/kg; *stable:* vagal maneuvers (ice water, Valsalva's)
Ventricular tachycardia	Structural disease, hypoxia, acidosis, electrolyte imbalance, toxic ingestion	Rate ≥120 bpm, wide QRS, no P waves	Oxygen; if unstable, synchronized cardioversion, 0.5-1.0 J/kg (pretreat with lidocaine, 20-50 μg/kg)
SLOW RHYTHMS			
Sinus bradycardia	Hypoxemia, hypotension, shock	Sinus rhythm; slow rate (<80 beats/min in infants, <60 beats/min in children)	Ventilation, oxygenation, cardiopulmonary resuscitation (CPR); atropine 0.02 mg/kg; minimum dose of 0.1 mg; epinephrine 1:10,000 solution, 0.1 ml/kg
Junctional rhythm, heart blocks	Hypoxemia, hypotension, acidosis	Rare in children, slow rate, P waves may or may not be present	Ventilation, oxygenation, CPR, atropine 0.02 mg/kg; minimum dose of 0.1 mg; epinephrine 1:10,000 solution, 0.1 ml/kg
ABSENT/DISORGANIZED/NONPERFUSING RHYTHMS			
Asystole	Hypoxia, hypovolemia, acidosis	Flat line on electrocardiogram (ECG), absent pulse, absent respirations	CPR, advanced life support (ALS) procedures
Ventricular fibrillation	Rare in infants and children; hypoxia, acidosis	No identifiable P, QRS, or T waves; wavy line on ECG	CPR, ALS procedures (defibrillation dosage 2 J/kg, doubled to 4 J/kg and repeated)
Electromechanical dissociation	Hypoxia, acidosis, tension pneumothorax, hypovolemia	Pulselessness, with organized electrical activity on ECG	CPR, determine and correct underlying cause

of the femur. This procedure was used extensively in the 1940s and has recently been revived. This procedure has been found to carry little risk when left in place for less than 24 hours. Intraosseous infusion should be considered a temporary measure for use when other vascular access is unavailable. Although fluid administration is slower through an intraosseous line, sufficient fluid and most drugs may be given through this route until other access is obtained. Rate of fluid infusion is calculated on the basis of the child's weight and degree of dehydration.

Diagnostic tests, usually CBC, electrolytes, glucose, blood urea nitrate (BUN), and urinalysis, are needed to assess hydration status, to guide treatment and to help determine the reason for dehydration. Patients requiring ad-

mission are those who are more than 5% to 10% dehydrated (evidenced by weight loss, dry mucous membranes, tachycardia, oliguria, urine specific gravity >1.030, and elevated BUN), or who are unable to retain oral fluids. Patients who are only slightly dehydrated and whose laboratory results are within normal limits are discharged with home care instructions unless there are other reasons for admission.

Distributive Problems

Septic shock. The child with sepsis is at risk for or may be in septic shock, and management in the ED must focus on preservation of vital functions. Adequate ventilation and oxygenation is the first priority: give the patient oxygen and assist with breathing if ventilation is inadequate. A pulse oximeter should be used and/or arterial blood gases drawn to determine oxygenation and respiratory status. An IV line (preferably two) of normal saline solution should be inserted, and 20 ml/kg given until improvement is seen. If peripheral access is not obtained in 90 seconds, an intraosseous line may be used. Laboratory tests include CBC; electrolyte, glucose, BUN, and creatinine determinations; blood gas analysis; blood cultures; serum glutamic-oxaloacetic transaminase (SGOT) and serum glutamic-pyruvic transaminase (SGPT) measurement; and urinalysis. Prothrombin time, partial thromboplastin time, and platelet count are also necessary because the patient is at risk for disseminated intravascular coagulation. The infection is treated with IV antibiotics.

Anaphylaxis. Anaphylaxis is both a respiratory and cardiovascular emergency. Systemic reaction to an antigen (penicillin is probably the most common) results in release of histamine, causing urticaria, laryngeal edema, and cardiovascular signs. In an acute anaphylactic reaction the airway is the first concern. After assuring airway patency and adequacy of ventilation and oxygenation, start two IV lines with large-bore needles. If the patient is in shock, give a fluid bolus of 20 ml/kg of normal saline solution. Ongoing intervention also includes antihistamines, steroids, and possibly bronchodilators. A thorough history is important to isolate the cause of the anaphylactic reaction.

Sickle cell disease. Sickle cell disease is a hereditary blood disorder found mostly in the black population. In patients who manifest the disease, sickled hemoglobin molecules are produced, causing irregularly shaped red blood cells. The sickle cells clump together, occluding small blood vessels and causing tissue ischemia.

There are three major categories of sickle cell crisis. *Vasoocclusive crisis* occurs when small vessels in bone, soft tissue, and organs (liver, spleen, brain, lungs, penis) are occluded, resulting in ischemia, pain, and swelling. The first presentation of vasoocclusive crisis is usually after 2 or 3 months of age and is precipitated by infection, exposure, dehydration, or other stress. The first signs of vasoocclusive crisis in the very young child may be warmth and swelling of one or both hands or feet. Older patients have pain in affected organs, visual disturbances, respiratory distress, and priapism.

Another problem resulting from sickle cell disease is *aplastic crisis,* when anemia caused by red blood cell destruction is coupled with impaired red blood cell production in the bone marrow. This increases the anemia and leads to high-output CHF.

Sequestration crisis is the most fulminant manifestation of sickle cell disease. Sequestration crisis is less common but may be rapidly fatal and is seen in young children (6 months to 6 years of age). Blood suddenly pools in the spleen and other visceral organs and results in severe anemia and hypovolemic shock.

Patients with sickle cell disease are susceptible to infec-

tions, including *Pneumococcus* and *Salmonella;* infection in turn causes increased sickling. Because of the need for close monitoring, most of these patients are cared for by specialists, but those who are having either the first crisis or a severe crisis are often seen in the ED. Treatment of severe sickle cell crisis requires oxygen administration for treatment of hypoxia and acidosis. Most patients require IV hydration with normal saline solution and pain medication, preferably with a narcotic analgesic (meperidine or morphine). Fluid boluses (20 ml/kg) are given if the patient is showing signs of shock. Hemoglobin and hematocrit levels should be determined, and administration of packed cells may be required, especially in aplastic crisis, when anemia can be profound.

NEUROLOGIC EMERGENCIES

Head trauma is the most common cause of neurologic emergency in children, but seizures, obstructive problems such as shunt malfunction, and, rarely, brain tumors and congenital vascular malformations also affect mental status in the pediatric age-group, as do infectious processes such as meningitis and sepsis.

Neurologic Assessment

When a child has altered mental status, it is especially important to remember that the first priority is the patient's airway and ventilation. Neurologic assessment of pediatric patients presents special challenges, especially for the preverbal child. Whenever caretakers describe their child as "not acting normally," this should be taken seriously. Early signs and symptoms of increased intracranial pressure include altered mental status, restlessness, irritability, headache, and vomiting. Constricted or dilated pupils and decorticate or decerebrate posturing are late signs of increased intracranial pressure.

Many methods of assessing neurologic status of children have been proposed, including various adaptations of the Glasgow coma scale. The simplest and probably most useful in the emergency setting is the following mnemonic, the *AVPU* method:

A (*a*lert)
V (responds to *v*erbal stimuli)
P (responds to *p*ainful stimuli)
U (*u*nresponsive)

Serial assessment with this mnemonic, together with a description of the patient's behaviors, is the clearest means of documenting changes. An accurate history from caretakers is also helpful, and when a child is brought in with altered mental status, ask about possible trauma, previous medical problems, possible ingestions, headache, and signs and symptoms of infection.

Seizures. A seizure is involuntary movement and/or alteration in sensation, behavior, or consciousness caused by abnormal electrical activity in the brain. About 5% of chil-

Table 48-4   Seizure medications

	Dose	Method	Side effects
Ativan,* lorazepam	0.03-0.05 mg/kg; status epilepticus, 0.1 mg/kg; has longer half-life and faster onset than diazepam	IV	Respiratory depression
Diazepam*	0.2-0.5 mg/kg	IV, intramuscular, endotracheal, rectal	Respiratory depression
Paraldehyde*	0.3 mg/kg in equal amount of mineral oil	Rectal	Respiratory depression
Phenytoin*	15-20 mg/kg	Slow IV push 50 mg/min; only with normal saline solution; monitor patient	Hypotension, respiratory depression, cardiac rhythm disturbance
Phenobarbital*	15-25 mg/kg; maximum dose 600 mg/day	Slow IV push, 50 mg/min; only in NS	Hypotension, drowsiness, respiratory depression

*Ativan, diazepam, and paraldehyde are used in emergency situations to treat status epilepticus. Phenytoin and phenobarbital have more long-term use in preventing recurrence.

dren have at least one seizure before the age of 16, and many if not most of these patients are seen in the ED. In young children many seizures are associated with fever and are of little long-term consequence. Epilepsy is the diagnosis used when seizures are recurrent and when there is no apparent cause for the seizures. The seizure patient may exhibit a wide range of behaviors, from lip-smacking and staring to violent muscular contractions or sudden loss of consciousness. Status epilepticus occurs when seizure activity is prolonged or when the patient has sequential seizures without regaining consciousness in between. Care of the seizure patient requires airway management, prevention of injury, and cessation of seizure activity by means of drug therapy (Table 48-4).

In the emergency setting the major issue is to distinguish febrile from nonfebrile types of seizures. A child who has had a simple febrile seizure may be discharged home with a responsible caretaker, but the child who has had a nonfebrile seizure for the first time requires admission to the hospital and extensive testing to pinpoint the precise cause of the seizure. The febrile seizure has the following characteristics:

1. Occurs in an otherwise normal child (no neurologic disease)
2. Occurs between 6 months and 6 years of age
3. Occurs on the rise of a high fever; usually less than 1 day in duration
4. Has generalized seizure activity, without focal findings
5. Has no postictal phase
6. Is not associated with loss of consciousness

Standard laboratory analyses include CBC, urinalysis, and measurement of electrolytes. A lumbar puncture (LP) is performed in children less than 18 months of age or when the seizure does not have the characteristics of a febrile

seizure. When a child has had a febrile seizure, parents need reassurance. They should be told that febrile seizures, although frightening to observe, are not uncommon, that less than half the children who have febrile seizures have another, and that this event in all probability does not signal the beginning of a long-term disease.

Status epilepticus. Prolonged and continuous seizure activity, status epilepticus, may be a manifestation of anoxia, infection, trauma, ingestion, or metabolic disorder. For about half the children in whom status epilepticus develops, the cause is not identified. Sustained seizure activity produces cerebral anoxia and possible ischemic brain damage, so airway maintenance, oxygenation, and rapid termination of convulsive activity are the priorities. Assure the child's safety and insert an oral airway to keep the airway open. It is not advisable to attempt insertion of the airway (or tongue blade or bite block) if the child's teeth are clenched. If the child is in severe respiratory distress or stops breathing, bag-valve-mask ventilation should be used until intubation is possible. A large-bore IV catheter should be inserted for administration of fluids and medication. Anticonvulsant medications are given (usually IV) until seizure activity ceases. Laboratory tests include CBC; determination of electrolyte, glucose, calcium, magnesium and BUN levels; urinalysis; and toxicology screening.

GASTROINTESTINAL AND GENITOURINARY EMERGENCIES
Vomiting and Diarrhea

Innumerable children are brought to the ED with complaints of nausea, vomiting, diarrhea, and poor feeding. Most often the problem is viral gastroenteritis or viral syndrome, and the patient is discharged. If the child has abdominal pain, the possibility of an acute abdominal condition must be ruled out and the child should not be allowed to drink any fluid in the ED until this is done. A CBC; electrolyte, glucose, and BUN determinations; and urinalysis are usually taken. Patients whose laboratory analyses are within normal limits, who are only mildly dehydrated, and who are able to take fluids by mouth can be discharged. Instruct the caretakers to give the child small, frequent amounts of clear liquids (a teaspoon at a time), progressing to the BRAT (bananas, rice, applesauce, and tea or toast) diet. Apple juice should not be used because of its hyperosmolarity, which may worsen diarrhea. Also instruct them to return to their physician or to the ED if the patient does not show improvement within 24 hours, if there is increasing abdominal pain, or if the child appears to be acting strangely in any way.

Abdominal Pain

Other illnesses causing gastrointestinal upset and/or abdominal pain are infections with bacterial agents and parasites; surgical emergencies such as appendicitis, strangulated hernia, intussusception, testicular torsion, and bowel obstruction; urinary tract infection; and toxic ingestion. Frequencies of the various causes of abdominal pain by age are listed in Table 48-5.

For the most part, ED treatment of the stable patient with abdominal pain focuses on (1) assessing the patient, including obtaining an accurate history and vital signs; (2) deciding whether the patient can be discharged or will require hospitalization; and (3) determining whether the problem needs medical or surgical management. In general, the possibility of a surgical abdomen should be considered for any patient having abdominal pain on palpation or on movement. Surgical consultation should be obtained as quickly as possible; basic diagnostic tests include CBC, urinalysis, and chest and abdominal radiographs. In all adolescent female patients ask about the possibility of pregnancy before any radiographs are obtained. It is probably wise to assume that a female of childbearing age is pregnant until proved otherwise, so a pregnancy test will be needed. If the patient goes directly to the operating room from the ED, a surgical panel including CBC; electrolyte, glucose, BUN, and amylase determinations; and blood type and cross-match (among others) will be required.

Appendicitis

The signs and symptoms of appendicitis vary greatly but may include midepigastric pain or lower right quadrant pain, possibly with nausea and vomiting. If nausea occurs before pain, the cause is more likely to be medical.[2] The most important diagnostic test is a white blood cell count, which with appendicitis is usually in the range of 15,000 to 20,000 cells/ml. When appendicitis is suspected, the patient should be given nothing by mouth. Preoperative antibiotics may also be ordered.

Incarcerated (Strangulated) Hernia

Incarceration may occur when a portion of bowel protrudes through an opening in the abdominal wall. In girls the ovary rather than the bowel may be incarcerated. When the opening is constricted, circulation to the protruding bowel or ovary is impaired, resulting in ischemic damage. The hernia can often be manually reduced in the ED; giving pain medication (morphine or meperidine), placing the patient in Trendelenburg's position, and applying ice to the area may assist in this process. Surgical intervention is usually required eventually.

Intussusception

Intussusception occurs when a portion of intestine telescopes into a more distal portion. This occurs in infancy,

---

Table 48-5   Causes of pediatric abdominal pain by age

Under 2 years	2 to 5 years	5 to 16 years
COMMON		
Gastroenteritis, viral syndrome, bowel obstruction	Gastroenteritis, appendicitis, urinary tract infection, pneumonia, asthma, viral syndrome, otitis, trauma or abuse	Gastroenteritis, appendicitis, urinary tract infection, constipation, viral syndrome, otitis, pelvic inflammatory disease, sickle cell crisis
LESS COMMON		
Sickle cell crisis, strangulated hernia, trauma or abuse, lead poisoning	Strangulated hernia, intussusception, pyelonephritis, Meckel's diverticulum, hepatitis, diabetic ketoacidosis, bowel obstruction, lead poisoning	Pneumonia, asthma, ectopic pregnancy, ovarian cyst, cholecystitis, diabetic ketoacidosis, gastritis
LEAST COMMON		
Appendicitis, volvulus, ovarian torsion	Strangulated hernia, rheumatic fever, myocarditis, pericarditis	Rheumatic fever, ovarian or testicular torsion

From Reynolds S, Jaffe D: Quick triage of abdominal pain, *Emerg Med.*

most often between 3 months and 1 year of age. Although the onset may be gradual, the pain caused by obstruction becomes severe and colicky in nature, with intermittent spasms. "Currant jelly" stool is not seen until late in the disease.

Volvulus

Volvulus, rotation of the bowel on itself, is a dangerous problem that occurs early in infancy. The rotation causes obstruction of the blood supply and leads to bowel necrosis. Volvulus has an acute onset with vomiting and cramping abdominal pain.

Testicular Torsion

A prepubertal male with sudden onset of severe scrotal pain radiating to the abdomen may have testicular torsion. The twisting of the spermatic vessels causes ischemia, swelling, and a high-lying testis. Rapid diagnosis is essential, because even partial obstruction to the blood supply for an extended period may cause necrosis.

Other common genitourinary problems seen in the ED are urinary tract infections, phimosis, dysmenorrhea, and pregnancy-related problems. Treatment for these illnesses is essentially the same as for adults.

Infectious Disease Emergencies

Children with upper respiratory infections such as colds, sore throats, sinusitis, otitis, and croup are often brought to the ED. For the most part they are rapidly discharged and followed by their physicians. Some of the more serious infectious diseases are described below and in Table 48-6.

Bacteremia. The effects of bacterial invasion of the bloodstream may range from relatively mild signs and symptoms of infection (bacteremia) to overwhelming, life-threatening infections (sepsis or septicemia). Bacteremia and septicemia represent the two extremes on a continuum of severity rather than disparate entities.

Bacteremia may occur in association with an infection such as meningitis, cellulitis, or kidney infection. It may also occur without localized findings (occult bacteremia). Bacteremia is most common in children younger than 2 years old and may be difficult to detect in the child less than 2 months of age. Any child less than 2 years of age should be suspected of bacteremia when there is fever and a documented infection (white blood cell count >15,000 cells/mm²) without observable focus of infection. Bacteremia occurs rarely in infancy and may be especially difficult to detect at this age because infants often do not respond to infection with fever. Bacteremia should be suspected when a child has a fever with malaise, poor feeding, and irritability, and is not playful or easily consoled. The diagnostic workup includes CBC, blood cultures, sometimes a chest radiograph, and a complete septic workup, including lumbar puncture if indicated.

In the ED the child with a fever of more than 38.4° C

(101.1° F) may be given acetaminophen (10 to 15 mg/kg) to lower the temperature. Although a tepid bath is still used in many EDs to lower temperature, the benefits of this procedure are currently being questioned and many EDs have eliminated it from fever protocols. Frequently, oral antibiotics are prescribed; if the patient is discharged, careful attention should be given to the caretaker's ability to give the medication on schedule and clear directions given concerning danger signs of sepsis. The child should be reevaluated within the next 24 to 48 hours. Bacteremia has the potential of progressing to sepsis if the patient is not adequately treated.

Sepsis. Sepsis is an overwhelming, life-threatening infection of the bloodstream with an overall mortality rate of 15% to 50%, depending on the infectious agent. The younger the child, the higher the risk. The child with sepsis appears very ill. A child less than 3 months old may be afebrile, but older children more often have a high fever with tachycardia, abnormal skin signs, altered mental status, and sometimes petechiae or purpura. Intervention for sepsis requires immediate assessment and intervention for shock (described previously) and determination of the cause of infection by laboratory analysis: CBC; electrolyte, glucose, BUN, and creatinine determinations; blood cultures; prothrombin time and partial thromboplastin time; and SGOT and SGPT determinations. IV antibiotics are given and may cause deterioration because of release of endotoxin, so the patient's vital signs and skin signs should be carefully monitored throughout the stay in the ED. The patient with sepsis requires a high level of care and is admitted to an intensive care unit.

Meningitis. Meningitis, an acute inflammation of the meninges, is a common cause of death and disability in children. The incidence of meningitis is one case per 2000 children yearly; 90% of these infections occur in children from 1 month to 5 years of age. The causative organism is often bacterial, but viral (aseptic) meningitis also occurs. In bacterial meningitis the organism enters the bloodstream (through focal infection or by routes such as open wounds, skull fractures, and surgical procedures) and spreads into the cerebrospinal fluid (CSF), which spreads the infection throughout the subarachnoid space, causing swelling and pain. Recognition and thorough treatment is essential in preventing death and residual damage from this dangerous disease.

Increased intracranial pressure is a major concern in meningitis. As inflammation increases, expansion within the rigid skull causes direct pressure on the brain and its vessels and may occlude the narrow passageways to the ventricles, obstructing CSF outflow and producing an altered sensorium.

In many children the presentation of meningitis is nonspecific: headache, nausea, and vomiting or poor feeding. Most children have an elevated temperature, but infants may have normal temperatures, even hypothermia. The classic

Table 48-6 Infections with skin rashes

	Measles (rubeola)	Chickenpox (varicella)	Scarlet fever	Roseola (exanthem subitum)	Petechial rash (from meningitis)
Incubation	10-11 days	10-20 days	2-4 days	10-15 days	None
Signs and symptoms	3-5 days fever, cough, coryza, toxic appearance, conjunctivitis; Koplik's spots (mucosal lesions) appear 2 days before body rash	Fever and cough, simultaneously with rash; headache; malaise	Fever for 1-2 days, sore throat, strawberry tongue, vomiting, chills, malaise	Rapid rise of high fever lasting 3-4 days, in otherwise well child	May be sudden onset or preceded by fever and malaise; if sudden onset and accompanied by fever, may indicate sepsis
Exanthem (rash)	Reddish brown; begins on face, spreads downward; confluent high on body, discrete lesions in lower portions; lasts 7-10 days	Vesicles appearing in crops: trunk, scalp, face, extremities; lesions in all stages of development	Punctate, sandpaper texture; blanches on pressure; appears first in flexor areas; rash lasts 7 days	Appears discrete, rose-colored; appears after fever; begins on chest and spreads to face	Reddish purple vascular, *nonblanching* rash
Complications	Pneumonia, encephalitis, otitis media	Pneumonia, encephalitis, Reye's syndrome	Rheumatic heart disease	None	Sepsis, septic shock, long-term sequelae from increased intracranial pressure
Management	Supportive: acetaminophen, isolate; prevention by vaccination	Supportive: acetaminophen, calamine lotion, diphenhydramine, isolate	Supportive: antibiotics, isolate	Supportive: acetaminophen, possibly antibiotics	Basic life support, advanced life support, immediate physician evaluation, liver function tests; isolate; if gradual onset and no fever, may be from blood dyscrasia or prolonged Valsalva's maneuver (cough, vomiting)

sign of meningitis, nuchal rigidity, is also rarely seen in infancy. Common signs and symptoms of increased intracranial pressure may be evident: irritability or restlessness, altered mental status, and seizures. Bulging fontanelles are a late sign. A severely ill child may be in respiratory distress and/or cyanotic, and have a rash or petechiae.

In the late stages meningitis requires aggressive intervention: airway management and hyperventilation to prevent increased intracranial pressure, IV medication (mannitol, steroids, diuretics, antibiotics), and admission to an intensive care unit. Strict isolation is required. Seizures are treated with anticonvulsant medication until seizure activity ceases. Definitive diagnosis requires an LP and laboratory analysis of CSF, but if meningitis is suspected, antibiotics are given before culture results are obtained. Other laboratory tests include serum electrolyte and glucose determinations (to be obtained before the LP because the stress of the procedure may raise the glucose level).

Meningococcemia. Meningococcemia is caused by invasion of the bloodstream with *Neisseria meningitides* and may occur with or without meningitis. The child with meningococcemia has fever, headache, and rash (maculopapular rash, petechiae, purpura). Shock and disseminated intravascular coagulation may quickly progress. An IV line should be established immediately, because meningococcemia can be rapidly fatal. Diagnostic tests should include CBC, electrolytes, glucose, and urinalysis. An LP, blood cultures, and clotting studies are also necessary.

Encephalitis. Acute encephalitis, inflammation of the brain parenchyma, may be caused by direct invasion of a virus or it may follow an infection such as measles. Herpes encephalitis, an inflammation of the brain parenchyma caused by the herpesvirus, has a very high mortality rate (70%).[1] Symptoms and treatment of encephalopathy vary by cause. Supportive measures with fluid restriction and monitoring of electrolytes may be all that is required for acute encephalitis, but herpes encephalitis is a life-threatening disease requiring aggressive intervention.

Reye's syndrome. Reye's syndrome, an encephalopathy associated with fatty infiltration in the liver, is rarely seen today. This illness develops a few days after the onset of what appears to be a mild viral illness. The cause is unknown, but genetic predisposition, use of aspirin during the course of a viral illness, and an intrinsic toxin affecting mitochondrial metabolism have all been proposed. Symptoms of Reye's syndrome are recurrent vomiting and altered mental status, progressing rapidly to coma. Reye's syndrome requires rapid diagnosis and aggressive and complex intervention to prevent death or devastating sequelae. Many of the standard diagnostic tests as well as SGOT and SGPT determinations are required, but presumptive diagnosis is initially made by elevated blood ammonia level, usually with a normal bilirubin level.

Infectious diseases with skin rashes: measles, chicken pox, scarlet fever, roseola, and meningitis with petechiae. Children are brought to the ED with many types of rashes. Most rashes, such as neonatal acne, diaper dermatitis, and viral exanthem, are not life threatening. Other diseases may have long-term consequences and should be taken seriously. Some of the infectious diseases that present with a skin rash are shown in Table 48-6.

Other Diseases With Skin Lesions

Scabies. The major symptom of scabies, caused by the itch mite *Sarcoptes scabiei,* is extreme itching. Infestation results in an eruption of wheals, papuloses, vesicles, and often visible threadlike burrows. It is transmitted by direct contact and is treated by application of lindane (not for use in children under 1 year of age) or crotamiton. All bedding and clothing should be removed and washed.

Impetigo. Impetigo, a skin infection caused by group A streptococci, is typically found in the child less than 6 years of age. The patient has skin lesions that ooze serous fluid and may crust when dry. Most cases of impetigo can be treated on an outpatient basis with oral or intramuscular antibiotics.

Cellulitis. An injury that breaks the skin barrier, such as an insect bite, abrasion, laceration, or surgical procedure,

may allow the entry of organisms causing cellulitis (usually *Staphylococcus aureus* or group A streptococci). Inflammatory response causes edema and swelling, usually without fever. Most of these patients are treated on an outpatient basis. Children less than 3 years of age with facial cellulitis are more likely to have bacteremia and may require IV antimicrobial therapy.

SUMMARY

This chapter gives only a brief overview of a small number of medical emergencies seen in the pediatric age-group. Many other illnesses not discussed here also appear in adults and are treated in a similar fashion. In caring for all pediatric illnesses, however, it is important to remember that the child's medical care is only one aspect of treatment. Recognition of the fundamental importance of the parent-child relationship is essential for both parent and child, however difficult this may be in an emergency. Showing concern and offering support for the family, including the family in the child's care whenever possible, and giving thorough and clear discharge instructions for the child lays the groundwork for ongoing care of the child once the emergency is over.

REFERENCES

1. Fleisher GR, Ludwig S: *Textbook of pediatric emergency medicine*, ed 2, Philadelphia, 1988, Williams & Wilkins.
2. Jaffe DM: Quick triage of children with abdominal pain, *Emerg Med* 22(14):39, 1988.

SUGGESTED READINGS

American Association of Critical Care Nurses: *Critical care nursing of children and adolescents*, ed 1, Philadelphia, 1981, WB Saunders.

American Heart Association and American Academy of Pediatrics: *Textbook of pediatric advanced life support*, ed 1, 1988, American Heart Association.

Barkin RM, Rosen P: *Emergency pediatrics, guide to ambulatory care*, ed 2, St Louis, 1987, Mosby–Year Book.

California EMSC Project, L.A. Pediatric Society: *Prehospital care of pediatric emergencies: management guidelines*, 1986, American Academy of Pediatrics.

Kelley SJ: *Pediatric emergency nursing*, Norwalk, Conn, 1988, Appleton & Lange.

Krugman S, Ward R: *Infectious diseases of children and adults*, St Louis, 1973, Mosby–Year Book.

Mayer TA: *Emergency management of pediatric trauma*, Philadelphia, 1985, WB Saunders.

Whaley LF, Wong DL: *Essentials of pediatric nursing*, ed 3, St Louis, 1989, Mosby–Year Book.

Pediatric Trauma

Lisa Marie Bernardo and **Theresa Waggoner**

EPIDEMIOLOGY AND STATISTICS OF PEDIATRIC TRAUMA

Injury is the leading cause of death in children and youth 1 to 24 years of age.[14] In 1986 more than 22,000 children from birth to 19 years of age died of injuries in the United States. The leading causes of death from injury in children are motor vehicle crashes (occupant) (47%), homicide (12.8%), suicide (9.6%), drowning (9.2%), pedestrian (leading cause of death in children aged 5 to 9 years) (14.2%), and fires and burns (7.2%).[16]

Every year an estimated 600,000 children are hospitalized for injuries; almost 16 million children are treated for injuries in EDs. Furthermore, annually an estimated 30,000 children have permanent disabilities from injuries.[6]

Because of the frequency and severity of childhood injuries, it is imperative that the emergency nurse recognize and intervene appropriately to reduce the morbidity associated with trauma. Timely assessments and interventions are based on understanding the differences between children and adults with respect to mechanisms of injury and physiologic and psychosocial principles.

MECHANISMS OF INJURY

The most common agent of energy that causes injury in children is kinetic energy, which results in blunt trauma. The major causes of blunt trauma are related to motor vehicle accidents (passenger and pedestrian) and falls.

Injuries from motor vehicles occur when the child is a restrained or unrestrained passenger, pedestrian, or cyclist. The infant and young child restrained in car seats are susceptible to high cervical spine injuries during sudden deceleration. This susceptibility results from the following anatomic factors[7]:

1. The child has a heavy head on a small body, which can result in a high susceptibility to flexion-extension injury.
2. The degree of spinal mobility is greater because of lax spinal ligaments.
3. The infant has undeveloped cervical musculature.

4. Horizontal facet joints in the cervical vertebrae (C1-3) result in subluxation from minimal force.
5. Immature uncovertebral joints at card level C2-4 may not withstand flexion-rotation forces.
6. The higher fulcrum of cervical movement at C2-3 is more susceptible to high cervical spine injuries.

The child from 4 to 9 years of age who is restrained with the adult restraint system (lap belt and shoulder harness) is susceptible to certain injuries as a result of a number of developmental and anthropometric features. These features include the shorter sitting height of the child as compared with the adult and a center of gravity located on the torso above the level of the lap belt. A greater proportion of body mass is located above the safety belt, which may cause more forward motion and increase the risk for head injury from striking a dashboard or other parts of the car interior. Also, the child may jackknife over a lap belt restraint or the shoulder restraint may cross over the child's face and neck, causing an airway injury.[1] Finally, the belt portion of the restraint may ride over the abdomen of the child, causing abdominal injuries.[1] "Seat belt syndrome" (lumbar spine fracture and small bowel injury), as well as high cervical cord injury and lower extremity fractures, can result,[9] because the underdeveloped anterior iliac crests are not an appropriate anchor for the seat belt.[1]

The restrained child in an infant seat can be projected from the vehicle if the car seat is not secured properly. This can result in multisystem trauma to the infant or young child.

The unrestrained child in a vehicle becomes a missile that can be ejected from the vehicle through the windshield or side windows. As a missile, the child also can be pinned under the dashboard, impaled on the gearshift, and bounced against the doors, seats, and other passengers. The child held on an adult's lap can be crushed between the adult holding the child and the point of impact (dashboard, steering column, or front seat). All these events can result in severe multisystem injuries.

Children riding in the back of pickup trucks or in the back of open station wagons can be thrown from these vehicles into oncoming traffic, stationary or moving objects (trees or moving cars), or the road. Young children riding as passengers on all-terrain vehicles (ATVs) are in danger of being ejected from the vehicle and being crushed by the adult rider or by the ATV itself. Older children can crash into stationary or moving objects; older children who are not the appropriate size or weight to operate an ATV can flip the vehicle over onto themselves, thus sustaining multisystem injuries.

As a pedestrian, the child can be struck by a vehicle while playing, walking or running, crossing the street, or exiting a school bus. The child's age and size are factors for consideration in pedestrian motor vehicle accidents. The child struck by a car sustains injuries at two points of impact—the car bumper and the hood; such force causes injury to the thorax, abdomen, and femur. The child then is propelled into the air, lands on the ground (third point of impact), and sustains injuries to the head. This triad of injuries is known as Waddell's triad, which refers to the sustained extremity, thoracic and abdominal, and head injuries.[8]

Children riding bicycles, tricycles, skateboards, and low-to-ground cycles (such as Big Wheels) can collide with moving vehicles. Smaller children on cycles are not easily seen by drivers and can be run over by the vehicle, resulting in severe trauma to the child. Older children on cycles may be easily spotted by drivers; these children may collide with the moving vehicle and be thrown from their cycles. Severe head injuries can occur if a helmet is not worn; abdominal injuries can occur if the child strikes the handlebars while being thrown from the cycle.

Falls in the pediatric population are related to falling down steps in walkers, falls from heights (second-story windows, porches, playground equipment, and roofs), and falls from riding toys with wheels (bicycles). The most common injury is to the head.

DEVELOPMENTAL CONSIDERATIONS

Children differ from adults developmentally, anatomically, and physiologically. Recognizing these differences and implementing the appropriate interventions to support these differences can result in increased survivability of the pediatric trauma patient.

Airway

There are a few crucial anatomic and physiologic differences between the adult and pediatric airway. The child's oropharynx is relatively small, and the airway is easily obstructed by the large tongue. The epiglottis is U-shaped and protrudes into the pharynx. The tonsils and adenoids are often enlarged. The vocal cords are short and concave. The larynx is relatively cephaloid in position and is easily collapsible if the head is hyperflexed or extended. In the child less than 8 years of age the narrowest portion of the child's airway is the cricoid cartilage. Lower airways are smaller and their supporting cartilage is less developed in infants and small children, and the airways are easily obstructed by mucus and edema.[3,22]

Breathing

In the child, pliable ribs do not provide adequate support for the lungs. Therefore, in blunt force trauma to the chest, pulmonary contusions result rather than rib fractures. If rib fractures are present, a high index of suspicion for severe internal trauma should be considered. The mediastinum is more mobile, resulting in a greater susceptibility to great-vessel damage. Retractions are more likely to be observed when the child is in respiratory distress. These retractions can be suprasternal, supraclavicular, infraclavicular, intercostal, or substernal. Breathing is primarily diaphragmatic or abdominal in children less than 7 or 8 years of age.[18] Crying children are more prone to swallowing air, resulting in gastric distention, which also hampers adequate respiratory excursion. Because of the thin chest wall, breath sounds are easily transmittable, making an accurate respiratory assessment difficult. Respiratory rates are higher in children because of their higher metabolic rates. Finally, the presence of congenital or acquired health conditions should be considered, such as bronchopulmonary dysplasia, cystic fibrosis, or asthma.

Circulation

The child's estimated blood volume is 80 ml/kg, regardless of age or size.[13] Because of their large cardiac reserves and catecholamine response, children can maintain a high to normal blood pressure even with blood loss. Falling blood pressure is a *late* sign of hypovolemia in children and is a signal that cardiac arrest is imminent. The best assessment for cardiac perfusion is capillary refill, which should take less than 2 seconds. Other assessment factors are the child's level of consciousness, the presence of tachypnea or tachycardia or both, and decreased urinary output.

Children can have a variety of congenital heart defects that may impair their circulatory status in the event of an injury (tetralogy of Fallot, truncus arteriosus, and large ventricular septal defects). If a child has had a Blalock-Taussig shunt, blood pressures are unattainable in the arm from which the subclavian artery was used for the shunt; that arm is perfused by collateral circulation. Children may also have functional or nonfunctional heart murmurs. Finally, dextrocardia (heart on the right side) or situs inversus (transposition of all thoracic and abdominal organs) may be present.

Neurologic System

The infant's head is larger in proportion to the rest of the body. The skull is more malleable, thus providing less protection to the brain tissues. The posterior fontanelle closes at 4 months of age, and the anterior fontanelle closes at approximately 9 to 18 months.[20] Although the open fontanelles allow for release of increased intracranial pressure (ICP), they may allow for direct injury to the brain or may cause extensive bleeding. The infant can bleed significantly from a scalp laceration because of the large surface area and increased vascularity of the scalp.[22] Finally, the young child has a higher center of gravity, which, together with the larger head, makes the child prone to head injuries.

Cerebral tissues are thin, soft, and flexible as compared with those of adults.[18] This difference renders the brain tissues more easily damaged, especially from shearing injuries. The sulci are still deepening during childhood, and myelinization is still occurring.

Because the vertebral ligaments are not strong enough to adequately support the spinal column, the spinal cord can be stretched during an acceleration-deceleration or flexion-extension episode. On radiographs the spinal column appears intact, but the child shows signs of spinal cord injury. This syndrome is known as SCIWORA (*s*pinal *c*ord *i*njury *with*out *r*adiographic *a*bnormality).

Congenital subluxation of C1 and C2 may be present in a child and may be mistaken for a cervical spine injury. Children may also have a ventriculoperitoneal shunt for congenital or acquired hydrocephalus. The shunt runs subcutaneously from the scalp through the neck and chest, into the abdominal cavity.

Abdomen and Genitourinary Tract

Younger children have protruding abdomens as a result of their underdeveloped abdominal musculature. This protrusion leaves their abdominal organs vulnerable to blunt trauma. The pliable rib cage does not afford adequate protection to the abdominal organs and can predispose children to further internal injuries. Even though it is partially protected by the rib cage, the liver is still vulnerable to injury because of its large size and fragility.[11] Children have less perinephric fat, and the relatively larger kidneys are positioned more anteriorly in the abdomen. Congenital abnormalities such as hydronephrosis, horseshoe kidneys, and ectopic kidneys can make the child more susceptible to renal trauma. Many of these congenital anomalies are not diagnosed until abdominal trauma has occurred. The greater elasticity of the child's spine makes ureteral tearing injury possible, although rare.[22] Ureteral injuries are suspected with penetrating trauma to the abdomen or flank area. The bladder is less protected when full in children because it becomes an abdominal organ; in girls the bladder neck is less protected. The tissues of the prepubescent girl are more rigid because of the lack of estrogen; they do not become more pliable until adolescence, when estrogen is released. Serious internal injuries may result from what appears to be a mild external trauma (internal extension).[4]

Musculoskeletal System

The child's developing musculoskeletal system is vulnerable to injury from blunt or penetrating trauma. Children are more prone to fractures than to muscle sprains or ligament tears because the ligaments, muscles, and tendons are strong and are able to withstand injury forces. Children can bleed significantly from injuries to the chest, abdomen, retroperitoneal spaces, pelvis, and thigh because of a lack of anatomic structures that would tamponade bleeding in these areas.[10] For example, a child with a femur fracture can lose 300 to 400 ml of blood into the thigh, causing a 15% to 25% loss of total circulating blood volume relative to the child's weight.[11] Children may also have congenital anomalies such as osteogenesis imperfecta, muscular dystrophy, cerebral palsy, or scoliosis.

Integumentary System

Children have a larger ratio of body surface area to weight, which makes them prone to hypothermia. Also, infants less than 6 months of age do not have the fine-motor coordination to shiver and are unable to keep themselves warm. Children have less subcutaneous fat to insulate them and can lose heat through radiation, convection, conduction, and evaporation. Therefore external heat sources must be readily available to help injured children maintain thermoregulation.

Psychosocial Considerations

Normal developmental characteristics render children vulnerable to injury. Infants rely on their caregivers to provide them with a safe environment. As they grow, they learn how to roll, sit unsupported, crawl, creep, and "cruise." At each of the stages the environment must be adapted to keep them safe. Toddlers and infants require close supervision at all times. Toddlers are becoming autonomous and are interested in exploring their environment. They begin to climb, crawl into hiding places, and run. They enjoy tasting new foods and will put anything into their mouths, and are therefore vulnerable to poisoning. Preschool-aged children like to imitate their caregivers and try to perform adult activities (reach for a pot on the stove, light matches), leaving them vulnerable to many injuries. They are learning how to ride tricycles and other low-to-ground vehicles. School-aged children are more independent and less supervised. They like playing organized sports and games. They may try to "dare" each other in different activities, which may lead to a serious injury. Their proficiency at bicycle riding and swimming may lead them into dangerous situations. They want to be one of the group and may go against better judgment to be accepted (for example, not wearing a helmet or swimming in deep water). Adolescents are searching for their identities, and peer group acceptance, as well as body images, is their major concern. Operating motor vehicles and boats creates new ways for them to become injured, especially when alcohol or drugs are involved.

INTERVENTIONS FOR THE CHILD WITH MULTIPLE INJURIES

EDs must be equipped with the personnel and supplies necessary to treat the injured child effectively and efficiently. The trauma resuscitation room must be prepared to receive the injured child before his or her arrival. Equipment should be prepared before arrival, and the equipment should be readily available.

The assessment of the injured child consists of the same primary and secondary surveys used in cases of adult trauma. However, there are differences in the interventions used to treat the injured child during the trauma resuscitation.

Airway and Cervical Spine

The tongue is the most common cause of airway obstruction in the child. The first maneuver to relieve airway obstruction is to open the airway by using the jaw-thrust or chin-lift technique. Both maneuvers prevent hyperextension of the cervical spine. The oropharynx can be suctioned with a tonsillar suction if vomitus, blood, or teeth are present. Placement of an oropharyngeal airway adjunct helps maintain airway patency in the obtunded child. The oropharyngeal airway is measured from the corner of the mouth to the tragus of the ear. An oropharyngeal airway adjunct that is too small or too large will obstruct the airway. A nasopharyngeal airway adjunct may also be used to maintain airway patency if there is no evidence of a basilar skull fracture. The nasopharyngeal airway is measured from the naris to the tragus of the ear.

Endotracheal intubation is considered if the child is not breathing spontaneously, is obtunded, or has a severe head injury. Endotracheal intubation must be undertaken by a physician who is skilled in pediatric intubation. Atropine must be administered to prevent bradycardia resulting from the vagal response during intubation. Paralytic and sedative agents may be given at the discretion of the physician. These medications should be prepared ahead of time. After intubation is completed, breath sounds should be auscultated over the trachea, bilateral anterior aspect of the chest, and epigastrium and high in the axilla regions because breath sounds are easily transmittable across the thin chest wall. Because right mainstem bronchus intubations are a common complication with pediatric intubation, bilateral chest wall movement should be observed during ventilation with a bag-valve-mask device that is set at 100% oxygen. This movement is best assessed by standing at the foot of the bed and watching the child's chest rise and fall during ventilation. After endotracheal tube placement is confirmed by auscultation, a chest radiograph must be obtained. In the meantime the tube must be securely taped with benzoin and adhesive tape. The tube must not press on the corner of the mouth (or naris if nasotracheal intubation is performed) because pressing will cause tissue breakdown. A nasogastric or orogastric tube should be inserted and connected to suction before intubation, to prevent aspiration of stomach contents.

Cricothyrotomy and tracheostomy are reserved for severe cases of airway instability from facial trauma or head and neck trauma.

Maintaining cervical spine stability in the young child is a challenge. If the infant or young child who has been traumatized is still in the car seat, the child can be immobilized in the car seat; the child should not be removed from the car seat until a lateral cervical spine radiograph has ruled out the possibility of cervical injury. One method used to immobilize the infant or child in a car seat is to place towel rolls on either side of the head and secure them with wide tape. A towel can also be placed around the neck of the infant or child for cervical immobilization.

Pediatric spinal immobilization devices are now on the market. These are more in keeping with the child's size and need for total body immobilization. When a cervical collar is placed, the appropriate size must be used. A collar that is too large pushes the jaw backward and causes an airway obstruction, and the child will be able to move the head from side to side, thereby preventing any cervical spine control. A collar that is too small does not provide appropriate alignment and may cause airway compromise as a result of being too tight around the neck.

The cervical collar fits properly if the chin rests securely in the chin holder and if the collar is beneath the ears and is not covering the upper part of the sternum.

Breathing

Before the chest is examined, the cervical collar is opened to check for jugular vein distention or tracheal deviation and then closed. Next, the child's respiratory status is assessed by auscultating for breath sounds high in the axillae and the anterior aspect of the chest. The rate, rhythm, and depth of respirations are assessed to identify any life-threatening injuries. The chest is observed for contusions, penetrations, abrasions, and paradoxic movements.

A supplemental oxygen source must be given to any child who sustains multiple trauma. The nasal cannula can be set at a rate 4 to 6 L/min of oxygen; flow rates higher that 6 L/min cause irritation to the nasopharynx. A cannula is used in children whose oxygen requirements are minimal. In infants and young children it is best to secure the cannula into the nares and then start the flow of oxygen because the oxygen flow may frighten the child. A partial rebreathing mask set at a flow rate of 10 to 12 L/min of oxygen delivers an inspired oxygen concentration of 50% to 60%.[3] These masks are not well tolerated in the pediatric population because children do not like to have anything near their faces. Telling the child that it is a "space mask like the astronauts use" may gain his or her cooperation.

Circulation

The apical pulse is assessed for rate, rhythm, and quality. Capillary refill time should be less than 2 seconds. When a blood pressure reading is obtained, it should be considered together with the other vital signs. The blood pressure cuff should fit two thirds of the upper part of the arm; a smaller cuff gives a falsely high reading, whereas a larger cuff gives a falsely low reading. A decreased blood pressure is a *late* sign of hypovolemia and indicates that the child is in extremis. Children can maintain normal blood pressure despite 25% to 30% blood loss.

Pneumatic antishock garments are used in children with hypovolemia or with pelvic or femur fractures. These garments are not usually used in infants or small children because of the lack of small trousers. Also, for children the abdominal compartment should be inflated carefully because the pressure could impinge on the diaphragm and hamper respiratory excursion. Pneumatic antishock garments are inflated and deflated by using the same procedure that is used with adults.

Chest tubes are inserted if there is an indication of a hemothorax, pneumothorax, or hemopneumothorax. As with adults, local anesthetic (and preferably sedatives) must be administered before the insertion of chest tubes.

Disability (Neurologic Status)

The injured child is frightened: strange, painful things are happening. The patient may feel that he or she is being punished for a real or imagined wrongdoing. Talking with the child in language he or she understands is paramount in relieving anxiety and assessing neurologic status.

The Glasgow coma scale, although appropriate for adults and older children, is not appropriate for infants and preverbal children. The infant coma scale is a more reliable measurement of neurologic status in these age-groups.

Serial neurologic assessments are necessary to identify any changes in mental status. A change in the child's level of consciousness can indicate increased ICP or hypovolemia. In the adult and older child the first signs of increased ICP are disorientation first to time, place, and familiar persons, then to self; however, this description is not applicable to the younger child, who has no concept of time or place. The younger child's emotional status is assessed by answering such questions as the following: Is the child easily consolable? Does the child answer when spoken to, or does he or she appear interested in the environment? Can he or she recognize a familiar object such as a favorite toy? Children should be given neurologic tests that they are developmentally able to answer; a preschool-aged child would not be able to give the time of day, the day of the week, or the name of the President of the United States. However, this child may be able to recognize Bert and Ernie or a picture of Mister Rogers.

The child's pupils are assessed for reactivity and size. The scalp is palpated for lacerations or impaled objects. The multiply injured child should be checked for the presence of otorrhea and rhinorrhea that tested positive for glucose.

Early signs of increased ICP in an infant are vomiting and irritability; a *late* sign is a bulging fontanelle. With a severe head injury, intubation and hyperventilation with 100% oxygen to maintain an arterial carbon dioxide pressure of 20 to 25 torr are recommended.[15] Medications such as mannitol and furosemide (Lasix) decrease ICP by their diuretic effect, and methylprednisolone sodium sucinate preparations (Solu-Medrol) decrease ICP through their antiinflammatory effect.

Exposure (Thermoregulation)

The injured child must be undressed so that all injuries can be identified. Because of the large ratio of body surface area to weight, hypothermia is a major concern. The use of radiant warmers, warm blankets, and warm IV fluids and blood products prevents the possibility of hypothermia. Because the child may be in a state of exposure (during a prolonged extrication), a reading of rectal temperature must be obtained as early as possible.

Being undressed and naked may be embarrassing for young children, as well as for older children and adolescents. As soon as the injuries have been identified, the child or adolescent should be covered with a sheet or blanket to protect his or her modesty.

Fluids

Two large-bore IV lines, preferably in the upper extremities, are necessary to begin adequate fluid resuscitation. Blood is obtained for laboratory analyses as warranted by the child's condition and the mechanism of injury. Analyses include complete blood cell count and differential; determinations of electrolytes, blood urea nitrogen, glucose, and creatinine; type and hold for 2 pediatric units; toxicologic screening; and determinations of amylase, lipase, creatine kinase, lactate dehydrogenase, aspartate aminotransferase, and alanine aminotransferase. Lactated Ringer's solution (preferably warmed) is the fluid of choice in pediatric trauma resuscitation, and administration should be initiated immediately. If symptoms of hypovolemia are present (tachypnea, tachycardia, decreased level of consciousness, decreased urinary output, and decreased capillary refill), fluid resuscitation is performed as follows. A bolus of lactated Ringer's solution at 20 ml/kg is given as rapidly as possible. A favorable response should be almost immediate. If no change is seen, a second bolus of 20 ml/kg is indicated; no response to the second bolus indicates active bleeding, and the administration of packed red blood cells should be considered. Blood is administered at a rate of 10 ml/kg. Fluid resuscitation in children is based on body weight, to prevent fluid overload. Up to 25% of the child's blood volume (80 ml/kg) may be replaced with a crystalloid solution.[12]

If the child is hemodynamically stable or has a head injury, the IV rate may be decreased accordingly. Excessive fluid administration in the child with a head injury may result in increased ICP.

If after three attempts peripheral venous access is not established, alternate methods of access are employed. The intraosseous route should be considered in children less than 6 years of age; the bones in older children are calcifying and make intraosseous access difficult. Access to a central line through the jugular, subclavian, or femoral vein by an experienced physician is the next possibility. Venous cut-downs in the saphenous or brachial vein, again by an experienced physician, are the last choice. Central venous pressure monitoring or arterial pressure monitoring is reserved for the severely injured child and should be performed only under controlled circumstances by experienced personnel.

Gastrointestinal and Genitourinary Intervention

The abdomen is assessed for tenderness, distention, and signs of injury (tire marks, stab wounds). A nasogastric tube is placed if the child is intubated or has significant abdominal trauma. If a basilar skull fracture is evident, the gastric tube must be inserted orally. This decompression of the stomach prevents aspiration, leakage of stomach contents into the abdominal cavity, and impingement of the full stomach on the diaphragm. These contents should be checked for blood; the presence of blood may indicate active gastrointestinal bleeding, oral trauma, or traumatic nasogastric tube insertion. Nasogastric output must be measured to keep an accurate record of output. Peritoneal lavage is indicated with severe abdominal trauma; however, abdominal computed tomography (CT) scan is preferred over lavage because of its accuracy in predicting the presence of abdominal trauma.

An indwelling urinary catheter is placed if there is no sign of genitourinary trauma, such as blood at the meatus. The placement of a urometer on the urine collection bag allows for careful monitoring of the child's urinary output. A decreased output can indicate hypovolemia, whereas an increased output can indicate fluid overload. Hematuria indicates genitourinary trauma; however, the first urine specimen may test negative for blood because of the presence of urine in the bladder before the injury. Therefore it is necessary to test subsequent urine output. Normal urinary output for children less than 1 year of age should approach 2 ml/kg per hour; for children more than 1 year of age, 1 ml/kg per hour is optimal.[21]

Musculoskeletal Intervention

The pelvis is assessed for any instability, and the legs are assessed for any deformities or other injuries. Pulse rates are palpated in the dorsum of the foot, and neurovascular status is also assessed. Asking the child to wiggle the toes or to "push on the gas pedal" permits the child to participate in the examination.

Frequent monitoring of the neurovascular status of an injured extremity is necessary to identify impairment of circulation or possible compartment syndrome. An injured extremity can be splinted for protection and comfort until definitive care is provided. Once the extremity has been splinted or casted, frequent reevaluation is necessary because edema may develop and impede circulation.

Finally, the child is rolled over as a unit, and the back is assessed for tenderness along the spine and in the flank region. Tetanus status is determined, and appropriate pro-phylaxis is given. Administration of antibiotics may be initiated for large, open, contaminated wounds.

INJURY SCORING

Once the initial assessment has been completed, the severity of the child's injury is quantified; the Pediatric Trauma Score (PTS) is used as a method of determining severity of injury. The PTS assesses each of the six components important in the outcome of pediatric trauma: weight, airway control, central nervous system response, systolic blood pressure, open wounds, and skeletal deformities. Each component is graded into one of three categories ($+2$, $+1$, -1) and the grades are added together: the result is the PTS. The higher the PTS ($+9$ to $+12$), the greater the probability for survival (0% mortality); the lower the PTS ($+8$ to -6), the greater the probability for death (2% to 100% mortality).[17]

PSYCHOSOCIAL CONSIDERATIONS

The injured child has a number of fears: fear of mutilation, fear of losing control, fear of getting into trouble with his or her parents for engaging in a forbidden activity, fear of death, fear of disfigurement, and fear of pain. It is the responsibility of the emergency nurse to help the child cope effectively during the trauma resuscitation.

It is helpful to assign one nurse (or a child life specialist, if that luxury exists) to serve as that child's support person. When the child has cervical and spinal immobilization, it is best to stand at the child's side and down from his or her face (about chest level) so the child is able to see the nurse. Standing directly over the child's face is frightening, especially when different faces keep appearing and reappearing. Hold the child's hand or stroke his or her hair to provide tactile comfort. Talk softly and slowly to the child, using words he or she can understand ("The doctor is going to listen to your heart beat," "You will feel a pinch in your right arm: you can scream, but you must keep your right arm still"). Avoid words such as "take" or "cut out" because they imply mutilation; use words such as "make it better." If the child requires general anesthesia, avoid telling the child that he or she will "be put to sleep"; the child may have had a pet that was "put to sleep," and this statement may create death fears. Instead, tell the child that he or she will get "special medicine to help him or her take a short nap" because the child understands "nap" to be a short time. Tell the child what will happen before it happens; children do not like surprises any more than adults do. Prepare them by using feeling terms ("This will feel cold; this will feel heavy; this will smell sweet"). If a procedure will hurt, tell the child; lying to the child will only cause him or her to mistrust you.

Children cope in a variety of ways. Because young children are mobile, crying and kicking are ways for them to cope; to them, being restrained may mean not being alive.[19] School-aged children and adolescents cope by seeking information[16]; they may ask the same questions over and over again. Be patient with the child; scolding or theatening the child is fruitless and will only increase his or her fear and resistance.

If the child has a severe mutilating injury, shield the child so that the deformity is not readily visible to the child. Refrain from discussing how "horrible" the injury is in front of the child because children's reported fantasies are worse than reality, and the child will imagine terrible things.

For the child who is comatose or unresponsive, talk to him just as with the awake child. It is not known how much information unconscious children remember: avoid talking about other family members or the child's condition in his or her presence.

Children have pain, and their pain should be acknowledged and treated appropriately. Although pain medication should be given judiciously in the child with a head injury, pain medication should be considered with the same frequency as with adults. Never tell a child he or she does not have pain or that it does not hurt; this kind of statement will cause the child to mistrust you. If pain medication is not an option and the child does have pain, some alternative techniques for pain control should be considered. These include telling a story, deep-breathing exercises, guided imagery, or distraction techniques. Allowing the infant to suck a pacifier promotes comfort, whereas allowing the toddler to hold a transitional object (blanket or toy) promotes security.

The presence of a supportive parent does wonders for the frightened child. Have the parents see the child as soon as possible after stabilization is complete. Explain to the parents before their seeing the child what they will see and why; this explanation prevents any surprises. The parents may need permission to touch or talk to their child; encourage them to do so. Controversy exists as to whether parents should be present during resuscitations; if the parents are present, one nurse must stay with them and explain what is happening to their child.

While the parents are waiting to see their child, a social worker or an emergency nurse should keep them apprised of the situation and serve as the support person for them. If the decision is made to transfer the child to another facility, the parents should see their child before his or her departure; if the child dies before the parents arrive at the accepting institution, they may have guilt that they were not able to see the child or that they agreed to have him or her transferred. When the child leaves, it is better to say "Mommy will see you later" than to say "goodbye" because "goodbye" implies that they may never see each other again.

INJURIES UNIQUE TO PEDIATRIC PATIENTS
Head Injuries

Approximately 30% of all injury-related deaths in children are the result of head injuries.[6] Head and spinal cord injuries unique to children are related to skull fractures and SCIWORA.

Diastatic skull fractures occur in the first 4 years of life and are traumatic separation of the cranial bones at the suture sites. They are most often seen with depressed and linear skull fractures.[5] Pediatric concussion syndrome is seen in children who have sustained a minor head injury with a subsequent loss of consciousness. Within minutes or hours, progressive neurologic deterioration develops, including loss of consciousness, pupillary dilation, positive Babinski sign, and decerebrate posturing.[5] It is strongly recommended that any child who loses consciousness after a head injury be admitted to the hospital for 24-hour observation and be observed for pediatric concussive syndrome.

Epidural hematomas are rare in children less than 2 years of age; however, when an epidural is present, children do not always have the lucid period that occurs in adults.[5] Subdural hematomas are frequently the result of child abuse.

SCIWORA is seen frequently in the pediatric population. This spinal cord injury occurs without fracture or dislocation because the vertebral column is spared from disruption, whereas the spinal cord itself is vulnerable to injury. This vulnerability is seen in children less than 8 years of age.[15]

Facial Injuries

Although facial injuries are rare in children, particular attention must be given to the child's dentition. Dental trauma in the young child must be treated by appropriate pediatric specialists to avoid growth disruption in later life.

Chest Injuries

Chest injuries are not as frequently seen in children as in adults. Particular attention should be made to assess for pulmonary and cardiac contusions caused by the pliant chest wall, leading to blunt force injury to these organs.

Abdominal and Genitourinary Injuries

Injury to abdominal and genitourinary organs must be suspected even with low-force blunt injury because less protection is offered to these organs by the abdominal wall.

Musculoskeletal Injuries

Because the child's bones are still growing, injuries to the growth plate can occur. A number of fractures are unique to the pediatric population. Greenstick fractures are common in young children because of their soft bones. The growth plate (epiphyseal plate) can be injured from compression, torsion, or other mechanisms. The severity of these fractures is assessed according to the Salter-Harris classification, on a scale of 1 to 5, with 1 being the least severe. Complications of growth plate injuries are growth disruption or growth arrest.

One common minor musculoskeletal injury in children is radial head subluxation, or nursemaid's elbow. This is seen in the younger child and is caused by the sudden pull on the pronated arm when the mother pulls her child away from danger. The child has a pronated arm that he or she is not able to use. Management involves reduction of the arm by an experienced physician.

PREVENTION OF INJURIES

The emergency nurse is in a unique position to offer anticipatory guidance to families concerning prevention of injuries. Becoming actively involved in trauma prevention and safety education is another way for nurses to promote safety. Talking with school groups about safety (wearing bicycle helmets, safe water play, wearing safety belts) enhances the image of emergency nursing and educates children and their families. Becoming politically aware and supporting legislators who favor trauma legislation is another way for emergency nurses to contribute to injury prevention.

In conclusion, although pediatric trauma is a preventable disease, emergency nurses can minimize the effects of pediatric trauma by providing quality patient care to injured children and their families. Participating in injury prevention activities helps reduce the incidence of pediatric trauma and enhances the professional image of nursing.

REFERENCES

1. Agran P et al: Injuries among 4- to 9-year-old restrained motor vehicle occupants by seat location and crash impact site, *Am J Dis Child* 143:1317, 1989.
2. Bruce DA et al: Neurosurgical emergencies. In Fleisher G, Ludwig S, eds: *Textbook of pediatric emergency medicine*, ed 2, Baltimore, 1988, Williams & Wilkins.
3. Chameides L: *Textbook of pediatric advanced life support*, Dallas, 1988, American Heart Association, American Academy of Pediatrics.
4. Davis HW: Child abuse and neglect. In Zitelli BJ, Davis HW, eds: *Atlas of pediatric physical diagnosis*, St Louis, 1987, Mosby–Year Book.
5. DeJong SB: Traumatic head injury. In Joy C, ed: *Pediatric trauma nursing*, Rockville, Md, 1989, Aspen Publishers.
6. Division of Injury Control, Center for Environmental Health and Injury Control, Centers for Disease Control: Childhood injuries in the United States, *Am J Dis Child* 144:627, 1990.
7. Fuchs S et al: Cervical spine fractures sustained by young children in forward-facing car seats, *Pediatrics* 84:352, 1989.
8. Halpern JS: Mechanisms and patterns of trauma, *J Emerg Nurs* 15:380, 1989.
9. Hoffman MA et al: The pediatric passenger: trends in seatbelt use and injury patterns, *J Trauma* 27:975, 1987.
10. Joy C: Musculoskeletal trauma. In Joy C, ed: *Pediatric trauma nursing*, Rockville, Md, 1989, Aspen Publishers.
11. Kelley SJ: Multiple trauma. In Kelley SJ, ed: *Pediatric emergency nursing*, Norwalk, Conn, 1988, Appleton & Lange.
12. Manley LK: Pediatric trauma: initial assessment and management, *J Emerg Nurs* 13:84, 1987.
13. Matlak ME: Initial management of the injured child. In Hazinski MF, ed: *Nursing care of the critically ill child*, St Louis, 1984, Mosby–Year Book.
14. National Safety Council: *Accident facts*, Chicago, 1988, National Safety Council.
15. Pang D, Pollack IF: Spinal cord injury without radiographic abnormality in children—the SCIWORA syndrome, *J Trauma* 29:654, 1989.
16. Ritchie J, Caty S, Ellerton M: Coping behaviors of hospitalized preschool children, *Matern Child Nurs J* 17:153, 1988.
17. Tepas JJ et al: The pediatric trauma score as a predictor of injury severity in the injured child, *J Pediatr Surg* 22:14, 1987.
18. Thompson S: Developmental considerations influencing assessment and intervention. In Thompson S: *Emergency care of children*, Boston, 1990, Jones and Bartlett.
19. Thompson S: Emotional and psychological support of the child and family. In Thompson S: *Emergency care of children*, Boston, 1990, Jones and Bartlett.
20. Vaughan VC, Litt IF: Developmental pediatrics. In Behrman RE, Vaughan VC, eds: *Nelson textbook of pediatrics*, ed 13, Philadelphia, 1987, WB Saunders.
21. Ziegler MM: Major trauma. In Fleisher G, Ludwig S, eds: *Textbook of pediatric emergency medicine*, ed 2, Baltimore, 1988, Williams & Wilkins.
22. Zwick H: Initial assessment and stabilization of the critically injured child. In Joy C, ed: *Pediatric trauma nursing*, Rockville, Md, 1989, Aspen Publishers.

Marilyn Johnson

A child is a person who is going to carry on what you have started. He is going to sit where you are sitting, and when you are gone, attend to those things which you think are important. You may adopt all the policies you please, but how they are carried out depends on him. He will assume control of your cities, states, and nations. He is going to move in and take over your churches, and schools, universities, and corporations . . . the fate of humanity is in his hands.

ABRAHAM LINCOLN

In the 1990s, emergency nurses have become more aware of the need to gain knowledge about child abuse and neglect. The attention given to the topic and the overburdening of our social systems give everyone the responsibility to understand what constitutes abuse. Nurses are legally responsible to report their suspicions of abuse to the authorities. In addition, reporting, documenting factual data, acting as an advocate for the child, and focusing on prevention are valued roles. The combination of educational background, expertise in understanding human dynamics, and care-giving ability provides the nurse with a unique background for addressing the problem of child abuse.

The cost of child abuse and neglect is great. Emotional and physical costs to the child and long-standing problems can be created. The cost to taxpayers is rising with the increase in difficult cases. The U.S. National Center on Child Abuse and Neglect estimates that each case of reported child abuse costs approximately $2000 for investigation and short-term treatment. If the child is hospitalized or placed in foster care, the amount increases dramatically. When this amount is multiplied by the 2.4 million reports of child abuse that were filed in the United States in 1989, the financial implications are staggering. (Data from the National Committee for Prevention of Child Abuse, Chicago, Ill.)

The long-range problems that child abuse creates for the individual also become problems to society. Many of the victims have multilevel needs that may result in "acting-out" behaviors such as prostitution, substance abuse, crimes against society, and infliction of harm to others. The mistakes we make today, by failing to intervene or to take responsibility, have an impact on tomorrow's generation. Each of us must accept accountability for today's children.

DEFINITION

Child abuse and neglect have existed since the beginning of human history. This complex problem can be defined as harm to a child by a caretaker that results in emotional or physical harm. Repeated injury places the child at great risk.

The four types of abuse are neglect and physical, emotional, and sexual abuse (Table 50-1). Many children are abused in more than one way. Some developmental levels

Table 50-1 Types of child abuse

Type of abuse	Definition
Physical abuse	Nonaccidental trauma resulting in bruises, marks, burns, fractures, or other physical harm
Sexual abuse	Molestation by an adult or significantly older child or adolescent for gratification of the perpetrator; may include nontouching, touching, or violent acts
Emotional abuse	Abnormalities in care-giving behavior, such as aggression or unusual punishment, that damage psychologic well-being
Neglect	Failure of the caretaker to adequately provide basic human needs of clothing, food, shelter, education, or medical care

From Bittner S, Newberger E: Pediatric understanding of child abuse and neglect, *Pediatr in Rev* 2, 1981; *The nurse's role*, Pub No (DHDS) 79-30202, Washington, DC, 1981, US Department of Health, Education and Welfare.

create more parental challenges than others do, and abusive behavior may result. Symptoms vary because of the different ways the child may adapt to the abuse. Behavioral indicators may be the only clues that lead to a more complete investigation by the authorities. Nurses must be aware of the subtle signs that should lead them to suspect abuse. If a report is made because of this suspicion, the laws in all states protect the nurse (and all reporters), if the report is made in good faith. Abuse is often a generational phenomenon and is a reaction, without thought, directed toward a child. If the nurse intervenes, those careless acts that produce harm can be replaced with appropriate parenting skills. Parent teaching should include realistic expectations of the child at his or her developmental level. All parents occasionally lack self-control, but no child should be a victim of nonaccidental bruises, fractures, emotional harm, neglectful situations, or sexual abuse at the hands of a caretaker or other person.

HISTORY

It is easy to imagine that child abuse may be a problem resulting from today's stressful environment. In reality, child abuse has been noted throughout historical literature. What is different today is how we can recognize it and what we can do to prevent it. Some perspective related to history and current developments may be found in the box below.

DYNAMICS AND CAUSES OF CHILD ABUSE

The dynamics of abuse must be viewed as multidimensional. Many theories are available to help us understand why abuse occurs. One theory recognized by Bittner and Newberger[2] suggests that we study the following:

1. Sociologic and environmental factors
2. Parent-produced stressors
3. Child-produced stressors
4. Triggering situation
5. Result of maltreatment

Most individuals who abuse children are not psychologically impaired. Individuals who purposely want to hurt or inflict harm require intervention. Medical intervention is the beginning of the healing process, the treatment of wounds and emotional issues. The positive and nonblaming attitudes we demonstrate when caring for victims and their families are the building blocks for additional assistance from legal authorities and social service agencies. We must remember that punitive measures such as prison sentences are short-term solutions. The family and the perpetrator must have

---

CHILD ABUSE: HISTORY AND CURRENT DEVELOPMENTS

1874
Eight-year-old Mary Ellen was taken from a United States foundling home by a woman named Ethel Wheeler. A court case ensued; Mary Ellen's natural father sued for custody, and Mrs. Wheeler lost because of an ancient Roman law of *patriae postestas* (father as absolute authority). This law gave the father the right to absolute control (slavery, mutilation, or killing). Frustrated, Ethel turned to the head of the Society for Prevention of Cruelty to Animals.[7]

1875
The Society for Prevention of Cruelty to Children was founded in the United States.

1946
The medical community (Dr. John Caffey) began to recognize how children were mistreated. The principal mark of abuse was subdural hematoma, but radiographs also disclosed fresh, healing, and healed long-bone fractures in many abused children.

1961
Dr. C. Henry Kempe wrote about the battered child syndrome.

1963
The Model Child Protective Services Act was developed. The terminology defined protection of children and assisted states in adopting policies.

1964
The first state laws concerning child-abuse reporting appeared.

1970
All states had laws governing policies dealing with reporting of child abuse and neglect.

1971
Dr. Vincent Fontana expanded the definition of destructive child care to include all forms of child abuse.

1972
The National Committee for Prevention of Child Abuse (NCPCA) was established. This group enlists volunteers to prevent child abuse through advocacy, education, research, and hard work. The group's call to action is to ensure that "it doesn't hurt to be a child."

1974
The federal Child Abuse Act was passed, and the National Center on Child Abuse and Neglect was formed. Financial assistance for projects identifying the treatment of child abuse was provided.

1980
Trust funds for children began appearing in many states, initiating a movement for strong development of prevention programs directed toward community needs.

time and opportunities to replace negative behaviors with positive ones. The goal is to prevent negative behaviors from happening again and to prevent such behaviors from being passed on from one generation to another. This "disease" can be prevented, and the emergency nurse plays a key role.

Research on child abuse is continuing, and many theories related to the causes and effects are being studied. Attention to this problem has increased in the medical, social service, judicial, legislative, and lay public communities.

RECOGNITION OF CHILD ABUSE

Recognizing subtle clues of child abuse in the ED requires the use of a variety of nursing assessment skills. Each case has unique variables. Behavior indicators may be the only clues that warrant further assessment. Areas of concern that the nurse must take into consideration are the historical perspective, physical assessment, and behavioral indicators.[6]

When a child enters the ED, the information shared by the parents or caretakers and the child, from the time of triage through the departmental stay, may have relevance for investigators. Accurate documentation of statements made by parents or caretakers to different caregivers frequently shows a change of stories and points to implausible circumstances surrounding the injury or event. Information should be elicited with concern and compassion because of the desire to give the best care to the child. All questioning must be done with open-ended statements such as, "Tell me what happened."

The approach to dealing with a victim of abuse should be systematic. Each case has its own degree of crisis. The nurse plays a vital role in early recognition of abuse and neglect.

Physical Abuse

Emergency nurses should become astute in recognizing many signs of physical abuse.[1] Physical injury or trauma resulting from injury is also known as nonaccidental trauma. Such an injury could result from negligence or action of the caretaker. Confusing or conflicting histories of the mechanism of injury are often given. The stories told to the triage nurse, the primary nurse, and the physician may differ. The primary nurse, as the manager of patient care, should be observant for and should note discrepancies. Implausible histories from the child and the caretakers and significant behavioral or physical signs should lead the nurse to suspect that maltreatment may exist. The developmental level and age of the child should be considered when the mechanism of injury is evaluated.[2]

Bruises and welts. Varying stages of healing point to repeated injury at different times. These bruises may include imprints of hands, fingers, or the object that inflicted the injury. Grab marks (indicated by round finger-tip bruises), slap marks that leave a characteristic linear mark where blood collects between the fingers, or occasionally, an actual imprint of the hand may be seen. The emergency nurse should consider the amount of force and what such force may have done to the rest of the body on impact. The mechanism of injury must prompt the nurse to evaluate other body systems. For instance, a slap to the face and over the ear may rupture the tympanic membrane. Other manifestations may include retinal hemorrhage or cervical spine injury. Pinch marks or imprints left by implements such as belts, cords, or boards may be seen about the trunk, abdomen, buttocks, extremities, face, or head. The use of implements can point to the degree of lethality and help authorities to decide whether the child should be removed from the home because of the risk of further injury or death.

Fractures. Inconsistent history or discrepancies about the mechanism of a fracture should raise suspicion of intentional harm. Other bone injuries may include periosteal elevations, calcifications, multiple fractures at different stages of healing, and anterior or posterior rib fractures in infants (created when the trunk is squeezed). Subtle epiphyseal and metaphyseal (chip, corner) fractures caused by pulling or twisting of an extremity, spiral fractures, transverse fractures, and sternum, scapula, pelvis, or femur fractures result from great external force in children. Radiographic studies can be conclusive proof of repeated injury. Skeletal surveys (including anteroposterior and lateral long-bone studies and chest, skull, pelvis, and spine radiographs) can identify fractures that are not found during physical examination. These radiographs are generally useful for children under 2 years of age. When a high degree of suspicion exists in cases in which there are no positive fractures, follow-up studies in 10 to 14 days may show callous formations or metaphyseal fragments. Sometimes a single fracture is enough to point toward abuse.

Abdominal injuries. A traumatic blow to the abdomen can be life threatening. Hollow organs such as the liver or spleen, intestines, duodenum, or jejunum, pancreas, and kidneys are at risk when a child is kicked, thrown, or punched. The history of the mechanism of injury should be carefully documented in quotes of the caretakers' claims. The story often changes when a different member of the medical team asks the same question.

Head injuries. A large percentage of infant deaths are caused by head injuries. A child's head is large in relationship to the rest of his or her body until the child is approximately 10 years of age. The mechanism of many subdural hematomas in infants is shaking, which causes the shearing of vessels. Even if the child is thrown in the air forcefully or thrown down on a soft surface such as a bed, bleeding may result because of the sudden deceleration force. This syndrome is called the shaken baby syndrome and was first documented in 1972. Subdural hematomas are assumed to have been inflicted until proven otherwise. Subarachnoid hemorrhages, periorbital ecchymoses (black eyes), subgaleal hematomas, and scalp bruises that suggest nonaccidental origin must be considered as resulting from abuse until proven otherwise.

Burns. Inflicted burns indicate dysfunctional thinking on the part of the caretaker. Types of burns include cigarette burns, which are circumferential and vary in depth depending on the length of exposure to the heat. Differentiating a cigarette burn from impetigo may require observation of the lesion over time. Impetigo usually has irregular borders. Circumferential, scald, or submersion burns result when a child is placed in a hot liquid or when the hot liquid is poured over a body part. Children sometimes do pull hot liquids over onto themselves when pot handles or vessels that contain hot fluids are within their reach. Depending on the history and the behavior of the child or caretakers, the need for a report to Child Protective Services (CPS) may be considered if concern about intentional harm or neglect is present. An investigator will be able to assess how an incident occurred in the accident setting.

Guidelines are the same for dry contact burns caused by contact with radiators or other heated implements. Remember, *the medical team does not have to prove that child abuse exists. The suspicion is enough to mandate a report.* Only those entities defined by state law, such as CPS or police officers, have the right to investigate and substantiate abuse.

Traumatic alopecia. Traumatic alopecia is manifested by healthy hair found at varying lengths with petechial hemorrhages on the scalp. This condition is a result of the hair shaft being pulled from the follicle and may occur because the caretaker has pulled the hair or because the child has pulled his or her own hair. If the child inflicts harm on himself or herself, he or she may have depression caused by the home environment or other external factors. Either cause of alopecia is reason enough to request further intervention.

Eye injuries. Inflicted or nonaccidental eye injuries should raise concern. Once again, the mechanism of injury is an important qualifier for establishing suspicion. Eye injuries such as a hyphema, retinal detachment, scarring, or periorbital ecchymosis in children, especially children under the age of 3 years, should raise the suspicion of abuse. Retinal hemorrhages in children under 3 years of age (shaken baby syndrome)[5] constitute an automatic referral. These hemorrhages are created when there is a temporary obstruction of venous return. Frequently these injuries are seen in a child who may also have a subdural hematoma. Blood within the globe may create a long-lasting problem; as a result glaucoma may develop at an early age. Staining of the lens can also create permanent visual deficits.

Near-drowning and drowning. Near-drowning or drowning incidents may indicate intentional harm or neglect. Leaving babies and children unattended in the bathtub results in many deaths each year in the United States. Preventive teaching is a key responsibility of the emergency nurse.

Poisoning. Intentional poisoning warrants a report and a request for an investigation into family dynamics. Examples of this concern include caretakers who give children alcohol or drugs (over-the-counter medications, prescription drugs intended for use by another person, or illicit drugs) for the purposes of sedation, curiosity, punishment, or intentional harm.

Munchausen syndrome by proxy. Munchausen syndrome is a complex condition exhibited when a child is knowingly kept ill by a caretaker who enjoys the complexity of care. The child is subject to threatening illnesses caused by the caretaker. Some caregivers have been known to give children syrup of ipecac or other drugs. Mimicking hematuria by introducing a caretaker's blood from tampons or another source or introducing a pathogen such as *Escherichia coli* into a central line are known methods of tampering with medical evidence. These caretakers falsify symptoms and medical history to gain medical attention for their children. This serious problem can baffle experts, and approximately 10% of these children die as a result of misdiagnosis resulting from falsified evidence.

Petechia. A rash on the entire face and head may be caused by choking. Petechia on the pinna of the ear may be caused by direct twisting or trauma.

Laceration of the frenulum. When a frenulum is lacerated, the mechanism may be forced feeding. Some children may lacerate the upper-lip area by an accidental "faceplant" fall. The history (that is, difficult feeding problem such as cleft palate) and behavior of the child and caretakers are a vital part of the determination of possible abuse.

Human bite marks. Bite marks may appear on children as a result of inappropriate discipline measures. A spread of more than 3 cm between the canine teeth demarcation indicates that someone with permanent teeth (possibly an adult caretaker) made the bite. Animal and human bites may be distinguished by their appearance.

Frequent or repeated injuries. Consistent or repeated injuries to a child should raise concern. Once again, the alert emergency nurse may remember taking care of that child or family previously. A quick reference check with the medical records department can assist in making the decision for appropriate care of the child and the need to report a suspicious injury.

Unexplained injury. Possible neglectful inattentiveness or the potential for it should be suspected when the child is not able to injure himself or herself because of behavioral or physical limitations but has an injury. This situation should raise suspicion and alert the nurse to make a report.

The history of using multiple physicians and medical facilities may be a family's means to avoid "being found out." Abusive families are often isolated. Because of their dysfunction, they may not allow anyone to know them too well. EDs are frequently used because historical facts that could be used to judge the past are usually not readily available, and these brief encounters offer treatment only to the observable injury, not usually to the total problem. Abusive families may count on you to have tunnel vision. Do not be surprised if they become threatened when more than the observable injury is discovered. It takes a talented medical team to look at broader issues and employ tactics to begin the healing process not only of the injury but also of the mind and the family dynamics. The mind-set of the medical team that "discovers" the abuse and how the team deals with the family can set the stage for the family's desire to change behavior or resist any help. Evaluation of suspected physical abuse is described in the box below.

Behavior. The medical team should be alert to the following behaviors of abused children:

1. Deserving of punishment. A child's statement that he or she deserves maltreatment may signify a significant

---

EVALUATION OF SUSPECTED PHYSICAL ABUSE

History
1. Interview the child and parent(s) separately, if the child is old enough to talk. Do not ask leading questions; use open-ended questions when possible.
2. Is the history consistent with the child's age and the nature of the injury?
3. Obtain a detailed history. Pay close attention to the sequence of events.
4. Is the parent at high risk for abuse (for example, isolated, abused as a child, has low self-esteem)?
5. Is the child at high risk for abuse (for example, "difficult child," difficult developmental stage, premature infant)?
6. Is there a crisis—financial, social?
7. Are other children at home also at risk for abuse?
8. Is there alcohol or drug abuse in the family?

Physical examination
1. Are there old or new injuries or both?
2. Is the injury consistent with the history?
3. Measure, draw, and describe (location, color, induration, scarring) all lesions.
4. Is there evidence of old fractures, such as limited range of motion?

Laboratory and radiographic evaluation
1. Complete a workup for bleeding if there are multiple bruises.
2. Obtain a radiographic skeletal survey in children under 5 years of age. (The survey is most conclusive in patients under 2 years of age.)
3. Photograph the injury with consent of police officer or CPS. (Check your state statutes to determine whether consent is needed.)
4. Consider the use of advanced imaging techniques, when indicated.

Courtesy of Helen Britton, MD, Primary Children's Medical Center, Salt Lake City, Utah.

---

care-taking problem. If harm to the child creates physical or emotional signs of a problem, a need for help exists.
2. Fear and distrust of adults. If the child exhibits fear and distrust, especially around caretakers, there is cause for concern. Why has the behavior developed? Children who have a fear of further harm generally withdraw from the offending source, just as an adult would.
3. Manipulative behavior. Manipulative behavior could be a method of attention seeking or an indicator of needs that are not being met.
4. Poor self-esteem. Poor self-esteem is a major component of an abusive environment and is frequently displayed in a victimized child and other family members.
5. Vacant stare. This stare may be present in a child who has truly "given up." His or her needs are not being met, and a sense of futility exists.
6. Compliance or extremes of behavior. These behaviors may be signs of a child's coping method or adaptation to the environment in which he or she lives. It is normal for children to have a sense of mistrust for strangers until their fears are allayed.
7. Seeking affection from anyone. A child who has not been taught or has not defined any personal boundaries often seeks affection from anyone. This kind of behavior is frequently found in sexually abused children.

Neglect

When caretakers fail to provide the basic needs of the child, their behavior is deemed neglect. In some states, the issue of neglect is being addressed by the use of public health nurses in the home. If there is a consistent lack of parental concern or if there is imminent concern for the child's safety, the investigatory arm of the CPS takes action. In other states, the first line of assistance is CPS. Become familiar with your state's recommended approach.

Failure to thrive. Inadequate nutrition with resulting failure to thrive is considered neglect. The cause of failure to thrive is impossible to determine unless there is close medical supervision or hospitalization. A study of the baby's weight, length, occipital and frontal circumference at birth, and any measurements taken before the time of presentation must be compared on a nomogram. Progressive decline in the rate of weight gain suggests nutritional inadequacies when no medical problems are found. In severely malnourished infants, the rates of growth in height and head circumference decline after initial drop in weight. If a child falls below the average in all three areas and appears to be thriving, the facts may simply suggest that this is a "little baby with little parents." In cases of true failure to thrive, babies lack fat deposits and subcutaneous tissue; they also exhibit deprivational behavior of ravenous hunger but show little interest in eating. When a baby has no medical condition that could cause lack of growth and he or she fails to gain weight in the home setting, immediate care is needed. The diagnosis of failure to thrive is confirmed when the child is placed in a controlled environment and gains weight when the only treatment given is an appropriate diet for age. When lack of nurturing extends beyond feeding inadequacies, longer-term problems with behavior and development can occur. Appropriate feeding in a controlled environment is a rapid "fix" to a condition that can leave a child retarded or can cause long-term physical consequences if not corrected.

Psychosocial dwarfism. Psychosocial dwarfism is another form of failure to thrive that occurs between the ages of 3 and 12 years. It is characterized by failure of growth in height, weight, and mental development. Psychosocial dwarfism is a result of a seriously disordered relationship between parent and child.[3]

Lack of concern. Parenting is a large responsibility, and the medical community should be concerned when there is a lack of concern over the child's welfare: inadequate medical care (for example, care is not sought when medically indicated or child does not have appropriate immunizations) or dental care, delayed development as a result of deprivation, inadequate supervision, absence of a safe environment, or inappropriate clothing for the environment. Educational neglect should also be reported.

Bald patches on the scalp. An infant who rubs his or her head while lying or sitting in one place for long periods of time may be indicating that he or she has received improper nurturing. A flat molding of the back of the head may also be an indication of inadequate nurturing.

Behaviors. Neglected children may beg for or steal food, seek affection indiscriminately, exhibit role reversal (that is, assume adult responsibilities), vandalize, or steal. Medical evaluation of suspected neglect and failure to thrive is described in the box below.

Emotional Abuse

Caretakers must provide an environment that allows nurturing and growth. Failure to provide this important environment is categorized as abuse. This is a difficult type of abuse for investigating agencies to prove. Examples of emotional abuse are constant criticism, verbal abuse, threats to safety, unrealistic expectations of the child by the caretakers, or use of the child in custody battles. Some behaviors that the child may exhibit include depression (environmentally induced), behavior extremes (for example, overly compliant, passive, aggressive, or demanding), habit disorders (such as sucking, biting, rocking, enuresis, or eating disorders), neurosis (such as sleep disorders, unusual fearfulness, or a suicide gesture), conduct and learning disorders (such as withdrawal, antisocial behavior, cruelty, or stealing), anxiety, and delays in emotional and intellectual development.

Sexual Abuse

Sexual abuse is the use of a child for sexual gratification or financial benefit by an adult or significantly older child or adolescent. Different types of sexual abuse are nontouching, touching, and violent acts.

Frequently there are concerns about the legal responsibilities associated with the examination of a sexually abused child, and the focus can become misdirected. We need to attend to the patient's physical and emotional needs first. Medical needs must be addressed as for any other patient entering the ED.

Behaviors. Signs that a child has been sexually abused may include sexualized or seductive behavior and dress or interest that is inappropriate to the child's age. Children act out what is familiar to them. A child's vocabulary may also be inappropriate. Some children begin showing troubling behaviors suddenly because of the need to redirect their discomfort. Changes in school performance, running away, delinquency, or withdrawn behavior are signs that the child needs help.

Physical complaints. If a child has bowel or bladder problems or complains that his/her "bottom" hurts, physical evaluation should be performed to rule out medical causes. Such problems may be caused by frequent use of bubble bath, pinworms, lack of cleanliness, or a physiologic condition. Sleep disturbances, eating disorders, or drug or alcohol abuse may be "red flags" that indicate sexual abuse.

Medical indicators. A report to CPS or police officers

MEDICAL EVALUATION OF SUSPECTED NEGLECT AND FAILURE TO THRIVE

History
1. Lack of parental concern about physical illness, delayed development, or failure to thrive
2. Bizarre dietary or feeding history
3. Isolated or depressed parent
4. Financial or social crisis
5. Alcohol or drug abuse in parent
6. Any evidence of organic failure to thrive
7. Possible physical abuse

Physical examination
1. Lack of subcutaneous tissue
2. Developmental delay
3. Evidence of organic disease
4. Signs of physical abuse

Laboratory evaluation
1. Complete blood cell count
2. Renal assessment, including measurement of electrolytes and urinalysis
3. Does baby gain weight when adequate intake of a regular diet is established?

Courtesy Helen Britton, MD, Primary Children's Medical Center, Salt Lake City, Utah.

TYPES OF SEXUAL ABUSE

Nontouching
Verbal abuse
Obscene phone calls
Frank or shocking discussions of sexual acts to arouse
    interest or stimulation in the child (not to be confused
    with appropriate sex education)
Exhibitionism
Voyeurism
Purposeful exposure (visual or auditory) of child to
    sexual activity

Touching
Fondling
Genital stimulation
Oral stimulation
Pornography
Intercourse
Presence of a sexually transmitted disease

Violent acts
Rape
Physical injury
Murder

EVALUATION OF SUSPECTED SEXUAL ABUSE

History
1. Interview the child and parent(s) separately, if child
   is able to converse. Do not ask leading questions.
   Ask open-ended questions, when possible.
2. Does the child describe sexual events beyond
   appropriate knowledge for his or her age?
3. Specifically, ask what sexual acts occurred? Coitus?
   Sodomy? Fondling? Digital penetration? Fellatio?
   Cunnilingus? (Use language appropriate to child's
   age and stage of development.)
4. When did the events occur and who was the
   perpetrator?
5. Could the child be pregnant? By whom?
6. Is there a role reversal in this family?
7. Have other children in the family been molested?

Physical examination
Check for the following:
1. Injuries to or in the mouth
2. Damage to hymen, vaginal discharge, tears,
   lacerations
3. Laxity of rectum, rectal tears or lacerations
4. Evidence of other physical maltreatment

Laboratory evaluation
1. Culture the throat, rectum, vagina, or urethra, or a
   combination of these.
2. Obtain a smear for examination of sperm if
   intercourse occurred less than 96 hours before the
   examination.*
3. Obtain syphilis serologic study.
4. Evaluate acid phosphatase level of secretions, if
   ejaculation occurred less than 24 hours before the
   examination.*
5. Obtain forensic examination, if molestation or rape
   occurred less than 72 hours before the examination.*
6. Evaluate urine for the presence of urinary tract
   infection, in selected cases.

*Specimen must be sent to the police department's crime laboratory, and an official "rape" kit must be used. If uncertain about technique, consult an experienced professional (usually at a regional pediatric facility).
Courtesy Helen Britton, MD, Primary Children's Medical Center, Salt Lake City, Utah.

for further investigation should be made for bruises, injury, or swelling of the genitals (not consistent with the history), bites or petechial suction marks on the breasts, inner thighs, or in the genital area, sexually transmitted diseases, or blood stains or discharge on underwear. Pain in anal, genital, gastrointestinal, and urinary areas is a frequent complaint. Frequent urinary tract infections, encopresis, and enuresis may also be signs of sexual abuse. Children who complain of frequent stomachaches without medical cause may be using that complaint in the hope of discovery of the sexual abuse. Grasp marks can result from force. However, most sexual abuse is inflicted over time, with misdirected trust in or coercion by the perpetrator. Hyperpigmentation of the mucosa around the anus or laxity of the musculature of the anal opening can be a result of penile or object insertion. Pregnancy in children is an obvious need for a referral.

The saddest stories come from children and adults who have had problems with medical personnel who did not listen or believe when told about the abuse. Every person who becomes aware of abuse and reports it to CPS or the police department has unlocked the potential for healing devastating psychologic wounds.

There is a great need to stop sexual abuse and initiate therapy. There are many adults, who were victims themselves as children, who have not received psychologic help; such a dark secret may lead to a deep depression, dysfunctional living, and occasionally, suicide. In the ED, to work quickly to stop the cycle of abuse that may cripple a child for life emotionally or physically is just as important as to prevent a myocardial ischemia from causing further cell damage.

Types of sexual abuse are listed in the box above left; medical evaluation of suspected sexual abuse is described in the box above.

IMITATORS OF ABUSE

Some signs, symptoms, diseases, or situations may appear to indicate that abuse has occurred. It is important that these be distinguished from nonabusive phenomena. Several examples follow, but this is not an all-inclusive list.[5]

Failure to thrive. Metabolic or physiologic causes should be distinguished from environmental causes or inadequate calorie intake. Remember, a child may normally have a short stature or tendency toward leanness or may be in a normal, linear growth period. For physically threatened children, hospitalization and careful testing and monitoring are required for evaluation and treatment. Some states require a report to CPS on all children with failure to thrive. (Check your state statutes.)

Sudden infant death syndrome. Death resulting from child abuse is often thought to be caused by sudden infant death syndrome. In cases of apparent sudden infant death syndrome the appearance of pooled blood, mottling, or other discoloration should raise the suspicion of child abuse. If other factors clearly raise suspicion of child abuse, a report should be made. Because of the appearance of sudden infant death syndrome, a definitive cause of death will be determined by the medical examiner or coroner's office. It is difficult enough for parents to lose a child from this syndrome without being accused of abuse by medical personnel. It is important to recognize our role as supportive (not punitive), no matter what the cause of injury may be.

Clotting disorders. Clotting disorders such as Wiskott-Aldrich syndrome, hemophilia, and thrombocytopenic purpura can result in bruises of varying stages on a child. These conditions may cause chronic bruising.

Ehlers-Danlos syndrome. Ehlers-Danlos syndrome is a condition in which bruising and scarring occur easily, and poor healing occurs. When attention is drawn to conclusive testing, the syndrome may be diagnosed and conditions that could be life threatening can be treated.

Mongolian spots. Distinguishing these birth marks from bruises is sometimes confusing. The difference is that over time, mongolian spots do not change in coloration and size; they generally have a grayer appearance than bruises do. Ten percent of the Caucasian population have mongolian spots. These spots are found predominantly in Spanish-Americans, Southeast Asians, Southern Europeans, Indians, or in anyone who has a tendency toward dark pigmentation. Parents who have children with these spots may want to carry a letter from their pediatrician or health care provider that indicates the presence of these bruises.

Unusual but realistic mechanism of injury. The report of sports injuries, falls, or accidents may cause concern until you review the history and recreate the mechanism of injury in your own mind.

Phytophotodermatitis. When a person has phytophotodermatitis, the skin has increased melanin production. Increased melanin production may be caused by rubbing the skin with lime, lemon, fig, celery, or parsnip and by exposure to sunlight. Phytophotodermatitis can look like a burn or a bruise.

Maculae ceruleae. Maculae ceruleae are bluish spots on the skin that occur primarily in the pubic area, when it is infected with lice.

Multiple petechiae and purpura of the face. Multiple petechiae and purpura of the face may result from vigorous crying, retching, or coughing, which cause increased vena cava pressure. The condition is distinguished from intentional choking because there are no markings around the neck.

Bullous impetigo. This condition may be mistakenly diagnosed and may actually be an infected abrasion or burn. The condition constitutes neglect if the caretakers exhibit a lack of concern regarding care of the lesions.

Cultural or ethnic practices. Misinterpretation as a result of Western traditional thinking is possible. Practices that do physical harm may be addressed as educational issues. Several CPS agencies have culturally oriented workers who teach families about physically dangerous cultural practices. Some cultural practices include cupping (Chinese), *Cao gio,* that is, rubbing coins on the skin (Vietnamese), moxibustion (Asian), and intentional scarring (East African tribal). It is wise to be aware of cultural and social patterns of those who may live in your area. In Western culture, eye contact is common. In some cultures, eye contact may be considered disrespectful. Some families have an appointed health person. This is the person to whom you should direct health teaching.

There are many illiterate individuals who may be ashamed to admit that they cannot read. In these cases written instructions are not appropriate or understood. Visual teaching or drawings may be more helpful.

REPORTING REQUIREMENTS

Every state has a reporting law that requires anyone to make his or her *suspicions* of abuse known to a designated social service agency or the police department. First-time reporters often have difficulty because they may doubt their assumptions and wonder about repercussions or question what they may be doing to the family unit. Be assured that the laws have been enacted in the best interest of the child. Become familiar with your state's statute on child abuse and the reporting requirements.

Document your report. Record the name of the person to whom the report was given and a description of the information shared. Date and time of the report should also be a part of the record. Information given to the designated agency is described in the box on the next page.

TREATMENT AND MANAGEMENT

Medical treatment and management for victims of child abuse or neglect should not differ a great deal from that for an accidental injury. We must be clear about addressing legal and social issues as required by law. It is important

---

INFORMATION TO BE SHARED WITH DESIGNATED SOCIAL SERVICE AGENCY

1. Report as soon as suspicion is raised, preferably while the child is still in the ED. Allow the social service agency or police officers the opportunity to make their confrontation when "evidence" is fresh.
2. Write a concise reason for your suspicion that the child has been abused. Make the information clear, and use lay terms because not all who receive the information are medically knowledgeable. If the child has received care at your ED many times, share the background information. If there is an expected follow-up, explain the reason, explain what would happen in case of failure to comply, and provide any other pertinent information.
3. Provide the following information:
   a. Child's name
   b. Address of child's residence and address at which the incident may have occurred (if known)
   c. Telephone number of child's residence
   d. Mother and father's full names (Frequently the last name of the child may not be the same; many states list families by the mother's name.)
   e. Your name and telephone number (work number, unless this is a report unrelated to your work), which allow the investigators the opportunity to clarify information after the original referral
4. If the investigators (CPS or police agency) request a copy of the information, check your local statute to make certain that you have a policy and procedure in place to accommodate this issue. Many states allow information to be released without a subpoena. Your local county attorney's juvenile office can be a resource to you.
5. Document, on the medical record, that this report has been made. List who received the report and the time and date of the report. Many institutions have separate forms to complete for the housing of this information.
6. Inform appropriate supervisory or administrative personnel, as determined by your institution's policies and procedures.

---

that we ensure privacy when possible: confidentiality must be maintained. It is in the interest of the child and his or her family that rather than labeling them, we clearly act as their advocate and support them. As difficult as this may be, we may offer them the opportunity to take the first step in the healing process when we file a report. Treatment and management of child abuse and neglect are described in the box on the next page.

LEGAL ASPECTS
Documentation

Written information must be accurate, clear, and concise. What is not written is considered not done, as in all areas of medical care. Good documentation may prevent the medical team from having to go to court. If you are called as a witness, the written records will be extremely valuable to you.

Statements made by caretakers that relate to suspicion of nonaccidental trauma or sexual abuse should be quoted in the medical record. Avoid suppositions: document only factual data. Descriptions should be clear. Bruises, lacerations, swellings, or other visual signs should be documented, including size (in millimeters or centimeters), colorations, odor, and any physical or identifying characteristics.

Photographs taken with a 35 mm camera provide good evidence of visible injuries. Photographs must be marked with the date, time taken, person who took the photograph, chart identification number, and the child's name. Be clear about your state statutes: know whether you need a CPS or police request before photographs may be taken.

Anatomic diagrams are good visual aids with which to identify the location of injuries on the body. Many states have diagrams that are a part of the sexual assault evidence kit paperwork.

Behavior must be documented as well. The child's and caretaker's demeanor, affect, and reactions to specific procedures or questions can assist the investigating team. Descriptions of clothing, body hygiene, type of care given before arrival at the medical facility, and the length of time between the injury and the request for medical intervention are indicators that can make the diagnosis more complete.

Protocol

It is important to follow the protocol for a sexual assault examination as defined by your hospital and the legal requirements of your state. Many municipalities have designated facilities for specific examinations (that is, for children and adults). When triage or medical interviewing is performed, be sure to use only open-ended questions to elicit information. Do not display shock or horror. If you put leading statements or thoughts into a child's or an adult's mind, these could invalidate the investigation. Acceptance and caring are attributes that assist victims. Allow the investigators to interview the victim to obtain information before the examination when possible. This part of the process should be performed in a confidential setting. Allowing victims to remain dressed is appropriate. Anatomically correct dolls are rarely used in the ED. If used, they should be used only by someone who is therapeutically skilled in interviewing with this technique.

TREATMENT AND MANAGEMENT OF CHILD ABUSE AND NEGLECT

Emergencies

CHIEF COMPLAINT

1. Care of the injury is the primary medical concern.
2. All queries should be addressed with open-ended statements to the child and caretakers.
3. Judgments of possible perpetrators or reasons that the injury occurred are to be avoided.
4. The *investigations* are to be performed only by the police or division of family services. The medical team merely *suspects* and *reports specific concerns* and the reasons for those concerns.

PROVIDE REASSURANCE AND ESTABLISH TRUST

1. Assure the child that you are there to help. Allay fears and lay groundwork for trust and concern.
2. Give some degree of control to the child by giving him or her choices that still allow you to provide care. ("Which color gown, blue or green?" "May I listen to your heart, or do you want to listen to it first?")
3. Be clear, and explain what you do.
4. If something will hurt, be honest.

REPORT

1. When the suspicion of nonaccidental trauma or sexual abuse is raised, appropriate agencies must be alerted immediately.
2. The immediate report of suspicion allows the agencies to act appropriately.
3. If the child is in danger of further trauma should he or she be released to the caretakers, the child should be taken into protective custody. (Be familiar with your state statutes and method of employing this right.)

SEXUAL ASSAULT EXAMINATIONS

1. Sexual assault examinations are performed at designated facilities with specific protocols to preserve the chain of evidence.
2. The examination should not be performed against the patient's will.
3. If there is concern of physical harm or a strong suggestion of positive evidence collection, sedation may be considered if other comfort measures fail. Another "assault" on the victim, even though medical, can have a long-standing emotional impact.
4. Gathering positive evidence for sexual assault examinations is best accomplished within 48 hours of the incident.

5. Consult your hospital and community protocols for sexual assault examinations.

INFORMING CARETAKERS OF A REPORT

1. Reasonable judgment should be used when the decision is made to tell the caretakers that police agencies or CPS are involved.
2. Inflammatory reactions or responses on your part are to be avoided.
3. Factual statements of your legal responsibility to report suspicions are best.
4. Present your information at a time close to the arrival of the outside agencies.
5. If outside agencies will not see the family in the ED, reassure the caretakers that these are persons who are concerned about the welfare of children and families and will assist them.

DIAGNOSTIC TESTS

1. Prothrombin time, partial thromboplastin time, factor 13, fibrinogen level, platelet count, bleeding time, to rule out blood dyscrasias
2. Skeletal surveys—up to the age of 2 years, to rule out the presence of current and old fractures
3. Height, weight, and head circumference compared to nomogram, to rule out failure to thrive or to document a baseline
4. Developmental level of functioning
5. Eye and fundoscopic examination, to rule out the possibility of retinal hemorrhage

Nonurgent conditions

A child with no acute distress physically or emotionally who is in no danger of further harm when he or she leaves the medical setting with the caretakers is considered to have a nonurgent condition.

FOLLOW-UP CARE

1. Continuity of medical follow-up care is important, to ensure the return to health and to determine that caretakers are responsible.
2. If a follow-up examination is not scheduled, a phone call is appropriate, to remind the caretakers to make an appointment.
3. When a caretaker fails to follow through with expected medical care, a report to CPS is expected, especially if lack of that care jeopardizes or compromises the health of the child.

Reporting

Report your suspicion to the appropriate protective services or local police agency as soon as possible. If you are alone in your suspicion, possibly without the backup of the medical team, you must still report your suspicion. Contact CPS or the police department for consultation if you are in doubt about the procedure or about your suspicion (Fig. 50-1).

PREVENTION
Role

The nurse's role in education and prevention must be underscored. All nurses should have some education in the dynamics of potential abuse and should know how to recognize the symptoms. The next step is to act on that knowledge with appropriate intervention.

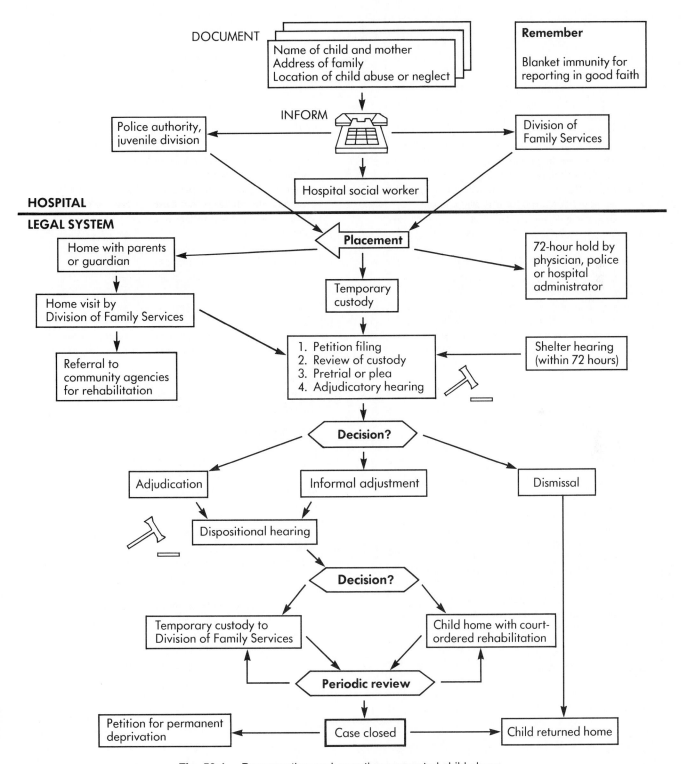

Fig. 50-1 Documenting and reporting suspected child abuse.

	2 weeks	2 months	4 months	6 months	9 months	12 months
Parent education	Safety, car seat Sibling interaction Mom and Dad's mental health, birth control Burping, gas "1st Year of Life" pamphlet Interpreting cries Colic (2 wk–5 mo) Bonding Postpartum blues	Safety, heights Growth spurt (6 wk, 3 mo, 6 mo) Vitamins, fluoride Instruct when to give bottle, what to put in it Diarrhea Spitting up Immunization side effects Fever treatment, how to use thermometer Sleep patterns	Safety, small object ingestion, rolling Teething URI and otitis media "First Foods" pamphlet Diet: fruit, cereals (amounts) Allergies	Safety, crawling, pulling, electrical burns, shoes, choking Vomiting Diet: vegetables, meats, finger foods Table manners Home-prepared foods Genitalia exploration Stranger anxiety Bottle propping	Safety, walking, baby-proofing home Delay toilet training Discipline: how and why Ipecac (syrup) Electric cords Diet: bottle, cup, spoon, nonfood rewards	Safety, toys, stairs, burns Limit setting Diet: appetite decreases, give smaller amounts of food
Immunization and laboratory screening	Ht, Wt, OFC Immunization PKU Thyroid screen	Ht, Wt, OFC DPT, OPV	Ht, Wt, OFC DPT, OPV	Ht, Wt, OFC DPT, third TOPV is optional Hct based on history and diet	Ht, Wt, OFC	Ht, Wt OFC, PPD
Development	Regards face Equal movements Can lift head when in prone position	Smiles as a response Eyes follow figure past midline Hands together Laughs Squeals (50%) Prone, head up 45 degrees Prone, head up 90 degrees (50%) Sits with head steady (50%) PDQ	Smiles spontaneously Grasps rattle Notices a raisin Reaches for objects Follows 180 degrees Squeals Bears some wt on legs (50%) Prone, chest up Sits with head steady Rolls over, PDQ	Feeds self cracker Resists toy pull Sit-looks for yarn Attempts to pick up raisin with fingers Passes cube hand to hand Turns to voice Bears weight on legs Can sit up with head and neck in alignment Sits unsupported Stands, holds on PDQ	Gets to sitting Pincer grasp Initiates speech Pulls to stand DDST	Plays "pat-a-cake" Stands for a moment Walks while holding on well Stands alone well PDQ
Speech and language	Startles to loud noise Quieted by familiar voice	Locates speaker with eyes	Uses sounds, "p," "b," "m" Repeats series of same sounds	Stops babbling to vocal stimulation Stops or withdraws to "no" Distinguishes general meaning: warning, anger, friendship Some word-like impressions Gestures to "come," "bye-bye"	Plays gesture games: "peekaboo," "pat-a-cake" Recognizes names of familiar objects Uses some gesture language: "no," "yes" Follows simple verbal request	Uses three or more words consistently

BP, Blood pressure; DDST, Denver Developmental Standardized Tests; DPT, diphtheria–pertussis–tetanus (vaccine); DPT, diphtheria–pertussis–tetanus (vaccine); Hct, hematocrit; Ht, height; MMR, measles-mumps-rubella (vaccine); OFC, occipital frontal circumference; OPV, oral polio vaccine; PKU, phenylketonuria; PPD, purified protein derivative (test for tuberculosis); TD, tetanus–diphtheria (vaccine); UA, urinalysis; URI, upper respiratory tract infection; Wt, weight.

	15 months	18 months-2 years	3-5 years	6-8 years	9-12 years	13-18 years
Parent education	Safety, car seat, fall, stairs / Tantrums / Fears / Diet, discontinue bottle feeding / Milk limit	Safety, poisons, street, yard, use of wide-wheeled and toddler tricycles / Independence / Toilet training / Separation anxiety / Visit to dentist / Home and day care / Diet: "picky" eater	Safety, trike, water, pedestrian, seat belts / Diet: gum, low-sugar snacks / Preschool / Peer play / Night terrors / Lying / Swearing / Body exploration (of others)	Safety, seat belts, skateboard / Dental hygiene / Television / Enuresis / School / Masturbation / Diet: gum, low-sugar snacks / Household chores / Place for privacy	Safety, drugs, alcohol, tobacco / Sexuality, menarche, masturbation, wet dreams / Diet: gum, snacks, iron, foods / School / Independence / Acne / Contact with other adults / Peer contact outside of school / Self-care responsibility: clothes, hygiene	Safety, seat belts, drugs, alcohol, tobacco / Sexuality / Acne / Diet: diets (reduction and sports) / Breast self-examination
Immunization and laboratory screening	Ht, Wt, OFC / MMR, Hct	Ht, Wt, OFC / DPT, OPV	Ht, Wt, BP, DPT, OPV, PPD, Hct, UA, speech and hearing screen / Scoliosis screen (5 yr)	Ht, Wt, BP, PPD / Vision screen / Speech and hearing screen / Conners parent questionnaire	Ht, Wt, BP, PPD, Hct / Cholesterol, triglycerides, both based on history / Scoliosis screen (12 yr)	Ht, Wt, BP, TD, Hct, PPD / Vision screen / Speech and hearing screen / Scoliosis screen (14 yr)
Development	Plays ball with examiner / Drinks from cup / Says Dada, Mama / Stands alone well / Stoops and recovers / Walks well (50%)	Imitates housework / Uses spoon well / Removes garment / Scribbles spontaneously / Tower of two cubes / Tower of four cubes / Can dump raisin from bottle / Walks upstairs / "Mama, Dada," three words / Points to one body part / Walks backwards / PDQ (18 mo)	DDST (3 yr) / DDST and Conners parent questionnaire (3-6 yr)	Conners parent questionnaire	Conners parent questionnaire	
Speech and language	Recognizes objects when named; seven or more true words	Recognizes body parts / Uses consonants, t, d, w, n, h / Begins repeating words / Repeats whisper using phrases				

IMMUNIZATION RECORD

DPT	TOPV	TD	PPD	Other
1st date	1st date	Booster	1st date	
2nd date	2nd date	Booster	2nd date	
3rd date	3rd date			
Booster	4th date			
Booster				

Measles Date given	Mumps Date given	Rubella Date given

Fig. 50-2 Care checklist for well child. (From Primary Children's Medical Center, Salt Lake City, Utah.)

Education

The most appropriate method of solving the problem of child abuse is *prevention*. A great deal can be accomplished in prenatal education, by addressing the important areas of bonding of the parents to the child and of parenting through all the phases of growth and development (Fig. 50-2).

Modeling behaviors is one method to teach parents caring, appropriate touch, positive, esteem-building, and nurturing care of the child. While we care for our patients we are critically observed. This is a good time to share parenting tips in a nonthreatening way. This kind of information is usually accepted and expected from nurses.

During assessment, we listen to the needs of children and families. It is our job to assist the medical team in delivering appropriate care on the basis of those needs.

If cultural differences are present, clarify the family's understanding of follow-up care. If there is a family spokesperson for medical care, be sure that that person receives and understands the education.

Discharge instructions are valuable tools. Clear, realistic expectations of care and expected results foster mutual respect and better outcomes. It is important that referral is made to community resources. Some resources that are valuable may include crisis nurseries, mental health centers, parenting classes, and hotlines.

Multidisciplinary Teams

Multidisciplinary approaches are methods of assuring that a global view of child and family care is obtained. Teams of physicians, nurses, social workers, CPS workers, lawyers, and police officers assist with decisions about the welfare of children who have been abused or neglected. Ask to be involved and contact your local CPS. Nurses are valuable assets to the team because they can demystify and explain medical procedures and language and provide holistic approaches that blend social and medical needs.

SUMMARY

The ability to make changes in the best interest of children and families is not impossible to acquire. Every city has community councils that deal with youth issues. Nurses are a welcome addition and are given appointments readily if interest is displayed. Of a variety of approaches, any one of them may be what best suits your interest and capability. Clearly the need for a global perspective in making assessments, rather than a "tunnel vision" approach, offers the opportunity to break the cycle of abuse in a family.

Many committee activities are the beginning of legislative changes. The use of informed people, at the grassroots level, assists with the development of reasonable and workable legislation.

Opportunities for community involvement include the following:

1. Parent and teachers associations
2. Community councils for youth
3. Local prevention teams
4. State prevention teams (Every state has a chapter of the National Committee for the Prevention of Child Abuse.)
5. Division of Family Services child abuse councils
6. Legislative committees of local and state nurses' associations and local and state child advocacy committees

REFERENCES

1. American Medical Association: Diagnostic and treatment guidelines concerning child abuse and neglect, *JAMA* 254:796, 1985.
2. Bittner S, Newberger E: Pediatric understanding of child abuse and neglect, *Pediatr Rev* 2:197, 1981.
3. Bross D et al: *The new child protection team handbook,* 1988, Garland.
4. Helfer R, Kempe H, Schmitt B: *The battered child,* ed 4, Chicago, 1988, University of Chicago.
5. Giangiacomo J, Barkett K: Ophthalmoscopic findings in occult child abuse, *Pediatrics* 22:234, 1985.
6. Green F et al: Child abuse: handling its challenges, *Patient Care* 17:160, 1983.
7. Nakou S et al: Health status of abused and neglected children and their siblings, *Child Abuse and Neglect: Int J* 6:279-84, 1982.

SUGGESTED READINGS

Castiglia PT: Sexual abuse of children, *J Pediatr Health Care* 4(2):91, 1990.

Chadwick DL: *Color atlas of child sexual abuse,* California Medical Association's Maternal Perinatal and Child Care Subcommittee on Child Abuse and Neglect, Chicago, 1989, Mosby–Year Book.

deChesnay M: Child sexual abuse as an international health problem, *Int Nurs Rev* 36(5):149, 1988.

DeJong AR: Maternal responses to sexual abuse of their children, *Pediatrics* 8(1):14, 1988.

Dykes LD: The whiplash shaken infant syndrome: what has been learned? *Child Abuse and Neglect* 10:211, 1986.

Elvik SL: From disclosure to court: the facets of sexual abuse, *J Pediatr Health Care* 1(3):136, 1987.

Guidelines for the Evaluation of Sexually Abused Children, *Amer Assoc Pediatr News* Nov 1990, p 20.

Heger A: *Response to child sexual abuse: a medical view,* Los Angeles, 1985, Guilford Publications.

Kelley S: Interviewing the sexually abused child: principles and techniques, *J Emerg Nurs* 11:234, 1985.

Kelley SJ: Learned helplessness in the sexually abused child, *Issues Comp Pediatr Nurs* 9(3):193, 1986.

Kelley SJ: Child abuse and neglect, *Pediatric emergency nursing,* 1988, Appleton & Lange.

Krugman RD: Recognition of sexual abuse in children, *Pediatr Rev* 8:25, 1986.

Muram D: Child sexual abuse: relationship between sexual acts and genital findings, *Child Abuse and Neglect* 13:211, 1989.

Paradise JE: The medical evaluation of the sexually abused child, *Pediatr Clin North Am* 1990.

Schetky D, Green A: *Child sexual abuse: a handbook for health care and legal professionals,* New York, 1988, Brunner/Mazel.

Sgroi S: *Handbook of clinical intervention in child sexual abuse,* Lexington, Mass, 1985, D C Health.

Strickland S: Sexual abuse assessment, *Pediatr Ann* 18:495, 1989.

Wilson EF: Estimation of the age of cutaneous contusions in child abuse, *Pediatrics* 60:750, 1977.

Index

A

Abdomen
  chest pain originating from, 494
  organs of, 349-350
  penetrating injuries of, 348-349
  trauma to, 347-350
    assessment and management of, 281
    in children, 685, 689
    incidence of, 347
    as indicator of child abuse, 693
    in pregnant patient, 350
    signs and symptoms of, 347-348
Abdominal emergencies, 517-527; *see also* Pain, abdominal
  laboratory tests and radiographic examinations, 519-520
  physical examination and laboratory tests and, 519
Abortion
  assessment for, 633
  defined, 633
  intervention for, 633-634
  types of, 633
Abrasions
  characteristics of, 256
  corneal, 315, *320*
  defined, 354
  of extremity soft tissue, intervention for, 354
  management of, 256-257
Abruptio placentae
  symptoms and differential diagnosis of, 636t
  symptoms and intervention, 635
Abscess
  Bartholin's gland, 644
  characteristics of, 257
  of extremity soft tissue, intervention for, 354
  management of, 257
  ovarian, 643
  perinephric, symptoms and intervention, 524
  peritonsillar and retropharyngeal, in children, 673
Abuse
  child; *see* Child abuse and neglect
  domestic violence, 606-608
  of elderly, 605
  emotional, in children, 696
  sexual; *see* Sexual abuse
Acceleration forces, effects of, 439
Accidents
  deaths from, by race and age, 467t
  falls, 467
  incidence of, by geographic region, 463-465
  from motor vehicle crashes, 465-467
  number and age-specific death rates for, 465t
  number and death rates for, by gender, 465t

Accountability, nursing diagnosis and, 78
Accreditation Manual for Hospitals, 223
Acetaminophen, overdose of, 559
  clinical effects of, 560
  laboratory tests for, 559
  mechanism of, 559-560
  treatment of, 560
Acetazolamide, brand names and action of, 322t
Achilles tendon, ruptured, 356
Achromycin; *see* Tetracycline
Acidosis
  metabolic, conditions indicated by, 219
  respiratory, conditions indicated by, 219
  as transfusion complication, 271
Acquired immunodeficiency syndrome, exposure to, 573
Acrilan, toxic products from combustion of, 503t
Acrylic, toxic products from combustion of, 503t
Acute adrenal crisis, 541-542
  assessment of, 541
  management of, 541-542
  nursing diagnoses in, 542
  pathogenesis of, 541
Acute myocardial infarction
  diagnostic criteria for, 143
  initial management of, 146-147
  medications for, 147t-149t
  pain relief for, 146-147
  patient history in, 143, 145
  signs and symptoms of, 143
Acute organic brain syndrome
  characteristics of, 620
  intervention for, 620
Adaptation syndrome, physical and psychologic changes in, 587t
Adenocard; *see* Adenosine
Adenosine for dysrhythmias, 489-490
Administration, systems management and, 39-41
Adrenal crisis, acute; *see* Acute adrenal crisis
Adrenal emergencies, 541-542
Adrenalin; *see* Epinephrine
Adult respiratory distress syndrome
  intervention for, 509-510
  signs and symptoms of, 509
Advanced life support, 9, 143-191
  airway management in, 150-154
  assessment in, 143-146
  assisted breathing in, 154-158
  automatic implantable cardioverter defibrillator in, 160
  cardioversion in, 159
  chest compressions in, 158
  dysrhythmia recognition and management in, 161-188
  pacemakers in, 159-160
  thrombolytic therapy in, 160-161
Adventitious sounds, auscultation of, 118
AEIOU TIPS mnemonic in level of consciousness assessment, 662t

---

Page numbers in italics indicate illustrations; *t* indicates tables.

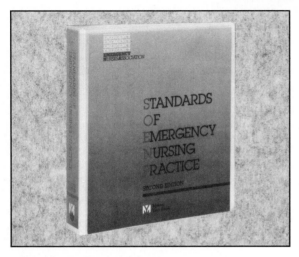
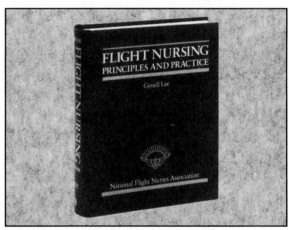
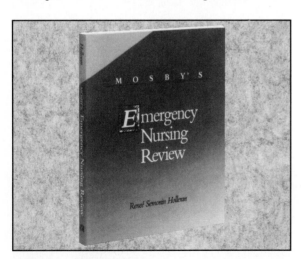
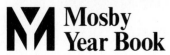